Combined Textbook of
Obstetrics and Gynaecology

Combined Textbook of Obstetrics and Gynaecology

Edited by

James Walker, C.B.E., B.Sc., M.D., F.R.C.P.G., F.R.C.O.G.
Professor of Obstetrics and Gynaecology, University of Dundee;
Honorary Consultant, Tayside Health Board.

Ian MacGillivray, M.D., F.R.C.P.G., F.R.C.O.G.
Regius Professor of Obstetrics and Gynaecology, University of Aberdeen;
Honorary Consultant, Grampian Health Board.

Malcolm C. Macnaughton, M.D., F.R.C.P.G., F.R.C.O.G.
Muirhead Professor of Obstetrics and Gynaecology, University of Glasgow;
Honorary Consultant, Greater Glasgow Health Board.

Foreword by
Sir Dugald Baird, B.Sc., M.D., D.P.H., F.R.C.O.G., LL.D. (Hon.), D.Sc. (Hon.), D.C.L. (Hon.)
Professor Emeritus of Obstetrics and Gynaecology, University of Aberdeen.

Ninth Edition

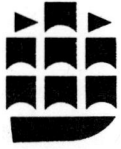

CHURCHILL LIVINGSTONE
Edinburgh London and New York 1976

CHURCHILL LIVINGSTONE
Medical Division of Longman Group Limited

Distributed in the United States of America by
Longman Inc., 19 West 44th Street, New York,
N.Y. 10036 and by associated companies,
branches and representatives throughout
the world.

First Edition   1923
Reprint   1928
Second Edition   1933
Reprint   1936
Third Edition   1939
Reprint   1941
Fourth Edition   1944
Reprint   1946
Fifth Edition   1950
Sixth Edition   1957
Seventh Edition   1962
Eighth Edition   1969
Ninth Edition   1976

ISBN 0 443 01072 2

**Library of Congress Cataloging in
Publication Data**

Main entry under title:

Combined textbook of obstetrics and
gynaecology.

   First–4th editions by J. M. M. Kerr and
others; 5th–8th editions by D. Baird; all under
title: Combined textbook of obstetrics and
gynaecology for students and practitioners.
   Includes index.
   1. Obstetrics.   2. Gynecology.   I. Walker,
James, 1916–   II. MacGillivray, Ian.   III.
Macnaughton, Malcolm C.   IV. Kerr, John
Martin Munro, 1868-1956.   Combined
text-book of obstetrics and gynaecology for
students and medical practitioners.   V. Baird,
Dugald, Sir, 1899–   ed. Combined textbook of
obstetrics and gynaecology for students and
practitioners.   VI. Title: Obstetrics and
gynaecology.

RG101.K53   1976   618   76-8406

Printed in Great Britain

Foreword

The first edition of the Combined Textbook of Obstetrics and Gynaecology, published in 1923, resulted very largely from the efforts of its first editor, Professor J. M. Munro Kerr. His aim was to produce a Scottish Textbook which would promote integration of the teaching of obstetrics and gynaecology to undergraduates and at the same time serve as a book of reference for general practitioners interested in practical obstetrics.

During this half century most of the contributors have been Scottish graduates, predominantly from Glasgow, which is perhaps not surprising in view of the unsurpassed variety of serious complications of pregnancy and labour which filled, and still fill, the maternity hospitals in this densely populated area of Scotland, and which created by necessity a high degree of obstetrical skill.

No one in his day did more than Munro Kerr by his writings and his example to inspire young men and women to specialize in obstetrics. He edited the first three editions of the Combined Textbook and invited me to edit the fourth edition, which was published in 1944, and I continued as editor until the eighth edition in 1969.

It gave me great satisfaction to hand over the editorship of the ninth edition to James Walker, Ian MacGillivray and Malcolm Macnaughton, all graduates of Glasgow and former members of my staff.

Aberdeen, 1976   Sir Dugald Baird

Preface

The Combined Textbook was first published in 1923 and in the half century spanned by its first eight editions the practice of Obstetrics and Gynaecology has changed profoundly.

Childbearing in the advanced countries of the world no longer carries a serious risk of death or of major damage to the mother. A maternal mortality rate of 12·9 per 100 000 in England and Wales in 1970–72 aptly summarizes the new situation. Despite this low rate, however, abortion, pulmonary embolus, haemorrhage, toxaemia, ectopic pregnancy, sepsis and anaesthetics still claim lives which could, with better care, be saved. This steady improvement in maternal care has paralleled the greatly increased safety of surgical procedures in general and major gynaecological surgery has therefore become relatively safe.

It must not be forgotten, however, that those fortunate states do not universally exist. Human reproduction in many communities and peoples is difficult and dangerous for mother and child and the problems of gynaecology, post pregnancy, infective and neoplastic, are serious and diverse.

Since the end of the Second World War, there has been a steady improvement in the perinatal mortality rate (now well under twenty in some centres) and in the short and long term prognosis for the prematurely born or the child of low birth weight. These improvements have been made possible by the application to clinical practice of the imaginative studies of the physiology of human and mammalian reproduction which developed extensively in the period from 1950 and which fortunately still continue. Reference to these studies is made throughout the relevant chapters.

The increasing understanding and availability of more reliable contraceptive techniques allowing women to have control over their fertility has greatly changed reproductive behaviour of western communities. The emancipation of women and their realization that sexual relations should be enjoyed has led to increasing demands for the provision of facilities for the study and treatment of sexual problems.

We are now, in the United Kingdom, in a period of low birth rates, very low maternal and perinatal risks and perhaps beginning a new era where not only will quality of care in these terms be excellent, but we can turn our attentions to improving the quality of the babies produced and also to ensuring that the mothers can look on the pregnancy and labour as an enjoyable experience.

In this edition we have attempted to compile a text which will encompass and act as a reference over the whole likely range of practice anywhere in the world. Written primarily as a basic text for the advanced undergraduates and trainee specialist, it is also designed for the practitioner in the more remote and in the less favoured parts of the world and much technical obstetrical detail has been retained for that reason. More time and effort can now be spent on the major problems of infertility, undue prematurity and fetal anomaly which have now assumed proportionally greater importance.

The Combined Textbook expresses the beliefs and practice of the Scottish Medical Schools and the writers have mainly therefore trained in Scotland or practice there. Our contributors have, however, been selected for their special knowledge and ability in the fields covered by their text.

Inevitably we have lost from previous editions by retiral some of our most valued contributors but we are fortunate that, although the book is almost entirely rewritten and remodelled now, much of the valued text from the previous chapters has been retained. This is especially true of the 'Labour' (Chapter 19) where the original texts of Emeritus Professor Sir Dugald Baird and of Emeritus Professor W. I. C. Morris have been, with permission, heavily borrowed. This debt is freely acknowledged.

New chapters in Genetics in relation to the practice of obstetrics and gynaecology; blood coagulation and fibrinolysis; immunology and incompatibility; risk to mother and child; sonar and X-rays in obstetrics and gynaecology; tropical gynaecology; termination of pregnancy and sexuality, sexual difficulties and sex education have been added. We are very greatly indebted to those who contributed to these new chapters which so greatly increased the value of the text.

We decided early that there would be few half-tone illustrations and certainly no colour, and have concentrated heavily on line drawings. For the illustrations we are indebted to Mr Edward Smith of the Department of Medical Illustration of the University of Aberdeen, who has done a magnificent job to our instructions. To Messrs Churchill Livingstone and especially to Mr Richard Zorab, Mrs Lyn Stubbs and Mr Andrew Walker, we give thanks for much help and great forbearance, and to Dr Isobel Leitch who has contributed so much to the science of our speciality, our special thanks for her magnificent work in compiling an index.

Dundee   James Walker
Aberdeen   Ian MacGillivray
Glasgow, 1976   Malcolm Macnaughton

Contributors

James Walker, C.B.E., B.Sc., M.D., F.R.C.P.G., F.R.C.O.G.

Professor of Obstetrics and Gynaecology, University of Dundee; Honorary Consultant, Tayside Health Board.

Growth and Development of Fetus and Placenta (Fetus); Medical Disorders (Diseases of the Respiratory System); Antenatal Care; Antenatal and Intrapartum Assessment of Fetal Growth, Maturity and Wellbeing (Antenatal); Labour; Risk to Mother and Child; Tumours; Pre-operative, Operative and Post-operative Care.

Ian MacGillivray, M.D., F.R.C.P.G., F.R.C.O.G.

Regius Professor of Obstetrics and Gynaecology, University of Aberdeen; Honorary Consultant, Grampian Health Board.

Hypertensive Disorders of Pregnancy; Other Specific Diseases of Pregnancy; Surgical Conditions in Obstetrics; Puerperal Infection; Multiple or Plural Pregnancy; Obstetric Operations; Infections of the Reproductive Organs; Endometriosis; Other Gynaecological Conditions; Surgical Conditions in Gynaecology; Termination of Pregnancy.

Malcolm C. Macnaughton, M.D., F.R.C.P.G., F.R.C.O.G.

Muirhead Professor of Obstetrics and Gynaecology, University of Glasgow; Honorary Consultant, Greater Glasgow Health Board.

Anatomy of the Female Pelvis and the External Genitalia; Bleeding During Pregnancy; Disturbances of the Reproductive System Complicating Pregnancy; Abnormalities of Menstruation; The Menopause and Post-Menopause; Displacements of the Uterus; Family Planning and Population Control.

David R. Abramovich, M.B., B.S., D.G.O. (Syd. Univ.), Ph.D., M.R.C.O.G.

Senior Lecturer, Obstetrics and Gynaecology, University of Aberdeen; Honorary Consultant, Grampian Health Board.

The Trophoblast, the Membranes and the Amniotic Fluid (Amniotic Fluid).

Sir Dugald Baird, B.Sc., M.D., D.P.H., F.R.C.O.G., LL.D. (Hon.), D.Sc. (Hon.), D.C.L. (Hon.)

Professor Emeritus of Obstetrics and Gynaecology, University of Aberdeen.

Human Reproduction.

John W. Crawford, M.B., Ch.B., F.R.C.O.G.

Consultant Obstetrician and Gynaecologist, Tayside Health Board; Honorary Senior Lecturer, University of Dundee.

The Trophoblast, the Membranes and the Amniotic Fluid (Trophoblastic Disease); Antenatal and Intrapartum Assessment of Fetal Growth, Maturity and Wellbeing (Assessment of Fetal Wellbeing in Labour).

K. John Dennis, M.B., Ch.B., F.R.C.S.E., F.R.C.O.G.

Professor of Human Reproduction and Obstetrics, University of Southampton.

The Puerperium.

Ian Donald, C.B.E., M.D., B.A., F.R.C.S.G., F.R.C.O.G., F.C.O.G. (S.A.)

Regius Professor of Midwifery, University of Glasgow; Honorary Consultant, Greater Glasgow Health Board.

Sonar and X-rays in Obstetrics and Gynaecology.

Alexander S. Douglas, B.Sc., M.D., F.R.C.P. (Lond., Edin., Glas.)

Regius Professor of Medicine, University of Aberdeen; Honorary Consultant, Grampian Health Board.

Blood Coagulation and Fibrinolysis.

Alan E. Emery, M.D., Ph.D., D.Sc., F.R.C.P.E., M.R.C.M., F.R.S.E.

Professor of Human Genetics, University of Edinburgh; Honorary Consultant in Medicine Genetics, Lothian Health Board.

Genetics in Relation to the Practice of Obstetrics and Gynaecology.

Henry B. Goodall, M.D., F.R.C. (Path.)

Senior Lecturer in Pathology, University of Dundee; Honorary Consultant Haematologist, Tayside Health Board.

Medical Disorders (Haematological System).

Peter W. Howie, M.D., M.R.C.O.G.

Senior Lecturer, Obstetrics and Gynaecology, University of Glasgow; Honorary Consultant, Greater Glasgow Health Board.

Shock and Maternal Injury.

Frank E. Hytten, M.D., Ph.D., F.R.C.O.G.

Head, Division of Perinatal Medicine, Clinical Research Centre, M.R.C. Northwick Park, Middlesex.

Physiological Changes of Pregnancy.

Geoffrey B. James, M.B., Ch.B., M.R.C.O.G.

Senior Lecturer, Obstetrics and Gynaecology, University of Dundee; Honorary Consultant, Tayside Health Board.

Growth and Development of Fetus and Placenta (Placenta and Membranes).

Arnold Klopper, Ph.D., M.D., F.R.C.O.G.

Professor of Reproductive Endocrinology, University of Aberdeen; Honorary Consultant, Grampian Health Board.

The Endocrine Physiology of the Reproductive System.

John Lawson, M.B., B.Chir., F.R.C.O.G.

Honorary Consultant, Area Health Authority (Teaching), Newcastle upon Tyne; (Formerly) Professor of Obstetrics and Gynaecology, University of Ibadan, Nigeria.

Tropical Obstetrics; Tropical Gynaecology.

Malcolm MacLeod, M.D., F.R.C.P.

Reader in Medicine, University of Aberdeen; Honorary Consultant, Aberdeen Royal Infirmary.

Medical Disorders (Renal System and Nervous System).

William M. Millar, C.B.E., M.D., F.R.C.P.E., F.R.C. (Psych.)

Crombie Ross Professor of Mental Health, University of Aberdeen; Honorary Consultant, Grampian Health Board.

Psychological, Psychosomatic and Psychiatric Aspects.

Ross G. Mitchell, M.D., D.C.H., F.R.C.P.E.

Professor of Child Health, University of Dundee; Honorary Consultant, Tayside Health Board.

The Newborn Infant.

Peter C. Olley, M.B., Ch.B., B.Sc., Dipl. Psych. (Edin.), M.R.C. (Psych.)

Senior Lecturer in Mental Health, University of Aberdeen; Honorary Consultant, Grampian Health Board.

Psychological, Psychosomatic and Psychiatric Aspects.

Philip Rhodes, M.A., M.B., B.Chir., F.R.C.S.E., F.R.C.O.G.

Dean, Faculty of Medicine, University of Adelaide; Professor of Gynaecology, University of Adelaide; (Formerly) Dean and Professor of Obstetrics and Gynaecology, St Thomas's Hospital Medical School, London.

An Approach to Gynaecology.

James K. Russell, M.D., F.R.C.O.G.

Professor of Obstetrics and Gynaecology, University of Newcastle upon Tyne; Honorary Consultant, Area Health Authority (Teaching), Newcastle upon Tyne.

Signs and Symptoms in Obstetrics; Signs and Symptoms in Gynaecology.

James S. Scott, M.D., F.R.C.S.E., F.R.C.O.G.

Professor of Obstetrics and Gynaecology, University of Leeds; Honorary Consultant, Leeds Area Health Authority (Teaching), Western District.

Immunology and Incompatibility.

John M. Stowers, M.A., M.B., B.Ch., M.A. (Harvard), F.R.C.P., F.R.C.P.E.

Honorary Consultant Physician, Grampian Health Board; Honorary Senior Lecturer, University of Aberdeen.

Medical Disorders (Alimentary and Endocrine System).

Hamish W. Sutherland, M.B., Ch.B., D.Obst.R.C.O.G., M.R.C.O.G.

Senior Lecturer in Obstetrics and Gynaecology, University of Aberdeen; Honorary Consultant, Grampian Health Board.

Sexuality, Sexual Difficulties and Sex Education.

Angus M. Thomson, B.Sc., M.B., Ch.B., D.P.H., F.R.C.O.G.

Director, M.R.C. Reproduction and Growth Unit, Newcastle upon Tyne.

The Epidemiological Perspective.

Michael E. Tunstall, M.B., B.S., D.Obst.R.C.O.G., F.F.A.R.C.S.

Honorary Consultant Anaesthetist, Grampian Health Board; Clinical Senior Lecturer, University of Aberdeen.

Analgesia and Anaesthesia in Obstetrics and Gynaecology.

Hamish Watson, T.D., M.D., F.R.C.P.E., F.R.C.P., F.A.C.C.

Chairman, Section of Cardiology, Department of Medicine, University of Dundee; Postgraduate Dean and Director of Postgraduate Medical Education, University of Dundee; Honorary Consultant Cardiologist, Tayside Health Board.

Medical Disorders (Cardiovascular System).

Contents

I. Human Reproduction

THE BIOLOGICAL AND EPIDEMIOLOGICAL BEHAVIOUR OF HUMAN COMMUNITIES

Great changes have occurred in the practice of obstetrics and gynaecology in the developed world in the last 50 years. Such changes reflect, to a large extent, the higher standard of living brought about by modern technology and the consequent improvement in health. The small family of one, two or three children is now the 'norm'; childbearing is usually completed by the age of 30 and more women return to work outside the home. The expectation of life has increased steadily, especially in women. These social and economic developments make new demands on the obstetrical and gynaecological services which are now required to be more closely integrated with preventive medicine and the social services.

The pre-requisites of successful childbearing

The basic requirements for successful childbearing are simple—i.e. youth, health, a high standard of obstetric care and positive imitation of family size. There is good evidence that the outcome of a first pregnancy is best when the mother is between the ages of 18 and 20 and is well grown and well nourished as a result of a good environment from birth to maturity. Such women have grown to the limit of their genetically determined height and are in consequence taller on average than those whose environment has not been so good. A rough but fairly reliable index of the state of health of any community in the developed world can be established from a distribution curve of the heights of a representative sample of young adults. If the skeleton is fully grown it is likely that all other tissues and organs will also be fully developed and functioning efficiently.

A National Survey in Britain in 1958 showed that the highest percentage of tall women (65 inches or more) was found in social classes I and II and the lowest percentage in social classes IV and V (Baird & Thomson, 1969). The lowest perinatal mortality rate in primigravidae (19 per 1000) was found in tall women (65 inches or more) in social classes I and II and the highest rate (49 per 1000) in short women (less than 62 inches) in social classes IV and V. The excess perinatal mortality rate in short women in social classes IV and V occurred in all clinical cause groups.

The basic requirements for successful childbearing are the same everywhere, although cultural differences may affect the pattern. Genetic differences are also found, for example, in the predisposition to congenital malformations or differences in the prevalence of blood groups.

In many under-developed countries today, where death rates in children are high, large families are still necessary for survival and childbearing starts soon after the onset of menstruation. At this early age the mother is not fully grown and during pregnancy her needs may conflict with those of the fetus. Whatever the reason, very young women tend to have small babies. In general, the younger the mother the shorter the stature and the higher the percentage of babies weighing less than 2500g. However, the small size of the baby and the extreme youth of the mother, which ensures elasticity of the pelvic ligaments, lessen the risk of dystocia which could be very dangerous in circumstances where skilled obstetric help is not available. Youth also improves the chance that lactation will be satisfactory, a necessity for the child's survival where there is no artificial substitute. Hytten (1954) found that youth is of great importance in Caucasians for successful lactation. In primigravidae breast enlargement, in response to pregnancy, output of breast milk and fat content are greatest between the ages of 18 and 20. Both the volume and fat content fall with increasing age of the mother. The practical importance of this was clear in the days when breast feeding was the rule rather than the exception that it is today. For example, in the 1930s many upper social class women postponed childbearing for economic reasons. They were usually anxious to breast feed but often failed to produce enough milk. Those in the lower social classes did not postpone childbearing and being young had little difficulty in initiating lactation. However, many were disinclined to persist with it and changed to artificial feeding within a short time. Babies grow quickly on cow's milk but the risk of infection and other complications is higher. In addition it has been suggested that the dietary content of artificial feeding based on cow's milk may predispose to degenerative and circulatory diseases in later life.

Birth rates

As already pointed out a high birth rate is essential for survival when death rates are very high. Today in under-developed countries death rates are falling quickly due to modern methods of control and treatment of infectious diseases while birth rates fall much more slowly because of long standing traditional attitudes to family size. Successful lactation is essential for the child's survival and it may be continued for a year or longer during which time coitus is forbidden. A high national birth rate may even be maintained by the practice of polygamy.

In England and Wales the population more than doubled between 1851 and 1950 because although the infant mortality rate was 150 per 1000 and remained at this level till the end of the century, the birth rate rose from 32 per 1000 in 1850 to 35 in 1881–90. As so many young children died, large families were thought to be necessary and indeed in Victorian society, from the Queen downwards, the large family was regarded as the ideal. Many factors contributed to this; the low status of women, the high child death rate, the poverty of the working classes in the slums of the large cities and the fact that children contributed to the family income. However, with Lord Shaftesbury's revelations of the conditions of employment of women and young children the national conscience was aroused and much social legislation was enacted. The most far-reaching was the Education Act of 1870 which made school attendance compulsory. Children were no longer a financial asset. The large family became the most important single cause of poverty. This led to a steady decline in the birth rate especially after 1900, despite the lack of knowledge of contraceptive methods amongst the majority of the population. The birth rate reached its lowest level in 1933 during the world slump in trade. However, despite this the population continued to increase steadily. In the 50 years between 1891 and 1940 the number of women in the reproductive age group in Britain increased by three million but in 1931 there were 322 000 fewer births than in 1901.

In 1933 when the economic depression was at its worst, the number of births was well below replacement level and the net reproduction rate had fallen to 0·74 compared to 1·5 in 1881. Great social class differences in family size had developed and were reflected in regional differences in the net reproduction rate. In London and the South of England, where a higher percentage of the population than average was in social classes I and II, the birth rate was well below replacement level but in the industrial North, where a higher proportion of the population than average was in social classes IV and V, it was well above. Many children, especially in industrial cities, were born and brought up in sub-standard conditions and were physically and intellectually deprived.

The writings of Booth and Rowntree show that, at the beginning of the present century, conditions were much worse for the population as a whole than in the economic depression of the 1930s. This was very clearly demonstrated by the medical examination of over two million men who were conscripted for military service in 1917–18. 'Out of every 9 examined, 3 were judged to be fit and healthy; 2 were inferior in health and strength; 3 were described as physical wrecks, and 1 was a chronic invalid with a precarious hold on life. Altogether 41 per cent were judged to be quite unfit for service.' (Burnett, 1966) In the Second World War young men called up for service in the armed forces were found to be much taller and healthier but considerable social class differences in health and physique still existed.

In the years 1946–48 the birth rate rose by about one-third, because of births postponed by the war. It rose again in 1951 in first births due to an increase in the marriage rate and to an earlier age at marriage. These changes were stimulated by a new social attitude based on full employment, a concept of social justice, and the 'welfare state' as envisaged by Beveridge. All social classes were affected and in social classes I and II, where the pre-war rate had been so low, families of three or four children became quite common. Large families remained relatively common in social classes IV and V. The variation in fertility in social classes I and II in response to changes in social circumstances and the lack of it in classes IV and V demonstrate the differing attitudes to family planning. This social class difference applies to many aspects of social behaviour.

Populations

Today the population of the UK is increasing at the rate of less than 0·5 per cent per annum, which seems small compared to the rates in many other countries but it must be remembered that Britain, more particularly England, is one of the most densely populated countries in the world (Taylor, 1969).

It has been calculated that the population of the UK will exceed 60 million by the end of the century, a conservative estimate in view of the increase in the last 10 years of approximately 2·7 million under the age of 30 and 1·5 million over the age of 55. The increase is confined almost entirely to the Midlands and the South of England, where the birth rate is lowest and is in fact due to emigration from Scotland, Ireland, the North of England, and from abroad.

This emigration has serious consequences for Scotland and the North of England. Scotland has been depressed economically since 1914–18 and this is reflected in higher unemployment rates, lower wages, higher infant mortality and perinatal mortality rates and the short stature which is a sign of chronic malnutrition and not an inherited characteristic. The emigration of so many energetic and intelligent young people has had a detrimental effect on the North, so that the South gets richer and the North poorer. The Republic of Ireland provides an interesting contrast of a population which despite a high birth rate (21·5 per 1000) remains static because of a high emigration rate. The Republic has the highest birth rate in Europe despite the low marriage rate and the high mean age at marriage and at the start of childbearing. She must pay a heavy price for this high emigration rate in the loss of so many of her more able young people. There is certainly an obstetrical disadvantage in the high proportion of elderly primiparae and 'grand multiparae'. Today 25 per cent of all births in Ireland are in women having a fifth or later child compared to 6 per cent in England and Wales.

There is much evidence that human beings, like the rest of the animal kingdom, need space, fresh air and quiet if their communities are to remain healthy in mind as well as in body. We should try to restrict numbers to a total for which this planet can provide the essentials for a good life.

It is more difficult to decide what the optimum population of the UK should be. Some say an increase to 60 million would be beneficial for the economy by increasing industrial production and the size of the home market. Others say that in view of increasing automation, the need for man power, especially semi-skilled and unskilled manual workers, will be much less and a more realistic figure would be 40 million. This would make Britain more self-sufficient for food—an important consideration in a hungry world. Clearly this question must be reconsidered in relation to our membership of the European Community.

Recent experience makes it clear that rapid changes in birth and death rates are undesirable. It would be difficult, even if it were advisable, for any Government in this country to regulate by decree the number of babies to be born. Parents in our society decide this for themselves and fortunately the majority are responsible citizens, but efficient contraception is essential for responsible parenthood. Children should be born because they are wanted. In the past the fear that not enough children would be born to maintain the population may have caused resistance to the provision of contraceptives. Parental instinct will probably prove strong enough to ensure that this does not happen, if economic and social conditions are favourable and seen to be just.

The determination of the women of this country to get proper advice on family planning and termination of unwanted pregnancy is a manifestation of their desire to control their own destiny and to raise the standard of living for themselves and their families. The chance of a child receiving higher education still depends largely on the relationship between the number of children in the family and the parents' income. For most parents this means careful regulation of family size.

These changing patterns of reproduction in the last 50 years have produced consequential changes in the practice of clinical obstetrics and gynaecology, in the research problems demanding investigation and in the training of obstetricians to meet these needs.

The evolution of obstetric practice during the last 50 years

In Britain 50 years ago childbearing was as hazardous as in many under-developed countries. Adverse environmental factors were a cold damp climate, lack of sunshine, pollution of the atmosphere and depressing slums in the poorer parts of the large cities. Such conditions were much worse in the industrial North of Britain than in the more prosperous South and in consequence the maternal mortality rate was much higher in the North. In Glasgow rickets was prevalent and obstructed labour very common. In the 1930s in the Glasgow Maternity Hospital 100 mothers died every year. Thirty per cent of those who died had six or more children and in many of them the previous obstetric history had been very abnormal. Most births took place in very overcrowded and insanitary homes with a 'handywoman' in attendance. A general practitioner was called to deliver the baby when the 'handywoman' thought that this was indicated, and if he failed the patient was sent to hospital.

The obstetrician in hospital was mainly engaged in emergency treatment of women admitted with serious complications of pregnancy and labour. The scope of his operative work in hospital was hampered by poor anaesthesia, inadequate facilities for blood transfusion and a very high risk of puerperal sepsis. The high mortality rate in the 1920s caused national concern and an Interdepartmental Committee was set up which reported in 1930. In 1929 the College of Obstetricians and Gynaecologists (now the Royal College) was founded. It played a vital part in raising the standard of clinical practice in the specialty by drawing up recommendations for the training of young obstetricians and gynaecologists and by granting Membership of the College to those who underwent this training and who passed a theoretical and practical examination conducted by the College. The resulting increase in the number of well trained specialists greatly eased the task of the National Health Service in 1948 in organizing a National Maternity Service.

The introduction of sulphonamides in 1936 and later the discovery of penicillin made maternity hospitals much safer and made it possible to introduce many new technical advances in diagnosis and treatment with safety. The development of blood banks came during the 1939–45 war. In these days the life of the mother was the main concern but very little attention was given to the primary cause of many of the deaths—namely excessive childbearing. Few doctors gave any advice on birth control and termination of pregnancy was only considered when the mother's life was in danger. The expressed attitude of the established churches was, at that time, so extreme that termination of pregnancy was rarely permitted even to save the mother's life.

The perinatal mortality rate was very high but this appeared relatively unimportant in the conditions existing at the time. However, between 1940–48 a dramatic and unexpected fall of 30 per cent in the national perinatal mortality rate occurred. The reduction in the rate was greatest in the most depressed areas where the pre-war unemployment rate had been highest, in South Wales for example. During the war years the National Food Policy of rationing, with special allocations to expectant mothers and children, and full employment ensured that everyone could have a good diet. The striking effect of this on the perinatal mortality rate focuses attention on the importance of good food during pregnancy, especially in chronically undernourished women, and stimulated interest in the influence of the mother's environment on reproductive efficiency.

On the recommendation of the Interdepartmental Committee on Medical Schools (1944) which was fully implemented after the introduction of the National Health Service in 1948 it became possible to plan a medical service to meet the needs of all. Professors and lecturers were appointed on a whole-time basis in the clinical departments of the Medical Schools which were greatly expanded with offices and laboratories adjacent to the hospitals to facilitate teaching and research. The overall standard of care improved more quickly in

Scotland than in England because the Teaching Hospitals were administered by the Regional Hospital Boards and were able to play a leading role in developing the Regional Service. This raised the standard of clinical care, provided better opportunities for clinical teaching and research and for evaluating the results of treatment. It also stimulated the clinicians to take responsibility for the standard of care in the whole region and to make the best use of available resources.

In obstetrics this improvement, as measured by the fall in the perinatal mortality rate, was easier to achieve in the smaller regions. In Scotland it fell more quickly in the North, North East and the Eastern Regions than in the South East and South West Regions.

In Aberdeen city a hospital confinement was offered to all expectant mothers from 1948 onwards and soon 85 per cent booked for hospital confinement. The remaining 15 per cent who still preferred a home confinement consisted very largely of women of high parity from social classes IV and V—a high risk group. Approximately 10 years later these women booked for hospital. Figure 1.1 shows the trend in the perinatal mortality rate in first and 4th+ births in two cause groups: (1) an 'environmental' group in which perinatal deaths are related to impairment of the mother's reproductive efficiency by the poor environment in which she was reared, and (2) an

'obstetrical' cause group consisting of deaths from complications of pregnancy and labour, many of which can be avoided by a high standard of obstetric and paediatric care. It will be seen that in the 'obstetrical' cause group in first pregnancies the death rate fell steadily from 1948 to 1970, particularly in the categories of difficult labour and 'unexplained' deaths of babies weighing more than 2500g. On the other hand there was no fall in the death rate from pre-eclampsia between 1948 and 1967 despite a uniformly high standard of antenatal care. It fell in the years 1968–70 mainly because mothers were younger. It has been shown by MacGillivray that the incidence and severity of pre-eclampsia increased steadily from south to north in Britain. The reason for this is not understood but it is clear that it cannot be explained by differences in standards of antenatal care. In 4th+ pregnancies little fall in the perinatal mortality rate occurred till 1963–67, when hospital confinement became the rule.

In the 'environmental' cause group perinatal death rates in primigravidae varied only slightly throughout the years 1948–70, being highest in 1948–52. In the 4th+ pregnancy group the rate was also high in 1948–52. It fell to its lowest level in 1953–57 and rose sharply again to reach its highest level in 1963–67. The probable explanation is that a cohort of women who started childbearing in 1948–52 had

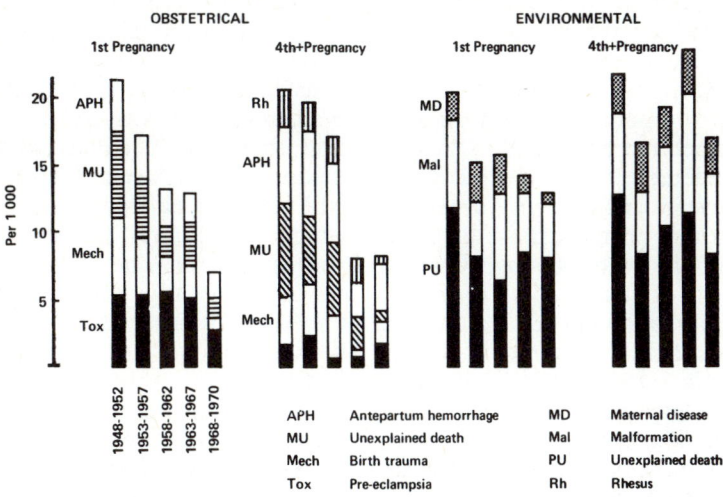

Fig. 1.1 The changes in the perinatal mortality rate from various causes in first and fourth or later pregnancies in Aberdeen between 1948–52 and 1968–70.

an unusually high death rate in each pregnancy from 'environmental' causes. Many of the women were born when the industrial depression was at its worst between 1928 and 1934 with an unemployment rate in Scotland of almost 30 per cent. Since many were undernourished and short in stature the high death rate from 'unexplained' causes in low weight babies was to be expected. The fact that high death rates from malformations also occurred suggests that the mother had received more specific damage at the fetal stage, possibly to her oocytes. The very high death rate from malformations of the central nervous system accounts very largely for the much higher perinatal death rate in the United Kingdom than in Holland, Denmark, Norway or Sweden.

This detailed examination of trends in perinatal mortality rates suggests that there may be limits to what can be done by improving standards of obstetric care and that these limits are set by the reproductive efficiency of the mother which is very much affected by her environment from birth to maturity.

It is not surprising that in Britain today the lowest perinatal mortality rate is in the Oxford Hospital Region where the health and physique of the mothers is good and the standards of obstetrics very high. However, the rate is not quite so low as the national rate for Sweden where the whole population is more socially advanced and the national provision of education and health services is at a very high level. To attain the same level in Britain will take time because although the standard of obstetrics can be improved fairly quickly, higher standards of health, physique, education and sophistication in the population can only be brought about much more slowly.

Political considerations are obviously involved since the standard of living necessary to bring about these changes must be more equal throughout the whole country instead of the present state of affairs which results in migration from poor to affluent areas. Although the national perinatal mortality rate in Britain has been falling since 1958 there has been no narrowing of the gap between the rates of North and South. The excessive death rate in the North continues to be largely in what are described in the Registrar-General's Reports as 'conditions of the fetus', corresponding approximately to environmental causes as described earlier.

Changing status of women in society

In Britain, replacement of the population requires an average of slightly over two children per family and most young people today plan their families carefully to give their children 'the best chance in life'. Since the great majority marry before the age of 25 it is clear that contraception has become the rule for almost everyone. With the discovery of oral contraception women now have a method within their own control and in future need have a child only when they want to have it. However, Garrett Hardin (1966) has said that 'short of the millennium it is difficult to imagine that the failure rate for a total population will ever fall below one pregnancy per 100 years of exposure'. He calculated that on this basis there would be about 225 000 unwanted pregnancies amongst married women every year in the USA (equivalent to approximately 50 000 in the UK) and he thought that the failure rate had been about 10 times this figure during the last two generations.

It seems incredible on humanitarian grounds that in Britain there should have been so little urgency on the part of the medical profession and the Government to include in the National Health Service free comprehensive provision of family planning, sterilization (both male and female) and abortion. It has only been the persistence of voluntary agencies such as the Family Planning Association, the Abortion Law Reform Association and the Simon Trust, that progress has been made in providing a service. Some enabling legislation has been enacted but the service is far from comprehensive except in a few enlightened areas. With regard to both abortion and contraception there has been an attempt to draw a distinction between 'medical' indications, which would be legal, and social indications, which would not. This is in practice artificial and unrealistic. The majority of women want contraceptive advice and abortion not because they are physically unfit to have a child but because they do not wish to have one. With justification they think seriously about the 15 years' commitment to the care of the child which would be involved. Many women now wish to return to work outside the home or to continue a professional career when they have completed childbearing. Not enough is done for such women to enable them to make this double contribution. High ability is not unlimited in any community and we cannot afford to under-employ one half of our most able citizens.

Changes in sexual mores have resulted in an increase in illegitimacy especially in single women in the non-manual occupational groups. It may be that well educated and intelligent young women and men, who come from homes where sex and marriage can be freely and intelligently discussed, may avoid many of the pitfalls of the new freedom characteristic of the so-called 'permissive society', but it is clear that many who do not have these advantages are much too immature to cope with it. The great increase in pregnancies in single women is evidence of this.

The place of the family doctor in the obstetrical and gynaecological service

Without minimizing the importance of a high standard of skill in the obstetrical services it must be kept in mind that at least 70 per cent of pregnancies and labours are uncomplicated and can be safely and efficiently conducted by the general practitioner obstetrician (Baird, 1969). In cities both normal and abnormal deliveries should take place in the same hospital in accommodation suitable for the particular needs of each case. General practitioners are gradually forming themselves into groups working from Health Centres and supplying a complete service both preventive and curative for the area in which they are situated. General practitioner obstetrics would involve some degree of specialization amongst general practitioners so that in addition to being personal doctors to their own particular patients they would be able to give advice to their colleagues on aspects in which they were specially qualified. The GP obstetrician could be responsible for the organization of the obstetrical service for all expectant mothers in the group practice, and refer high risk cases (some 30 per cent) to be under the immediate care of obstetric specialists. He could also undertake minor gynaecology and be responsible for organizing routine checks such as screening for cervical cancer. He would be interested in the field of sex education, contraception and abortion. He would be a member of the obstetrical and gynaecological department or division of the district or teaching hospital. The specialist would be relieved of much routine work and would have more time to devote to the care of complicated cases, to research, and to undergraduate and postgraduate teaching.

The obstetrical and gynaecological specialist

The changing problems in obstetrics and gynaecology brought about by the changing social conditions and the rapid increase in knowledge require changes in emphasis in the training of undergraduates and postgraduates. They need more knowledge of reproductive physiology, endocrinology, epidemiology and genetics. Clinical training should take place ideally in teaching hospitals with the responsibility for the care of patients in a total population of adequate size. As well as being equipped to meet modern needs of scientific medicine the specialist obstetrician must understand the psychological needs of the individual.

Career posts should be available for research workers who may or may not be medically qualified and who wish to work on long term research projects in co-operation with consultants in the National Health Service and with the staff of the University Clinical department. It is most important to have a post of Chairman of a division of Obstetrics and Gynaecology whose function is to act as a leader in his specialty and to co-ordinate the work of the various types of clinicians and research workers.

With the improvement in the health and physique of the population, the younger age at marriage and the much higher standard of obstetric and paediatric care, the perinatal mortality rate is falling steadily so that today the rates need be high only in those who have been reared in the depressed areas of the large industrial cities, and as such depressed areas disappear the perinatal deaths which are dependent basically on this faulty environment will also disappear. The problems which will remain are more likely to be related to genetic defects.

REFERENCES

Baird, D. (1969) Perinatal mortality. *Lancet*, **i**, 51–54.

Baird, D. (1969) An area maternity service. *Lancet*, **i**, 515–18.

Baird, D. & Thomson, A. M. (1969) *Perinatal problems. Second Report of the 1958 British Perinatal Mortality Survey.* Eds: R. Butler & Eva Alberman. Edinburgh and London: E. & S. Livingstone Ltd.

Baird, D. (1971) The Galton Lecture 1970—'The Obstetrician and Society'. *J. biosoc. Sci. Suppl.* **3** (1971), 93–111.

Burnett, J. (1966) Plenty and Want. *A Social History of Diet in England from 1815 to the Present Day.* London: Nelson.

Hardin, G. (1966) The History and Future of Birth Control. *Persp. Biol. Med.* **10**, 1.

Hytten, F. E. (1954) Clinical and chemical studies in human lactation. *Brit. med. J.*, **i**, 249.

Taylor, L. R. (1969) The Optimum Population for Britain. *Symposia of Institute of Biology*, **19**, London and New York: Academic Press.

2. The Epidemiological Perspective

There are lies, damned lies, and clinical impressions—Professor Sam Shuster (*British Medical Journal*, 29 April, 1972).

Even a well-read and experienced doctor may acquire a limited view of his profession, the only things that may appear to matter being the diagnosis and treatment of abnormalities in individual patients. Through his own clinical practice and discussions with colleagues, he builds up experience which is sufficient to guide him in everyday work and which may even lead to respectable seniority. Yet his judgement, like that of all of us, is likely to be swayed by prejudice and by personal experience, as well as by the current climate of opinion. Certainly, what doctors believe, practice and teach is not necessarily lastingly true: consider for example the fact that within living memory blood-letting and purgation were considered to be beneficial in many forms of illness.

As explained in Chapter 1, the practice of obstetrics and gynaecology is changing with great rapidity under the influence of social and economic events which would be of fundamental importance even if there were no concurrent changes in medical techniques of diagnosis and methods of treatment. The specialist and the general practitioner should be able to give competent advice on the development of the services they provide, so that the needs of the community are adequately met. The second 'Cogwheel' report (Department of Health and Social Security, 1972) observes that: 'The management of services is greatly affected—and sometimes made difficult—by decisions of doctors.' General clinical impressions provide an inadequate basis for planning, especially during a time of rapid technical change and increasing social complexity.

Professional competence therefore needs to be enhanced by a wider understanding of clinical and organizational problems than can be gained from personal experience in the consulting room, the hospital ward and the operating theatre. Properly collected and collated statistics summarize events in large populations over periods of time. They help the practitioner to discern trends, to weigh up the efficiency of current practice in his area, and above all to see where improvement is most needed. The obstetrician and gynaecologist is particularly fortunate, since he is intimately concerned with all three of life's landmarks— birth, marriage and death*—and information on each of these events is systematically recorded and regularly published in many countries.

Epidemiology seeks to measure the incidence or prevalence of specified events in defined communities and, by studying distributions in relation to time, space or social characteristics, to uncover clues about their nature, causes and means of control or prevention. Vital statistics are to a medical service what a balance sheet is to a business enterprise.

The word 'statistics' discourages many doctors, but it should be remembered that most professional statisticians have no medical experience and that a great deal can be achieved by good organization, common sense and simple arithmetic. When planning or interpreting vital statistics, it is useful to ask a few basic questions.

1. *Is the condition under examination clearly defined?* A birth or a Caesarean section is a definite event about the occurrence of which different observers are likely to agree (though there may be disagreement over marginal cases, e.g. whether the event was a 'birth' or an 'abortion'). But reported differences in the incidence of 'haemorrhage' or 'toxaemia' could easily be due to differences in the criteria used.

2. *Are all examples of the condition being*

---

* Anyone who doubts that the obstetrician is concerned with death should note that in England and Wales in 1969 there were 18 883 perinatal deaths, i.e. about the same number of deaths as occurred in adults of both sexes aged 15–54.

recorded? Doctors usually record what they consider to be relevant to the management of an individual patient, but may not record all information that may be essential for valid statistics. Some years ago a large increase in the incidence of 'fetal distress' was reported from one hospital. The increase was due almost certainly to the fact that growing realization of the importance of the condition had led to it being looked for more carefully, and recorded more frequently.

3. *What kinds of patients are included in the groups being studied?* There were, for many years, heated arguments about the relative safety of domiciliary or hospital maternity services. Advocates of delivery at home pointed to the fact that the death rates were nearly always lower than those obtained in hospital. What they ignored was that patients in whom difficulty was anticipated were (or should have been) booked selectively for delivery in hospital, whereas 'normal' patients were booked for delivery at home. It is always desirable to consider very carefully, what *kinds* of women are included in any two groups being compared.

4. *Are there any other snags in the data?* Statistical advice is often very helpful, but the uninitiated can at least look for obvious snags, such as reliance on percentages based on ridiculously small numbers or differences and trends which clearly do not accord with clinical reality and which may be artefacts of the method of selection, classification or analysis.

Ideally, vital statistics would be based on accurate information gathered from the whole of a defined geographic community. This is the situation in statistics of births and deaths compiled by the Registrar-General, and has been achieved in a number of national and local clinical surveys. Incidences in such data show what is happening in the community under consideration. Statistics drawn from a hospital or a medical practice may be far from representing any defined community. For example, in the hospital where the writer works there are far more cases of Rh disease than in the local community, because cases (but not all such cases) are referred to the hospital from a wide surrounding area. This is not to say that hospital statistics are useless: they can in fact be of enormous value, properly interpreted. But the mistake should not be made of confusing hospital experience with

general experience nor, for that matter, of comparing 'results' in one hospital with those of another, without taking into account the fact that the two institutions may be dealing with different types of patient.

Fortunately the limited value of the 'maternity hospital report' is now being recognized by most obstetricians. Most reports of the past attempted little more than a catalogue of activity and resulted in a situation where (to quote a recent comment), 'Statistical analysis of medical information became limited, for most clinicians, to analyses of the characteristics of series of patients, the authors being unaware of, or having forgotten, the basic principles of relating cases to population at risk'.

Finally, it should be remembered that the characteristics of populations are not static. As was pointed out in the last chapter, social conditions in industrialized countries have changed enormously during the past century. In Britain, at the time of writing, altered attitudes to sex, better control of fertility and legalized abortion are engendering such rapid changes in reproductive habits and therefore in the nature of the practice of obstetrics and gynaecology that it is already becoming necessary to be cautious about comparing contemporary vital statistics with those of even a few years ago.

SOURCES OF INFORMATION

In Britain, the main sources of official vital statistics are the reports of the Registrars General of England and Wales, and of Scotland. Each publishes two annual reports, one giving population and the other mortality statistics. Commentary volumes appear also, somewhat later than the tabulations on which they are based, together with reports on special subjects. Further statistical information is to be found in the reports of the Chief Medical Officer to the Department of Health and Social Security, numerous other official reports from central government departments, and in the annual reports of local medical officers of health. Census statistics are valuable for many purposes, but are often obsolescent by the time they are published. International vital statistics are published by the United Nations and its agencies, notably the World Health Organization. International comparisons are, however, made hazardous by differences of definitions and by incomplete or inaccurate returns from some countries.

POPULATIONS

Until the twentieth century deaths nearly balanced births, and populations were increasing rather slowly; the extra numbers were assimilated without much difficulty, or could move into sparsely populated and unexploited territories. During recent decades, death rates have fallen sharply while birth rates, especially in the less developed regions which include a majority of the world's population, have remained more or less at their previous high level. The result has been the notorious 'population explosion'. Figure 2.1,

been exaggerated in the past (food production has, to date, kept slightly ahead of population increase, thanks to the 'green revolution' and other advances in agricultural productivity) but even so, the uncomfortable consequences of rapid growth in numbers—such as increases in the ratio of 'dependant' to 'productive' members of society; the widening economic gap between rich and poor countries; collisions between peoples of varying races and creeds—are already clearly apparent. Even if, miraculously, some means were available of quickly reducing birth rates to a maintenance level, the above uncomfortable consequences would remain with us for a long time to come. But the fact is that no such quick solutions to the problems of excessive fertility are in sight. *The control of fertility is* **the** *human problem beside which all the other, more traditional,*

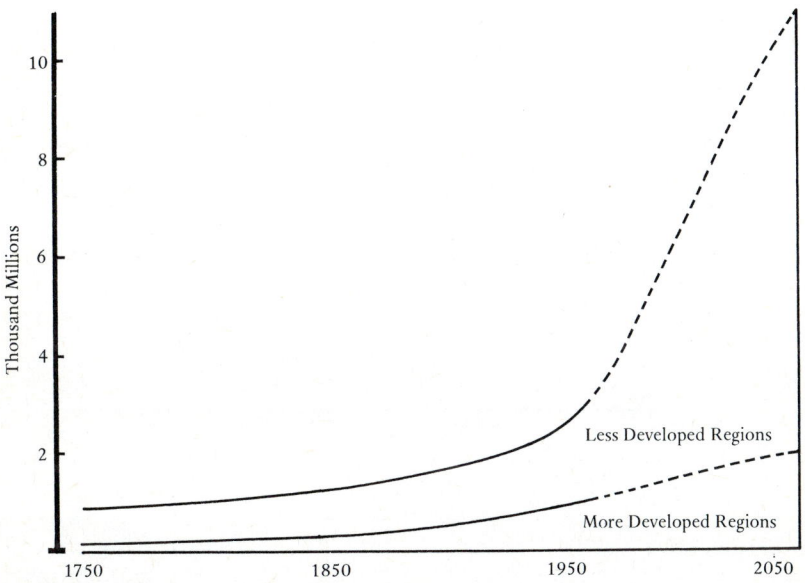

Fig. 2.1   Estimates and conjectures of past and future population of the world, and of the currently more developed and less developed regions, 1750–2050.
(Source: *United Nations Population Studies* No. 49, 1971.)

based on recent estimates and predictions by the United Nations, shows that the world's population has more than doubled since 1900. Since the rate of growth follows the laws of compound interest, currently at about 2 per cent per year, there will be roughly four times as many people alive in the year 2000, compared with the year 1900, even if current family planning programmes have some impact. Fears of world-wide starvation have

concerns of obstetricians and gynaecologists are insignificant. Potts (1971) has written: 'The magnitude of the problem is fearful...the battle against human fertility is going very badly ... Basically I think there has been a lack of realism in looking at the sociology of human family limitation practices. In the second part of the twentieth century, family planning must be undertaken with a set of second-rate reversible methods of contraception, a female irrevocable method which demands moderate medical skill, and perhaps only vasectomy is not open to medical improvement. Most important of all, there is a reluctance on the part of doctors and administrators to face the problem of abortion. Here, public and private attitudes are often in tragic conflict. The termination of pregnancy is one of the oldest and one of the commonest forms of fertility control. No nation has ever shown a marked fall in its birth rate without a considerable recourse to abortion . . . In summary, if the global population is to be dealt with there must be a total committal to the use of simple contraceptives, an honesty and realism about sterilization and a compassion about abortion.'

Europe has the slowest-growing population, by far, of any continent, partly because it was until recently able to export 'surplus' people

later marriage and motivated by a fashion for smaller families'.

There is no doubt about the trend towards smaller families. In England and Wales, the average woman married in 1860 at age 20–24 had seven children. This had fallen to 2·4, 2·2 and 2·3 children for similar women married in 1930, 1940 and 1950, respectively. There may be some increase in the size of completed families in subsequent marriage cohorts. For example, women aged 20–24 married in 1960 had an average family size of 2·11 children after 10 years of marriage, compared with 1·89 among those married in 1950. This may, of course, merely indicate closer spacing of births without implying that the completed family will be larger. We must wait and see. Whatever the result, it implies that modern women in Britain spend much less

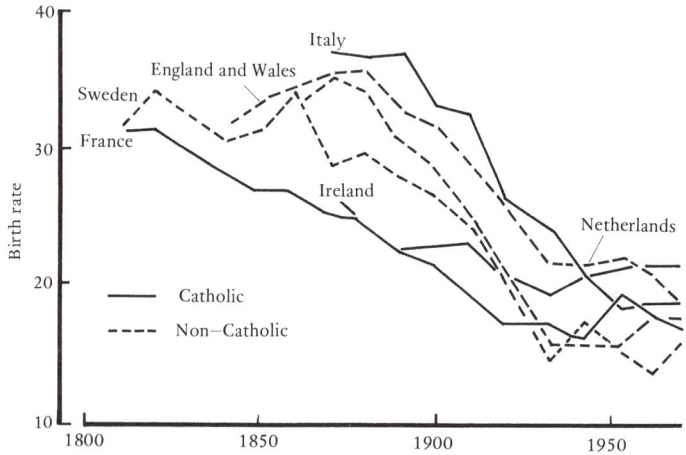

Fig. 2.2   Birth rates in selected European countries, showing differences in time and rate of decrease over 150 years. (Source: Parkes, *J. Biosoc. Sci.* 1971, Suppl. 3, p. 21.)

to other continents, and partly because it pioneered industrialization and a desire for smaller families that seems to be associated with a rapidly rising standard of living in industrial society. Figure 2.2 illustrates the interesting fact that birth rates in six European countries have fallen steadily since the beginning of the present century, long before mechanical or other contraceptive devices became available on a large scale. The rate of fall has been much the same in all these countries, irrespective of law or religion.* Parkes comments that 'presumably, therefore, it was due to birth control by some means or other, supplemented in the later stages by

time bearing and rearing children than their grandmothers. The gradual disappearance of the worn-out 'grand multipara' has obvious implications for the obstetrician.

MARRIAGES AND BIRTHS

In Britain, at this time a 'birth' usually refers to a fetus of more than 28 weeks' gestation; fetuses born earlier are regarded as abortions if dead. Twenty-eight weeks of gestation corresponds to an average birth weight of about 1kg, and uncertainty arises since some babies born sooner and lighter survive well

* There is however a tendency to plateau in the last 30 years.

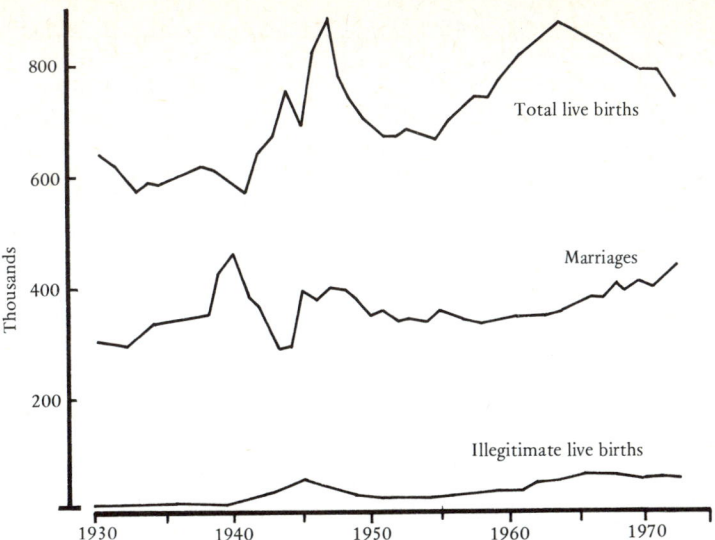

Fig. 2.3   Marriages and births, England and Wales, 1930–72. (Source: *Registrar-General's Statistical Review*, 1972, Part II.)

enough to be registered as live births. Crude birth rates are births per 1000 population of all ages and both sexes. Since the proportions of fertile women may differ considerably in various populations, fertility is better indicated by 'births per 1000 women aged 15–44'.

Figure 2.3 shows the numbers of marriages, total live births and illegitimate live births in England and Wales from 1930 to 1972. Rates per 1000 women aged 15–44 show much the same patterns. It is obvious that socio-economic factors play a considerable part. Thus, marriages fell during the great industrial depression of the early 1930s, and rose (together with births) during the pre-war economic recovery. The onset of the Second World War (1939–40) was associated with a sharp peak of marriages; and though the number of marriages fell steeply until 1943–44 there were many more births. Marriages increased again at the end of the war, followed by a striking peak of births, which settled to what seemed to be a fairly stable level during the early 1950s, in association with a gradual fall in the number of marriages. However, numbers of births increased steadily from 1956 to 1964, without an appreciable rise in the number of marriages, presumably because of economic prosperity. Those were the years, the Prime Minister of the time said, when the country had 'never had it so good'. From 1965 to date, numbers of marriages have increased but births have fallen steadily, presumably

because times have been harder and because 'the pill' has been widely used. Nevertheless, one cannot predict with confidence that numbers of births will continue to fall. The steady increase of births from 1955 reached a peak in 1964 that was as high as the peak of the

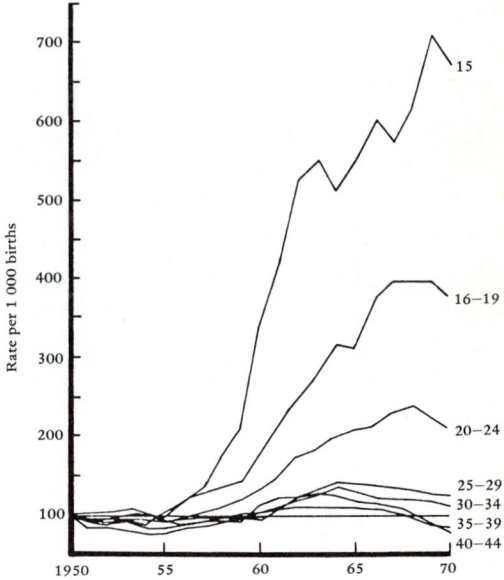

Fig. 2.4   Number of illegitimate births in England and Wales, 1950–1970, by age of mother, expressed as a percentage of the number in 1950.

(Source: Russell, *Clins. Obstet. Gynaec.*, 1974, **1**, p. 683.)

notorious post-war 'bulge' in 1947. Those babies will attain the age of fertility by the end of the present decade, and we have no reason to believe that their philoprogenitive instincts will be less strong than those of their mothers.

The lowest part of figure 2.3 shows numbers of illegitimate births. As might be expected, there was a rise during the Second World War, and there has been a slower but even greater increase during the 1960s, now showing some sign of a decline. This, presumably, has been one result of the 'permissive society'. The recent slight fall in illegitimate births is not necessarily a cause for complacency; it may simply mean that a higher proportion of illegitimate pregnancies are being terminated under the provisions of the Abortion Act. A fact which must give rise to serious concern is a five-fold increase in the number of illegitimate births in girls under 16. Figure 2.4 shows that the general increase of illegitimate births has occurred predominantly among young girls and women. Russell (1974) describes some of the consequent problems that arise in the practice of an obstetrician/gynaecologist.

PERINATAL MORTALITY

Definitions

A stillbirth, in Britain, is 'the birth of any child which has issued forth from its mother after the twenty-eighth week of pregnancy and which did not at any time after being completely expelled from its mother breathe or show any other signs of life'. Since it may be to some extent a matter of chance whether a baby dies just before or soon after birth, 'perinatal' death rates have been much used during the past 20 years. In Britain and most other countries perinatal deaths comprise stillbirths plus deaths during the first week of life, and the rate is per 1000 total (live and still) births. International comparisons should, however, be made with caution, since in some places babies born dead between 20 and 28 weeks of gestation are counted as stillbirths and perinatal deaths may include all deaths during the first 28 days after birth.

Secular trends

Figure 2.5 shows trends in the stillbirth, first-week death and perinatal mortality rates in England and Wales and in Scotland since 1930 and 1939, respectively. The rates are plotted on a logarithmic scale, so that the same relative change (e.g. halving the rates) occupies the same vertical space at any level.

1. *The years of industrial depression, 1930–33.* During these years the stillbirth and first-week death rates in England and Wales rose slightly, no doubt because unemployment and poverty were widespread and had deleterious effects on maternal health.

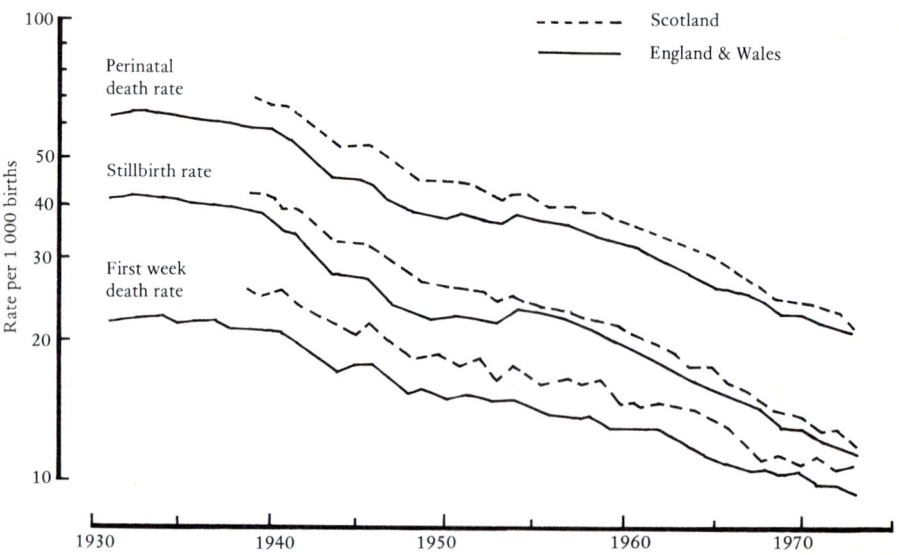

Fig. 2.5   Perinatal, stillbirth and first week death rates, England and Wales 1930–73, and Scotland 1939–73. (Source: *Registrar-General's Annual Review.*)

2. *The pre-war recovery period*. From 1934 to 1940 economic conditions improved, and perinatal mortality rates in England and Wales dropped slowly, the stillbirth rate slightly more than the first-week death rate. Thus, at the time when war broke out things were slightly better than they had been at the start of the industrial depression. Nevertheless, progress had been disconcertingly slow considering that considerable expansion of local authority and other maternity services had taken place.

3. *The war and immediate post-war period*. Perinatal mortality rates fell sharply in both countries from 1941 to 1944, despite the disruption of life caused by the war: indeed, this is the most dramatic improvement on record. It cannot be attributed to any major improvement in the organization of maternity services, nor to an important advance in obstetrical technique. The most probable explanation is that during the war years unemployment and the more severe manifestations of poverty disappeared; and an enlightened national food policy gave priority to pregnant women, who received special allowance of the 'protective foods', a supply of cheap milk, and free vitamin supplements (Duncan, Baird and Thomson, 1952).

The fall in the perinatal mortality rate was interrupted during 1945 and 1946, when a sharp increase in the birth rate (Fig. 2.2) caused considerable overloading of the maternity services. This was overcome, and progress was resumed during 1947 and 1948.

4. *The years 1949–57*. The establishment of the National Health Service in 1948 might have been expected to be followed by a further reduction in perinatal death rates. Disconcertingly, the stillbirth rate in England and Wales remained almost stationary during the years 1948–57, and the first-week death rates fell much more slowly than during the war years. In Scotland, both rates fell, but also slowly. This situation caused a great deal of concern, and in 1958 a nation-wide Perinatal Mortality Survey was organized by the National Birthday Trust. Some of the findings will be discussed below.

5. *Since 1958* perinatal mortality rates in both countries have declined much more steeply, largely as a result of an accelerated fall in the stillbirth rate. The reasons are not entirely clear. Improvements in the maternity services and in standards of care during pregnancy and labour have no doubt played an important part, but an equally important factor may be the influx of a new generation of mothers—those that have grown up in the much more favourable economic and social conditions that have prevailed since about 1940, and who in consequence are more healthy and better informed. As has already been indicated, the reduction in average maternal age and the gradual decline in the proportion of high parity births has also played a part.

Causes of perinatal deaths

The Eighth Revision of the International Classification of Causes of Death (WHO, 1967) gives a special list of 100 causes for tabulating perinatal morbidity and mortality; this is used in the statistics published annually by the Registrar-General. Unfortunately it is not very informative. In cases of stillbirth and death during early infancy the causes are often obscure and frequently multiple, so that errors of certification are easy to make. Furthermore, even if causes of deaths were uniformly recorded on the basis of complete information, the results would not be easy to interpret from the point of view of prevention. In England and Wales, the main causes registered were conditions of placenta (mainly premature separation) and umbilical cord, 20 per cent; congenital anomalies, 18 per cent; anoxic and hypoxic conditions, 17 per cent; 'other conditions of fetus and newborn' (mostly immaturity), 16 per cent; complications of pregnancy (mainly toxaemias and multiple pregnancy), 12 per cent; birth injury, 4 per cent; and haemolytic disease of the newborn, 3 per cent.

Changes in the official classifications, and the absence of any information on the causes of stillbirth in England and Wales before 1961, make it difficult to obtain a reliable picture of which causes of perinatal death have been most reduced; some idea can be obtained from the reports of the Registrar-General for Scotland. Birth injury, the classic cause of stillbirth many years ago, is now much less common, thanks to improvements in methods of delivery and to the gradual reduction of gross distortion of the maternal pelvis caused by rickets. Improvements in antenatal management have greatly reduced losses due to the toxaemias of pregnancy, placenta praevia, rhesus isoimmunization and many maternal diseases. Congenital malformations cannot yet be prevented, except for the small group (not necessarily lethal) due to such causes as rubella and teratogenic drugs. The official records indicate a reduction of deaths attributed to immaturity and ill-defined causes, but how much this is due to more accurate registration of causes and how much to a genuine improvement is difficult to say.

A fundamental difficulty is that even when it is possible to arrange for expert examination at autopsy, the pathologist is frequently unable to provide information that is useful from the point of view of prevention. At best, the pathologist can say *how* the fetus or neonate died, but he can seldom say *why*. In the 1958 Perinatal Mortality Survey (Butler and Alberman, 1969) over 90 per cent of the deaths were specially investigated by pathologists, and the following causes were found in 2210 perinatal deaths:

	%
Congenital malformation	16·0
Rh incompatibility	3·9
Birth trauma	2·9
Trauma+asphyxia	6·5
Asphyxia { prior to labour	10·2
Asphyxia { other	21·3
Hyaline membrane disease	5·0
Infection	4·4
Miscellaneous	4·9
No cause found	15·7
No autopsy	9·2
	100·0

Thus, in nearly half the deaths, no cause was found or it was a non-specific condition such as asphyxia which could be due to many different underlying causes. Some of the apparently more specific causes were closely associated with premature birth, and indicate little more than the manner in which very small babies die. More can be learnt from a pathological classification of causes such as the above if the material is cross-tabulated against a list of underlying clinical conditions, but the result is then a rather complicated two-way table with which it is difficult to compare different groups of cases—e.g. series taken from different areas or at different periods of time. The situation is not made easier by the fact that several different causes may have been present in one case, so that it is difficult to decide which should be regarded as the most

important. For example, if the mother was suffering from anaemia and pre-eclampsia, had a lengthy labour, and the baby died within minutes of birth from asphyxia, what was the prime cause of death?

Baird and his associates made an attempt to overcome some of these difficulties by devising a single classification which took account of both the pathological findings and the underlying clinical situation (Baird *et al.*, 1954; Butler and Alberman, 1969). Rules were devised to deal with multiple factors, and common sense was held to be as important as the features discovered at autopsy. For example, if cerebral haemorrhage ('birth trauma') was reported but the labour had been perfectly normal, it was held that from the point of view of prevention nothing would be gained by choosing a 'cause' which suggested that the nature of delivery was at fault: the defect was more probably in the child, and since its nature remained a matter of guesswork it would be realistic to label the death as being of unknown aetiology. Unexplained deaths (a high proportion of which were associated with signs of asphyxia) were subdivided into those in babies which were mature by weight (over 2500g birth weight) and those that were of low birth weight.

The general principle was that the 'cause' should be defined in terms of the feature which started the train of events culminating in death. Thus, where the history began with severe pre-eclampsia leading to the delivery by forceps of an immature baby which showed signs of cerebral damage or asphyxia at autopsy, the cause was held to be 'toxaemia'.

The data of the 1958 Perinatal Mortality Survey were so classified with the results shown in Table 2.1.

In theory, death rates from causes in the 'obstetrical' category can be reduced by improved standards of care, whereas those in the 'environmental' category are primarily influenced by the types of mothers involved. It may seem surprising that deaths classified as being essentially of unknown origin (the term 'placental insufficiency' is not very explanatory) should be allocated to the 'obstetrical' group. But the great value of epidemiological research is that it sometimes indicates means of prevention even when the aetiology is unknown (just as the association between cholera and the water-supply could be put to use before the causative organism had been

Table 2.1   1958 Perinatal Mortality Survey

'Obstetrical' causes	%	'Environmental' causes	%
Toxaemia	12·6	Unexplained prematurity	17·9
Mechanical causes	13·1	Malformations	18·8
'Placental insufficiency' (Mature		Antepartum haemorrhage	14·2
babies, cause unknown)	14·1	Miscellaneous causes	5·1
Rh incompatibility	4·3		
	44·1		56·0

discovered). Perinatal deaths in this group were found to be relatively common in pregnancies which continued beyond term, especially in elderly primigravidae, and to have a number of epidemiological characteristics which resembled those in deaths from mechanical causes. Clinically, many of them occurred with little warning or after a short period of fetal distress, and a common finding at autopsy was signs of asphyxia (Walker, 1954). Baird used these findings as the basis of a new policy in the Aberdeen Maternity Hospital, whereby postmaturity was prevented in selected cases by surgical induction of labour; in addition, signs of fetal distress were watched for more carefully, and Caesarean section was used more freely in the interests of the baby. His data indicate that these and later measures resulted in a considerable reduction of perinatal mortality in the city, which now has one of the lowest rates in Britain (Baird, 1963, 1971).

Factors influencing perinatal mortality

The illustrative material used below is derived from the Perinatal Mortality Survey (1958) (Butler and Bonham, 1963; Butler and Alberman, 1969). Special records were prepared for nearly all births in England, Wales and Scotland during one week in March 1958, and records were continued for stillbirths and neonatal deaths for three months. In addition to fairly detailed clinical information, an autopsy report was available for most of the deaths.

1. *Age and parity.* Figure 2.6 shows the perinatal mortality rates by the ages and parity of the mothers. In all parity groups, the rates rise with age after the age-group 25–29 at least. The rates are relatively high in the mothers under 20, probably because this age-group includes a high proportion from the poorest and least-educated social classes. Women having second babies have the lowest

rates of any parity group; it appears that a 'practice run' is needed for maximum efficiency. Thereafter, rates increase with rising parity, and are notably high after the fourth pregnancy.

When interpreting such information, it should be remembered that the mothers are not distributed equally in the various subgroups. Thus, primigravidae over 35 and women of exceptionally high parity are relatively few in number. Even a large reduction in the perinatal deaths occurring among such groups will accordingly have a relatively small influence upon the overall perinatal mortality rate. More benefit may be obtained by achieving a small improvement in the rates in the 'common' categories, say all parities between 20 and 30 years of age, than a much larger improvement in the 'rare' categories. This is not an argument against seeking improvement in the elderly primigravidae and high multi-

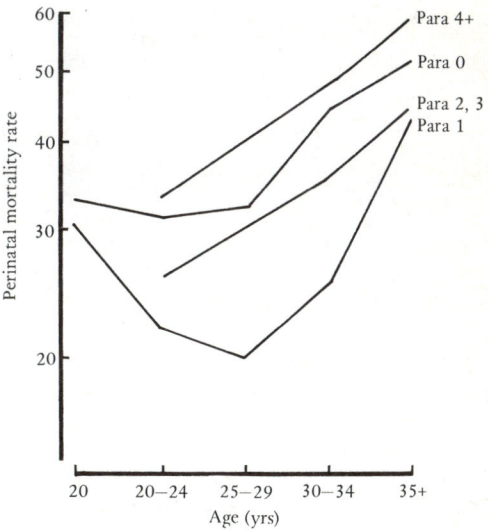

Fig. 2.6 Perinatal mortality rates by maternal age and parity; 1958 *British Perinatal Mortality Survey.* (Source: *see* Butler and Alberman, 1969, p. 22.)

parae—they may well be the categories in whom improvement is most easily achieved— but a warning that the effect on overall mortality is proportional to the size of the group as well as the extent of the improvement achieved.

Consideration of age and parity differences in terms of the clinico-pathological classification of causes of death (devised by Baird *et al.*, 1954) shows that primigravidity was associated with relatively high rates of perinatal mortality from toxaemia and to a lesser extent from mechanical causes and 'placental insufficiency'. Deaths from antepartum haemorrhage and Rh incompatibility were particularly common in women of high parity. High maternal age seems to be associated with increased death rates from most causes. Relatively high death rates in the youngest group of mothers are particularly noticeable in the group 'premature cause unknown', probably a reflection of the relatively poor social status of many women in that group.

various ways to yield information on employment, industrial and socio-economic groups. The classification most commonly used in medical statistics is 'Social Class', which distinguishes five main groups:

I   Professional etc. occupations, e.g. doctors, managing directors.
II   Intermediate.
III   Skilled occupations, mainly manual.
IV   Intermediate.
V   Unskilled occupations.

Class III, which is by far the largest, is sometimes divided into non-manual and manual categories. Three points should be noted: 1. Married women are usually classified by the occupations of their husbands; 2. The allocation of specific occupations to each of the social classes has been defined in detail by the Registrar-General; 3. Social class reflects income in a general way only; it is, in effect, a classification of occupations according to their standing within the community as a whole.

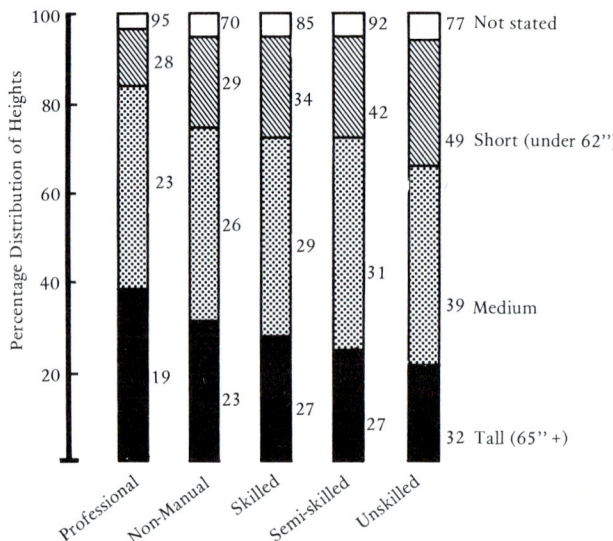

Fig. 2.7   Distribution of maternal heights, by socio-economic status of husbands (columns); and perinatal death rates by height and socio-economic group (figures).
(Source: *see* Butler and Alberman, 1969, p. 24.)

2. *Socio-economic status and physique.* Figure 2.7 shows death rates by maternal socio-economic status and height, and also indicates the distribution of heights within each socio-economic group. Since the 1911 Census, the Registrar-General has collected information on occupations, which has been classified in

There is obviously a gradient of perinatal mortality both with height and with socio-economic group. The lowest rate, under 20 per 1000, is in tall women in the professional group and the highest rate, nearly 50 per 1000, among short women married to unskilled manual workers. Although short women form a high-risk group and are commoner in the poorer classes, differences of stature explain only a small part of the difference in mortality between socio-economic groups, so that more than the physique of the mother seems to be involved.

As would be expected, the excess mortality in the poorer classes is to be found mainly in the 'environmental' category of causes.

3. *Regional differences.* Figure 2.8 shows variations of perinatal mortality in different parts of Britain during 1972. Though differences are less marked than they have been in the past, an association between relatively high rates and poverty, particularly where there is much heavy industry, is still apparent.

Only the most affluent areas of the UK have achieved rates comparable to those in some socially advanced countries as a whole; for example, Sweden, 16; Denmark, 18; Norway, 19; and Holland, 18 (all rates in 1970–71).

Only part of the regional differences in the UK can be explained by variations in age, parity, maternal physique and socio-economic status. It is probable that the maternity services also differ in effectiveness. Probably the lack of complete statistical 'explanation' in such terms is mainly due to the crudity of the statistical categories themselves. There is no evidence that regional differences are caused to any appreciable extent by climatic and genetic variations. The most plausible, as well as the most hopeful hypothesis is that where women are generally well grown and healthy, live in favourable conditions and receive a high standard of obstetric care, perinatal mortality rates are low. (All factors are needed for the best results.) Conversely, mortality is high where conditions are adverse, and particularly where several factors are adverse simultaneously. It should be noted that a very high standard of obstetrical care is most needed where mothers are commonly of inferior health and physique and live in poor conditions, whereas a moderate standard of care may suffice where mothers are basically healthy and are educated enough to make good use of the services available.

4. *Obstetrical care.* It is extremely difficult to provide satisfactory statistical evidence on the extent to which perinatal mortality rates are affected by the nature of the maternity services available. The situation is quite different from that with maternal mortality, where major causes of death, such as infection and haemorrhage, have been greatly reduced by specific advances in treatment. The main causes of perinatal mortality are non-specific, and only a few specific forms of treatment, for example, with regard to rhesus iso-immunization, have had effects that can be calculated with fair precision. The rest seems to be a matter of general tightening-up of the maternity services in a host of different ways, and of educating patients so that they make the best use of services.

The incidence of confinements in hospitals has increased rapidly in recent years, in 1970 to about 85 per cent in England and Wales, and to about 95 per cent in Scotland. Unfortunately, published figures do not differentiate between fully equipped maternity units with a full range of specialist services and small units with limited facilities. Fryer and Ashford (1972) found that until about 1966 there was a general correlation between increasing proportions of hospital confinements and decreasing perinatal death rates, but since

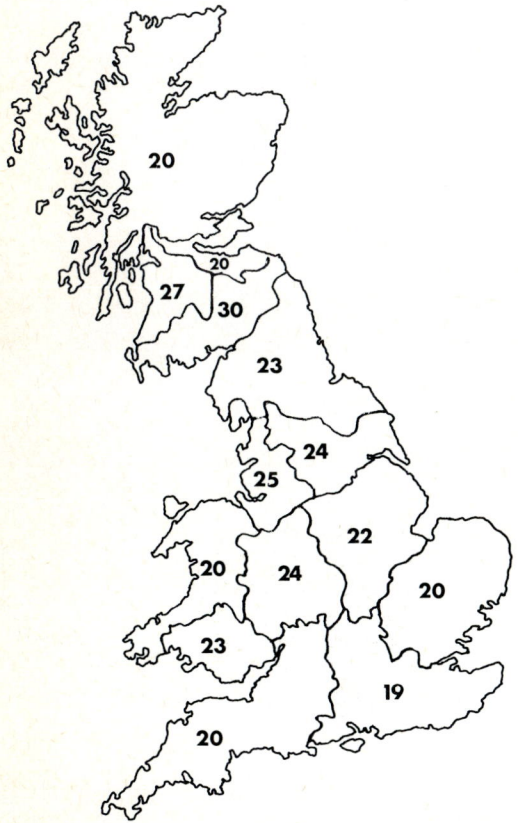

Fig. 2.8 Perinatal mortality rates by standard regions of England and Wales and Scotland, 1972.

(Source: *Registrar-General's Annual Review.*)

then local authorities with higher hospitalization rates (all forms of hospital) no longer tended to have the lower mortality rates. This, they suggest, supports the view that more is likely to be achieved by a sensible selection of high-risk patients for the higher and more expensive standards of care than by spreading the available resources more thinly in an attempt to increase the proportion of institutional births. Indeed, unless the hospital is adequately staffed and equipped and efficiently managed a false sense of security may be engendered.

Undoubtedly there is still much to be improved in selection of 'high-risk' cases for confinement in specialist hospitals or joint specialist, general-practitioner units. The Chief Medical Officer in England and Wales notes, for example, that in 1970 some 1166 women who were 35 years of age or more and who were known to have four or more previous live-born children had their babies at home. And many others were undoubtedly confined in institutions unable to cope efficiently with dangerous emergencies.

As has already been indicated, appeals to statistics in support of a domiciliary service are misleading if the argument is one of safety. The arguments in favour of domiciliary midwifery are social and psychological rather than medical; for example, reduction in the amount of travelling by the patient, who may have to go some distance to attend a hospital clinic; the advantage of supervision by a well-known and trusted family doctor or midwife; and, perhaps, the greater satisfaction of having the baby in familiar surroundings. It is possible that, as more modern hospitals are built and as hospitals learn to organize their attitudes of care, so that the convenience and the comfort of patients are important considerations, the stated advantages of domiciliary midwifery will become cancelled out. Similarly, the general-practitioner obstetrician might be most effective if his personal knowledge of the case were applied to a practitioner unit within the framework of a specialist division where experts could take over without delay in the event of a sudden emergency.

MATERNAL MORTALITY

By international agreement, deaths occurring during pregnancy or within six weeks of delivery, and attributable to complications of pregnancy, childbirth or the puerperium, are classified as maternal deaths. To these may be added 'associated maternal deaths', those not attributed to the specified list of 'maternal

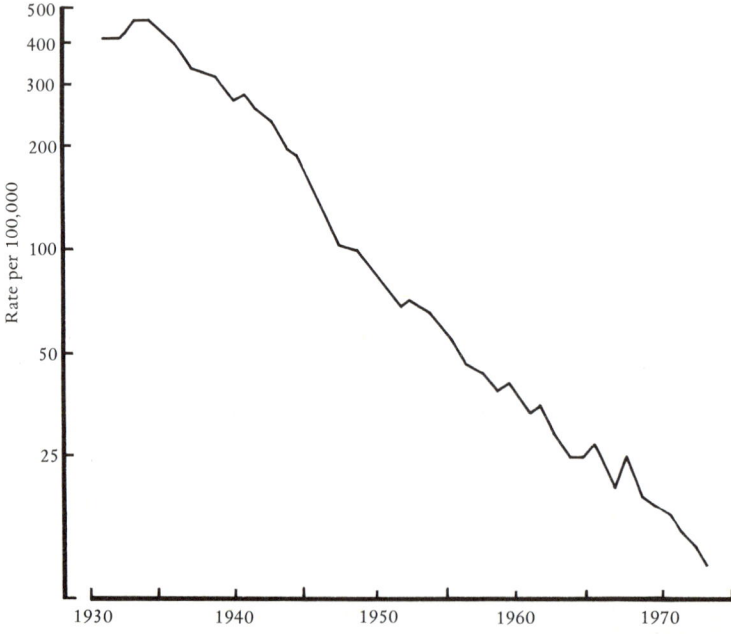

Fig. 2.9   Maternal mortality rates, England and Wales, 1931–73. (Source: *Registrar-General's Annual Review*.)

causes' but occurring coincidentally during pregnancy or the puerperium. It should be noted that in England and Wales (but not in Scotland) the international convention is modified by extending the puerperal period to 12 months; in practice, the difference is of little importance.

Until the 1930s, the chances of a mother dying during pregnancy, in labour, or during the puerperium were greater than one in two hundred, and obstetricians were often more concerned about saving the mother than the baby. Figure 2.9 shows that the maternal mortality rate in England and Wales is now less than one-twentieth of what it was in the early 1930s. One of the great killers—puerperal sepsis—the epidemic nature of which was emphasized by Semmelweiss and, before him, by Alexander Gordon of Aberdeen (*see* Chapter 21)—has been nearly eliminated by the sulphonamides and antibiotics. The dangers of haemorrhage have been greatly reduced by blood transfusions and other forms of treatment. In fact, as Table 2.2 shows, the numbers of maternal deaths have been sub-

assessor records his views on the causes of death and on the presence of any avoidable factor in the clinical care or administrative management. Specifying an avoidable factor is not an allocation of blame, nor is it an indication that the death could have been prevented; it only signifies that, in the assessor's opinion, the management fell short of the highest standard in some way.

These reports are strictly confidential, but at intervals the Department of Health and Social Security publishes a 'Report on Confidential Enquiries into Maternal Deaths in England and Wales'. The latest report was published in 1972 and covers the years 1967–69. Coverage was not complete, but reports on 87 per cent of maternal deaths known to the Registrar-General were available. There were 455 reports on deaths considered to be directly due to complications of pregnancy, childbirth and the puerperium and 243 deaths attributed to incidental diseases which occurred in association with pregnancy and its aftermath. The four main causes of maternal deaths in numerical order of importance were abortion,

Table 2.2 Numbers of maternal deaths from principal causes, England and Wales, 1940 and 1972

	Numbers of maternal deaths	
	1940	1972
Puerperal phlebitis, thrombosis and embolism	134	13
Puerperal sepsis	195	3
Antepartum and post-partum haemorrhage	286	11
Toxaemia	398	21
Complications of delivery	236	12
Other maternal causes	124	26
Criminal abortion	76	7
Other abortion	192	19
Total deaths from maternal causes	1641	112
Associated maternal deaths	424	28
All	2065	140

stantially reduced in all cause groups. This has been one of the great triumphs of medical science.

Although the maternal mortality rate is now very low and still seems to be falling (Fig. 2.9), a maternal death is such a serious event that the utmost vigilance remains necessary and each one is therefore carefully investigated. The inquiry was initiated by the local medical officer of health until 1974 but since then it will be the responsibility of the district or area administrative medical officer. The

pulmonary embolism, toxaemia and haemorrhage. (The list, and its order, differs somewhat from that indicated by causes on death certificates, summarized in Table 2.2.) In 56 per cent of all the maternal deaths, one or more avoidable factor was considered to be present. These range from faults for which the patient was primarily responsible (e.g. seeking an illegal abortion), through administrative failures (e.g. in following up defaulters, or delays in making appointments), to errors in the medical management of cases. The antenatal period was considered to be specially important, and the general practitioner had a particular responsibility as the doctor with whom the patient first made contact. Attention was drawn to one area where greater improvement is possible: the number of maternal deaths attributed to anaesthesia. Regional assessors in anaesthetics are being appointed. The incidence of confinements in hospital continues to rise, but in 28 per cent of women so booked who subsequently died, unsuitable booking arrangements were considered to have been made.

INDUCED ABORTIONS

The Abortion Act, 1967, took effect in England and Wales in April 1968. In discussions leading up to the Act, estimates of the frequency of illegal abortions in Britain ranged from 10 000 to 250 000 cases a year, the most-quoted figure being 100 000. Goodhart (1969) considered this estimate to be 'little more than a good round number arrived at by guesswork', and concluded, on the basis of data collected in Aberdeen, that the true figure for the whole of Britain probably did not exceed 20 000. In addition, over 6000 therapeutic abortions were undertaken in National Health Service hospitals in England and Wales in 1966, and it has been estimated that at least as many were being undertaken in private practice.

Since 1968, accurate statistics of notified legal abortions have been available. The Registrar-General for England and Wales publishes annual Supplements on Abortion in his Statistical Reviews. These show that the number of terminations under the Act increased steadily from 54 819 in 1969 to 167 149 in 1973; more recently the rate of increase has tended to fall off. One-third of the cases in 1973 were women not resident in England and Wales, among whom practically all abortions were undertaken in non-NHS hospitals. The proportion (but not the absolute number) of legal abortions undertaken in NHS hospitals fell from 61 per cent in 1969 to 33 per cent in 1973, with a corresponding rise in the proportion undertaken in other 'approved places'. The proportions of abortions performed on single women (49 per cent), married women (43 per cent) and on widowed, divorced or separated women (8 per cent) have remained fairly constant. A much lower proportion of

single women were terminated in NHS hospitals than in 'approved places', probably signifying that the two types of institution are dealing largely with different groups of women.

In 1973, among women resident in England and Wales, 52 per cent of abortions were on multiparae and nearly 10 per cent on women with four or more previous live-born children. About 40 per cent of the latter were sterilized at the same time.

There are large variations from area to area in the numbers of abortions performed and in the proportions undertaken in NHS hospitals. A report of the Royal College of Obstetricians (1972) notes that the Act permits, and receives, a very wide range of interpretation, which is confusing both to the public and to the medical profession.

Though increasing skill in the performance of abortions should further reduce the low incidence of immediate morbidity, there are indications that the operation may not be without long-term hazards. Wright *et al.* (1972) have reported a ten-fold increase in the incidence of second-trimester abortion in pregnancies which followed vaginal termination of pregnancy. In some countries, such as Hungary, where the number of legal abortions has exceeded the number of births, a rising incidence of low-birth-weight babies has been reported (Czeizel *et al.*, 1970). Whatever one's views on the ethics of abortion, it is clearly desirable for vigilance to be maintained and for more use to be made of epidemiological methods in a study of the interpretation of the Act and the risks of the procedure.

BIRTH WEIGHT

Maternal and perinatal death rates are now so low in Britain that they have become less useful than they used to be as indicators of the 'quality' of reproduction in a community. The incidence of babies of low birth weight has been used increasingly as such an indicator.

About half a century ago, international agreement was reached that 'premature' babies should be defined as those of birth weight 2500g or less, and 'prematurity rates' per 100 births were widely reported. At that time, there was little interest in gestational age (which is, in any event, often unknown or uncertain), so the ambiguity due to defining prematurity in terms of birth weight was ignored for many years. It gradually became apparent that a high proportion of 'premature' births were not, in fact, premature by dates, and in 1961 the World Health Organization recommended that babies weighing less than 2500g at birth should be described, more correctly, as of 'low birth weight'. About the same time interest in gestational age as a separate variable increased, and in 1963 Lubchenco and others published the first fetal growth standard, in which the distributions of birth weight at different weeks of gestation were specified. (Because it was the first, the Lubchenco standard is still rather widely used, but it is based on selected births in a city about a mile above sea level, and should not be regarded as a reliable guide to normality in other communities.)

With the availability of fetal growth standards, a new concept arose: that of the 'light for dates' baby, e.g. one where weight is below the 10th percentile of birth weight at any gestational age. While it is clinically useful, and has been taken to imply 'intra uterine malnutrition', this concept has disadvantages from the point of view of vital statistics, both because of a multiplicity of standards in use, and because it may be difficult or impossible to distinguish the effects of the two basic elements involved, i.e. birth weight and gestational age. The latter disadvantage may to some extent be reduced by distinguishing 'preterm' (less than 37 completed weeks), 'term' (37–41 completed weeks) and 'post-term' (42 completed weeks or more) babies.

A general discussion of fetal growth and birth weight will be found in Chapter 10 of Hytten and Leitch (1971) and Chapter 6 of this textbook; and a brief account of some physiological determinants of birth weight in a paper by Thomson (1971). Here, it will suffice to summarize one example of an epidemiologically satisfactory fetal growth standard, that of Thomson, Billewicz and Hytten (1968).

The data were those of a defined geographical community, namely, 52 004 legitimate, single births in the city of Aberdeen during the years 1948–64. Since the great majority of the births took place in one hospital, the recorded weights were exceptionally reliable and precautions were taken to estimate gestational ages at birth as accurately as possible. About 10 per cent of records had to be rejected, mostly because the gestational ages could not be determined with reasonable accuracy; and it was decided to exclude macerated stillbirths and babies which died because of malformations. Figure 2.10 shows the smoothed median

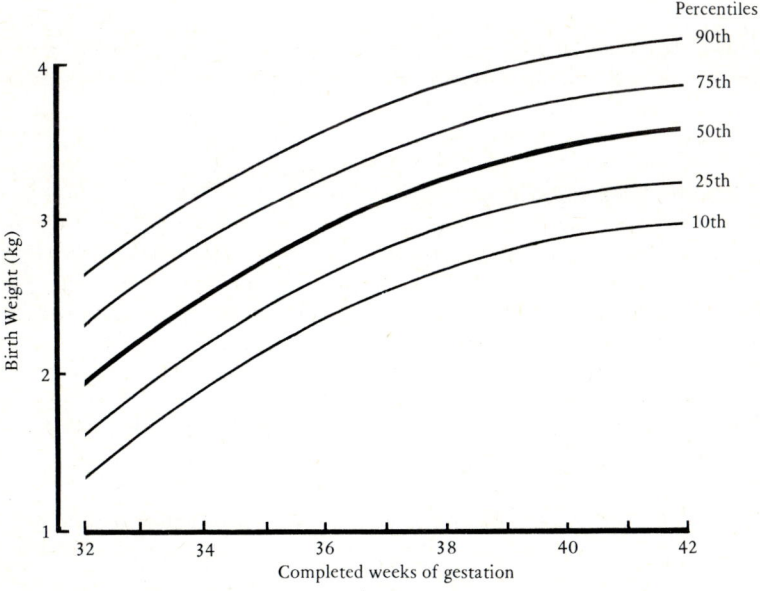

Fig. 2.10   Percentiles of birth weight, 32 to 42 completed weeks of gestation. (Source: Thomson *et al.*, 1968, *J. Obstet. Gynaec. Brit. Cwlth*, **75**, 903.)

values and the 5th, 25th, 75th and 95th percentiles of birth weight for all babies, from 32 to 42 completed weeks of gestation.

It should be noted that the curves are based on cross-sectional data; each baby could be weighed once only, after birth, and the curves therefore do not necessarily describe the pattern of growth in any given baby. A baby below, say, the 10th percentile is correctly described as 'light for dates', but we have no means of knowing whether it became 'light for dates' because of restricted growth during a limited period before birth, or whether it was 'light for dates' throughout gestation.

Unfortunately, there is as yet no fully organized system in England and Wales for reporting trends in average birth weights or in the incidence of low-birth-weight babies. Information on birth weight distributions by length of gestation from the records of the Hospital In-Patient Enquiry (see later) has been published by Milner and Richards (1974). Babies weighing 2·5kg or less (irrespective of gestational age) are notified to local health authorities, which supply annual returns to the Department of Health and Social Security. The Department publishes a summary in the Annual Reports of the Chief Medical Officer. In 1970, the incidence of live-born babies of low birth weight was 6·8 per cent of all live-born babies.

Fryer and Ashford (1972) have shown that the incidence of low birth weights in England and Wales fell slightly from 1960 until 1965, and since then has tended to rise. The reasons are by no means clear; Fryer and Ashford think the trend is more likely to be due to an accumulation of many factors than to any single dominant factor.

Mention may be made of one specific factor that obstetricians can do something about: cigarette smoking. The results of the 1958 Perinatal Mortality Survey (Butler and Alberman, 1969) confirmed several previous investigations by showing a significant reduction, 170g on average, in the birth weights of babies of mothers who smoked during pregnancy. This reduction in weight was accompanied by a significant increase in stillbirth and neonatal mortality rates. Butler and Alberman conclude that 'smoking in the latter part of pregnancy is definitely prejudicial to the normal growth and consequently to the survival of the fetus, particularly in mothers who are for other reasons in groups of higher than average risk. Every effort should be made to discourage this habit during pregnancy.'

MORBIDITY

Births and deaths are registered by law, and there is official machinery, tested by long experience, which ensures that information is properly recorded, analysed and published. The situation with regard to morbidity is not nearly so satisfactory; firstly, because methods are still in the stage of development; secondly, because the necessary facilities and organization are often inadequate; and thirdly, because many doctors fail to provide reliable basic information.

Acheson (1967) has observed that: 'The vast bulk of the information recorded about sickness consists of narrative notes written in longhand at the bedside or in the clinic. Stored in this form, unclassified, without summaries and unindexed, the information is almost as inaccessible for systematic study as if it had been destroyed.' The information itself may be seriously inadequate. Anyone who has worked through hospital case records in an attempt to determine, for example, the exact reasons for emergency admissions, or for surgical induction of labour, or for delivering babies by Caesarean section, soon becomes aware that medical records say more about what happened than about why it happened. Records in general medical practice may be even more perfunctory: in a survey of eight practices, Dawes (1972) found that a diagnosis was recorded in little over half the episodes and the dosage used in less than one-fifth. 'A general air of guiltless acceptance of the inadequacy of the records was apparent among those who co-operated.'

Even where records are reasonably well kept and where there are systems for filing and indexing, it is usually difficult and sometimes impossible to bring related items of information together because they are on different and uncoordinated record systems: for example, those of a general practice, a hospital, a local health authority and a registrar of births and deaths, all of which have had dealings with the same patient.

Data processing and record linkage on a large scale was extremely slow and cumbersome before the advent of electronic computers. Though formidable difficulties remain to be overcome, recording medical information for computers already forms part of many doctors' duties. It will still be their responsibility even if they succeed in delegating many of the chores to lay clerks.

The practical value of clinical records, carefully prepared and systematically analysed, needs no emphasis. It may, however, be less readily apparent that the value of clinical analyses is greatly increased when the statistics can be broken down by types of patient as well as by types of abnormality: for example, by marital status and duration of marriage, age, parity and previous history of pregnancies; by husband's occupation, which indicates socio-economic status; by height, weight, and so on. Information along these lines is essential if clinicians are to identify 'high-risk' categories which require exceptional vigilance or special types of service.

It may be even less apparent to clinicians that they have managerial as well as clinical responsibilities, which can be exercised intelligently only if they are based on reliable information. The second 'Cogwheel' report (Department of Health and Social Security, 1972) points out that without collaborative arrangements for consultation and dissemination of information, decisions of vital concern to clinicians 'will be made by other, non-medical, machinery or go by default'. Administrative matters of vital concern to obstetricians and gynaecologists range from the general organization of regional or local medical services to such details as the clinical safety and cost–effectiveness of a policy for early discharge of patients from hospital, the need for an obstetrical 'flying squad' and the best way of reducing the length of waiting-lists. Again, as patients become increasingly vocal about the merits or defects of what they rightly regard as *their* service, doctors will be under greater pressure to ensure that the organization is convenient and humane, as well as technically efficient.

HOSPITAL STATISTICS

The first official attempt to provide regular statistics of morbidity in NHS hospitals was the Hospital In-Patient Enquiry (HIPE), initiated in England and Wales in 1949, and now covering a 10 per cent sample of all discharges from non-psychiatric hospitals. Though HIPE data proved useful for central administrative and long-term planning purposes, they are less satisfactory from the point of view of local clinical services. Hospital Activity Analysis (HAA) was subsequently introduced, primarily to cover 100 per cent of hospital discharges with rapid feed-back to the periphery. Ashley (1972) has described some of the current limitations and uses of these two monitoring services.

In Scotland, the situation has developed more rapidly and further than in England and Wales. After preliminary trials, Scottish Hospital In-Patient Statistics (SHIPS) in 1963 covered all discharges from NHS hospitals except maternity hospitals, which however have been included since 1969. In addition to published tabulations (not available without some delay; statistics for 1970 were published in 1972), regional and hospital tabulations are sent as quickly as possible to all hospitals in Scotland; and since 1967 Scottish Consultant Activity Review Statistics (SCARS) have been sent to each consultant responsible for in-patient care, describing his case-load for the year under review. Finally, a diagnostic index is sent to each hospital or Board of Management, to enable easy identification of cases for purposes of review and research and to facilitate the preparation of simple tabulations for local clinical or administrative use; and a National index is held in the central Department to facilitate tracing of cases or investigations on a large scale.

As already noted, maternity hospital statistics lagged behind those from general hospitals, partly because the relationship between diagnosis and complications is not the same as that in other reasons for admission to hospital. In Scotland, a maternity discharge record form (SMRM) was introduced in 1969. In England, a similar form is being tested in a few maternity hospitals, with a view to eventual introduction on a wider scale.

A report by Lockwood (1971) probably gives the best view so far available of the scope of hospital morbidity records. Their value for administrative and planning purposes has already been proved, and future advances should make their clinical utility more evident. The fact that the statistical unit is the discharge from hospital, and not the individual patient or episode of disease, is a serious limitation which may in due course be overcome by suitable forms of record linkage.

Cancer

Since 1962, all patients diagnosed as suffering

from cancer and seen at a hospital in England and Wales have been, or should have been, registered, the Registrar General being responsible for collection and analysis. Regional Hospital Boards are responsible for follow-up, and survival rates are computed by comparing notifications with death certificates. The supplements on Cancer to the Annual Reviews of the Registrar-General form an important source of information on survival rates, but the range of data collected is limited.

A chapter on epidemiology should not fail to mention recent studies of cancer of the uterine cervix. This cancer has features which point strongly towards an environmental cause or causes acting on susceptible individuals: for example, it is rare among nuns and Jews, and relatively common in women of the poorer classes. In Aberdeenshire, Aitken-Swan and Baird (1966) found higher rates in city than in country women, in widowed and divorced women, and in the lower socio-economic groups. Their evidence suggested that it was some attribute of coitus, perhaps a low standard of penile hygiene, that induced malignant change in susceptible individuals.

Cancer of the cervix is one of the few cancers that is detectable in the pre-invasive stage, through exfoliative cytology. The efficient use of screening methods in populations would be expected to lead, eventually, to a fall in the death rate from cancer of the cervix. But this mortality rate has been declining for a long time (Adelstein, Hill and Maung, 1971), and in British Columbia the recent rate of fall has so far been no greater than in other parts of Canada where cytological screening has been used much less extensively (Ahluwalia and Doll, 1968). In Aberdeen, Macgregor (1967) thought that screening had produced a definite reduction in mortality from cancer of the cervix in women aged under 60, but not in older women. There have been suggestions that there are two forms of the disease: 1. slow-growing, slow to metastasize, occurring in younger women, and likely to be preceded by a long pre-invasive stage, hence amenable to diagnosis and prevention by cytological screening: 2. rapidly growing, occurring in older women, and less susceptible to cure. Such suggestions are still speculative. The value of cytology screening is further discussed in Chapter 38.

Congenital malformations

Congenital malformations in newborn babies are notified on a voluntary basis by many local health authorities (174 in England and Wales, 1970) to the Office of Population Censuses and Surveys, and summaries are presented in the Annual Reports of the Chief Medical Officer. In 1970, more than 17 000 malformations were reported in just over 14 000 babies, the most common being talipes, spina bifida or hydrocephalus or both, anencephalus and cleft lip or cleft palate or both. There were 17·6 malformed babies (as reported) per 1000 live and stillbirths. Baird (1974) has reviewed the epidemiology of the congenital malformations of the central nervous system in Scotland.

REFERENCES

Acheson, E. D. (1967) *Medical record linkage*. London: Oxford University Press.

Adelstein, A. M., Hill, G. B. & Maung, L. (1971) Mortality from carcinoma of the uterus: an international cohort study. *Brit. J. prev. soc. Med.*, **25**, 186.

Ahluwalia, H. S. & Doll, R. (1968) Mortality from cancer of the cervix uteri in British Columbia and other parts of Canada. *Brit. J. prev. soc. Med.*, **22**, 161.

Aitken-Shaw, J. & Baird, D. (1966) Cancer of the uterine cervix in Aberdeenshire. *Brit. J. Cancer*, **20**, 624, 642.

Ashley, J. S. A. (1972) Present state of statistics from hospital in-patient data and their uses. *Brit. J. prev. soc. Med.*, **26**, 135.

Baird, D., Walker, J. & Thomson, A. M. (1954) Causes and Prevention of Stillbirths and First Week Deaths. III. A Classification of Deaths by Clinical causes. *J. Obstet. Gynaec. Brit. Emp.*, **61**, 433.

Baird, D. (1963) The contribution of operative obstetrics to the prevention of perinatal death. *J. Obstet. Gynaec. Brit. Cwlth.*, **70**, 204.

Baird, D. (1971) The obstetrician and society. *J. Biosoc. Sci.* Suppl. 3, 93.

Baird, D. (1974) Epidemiology of congenital malformations of the central nervous system in (a) Aberdeen and (b) Scotland. *J. Biosoc. Sci.*, **6**, 113.

Butler, N. R. & Alberman, E. D., Editors (1969) *Perinatal problems: The second report of the 1958 British Perinatal Mortality Survey*. Edinburgh: E. & S. Livingstone Ltd.

Butler, N. R. and Bonham, D. G. (1963) *Perinatal mortality: The first report of the 1958 British Perinatal Mortality Survey*. Edinburgh: E. & S. Livingstone Ltd.

Czeizel, A., Bognar, Z., Tusnady, G. & Revesz, P. (1970) Changes in mean birth weight and proportion of low-weight births in Hungary. *Brit. J. prev. soc. Med.*, **24**, 146.

Dawes, K. S. (1972) Survey of general practice records. *Brit. med. J.*, **iii**, 219.

Department of Health & Social Security (1972) *Second report of the Joint Working Party on the Organisation of Medical Work in Hospitals.* London: H.M. Stationery Office.

Department of Health & Social Security (1972) *Report on Confidential Enquiries into Maternal Deaths in England & Wales, 1967–69.* London: H.M. Stationery Office.

Duncan, E. H. L., Baird, D. & Thomson, A. M. (1952) The causes and prevention of stillbirths and first week deaths. I. The evidence of vital statistics. *J. Obstet. Gynaec. Brit. Emp.*, **59**, 183.

Fryer, J. G. & Ashford, J. R. (1972) Trends in perinatal and neonatal mortality in England & Wales, 1960–69. *Brit. J. prev. soc. Med.*, **26**, 1.

Goodhart, C. B. (1969) Estimation of illegal abortions. *J. Biosoc. Sci.*, **1**, 235.

Hytten, F. E. & Leitch, I. (1971) *The physiology of human pregnancy*, 2nd ed. Oxford: Blackwell Scientific Publications.

Lockwood, E. (1971) Scottish hospital morbidity data. 1961–68. *Scottish Health Science Studies*, No. 20.

Lubchenco, L. O., Hansman, C., Dressler, M. & Boyd, E. (1963) Intrauterine growth as estimated from liveborn birth-weight data at 24 to 42 weeks of gestation. *Paediatrics*, **32**, 793.

Macgregor, J. E. (1967) Cervical carcinoma: the beginning of the end? *Lancet*, **ii**, 1296.

Milner, R. D. G. & Richards, B. (1974) An analysis of birth weight by gestational age of infants born in England and Wales, 1967 to 1971. *J. Obstet. Gynaec. Brit. Cwlth.*, **81**, 956.

Parkes, A. S. (1971) Environmental influences on human fertility. *J. Biosoc. Sci.* Suppl. 3, p. 13.

Potts, D. M. (1971) Human fertility in global perspective. *J. Biosoc. Sci.* Suppl. 3, p. 41.

Russell, J. K. (1974) Sexual activity and its consequences in the teenager. *Clins. Obstet. Gynaec.*, **1**, 683.

Thomson, A. M. (1971) Physiological determinants of birth weight. *Proceedings of the 2nd European Congress of Perinatal Medicine.*, p. 174. London: Basel, Karger.

Thomson, A. M., Billewicz, W. Z. & Hytten, F. E. (1968) The Assessment of fetal growth. *J. Obstet. Gynaec. Brit. Cwlth.*, **75**, 903.

United Nations, Department of Economic & Social Affairs (1971) The world population situation in 1970. *Population Studies* No. 49.

Walker, J. (1954) Fetal Anoxia. *J. Obstet. Gynaec. Brit. Emp.*, **61**, 162.

World Health Organization (1961) Public health aspects of low birth weight. *Wld. Hlth. Org. techn. Rep. Ser.*, No. 217.

World Health Organization (1967) *Manual of the international statistical classification of diseases, injuries and causes of death.* 8th Revision, Vol. 1.

Wright, C. S. W., Campbell, S. & Beazley, J. (1972) Second trimester abortion after vaginal termination of pregnancy. *Lancet*, **i**, 1278.

3. Anatomy of the Female Pelvis and the External Genitalia

The physical process of labour and the detail of gynaecological examination, disease or operation require a clear knowledge of the clinical anatomy of the female pelvis and of the pelvic contents as well as the external genitalia.

FEMALE PELVIS

The iliopectineal line runs forward from the apex of the auricular surface of the innominate bone and demarcates the true from the false pelvis (Fig. 3.1). It forms the pelvic brim and above the brim is the false pelvis, while below it is the true pelvis. The shape and diameters of the true pelvis are supremely important from the standpoint of childbearing since it forms the bony canal through which the child must pass during the birth process.

The whole pelvis, true and false, consists of four bones—the two innominate bones, the sacrum and the coccyx.

The innominate bone

This consists of three bones—the *ilium*, the *ischium* and the *pubis*. These fuse into one after puberty.

a. The ilium : The alae of the iliac bones on each side form the side walls of the false pelvis. The iliac crest ends in front in the anterior superior spine.

b. The ischium forms part of the lateral wall of the true pelvis. The body of the ischium bears the ischial spine on its posterior border. This demarcates the upper and lower sciatic notches, inferiorly the body bears the ischial tuberosity and projects forward into the ischial ramus which meets the inferior pubis ramus.

c. The os pubis, with its fellow of the opposite

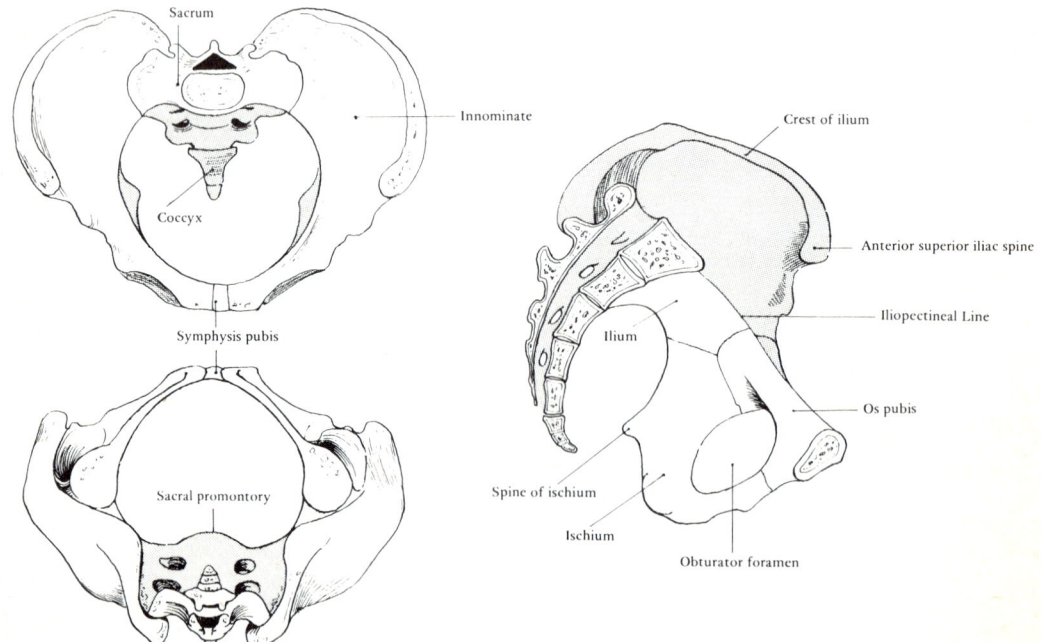

Fig. 3.1 Bony pelvis.

side, forms the front portion of the true pelvis. This junction is termed the symphysis pubis and is a joint whose structures expand to a small extent during pregnancy and labour. The upper and lower parts of the os pubis fuse with the ilium and ischium respectively by means of the superior and descending rami. These complete the pubic arch which forms the front and part of the lateral margin of the pelvic outlet.

The sacrum

This is made up of five fused vertebrae and forms with the coccyx the posterior wall of the bony pelvis. The anterior border of its upper part is termed the sacral promontory and forms the posterior margin of the pelvic brim. The normal sacrum is concave from above downwards and from side to side. It joins with the ilium on either side at the sacro-iliac joint which, like the symphysis pubis, softens during pregnancy.

The coccyx

This is made up of between three and five fused vertebrae which articulate with the sacrum. It represents, in man, the tail of more primitive animals. During delivery of the child some backward rotation occurs owing to the softening of the articular structure during pregnancy.

CLINICAL OBSTETRIC ANATOMY

There are two main differences between the male and female pelvis. The heavier build and stronger muscles of the male account for the stronger bone structure while in the female, the cavity is more capacious and cylindrical, thus making it well adapted to the process of parturition.

The normal pelvic brim is virtually round in both the male and the female. Differences in the sexes are mainly in heaviness of bone structure. The 'android' pelvic brim is not due to the influence of male hormones but is a growth defect arising from poor living

conditions and diet in the growing years (Bernard, 1951).

During its descent through the pelvis, the fetal head follows a curved course, usually described as the axis of the pelvis (Fig. 3.2). This is an imaginary line joining the central

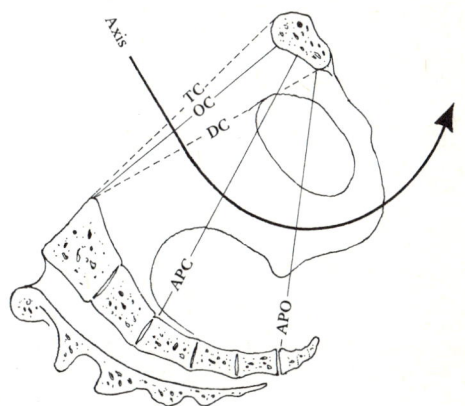

Fig. 3.2   Diameters of the true pelvis.

points of the anteroposterior diameters from the inlet to the outlet. When the patient is on her back, the plane of the inlet is inclined about 30 degrees to the horizontal. When the patient is standing, the inclination is to 50 to 60 degrees.

The pelvic brim or inlet of the true pelvis is normally round or slightly oval. The obstetric conjugate and the widest transverse diameter are the important obstetric measurements.

The anteroposterior diameter or true conjugate —from the sacral promontory to the top of the symphysis pubis, is not usually considered in obstetric measurements.

The obstetric conjugate—from the sacral promontory to the nearest point on the upper part of the symphysis pubis, is usually referred to as the 'conjugate' or the 'A. P. diameter'.

The widest transverse diameter needs no explanation.

The measurements of the inlet, mid-cavity and outlet of the true pelvis are shown in Table 3.1. The size of the pelvis is, in general,

Table 3.1

	Transverse	Oblique	Antero-posterior
Inlet	5 (12·7cm)	$4\frac{1}{2}$ (11·2cm)	4 (10cm)
Mid-pelvis	$4\frac{1}{2}$ (11·2cm)	$4\frac{1}{2}$ (11·2cm)	$4\frac{1}{2}$ (11·2cm)
Outlet	4 (10cm)	$4\frac{1}{2}$ (11·2cm)	5 (12·5cm)

related to the stature of the mother. In some countries, e.g. China, anteroposterior measurements vary much more with maternal stature than do the transverse. This may be related to the fact that small adult stature is frequently related to undernutrition during the period of growth. This results in stunting and flattening of the pelvis. In the case of a woman, however, who has grown to her genetically determined height but is nevertheless very small it seems likely that both the transverse and anteroposterior diameters will be short and thus the shape of the pelvic brim will remain round. While many women with small brim conjugates produce small babies by vaginal delivery, this is not always the case. It is not, therefore, possible to lay down a minimum normal measurement for safe passage of any infant. Disproportion at the brim, however, is not often seen with a conjugate measurement of $4\frac{1}{2}$ inches (11·2cm) or more and this is often considered the lower limit of 'normal'. Similarly, a transverse diameter of $5\frac{1}{4}$ inches (13·2cm) may be considered 'normal'. It is unusual for other pelvic diameters to be unsatisfactory when the A. P. at the brim is adequate.

The diagonal conjugate—the distance from the sacral promontory to the lower margin of the symphysis pubis, can be assessed clinically. It is not usually possible in the 'normal' pelvis to reach the sacral promontory on vaginal examination or without discomfort to the patient. An estimate of the obstetric conjugate can be obtained from the diagonal conjugate.

The cavity of the pelvis lies between the brim and the outlet. It is generally more capacious than the brim owing to the sacral concavity. An anteroposterior diameter from the upper border of the third sacral vertebra to the mid-point on the internal aspect of the symphysis pubis usually measures about 5 inches (12.5cm). Transverse measurements between the side walls at this level are difficult to take since there are no clearly defined end points but deep in the cavity the distance between the projecting ischial spines—the interischial-spinous diameter—can be accurately measured by X-ray or assessed clinically. It is usually 4 inches (10cm) but measurements as low as $3\frac{1}{2}$ inches (8·75cm) are not uncommon.

The outlet is bounded in front by the apex of the pubic arch, laterally by the ischial tuberosities and behind by the sacral tip.

These structures do not lie in the single plane but form two planes with a common base between the ischial tuberosities. The anteroposterior diameter of the outlet is measured from the lower margin of the symphysis pubis to the tip of the sacrum. As a rule it measures about 5 inches (12·5cm). The available anteroposterior diameter is less than this and is the real diameter available to the fetal head. It can be measured radiologically by a line joining the sacral tip and the point of contact with the parietal bones of the fetal skull on the pubic rami—the parietal touch points—lies in the plane of the pelvic outlet. The method is described by Gillanders (1959) and details of its calculation can be obtained from Gillanders' paper. The subpubic angle is conveniently described as the angle between the lines drawn from the symphysis pubis to the ischial tuberosities. It is normally about 85°. The intertuberischial diameter is the distance between the inner margins of the tuber ischii—it usually measures 4 inches (10cm) at least, but is difficult to define exactly.

Abnormalities in shape and size of the pelvis

Changes in shape and size of the pelvis are important in clinical obstetrics because of their effect on labour and the passage of the child through the birth canal. Major degrees of contracted pelvis have long been recognized as an important cause of difficult labour (dystocia). Grossly contracted pelvis is now found much less commonly than previously owing to the decline in such diseases as rickets and gross malnutrition. The obstetrician now has to direct his attention increasingly to minor variations in pelvic size and shape and their influence on labour. More than fifty years ago, Turner, the Anatomist, studied dried pelves in anatomical museums and classified them according to the shape of the brim into three broad groups, i.e. long oval, round and flat. Since then many more complicated classifications and terminologies have been used but, in clinical practice, Turner's terminology with a fourth category added, the triangular or wedge-shaped brim, is most descriptive and will be used in this book. Caldwell and Moloy classified pelvic brim shapes into four types, the gynaecoid (round), anthropoid (long oval), platypelloid (flat) and android (wedge-shaped) and these terms are used by some writers. First of all, the obstetrically 'ideal' pelvis will be described.

The brim of the true pelvis should be rounded or slightly oval, without undue projection of the sacral promontory (Fig. 3.1). In the erect posture, the plane of the brim should incline at an angle of 50–60 degrees to the horizontal. The pelvic cavity should be shallow with straight side walls: not deep or funnel-shaped. The sacrum should have a smooth curve both longitudinally and transversely. The shape of the sacro-sciatic notch is an important guide to the adequacy of the outlet, and should be wide and shallow. The sacrum should not be inclined or curved too sharply forwards, and the ischial spines should not project unduly into the pelvic cavity. The pubic arch should be wide and well curved so that the fetal head can make full use of the available space as it extends under the arch. Finally, the transverse diameter of the outlet—the distance between the ischial tuberosities—should be wide.

Departures from this ideal shape make the pelvis less suitable for labour. The gross deformities due to such diseases as rickets and osteomalacia are easy to diagnose and classify and their effect on the course of labour is obvious. Classification of minor variations in shape and size of the pelvis has only been possible since the advent of X-ray pelvimetry, and although we now have considerable information, their aetiology and effect on the course of labour is not yet fully understood.

Broadly speaking, a satisfactory brim area and shape indicates that the pelvis is satisfactory, generally, and most classifications are based primarily on the shape and size of the brim. Usually, also, unsatisfactory shape tends to be associated with unsatisfactory size. Shape is most simply expressed in terms of the relative length of the anteroposterior and widest transverse diameters—e.g. the brim index is:

$$\frac{\text{Anteroposterior diameter of the brim}}{\text{Widest transverse diameter of the brim}} \times 100$$

If the index is about 100, the pelvic brim shape is nearly round; if the index is less than 100, there is some flattening anteroposteriorly; and if it is more than 100, the shape is 'long oval'. Brim index does not define the triangular or wedge-shaped pelvic brim (the so-called android or male type) in which, however, the brim index is usually much less than 100.

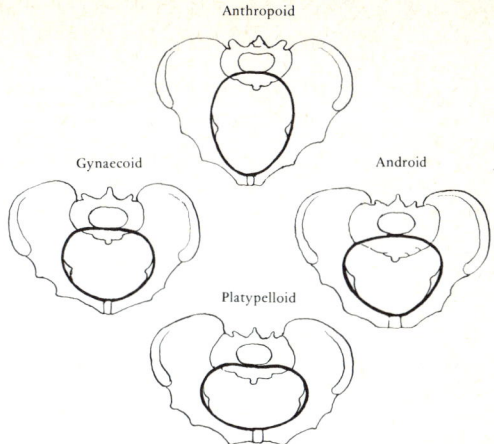

Fig. 3.3   Four types of pelvic brim shapes (Caldwell and Moloy).

There are four main pelvic brim shapes of which the 'normal round brim' is the most common (Fig. 3.3). Average measurements for a normal pelvis are shown in Table 3.2.

Table 3.2   Average measurements for a normal pelvis

True conjugate diameter	12·2cm
Widest transverse diameter	13·5cm
Interischial spinous diameter	11·2cm
Brim index	90 per cent

The long oval pelvis may be regarded as a variant of the normal. The flat and triangular types are liable to give rise to difficulty in labour and may be regarded as abnormal. The incidence of the various types depends to some degree upon the growth and nutrition which is measured by the height of the woman concerned. Thus in a well-grown and tall population there are relatively few flat and triangular pelves; and the higher the proportion of small women, the more common are the flat and wedge-shaped types. It is possible that these last two types are minor degrees of the true rachitic pelvis.

Factors determining the shape and size of the female pelvis

It is well known that rickets and osteomalacia can cause gross deformity of the pelvis but much less is known about other factors like heredity which may affect pelvic shape. Skeletal growth is influenced by standards of living and diet and the sex hormones and these are likely to be important in determining pelvic size and shape.

Tall women 5ft 4 in. or more (163cm) were found by Bernard (1952) to have much bigger pelves as judged by the brim area and the length of the true conjugate than small women under 5ft 1in. in height (157cm). Tall women also have less flattening of the pelvis than small women. More than one-third of small women assessed as being of inferior physique showed flattening of the pelvic brim, mainly in the posterior segment. Caesarean section for disproportion is very seldom necessary in women of 5ft 4 in. (163cm) or over with normal sized babies. Bernard examined a group of tall men (medical students) and a group of small men (from the lower income groups) and showed that the distribution of shape of pelvic brim was almost identical with that found in tall and small women respectively. In most instances the sex cannot be diagnosed from the X-ray picture of the brim. If conditions in Britain were favourable enough to allow all women to grow to their maximum genetic potential probably not more than about 5 per cent would be under 5ft 1in. (157cm) tall. Women who are small genetically have smaller brim areas than tall women even though there is little or no distortion of shape so that labour might be difficult if the baby proved to be large; however, with good pelvic shape the chances of serious difficulty are less likely. Difficult labour due to contracted pelvis will become less common in the future since the mean heights of school children are increasing. The average height of a girl aged 13 in Glasgow in the period 1910–1914 was 55in. (135cm) whereas at the same age in 1965–1969 the average height was 60·2in. (153cm).

The evidence so far suggests that the standards of living, probably of nutrition especially, are the most important factors influencing the shape and size of the pelvis. Size is of more practical importance than shape and, in any case, where the brim area is large the shape is almost always round or oval. On the other hand, with smaller brim areas all shapes may occur and play an important part in determining the outcome of labour.

Normal and abnormal pelvic types

Gross deformities of size and shape are relatively uncommon, but have been included in the following comprehensive classification of pelvic abnormalities:
1. Pelves with 'Normal' Shape and Bone

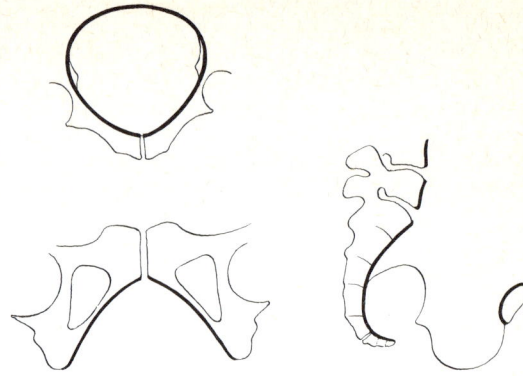

Fig. 3.4   Brim, outlet and sacrum in normal (gynaecoid) pelvis.

Development: Round or long oval (measurements usually ample but occasionally small).
2. Pelves with Abnormality of Shape and Bone Development (usually also decreased measurements).
  a. Defects of Nutrition and Environment:
   (i) Minor (triangular and flat pelvic brim).
   (ii) Major (rickets and osteomalacia).
  b. Disease and Injury:
   (i) Spinal:
    Kyphosis.
    Scoliosis.
    Spondylolisthesis.
   (ii) Pelvic:
    New growths.
    Tuberculosis.
    Fracture of the pelvis.
   (iii) Lower Limbs:
    Tuberculosis, poliomyelitis, coxalgia, congenital dislocation of the hip.

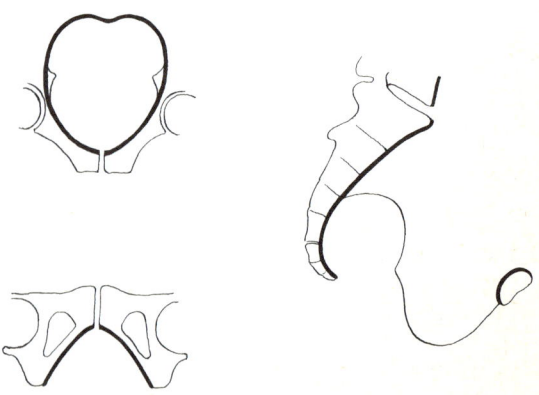

Fig. 3.5   Brim, outlet and sacrum in long oval pelvis.

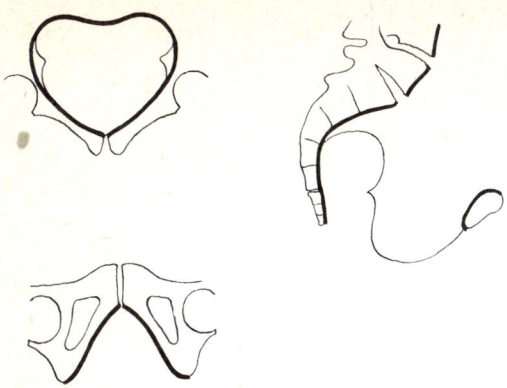

Fig. 3.6 Brim, outlet and sacrum in triangular (android) pelvis.

show the stigmata of having had rickets in childhood. In such cities, there has also, in recent years, been a recurrence of rickets in some immigrant populations due to flour used for cooking being unleavened thus making the calcium unavailable. In some developing countries the problem may still be of significance.

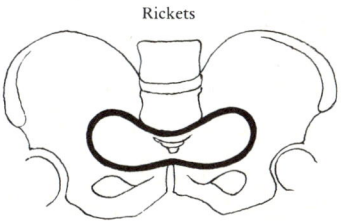

Rickets

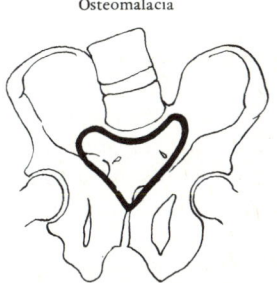

Osteomalacia

Fig. 3.8 Brim shapes in rickets and osteomalacia.

c. Congenital Defects:
  (i) Nägele's pelvis.
      Robert's pelvis.
  (ii) Split pelvis.
  (iii) Assimilation.

DEFECTS OF NUTRITION AND ENVIRONMENT

(i) *Minor*—It has already been shown that defective environment, insufficient to cause recognizable illness, may cause a tendency to flattening of the pelvic brim. Although the exact mechanism of these changes is not understood it is probable that they differ only in degrees from those resulting from such conditions as rickets.

(ii) *Major*—Rickets and osteomalacia are the only examples in this category and indeed in the more advanced countries they are seldom seen. Even in large industrial cities such as Glasgow and Manchester, rickets in childhood is now rarely seen but there are still occasional women of childbearing age who

In a young child suffering from rickets, the weight of the trunk is said to press the promontory of the sacrum downwards and forwards while the sacrum itself is inclined backwards. At the same time, the antero-superior iliac spines tend to flare out, becoming the most widely separated points of the crests. The tuberosities of the ischia are pressed outwards by the weight of the child and the subpubic angle and transverse diameter of the outlet become wide. As the sacral promontory is pushed forwards, the brim becomes flattened or kidney-shaped and in severe cases may even assume the shape of a figure of eight, the symphysis being pulled backwards by the action of the abdominal muscles. The true conjugate may be reduced to below 2in. (5cm); the transverse diameter of the brim also is usually smaller than normal although it will appear large by comparison with the narrow anteroposterior diameter. In the typical rachitic pelvis the anteroposterior diameter of

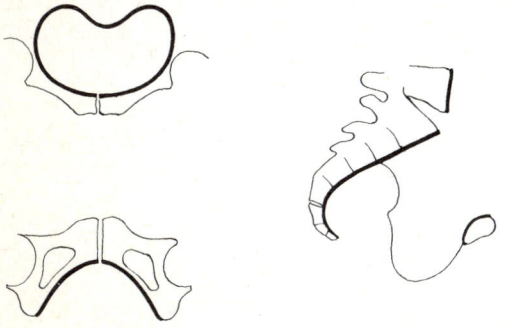

Fig. 3.7 Brim, outlet and sacrum in flat (plattypelloid) pelvis.

the brim is the smallest dimension of the pelvic passage so that if the head passes this point the rest of labour and delivery is often easy. Sometimes the anterior surface of the sacrum may bulge forwards, reducing the anteroposterior diameter of the cavity; or a sharply angulated sacral tip may cause difficulty at the outlet.

Osteomalacia is a disease of adult life which affects women, usually multiparae, during the reproductive period. The disease, which is associated with gross deficiency of minerals and of vitamin D in the diet, is practically confined to certain localities in China, India and the more backward areas of Europe, although a few cases have been reported in the UK. The symptoms often appear for a first time during pregnancy. The patient, who has probably had several normal pregnancies and labour, complains of muscular weakness and difficulty with walking, and labour may be obstructed. The sacrum is pushed downwards and forwards and the lateral pelvic walls are also pushed back inwards. This makes the pelvis 'beak' shaped. The subpubic angle is narrowed, the ischial tuberosities are approximated and the acetabula are turned more forward, leading to a peculiar swinging gait. Caesarean section is usually necessary.

DISEASE AND INJURY:
(a) *Spinal*
    Kyphosis—In the upper dorsal region only severe kyphosis alters pelvic shape. With lower dorsal or lumbar kyphosis dating from childhood the upper sacrum is often displaced backwards and the lower part forwards. The side walls of the pelvis slope inwards, the subpubic angle is narrow and the ischial spines are close together. Typically, the brim is long and narrow and the cavity funnel-shaped, so serious outlet obstruction is likely to occur. It is important to anticipate this, for patients with this type of deformity are often in poor general condition and unfit to stand a difficult labour. There is much to be said for delivering them by elective Caesarean section.
    Scoliosis—Pronounced lateral curvature is usually rachitic in origin and may cause the bays on either side of the sacral promontory to be asymmetrical—i.e. of different size and shape. In this 'scolio-rachitic' pelvis the outcome of labour may depend on which of the bays the head enters.
    Spondylolisthesis—The fifth lumbar vertebra is displaced forwards and projects beyond

the sacral promontory. Severe displacement is rare and is usually due to faulty development of the articular processes of the lumbar vertebrae. Less marked displacement due to subluxation of the joints may occur during pregnancy or as a result of debilitating disease. The available conjugate diameter of the brim is shortened by the forward thrust of the vertebrae. Diagnosis is possible only by X-ray.
(b) *Pelvic:*
    New Growths—Osteomata are occasionally found on the symphysis pubis, the sacro-iliac joints and the iliopectineal eminences. These may obstruct the labour and may indent the fetal skull. The uterus may tear if it is nipped between the tumour and the fetal head. Large tumours are very rare and usually malignant. In these cases, Caesarean section is usually required.
    Tuberculosis—This is now a relatively rare condition in the UK. The acetabula may be perforated in tuberculous disease and there may be irregular bone formation on the inner surface of the lateral pelvic wall. Caries of the sacro-iliac joint may interfere with the development of one sacral ala and may result in oblique deformity (the Nägele type).
    Fractures of the Pelvis—This is the commonest cause of gross deformity in UK now. They usually occur as a result of a motor accident or a fall from some height. Ankylosis of the coccygeal joint after dislocation is more common, and if the coccyx is directed forwards it may obstruct the second stage of labour and again be fractured. In any pregnant woman where there is a history of fracture of the pelvis, X-ray pelvimetry is essential.

(iii) *Lower limbs*—Congenital dislocation of the hip or poliomyelitis may cause pelvic deformity if it shortens one leg in childhood. The longer leg bears most of the weight and that side of the pelvis is pressed in and flattened.

CONGENITAL DEFECTS:
(a) *Nägele and Robert's Pelves*—These are very rare deformities of the pelvis found in association with congenital deformities or resulting from sacro-iliac disease in infancy. The entire pelvic cavity is usually narrowed and the reason for this can only be shown by X-rays. Caesarean section is invariably required for delivery in these patients.
(b) *Split Pelvis*—The pubic bones are united

by fibrous tissue; the condition is often associated with ectopia vesicae and other urogenital malformations. This is an extremely rare condition.

(c)   *Assimilation*—The 'high assimilation pelvis' is one in which the fifth lumbar vertebra is incorporated with the sacrum so that the conjugate diameter and the inclination of the brim are increased. This type of pelvis favours the occipito-posterior position of the fetal head. In the less common 'low assimilation pelvis' there are only four sacral vertebrae. These abnormalities of pelvic shape are relatively rare in this country but in areas where nutrition, for example, is poor they may be more common and certainly have to be considered as possible difficulties applied to labour.

THE FEMALE GENITAL ORGANS

The Vulva

The vulva is the term applied to the female external genitalia and consists of the— Mons Pubis or Mons Veneris, Labia Majora,

is covered by skin which after puberty is covered by hair limited to a line one inch above the symphysis and below extending to the labia majora. The labia minors lie between the labia majora and are lips of soft skin which meet posteriorly in a sharp fold, the fourchette. Anteriorly, they split thus enclosing the clitoris and forming a prepuce anteriorly and a frenum or frenulum posteriorly.

The area enclosed by the labia minora and containing the urethral orifice and the vaginal orifice is known as the *vestibule*.

The vaginal orifice itself is surrounded in the virgin by a thin skin fold known as the *hymen*. This is usually perforated to allow the drainage of the menses. It usually has an annular appearance in the virgin but following first coitus the hymen becomes torn and after childbirth particularly, nothing is left of it but a few tags known as the *carunculae myrtiformes*. Sometimes the hymen is imperforate and menstrual blood then distends the vagina (haematocolpos). This condition of hidden menses is known as *cryptomenorrhoea*.

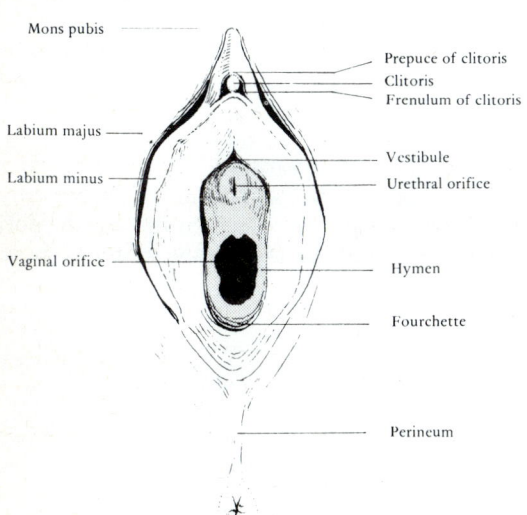

Fig. 3.9   Female external genitalia.

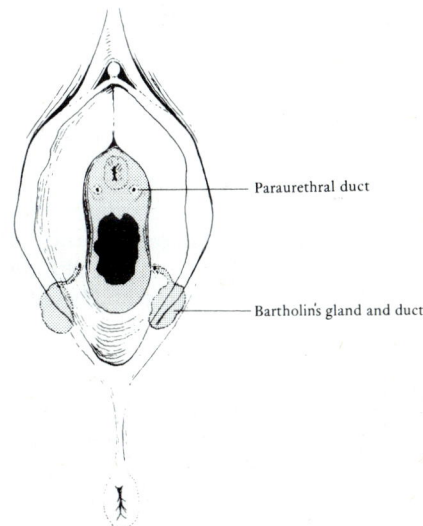

Fig. 3.10   Paraurethral (Skene's Ducts) and Bartholin's gland showing ducts.

Labia Minora, Clitoris, External Urethral Orifice, Hymen and Vaginal Orifice.

The labia majora are prominent hair-bearing folds which extend backwards from the mons pubis to meet in the mid-line of the perineum. The mons pubis is a pad of fat which lies in front of the symphysis pubis and

Bartholin's Glands (Fig. 3.10) which are a pair of lobulated mucous-secreting glands lying deep to the posterior part of the labia majora, are normally not palpable but may become inflamed or cystic resulting in the well known condition of Bartholinitis or a cyst of Bartholin's gland. Bartholin's glands drain by a duct which opens into the groove between the hymen and the posterior part of the labium minus. The lining of the duct is formed by transitional epithelium except in its deeper part where it consists of a single layer of columnar cells.

The paraurethral or Skene's Ducts run parallel to the urethra and open into the vestibule close to and just below the urethral orifice. The perineum itself consists of the perineal body which lies between the vagina and the rectum and is wedge-shaped on sagittal section (see p. 45).

The Vagina

The vagina surrounds the cervix of the uterus and then passes downwards and forwards transversing the pelvic floor to open into the vestibule. When the woman is standing the vagina makes an angle of about 50 degrees with the horizontal (Fig. 3.11). The annular fossa in the vaginal vault surrounding the cervix is divided into four regions or fornices anterior, posterior, right and left. This is a convenient description to denote the position and relationship of the structures felt through the vaginal vault during an examination with the fingers.

RELATIONS OF THE VAGINA
Anteriorly, the base of the bladder and the urethra are closely related to the vagina, the latter being imbedded in the anterior vaginal wall. Posteriorly, the relations of the vagina are the anal canal separated from the vagina by the perineal body rectum and then peri-

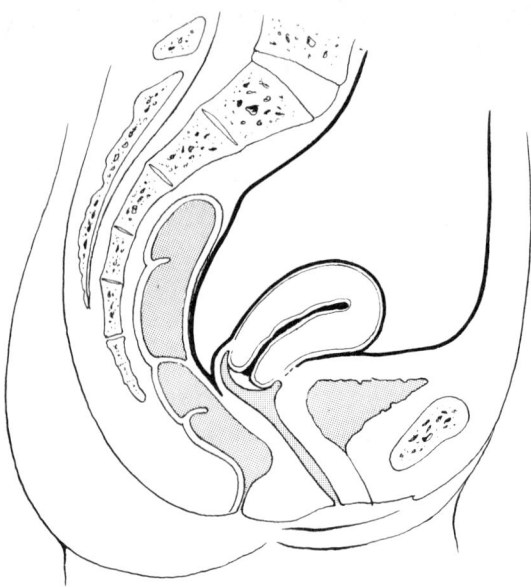

Fig. 3.11   Position of uterus in pelvis showing peritoneum.

toneum of the Pouch of Douglas, the latter of which covers the upper fourth of the posterior vaginal wall, and is directly related to the peritoneal cavity and any structures therein. Laterally, the vagina is related to the levator ani, pelvic fascia and ureters, which lie close to the lateral fornices (Fig. 3.12).

STRUCTURES OF THE VAGINA
The vagina and the vaginal cervix are lined by stratified squamous epithelium. It is not, therefore, a mucous membrane and it is more

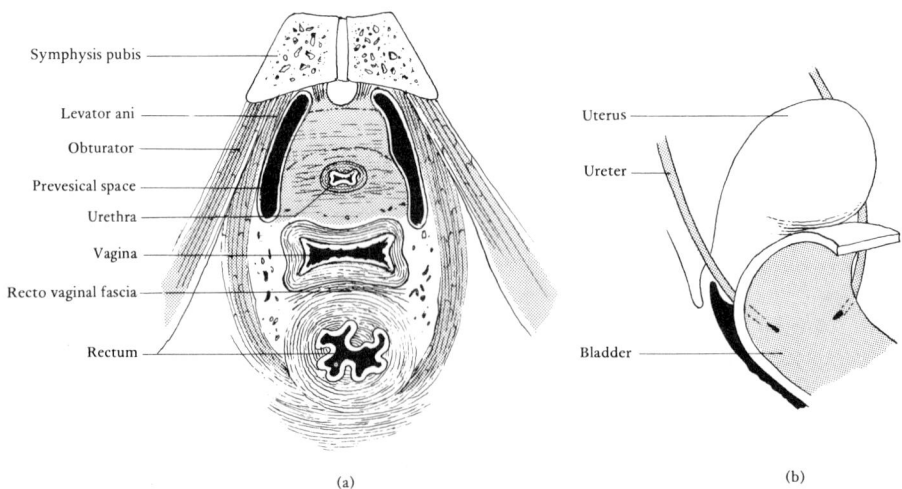

(a)   (b)

Fig. 3.12   (a) Transverse section of pelvis showing relations of the vagina. (b) Relation of ureter to cervix.

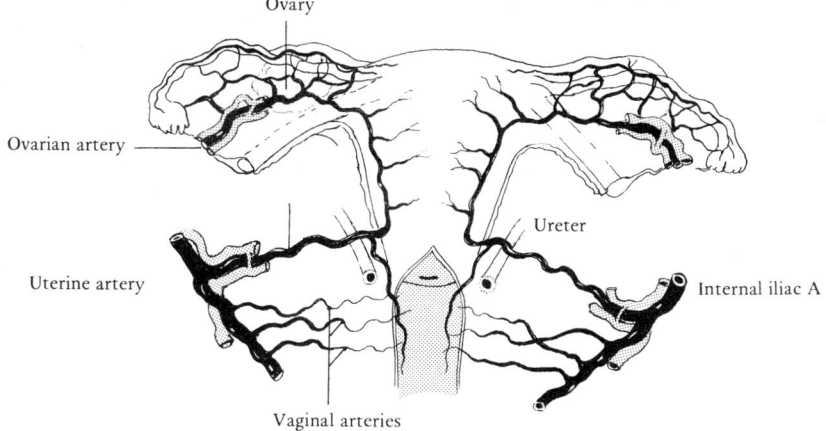

Fig. 3.13   Arterial blood supply to pelvic organs.

correct to talk about the vaginal skin rather than the vaginal mucosa. The vagina contains no glands and is lubricated partly by mucous from the endo cervical glands and partly by desquamated vaginal epithelial cells. The vaginal wall is rugose in nulliparous women but frequently becomes smoother after childbirth. It may become atrophic following the menopause. There is a thin areolar layer beneath the epithelial coat and below this is the muscular wall which is made up of criss-crossing involuntary muscle fibres. The muscle layer is ensheathed by its own fibro-elastic fascia derived from the main layers of pelvic fascia thus the vagina is firmly supported in its place.

BLOOD SUPPLY

(Fig. 3.13) The arterial blood supply is from the internal iliac artery via its vaginal, uterine, internal pudendal, and middle rectal branches. Venous drainage is via the vaginal vein into the internal iliac vein.

LYMPHATIC DRAINAGE

The upper third of the vagina drains to the external and internal iliac nodes, the middle third to the internal iliac nodes and the lower third to the superficial inguinal nodes thus the lower third of the vagina drains similarly to the vulva whereas the middle and upper thirds drain in a similar manner to the cervix (Fig. 3.14).

The uterus

The uterus is a pear-shaped organ about 3 in. (7·5cm) in length, the larger end of the pear being uppermost where it projects free into the peritoneal cavity. The uterus is made up of the fundus, body and cervix. The Fallopian tubes enter the uterus at the superolateral angle—the cornu. Above this lies the fundus of the uterus.

The body of the uterus narrows to a waist known as the isthmus which lies between the cervix of the uterus and the body (Fig. 3.15). The cervix is joined about its middle by the vagina and this attachment divides it into a vaginal and supravaginal portion.

The cavity of the uterus is triangular in shape in coronal section but in the sagittal plane it forms a slit. The cavity communicates with the cervical canal via the internal os and the cervical canal opens into the vagina via the external os. In a nulliparous woman the

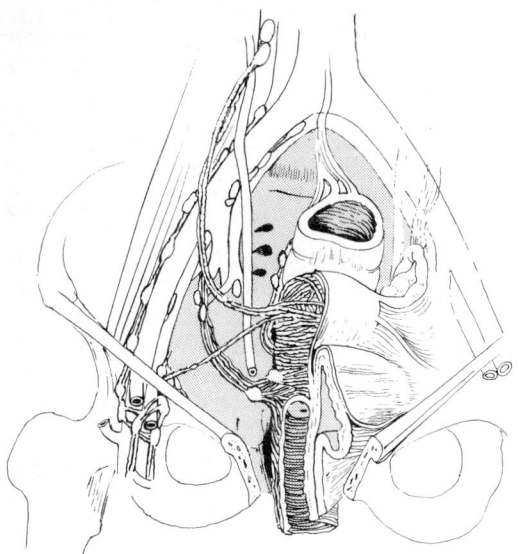

Fig. 3.14   Lymphatic drainage of pelvis.

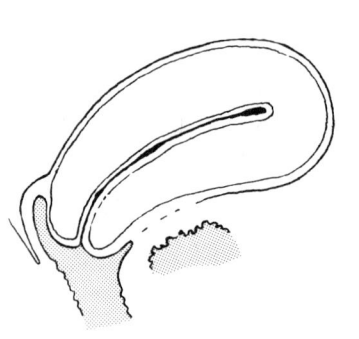

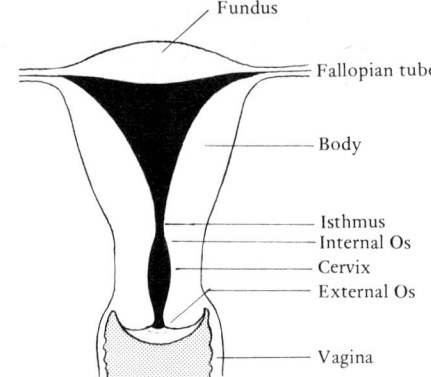

Fig. 3.15   Anatomy of the uterus.

external os is circular but after childbirth it becomes a transverse slit and with an anterior and posterior lip. The non-pregnant uterus of the adult woman occupies a central position in the pelvis, with its fundus just below the plane of the pelvic brim. Its anterior surface rests on the bladder. The organ is fairly mobile unless fixed by adhesions or other abnormal conditions in the pelvis. For example, when the bladder distends it is lifted upwards and backwards, but when the pelvic colon distends

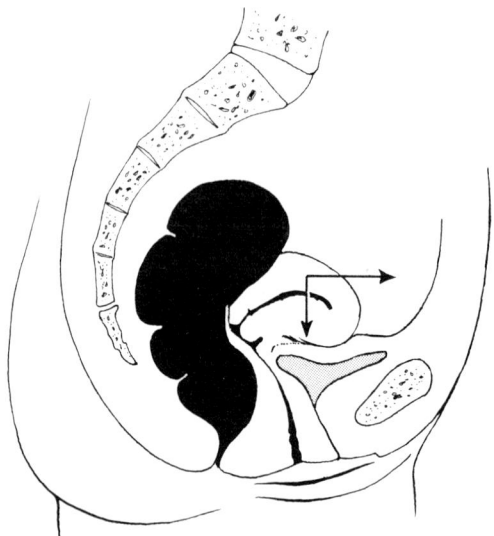

Fig. 3.16   Pelvic colon pressing uterus downwards and forwards.

it is pressed downwards and forwards (Fig. 3.16). Likewise the uterus moves up and down with the pelvic floor during respiratory movements.

In fetal life the cervix is larger than the body and in the prepubertal child the cervix is still larger than the uterine body. At puberty the uterus enlarges to its adult size and proportions when the body becomes relatively larger than the cervix.

The uterus is not in a vertical position but has a forward pitch—'anteversion'. The adult uterus is bent forward on itself at about the internal os, forming an angle of about 170 degrees—'anteflexion'. In the erect position with the bladder empty, the long axis of the uterus is approximately horizontal. When the uterus is retroverted the axis of the cervix is directed upwards and backwards. In the retroflexed position, the axis of the body of the uterus passes upwards and backwards in relation to the axis of the cervix. Both retroversion and retroflexion are abnormal but may occur frequently in women without causing symptoms. Sometimes, due to disease such as endometriosis or pelvic inflammatory disease, the retroversion becomes fixed and then symptoms may result.

MEASUREMENTS OF THE UTERUS
Externally, the total length (in the adult) from the tip of the fundus to the external os is 3in. (7·5cm). Of this 2in. (5cm) are formed by body, 1in (2·5cm) by cervix. The antero-posterior thickness is 1in (2·5cm). The thickness of each wall is $\frac{1}{2}$in. (1·2cm). The length of the cavity is $2\frac{1}{2}$in. (6·2cm) of which the body accounts for $1\frac{1}{2}$in. and the cervix 1in. All measurements are fractionally greater in a woman who has borne a child.

RELATIONS OF THE UTERUS
Anteriorly—Immediate relation of the body is to the uterovesical pouch of peritoneum and lies either on the upper surface of the bladder or on coils of intestine. The supravaginal cervix

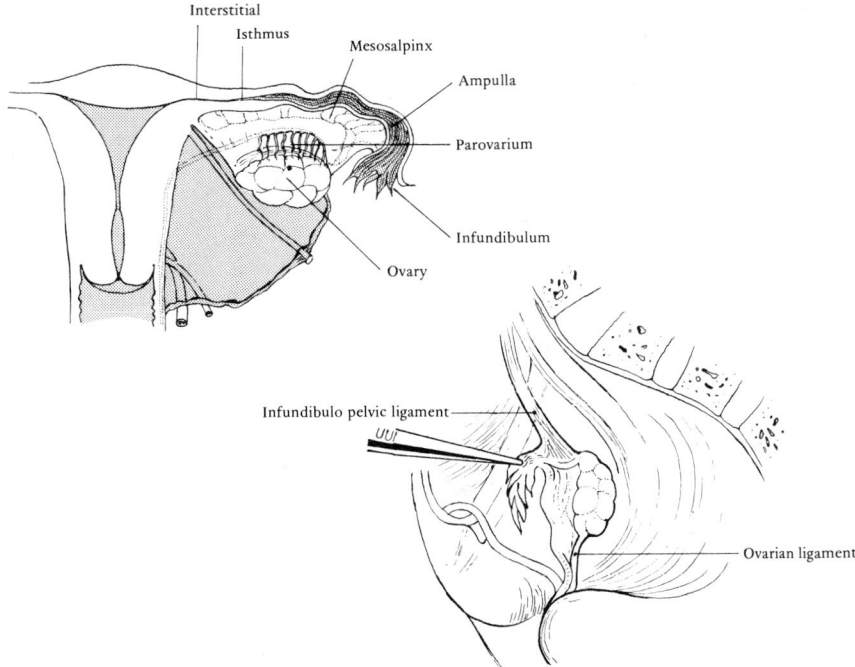

Fig. 3.17   Relations of the Fallopian Tubes.

is related directly to the bladder, the intra-vaginal cervix to the anterior fornix which lies in front.

Posteriorly—The Pouch of Douglas with coils of intestine.

Laterally—The broad ligament and its contents, which include the uterine vessels. In this situation, the ureter lies ½in. laterally to the supravaginal cervix. This is a particularly important relationship in any operation dealing with the uterus in obstetrics or gynaecology, such as Caesarean section or hysterectomy (Fig. 3.17).

STRUCTURE OF THE UTERUS

The uterus is covered with peritoneum which invests the body completely except anteriorly where it is reflected on to the bladder at the uterine isthmus and laterally between the two leaves of the broad ligament. The muscle of the uterus or myometrium is thick and is made up of criss-crossing fibres, involuntary fibres mixed with connective tissue. There are three layers of muscle; an outer layer which runs longitudinally, an intermediate layer in which the fibres run irregularly and an inner layer which runs circularly. The inner layer is especially developed around the orifices of the Fallopian tubes and the internal os.

The lining of the cavity of the uterus is known as the endometrium. It comprises a single layer of cuboidal ciliated cells forming simple tubular glands which dip down into the underlying muscle wall. Below the epithelium there is a stroma of connective tissue containing blood vessels and round cells. The epithelium of the cervical canal is composed of tall columnar cells which secrete an alkaline mucous. This forms a protective cervical plug which fills the canal and is particularly prominent during pregnancy when it is known as the operculum. The vaginal surface of the cervix is covered with stratified squamous epithelium which is continuous with that lining the vagina. The endometrium undergoes extensive change during the menstrual cycle and this will be described under the physiology of the menstrual cycle.

BLOOD SUPPLY

The uterine artery (Fig. 3.13)—A branch of the internal iliac artery runs in the base of the broad ligament and crosses above the ureter to lie alongside the uterus at the level of the internal cervical os. The artery then ascends in a tortuous way alongside the uterus between the leaves of the broad ligament and supplies the corpus before anastomosing with the ovarian artery. The uterine artery gives off a descending cervical branch and also branches to the upper vagina. The veins accompany the arteries and drain into the internal iliac veins. They also communicate via the pelvic plexus with the veins of the vagina and bladder.

LYMPH DRAINAGE

Fundus (Fig. 3.14)—The lymph drainage of the fundus is mainly along the ovarian vessels to the aortic nodes. Some lymphatics, however, pass along the round ligament to the inguinal nodes and these, therefore, may be enlarged in some cases of carcinoma of the body of the uterus where the lesion lies in the fundus.

THE BODY

Drains via the broad ligament to glands lying alongside the external iliac vessels.

CERVIX

Drains—(1) laterally in the broad ligament to the external iliac nodes; (2) posterolaterally along the uterine vessels to the internal iliac nodes and (3) posteriorly along the uterosacral folds to the sacral nodes. The lymphatics from these nodes then ascend along the vessels to the region of the bifurcation of the aorta.

The Fallopian tubes

The Fallopian tubes or oviducts convey the ova from the ovary to the uterus and the sperm-cells upwards to meet them. Fertilization normally occurs in the Fallopian tube.

They extend, one on each side, from the cornua of the uterus outwards for a distance of 4 or 4½in. (10–11cm). The course of the tube is tortuous, firstly, passing outwards and then turning backwards and downwards and inwards, partly encircling the ovary. The outer end of the tube embraces the ovary at or about the time of ovulation but is free and mobile at other times (Fig. 3.17).

The tube is situated within the upper edge of the broad ligament during the first part of the course. When it turns backwards it leaves the broad ligament, though it carries with it a peritoneal investment derived from the posterior layer of this ligament.

Each tube comprises—

1. *the infundibulum*—a horn-shaped extremity extending beyond the broad ligament and opening into the peritoneal cavity via the tubal ostium. The ostium is surrounded by a loose radiating series of fimbriae or tapering tags of mucous membrane.

2. *the ampulla*—which is wide, thin-walled and tortuous.

3. *the isthmus*—which is narrow, straight and thick-walled.

4. *the interstitial part*—which pierces the uterine wall and enters the uterine cavity.

The tube consists of a muscular channel lined by mucous membrane. Its isthmal and ampullary portions are invested with the peritoneum of the broad ligament, which is related to the tube like the mesentery of the bowel and for this reason is called the mesosalpinx.

The tubes are composed of an outer serosal layer, a muscular layer and an inner layer of mucous membrane which is lined by columnar epithelium. The majority of the cells are ciliated and the cilia extend on to the tubal fimbrae. Their function is to produce ciliary current which transports ova from the ovaries towards the tubes. There are also secretory cells in the tubes but very little is understood of their secretions. The mucous membrane lining the tubes forms a very complicated system of longitudinal folds which make the lumen resemble a maze.

The ova are propelled to the uterus along the tube, in part, by the action of peristalsis and, in part, by ciliary action.

BLOOD SUPPLY (Fig. 3.13)

The blood supply of the tubes is from the ovarian arteries which anastomose with the branches of the uterine arteries.

Ovaries

The ovaries are two almond-shaped bodies about 1½in. (3·7cm) long attached to the back of the broad ligament by the mesovarium (Fig. 3.17). The position of the ovary varies somewhat in different individuals and in the same individual at different times. The ovary has two other attachments (1) *the infundibulo pelvic ligament* which carries the ovarian vessels and lymphatics from the side walls of the pelvis and (2) *the ovarian ligament* which passes to the cornu of the uterus and is a rounded cord of fibromuscular tissue recognizable by its whitish appearance.

Up to puberty, the surface of the ovary is smooth and shining. After the commencement of menstruation the surface becomes roughened and puckered by the repeated rupturing of the follicles with the escape of the ova, and this puckering increases as the woman gets older. When menstruation ceases at the time of the menopause the ovaries become small and fibrotic.

The ovary is divided into three regions: (1) the hilum; (2) the medulla; (3) the cortex (Fig. 3.18).

of the organ. It is composed of (a) connective tissue stroma; (b) epithelial structures.

The connective tissue stroma consists of closely packed fibres which form a dense matrix for the vessels and Graafian follicles. Just under the covering epithelium it is thickened to form the tunica albuginea, a dense connective tissue layer which encloses

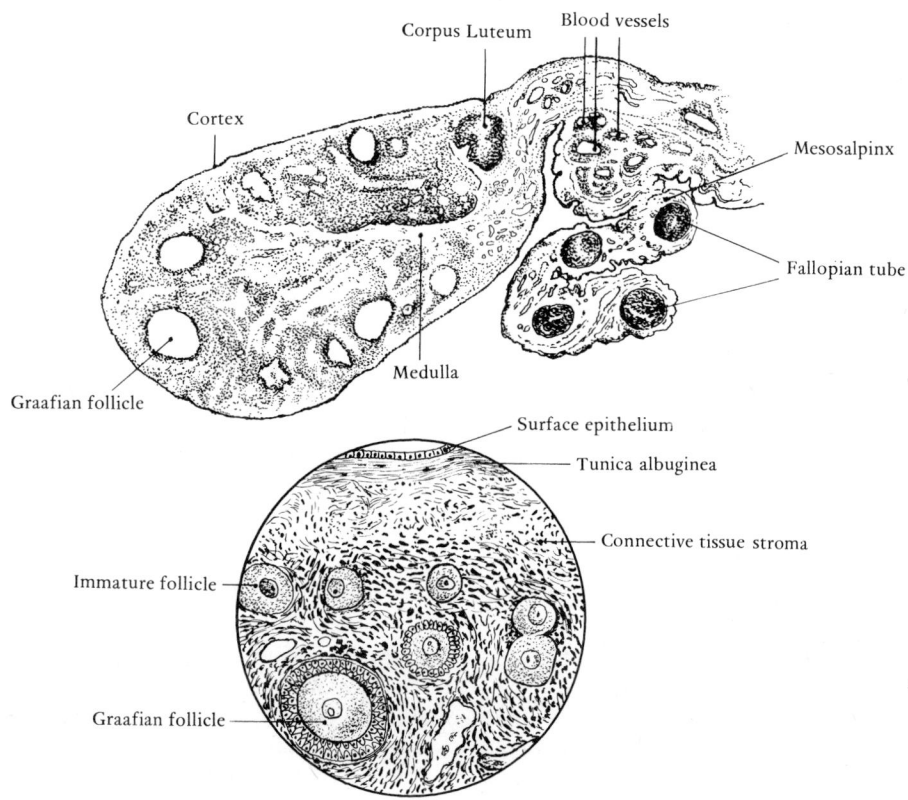

Fig. 3.18   The ovary showing Graafian follicle.

1. *Hilum*—The small area which adjoins the mesovarium and which receives the twigs of the ovarian vessels, lymphatics and nerves which enter from the broad ligament. In addition it contains some scattered tubules—rete ovarii: the significance of which will become apparent later. The hilum possesses connective tissue and some unstriped muscle fibres continuous with the similar structures of the broad ligament.

2. *Medulla*—This subtends the hilum as a semilunar area enclosed by the cortex. Its structure is similar to that of the hilum.

3. *Cortex*—This is the specialized functioning part of the ovary forming the main mass

the ovary, and the presence of which gives the whitish colour to the surface of the organ.

EPITHELIAL STRUCTURES
These are: (a) The germinal epithelium—a sheet of cubical cells one layer deep which covers the free surface of the ovary as far as the hilum, where transition into the endothelium of the peritoneum takes place. (b) The interstitial gland of the ovary—this consists of patches of epithelial cells scattered irregularly throughout the stroma which are inconspicuous. (c) The Graafian follicles—formed round the ova which they enclose and nourish throughout their ovarian existence. The germ

cell is surrounded by the granulosa cell layer and the stroma cells immediately related to this form the theca interna.

FUNCTIONS OF THE OVARIES

The ovaries perform two intimately related functions—(1) gametogenic and (2) endocrine. These follow a strictly repetitive sequence known as the ovarian cycle. This cycle is based on the growth changes which occur around the female germ cells. When the ovary is cut open a number of rounded spaces of varying size filled with a clear fluid are visible to the naked eye. These are ripening follicles. The smaller follicles are recognizable by the unaided eye. In the infant ovary, there are about 100 000 follicles, but by puberty this number has diminished to about 30 000 by a process of atresia. This continues until at age 45 about 10 000 follicles remain which undergo atresia at the menopause. The follicle develops through four stages: (1) the primordial follicle; (2) the developing follicle; (3) the mature follicle; (4) the corpus luteum. This cycle occurs each month when successive numbers of primordial follicles undergo the process of maturation and regression. During the cycle the granulosa and theca interna proliferate and a small cavity forms containing follicular fluid. At this stage one or sometimes two of the group of follicles continue to develop while the others regress. The mechanism by which the single follicle matures each month is not understood. It does, however, become less efficient with older age of the mother.

The follicular fluid volume increases and displaces the germ cell to one side of the follicle where it lies in an area of granulosa cells known as the cumulus oophorus. The cells which immediately surround the germ cells are arranged in a radial fashion and known as the corona radiata. As the follicle enlarges the ovarian stroma is compressed into a false capsule known as the theca externa. This structure is now known as the Graafian follicle after the Dutch scientist Reinier de Graaf who was first to describe it. The diameter of the original primordial follicle is about 30mm whereas that of the mature follicle varies from 10 to 30mm in diameter, a very large relative increase in size.

OVULATION

When the follicle reaches maturity it ruptures through the surface of the ovary and discharges the germ cell with its attached cumulus into the peritoneal cavity. The mechanism responsible for this is unknown.

When rupture of the follicle occurs the fimbriae of the Fallopian tubes is approximated to the ovarian surface and, therefore, entry of the ovum into the abdominal ostium is facilitated. The ovum is then carried toward the ampulla by the ciliary activity of the tubal epithelium. Fertilization usually occurs in the ampulla of the tube. Direct entry of the ovum into the tube is not the rule since in some tubal pregnancies the corpus luteum is found in the contra lateral ovary. Cases have also been described where as a result of surgery the patient has a tube on one side and an ovary on the other and fertilization has occurred in the tube.

LUTEINIZATION

After rupture and ovulation collapse of the follicle occurs, the granulosa cells proliferate and become vascularized. These granulosa cells form the corpus luteum (yellow body), the yellow colour of which is due to the presence of carotene in the luteinized granulosa cells. The corpus luteum in the human synthesizes sex steroid hormones for 8–10 days. If fertilization does not occur during this time it undergoes degeneration or luteolysis and the endocrine activities cease. Thereafter, it slowly degenerates into a structureless mass, the corpus albicans.

If pregnancy occurs, the corpus luteum enlarges progressively for about eight weeks when it reaches its maximum. This is termed the corpus luteum of pregnancy which is concerned with embedding and development of the ovum during the early stages of pregnancy.

BLOOD SUPPLY OF THE OVARY (Fig. 3.19)

The ovarian artery rises on each side from the abdominal aorta. It enters the pelvis by crossing the upper part of the external iliac artery and passes between the layers of the outer end of the broad ligament. It runs in the upper part of the broad ligament to the uterine cornu, where it anastomoses with the terminal branch of the uterine artery. On the way it supplies the ovary and the Fallopian tube. The accompanying veins form the pampiniform plexus which is specially developed during pregnancy. From this plexus two ovarian veins emerge, only one of which drains the ovary. These later fuse to form a single ovarian vein but, while the right vein passes into the vena cava, the left passes

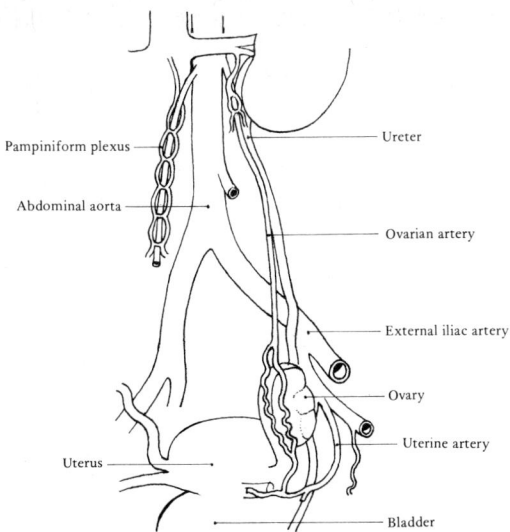

Fig. 3.19   Blood supply to the ovary.

into the left renal vein. These veins form the main drainage channels from the uterus especially in pregnancy.

NERVES OF THE OVARY

The ovary is supplied from a plexus which is continuous at its upper end with the renal plexus and which accompanies the ovarian artery. Some fibres join the ovarian plexus from the aortic plexus. The afferent nerves of the ovary are believed to reach the spinal cord through the posterior routes of the tenth thoracic nerve.

LYMPH DRAINAGE OF THE OVARY

The lymph drainage of the ovary is into the para-aortic nodes.

Endopelvic fascia and pelvic ligaments

The connective tissue making up the floor of the pelvis and covering the levator ani and obturator internus is known as the pelvic fascia. The extraperitoneal cellular tissue of the uterus (the parametrium), vagina, bladder and rectum is known as the endopelvic fascia. This fascia is condensed into three important ligaments which support the pelvic viscera from the pelvic walls. These are—(Fig. 3.20)

1. The cardinal ligaments (transverse cervical ligament or Mackenrodt's ligament); these pass laterally from the cervix and upper vagina to the side walls of the pelvis. They consist of white fibrous connective tissue and are pierced in the upper part by the ureters. They form

the main supports of the uterus and vaginal vault, and laxity of them allows descent with resultant prolapse of the uterus.

2. The utero-sacral ligaments; these pass backwards from the postero-lateral aspect of the cervix at the isthmic level and from the lateral vaginal fornices and are attached to the periosteum in front of the sacro-iliac joints and the third piece of the sacrum. They are of importance in maintaining the uterus in a position of anteversion.

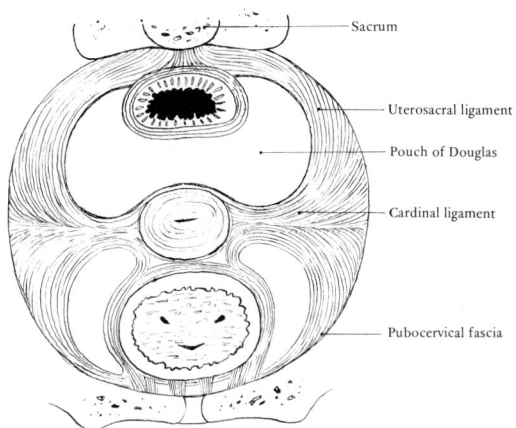

Fig. 3.20   Ligaments supporting the uterus.

3. The pubo-cervical fascia; this extends forward from the cardinal ligament to the pubis on either side of the bladder for which it acts as a sling.

Two other pairs of ligaments are attached to the uterus (Fig. 3.21).

4. The broad ligament; this a fold of peritoneum which connects the lateral wall of the uterus with the side wall of the pelvis on each side. The pelvic floor is, therefore, divided by the uterus and its broad ligaments into an anterior compartment containing the bladder and a posterior compartment containing the rectum. Within the broad ligament are found the Fallopian tube, the ovary, the round ligament, the ovarian ligament, the uterine vessels and branches of the ovarian vessels and lymphatics and nerve fibres. The ureter passes forwards to the bladder deep to the broad ligament and is found just lateral to the lateral fornix of the vagina. In this position it is always in danger during operations such as hysterectomy and Caesarean section.

5. The round ligament; this is a fibro-muscular cord which passes from the lateral

angle of the uterus running in the anterior layer of the broad ligament to the internal inguinal ring. It is the female equivalent of the male gubernaculum testes. It contains some

it usually disappears. In some rare instances, however, it may be traced along the anterior vaginal wall as far as the vulva and vaginal cysts may form from remnants of the ducts.

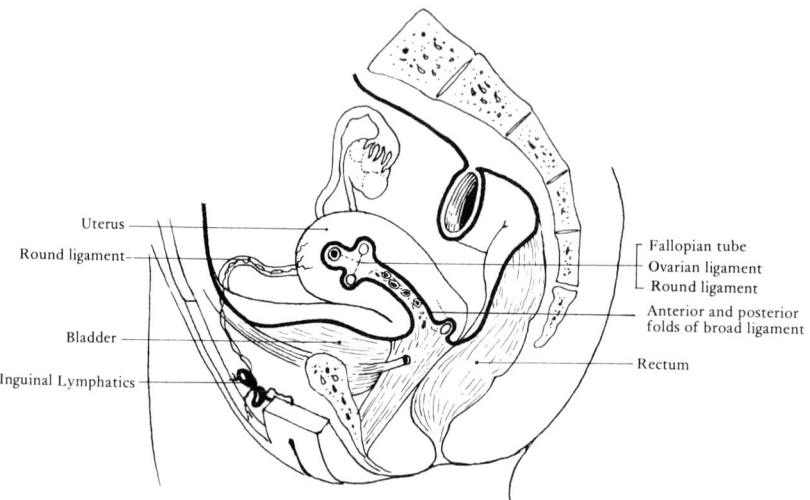

Fig. 3.21   Section of pelvis to show round and broad ligaments.

lymphatics. This point is of some importance since carcinoma of the body of the uterus situated near the origin of the round ligaments may spread via these lymphatics to the inguinal glands which become enlarged in some cases of carcinoma of the body of the uterus.

Parovarium

The parovarium or epoophoron is a vestigial structure in the female derived from the mesonephros and its duct corresponds in development to the epididymis and vas deferens of the male. It lies in the upper part of the broad ligament and its general structure can be readily seen, if the broad ligament be put on the stretch between tube and ovary (Fig. 3.17). It is then seen to consist of 10 or 12 vertical tubules, which pass upwards close to one another from the hilum of the ovary to unite with a single transverse duct—the duct of the epoophoron (formerly called the duct of Gartner). This duct is blind at its outer end where it often splits into a number of tubules. These sometimes dangle free from the broad ligament and may become transformed into small cysts. The inner end of the duct turns downwards along the side of the uterus, where

These cysts may give rise to discomfort and require removal.

Pelvic floor

The pelvic floor consists of soft tissues which close the outlet of the bony pelvis, namely, the peritoneum, pelvic fascia with vessels, lymphatics and nerves, levator ani and coccygeus muscles, and skin and mucous membrane. The pelvic viscera—bladder, uterus and rectum—which channel the pelvic floor by means of their respective canals, urethra, vagina and anal canal, form a component part of the pelvic floor.

PERITONEUM OF THE PELVIS

The pelvic peritoneum is continued down into the pelvis from the abdomen (Fig. 3.11). Leaving the anterior pelvic wall at the back of the symphysis pubis, it arches over the fundus of the bladder to the isthmus of the uterus, from which it is reflected upwards to enclose the body of the uterus. The shallow pouch between the bladder and uterus is called the uterovesical pouch. The peritoneum is laid loosely over the bladder, an arrangement which allows of ready distension of this organ.

After enclosing the body of the uterus in

front and behind, the peritoneum is continued downwards over the posterior surface of the supravaginal cervix and uppermost part of the posterior vaginal wall. From this it is carried on to the anterior rectal wall, the deep pouch between the vagina and rectum being called the Pouch of Douglas. In its lower part it covers only the anterior wall of the rectum, whilst higher up it encloses the lateral walls as well. From the rectum it passes directly on to the front of the sacrum.

The fold formed by the broad ligament on each side and containing the uterus acts as a transverse septum, dividing the pelvic cavity into two compartments, one in front and one behind the uterus. In the anterior compartment, the peritoneum extends from front to back, as already described. From side to side it extends as a shallow pouch rising in the middle over the bladder. Under this sheet on each side the round ligaments course obliquely forwards and outwards from the uterine cornue to the internal abdominal rings.

Passing inwards from the side wall of the pelvis on each side the peritoneal sheet covers the uterosacral ligament and just within this dips down abruptly to line the deep Pouch of Douglas.

THE MUSCLES OF THE PELVIC FLOOR AND PERINEUM (Fig. 3.22)

The cavity of the bony and ligamentus pelvis is closed by a diaphragm of muscles and fascia through which the rectum, urethra and vagina pass to reach the exterior.

The levator ani is the most important muscle of the pelvic floor. Arising from the back of the pubis, the fascia of the side wall of the pelvis and spine of the ischium it sweeps down in a series of loops, (a) to form a sling around the vagina being inserted into the perineal body; (b) forming a sling around the rectum and reinforcing the deep part of the external anal sphincter; (c) being inserted into the coccyx.

This muscle is the principal support of the pelvic floor and also has a sphincteric action on the rectum and vagina. It helps to increase intra-abdominal pressure during defaecation, micturition and parturition. On its deep aspect it is related to the pelvic viscera and its perineal aspect forms the inner wall of the ischio-rectal fossa.

PERINEAL MUSCLES

In obstetrics the structure referred to as the perineum or perineal body is the triangular mass of fibromuscular tissue between the vagina and the lowermost portion of the rectum. The true anatomical perineum is a more extended area, which is divided into an anterior and a posterior section by the vaginal canal. The muscles include the sphincter ani externus, the transversus perinei, the bulbocavernosus and ischiocavernosus. All except the ischiocavernosus have one insertion in the central part of the perineal body. They contract during coitus and defaecation; and are greatly stretched and may be torn during delivery.

The ischio-rectal fossae lie at each side of the anus. These fossae contain coarse fat and

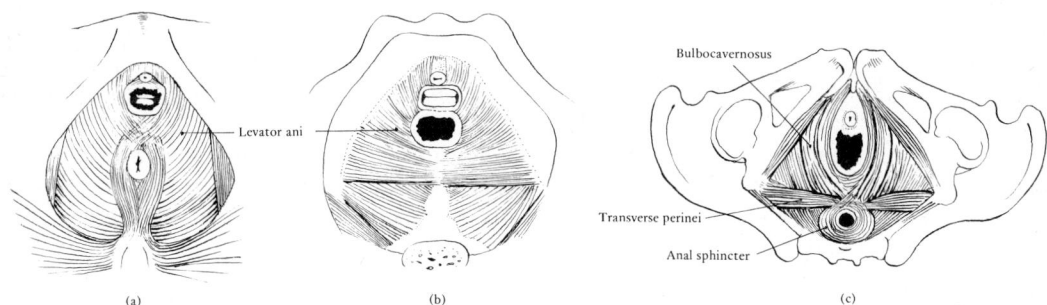

Fig. 3.22   Pelvic floor: (a) From below; (b) From above; (c) Muscles of pelvic floor.

The muscles are divided into: (1) the pelvic diaphragm consisting of the levator ani and coccygeus muscles; (2) the superficial muscles —(a) the anterior (urogenital) perineum, and (b) the posterior (anal) perineum.

communicate with each other behind the anus. They sometimes become infected after delivery or may become the site of a haematoma after an episiotomy or a perineal tear. They contain no important structures and can, therefore, be incised if infected. The boundaries of the ischio-rectal fossae are laterally: the side wall of the pelvis and the fascia over the obturator internus muscle. In this area, inside a fascial tunnel, called Alcock's canal, the pudendal vessels and nerve run (Fig. 3.23). These give

in the interval between them it is surrounded by the sphincter urethrae membranaceae. Its lower part is intimately incorporated in the vaginal wall.

The urethra has a muscular, a submucous and a mucous coat. The muscular wall is

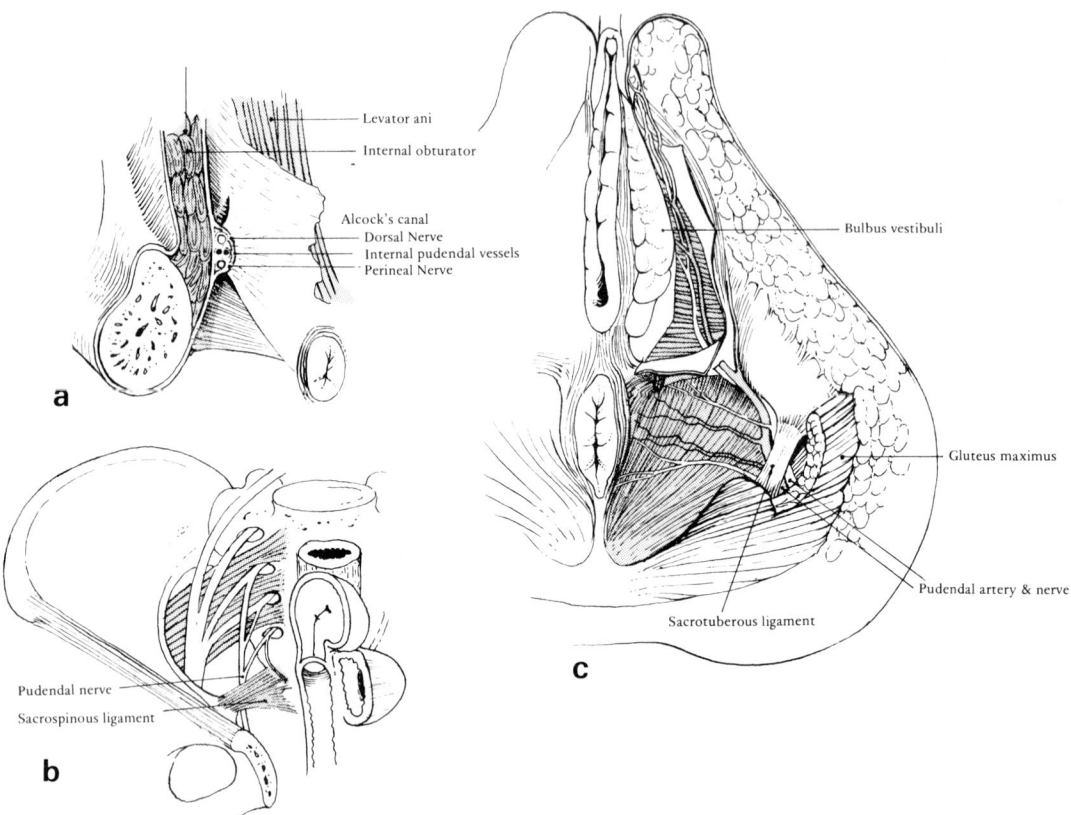

Fig. 3.23 Pelvic anatomy showing: (a) Alcock's canal; (b) Relations of pudendal nerve; (c) Course of pudendal vessels and nerve.

off the inferior haemorrhoidal vessels and nerves to the anus and then pass forward to supply the perineal tissues. The pudendal nerves can be blocked at this site by an injection through the vaginal wall and this forms the site of anaesthesia for pudendal nerve block which is used for regional anaesthesia in forceps delivery.

URETHRA

The urethra in the female is 1½in. (3·7cm) long. After leaving the base of the bladder it passes downwards and forwards to the external urethral orifice. During its course it pierces the two layers of the triangular ligament, and

composed of an outer circular and an inner longitudinal layer. The submucous coat consists of loose fibrous and elastic fibres. The mucous membrane is thrown into longitudinal folds. It is lined by transitional epithelium near the bladder and by squamous epithelium near the meatus. The urethra possesses numerous glands, especially near the meatus. Two comparatively large ducts, open one on each side of the posterior wall of the urethra within the meatus and are known as Skene's ducts. The urethra of the female is dilatable and for purposes of examination can be expanded to a diameter of ½in. (12mm) without damage. The sphincter urethra is a tenuous structure and bladder control seems to depend mainly on the intrinsic sphincter of condensed circular muscle fibres of the bladder.

BLADDER (Fig. 3.16)
The bladder in the fetus and infant is an abdominal organ but in the adult is normally within the pelvis, where it lies between the pubes and the uterus. When the bladder is distended the uterus is lifted upwards more into the erect position. The normal capacity of the bladder is about 12–14 ounces. When fully distended, it forms an elastic swelling of a flat ovoid shape felt distinctly above the symphysis pubis.

The upper wall and sides of the bladder are covered by peritoneum which, behind, is reflected on to the uterus at the level of the isthmus. The shallow peritoneal fossa between bladder and uterus is the uterovesical pouch. In front, the bladder is related to the back of the pubis, from which it is separated by loose tissue. Behind, it lies against the supravaginal cervix and upper part of the anterior vaginal wall. With each of these it is only loosely

descends along the front of the internal iliac artery to the level of the ischial spine. It then turns inwards and coursing forwards and downwards it passes beneath the base of the broad ligament. At this point it is crossed by the uterine vessels. It then crosses the lateral fornix and upper part of the front wall of the vagina to reach the side of the bladder about 2in. (5cm) from its fellow of the opposite side. As the ureter approaches the bladder its oblique course brings it nearer and nearer to the supravaginal cervix, and just before it reaches the bladder it is only $\frac{1}{2}$in. (1·2cm) from the cervix. It is in this position that it is very liable to damage either in gynaecological surgery of the uterus or, in some instances, during lower uterine segment Caesarean section.

THE DEVELOPMENT OF THE FALLOPIAN TUBES, UTERUS AND VAGINA

The Mullerian or paramesonephric ducts develop, one on each side, near the mesonephric

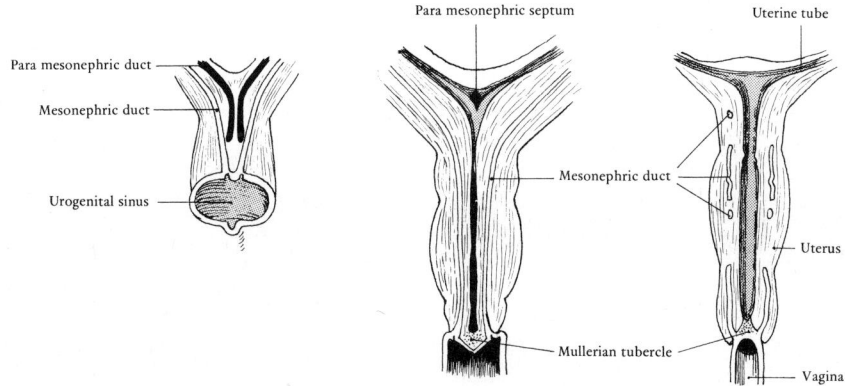

Fig. 3.24   The development of the Fallopian tubes, uterus and vagina.

incorporated. Below, the bladder is supported by the visceral layer of the pelvic fascia and by the levatores ani muscles.

URETER
The pelvic portion of the ureter has an important relation to the pelvic organs and its exact position must be kept constantly in mind by the gynaecological surgeon. The ureter enters the pelvis by crossing the brim at the level of the lower end of the common iliac or the upper end of the external iliac artery. It

(Wolffian) ducts in the posterior abdominal wall and are mesodermal in origin (Fig. 3.24).

The paramesonephric duct appears in embryos at about five weeks after fertilization. The two paramesonephric ducts meet and fuse into the urogenital septum in the mid-line. At first, the fusion is partial resulting in a septum being present between the two lumina. The septum eventually disappears and a single mid-line cavity is established. These fused segments of the paramesonephric ducts form the uterovaginal canal. The free parts of the ducts above the urogenital canal give rise to the uterine tubes.

The caudal end of the uterovaginal canal remains solid and reaches the posterior wall of the urogenital sinus. Where it reaches the urogenital sinus it produces an elevation called the Mullerian tubercle.

Outgrowths from the Mullerian tubercle push back the wall of the urogenital sinus and constitute the vaginal plate. The vaginal plate is canalized by extension of the uterovaginal canal from above and by the breaking down of the epithelium of the sinovaginal bulb from below. This process is completed late in fetal life.

The junction between the body of the uterus and cervix becomes recognizable at about 10 weeks, but the uterine portion of the utero-vaginal canal does not separate from the vaginal portion until about five and a half months.

Developmental abnormalities of this system comprise mainly failure of union of the two Mullerian ducts resulting in persistence of a double tube. This may cause all abnormalities from a bicornuate uterus to complete redupli-cation of the uterus and vagina. A further common abnormality is failure of canalization of the original solid caudal end of the duct and this results in accumulation after puberty of menstrual blood above the obstruction giving rise to the clinical condition of cryptomenor-rhoea (see Chapter 34).

DEVELOPMENT OF THE EXTERNAL GENITALIA

At about the fifth week of intra-uterine life the urethral plate forms. The mesenchyme along each side of the urethral plate proliferates and raises the overlying ectoderm to form primitive urethral folds. The phallus and its glans develop but the urethral folds do not unite, as they do in the male. The genital folds form labial swellings which flank the base of the phallus.

The phallus forms the clitoris, the labial swellings become the labia majora and the unfused urethral folds become the labia minora. The definitive form of the external genitalia is achieved at about $4\frac{1}{2}$–5 months of intra-uterine life.

DEVELOPMENT OF THE OVARY

The early gonads appear about five weeks after fertilization as thickenings of coelomic epithelium—the genital ridge on the medial aspect of the mesonephros. As the ovary enlarges it projects more and more from the medial aspect of the urogenital ridge. The ovary eventually comes to occupy a final position very different from its original site in the embryo. It descends from its para-mesonephric situation into the pelvis. This descent explains the blood supply and lymph drainage of the ovary both of which are established before descent. The gubernaculum of the ovary becomes attached to the fused uterovaginal segments of the paramesonephric ducts at their junction with the free tubal portions. This attachment of the true guber-naculum to the uterus causes the ovary to enter the true pelvis where it lies on the dorsal surface of the urogenital mesentery which has descended from the ovary and now forms the broad ligament. The part of the gubernaculum persisting between the ovary and the uterus becomes the ligament of the ovary and the part between the uterus and labium majus becomes the round ligament of the uterus.

THE INNERVATION OF THE FEMALE GENITAL TRACT

Apart from the vulva, the innervation of the genital tract is by the autonomic nervous system.

Post ganglionic fibres from the thoracic sympathetic duct and prevertebral ganglions run to the pelvis along the visceral branches of the abdominal aorta especially the ovarian and uterine arteries. Some fibres are derived from the hypogastric plexus and these descend to the pelvic plexuses where they join with the parasympathetic component.

These pelvic plexuses are situated on each side of the rectum and fibres run forwards along the utero-sacral ligaments to the cervix and from there to the uterus and vagina.

Afferent fibres from the ovaries return via the ovarian arteries. The uterine sensory fibres run towards the pelvic plexuses. These fibres enter the spinal cord between segments T10 and L1. Sympathetic motor fibres arise from the lower thoracic segments and para-sympathetic fibres from S2–4. The final site of termination of these afferent fibres in the uterus is not known and their motor function not understood.

The innervation of the external genitalia is primarily by the branches of the pudendal nerve. Further innervation is obtained from the perineal branch of the posterior cutaneous nerve of the thigh, the genital branch of the genito-femoral nerve, and the ilio-inguinal nerve.

THE ANATOMY OF THE MALE SEXUAL ORGANS

In view of the importance of the male in infertility investigations it is necessary to give a description of the male sexual organs (Fig 3.25).

These may be considered under two headings: (1) those concerned with the production of semen, namely, the testes, epididymis, the

complex convolutions form the globus major or head of the epididymis. There the vasa efferentia open into a single convoluted tube which forms the body and globus minor of the epididymis and continues as the vas deferens. The vas deferens passes upwards into the spermatic cord, enters the abdominal cavity through the inguinal canal and then passes downwards behind the bladder, uniting with the duct of the seminal vesicle to form the ejaculatory duct which passes through the prostate to enter the first portion of the urethra.

Spermatogenesis takes place in the seminiferous tubules. On section these tubules are seen to consist of a basement membrane and a lining epithelium containing several layers of cells. In the adult, certain cells of the epithelium constantly undergoing transformation into spermatozoa. These cells, as they

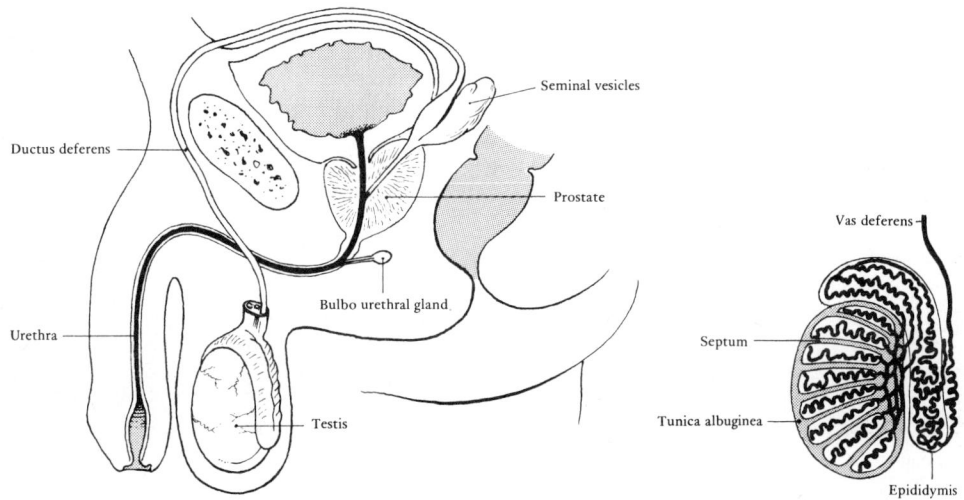

Fig. 3.25   Anatomy of the male sexual organs.

prostate and seminal vesicles; (2) those responsible for delivery of semen into the vagina, namely, the urethra and penis.

Nothing need be said here about the anatomy of the organs in group (2). Each testis consists essentially of large numbers of convoluted tubules (seminiferous tubules) and of interstitial cells (cells of Leydig) situated between the tubules. The convoluted seminiferous tubules pass towards the mediastinum testis and unite to form a smaller number of straight seminiferous tubules which open into the rete testis. From the rete testis run 15–20 narrow ducts (vasa efferentia), and these by their

transform, gradually pass inwards from the basement membranes towards the lumen of the tubule. From without inwards, these germinal cells are termed respectively spermatogonia, spermatocytes, spermatids and finally spermatozoa, which are shed into the lumen of the tubule. Occasional tall cells are seen stretching from the basement membrane almost to the lumen of the tubule. Many spermatozoa may be seen attached to the innermost ends of these cells (Sertoli cells).

The spermatozoa leave the seminiferous epithelium and pass to the rete testis and then via the efferent ducts to the epididymis. Here they may be stored especially in the tail of the epididymis for long periods, hence the need for other contraceptive measures to be adopted for some months after vasectomy.

Spermatozoa acquire their motility and fertilizing capacity in a final process of maturation as they pass through the epididymis. Further physiological changes called capacitation, take place during passage through the female genital tract.

REFERENCES

Bernard, R. M. (1951) The shape and size of the female pelvis. *Edin. med. J.* (Trans. Edinb. Obstet. Soc.) Session CIV, 1.

4. The Endocrine Physiology of the Reproductive System

Central to the modern concept of reproduction in all mammalia is *a blind life within the brain,* from which springs the function of all the rest. It is appropriate therefore to start this account of the physiology of reproduction with the role of the brain.

THE HYPOTHALAMUS

It has long been surmised that reproductive processes, such as the menstrual cycle or ovulation, must in some way be under nervous control, for many reproductive phenomena arise in consequence of environmental changes which could only be perceived by the nervous system. Thus, for instance, oestrus in a ferret is dependent on the length of daylight, and amenorrhoea in a woman can result from psychological stress. The elevation of the pituitary, at the beginning of this century, to leadership of the endocrine orchestra, put physiologists in a dilemma. On the one hand it was indisputable that gonadal activity was controlled by the pituitary, while on the other hand, the most sophisticated histological techniques could display no nervous connection between the brain and the anterior pituitary. True, there were nerve axons coming down the pituitary stalk from the supraoptic and paraventricular nuclei above, but all these ended in the posterior pituitary; a quite separate gland and one whose only connection with the anterior pituitary appeared to be a fortuitous juxtaposition. Further experimental work at first only complicated the matter. If the pituitary stalk was cut, pituitary function, and hence gonadal activity, declined but tended after a while, to recover again. If the pituitary were completely isolated from the brain above by inserting a wax plate between it and the brain, or by transplanting the pituitary to some other part of the body, a basal level of pituitary activity persisted, but not enough to restore ovulation or oestrus.

The mystery was solved by Geoffrey Harris, professor of anatomy at Oxford until his death in 1971. Harris pointed out that, while there was no nervous connection between the brain and the anterior pituitary, there was a direct vascular channel between the hypothalamus above and the pituitary below, which might well serve as a means to convey a biological signal from the nervous system to the gland. So it proved to be. The superior hypophysial artery which supplies part of the hypothalamus breaks into capillaries which drain into the hypophysial portal vein which runs down the pituitary stalk and then, in the anterior pituitary, divides into a second leash of vessels —the sinusoids of the anterior pituitary gland. One of the last major publications by Professor Harris was a review, together with Dr F. Naftolin, of modern concepts of hypothalamic function. It is noted in the list of recommended reading and would repay study.

The functional anatomy of the hypothalamus

The relationship between the hypothalamus and the pituitary is shown diagrammatically in figure 4.1. When parts of the hypothalamus concerned with reproductive function are experimentally damaged, pituitary gonadotrophin secretion stops. By means of localized lesions in the ventral hypothalamus it has been possible to map out areas which contain nuclei from which come the nerve fibres which end in the portal vessels supplying the anterior pituitary. Apart from the median eminence, the retrochiasmatic and ventromedial nuclei have been shown to be concerned in the control of gonadal function. It is not known which cells, whether glial cells, neurons or other neuroendocrine cells, produce the material which is transported via the portal circulation.

At first sight there is some similarity between the microscopic anatomy of the neuroendocrine apparatus of the anterior pituitary and that of

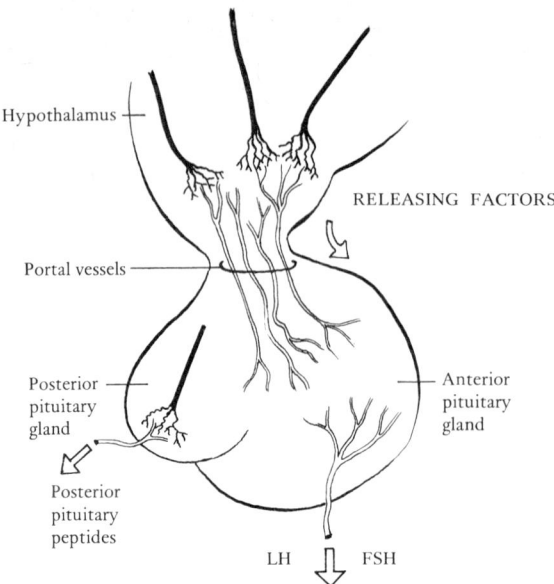

Fig. 4.1   The relationship between the hypothalamus and the pituitary.

the posterior pituitary. In the case of the posterior pituitary the supraoptic and paraventricular nuclei are concerned in the function of the gland. But the nerves from these nuclei convey material directly to the posterior pituitary, not via the circulation. The materials they convey are the very polypeptides secreted by the posterior pituitary, which is therefore an organ of storage, not of synthesis. On the other hand, the materials conveyed to the anterior pituitary from the hypothalamus are quite unlike the protein hormones of the anterior pituitary which is therefore a gland of synthesis, not storage.

The chemistry of hypothalamic hormones

As soon as it became clear that the hypothalamus produced materials which controlled the release of pituitary trophic hormones, great interest was engendered in trying to determine the nature of these materials. At first they were called releasing factors but when their true hormonal status became apparent, the name was changed to releasing hormones. Many laboratories all over the world competed for the great prize of being the first to work out the constitution of a releasing hormone, but gradually the lead came to be divided between two teams in the United States, those of Guillemin and of Schally. The work of

identification was made very difficult by the tiny amounts of releasing hormones present in the hypothalamus. Thus Schally extracted 50 000 pig hypothalami in order to obtain a few milligrams of crude LH releasing hormone. Happily it soon became clear that there was no species specificity for releasing hormones, and material from pigs or cattle was equally active in humans and vice versa.

As it happened, the first releasing hormone whose structure was determined was not concerned with gonadal function, but was the hormone which caused release of the thyroid stimulating hormone of the anterior pituitary. It fell to Guillemin to isolate and synthesize thyrotrophin releasing factor (TRF). It turned out to be an unusual polypeptide in which the N terminus was protected and the C terminus amidated. This gave the essential clue to Schally who, late in 1971, was able to announce that luteinizing hormone releasing hormone, LH-RH, was also a polypeptide. It proved to be a decapeptide with the following chain of amino acids:

(pyro) Glu-His-Trp-Ser-Tyr-

Gly-Leu-Arg-Pro-Gly-NH$_2$

A substance with this structure was soon synthesized and found to be indistinguishable, both in terms of physiochemical and of biological properties, from the natural hormone extracted from the hypothalamus.

For some years before the structure of LH-RH was elucidated and the hormone synthesized, another structural question had been puzzling biochemists. This arose from the finding that all highly purified extracts of LH-RH still contained some FSH releasing activity. Endocrinologists were obliged reluctantly to entertain the notion that there might not be, as hitherto supposed, separate FSH and LH releasing hormones but that both activities may reside in the same molecule. Even the synthesis of LH-RH has not fully resolved this question. It is true that pure LH-RH also has FSH releasing activity but this does not prove that another substance with FSH releasing power is not produced elsewhere in the hypothalamus. If one molecule contains both FSH and LH releasing powers, the beautiful simplicity of one particular releasing hormone causing the secretion of a single trophic hormone is lost. Endocrinologists then have to explain why a single releasing hormone can cause gonadotrophin secretion from the pituitary which at one time consists mainly of FSH and at another is predominantly LH. A hypothesis which is currently being examined is the suggestion that the response of the pituitary gland depends on the circulating level of ovarian hormones. Thus oestrogens could potentiate LH release by LH-RF and progesterone could suppress this.

The physiology of gonadal control by the hypothalamus

Not only are the hypothalamic nuclei known to elaborate releasing factors concerned in the control of pituitary function but so is the whole limbic system. In this way an input from other areas of the brain is ensured. This is the way in which the nervous control of reproductive function is achieved: whether it be the eye of a ferret sensing light or the mind of a woman rebelling against a burden of anxiety. This input from elsewhere in the brain is by way of an overriding factor, superimposed on another rhythm, derived from a second, basic signal. This second signal is the circulating level of the gonadal hormones, oestrogen and progesterone. In some mysterious way the hypothalamic nuclei are able to perceive the circulating levels of the steroid hormones of the ovary, testis and adrenal and, by way of the releasing hormones, to cause the appropriate pituitary response. This second input to the hypothalamus has

been aptly named a feedback mechanism and the details of its operation as applied to the ovary will be described later when the ovarian hormones are discussed.

Although hypothalamic function has been considered only in terms of the polypeptide hormones known to have the property of causing secretion of pituitary trophic hormones, there are other substances in nervous tissue, notably amines like dopamine, which affect pituitary function, and it may be that some of these play a role in their own right. It is not known how the releasing hormones cause the secretion of pituitary trophic hormones. It has been suggested that they may play some part in the biosynthesis of pituitary hormones, but the evidence is strongly in favour of the view that the releasing hormones simply cause release into the circulation of preformed pituitary hormones.

The pituitary response to releasing hormones is very rapid. Under experimental conditions the trophic hormones are secreted within seconds of the application of the corresponding releasing hormone. The inactivation of the gonadotrophin releasing hormones is also rapid. They disappear rapidly from the plasma, presumably as a result of enzymatic degradation.

The male hypothalamus discharges its gonadotrophic releasing hormones in a steady, tonic manner, whereas the female hypothalamus produces the same hormones in a rise and fall rhythm. In the last resort this is one of the most fundamental physiological differences between male and female and lies behind the periodicity of reproductive behaviour and capacity of the female mammal. This cyclicity of hypothalamic rhythm is imprinted on the female nervous system before birth, probably by the hormones secreted by the fetal gonads during intra-uterine life. It is a delicate process, easily interfered with in early post-natal life. Thus newborn female rats if injected with testosterone at birth, will lose their female hypothalamic rhythm and go into a state of permanent oestrus. It has been suggested that a similar mechanism may lie behind some of the aberrations of sexual function in the human.

Not all gonadotrophin releasing hormones act positively to cause discharge of the corresponding trophic hormone. Prolactin appears to be constantly produced and discharged by the anterior pituitary and the hypothalamic hormone controlling it acts negatively by inhibiting the discharge of prolactin. This hormone has therefore come to be known as prolactin inhibiting hormone (PIH).

Therapeutic application of hypothalamic releasing hormones

The gonadotrophin releasing hormones of the hypothalamus move a short distance in a small circumscribed volume of blood from their point of release to their target organ. They are rapidly inactivated in their highly diluted state in the general circulation. It might therefore be supposed that the possibilities of therapeutic application by parenteral administration are remote. Surprisingly this does not appear to be the case. It was found possible to induce ovulation in amenorrhoeic women by extracts from beef hypothalami and now that synthetic LH-RH has been shown to have the same action, the field is greatly extended. Extensive clinical trials are going on in many parts of the world and it is not too fanciful to suggest that it will soon be possible to produce a controlled ovulation in any woman capable of pituitary and ovarian response.

THE GONADOTROPHIC HORMONES OF THE ANTERIOR PITUITARY

Although the fanciful description of the adeno-hypophysis as the leader of the endocrine orchestra no longer appears in textbooks, it is still regarded as the final link in the control of gonadal function and, on this account, an understanding of pituitary physiology is necessary for the study of gynaecology.

In this section only the gonadotrophic hormones of the anterior hypophysis—follicle stimulating hormone (FSH), luteinizing hormone (LH) and prolactin, will be considered. Other hormones such as thyrotrophin and adrenocorticotrophin, produced by the same gland, will not be described.

Pituitary anatomy

The pituitary is a composite organ; its separate halves have quite different developmental origins. The anterior lobe with which we are here concerned develops from Rathke's pouch, an extension of the ectoderm of the oral cavity. The posterior lobe is a downgrowth from the diencephalon.

At first only three cell types—acidophiles,

basophiles and chromophobes—could be detected in the adenohypophysis, although it was clear from early on that at least six hormones are produced by the gland. As staining techniques became more sophisticated it became possible to identify subgroups of these cell types associated with particular hormones. Although thyrotrophs and gonadotrophs can now be distinguished with confidence, the differentiation of the gonadotrophs secreting FSH or LH is still a subject of controversy. The morphological differences between pituitary cells can now be clearly demonstrated by electron microscopy. The gonadotrophs in particular can be distinguished from cells producing other hormones by the characteristics of the granules in their cytoplasm. It has been claimed that ultra microscopic examination can differentiate between cells producing LH and those producing FSH, although it must be owned that from what is known about blood levels of these two hormones, they could well be produced by the same cells.

Chemistry of the gonadotrophins

Attempts to extract and purify the FSH and LH contained in the pituitary gland have been made in many laboratories. As methods have become more and more sophisticated purer and purer preparations have been achieved although it must be acknowledged that no absolutely pure material has been produced. Certainly the best preparations are good enough to give secure information about the chemical nature of gonadotrophins. Both LH and FSH are very large molecules, built, as is the case with all proteins, of long chains of amino acids. Like other proteins the gonadotrophins are species specific. Although the differences between LH or FSH from the sheep, the ox and man are subtle, techniques are already sufficiently advanced to detect the small chemical differences between them. The species specificity and the large size of gonadotrophin molecules have posed formidable problems in clinical application. In the first instance it has meant that gonadotrophins from animal pituitaries are of little use in man and the slaughterhouse which was the source of many hormones soon after the turn of the century proved to be of no use for the supply of gonadotrophins active in humans. Secondly, the large molecules with their complex structure and enormous permutations of amino acid sequence are exceedingly difficult to imitate artificially. Indeed, it is doubtful whether synthetic LH or FSH will ever be made.

Gonadotrophins readily aggregate into larger and larger molecules. It is to some extent an arbitrary question whether one regards a particular molecule as representing LH or prefers another some multiples larger. Not surprisingly estimates of the molecular weight both of FSH and of LH have varied greatly. Present-day findings suggest that FSH from human pituitaries has a molecular weight of about 41 000, while LH at 26 000 is somewhat smaller. The corresponding hormones which are excreted in urine are clearly somewhat degraded and have smaller molecular weights. The amino acids constituting the gonadotrophic hormones can readily be determined by hydrolysing the intact protein and many such analyses have been published for both FSH and LH. It turns out that, in addition to amino acids there is also a carbohydrate constituent in each, i.e. both FSH and LH are glycoproteins. The carbohydrate forms a larger part of the FSH molecule than of LH. In FSH there is 10·4 per cent hexoses, 9·6 per cent hexosamine and 8·6 per cent sialic acid while in LH the corresponding proportions are 5·9 per cent, 5·1 per cent and 0·7 per cent.

Recent work on the chemistry of the gonadotrophins has shown a curious similarity of structure in LH, FSH, chorionic gonadotrophin (HCG) and thyrotrophin (TSH). It appears that each of these consists of two sub-units, an α and a β chain. The α chain is in fact common to all four hormones and probably accounts for their immunological cross reactions. The β chain is hormone specific, e.g. the β chain of LH is different from the FSH and is the reason for the difference in biological activity of the two hormones.

The chemistry and physiology of prolactin has not been so thoroughly explored. Although it appears to have gonadotrophic activity in some animals there is no evidence that it does so in the human; here its main demonstrable effect is to cause lactation when the breast has been acted on by oestrogen, progesterone and corticotrophin. Just as LH, FSH, HCG and TSH form a group of chemically and immunologically related hormones, so prolactin and pituitary growth hormone appear to be related. Indeed it seemed doubtful at first whether they were entirely separate entities, but recently prolactin preparations without growth hormone activity, and vice versa, have been obtained. Research on the physiology of prolactin has for some time been in the doldrums but has now picked up and it is probable that in future a more important role in the physiology of reproduction will be assigned to it.

The secretion of pituitary gonadotrophins during the menstrual cycle

The events of the menstrual cycle which make up much of the substance of clinical practice in gynaecology, take their origin from the secretion of gonadotrophins by the pituitary. Gynaecologists have for some time concerned themselves with the pattern of secretion of gonadotrophins by the pituitary. At first, pituitary activity could only be roughly traced by estimating the urinary excretion of degraded fragments of the hormones but the introduction of radioimmunoassay techniques has made it possible to follow moment by moment the amount of gonadotrophin being secreted by the pituitary.

There is now a generally accepted concept of the pattern of changing concentration of FSH and of LH in blood during the menstrual cycle. It is widely accepted that these changes reflect the secretion of the hormones by the pituitary. In the first few days after the onset of menstruation the blood levels of FSH are high, being presumably concerned with stimulating the growth of a fresh set of follicles. After this initial peak the FSH values decline somewhat, reaching a nadir just before ovulation. Then a surge of FSH secretion takes place. These high values last only for a short period of time—a day or two at the most and coincide with a peak of LH secretion. After the mid-cycle peak FSH concentrations fall to a steady level, somewhat lower than those of the proliferative phase, and continue at this level until menstruation supervenes. The LH patterns during the menstrual cycle follow a somewhat similar course, the mid-cycle rise of LH being particularly pronounced. The average plasma levels found in 16 ovulatory cycles by Ross *et al.* (1970) are shown in figure 4.2.

Unlike FSH concentration the LH concentration does not fall to a pre-ovulatory nadir. On the contrary LH levels rise slowly throughout the follicular phase and are above the level of the onset of menses when the mid-cycle surge begins. After the pronounced

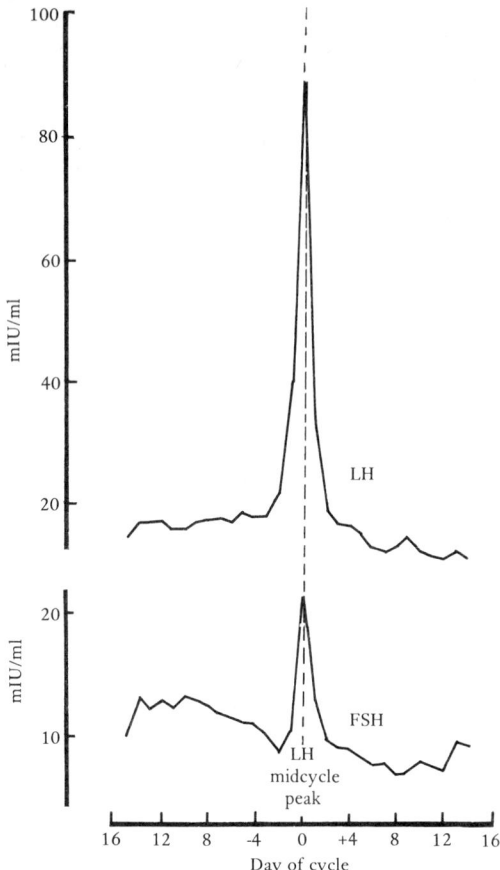

Fig. 4.2   The plasma levels (mean and 95% confidence limits) of LH and of FSH during the menstrual cycle, taking the mid-cycle peak of LH as day 0. Adapted from Ross *et al.* (1970).

mid-cycle peak LH concentration falls steadily until the onset of the next menses without the preliminary rise just before menses which occurs with FSH.

In the normal menstrual cycle, the mid-cycle LH peak, presumably related to ovulation, precedes ovulation by 24–36 hours, and is the fixed central event of the menstrual cycle. Menstrual cycles may vary greatly in length, almost always by variation in the length of time between the onset of menstruation and the subsequent ovulation. Although menstrual bleeding can readily be identified and ovulation cannot, the latter is really the dominant event of the cycle and it would be logical to measure and describe the cycle from one ovulation to the next. Although ovulation cannot be easily fixed in time, the LH surge which precedes it can be, so that it is becoming increasingly

common to see menstrual cycles compared, as in figure 4.2, in terms of days before and after the mid-cycle LH peak.

Mechanism of action of gonadotrophins

Although gonadotrophins have been used therapeutically for nearly a decade, very little is known about how they exert their effects upon the gonads. In part this is due to the fact that pure preparations are not available and it is therefore impossible to say whether a particular effect is due to FSH or to LH or to the two acting in concert. Some generalizations about the actions of gonadotrophins can be made by examining the changes in the gonads after the administration of gonadotrophins. In the case of LH, two results can be found. If LH or its biological equivalent is given to an animal or a woman having a ripe follicle in the ovary, ovulation will occur. The prime action of the mid-cycle spurt of LH secretion is probably to cause ovulation, although it is by no means clear how this effect is exerted on the ovary. The second action of LH is concerned with steroidogenesis. The ovary and the testis can make progesterone or testosterone out of simple two-carbon fragments—acetates. The gonads make their characteristic hormones by building the acetate radicals into increasingly large and more complex molecules, until, after several stages, a 27 carbon molecule, cholesterol, is reached. This molecule serves as the common precursor of all the steroid hormones. The first step in making sex hormones such as testosterone, the oestrogens or progesterone is to cut off enzymatically 6 carbon atoms in the side chain of cholesterol. This is done by first converting cholesterol to 20,22-dihydroxy-cholesterol and then removing the side chain by scission at the link between C20 and C22. It is probably at this point that LH exerts its action, by promoting this scission and thus making available to the gonad an increased supply of the more advanced C21 precursor, Δ^5-pregnenolone. The overall effect of LH on steroidogenesis can be observed by incubating ovarian or testicular tissue with radioactive acetate. It can be shown that under such circumstances, when LH is added to the incubation, the production, first of radioactive cholesterol, and ultimately of radioactive progesterone or testosterone as the case may be, is speeded up. Other generalizations about the mode of action of LH are possible. Cyclic-

3′,5′-AMP is a fundamental factor in the energy cycle of all cells and nearly all hormones exert their action by affecting synthesis of this material. It has been shown that LH causes an increase in cyclic-3′,5′-AMP formation in gonadal cells.

The mode of action of FSH is less easy to describe. There is no clear evidence that, like LH, it is directly involved in the processes of hormone synthesis in the ovary. Its role appears to be a morphological one. The biological signal which FSH carries to the ovary is one which starts the growth of the Graafian follicle. As FSH preparations are always contaminated to some extent with LH it is difficult to tell whether the effects upon the ovary of a particular injection are due to FSH or LH. It is likely that the action of FSH on the ovary is primary in the sense that FSH activity always precedes LH activity and that FSH action is necessary before LH can exert its characteristic action—ovulation. It is noteworthy that the actions of both FSH and LH centre on the first half of the cycle. The blood levels of both hormones are at their lowest during the luteal phase and it is doubtful whether FSH plays any part in the growth and function of the corpus luteum although there is some evidence that the progesterone production of the corpus luteum is regulated by circulating levels of LH. What, in the absence of pregnancy, causes the eventual involution of the corpus luteum and the cessation of its steroidogenic activity is a mystery as far as the human species is concerned. In some mammals, like the pig, the uterus itself produces a substance late in the luteal phase, which, when it reaches the ovary, causes the corpus luteum to disintegrate and cease to function. Attempts to identify this substance have not been entirely successful, but there is good reason to suppose that it is a prostaglandin. No uterine luteolysin, prostaglandin or otherwise, has been found in the human. The identification of the factor which causes involution of the human corpus luteum remains one of the great prizes of endocrinology.

The changing levels of FSH during the cycle—a high towards the end of menstruation, declining slightly, with a sharp peak at mid-cycle a few days before ovulation and low levels after ovulation—coincide with the morphological events of the ovarian cycle. It is tempting to suppose that the high levels at the end of menstruation cause the wave of follicular growth which takes place at this time and that the mid-cycle peak is associated with the spurt of rapid growth which transmutes one or two follicles into fully developed Graafian follicles capable of releasing a viable ovum. If this is the mode of action of FSH there is a fine point about the control of its secretion which disastrously escapes the understanding of the endocrinologist. In some mysterious fashion just enough FSH is secreted in the normal cycle to transform one or two follicles into fully grown Graafian follicles. When, in the treatment of anovulatory infertility, the gynaecologist sets out to imitate this process by the injection of FSH, he may get the dosage wrong and produce multiple ovulation with unwanted multiple pregnancies.

Therapeutic applications of gonadotrophins

In a large proportion of cases secondary amenorrhoea is due to a failure of gonadotrophin secretion. Occasionally this failure is caused by pituitary destruction as in Sheehan's syndrome or Simmond's disease. More commonly the failure is due to a lack of hypothalamic releasing hormones. Whatever the cause, the consequent infertility can sometimes be set to rights by the induction of ovulation with pituitary gonadotrophins.

The biological and immunological similarities between LH and HCG have already been remarked upon. HCG can easily be extracted from pregnancy urine or the placenta and a single injection of 5000 I.U. HCG will efficiently substitute for the mid-cycle surge of LH secretion. HCG will therefore, by itself, induce ovulation as long as the ovary contains a follicle capable of ovulation. But very few amenorrhoeic infertile women have follicles capable of ovulation. It is therefore necessary to pretreat them with FSH in order to induce follicular growth. At first the only source of FSH was human pituitaries removed at autopsy, and for some years ovulation induction was on the somewhat haphazard basis of local treaties between gynaecologists and pathologists. It was not until an alternative source of gonadotrophins—human menopausal urine—came to be exploited, that it was possible to induce ovulation in routine clinical practice.

Once expensive commercial FSH preparations from human urine became available they were widely used, and a few maternal deaths and many multiple pregnancies have not yet entirely driven home the lesson that this physiological substance needs to be used with care and skill, and that treatment with human menopausal gonadotrophin should only be undertaken when sophisticated laboratory services are available to monitor the ovarian response. The problem is largely one of dosage. An amount of FSH which fails entirely to stimulate any ovarian activity in one woman may cause gross overstimulation in another. The problem can to some extent be overcome by measuring the output of urinary oestrogen daily. If the oestrogens rise too high, the HCG injection, which often provokes the over-stimulation syndrome and is of course always the cause of multiple ovulation, is withheld.

Although the preliminary injections of the urinary extract are thought of as being FSH, all such preparations are in fact contaminated with LH. The most successful preparations are those containing the largest proportion of LH and it is clear that the action of this hormone is necessary, not only for ovulation, but for the growth and steroidogenesis of the follicle.

THE OVARIAN CYCLE

The onset of menstruation marks the end of a menstrual cycle, not its start. The fixed point in the cycle is the central event of ovulation which determines the onset of menstruation some 14 days later. Now that it is possible to determine the day of ovulation by hormone assay, endocrinologists are starting to locate the events of the cycle in terms of ovulation rather than menstruation but, because periodic bleeding is the only evidence of cyclicity readily available to the gynaecologist, it is convenient to describe the ovarian cycle from the onset of one bleeding phase to the next.

The development of the follicle

Although the human ovary loses the greater part of its reproductive potential during intra-uterine life, the female baby is born with many thousands of totipotent reproductive cells. These take the form of primordial follicles; an ovum surrounded by a ring of flattened epithelial cells. From time to time a further development of the primordial follicle takes place. The ovum enlarges and the surrounding cells become cuboidal and multiply so that they form several layers. The earliest stages of the developing follicle are shown in figures 4.3 and 4.4.

The cells surrounding the ovum continue to multiply until they form a thick sheath around it. At this stage they produce a watery

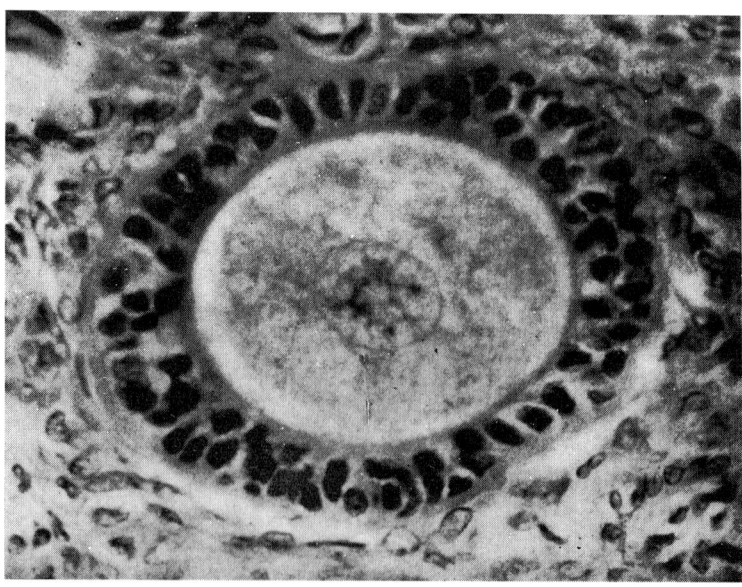

Fig. 4.3   Early stage of Graafian follicle.

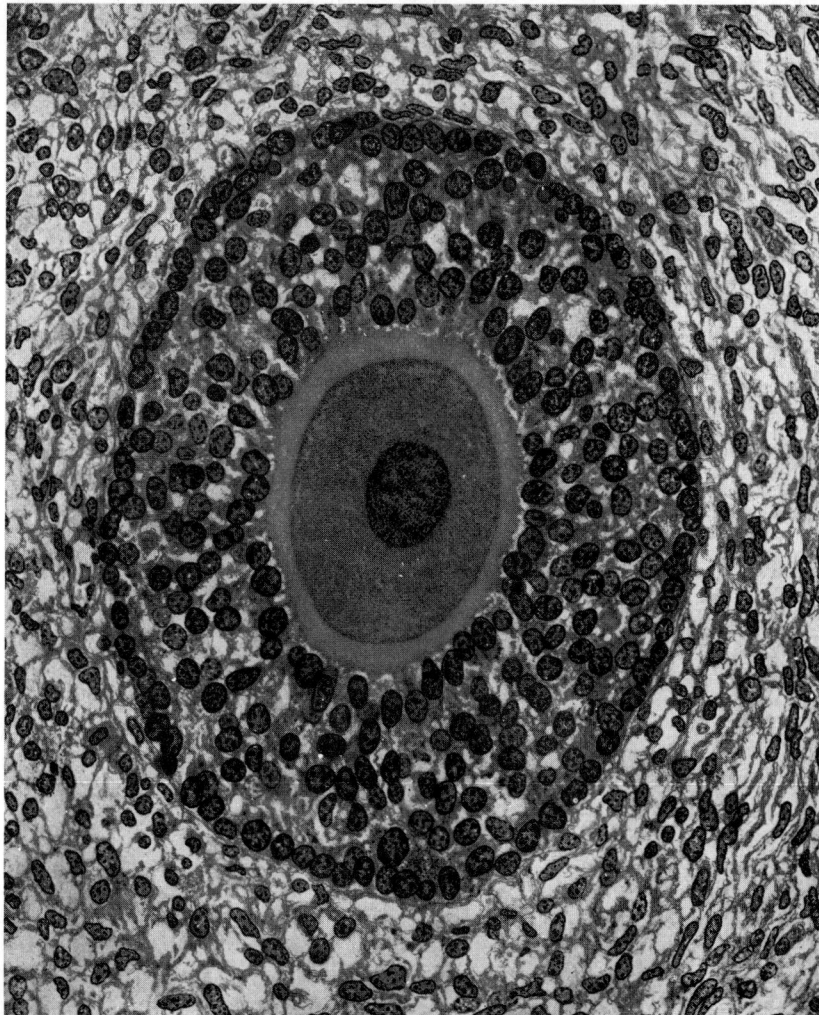

Fig. 4.4   Early developing follicle.

secretion, the liquor folliculi, which accumulates between the cells. This stage of follicular development is shown in figure 4.5, the follicular fluid having accumulated to a sufficient degree to form a distinct cleft in the follicle.

The accumulation of follicular fluid increasingly distends the follicle, with a small mound of follicular cells, the cumulus öophorus, covering the ovum at one pole. The ovum itself has meanwhile enlarged considerably as compared to the size of the ovum in a primordial follicle. It has developed at its outer margin a clear membrane, the zona pellucida, the beginning of which is indicated in figure 4.4. The zona pellucida remains as a kind of shell around the developing ovum during the first few cell divisions after fertilization. It is also of importance in reproductive physiology by virtue of the fact that the zona pellucida has to be penetrated by the sperm in effecting entry to the cytoplasm of the ovum in the act of fertilization.

In the last day or two before ovulation the follicle increases rapidly in size, mainly by increasing distention as a result of the accumulating follicular fluid. The ovum itself is the largest single cell in the body, measuring 0·13–0·14mm in diameter and barely visible to the naked eye. The mature Graafian follicle now presents the appearance first described 300 years ago by de Graaf looking down Anton

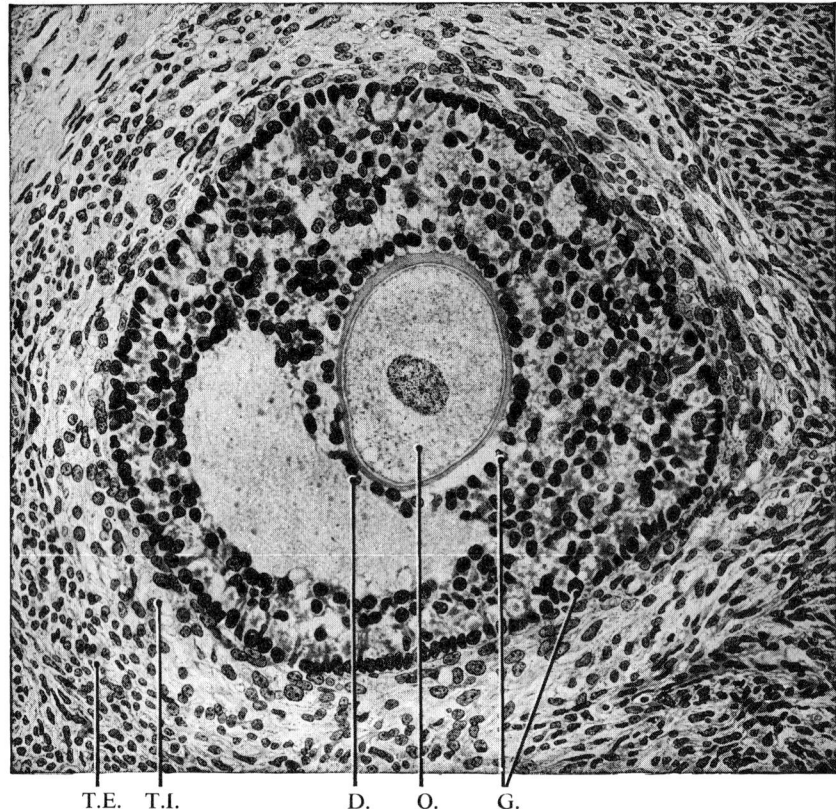

T.E. T.I.   D.   O.   G.

Fig. 4.5   The maturing Graafian follicle showing follicular cleft.

van Leeuwenhoek's microscope. The ovum, pressed to one side by the liquor folliculi, is covered by highly differentiated cells derived from the original sheath of follicular cells in the primordial follicle. These cells, the granulosa cells, are small round cells with darkly staining nuclei. The granulosa cells extend as a membrane several layers thick all round the cavity containing the liquor folliculi. On the outer periphery of the membrana granulosa, between it and the rest of the ovary, is a polymerized basement membrane which may play an important part in ovarian physiology, as it regulates the passage of molecules such as hormones between the liquor folliculi and the granulosa cells on one hand and the rest of the ovary on the other. The granulosa is surrounded by a sheath, the theca folliculi, formed by differentiation of the connective tissue stroma of the ovary. The theca has two layers of cells. The theca interna, consisting of several layers of large clear cells, is adjacent to the granulosa cells and separated from them by the basement membrane. In the mature

follicle the theca interna cells are evidently actively secreting cells. They appear granular; lipids and a yellowish pigment are found in their cytoplasm. On account of this faint yellow appearance the cells of the theca interna are referred to as theca lutein cells. They contrast sharply with the smaller darker granulosa cells. A further distinction between the theca lutein and the granulosa cells is, that in the mature Graafian follicle, the theca lutein cells are well vascularized, but the capillaries do not penetrate the basement membrane, so that the granulosa cells have no access to the circulation at this stage of their development. Surrounding the theca lutein cells is a capsule of ovarian connective tissue stroma arranged concentrically around the follicle, the theca externa. Figure 4.6 is a representation of a section through the wall of a mature Graafian follicle, showing the arrangement of the theca externa, the theca interna, the granulosa and the liquor folliculi.

It is possible to draw an analogy between the cells of the Graafian follicle and those of

Follicular fluid   Granulosa

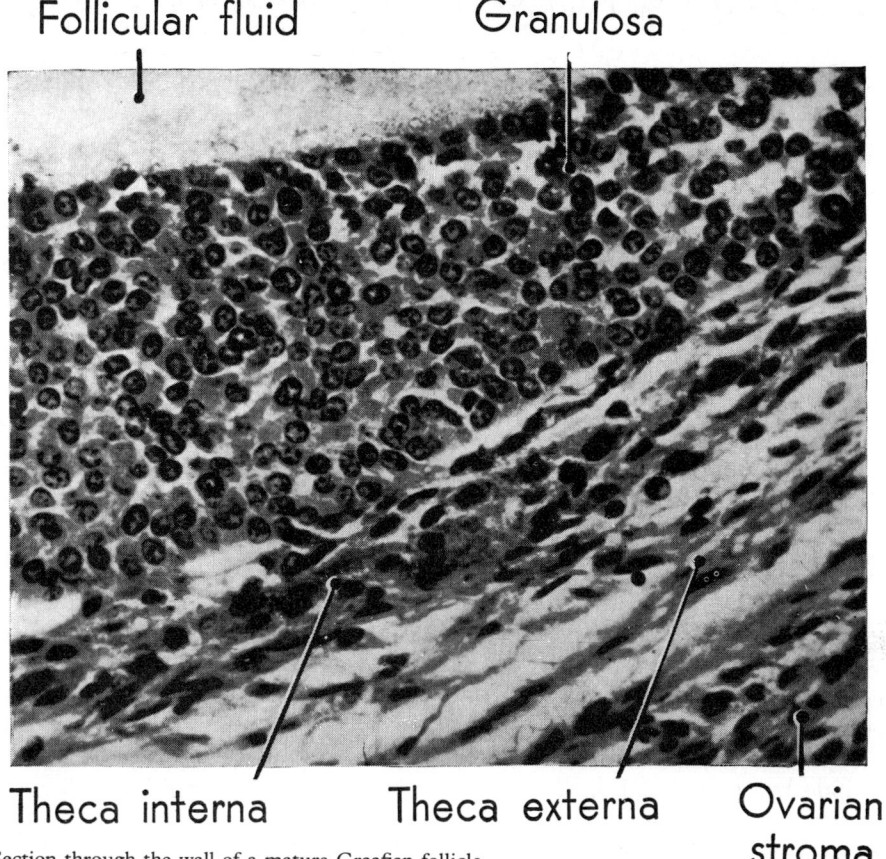

Theca interna   Theca externa   Ovarian stroma

Fig. 4.6   Section through the wall of a mature Graafian follicle.

Figs. 4.3 to 4.6 are reproduced from Williams Obstetrics (ed. Eastman, N. J. & Hellman, L. M.), 13th edn. (1966) by courtesy of the editors and publishers, Prentice-Hall International, USA.

the seminiferous tubules in the testis. In the first instance the spermatogonia, spermatocytes, spermatids and spermatozoa correspond to the ovum in its development from the primordial follicle to the mature öocyte. The Sertoli cells, in intimate contact with the male gametocytes and separated from the specialized connective tissue cells of the testicular stroma by the basement membrane of the seminiferous tubule, can be likened to the granulosa cells. Finally, the Leydig cells could be considered to be the male equivalents of theca lutein cells. Although such an analogy is feasible in the anatomical sense, it is less convincing in a physiological sense. Certainly the cells of the ovary and the testis manufacture their hormones by a common route which diverges only in its last stages, and it may be that corresponding gonadal cell types serve similar functions in steroidogenesis. It must be remembered, however, that the ovary makes

two hormones and has a cyclical secretory function, while the testis makes one hormone of a different structure and secretes continuously.

Ovulation

In a burst of rapid growth immediately before ovulation, the Graafian follicle reaches a size of 10–15mm in diameter. It protrudes above the surface of the ovary as a glistening fluid-filled bleb, covered by a thin layer of tunica albuginea. At the point of maximum stretching of the ovarian capsule, a pale avascular area, the stigma, can be discerned. Eventually the tissues give way at this point and the contents of the follicle are emptied into the Fallopian tube. The process which causes the wall of the follicle to give way is not clearly understood but two facts about it are established. The rupture of the wall is caused, not by increasing distention of the follicle with fluid, but by an active necrobiosis at the site of the stigma. Also, the release of the contents is not explosive, but a more gradual extrusion.

FOLLICULAR ATRESIA

In each menstrual cycle a wave of follicles starts the process of development from the primordial follicle stage. Only one or two follicles attain the final spurt of growth which leads to a mature Graafian follicle, capable of ovulation. The remainder cease growth at various stages, the granulosa cells involute and the ovum disintegrates. They become small fluid-filled vesicles lined by a flattened layer of theca interna and are gradually reabsorbed into the ovarian stroma. During intra-uterine life and to a lesser extent in the prepubertal girl, frustrated follicular growth, leading not to ovulation but to atresia, takes place. Thus it happens that by the time a woman reaches reproductive age, the greater part of her toti-potent reproductive cells have already been expended. Follicular atresia in prepubertal females can be explained on the grounds that they lack the integrated gonadotrophin secretion which causes the final maturation of the Graafian follicle and ovulation. But why should only one follicle respond by full maturation in the menstrual cycle when normal gonadotrophin secretion is present? The answer to this question so far completely eludes us. Until this problem is solved the diagnosis and therapy of menstrual disorders will be haphazard. For example, although it is at present possible to stimulate follicular growth in anovular patients, because the mechanism which causes atresia is unknown and not amenable to control, such patients often have a multiple follicular development.

Development of the corpus luteum

When the ovum is discharged at ovulation it takes with it a covering of granulosa cells—the corona radiata. The remaining granulosa cells stay behind, attached to the wall of the collapsed follicle. The wall of the follicle is thrown into folds by the loss of its fluid content. The folds are covered by granulosa cells, lying over the two layers of theca with a thin core of ovarian stroma. The exit hole of the ovum is sealed by a fibrinoid plug, and some haemorrhage takes place into the cavity. From the point of view of its endocrine function the most significant event in the early development of the corpus luteum is the fact that the capillaries of the theca interna penetrate the basement membrane and the granulosa becomes vascularized. *Pari passu* with the spread of blood vessels in the granulosa, the cells change their appearance. They become large clear cells with vacuolization of the cytoplasm—the granulosa lutein cells. The theca interna cells also show vacuoles which stain positively for lipid. Both cell types are evidently secreting actively. Meanwhile, the blood clot becomes organized and reabsorbed, leaving only a central pale coagulum.

At its maximal growth the corpus luteum is two or three times as large as the follicle from which it originated. It is easily recognized as an encapsulated structure bulging the surface of the ovary. The cut surface has a yellow colour (the 'yellow body') due to accumulated lipid. The microscopic structure of the corpus luteum is shown in figure 4.7.

The corpus luteum reaches its mature stage of development about seven days after ovulation. It continues in full function for four or five days and then begins to involute. The secretory vacuoles start to disappear from the cytoplasm of the granulosa cells. The central coagulum is replaced by connective tissue. The characteristic yellow colour fades, the theca interna cells disintegrate and can only be found here and there in clumps. When regression is well advanced menstruation takes place. Thereafter the degenerated lutein cells are absorbed and the whole structure replaced by fresh connective tissue. As the old corpora lutea age they present the appearance of white nodules, the corpora albicantia. Ultimately the corpora albicantia shrink to small areas of scar tissue.

If pregnancy supervenes the involution of the corpus luteum does not take place. At the time when degenerative changes should be starting it becomes hyperplastic and congested. Microscopic criteria suggest that it is in a very active secretory state and a study by Adams and Hertig (1969) shows that the corpus luteum of early pregnancy can readily be distinguished from that of the menstrual cycle. At about 20 weeks of pregnancy, degenerative changes appear in the corpus luteum of pregnancy. It usually becomes cystic and is partially reabsorbed by term, although on occasion structurally normal corpora lutea have been found at Caesarean section.

The manifestations of the ovarian cycle

The visible outward sign of this series of cyclical events in the ovary is, of course, the periodic occurrence of the menses. On the average this lasts 28 days from the first day of one bleeding phase to the first day of the next, although cycles as short as 25 days or as long as 35 days are not at all uncommon. Ovulation is the central event which divides the cycle into two, frequently unequal, halves. The growth and involution of the corpus luteum takes a relatively fixed time, and under normal circumstances the luteal phase which lasts from ovulation to the onset of menses, takes 14 days with a variation of a day or two at most. The growth spurt which leads to the development of a mature Graafian follicle takes only 3 or 4 days but it may start at any time after the first few days of bleeding. Thus the follicular phase which extends from the first day of bleeding to ovulation may vary from 7 to 20 days in length, accounting for most of the variability of the cycle.

Occasionally the peritoneal irritation caused by the escape of follicular fluid or even blood at ovulation gives rise to abdominal pain (Mittelschmerz) and some women are there-fore able to fix the day of their ovulation. It is said that the pain usually occurs alternately on one side or the other, suggesting that ovulation alternates from ovary to ovary month by month.

A further manifestation of the ovarian cycle can be seen in the cervix. As will be discussed later, the hormones produced by the Graafian follicle are somewhat different from those of the corpus luteum. They affect the mucus produced by the endocervical glands differently. As the Graafian follicle starts to grow and secrete its hormones in the late follicular phase, the mucus becomes clear and runny, so that on the day of ovulation the drop of mucus at the external os looks like an opalescent pearl. At this time the content of sodium chloride in the mucus is maximal and alters the physical characteristics of the mucus. When spread on a slide and dried the mucus crystallizes in an arborescent pattern of fern-like fronds. This 'ferning' is of course not a reliable sign of ovulation; merely an indication that there is a Graafian follicle producing its hormones. When the corpus luteum starts to secrete, the mucus becomes opaque and inspissated and ferning is no longer present.

Another manifestation of the ovarian cycle

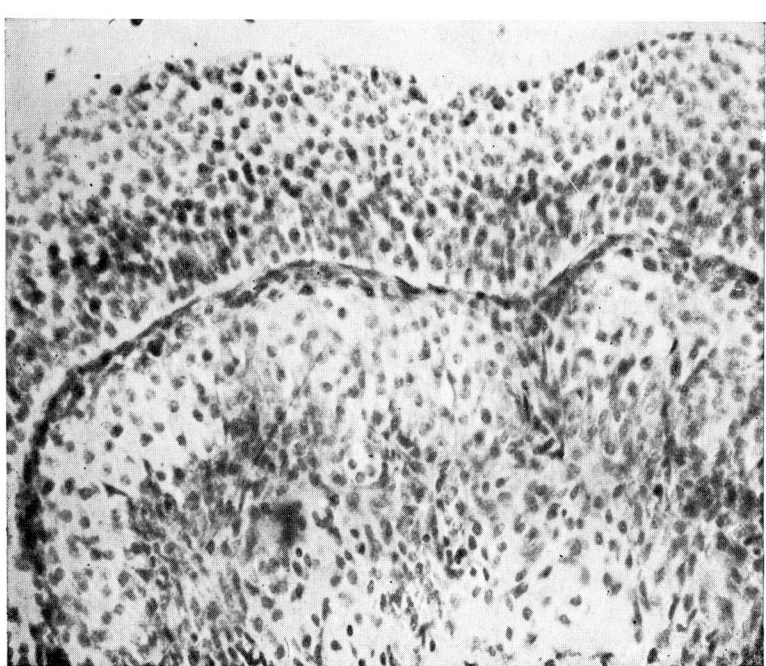

Fig. 4.7   Section through the wall of an early corpus luteum showing the granulosa cells separated from the folds of theca interna by a vascular layer. (By courtesy of Novak, E. R. & Woodruff, J. D. (1962) *Gynaecological and Obstetric Pathology*, 5th edn., Philadelphia, USA: W. B. Saunders Co.)

also results from the differential hormone production of the follicle and the corpus luteum. If a woman's temperature is recorded on wakening each morning before activity has any effect, it will be found that her temperature is generally around 36·5°C during the follicular phase. After ovulation the hormones from the corpus luteum cause an abrupt shift in temperature and in the luteal phase her basal temperature runs at about 37·0°C, falling towards follicular phase levels when the corpus luteum involutes.

The ovarian hormones

The hormones produced by the ovary are steroids. Steroids occur in many forms in the body, not only as hormones. In order to understand how the ovary makes its hormones and how they act, it is necessary to consider briefly the chemistry of the steroids. The steroid nucleus consists of a number of benzene rings fused together. Each benzene ring has six carbon atoms linked together in a six point ring. At each point, representing a carbon atom, are attached hydrogen atoms to satisfy the carbon valencies not taken up in forming carbon-to-carbon links. Four such benzene rings are combined together to form the steroid nucleus, the last ring having only five carbon atoms. The basic structure, called a cyclophenanthrene ring is shown in figure 4.8.

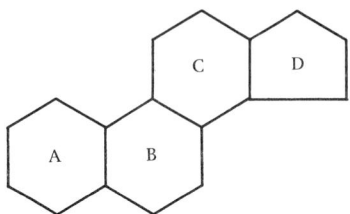

Fig. 4.8   The steroid nucleus showing the lettering system of the rings.

It can be seen that in order to identify them the rings of the steroid nucleus are designated alphabetically A, B, C and D. Ring D is five membered.

A particular hormone is formed by attaching substituents to one or other of the carbon atoms of the steroid nucleus. In order to identify the carbon atoms of the steroid nucleus each has been numbered. The numbering system is shown in figure 4.9. It can be seen that, although the four rings total only 17

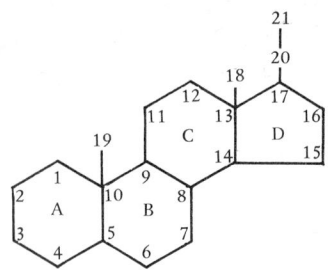

Fig. 4.9   The steroid nucleus showing numbering system of the carbon atoms and the angular methyl groups C18 and C19.

carbon atoms, there are two extra carbon atoms in the form of methyl groups (CH_3) attached to C10 and C13. These methyl groups are useful for indicating the location in space of substituents on other carbon atoms. The steroid nucleus is a somewhat flat elongated molecule and if it were regarded as lying in the plane of this paper the C18 and C19 methyl groups would stick up at right angles directly towards the eye of the reader.

The hormones of the ovary are of two types; oestrogens and progestogens. The basic structure common to all oestrogens involves an interesting and unusual transformation of the steroid nucleus. Ring A is aromatic, i.e. alternate bonds between the carbon atoms are double (unsaturated). In forming this aromatic ring A the C19 methyl group is lost so that oestrogens have not 19 but 18 carbon atoms. The individual oestrogens are formed by adding substituents, either hydroxyl (OH) or oxygen (O) to particular carbon atoms in this modified structure, commonly at C3, C17 and C16. Although 23 different oestrogens have been isolated from pregnancy urine, only three are of immediate clinical interest. The structure of these three 'classical' oestrogens is shown in figure 4.10.

Examination of figure 4.10 shows that oestrone has one hydroxyl (OH) group at C3 and a keto (=O) group at C17. Oestradiol has two hydroxyl groups; at C3 and C17. Oestriol has three hydroxyl groups; at C3, C17 and C16. The actual compound secreted by the ovary is oestradiol. It is, however, readily converted by a reversible reaction to oestrone. Oestriol is a metabolite of oestradiol and its formation is irreversible. In terms of ovarian hormone production it is mainly a relatively inert endproduct and as such is excreted in the urine in larger quantities than the other

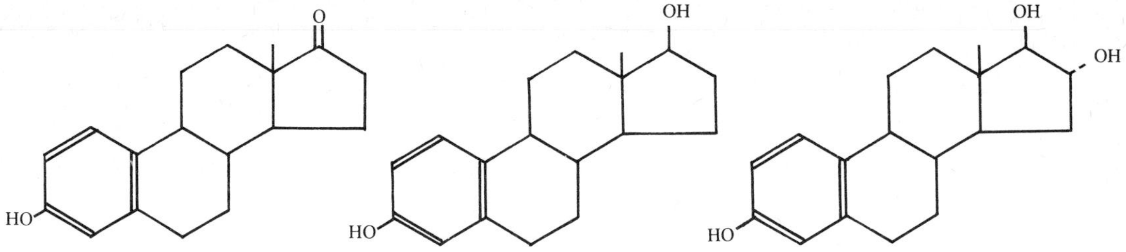

Fig. 4.10   The structure of the classical oestrogens, oestrone, oestradiol and oestriol.

two. In pregnancy the feto-placental unit produces large amounts of oestriol, not as a metabolite of oestradiol but as an original secretory product, whose physiological function has so far evaded all investigators. All three oestrogens have a very evanescent existence as the original active molecule. They are rapidly inactivated by having glucosiduronic acid or sulphuric acid attached to the hydroxyl groups and are excreted in urine as glucosiduronates and sulphates.

The structure of the second type of ovarian hormone, the progestogens, differs in several respects from that of the oestrogens. Although three different compounds, each having progestational activity have been isolated, there is every reason to believe that in the case of the hormones produced by the ovary we are dealing with a single compound—progesterone. The structure of progesterone and its inert urinary metabolite, pregnanediol, is shown in figure 4.11.

progesterone has a two-carbon side chain at C17 and is therefore a 21-carbon compound.

THE BIOSYNTHESIS OF OVARIAN STEROIDS
The problem of what substances the Graafian follicle and the corpus luteum use to make oestrogens and progesterone has long concerned endocrinologists. A likely line of investigation was to incubate possible raw materials with homogenates prepared from fresh follicles and see if any oestrogens or progesterone were formed. These researches gained impetus when it became possible to prepare a variety of possible precursors in a radioactive form. If, during incubation with ovarian tissues, radiolabelled oestrogens or progesterone were formed it could safely be assumed that they had come from the original radioactive raw material. It turned out that the biogenesis of ovarian hormones was a complicated process involving many intermediate compounds, but as a great many

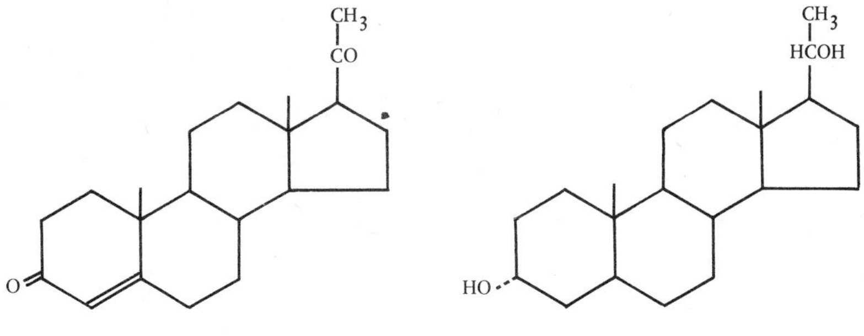

Fig. 4.11   The structure of progesterone and its urinary metabolite, pregnanediol.

Examination of figure 4.11 shows that progesterone, unlike the oestrogens, does not have an aromatic ring A. The methyl group at C19 is therefore intact and all 19 carbon atoms of the steroid nucleus are retained. Furthermore

ovarian disorders arise from faults in steroid manufacture it is necessary to consider the process briefly.

Many research workers have contributed to our knowledge of ovarian steroid synthesis;

notably an American obstetrician, Kenneth Ryan. His account (Ryan and Smith, 1965) makes interesting reading. It was known that the most widely distributed steroid in the human body, cholesterol, was made from simple acetate fragments containing only two carbon atoms, and Ryan soon showed that the ovary could make both progesterone and oestradiol from acetate. It next appeared that cholesterol was an obligatory intermediate, the ovary had first to make cholesterol and then to transform this into its own steroid hormones. The question then arose whether the ovary was obliged to start with acetate or whether it could simply use some of the large quantity of cholesterol present in the

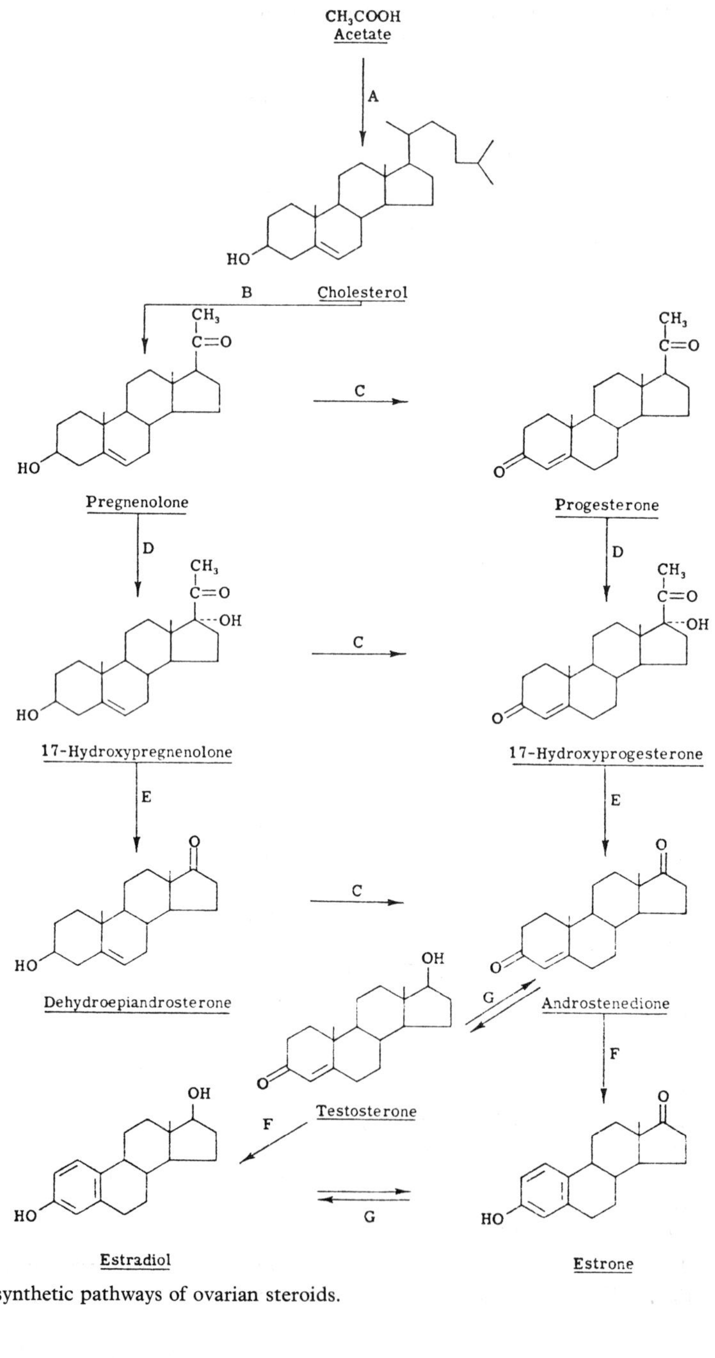

Fig. 4.12   The biosynthetic pathways of ovarian steroids.

circulation. This question is still not entirely resolved. Most likely the usual raw material is a special form of cholesterol although the ovary can start with a much simpler molecule if necessary.

Cholesterol is a surprising candidate as the raw material for ovarian hormones. It is bigger than either oestradiol or progesterone, having 27 carbon atoms. The first step in ovarian steroid synthesis is therefore to remove 6 carbon atoms to leave a C21 compound of the general type to which progesterone belongs. This removal of a 6 carbon side chain from cholesterol is done by specific enzymes contained in the ovarian cells. All the other steps in steroid synthesis are similarly enzymatic in nature. Like the ovary, the adrenal, the testis and the placenta have an array of these enzymes. All these glands, as a first step in the synthesis of their characteristic enzymes can make cholesterol from acetate or remove the side chain from cholesterol to leave a C21 compound, pregnenolone. This step and the succeeding ones in the biosynthesis of ovarian steroids are shown in figure 4.12.

Pregnenolone is the final common precursor of all the steroid hormones. Whether it be the adrenal making cortisol, the testis making testosterone, the placenta making progesterone or the ovary making oestradiol, they all start with pregnenolone. It is therefore of interest to look more closely at the structure of this steroid in figure 4.12. What changes does it have to undergo in being transformed into the characteristic ovarian hormones? Pregnenolone, like its precursor, cholesterol, has a hydroxyl group at C3 and an unsaturated bond in the B ring. In order to transform pregnenolone into progesterone therefore the hydroxyl group has to be oxidized to a keto group and the double bond switched from the B ring to the A ring. This is done in a single step by an ovarian enzyme, 3β-hydroxysteroid dehydrogenase. Many other steroid producing tissues possess this enzyme system. Indeed what hormones a gland produces and how much, is often dependent on the concentration of 3β-hydroxysteroid dehydrogenase.

It will be evident from figure 4.12 that after pregnenolone the synthesis of oestradiol can proceed in two ways. One pathway leads through progesterone to 17 hydroxyprogesterone. After this the 2 carbon side chain is removed to produce a weak androgen, androstenedione, which, like all the other androgens

has only 19 carbon atoms. Androstenedione can be directly transformed into oestrone which is converted to oestradiol, but it is likely that the main pathway from androstenedione to oestradiol goes via the characteristic male steroid testosterone. In the sense of steroid biosynthesis the main difference between male and female is that the testis mostly lacks the aromatizing enzyme system to transform testosterone to oestradiol. It is likely that some types of masculinization of the female are also due to a relative lack of this enzyme with the result that the ovary secretes some testosterone rather than transforming all to oestradiol.

Probably the main oestradiol biosynthetic pathway does not go through progesterone but through the alternative pathway shown in figure 4.12. In this case pregnenolone is transformed to 17 hydroxy-pregnenolone, from which the 2 carbon side chain is then removed to form another C19 androgen, dehydroepiandrosterone. This steroid is readily converted to androstenedione, thus joining the pathway through progesterone.

A further aspect of oestrogen biogenesis is worthy of note. This is that not only the ovary possesses the aromatizing enzyme system capable of converting androstenedione into oestrone. It exists also in other tissues, most likely the liver. It has become clear that a substantial proportion of the oestrone in the peripheral circulation is not secreted directly by the ovary but comes from the peripheral conversion of androstenedione.

THE CELLULAR ORIGIN OF OVARIAN STEROIDS

The first evidence concerning which cells in the ovary were responsible for the production of oestrogens came from the work of Bengt Falck (1959). He transplanted into the eyes of castrated rats small fragments of tissue from their ovaries and, immediately adjacent to this a strip of vaginal mucosa. If the transplanted ovarian tissue produced oestrogens, they could be detected by the appearance of cornified cells in the vaginal transplant. Using this model Falck concluded that both theca interna and granulosa cells were necessary for the production of oestrogens.

Falck was of course not able to say which oestrogens were being produced by the cell types in his transplants or to relate oestrogen production to the events of the ovarian cycle. Short (1962) carried the matter a stage further by analysing the steroids to be found in the follicles of the mare at various stages of follicular development. He also incubated various cell types with radioactive precursors to see what transformations of the steroid molecule they could do. From these studies Short (1962) evolved the 'two cell type' theory of ovarian steroidogenesis. The theory postulates that the theca interna cells have all the enzyme systems necessary for the synthesis of oestradiol from acetate or cholesterol, whereas the granulosa cells have only a weak 17-hydroxylase ability and cannot therefore convert pregnenolone or progesterone into their 17-hydroxylated derivatives. The granulosa cells also have no 17-desmolase enzyme system so that even if they could 17-hydroxylate the C21 precursors, they cannot convert them into the C19 androgens for oestrogen synthesis. During the growth of the follicle the theca interna cells are well vascularized and therefore supplied with all the requirements for steroid synthesis. By virtue of their full array of enzymes for oestrogen synthesis they complete the whole biogenetic sequence and are the source of the oestradiol secreted by the growing follicle. The granulosa cells, meanwhile having no access to a blood supply, are non-secretory. Once the follicle ruptures the granulosa cells acquire a blood supply and now start to produce steroids. But the deficient 17-hydroxylase and 17-desmolase of the granulosa cells mean they can carry the biosynthetic process only as far as progesterone. The theca interna cells, temporarily disrupted by ovulatory haemorrhage, soon resume their activity so that the corpus luteum produces progesterone from the luteinized granulosa cells and oestrogens from the theca lutein cells. It may be that not all the steroids in the theca lutein cells are fully transformed into oestrogens before being secreted. There are certainly intermediates such as androstenedione in ovarian vein blood and it is likely that a proportion of the ovarian production is only peripherally transformed into oestrogens.

Further investigations have disclosed that the follicle and the corpus luteum are not the only steroidogenic tissues in the ovary. Savard et al. (1964) have examined the capacity of the ovarian stroma to synthesize steroids. They have found that the cells of the ovarian stroma are capable of the full biogenetic sequence indicated in figure 4.12. There is no reason to suppose that the stroma makes a substantial contribution to ovarian steroidogenesis under normal circumstances, but this explains why one occasionally finds evidence of oestrogen production in the absence of either follicles or corpora lutea. A further feature of stromal steroidogenesis is worthy of note. It appears that the main pathway of stromal oestrogen biosynthesis is through the androgenic pathway, i.e. not involving progesterone but going through dehydroepiandrosterone, androstenedione and testosterone. If, therefore, there is any deficiency in the final conversion steps of androgens to oestrogens, the ovarian stroma may secrete significant quantities of androgens. This may account for the fact that postmenopausal women, who have no follicles or corpora lutea and have to rely entirely on the stroma for ovarian steroidogenesis, may occasionally show androgenic manifestations such as hirsuties.

The pattern of hormone production during the ovarian cycle

Until recently the only way in which hormone production during the normal cycle could be assessed was to measure the urinary output of steroid metabolites. The technique of radioimmunoassay has made it possible to measure the very small amounts of oestradiol and progesterone which exist in plasma, and bids fair to open a new era in our understanding of ovarian physiology. The first successful study of plasma oestradiol by Baird and Guevara (1969) was in fact not done by radioimmunoassay but by the much more tedious and laborious technique of double isotope dilution. Subsequent work with radioimmunoassay has confirmed their findings. Radioimmunoassay, and the related method of competitive protein binding, has found widespread application to clinical studies of plasma steroids. The pattern of plasma oestradiol during the menstrual cycle as measured by radioimmunoassay by Shaaban and Klopper is shown in figure 4.13.

This figure shows the mean and standard deviation of oestradiol concentration in eight women, day by day throughout the cycle. It can be seen that the plasma oestradiol concentration, like the urinary excretion of oestriol, rises to a peak in mid-cycle. This peak probably represents the maximal secretory activity of the Graafian follicle. It is the most constant fixed event of the hormone pattern in the normal cycle and is a convenient point from

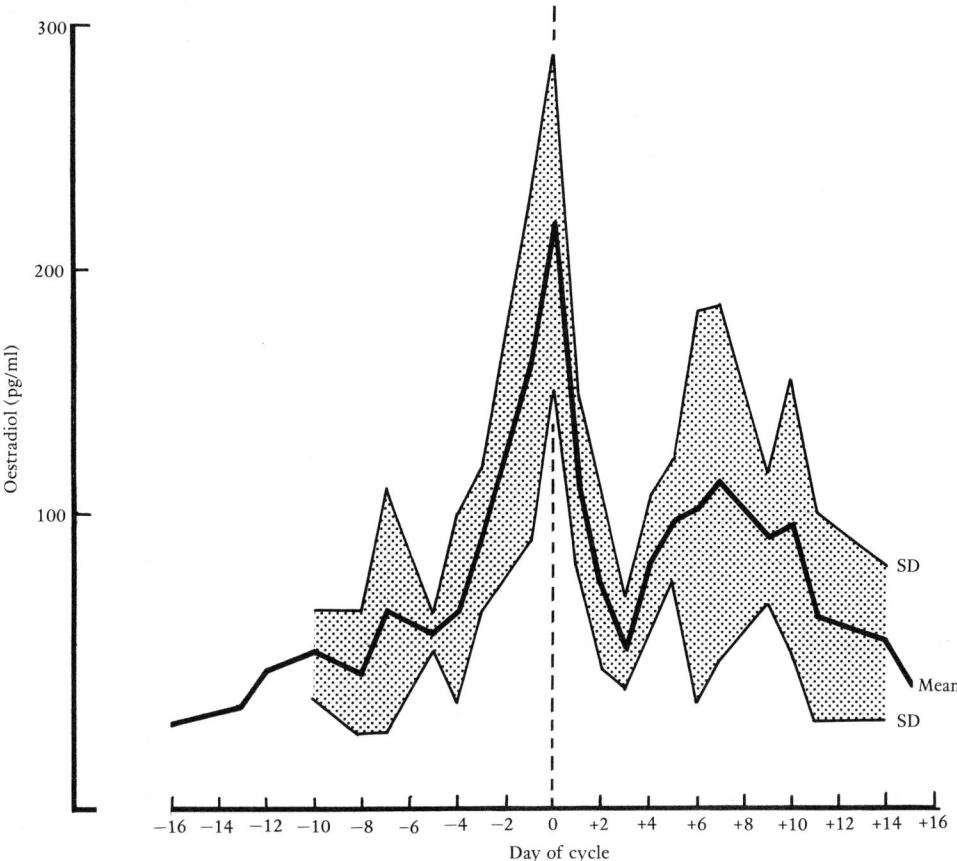

Fig. 4.13   The mean and standard deviation of plasma oestradiol concentration during the normal menstrual cycle. After Shaaban and Klopper (1973) *J. Obstet. Gynaec. Brit. Cwlth.*, **80**, 778.

which to time the changes of the rest of the cycle. In figure 4.13 the day of the oestradiol peak has been designated as day 0 for all eight women in this study. On the average in a 28-day cycle, the first day of menstruation would be 14 days before this peak (day −14) and the onset of the subsequent period would follow 14 days after the oestradiol peak (day +14). There is, however, a good deal of variability about these averages, particularly in the first half of the cycle.

The average plasma oestradiol starts to rise at the time the period ceases and it may be that the rising oestrogen levels provide the regenerative stimulus to the endometrium. There is not, however, a simple direct connection between plasma oestradiol concentration and the cessation of bleeding. Although plasma oestradiol rises steadily in the early part of the proliferative phase of the cycle, the sharp rise in mid-cycle takes only four days to reach its peak value. It is probable that this surge

of oestrogen represents the final growth spurt of the Graafian follicle, when one follicle grows to full maturity and the others regress. At the peak, oestradiol concentrations range from 200–400pg/ml of plasma while at their nadir during the menstrual period they average 30pg/ml.

It can be seen from figure 4.13 that the peak on day 0 is followed by a precipitous drop in oestradiol concentration over the next 2–3 days. It is likely that this drop represents rupture of the follicle with subsequent disorganization of steroidogenesis.

Although, for a day or two, the oestradiol level is low following the mid-cycle peak, the average concentration does not fall as low as that obtaining during the bleeding phase, and it soon rises to a sustained plateau, only slightly lower than the mid-cycle peak. It is presumed that this rise, which is sustained for about a week, represents oestrogen biogenesis by the corpus luteum. The onset of the subsequent period is always preceded by a fall in oestradiol concentration starting two or three days earlier. There is not a critical concentration below which bleeding is always precipitated, although oestradiol levels always reach their nadir at the onset of the period, and it appears very likely that withdrawal of the oestrogenic stimulus has some bearing on the onset of menstruation. The fall in oestradiol concentration which precedes bleeding coincides with a fall in plasma progesterone and it may be that it is the latter, or the combined withdrawal of both hormones which is responsible for the disintegration of the endometrium.

Before the mid-cycle peak of oestradiol the concentration of progesterone is low, seldom rising above 1ng/ml. As can be seen in figure 4.14, plasma progesterone starts to rise after

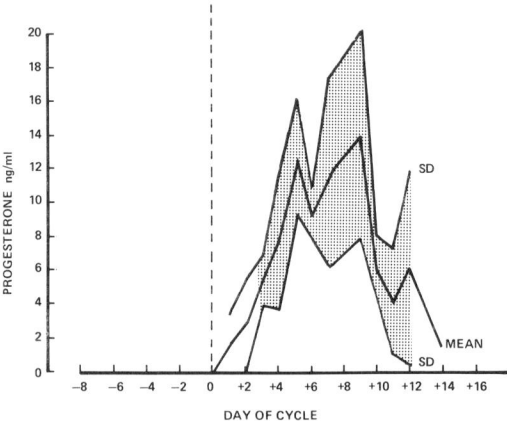

Fig. 4.14   The mean and standard deviation of plasma progesterone concentration during the normal menstrual cycle. After Shaaban and Klopper (1973) *J. Obstet. Gynaec. Brit. Cwlth.*, **80**, 780.

the mid-cycle oestradiol peak (day 0) and by day +4 averages above 5ng/ml plasma.

A value of 5ng/ml is a useful dividing line. A finding of plasma progesterone above 5ng/ml is good presumptive evidence of the existence of a corpus luteum and hence of ovulation having taken place. In the luteal phase plasma progesterone is maintained at an average of 11ng/ml for at least a week. Involution of the corpus luteum, as represented by the fall in plasma progesterone begins three or four days before the onset of the period.

The regulation of ovarian secretion

The pattern of pituitary secretion shown in

figure 4.2 and the pattern of ovarian secretion are linked phenomena. The hypothalamic centres are able in mysterious fashion to detect the levels of circulating ovarian hormones and to regulate the secretion of gonadotrophins accordingly; i.e. a feedback mechanism. At the onset of the menses FSH levels are high and oestrogen levels are low. This situation lasts for seven or eight days. During this time the high FSH levels stimulate fresh follicular growth. When, after the growth period, oestrogen secretion starts, the FSH secretion drops *pari passu* with the rise in plasma oestradiol so that FSH levels reach their nadir at the time of the preovulatory oestradiol peak. The rising oestradiol has a further effect in that it triggers off the ovulatory LH surge which follows 12–36 hours after the oestradiol peak. Numerous clinical experiments have demonstrated the association between oestrogen administration and subsequent LH secretion. It appears that the concentration of oestrogen is critical, about 150pg/ml of oestradiol being required to cause the LH surge—levels not attained in the normal cycle until the mid-cycle oestradiol peak.

If a mature follicle is present the LH surge will cause ovulation. Evidence has already been cited that the onset of progesterone secretion by the corpus luteum is the mechanical consequence of the granulosa cells acquiring a blood supply as the result of ovulation. Studies by Vande Wiele and his colleagues (1970) have shown that small doses of LH will maintain progesterone secretion, and it is well known that chorionic gonadotrophin (HCG) which resembles LH both physiologically and immunologically, will also stimulate progesterone secretion by the corpus luteum. LH levels are somewhat higher in the luteal phase than in the follicular phase and are probably high enough to account for the continued activity of the corpus luteum.

The involution of the corpus luteum in women lacks an explanation. The continued administration of LH or HCG will not maintain the corpus luteum for more than a few days beyond its allotted span. Nor is there any evidence of a fall in LH secretion triggering off luteal regression. In some other mammals, e.g. the guinea pig, it has been found that at a late stage in the secretory phase the uterus itself produces a substance which causes involution of the corpus luteum. In some cases this luteolytic hormone has been tentatively identified as a prostaglandin. There is no evidence of such a uterine luteolytic factor in women and administration of prostaglandins will not cause regression of the corpus luteum. Research into luteolytic factors is being vigorously pursued in the hope that such a compound will provide a safe physiological means of early abortion.

The pituitary, the uterus and the conceptus all influence ovarian hormone production and are in turn affected by the ovarian hormones. Such a complex interplay is not easy to set out simply. Figure 4.15 summarizes in diagrammatic form the interrelationships which have so far been discussed.

THE ENDOMETRIAL CYCLE

The ovarian cycle consists of two separate stages of secretory activity, divided by the central event of ovulation. The endometrial cycle, which is a reflection of the ovarian cycle, correspondingly shows two phases of cellular development, separated by ovulation. The first half, *the proliferative phase*, consists of three merging stages of tissue growth. The bleeding stage lasts for 4–6 days and is followed by a stage of rapid growth, the early proliferative stage. The late proliferative stage is marked by further endometrial growth and cellular differentiation.

The appearance of the endometrium during the bleeding phase has been described by

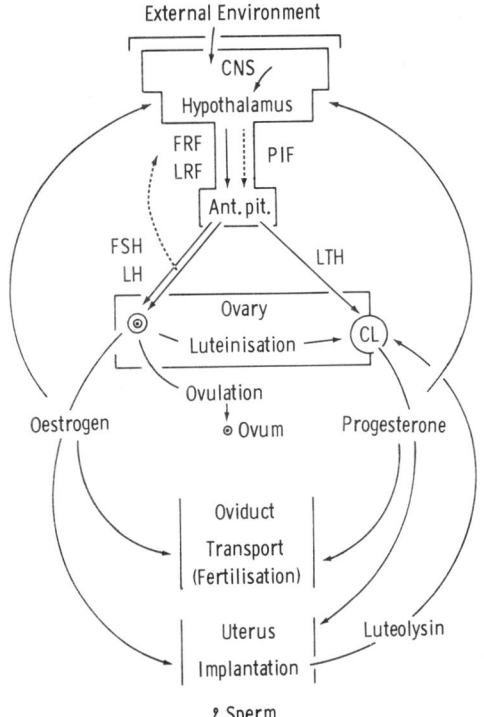

Fig. 4.15 A schematic representation of the control of ovarian hormone production. Reproduced with permission from Dr A. Walpole.

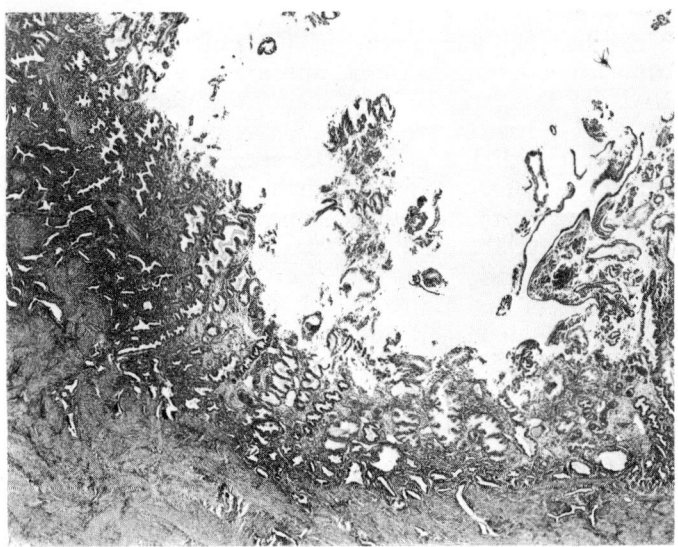

Fig. 4.16 Endometrium on first day of bleeding. (From McLennan, C. E. & Rydell, A. H. (1965) *Obstetrics & Gynaecology*, **26**, 605–621; by courtesy of Harper & Row, Publishers Inc.)

McLennan and Rydell (1965) and their findings on the first day or two are shown in figure 4.16. It can be seen that endometrial disintegration starts at the surface (Fig. 4.16), but soon extends down close to the non-functioning basal layer of the endometrium. Indeed, it was for some time a matter of controversy whether the whole functional layer of the endometrium was stripped off, leaving regeneration to take place from the stubs of the glands in the basalis which does not participate in the cyclical

In the late proliferative phase the endometrium is thicker, partly because of growth of the glands and surface epithelium, and partly because of increase in ground substance in the stroma which now appears much less dense in the superficial layers. The glandular epithelium which has grown taller presents a pseudo-stratified appearance.

The appearance of the endometrium in the proliferative phase is shown in figure 4.17a and b.

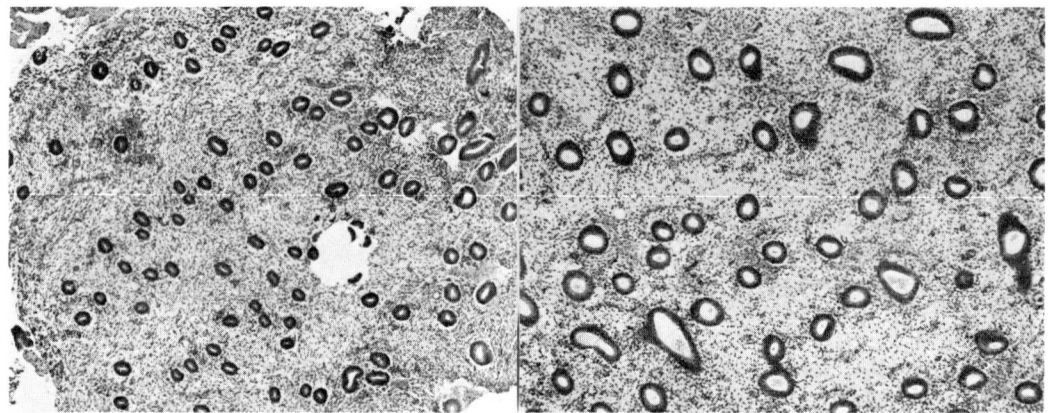

Fig. 4.17a.   Endometrium in early proliferative phase.   b.   Endometrium in late proliferative phase.

changes of the endometrium. It is now agreed that by day 3, new epithelial growth has started to cover the disorganized surface of the endometrium, coming mainly from the secretory glands in the fragments of the spongy functional layer left adhering here and there to the basalis, with a contribution of outgrowth from the unchanged glands of the basalis. The epithelium which by day 5–6 has covered the entire surface grows over small hillocks of remaining spongy layer so that by day 6 a few areas can be discerned where the secretory glands from the previous cycle have been incorporated and are being transformed. By day 5 the connective tissue of the stroma is also proliferating rapidly and collagen and ground substance containing acid mucopolysaccharides is accumulating.

During the early proliferative phase the endometrium is thin (1–2mm), and the glands are narrow tubular structures running straight to the surface. The glandular epithelium is columnar and the nuclei lie at the end of the cell away from the lumen. The stroma is dense with small dark nuclei.

The second half of the endometrial cycle, corresponding to the luteal phase of the ovarian cycle, can be divided into two stages; the early secretory stage and the late secretory stage.

Ultramicroscopic studies have detected the appearance of glycoprotein secretory granules below the nucleus on, or immediately after, the day of ovulation. The same process can be seen under the light microscope two or three days later when large clear vacuoles appear under the nucleus, pushing it towards the luminal border. This subnuclear vacuolation is characteristic of the early secretory phase and has come to be regarded as good histological evidence of recent ovulation.

In the late secretory phase the endometrium presents a characteristic appearance. It is thick (5–6mm) and succulent on curettage, and under the microscope the stroma is seen to be oedematous with coiled glands having a typical saw-toothed appearance of their luminal border. The epithelial cells are cuboidal, most of their peripheral cytoplasm having been discharged into the lumen, where it can be seen as abundant secretion giving positive reactions with glycogen stains. The microscopic appearance of the secretory phase endometrium is shown in figure 4.18a and b. When the corpus luteum starts to involute the

is peculiar. There are two types of arteries. The basal third of the endometrium which does not undergo histological changes during the endometrial cycle and is not shed at menstruation, is supplied by short straight

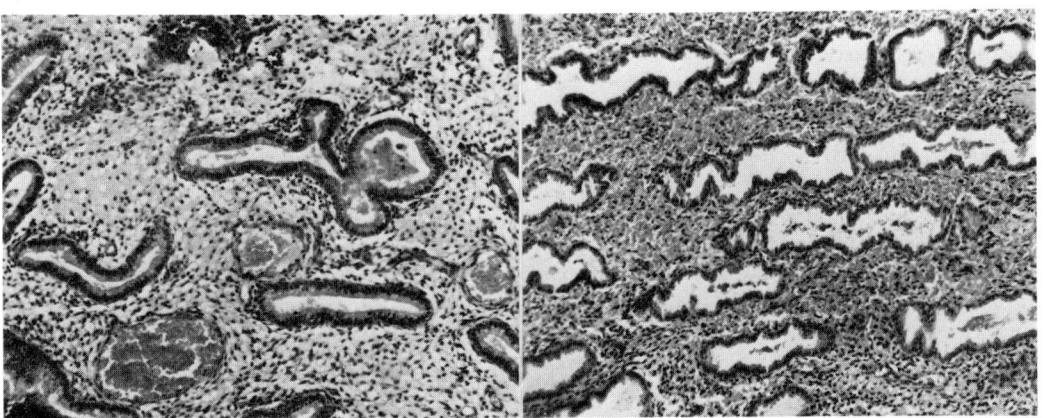

Fig. 4.18a.   Endometrium in early secretory phase.   b.   Endometrium in late secretory phase.

late secretory phase declines. A leucocytic infiltration takes place, the stroma starts to disintegrate and the oedema disappears so that the endometrium shrinks.

Vascular changes in the endometrial cycle

It has been known for more than 30 years that the precipitating cause of menstruation is change in the endometrial vasculature. Unfortunately work has not progressed beyond a description of the anatomical changes which can be observed in the blood vessels and the biochemical basis of these changes still remains to be explored. It is true that at one time toxic materials were thought to have been isolated from menstrual discharge which were capable of inducing a menstrual-like disintegration of the endometrium. This 'menotoxin' was thought to be a euglobulin, lethal to infantile rats, but later work showed that most of the effects of the so-called menotoxin could be ascribed to bacterial contamination of the crude extracts. It is now known that the endometrium is a rich source of prostaglandins which have marked effects on blood vessels. It is likely that an adequate explanation of the physiology of menstruation will involve a revival of a version of the menotoxin theory with prostaglandins cast in the chief role.

The vascular anatomy of the endometrium

arteries. The superficial, functioning two-thirds of the endometrium is supplied by a different set of highly coiled arteries, and it is the changes in these which result in menstruation.

Our knowledge of the changes in the spiral arteries of the endometrium comes from the classical work of Markee (1940), who transplanted fragments of endometrial tissue into the eyes of rhesus monkeys, where he could observe the vascular changes day by day in an animal having a menstrual cycle similar to that in women. Markee observed that during the proliferative phase of the cycle the spiral arteries grow faster than the thickening of the endometrium, so that these arteries become more and more coiled with their tips close to the surface epithelium. When, at the end of the late secretory phase, the stroma disintegrates and its oedema disappears, the coils are compressed and buckled by the shrinking of the endometrium, and a stasis of flow with vasodilation results. In the last day before the onset of bleeding vasodilation is succeeded by vasoconstriction and marked ischaemia of the superficial endometrium results. Eventually the damaged capillaries rupture and the endometrium is ploughed up by small haemorrhages.

There are no lymphatic vessels in the superficial half of the endometrium and it may be that inadequate lymph drainage reinforces the vascular effects. The suggestion is that the vascular stasis followed by vasoconstriction leads to tissue breakdown and that the proteins so liberated, not being removed by lymphatic drainage, trigger menstruation.

Biochemical changes during the endometrial cycle

During the proliferative phase, while growth is being stimulated by oestrogen; enzymes, glycogen and acid mucopolysaccharides accumulate in the endometrium. The enzymes, once formed in the glandular epithelium, are enclosed in subcellular particles called lysosomes, within the cytoplasm of the cell. Among other enzymes, increasing amounts of acid phosphatase, of β-glucuronidase and of lactic dehydrogenase form during the menstrual cycle. These are hydrolytic enzymes which, if they escape through the enclosing lipoprotein membrane of the lysosome, are capable of destroying the cell. The glycogen content of the cell cytoplasm also varies in response to the hormonal milieu. Glycogen is a biological form of stored energy and as such its function in the glandular epithelium is probably concerned with the energy for growth and differentiation, and its secretion into the gland lumen represents a source of energy supply for the implanting ovum.

During the period of stromal growth, collagen fibres are laid down and the ground substance increases. Important components of the ground substance, which can be measured, are the acid mucopolysaccharides such as hyaluronic acid, chondroitin sulphate and heparin. These acid mucopolysaccharides are carbohydrates which exist in an easily split complex with protein. Their production by the stroma is initiated by oestrogen.

The decline in ovarian production of oestrogen and of progesterone brought about by the involution of the corpus luteum affects all these endometrial constituents. The lysosomal membrane becomes more permeable, destructive hydrolytic enzymes are released into the cell cytoplasm, where they come into contact with their substrates. The secretion of progesterone blocks further synthesis of acid mucopolysaccharides. As these substances have a short biological half life they disappear from the ground substance which alters its physical characteristics. The ground substance

loses its gel-like consistency and becomes watery, hence the loose oedematous appearance of the stroma at the height of the secretory phase. When oestrogen support is withdrawn, water is lost, and the series of vascular changes resulting from stromal shrinkage is initiated.

Hormone deprivation

It is clear from the foregoing that the onset of menstrual bleeding is in large measure a direct consequence of the decline in oestrogen and progesterone. If oestrogens are given to an amenorrhoeic or to a castrate woman and then stopped, uterine bleeding—an oestrogen withdrawal bleeding—will usually result. Such bleeding is heavier and lasts longer than a normal period and it is unlikely that the normal menses is simply a consequence of declining oestrogen. Such a state of affairs may, however, well apply to pathological uterine bleeding. In some forms of menorrhagia the bleeding is not preceded by ovulation, but results from the decline in oestrogen production by unovulated follicles. Not surprisingly, the bleeding is often severe and prolonged.

If oestrogen deprivation alone is not enough to explain menstruation, it is fitting to examine the role of progesterone deprivation. In the normal cycle progesterone and oestrogen are secreted together after a period of oestrogen secretion. Under experimental conditions it was found that the prior action of oestrogen (oestrogen priming) was necessary for the induction of bleeding by progesterone withdrawal. If a woman is pretreated with oestrogen, and oestrogen and progesterone are then given together, the withdrawal of progesterone will result in bleeding even if oestrogen administration is continued. This suggests that in the normal cycle, progesterone withdrawal is an element in the onset of menstruation. It is likely that the dominant feature is oestrogen deprivation, but the nature of the bleeding is much altered by the endometrial changes brought about by progesterone.

The mechanism of action of ovarian hormones on the endometrium

In recent times some light has been shed on what happens to the oestrogen molecule once it enters the endometrial cell. Much of this came from the work of Jenson and Jacobson (1962). They were able to prepare oestradiol with a high degree of radioactivity so that they could follow the distribution of the oestrogen in the body of a rat when this animal was injected with the minute amounts of oestrogen produced under physiological circumstances. They found that the radioactivity was taken up in various organs such as liver, kidneys and uterus. The uterus differed in its pattern of oestrogen uptake from that of other organs. Organs such as the liver took the injected oestrogen up very rapidly and discharged it almost as quickly, so that within two hours no radioactivity could be detected in these organs. Uptake in the uterus was much slower, but once taken up, the oestrogen was retained so that the radioactivity in the uterus fell slowly over the next six hours. The molecule of oestradiol was not changed by its uptake into the uterus. Long after the series of intracellular events initiated by oestradiol was already begun, only unchanged oestradiol could be recovered from the uterus. Thus, although oestradiol is extensively metabolized by other tissues, metabolism to other compounds is not part of its activity in the endometrium.

Once oestradiol enters the endometrial cell it is bound to a specific receptor protein in the cytoplasm of the cell and it has become apparent that such intracellular protein binding is an essential first step in the action of an oestrogen. This protein (known as 9·5S protein from its sedimentation rate in sucrose solutions when spun in an ultracentrifuge) passes the oestrogen to a second smaller (5S) receptor protein in the cell nucleus. Within the nucleus the oestradiol fixes on to the cell chromatin. It is here concerned with the template for protein synthesis by affecting the production of messenger RNA. The accumulation of RNA starts within 6–24 hours of the administration of oestradiol and new protein synthesis follows in its wake. In essence, this is the process by which oestrogens stimulate growth and proliferation in the uterus.

The intracellular events resulting from the entry of progesterone into the endometrium have not been worked out, but there is every reason to believe that here too, binding to a receptor protein is an essential pre-requisite.

The menarche and the menopause

These aspects of menstrual life are more fully dealt with in Chapter 3 and only a few observations on the endocrinological basis are considered here.

THE MENARCHE

It has been noted in many countries that the average age at first menstruation has become younger in the last 40 or 50 years, although this trend has now probably halted in Britain and the United States. An adequate explanation of the decline in the age of menarche will not be forthcoming until the reasons for the onset of the menstrual cycle are fully known, but it is possible to offer a hypothesis based on present knowledge of the control of the menstrual cycle. The ovaries of the prepubertal girl are capable of responding to gonadotrophins and the reason why they are not active is presumably because they are not being stimulated by FSH and LH. Gonadotrophins are indeed in lower concentration in the circulation of the premenstrual girl than in the sexually adult woman, and the mid-cycle surge in particular is absent. On the other hand there appears to be plenty of gonadotrophin actually present in the substance of the prepubertal pituitary. The stimulus for their release into the circulation is not present. It has been demonstrated that the hypothalamic gonadotrophin releasing hormones are partially under cerebral control. It may be that cerebral influences affect the start of the hypothalamic function in this respect. In our society the media of mass communication and other cultural influences have placed increasing emphasis on the importance of sexual activity. Young girls are becoming sexually mature at an earlier age because their social environment puts sexual maturity at a premium.

Puberty itself shows several successive growth phases and the ovarian cycle, of which the menarche is an expression, does not start abruptly in its complete form. Waves of follicular growth with accompanying oestrogen synthesis precede the first bleeding and initiate the pubertal changes in secondary sex characters. When the oestrogen secretion is sufficient to stimulate appreciable endometrial proliferation it is not usually followed by ovulation at first. The first few periods are therefore frequently simply oestrogen withdrawal bleedings. Such periods are generally painless, which explains why dysmenorrhoea often starts only after some months of painless periods.

THE MENOPAUSE

The menopause may be a much more mechanically determined event than the menarche.

A woman sets out on her reproductive career with a limited number of ova and can form no more during her lifetime. When her stock of primordial follicles is exhausted, the means for steroidogenesis is gone and the whole basis of the ovarian cycle is lost. The pituitary, set free of the restraint of negative feedback from the ovarian hormones, secretes gonadotrophins continuously. The plasma and urinary levels of gonadotrophin are high in the postmenopausal woman but her ovaries are no longer capable of response.

Premenopausal women are less fertile than in their younger years. In part this is due to the fact that the incidence of anovular cycles increases as the menopause approaches. The fact that her periods may often result from oestrogen withdrawal also explains why irregular and prolonged bleeding is more common at the menopause.

All oestrogen production does not stop at the menopause. Small amounts of oestrogen can be found in the blood and urine of postmenopausal women. In part they may be derived from peripheral conversion to oestrogens of adrenal androgens and in part from the ovarian stroma. Many of the untoward symptoms of the menopause derive from the decline in oestrogen production and the continued synthesis of small amounts of oestrogen by postmenopausal women provides a sound physiological reason for the exhibition of oestrogens in the therapy of the menopause.

THE ENDOCRINOLOGY OF PREGNANCY

The hormones produced in pregnancy by the placenta alone, or by the fetus and placenta in combination, are best thought of as tools by which the fetus adjusts maternal physiology to ensure its own survival. These hormones are diverse and alter a variety of maternal functions, for example the ovarian cycle and carbohydrate metabolism. The hormones are of two sorts, proteins and steroids.

Protein hormones of the placenta

1. *Human chorionic gonadotrophin* (HCG)
The detection of this hormone in pregnancy urine nearly 50 years ago by Aschheim and Zondek (1927) greatly enlarged our understanding of the physiology of pregnancy but to this day the main clinical application for

assays of the hormone remains the diagnosis of pregnancy.

Chorionic gonadotrophin consists of at least two peptide chains loosely linked. The individual molecules tend to aggregate into larger units so that estimates of the molecular size have varied greatly. It is likely that the true molecular weight is between 30 000 and 40 000. One of the peptide chains (the α chain) consists of the same sequence of amino acids as occurs in luteinizing hormone and in thyroid stimulating hormone. One of the main antigenic components is therefore the same in all three hormones, and antisera to HCG will cross-react with LH and TSH. This common component also explains why HCG should have a similar action to LH and can, for instance, be used to induce ovulation when a mature Graafian follicle is present.

HCG is present in maternal blood and urine throughout pregnancy, and the detection of the hormone in these fluids is the basis of nearly all pregnancy tests, as HCG is to all intents and purposes only found in pregnancy. It can be detected soon after implantation, sometimes as early as the time of the first suppressed menstruation (i.e. day 28). The serum measurements are more reliable than the urinary assays and according to Teoh (1967) the levels rise rapidly to a peak at 61–70 days from the last menstrual period. During mid-pregnancy they drop to the lowest point in pregnancy and then rise again to a second lower broader peak at 33–36 weeks. The mean

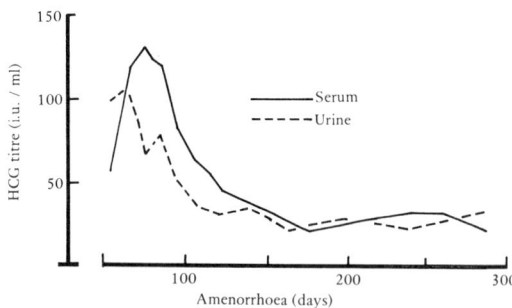

Fig. 4.19   The mean urinary and serum values of chorionic gonadotrophin during pregnancy. After Teoh (1971) *J. Obstet. Gynaec. Brit. Cwlth.*, **74**, 77.

values in serum and urine are shown in figure 4.19.

The first peak of HCG is easy to understand. The main function of the hormone is to stimulate the corpus luteum, preventing its involution and the subsequent drop in progesterone and oestradiol secretion which would result in menstruation. The fertilized ovum has a vital need to produce HCG to ensure its own survival, and, when only a speck of tissue, already produces enough of the hormone to be detectable in the mother's urine. After 10–12 weeks the function of the corpus luteum has declined and it is no longer necessary for the continuance of the pregnancy. HCG is produced in the placenta, probably in the syncitiotrophoblast. Why then does the syncitiotrophoblast continue to produce HCG long after its function has disappeared and indeed increase its production in late pregnancy? It may be that HCG has more functions than have yet been surmised. There is, for instance, some evidence that it is concerned in the control of the manufacture of the steroid hormones in the feto-placental unit.

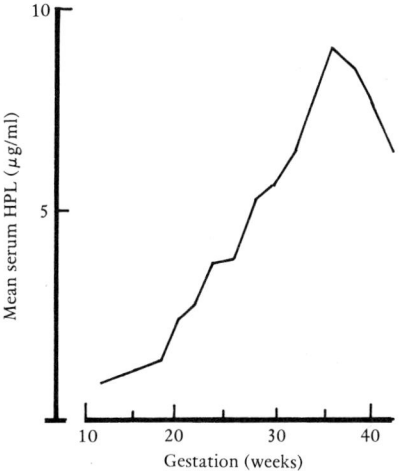

Fig. 4.20   The mean human placental lactogen concentration during pregnancy. After Teoh *et al.* (1971) *J. Obstet. Gynaec. Brit. Cwlth.*, **78**, 673.

2. *Human placental lactogen* (HPL)

This hormone has been known by a variety of names since it was first detected in placental extracts by Japanese workers in 1961. An alternative term, which is still widely used, is human chorionic somatomammotrophin (HCS). Here the designation of human placental lactogen will be used, if only because it is easier on the tongue.

HPL, like HCG, is produced by the syncitiotrophoblast. It is a somewhat smaller molecule than HCG, the molecular weight being in the range of 18 000–25 000. Like HCG, one of its peptide chains is the same as that of a pituitary hormone. In this case HPL and human growth hormone (HGH) have a common component. HPL therefore has antigenic similarities with HGH and it has growth-promoting properties.

The curve of HPL concentration in serum during pregnancy is, however, quite different from that of HCG. The mean normal HPL concentration throughout pregnancy is shown in figure 4.20.

The HPL concentration rises steeply during pregnancy until 36 weeks, after which it drops off. The curve of HPL concentration during pregnancy is similar to the curve for placental weight during pregnancy and it is likely that the HPL concentration is a reflection of the growth of the syncitiotrophoblast which produces it. This connection with placental growth has led to assays of serum HPL being used as a measure of placental function.

Very large amounts (about a gram per day at term) of HPL are produced by the placenta. This amount is probably the largest amount of hormone produced by any endocrine gland. In spite of this, very little is excreted in the mother's urine and the metabolic disposal of HPL is largely unknown. Although HPL is produced by a fetal organ, there is little of the hormone in the fetal circulation and the placenta clearly secretes it mainly into the mother's blood stream. The same applies to HCG, further supporting the thesis that these two protein hormones are aimed at the mother, adapting her physiology to the needs of pregnancy.

HPL will cause lactation when injected into animals but, by virtue of the fact that it disappears soon after the birth of the placenta, it is unlikely to have a lactogenic function in pregnancy. It has growth-promoting properties, but as most of it is secreted to the mother, it is unlikely to be the prime factor directly controlling fetal growth.

There is, however, one respect in which HPL has to do with fetal growth. This concerns its metabolic effects on the mother. It is an insulin antagonist and will therefore cause blood glucose to rise. This stimulates increased maternal insulin production so that the normal mother is able to control her fetus's demand for glucose, but the diabetic mother whose capacity to secrete additional insulin is limited, will require insulin supplementation in pregnancy to cope with the effects of HPL. HPL also has a lipolytic effect and will increase the maternal levels of free fatty acids and also of amino acids thus further increasing the supply of nutrients to the fetus.

3. *Other placental protein hormones*
From time to time placental extracts have been prepared which mimic the action of other protein hormones. Thus, for instance, material which stimulates the adrenal gland has been found, and it has been supposed that the placenta produces adrenocorticotrophin. Subsequent work has not supported this, but there is unchallenged evidence of the presence of thyroid stimulating material both in choriocarcinoma and in normal placentae. It may be that the changes in thyroid activity which occur in pregnancy, are engendered by the placenta.

The steroid hormones of the fetoplacental unit

Although the placenta, in common with other steroid producing glands, has the capacity to produce a great variety of steroids, it directs the biosynthetic processes mainly down pathways leading to two groups of steroids—the progestogens and the oestrogens. The placenta is peculiar among steroid producing glands in that it does not possess the full range of enzymes for all the steps in the making of its characteristic hormones. Some of the essential transformations are carried out in the fetus, mainly in its adrenals and liver. There is thus a constant to and fro traffic of steroids between fetus and placenta, functional groups of the molecule being altered in each location. In this sense the fetus and placenta together make a functional unit, the feto-placental unit—a concept pioneered by Diczfalusy and his colleagues in Stockholm (1969).

THE PROGESTOGENS
Although two other compounds (20α and 20β dihydroprogesterone) having progestational activity are found in the feto-placental unit, the major progestogen is progesterone itself.

During the first few weeks of pregnancy nearly all the progesterone is produced by the corpus luteum although there is evidence that the trophoblast starts to secrete progesterone as early as three weeks after ovulation. The functional life of the corpus luteum of pregnancy is short. Six weeks from the last menstrual period the corpus luteum is pro-

ducing its maximum amount of progesterone. It then declines and eight weeks from lmp a nadir in maternal plasma progesterone is found. By this time, however, the trophoblast is producing more and more progesterone so that maternal blood levels soon rise again. If the ovaries are removed after this time, abortion does not usually occur. If luteal malfunction is a cause of spontaneous abortion, it must be operative in the first eight weeks of pregnancy.

The site of steroid synthesis in the placenta is the syncitiotrophoblast. The question arises what raw materials this tissue uses for the synthesis of progesterone and whether these are derived from the mother or the fetus. The placenta can transform acetate to progesterone but does so in very small quantities. There is every reason to believe that the precursor to progesterone is preformed cholesterol. When the fetus dies *in utero*, or there is no fetus as in hydatidiform mole, the trophoblast still produces large amounts of progesterone. It seems therefore that the source of the placental progesterone is the abundant supply of cholesterol reaching it from the maternal circulation. The placenta does not make progesterone directly from cholesterol, it does so via pregnenolone. The synthesis of progesterone therefore involves two enzymic steps. The first is the removal of the 6 carbon side chain of cholesterol, a C27 compound, to leave pregnenolone, a C21 compound. This step is the essential preliminary to the synthesis of all steroids and pregnenolone is therefore the last common precursor of all steroid hormones. The transformation of pregnenolone into progesterone involves the shifting of the double bond between C5 and C6 in ring B to C4 and C5 in ring A and the transformation of the hydroxyl (OH) group at C3 into a keto ($C = O$) group. This is done by an enzyme system, 3β-steroid dehydrogenase, which plays an important role in steroid synthesis generally. The fetal adrenal, for instance, does not possess this enzyme and the fetus is therefore unable to make progesterone from pregnenolone or to make such adrenal steroids as involve this transformation. The placenta, on the other hand, has plenty of 3β-steroid dehydrogenase and readily transforms pregnenolone to progesterone.

The progesterone thus produced in the placenta is secreted both into the maternal and into the fetal circulation. There is no evidence that in the fetus, progesterone acts as a hormone in its own right. Its main function is to supply a reservoir of material having the Δ3-ketone structure in ring A, for the synthesis of other steroids. Not a great deal of fetal progesterone is used up in this way. Some of the progesterone is converted to pregnanediol by the fetus and this inert compound is eventually excreted by the mother. A further proportion of progesterone is converted to 20-dihydroprogesterone and returned to the placenta where it is once more changed back to progesterone. This to and fro conversion between progesterone and dihydroprogesterone in fetus and placenta serves as a means of conserving progesterone in the feto-placental unit until it can be secreted into the intervillous maternal blood to exert its function in restraining myometrial contraction.

The mean concentration of progesterone in plasma and the mean urinary excretion of pregnanediol throughout pregnancy is shown in figure 4.21.

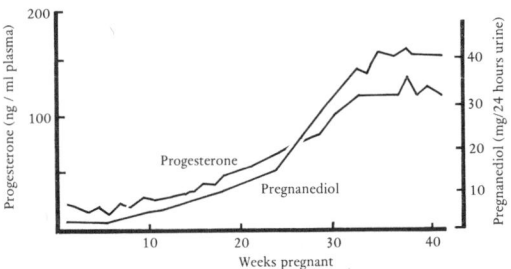

Fig. 4.21 The mean concentration of progesterone in plasma and the urinary excretion of pregnanediol during pregnancy.

These two curves have very similar shapes and resemble the curve of placental growth during pregnancy. It is likely that either of the steroid levels reflect the amount of active syncitiotrophoblast and their measurements have been used as a means of assessing placental function. Very often, however, the cause of fetal death is not in the placenta but in the fetus. In such cases the fetus may be very seriously affected without altering plasma progesterone or urinary pregnanediol.

THE OESTROGENS

During pregnancy the concentration of oestrogens in plasma increases greatly and 22 different oestrogens have been identified in pregnancy urine. The concentration of oestradiol-17β in the blood of a non-pregnant woman may reach 0·3ng/ml at the height of ovarian secretion; in late pregnancy it rises to 12·0ng/ml. The increase in oestriol is much greater, so that in pregnancy it forms a much larger proportion of all the oestrogens. Although no function attributable to the oestriol molecule only has been discovered, the high production of this oestrogen is so characteristic of pregnancy that its biogenesis and normal levels will be considered in some detail.

Much of our knowledge of how oestriol is made in the feto-placental unit stems from the classical work of an American obstetrician, Kenneth Ryan (1959). Oestrogens are 18 carbon compounds and have an aromatic ring A (three double bonds). Ryan showed that the placenta has an enzyme system capable of making this characteristic oestrogen structure from neutral 19 carbon precursors such as dehydroisoandrosterone, androstenedione and testosterone. The remarkable thing is that all these C19 compounds are androgens and that the major hormone of pregnancy is therefore made from an androgen.

Of course the androgens themselves are synthesized from other steroids and in order fully to trace the genesis of oestriol we have to go back to the fundamental raw material—pregnenolone whose biogenesis from cholesterol in the placenta was described in the section on progesterone. The first step in transforming pregnenolone to oestriol is the insertion of a hydroxyl group at C17, converting it to 17-hydroxy pregnenolone. This is a step for which the placenta does not possess the requisite enzyme system but the fetal adrenal does. Placental pregnenolone is therefore converted to 17α-hydroxypregnenolone in the fetus. The next step is also fetal. The fetal adrenal also has the enzyme system for removing the 2 carbon side chain of 17α-hydroxypregnenolone to yield a C19 androgen, dehydroisoandrosterone. This steroid is central to the synthesis of oestriol and other oestrogens and its supply by the fetus is likely to be an important rate-limiting step in determining how much oestriol is produced by the feto-placental unit and excreted in the mother's urine.

A characteristic feature of the structure of oestriol is that it has a hydroxyl (OH) group on C16. In the biogenesis of oestriol there have therefore to be enzyme systems which can introduce a hydroxyl group at C16. The placenta has no such 16-hydroxylating system,

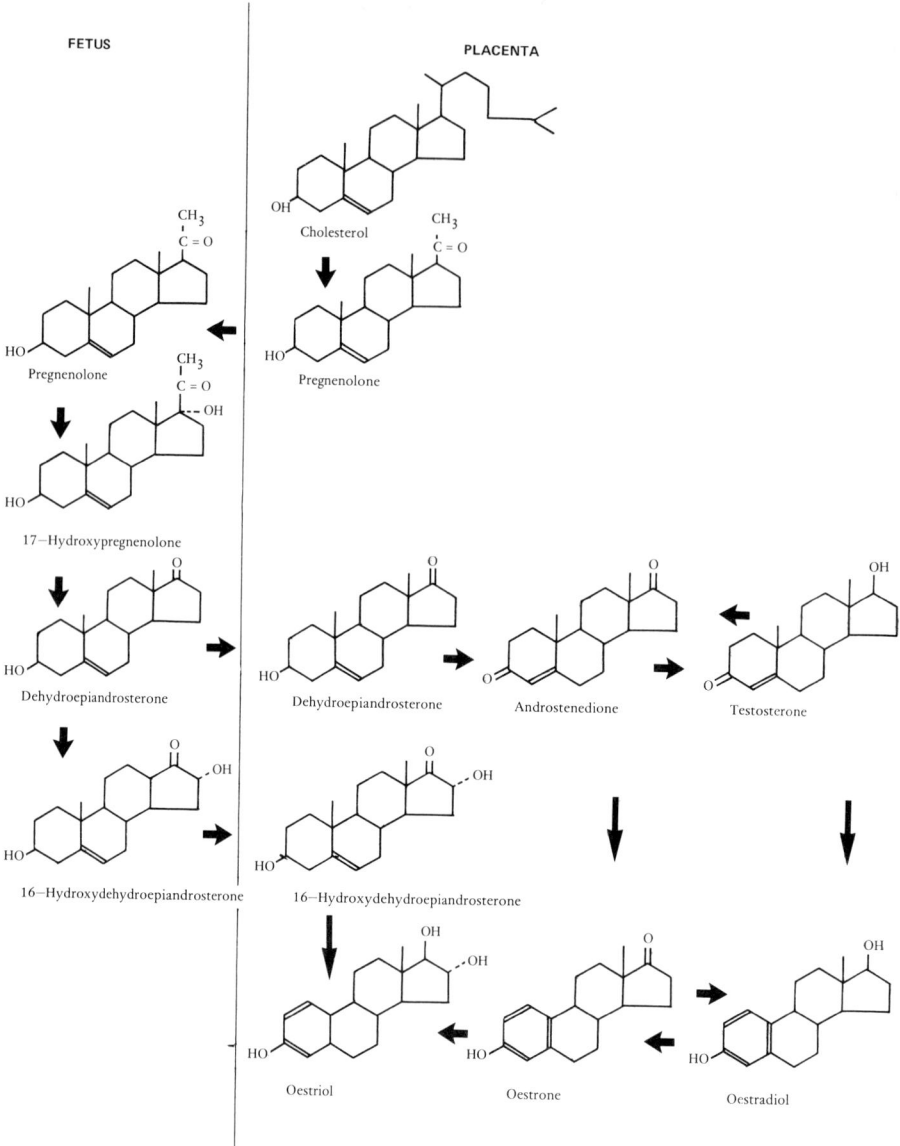

Fig. 4.22   Fetal and placental steps in the biogenesis of oestriol.

but enzymes capable of 16-hydroxylation, notably of pregnenolone or of dehydroiso-androsterone, are present in the fetal liver. The main precursor of oestriol is therefore 16-hydroxy-dehydroisoandrosterone formed in the fetus either from 16-hydroxypregnenolone or by 16-hydroxylation of dehydroisoandro-sterone. This also is a very important and essentially fetal step in oestriol biosynthesis. It may be that often when a decline in oestriol excretion signals fetal jeopardy, the fall in oestriol is due to a failure of 16-hydroxylation by the distressed fetus.

The final step, transformation of 16-hydroxy-dehydroisoandrosterone to oestriol, takes place in the placenta which alone possesses the aromatizing enzyme system. Again this is a critical step and oestriol production is liable to be adversely affected by any placental damage which interferes with aromatizing activity. The different roles of fetus and placenta in the biogenesis of oestriol are shown in figure 4.22.

In some ways the representation of oestriol biogenesis in figure 4.22 is an oversimplifica-tion. For one example the pathway shown is certainly not the only one by which oestriol is made in the feto-placental unit. A small proportion comes from progesterone via 17α-hydroxyprogesterone and some oestriol is also produced in the maternal side by conversion of oestradiol or oestrone from the placenta. The steroids are also not, by and large, present in the feto-placental unit as free steroids but as conjugates with sulphuric acid, e.g. pregnenolone sulphate. It may be that the true oestriol precursor is not dehydroisoandrosterone but dehydroisoandrosterone sulphate and that the final compound produced is oestriol sulphate. This is a point of some importance because such conjugates are, of themselves, biologically inactive and sulphurylation may be a mechanism by which the fetus protects itself against the biological activity of the steroids it is making. Unconjugated oestriol crosses the trophoblast readily and is rapidly transferred to the maternal circulation. Oestriol sulphate escapes much more slowly and most of it probably has to be hydrolysed to free oestriol in the placenta before transfer. There is a lot of sulphatase activity in the placenta and membranes and normally the hydrolysis of oestriol sulphate and the transfer of the free steroid goes rapidly but this could be a mechanism by which the placenta regulates access of the active oestriol to the mother.

The mean levels of oestriol in blood and urine through pregnancy are shown in figure 4.23.

It is noticeable that the rate of oestriol production increases sharply after 32–34 weeks. This suggests that at this stage in pregnancy some new additional process leading to the production of oestriol becomes operative. What this process is, or why the feto-placental unit should need to increase its oestriol production in late pregnancy, is unknown. One valuable clinical application stems from the rapidly rising oestriol output of late pregnancy. This arises from the fact that a steeply increasing output of oestriol is mainly a feature of a normal feto-placental unit. A variety of obstetric diseases which can affect either the fetus or the placenta interfere with oestriol production, and, if the levels in blood or urine are measured day by day, an assessment of fetal well-being is obtained. A particular advantage of oestriol assays over, say, progesterone or placental lactogen assays which are also used for this purpose, is that oestriol is a product of combined fetal and placental activity. It is therefore a direct reflection of fetal events, not indirectly through the placenta. Not all obstetric diseases affect the capacity of the feto-placental unit to produce oestriol. For instance Rh-incompatibility, even when the fetus is severely affected, does not lead to a fall in the urinary output of oestriol or in its plasma concentration. Even when oestriol production is affected not all obstetric diseases affect the same steps in oestriol synthesis or affect the process to the same extent. Different degrees of change in oestriol production (and therefore different oestriol levels) are found in different diseases. The decline in oestriol output is perhaps fortunately most clearly seen when fetal growth retardation is present; a condition which may present the obstetrician with extraordinary difficulty in diagnosis and treatment.

In rather general terms functions can be ascribed to the oestrogens produced by the feto-placental unit. As with the protein hormones and with progesterone, the oestrogens are a biological tool with which the fetus is resetting maternal physiology to fit its needs. Thus the oestrogens stimulate growth processes in the mother, notably in the breasts, as a preparation for lactation and in the uterus in order to allow for the accommodation of the growing conceptus. But these are properties inherent in all the oestrogens, most markedly in the biologically highly active oestradiol. No function peculiar to oestriol, the oestrogen produced in such abundance by the feto-placental unit, has been defined. It may be that oestriol is a kind of metabolic garbage, a

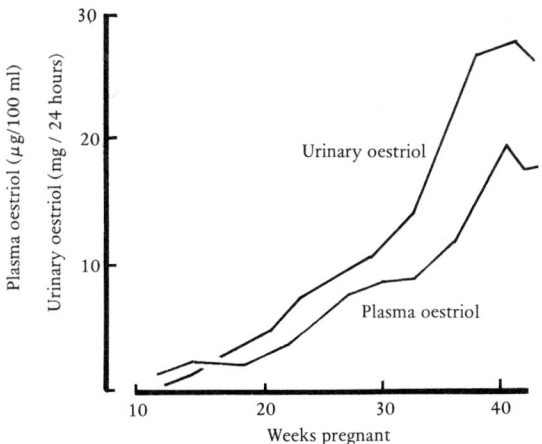

Fig. 4.23   The mean concentration of oestriol in blood and the urinary excretion during pregnancy.

way of inactivating and disposing of unwanted biologically active material. But why make it in the first place, and by a route not involving other oestrogens? The mystery deepens when other pregnant mammals are examined. Such large-scale oestriol synthesis appears to be peculiar to pregnancy in man and possibly some of the higher primates. At a time when our knowledge of the endocrinology of pregnancy is going forward by leaps and bounds, our understanding of the function of oestriol is at a standstill. Perhaps Goethe's dying words, 'Mehr licht', are applicable here too.

The endocrinology of lactation

There are three phases in the production of milk, each of which is under separate endocrine control. The first is a morphological phase, consisting of the build-up of the cellular apparatus for producing milk. During pregnancy marked growth changes take place in the breast. Part of this growth consists of the proliferation of milk ducts. This epithelial growth appears to result from oestrogenic stimulus. At the same time alveolar budding occurs. The alveolar growth is promoted by progesterone.

The second phase, the actual production of milk in the gland, is a complex process in which the steroid hormones oestrogen, progesterone and probably cortisol all play a part. Human placental lactogen, although it is capable of provoking milk production, does not play an important part as it is no longer produced when lactation is established in the puerperium. Two maternal pituitary hormones, growth hormone and prolactin have been implicated. Growth hormone and prolactin are biologically and immunologically related and it is likely that the primary agent is prolactin. Its concentration in the mother's plasma rises during pregnancy and reaches its maximum level in the puerperium. There is also a marked response to suckling.

The third phase is an active ejection of milk by the contraction of the myoepithelial cells of the alveoli and small milk ducts. This results from the action of yet another pituitary hormone, oxytocin. This polypeptide is released from the anterior pituitary on stimulation of the nipples by suckling.

REFERENCES

Adams, E. C. & Hertig, A. T. (1969) Studies on the human corpus luteum II. Observations on the ultrastructure of luteal cells during pregnancy. *Journal of Cell Biology*, **41**, 716.

Aschheim, S. & Zondek, B. (1927) Anterior pituitary hormone and ovarian hormone in the urine of pregnant women. *Klin. Wchr.*, **6**, 248.

Diczfalusy, E. & Mancuso, S. (1969) Oestrogen metabolism. In *Foetus and Placenta*. Edited by A. Klopper & E. Diczfalusy. Oxford: Blackwells.

Falck, B. (1959) Site of production of oestrogen in rat ovary as studied in micro-transplants. *Acta physiol. scand.*, Suppl., 163.

Harris, G. W. & Naftolin, F. (1970) Hypothalamus and control of ovulation. *British Medical Bulletin*, **26**, 3–9.

Jenson, E. V. & Jacobson, H. I. (1962) Basic guides to the mechanism of estrogen action. *Recent Progress in Hormone Research*, **18**, 387.

Markee, J. E. (1940) Menstruation in intraocular endometrial transplants in the Rhesus monkey. *Contributions to Embryology of the Carnegie Institution*, **28**, 219.

McLennan, C. E. & Rydell, A. H. (1965) Extent of endometrial shedding during normal menstruation. *Obstetrics and Gynaecology*, **26**, 605.

Ross, G. T., Cargille, C. M., Lipsett, M. B., Rayford, P. L., Marshall, J. R., Strott, C. A. & Rodbard, D. (1970) Pituitary and gonadal hormones in women during spontaneous and induced cycles. *Recent Progress in Hormone Research*, **26**, 1.

Ryan, K. J. (1959) The metabolism of C–16 oxygenated steroids by human placenta: The formation of estriol. *J. Bio. Chem.*, **234**, 2006.

Ryan, K. J. & Smith, O. W. (1965) Biogenesis of steroid hormones in the human ovary. *Recent Progress in Hormone Research*, **21**, 367.

Savard, K., Marsh, J. M. & Rice, B. F. (1965) Gonadotrophins and ovarian steroidogenesis. *Recent Progress in Hormone Research*, **21**, 285.

Short, R. V. (1963) Steroids in the follicular fluid and the corpus luteum of the mare. A two-cell type theory of ovarian steroidogenesis. *J. of Endocr.*, **24**, 59.

Teoh, E. S. (1967) Chorionic gonadotrophin in the serum and urine of Asian women in normal pregnancy. *J. Obstet. Gynaec. Brit. Cwlth.*, **74**, 74.

Van de Wiele, R., Bogamil, J., Dyrenfurth, I., Ferin, M., Jewelewicz, R., Warren, M., Rizkallah, T. & Mikhail, G. (1970) Mechanisms regulating the menstrual cycle in women. *Recent Progress in Hormone Research*, **26**, 63.

5. Physiological Changes of Pregnancy

In physiological terms pregnancy may be looked at as a complex nutritional exercise, the main objects being to acquire materials for the building of a baby, to arrange for their transport, to provide internal environmental conditions suitable for fetal growth and metabolism, and adequate provision for the disposal of fetal waste products; and to lay in stocks of nutrient against possible periods of deprivation and for eventual use in milk for the newborn baby.

Pregnancy represents the most profound physiological upheaval a normal woman will ever have to face; no system of the body is spared and homeostasis is so affected that the 'milieu interieur' which she has assiduously preserved all her non-pregnant life is almost totally changed. But unlike most physiological changes which represent 'post hoc' responses to an imposed stress, the adjustments of pregnancy are characteristically anticipatory, often taking place in the early weeks before any demonstrable need has arisen.

It is reasonable to assume that, in health, the body is preserving its homeostatic norms because they provide the conditions it needs for maximum efficiency of function. If so, then the greatly altered homeostasis of pregnancy cannot be equally advantageous to the mother and it must be assumed that it represents changes which allow maximum efficiency of fetal development. The fetus itself is largely responsible, reaching out with its hormones to over-ride and reset many of the mothers' control mechanisms in its own interests.

Exploration of the changes associated with normal pregnancy has only recently begun and in general the limits of normality have still to be established. The truly physiological range, often well outside the range which is considered normal for the non-pregnant subject, can only be determined by making measurements in carefully selected patients whose well-being is not open to question; even so the question of what is normal is likely to remain in dispute because the distinction between the normal and the abnormal is a matter of gradation.

Some of the physiological changes make obvious biological sense: the increased circulation to supply such new areas of demand as the pregnant uterus, the increased circulating haemoglobin to cover the increased need for oxygen carriage, and the reduced maternal pCO_2 which offers such a clear advantage to a fetus needing to dispose of it. Other changes, such as the reduced levels of nutrients in the blood, the increased concentration of lipids and the changes in the renin-angiotensin system are less easy to explain; and some such as the greatly increased excretion of nutrients in the urine are at present totally baffling. In this chapter it will be most convenient to consider the maternal adjustments system by system, although it should be remembered that many of the changes, occurring in concert, affect several systems simultaneously and changes initiated in one system are likely to lead to other changes in another system.

BLOOD VOLUME AND COMPOSITION

During pregnancy both plasma volume, and the total volume of red cells or 'red cell mass' increase, but not in the same proportion. The larger proportionate increase in the plasma leads to 'haemodilution', an unfortunate term which implies, for many clinicians an abnormality, and an important physiological principle must therefore be emphasized at the outset: the *ratio* between the plasma volume and the red cell mass, the 'haematocrit', characteristic of a healthy person living at sea level has not in itself any particular physiological significance. Plasma volume rises and falls in response to the need for plasma, for example it rises in high environmental temperatures when skin blood flow increases to dissipate heat; the red cell mass rises and falls in response to the quite independent need for oxygen carriage, for example it rises at high altitude. The change in pregnancy reflects alterations in both

Table 5.1   The blood in human pregnancy

	Non-pregnant	Weeks of pregnancy		
		20	20	40
Plasma volume, ml	2600	3150	3750	3850
Red cell volume, ml	1400	1450	1550	1650
Total blood volume, ml	4000	4600	5300	5500
'Body haematocrit', per cent	35·0	31·5	29·2	30·0
Venous haematocrit,* per cent	39·8	35·8	33·2	34·1

* Assuming a haematocrit ratio of 0·88.

components, plasma volume rises greatly in response to a greatly increased demand for circulating fluid (not needed to carry oxygen), i.e. to the kidneys and skin; the proportionately smaller increase in red cell mass provides more than enough additional total oxygen carrying capacity for the increased oxygen consumption of the mother.

Plasma volume

In a healthy first pregnancy plasma volume rises by about 1250ml, about 50 per cent of the average non-pregnant volume of 2600ml, although the rise is not related to the non-pregnant value and the percentage rise is a misleading concept. The rise begins towards the end of the third month and reaches a plateau during the final two months. The widely described fall in late pregnancy is almost certainly an artefact due to measurements made with the subject lying supine (*see* Cardiac output). The response is variable and correlated with clinical performance. For instance, the rise of plasma volume is related to the birth weight of the child, and women who give birth to underweight babies have, in general, much smaller increases in plasma volume than those with a normal pregnancy and a child of normal size.

Red cell mass

The total volume of red cells in healthy women who are not being treated with iron, rises by about 250ml from an average non-pregnant volume of about 1400ml, an increase of about 18 per cent. When supplementary iron is given the rise is considerably greater, as much as 400–450ml.

Haematocrit

With plasma volume rising by an average of about 50 per cent and the red cell mass by less than 20 per cent, it is obvious that the haemato-crit must fall and the 'whole body haematocrit' derived from these averages is shown in Table 5.1. Because of the uneven distribution of red cells in blood from small and large vessels, the whole body haematocrit is only about 88 per cent of the haematocrit measured in blood from a peripheral vein and the appropriate figure for peripheral venous blood is also shown. These derived figures are closely parallel to direct measurements of haemoglobin concentration and packed cell volume (PCV, haematocrit) which have been published.

Haemoglobin concentration and packed cell volume (PCV)

In healthy non-pregnant women the haemoglobin concentration in peripheral blood is usually between 13·5 and 14·0g per 100ml, the PCV about 40 per cent. As predicted by the changing volumes of plasma and the red cell mass, both fall to a minimum in the third trimester, typically between 11 and 12g/100ml for haemoglobin, with a PCV of between 33 and 34 per cent.

THE RED CELLS
Due to a fall in the plasma colloid osmotic pressure (*see* plasma proteins) the red cells imbibe water, become more spherical and have a slightly increased fragility. The mean cell haemoglobin concentration also falls slightly but remains well within normal non-pregnant limits.

THE LEUCOCYTES
The concentration of leucocytes in blood rises in pregnancy from about 7000 to 10 000/mm^3, chiefly by increase of neutrophil polymorphonuclear cells. The change appears to be due to the action of oestrogens.

PLATELETS
The platelet count is somewhat lower in pregnancy than in the non-pregnant woman (*see* Chapter 13).

The composition of the plasma

The term 'haemodilution', generally applied to the 'dilution' of red cells by the rising volume of plasma, is also sometimes used in reference to the plasma itself which has a somewhat higher water content in pregnancy. The term is equally misleading in this context, since the changes in plasma composition are extremely complex and in no sense due to the simple addition of water.

ELECTROLYTES

There is a small fall in the concentration of most electrolytes in pregnancy, although the change is little more than the error of the method of measurement and has not been found by all investigators. Sodium falls by about 2mEq/litre and potassium by less than 0·5mEq/litre. Calcium, both total and ionized, and magnesium fall slightly and these cation changes are matched by a fall in anion concentration which mostly affects bicarbonate (*see* Respiration) and phosphate; the concentration of chloride appears to remain at about the usual non-pregnant level.

OSMOLALITY

Plasma osmolality drops abruptly in early pregnancy by about 10mOsm/kg of water, from about 290 to 280. The reduced level which is considerably outside normal fluctuation, remains constant throughout pregnancy and is largely attributable to the lower concentrations of electrolytes although the reduced concentrations of many nutrients and non-protein nitrogen fractions (*see* Renal Function) will have some influence. The ability to tolerate and preserve a level of osmolality which for the normal non-pregnant person would cause a perpetual maximum diuresis, suggests that the osmoreceptors are in some way reset.

PROTEINS

The total protein content of plasma falls from a typical non-pregnant value of about 7g/100ml to between 6 and 6·5g/100ml by mid pregnancy after which little or no further fall occurs. That overall change is largely dictated by a fall in the concentration of albumin from about 3·5 to 2·5g/100ml during the first half of pregnancy. The globulin fractions tend to increase progressively in concentration, the α fractions by about 0·1g/100ml and the β group by some 0·3g/100ml. The immune globulins show little change but IgG may fall slightly

in concentration; fibrinogen concentration rises. That broad picture covers a huge range of change in many specific protein fractions such as enzymes and carrier proteins of many types, which is still to be fully described.

COLLOID OSMOTIC PRESSURE

In oversimplified terms a measure of the 'attraction' exercised by large molecules like protein on water movement across semipermeable membranes, falls dramatically in pregnancy from about 35cm of water to about 30cm of water. The change is dictated by and closely follows the changing concentration of plasma albumin.

ERYTHROCYTE SEDIMENTATION RATE (ESR)

Because of the changes in plasma protein concentrations, ESR is high in pregnancy, averaging in late pregnancy 78mm in the first hour for whole blood and 56mm for citrated blood, compared to upper limits of normality for the non-pregnant woman of 20 and 10mm. The ESR is therefore of no clinical value during pregnancy.

ENZYMES

Alkaline Phosphatase concentration rises progressively in pregnancy largely due to a heat stable iso-enzyme derived from the placenta. Its measurement enjoyed a short vogue as an index of 'placental function'.

Amylase activity does not change.

Cholinesterase activity is generally unchanged in pregnancy but in a minority of women it may fall to such an extent that the action of the muscle relaxant succinyl choline is unduly prolonged.

Caeruloplasmin, a copper containing oxidase, doubles in concentration in pregnancy.

Diamine Oxidase (DAO, histaminase) shows a large increase in concentration and has also been used as an indicator of 'placental function'.

Lactate Dehydrogenase (SLD); Iso citrate Dehydrogenase (ICD): L-Hydroxybutyrate Dehydrogenase (SHBD) remain within normal non-pregnant limits.

Leucine Aminopeptidase; Cysteine Amino Peptidase (Oxytocinase) two of a group of enzymes capable of splitting polypeptides and therefore destroying polypeptide hormones such as oxytocin. They are probably derived from the placenta and increase greatly in pregnancy.

Lipoprotein Lipase activity falls in pregnancy.

Glutamic Oxaloacetic Transaminase (GOT);

Glutamic-Pyruvic Transaminase (GPT) remain within the normal non-pregnant range.

Lipids. Most plasma lipid fractions rise during pregnancy. Cholesterol concentration increases progressively from under 200mg/100ml to between 250 and 300mg/100ml; the usual relation between free and ester cholesterol is maintained. Total phospholipid concentration also rises, preserving the usual ratio between cholesterol and phospholipid, but the various fractions behave in different ways: phosphotidyl-ethanolamine and lecithin rise both absolutely and as a proportion of total phospholipid; sphingomyelin increases less and the concentration of lysolecithin falls.

There is always a conspicuous rise in the concentration of triglyceride fat, and also of free or non-esterified fatty acids (NEFA) in late pregnancy.

Fats are carried in blood attached to proteins —the lipoproteins. There are two major fractions: α- and β-lipoprotein; in pregnancy the increase is predominantly of β-lipoprotein.

CARDIOVASCULAR DYNAMICS

Cardiac output

The evolution of understanding the pattern of cardiac output in pregnancy has been long and interesting. For many years it was accepted that basal cardiac output rose gradually to a peak at the end of the second trimester after which it declined towards non-pregnant values by term and the peak danger period for women with heart disease was confidently believed to be around 30 weeks of pregnancy. The development of more direct techniques of measurement by cardiac catheterization in the 1940s and 1950s led to the accumulation of evidence that the rise to peak cardiac output was much earlier, within the first trimester, remaining at a high level until the last weeks of pregnancy when it declined. Finally, within the last decade has come the realization that the terminal decline is an artefact seen only when measurements are made with the subject lying supine so that her uterus obstructs the vena cava and impedes venous return to the heart. Present evidence gives support to the idea that the basal cardiac output is raised from early in the first trimester to the end of pregnancy by about 1·5 litres/minute.

The increase in cardiac output is brought about by both an increased heart rate and a larger stroke volume.

Pulse rate

The resting pulse rate is raised above the non-pregnant level by about 15 beats/minute from early pregnancy.

Stroke volume

Few direct measurements have been made but the rise in resting pulse rate is not enough to provide the raised cardiac output, and stroke volume probably rises by about 10ml. The proportioning between pulse rate and stroke volume is flexible and it is of some interest in this context that normal pregnancy is possible when the mother has an artificial cardiac pacemaker giving a fixed heart rate of about 70/minute.

Central arterio-venous oxygen difference

Both cardiac output and circulating red cell mass rise more, proportionately, than oxygen consumption, and more oxygen is therefore returned to the heart unused than usual. The average non-pregnant difference of about 45ml O_2/litre, is reduced, particularly in early pregnancy, to less than 35ml O_2/litre.

Intra vascular pressure

Arterial blood pressure

Although numerous studies of blood pressure have been published, most are unsatisfactory for one reason or another, and since technique makes a considerable difference to the pressure recorded, there is little point in presenting average figures. In general, the systotic pressure may be a little below the non-pregnant average, but rises to the usual level in late pregnancy. Diastolic pressure is conspicuously lower than the non-pregnant level throughout most of pregnancy, so that the pulse pressure is consistently raised; it returns towards non-pregnant levels in late pregnancy. Since cardiac output is raised and blood pressure is not, it follows that resistance to flow, the peripheral resistance, is decreased. Posture has a more marked effect on blood pressure in pregnancy. If a woman in late pregnancy lies on her back the uterus compresses the aorta and femoral blood pressure in that situation is lower than brachial blood pressure. The vena cava is also compressed and in some women lacking an adequate collateral circulation there may be a profound fall in blood pressure and fainting—the 'supine hypotensive syndrome'.

Venous blood pressure

In the upper part of the body, pressures are

ordinarily unaltered, so that there is no change either in the arm veins or in central venous pressure. In the lower limbs there is a progressive rise in pressure during pregnancy and an associated slowing of blood flow. Femoral venous pressure rises from about 10cm of water to as much as 30cm of water. There are two likely causes: (a) Simple mechanical pressure by the growing uterus on the iliac veins, and (b) hydrodynamic obstruction due to the outflow of blood at relatively high pressure from the uterus.

High venous pressure in the legs, possibly helped by the reduced plasma colloid osmotic pressure, probably accounts for the common lower limb oedema of normal pregnancy, and to some extent for the increased incidence of varicosity of the saphenous vein system.

Heart signs

The heart enlarges during pregnancy and is pushed upwards and rotated forward by the diaphragm, producing a characteristic clinical and radiological picture. It is uncertain whether the enlargement is due to no more than the greater diastolic filling or whether there is also some true myocardial hypertrophy. The electrocardiogram shows a marked left axis deviation and there are other changes that may mimic minor degrees of heart disease.

Regional distribution of increased blood flow

The uterus

This may be regarded as the central target of the increased circulation of pregnancy, but techniques of measurement are particularly difficult and relatively few observations have been made. The information available suggests a progressive increase in uterine blood flow reaching about 200ml/minute at 28 weeks and about 500ml/minute at term.

The kidneys

Renal blood flow rises from a non-pregnant average of under 900ml/minute to about 1200ml/minute in early pregnancy and is maintained at that level throughout pregnancy.

The skin

There is abundant evidence of increased blood flow to the skin in pregnancy. The skin, particularly of the extremities, is characteristically warm and moist and skin temperature is raised; pregnant women themselves feel warm, often complain of the heat, and are more than usually tolerant of cold. Peripheral arteriolar vasodilatation is evident in the first few weeks of pregnancy and patients with Raynaud's disease have an immediate remission. The increase in blood flow is difficult to quantify. Hand and foot blood flow may increase 5- or 6-fold, forearm and leg blood flow somewhat less. For the whole body a total increase of the order of 500ml/minute seems realistic.

Other sites

The liver and brain have been shown to have no increase of blood flow; and there is no quantitative evidence of increased blood flow to any other part of the body although

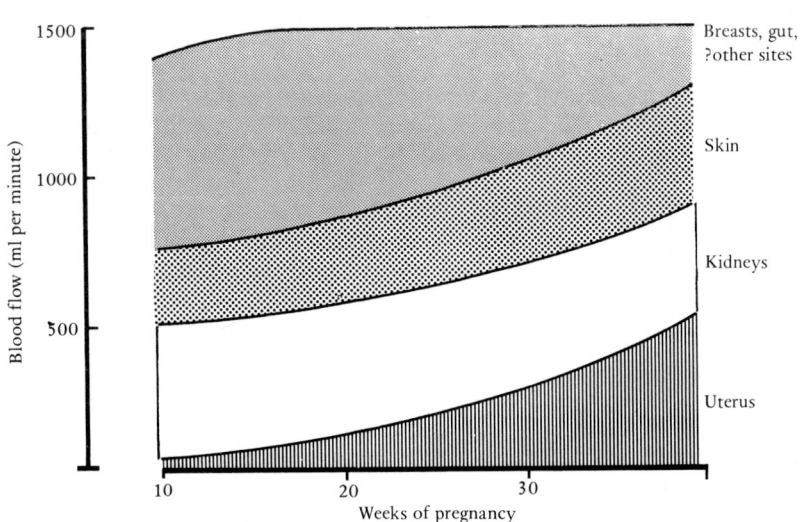

Fig. 5.1 Distribution of the increased cardiac output of pregnancy.

clinically it seems likely that the breasts and the gut at least have an increase.

Summary

Figure 5.1 shows the disposition, as far as is known, of the increased cardiac output of pregnancy. It should be noted that two major targets of increased blood flow, the kidneys and the skin, serve purposes of elimination, the kidneys of soluble waste, the skin of heat. Both processes require plasma rather than whole blood which gives point to the 'disproportionate' increase in plasma volume in the expansion of the blood.

The mechanisms controlling the major cardiovascular changes are not understood, but vasodilation is central to most of them. In the laboratory animal there is evidence that progesterone may modify the pressor effect of angiotensin, and oestrogen which in some areas appears to have a direct vasodilator effect may depress sympathetic tone. Both steroids may play a part in human pregnancy.

RESPIRATORY FUNCTION

Anatomical changes and the mechanics of breathing

Anatomical changes occur in the chest from early pregnancy; the subcostal angle increases, the lower ribs flare, and the transverse diameter of the chest increases. At the same time, and long before there can be any question of displacement by the uterus, the level of the diaphragm rises by as much as 4cm. Far from the old view that the diaphragm was 'splinted', breathing at all stages of pregnancy is more diaphragmatic and less costal than in non-pregnant women.

Lung function:

Ventilation

Ventilation rate rises progressively throughout pregnancy from about 7 litres/minute to about 10 litres/minute, an increase of more than 40 per cent. The increase is achieved almost entirely by an increase in tidal volume; there is little or no change in respiratory rate.

Lung volumes

Vital capacity is not affected by pregnancy but there is a rearrangement of its components. The increase in tidal volume is at the expense of the expiratory reserve volume; that is, the lung is more collapsed than usual at the end

of normal expiration. The residual volume is also reduced, so that the functional residual capacity is considerably smaller (Fig. 5.2). This has important consequences: the increased tidal volume of air is now taken into

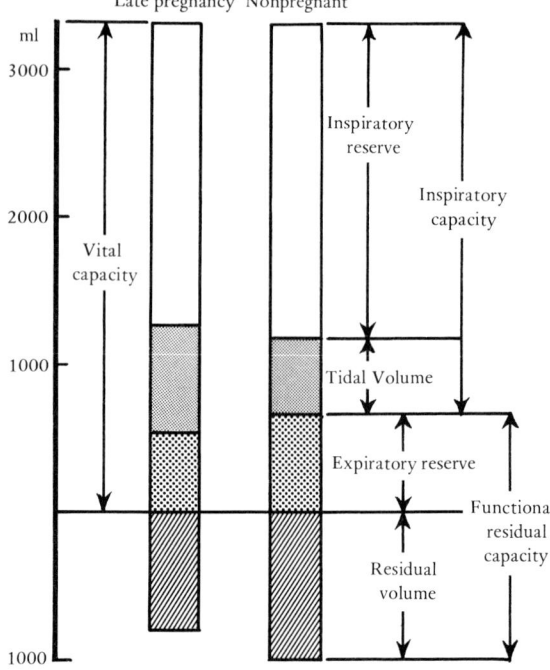

Fig. 5.2   The components of lung volume in late pregnancy compared with those of the non-pregnant subject.

a smaller residual volume of gas in the lung, giving much more efficient gas mixing. It can be calculated that alveolar ventilation increases by about 65 per cent.

Lung function tests

Maximum breathing capacity and timed vital capacity are not appreciably affected by pregnancy, but as would be expected from the greatly increased alveolar ventilation, gas distribution as measured by the 'pulmonary mixing index', is much more efficient. There appears to be no change with pregnancy in the pulmonary diffusing capacity.

Gas exchange

Oxygen consumption in pregnancy has been the subject of many studies, usually as 'basal metabolic rate'. It is clearly difficult to achieve truly basal conditions and most of the estimates are unsatisfactory; they range from about 14 per cent to nearly 50 per cent above the non-pregnant rate. The lowest estimates of about 14–15 per cent, or some 32ml of oxygen/minute above the non-pregnant oxygen consumption, best fit the facts; for example, the reduced arteriovenous oxygen difference associated with an increase in oxygen-carrying capacity of 18 per cent.

With oxygen consumption increasing by less than 20 per cent and minute ventilation increasing by more than 40 per cent—it is clear that there is considerable 'overbreathing', all the more pronounced because of the greatly enhanced gas mixing. The increase in alveolar ventilation is probably four times that of oxygen consumption.

The phenomenon of overbreathing begins in early pregnancy, indeed at the end of every menstrual cycle, and washes out carbon dioxide from the alveoli. Alveolar pCO_2 falls from a usual non-pregnant figure of about 38mmHg to about 30mmHg by about the twelfth week. The respiratory centre not only has the lower threshold that is indicated by these figures, it is also more sensitive. For example, the normal person increases ventilation rate by about 1·5 litres/minute for each 1mmHg rise in arterial pCO_2; in pregnancy the increase is about 6 litres/minute/mmHg. The lowered threshold is almost certainly due to the action of progesterone; the increased sensitivity may be an oestrogen effect. The reduced pCO_2 is accompanied by a parallel decrease in blood bicarbonate, a change which may be basically responsible for the fall in plasma osmolality; there is no change in pH.

Dyspnoea

The reduced alveolar pCO_2 may contribute to the common symptom of dyspnoea in pregnancy. The sensation of dyspnoea, a conscious need to breathe, may be paradoxical in pregnancy, present at rest but not on moving about. Many circumstances may lead to dyspnoea in non-pregnant persons and the most likely explanation is that some centre is continuously relating the demand for ventilation to the actual ventilation and that the sensation of dyspnoea arises when the ventilatory response is 'inappropriate' to the demand. This theory would fit the facts of pregnancy well. For a woman habituated to breathing at pCO_2 of 38mmHg, the compulsion to breathe much harder at pCO_2 of 30 may well seem inappropriate. Associated with the reduced pCO_2 is a slight rise in alveolar pO_2.

RENAL FUNCTION

Anatomical changes

Dilatation of the ureter above the level of the pelvic brim is characteristic of pregnancy; it is apparent from as early as the 10th week and may be extreme, with kinking. The traditional explanation, that the dilatation was the result of atony due to the action of progesterone on smooth muscle, is no longer tenable; ureteric tone and contractile pressure is not affected by pregnancy or may even be higher than usual. The phenomenon is therefore presumably due to a mechanical obstruction and there is some evidence that this may be caused by a leash of dilated ovarian veins which surround the ureter at the level of the pelvic brim. Bladder tone is unaffected by pregnancy.

There is some evidence of renal enlargement in pregnancy, presumably due to slight distension of the vasculature consequent on the raised renal blood flow.

Blood and plasma flow

Plasma flow appears to increase rapidly in early pregnancy from about 500ml/minute to a plateau at something above 700ml/minute. Blood flow behaves similarly, rising from a non-pregnant level of about 800ml/minute to more than 1200ml/minute. As with measurements of plasma volume and cardiac output, renal blood flow appears to fall in late pregnancy, on average by about 20 per cent, if the measurements are made with the subject supine.

Glomerular filtration rate

This is considerably raised throughout pregnancy. It rises within the first trimester from a non-pregnant average of about 90ml/minute to a plateau of about 150ml/minute for the whole of pregnancy. When measurements are made in late pregnancy with the subject supine there may be some reduction. Since glomerular filtration rate rises proportionately somewhat more than renal plasma flow, the proportion of plasma filtered, the filtration fraction, is also raised.

Clearance of waste products

Urea, creatinine and uric acid are all excreted more effectively by the enhanced renal clearance in pregnancy, and blood levels are considerably reduced. Plasma urea concentration falls from about 25mg/100ml in the non-pregnant woman to less than 20mg/100ml before mid pregnancy. Similarly, creatinine concentration falls from 0·6–0·7mg/100ml to less than 0·5mg/100ml, and uric acid from non-pregnant levels a little below 4mg to levels of less than 3mg/100ml. As a result of the reduced uric acid levels, gout has been observed to improve in pregnancy.

Sodium and water
The reduced plasma sodium and osmolality referred to above (p. 85) would in the normal non-pregnant woman call for a corrective water diuresis. That this does not happen in pregnancy suggests a resetting of the central osmoreceptors to accept and preserve the new homeostatic levels. Nevertheless, considerable changes occur in the mechanisms controlling sodium excretion. The filtered load of sodium rises with glomerular filtration rate in pregnancy but its recovery is well within the capacity of the normal kidney; at the same time there is an increasingly high level in the plasma of aldosterone reflecting a secretion rate which in late pregnancy may reach five times the non-pregnant rate, and when this is suppressed there is an immediate rise in sodium excretion leading to severe depletion. The augmented aldosterone secretion is therefore necessary to sodium conservation and supports a suggestion that there is some potent sodium-losing mechanism associated with pregnancy; there is evidence that it may be progesterone. Posture has long been known to affect sodium excretion and recent evidence indicates that the supine position in late pregnancy leads to a considerably increased active reabsorption of sodium by the proximal tubule; the mechanism is not known.

Water excretion behaves in a similar fashion to sodium, but the capacity to deal with a water load changes dramatically. Before mid-pregnancy the kidney is capable of prodigious rates of urine flow; 30ml/minute is not unusual. But this ability declines as pregnancy proceeds and in late pregnancy the ability to excrete a water load is much below normal; maximum rates of flow are commonly below 10ml/minute at term.

The high rate of loss in early pregnancy coincides with a period when most pregnant women admit to unusual thirst, but although frequency of micturition is common, polyuria has not been demonstrated. In late pregnancy it is possible that water may pool in the lower limbs and is only mobilized when the woman lies down. In any event there is some evidence that the normal pattern of urine output is reversed, tending to be higher at night than during the day.

Nutrient excretion
The kidney normally exhibits high efficiency in recovering filtered nutrients and it is one of the more bizarre and unexpected features of normal pregnancy that the efficiency of recovery declines. Every person excretes up to 150mg of glucose daily, that amount being undetectable by normal tests, but detectable glycosuria has always been recognized as a commonplace in pregnancy and about half of all healthy pregnant women will show it at some time. Losses of over 1g in 24 hours are common and can be as high as 10g without any evidence of abnormal carbohydrate metabolism. A characteristic feature of glycosuria is its intermittency, days or groups of days with almost continuous glycosuria interspersed with days or groups of days free of it. The ability of the tubules to reabsorb glucose may be somewhat reduced in pregnancy but the picture is more of intermittent tubular failure of unknown cause. Other sugars such as lactose and fructose behave in similar fashion.

Amino acids are also excreted in greater amounts than usual. The excretion of glycine, histidine, threonine, serine and alanine increases rapidly in early pregnancy and continues to increase until the end of pregnancy when losses are 4 or 5 times normal and an average of as much as 20 per cent of filtered glycine or histidine is lost in the urine. For lysine, cystine, taurine, tyrosine, phenylalanine, valine and leucine there is also a greatly increased excretion in early pregnancy but thereafter excretion tends to fall. Other amino acids show no obvious change. The mechanism is again quite unknown although a similar pattern can be induced in the non-pregnant person with cortisol and the high circulating levels in pregnancy may be responsible.

Water soluble vitamins are squandered in the same way; for example as much as $50\mu g$ of folate may be excreted daily by a normal pregnant woman who is not taking folic acid supplements.

The renin–angiotensin system
The circulating level of the enzyme renin is raised in pregnancy to five to ten times the level in non-pregnant women and the α_2-globulin substrate on which it acts to produce

angiotensin is similarly raised. Those two changes do not necessarily imply that there is an increased production of angiotensin although this is presumed. What is clear is that the pregnant woman has a greatly reduced sensitivity to the pressor action of angiotensin and its major effect in pregnancy may be to stimulate aldosterone production and so balance the sodium-losing tendency of the kidneys.

The raised levels of angiotensin may also be responsible for the pronounced thirst so common in pregnancy.

ALIMENTARY FUNCTION

Appetite and food habits
A majority of women report an obvious increase in appetite during the first trimester. It is not necessarily inconsistent with the common symptom of nausea in early pregnancy; many women feel ravenous once the wave of early morning nausea has passed. A noticeable thirst is even more common.

Increased appetite is probably secondary to a 'resetting' of the central control of body composition, the effect of progesterone in promoting storage of depot fat (see below), rather than to any direct effect on the appetite-satiety centres.

Qualitative changes are surprisingly common. Preferences even amounting to craving for, or aversions to certain foods may affect two-thirds of normal pregnant women, the most common cravings are probably for fruit or highly flavoured savoury foods; the most common aversions to tea, coffee and fried food.

Pica may develop in a few pregnant women; cravings for such things as coal or chalk are occasionally reported.

The mouth
The old belief, 'for every child, a tooth' is not supported by scientific opinion. Certainly no convincing evidence has been produced of demineralization of the teeth in pregnancy, nor of an increase in caries. The gums, on the other hand, appear often to be adversely affected. The primary lesion appears to be gingival oedema with infection, gingivitis, following, but the oedema itself is probably physiological and part of the general change in connective tissue ground substance induced by oestrogen (see oedema).

The oesophagus and stomach
The oesophagus is a focus of discomfort in many pregnant women as the site of heartburn, a reflux oesophagitis resulting from persistent regurgitation of gastric acid. The condition is due to a relaxation of the cardiac sphincter.

The stomach shows many signs of reduced function. Acid production after test meals and after histamine stimulation is depressed and there is less production of pepsin, features which may contribute to the well known clinical observation that peptic ulcer is rare in pregnancy.

Reduced gastric mobility has been demonstrated radiologically on many occasions, and while slow emptying may allow better digestion, the hypomotility probably has much to do with the tendency of the pregnant woman to nausea.

The intestine
There is no convincing evidence of an increased efficiency in the transport of nutrients through the gut. More iron is absorbed from a given dose but that represents no more than an extension of the mechanism which operates in the non-pregnant subject, increased absorption when there is increased demand. All other examples of apparently improved adsorption, particularly in such states as Crohn's disease or after extensive bowel resection probably rest on reduced mobility allowing longer time for absorption.

Reduced mobility of the large intestine, together with enhanced water reabsorption which may be due to the high circulating levels of aldosterone in pregnancy, leads to the common complaint of constipation.

The liver and gallbladder
The liver is undoubtedly involved in many of the adjustments in pregnancy such as changes in the pattern of plasma proteins, enzyme activity and in the metabolism of nutrients, but there is no direct evidence.

Liver function is essentially unchanged by pregnancy as far as can be judged by the few studies of it. The bromsulphthalein (BSP) test shows some curious features: the liver removes BSP more rapidly than usual from the plasma but seems unable to excrete it so quickly to the bile and returns it to the blood. The phenomenon can be simulated in non-pregnant women by oestrogen administration.

MATERNAL ENDOCRINE GLANDS

The pituitary gland

The pituitary gland enlarges in pregnancy but relatively little is known about any change of function, to a large extent because almost every pituitary hormone has an analogue produced by the placenta which confuses the assay.

Gonadotrophins are secreted by the pituitary gland throughout pregnancy but probably within the normal range of non-pregnant secretion; there is no evidence of cyclicity.

Adrenocorticotrophin (ACTH) might be expected to be secreted in greater amounts than usual because of the greatly increased secretion of adrenocortical steroids (*see below*) but there is no direct evidence.

Thyrotrophin (TSH) from the pituitary is probably not secreted in greater than usual amounts (*see* Thyroid Gland).

Sommatotrophin, growth hormone (HGH) secretion is not apparently affected by pregnancy and clinically normal pregnancy is possible in its total absence.

Prolactin appears to be secreted in increasing amounts, with plasma concentration rising some ten-fold during pregnancy.

Melanocyte—stimulating hormone (MSH) appears to be secreted in increased amounts during pregnancy and is responsible for the changes in skin pigmentation, chloasma and the darkening of the nipples and linea nigra, characteristic of pregnancy.

Posterior pituitary hormones. There is no information about possible changes in the secretion of either oxytocin or vasopressin in pregnancy.

The adrenal gland

The two hormones of major physiological importance, cortisol and aldosterone, are both secreted in increased amounts in pregnancy.

Cortisol. While there is some debate about the extent to which the secretion of cortisol may increase in pregnancy, there is general agreement about the considerable increase in excretion in urine of both cortisol and its metabolites, and about the greatly increased levels in plasma. Cortisol in blood is raised to particularly high levels largely because of an increase in protein binding, an oestrogen effect, but there is also a two- to three-fold increase

in the level of free cortisol in plasma. That may account for the fact that some diseases such as rheumatism remit in pregnancy and it may play a part in modifying the mother's immune responses, so assisting the toleration of the placental homograft. But to what extent it produces, as some have claimed, a mild Cushing's syndrome, is not clear. Skin striae, primarily due to stretching, may be provoked by it, and the tendency to excrete nutrients in the urine, amino acids and glucose, may also be due to high cortisol levels, but the similarity seldom extends beyond these signs. It is of some interest that women who have had a bilateral adrenalectomy are often able to have an apparently quite normal pregnancy without an increase in their usual corticosteroid replacement therapy.

Aldosterone is secreted in increasing quantities, perhaps up to ten times the non-pregnant amount by late pregnancy, and is excreted in the urine in similarly raised amounts; there is evidence of considerable changes in its metabolism. The mechanism responsible is presumably through the increased activity of the renin–angiotensin system and present evidence suggests that the increased amounts of aldosterone are necessary to combat the sodium-losing effect of progesterone on the renal tubules. On the other hand normal pregnancy after bilateral adrenalectomy has been described in women who were not given mineralocorticoid replacement.

Catecholamines. There is no convincing evidence of any change in catecholamine production or release in normal pregnancy.

The thyroid gland

Many aspects of thyroid metabolism are affected by pregnancy and they are indicated in figure 5.3. The gland itself may enlarge somewhat, due in part to hyperaemia and in part perhaps to some colloid storage, although the term 'goitre' which has been used to describe it is an exaggeration and inappropriate.

Clearance of inorganic iodine from the blood is raised but the plasma level is low so the combined effect may or may not result in an increased absolute uptake of iodine: Evidence is divided.

The total concentration of circulating thyroid hormone is greatly increased in pregnancy due to the effect of oestrogen in raising the amount and the carrying capacity of

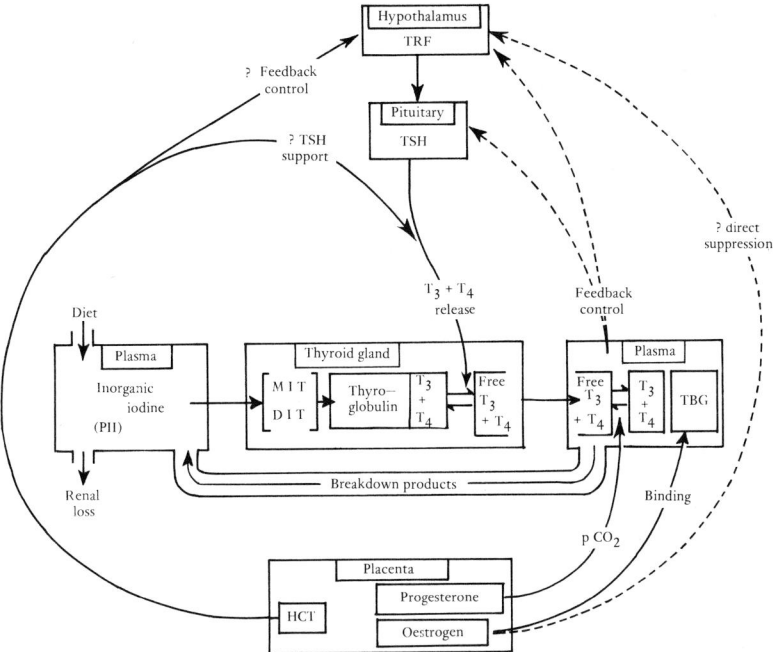

Fig. 5.3. A diagrammatic representation of thyroid metabolism and its modification in normal pregnancy.

thyroxine-binding globulin (TBG) but the concentration of free or effective hormone is somewhat lower than in the non-pregnant person due to the low pCO_2 (*see* page 89) of plasma which affects binding equilibrium. A reduced concentration of free thyroid hormone might be expected to induce a raised secretion of pituitary TSH but oestrogen tends to suppress secretion and the net effect may be one of no change; the role of chorionic thyro-trophin (HCT) is obscure, it may support the action of TSH.

In pregnancy the normal clinical criteria of thyroid malfunction may be misleading. The raised basal oxygen consumption (BMR), the fast pulse rate, the hot skin and tolerance of cold are all part of the normal adaptation of pregnancy. And the high level of circulating hormone (PBI) is no more significant of thyroid overaction than the high level of cholesterol is significant of thyroid under-action. The only meaningful tests of thyroid normality in pregnancy are those that measure the amount of free hormone, for example the uptake of T_3 or T_4 by red cells or by resin sponge from pregnancy plasma.

The parathyroid glands

There is some evidence of increased concen-trations of parathormone in the blood during the second half of pregnancy. The rise may be provoked by the fall in the level of plasma calcium.

WEIGHT GAIN IN PREGNANCY

The range of weight change in pregnancy is wide from a loss to a gain of 25kg or more. A normal clinical course is likely throughout the range but the incidence of complications increases at the extremes and is minimal at a gain of about 12·5kg. That represents an average gain of about 450g per week during the last two-thirds of pregnancy and, as well as being the gain associated with the best clinical outcome, is also about the average weight gained by healthy women eating to appetite. The period of most rapid weight gain is around 20 weeks of pregnancy and the rate of gain is generally falling in the last few weeks before term. Multigravidae gain rather less weight on average than primigravidae and women who are overweight before pregnancy tend to gain less weight than thinner women.

THE COMPONENTS OF WEIGHT GAINED
The major components of the weight gained by the average healthy pregnant woman are

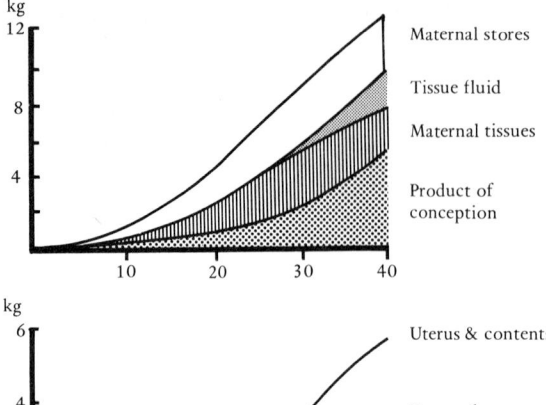

Fig. 5.4 The major components of weight gain in pregnancy.

shown in figure 5.4 and Table 5.2. All are subject to considerable individual variation.

The product of conception, fetus, placenta and amniotic fluid, accounts for only about 5kg of the 12·5kg gained; details are discussed in Chapter 4.

The uterus. The average non-pregnant weight ranges from under 50g in nulliparae to over 100g in high multiparae. Growth is rapid in pregnancy reaching a mean of about 1100g at term, a gain of about 1kg. While it is widely held that growth of the uterus by hypertrophy occurs only during about the first two-thirds

of pregnancy, after which growth in size is largely the result of stretching, there is no convincing evidence for that view; what little information there is about growth during the second half of pregnancy suggests that growth in weight is continuous.

The breasts. Evidence of breast growth in pregnancy (*see below*) suggests a mean increase in weight during pregnancy of about 450g for both breasts together, with most of that growth occurring before 30 weeks of pregnancy.

Blood. Increase of blood volume, an important component of weight gain, has been detailed on page 84 and in Table 5.1. At term it amounts to about 1·5kg.

The components of weight gain discussed so far are probably all related to fetal weight: the weight of the placenta and the volume of amniotic fluid are certainly related, it seems likely that the growth of the uterus will be influenced by the size of its contents, and the amount of increase in blood volume has been shown to be a function of fetal weight. What remains to be accounted for is more than a third of the total average weight gain, between 4·5 and 5kg, not in organs specifically concerned with reproduction but associated with generalized compositional changes in the mother's body: body water and depot fat.

MATERNAL BODY WATER

Total body water, as estimated by such tracers as deuterium oxide, increases by an average of some 8·5 litres in healthy pregnant women but with great variation due largely to differences of oedema (*see below*). 'Extracellular' water, usually determined as the sodium or thiocyanate space, increases by an average of about 6·5 litres. A large proportion of those

Table 5.2   An estimate of total and extracellular water added during pregnancy compared with measured increments

	Total water g	Extracellular water g
Fetus	2343	1360
Placenta	540	260
Amniotic fluid	792	792
Uterus	743	490
Mammary glands	304	148
Plasma	1150	1150
Red cells	163	0
Calculated total	6035	4200
Average measured increase	8500	6500
Difference	2465	2300

increments is in the water contents of the components listed above (Table 5.2) but some 2·5 litres remains to be accounted for, and all or about all of it appears to be extracellular.

The effect of oedema

As would be expected, women who develop obvious oedema in pregnancy accumulate more body water than those who have no oedema. The 'unaccounted-for' water which averages 2·5 litres (Table 5.3) amounts to only about

common in pregnancy, being noted during routine antenatal examinations in at least 40 per cent of normotensive women, in about one-third of whom the distribution was generalized; it occurs more commonly in women with hypertensive disorders. Moreover the presence of oedema is associated with babies of greater birth weight who may have a smaller, certainly not an increased perinatal mortality rate. The increased size of the infants is not associated with increased length of gesta-

Table 5.3 Analysis of weight gain

Tissues and fluids accounted for and total weight gained	Increase in weight (g) up to:			
	10 weeks	20 weeks	30 weeks	40 weeks
Fetus	5	300	1 500	3 400
Placenta	20	170	430	650
Amniotic fluid	30	350	750	800
Uterus (blood free)	140	320	600	970
Mammary gland (blood free)	45	180	360	405
Blood	100	600	1 300	1 500
Extracellular extravascular fluid				
(1) No oedema or leg oedema	0	30	80	1 430
(2) Generalized oedema	0	500	1 526	4 647
Total				
(1) No oedema or leg oedema	324	1 950	5 020	9 155
(2) Generalized oedema	324	2 420	6 466	12 372
Total weight gained				
(1) No oedema or leg oedema	650	4 000	8 500	12 500
(2) Generalized oedema	650	4 500	10 000	14 500
Weight not accounted for				
(1) No oedema or leg oedema	326	2 050	3 480	3 345
(2) Generalized oedema	326	2 080	3 534	2 128

1·5 litres in women who develop no clinical oedema and about 2 litres in women with no more than leg oedema, but averages almost 5 litres in women who develop more generalized oedema even though this is almost always clinically trivial, typically no more than a tight wedding ring. In general 'unaccounted-for' water is apparent only after 30 weeks; before that, all the water accumulated by the mother can be attributed to the water content of the product of conception, growth of reproductive organs, and blood. But in women with generalized oedema, 'excess' water is apparent from about mid-pregnancy.

Oedema is traditionally regarded as a serious sign of pathology even although most obstetricians are aware that it commonly occurs in healthy pregnant women. There is extensive epidemiological evidence that oedema is indeed

tion, nor apparently with oedema of the infants themselves; it appears to be due to a genuine increase in the rate of fetal growth.

Thus it seems that oedema in healthy pregnant women can be regarded as both common and normal, and it is physiological for the mother to store several litres of extracellular water in her own tissues. The interpretation of oedema in normal pregnancy depends on an understanding of where this excess water is lodged, how it is stored, and what its purpose might be.

The nature of oedema

The classic Starling concept of oedema as fluid escaping from the capillaries to the extracellular space seems a plausible explanation of leg oedema. The ordinary pitting ankle oedema is clearly gravitational and tends to disappear when the legs are raised. It would be provoked by increased venous pressure in the lower limbs due to pressure from the uterus on the pelvic veins and by the fall in colloid osmotic pressure due to the sudden drop in plasma protein concentration occurring in pregnancy. And yet the evidence suggests that oedema of the legs accounts for very little of the unaccounted-for extracellular water, probably no more than an average of about 300ml.

It is therefore necessary to account for upwards of 1·5 litres of body water which the normal pregnant woman stores even in the absence of clinical oedema, and a considerably greater amount in women with more generalized, though clinically slight, oedema. The key to understanding the widespread and variable water retention in pregnancy appears to lie in the ground substance of connective tissue, a highly complex mixture of chemicals with a large content of mucopolysaccharides. Among its many functions it has been described as the great reservoir of water and ions, determining their concentrations in the cellular environment, and constituting the chief mechanism for homeostasis of the cellular environment. A modern concept of the ground substance is as a two phase system having a dense colloid-rich, water-poor stroma in which small sub-microscopic droplets of watery, colloid-poor solution exist in osmotic equilibrium. In this system salt solutions can be taken up without 'diluting' the colloids and upsetting osmotic equilibrium, simply by increasing the number of small droplets, and the relative proportion of the two phases could vary within wide limits.

An increase in the water content of the ground substance causes it to swell and become softer; connective tissue becomes more stretchable. Such changes are known to take place under the influence of hormones, for example the cock's comb under the influence of androgen and the sex skin of the monkey under the influence of oestrogen. Local oedema has been induced by oestrogens in the skin of the mouse and it seems very probable that the normal pregnant woman also exhibits a physiological oedema due to oestrogens. A profound change in connective tissue occurs in the direction of increased softness and mobility; for example the cervix is more readily distensible, the pelvic joints become lax, and the anchorages of the nipple are more stretchable. The skin contains large amounts of connective tissue

and it is likely that much of the unaccounted-for extracellular water is held in it, leading often, though not always, to clinical oedema.

The postulated change in the consistency of the ground substance, which includes the basement membranes of cells, would increase the diffusibility of solutes and so facilitate the nutrition of cells.

Thus a physiological change which may be an important aspect of the maternal adaption to pregnancy may lead to an outward sign, swelling, which has been traditionally regarded as indicating a pathological condition. Such a change would explain the finding that otherwise healthy women with clinical oedema have an enhanced reproductive performance. If oedema in pregnancy is a normal phenomenon due to the effect of oestrogens on connective tissue ground substance it is difficult to understand why it is not clinically obvious in all pregnant women. Evidence suggests that the change in ground substance is universal in pregnancy but why the clinical manifestations are so variable remains a mystery.

MATERNAL BODY FAT

From figure 5.4 and Table 5.3, it is clear that a large part of the maternal weight gain, about 3·5kg is still unaccounted for, but contains no water; it can only be body fat.

The earlier suggestion that the pregnant woman stores protein can no longer be supported; not only because the balance studies which led to the idea were almost certainly fallacious but because the body has little capacity to 'store' protein, and that must in any case be stored with some four times its weight in water.

Evidence for extensive fat storage is, at present, indirect and circumstantial. But the hypothesis is supported by the fact that many women become ruefully aware of increasing adiposity, especially round the hips, during pregnancy and more objective support comes from the evidence of increasing skinfold thickness particularly around the thighs and abdomen, and from the fact that the 3·5kg of weight is still present several weeks after delivery.

Stores of fat laid down on such a scale during the first two-thirds of pregnancy represent the provision of a substantial energy reserve: 3·5kg of fat would be capable of supplying more than 30 000kcal, enough to sustain fetal growth during the last trimester or to subsidize the energy cost of lactation. It is the end point of a complex change in maternal energy balance in pregnancy.

Energy metabolism

The large positive energy balance which leads to the storage by the mother of 3·5kg of body fat in a few months is accomplished by a number of physiological adjustments. The primary change is probably the resetting by progesterone of the central control of body composition, the 'lipostat', which is adjusted to accept an extra 3·5kg of body fat. That new demand can be met either by a greater energy intake as food or by a reduced energy output, and the normal pregnant woman appears to use both approaches. Her appetite increases from early pregnancy and she eats an average of some 200kcal more than her normal intake throughout pregnancy. But she also economizes on energy output, resting more, remaining longer in bed, and perhaps more importantly, performing her usual tasks with greater economy of effort; the pregnant woman is much more 'relaxed'. She is helped in her general relaxation by a somewhat lower level of free thyroid hormone, voluntary muscle tone and metabolism generally is reduced.

uterine muscle, and almost 4kg of fat, mostly in the maternal depots but also in the fetus; and, (2) 'Running costs' which are represented mostly by the metabolic needs of the product of conception and the extra maternal tissue, and by the additional cardiac and respiratory work of the mother.

It is clear from the figure that the storage of fat is a large proportion of the total energy needs and that the amount accumulated in the first two-thirds of pregnancy could readily subsidize the running costs in the last trimester. The figure also demonstrates the relatively even distribution of energy needs throughout pregnancy, the increasing metabolic demands of late pregnancy balanced by the capital gains earlier in pregnancy.

Nutritient metabolism

Glucose. The complexities of glucose metabolism are not well understood in the non-pregnant person and there is little doubt that pregnancy complicates the picture still further. Some needless complication is added by an entrenched belief that pregnancy is 'diabetogenic' and although it must be admitted that the incidence of diabetes in late middle age is

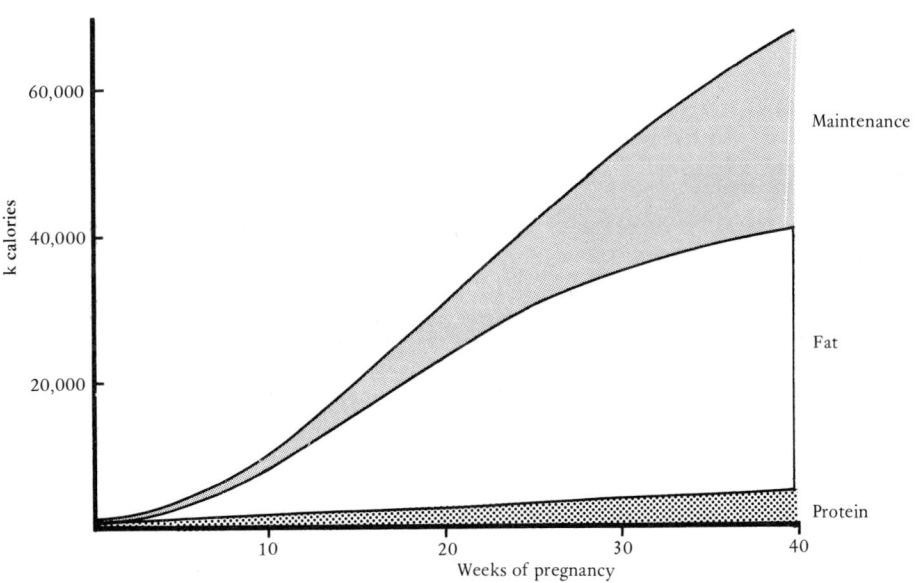

Fig. 5.5 The cumulative energy cost of pregnancy and its major components.

The total cumulative energy balance in pregnancy is shown in figure 5.5. It is made up of two major components: (1) 'Capital gains' represented by the storage of almost 1kg of protein, largely in the fetus, placenta and extra

related to parity and that established diabetes is worsened by pregnancy, the changes which occur during the course of normal pregnancy are difficult to interpret. Compared to the non-pregnant person fasting blood glucose is reduced throughout pregnancy by about 10mg/100ml, but blood glucose changes in response to an oral glucose load, although remaining well within normal limits, suggest a slight but progressive 'intolerance' in that the peak level is reached later and the blood glucose remains above fasting for longer. That change in blood glucose is accompanied by a more dramatic change in plasma insulin, the peak levels of which rise progressively in pregnancy to considerably above the usual non-pregnant response. That is to say the pregnant woman requires much more insulin than usual to maintain glucose homeostasis; she might be described as 'insensitive' to insulin, and is indeed less sensitive than usual to an injected dose. The basis of her insensitivity, or 'insulin antagonism' is not known. The growth hormone—like HCS has been suggested and may play some part, so may increased corticosteroid levels; there is no information about glucagon.

Glycosuria has been mentioned above; it is commonplace in pregnancy and so far inexplicable. It does not carry the same significance as glycosuria in the non-pregnant person.

Lipids. Lipid metabolism has been less investigated and is even less well understood than glucose metabolism. The levels in blood of all lipids rise considerably during pregnancy (*see* page 86) and some investigators have shown particularly high circulating levels of free fatty acids (NEFA) in late pregnancy. The levels of NEFA rise during the last few weeks of pregnancy when fat storage gives way to lipolysis.

Cholesterol metabolism also appears to be considerably altered and the conspicuous rise in plasma level has been found in many different populations, vegetarian and non-vegetarian. A diet low in saturated fatty acids and high in polyunsaturated fatty acids, which invariably reduces plasma cholesterol in the non-pregnant person, has no effect in pregnancy; and injected glucose, with or without insulin, which also usually reduces plasma cholesterol, appears to raise it in pregnancy.

Homeostasis of other nutrients. Like glucose, but unlike lipids, almost all other nutrients appear to be maintained at circulating levels well below those usual for the non-pregnant woman. That is true of most free amino acids and the water soluble vitamins, for example, ascorbic acid, pyridoxin, riboflavine, vitamin B_{12} and folate, although the amino acid levels, like glucose, characteristically fall to a new low level in early pregnancy while the vitamin levels tend to decline slowly throughout pregnancy.

The almost universal reduction in the blood levels of nutrients suggests a common mechanism or perhaps a common purpose. No mechanism is known; dietary deficiency or failure of absorption is certainly not responsible, at least for most of the low levels described, although many can be artificially raised by large dietary supplements. Nor is it likely that the kidney plays more than a marginal role: all women show a reduced fasting blood sugar but not all have increased glycosuria; and there is little relation between amino acid excretion and blood levels. For example, histidine which is lost in greatest amounts has raised blood levels in pregnancy.

It is perhaps worth stressing the general implausibility of dietary deficiency as a cause of reduced nutrient levels in normal pregnancy. First, it is hardly rational to claim that a phenomenon affecting all healthy well-nourished women having normal pregnancies and healthy babies is due to dietary inadequacy. Second, the reduced concentrations often occur in the presence of greatly increased total circulating quantities. Third, it also seems illogical to claim that reduced levels of some nutrients such as folate, vitamin B_6 and inorganic iron indicate dietary deficiency and require supplemental supplies when other nutrients with equally reduced levels such as glucose, taurine, ornithine and even bicarbonate are ignored. The changes in blood concentrations are so widespread and varied in detail that we are left with the impression that levels of many different nutrients are reduced by a resetting of many different homeostatic mechanisms, which suggests a common purpose.

It may be that a general lowering of nutrient levels in the blood produces a balance which favours transfer to the fetus rather than to the maternal tissues. The placenta is clearly able to take up nutrients with considerable efficiency from maternal blood and store within its cells particularly high concentrations of the nutrients we are discussing; it is perhaps better able to do so at the low levels in blood in pregnancy than are the maternal tissues.

It is reasonable to assume that, in health, the body maintains in its fluid environment the amounts and concentrations of the substance it needs for maximum efficiency of function; that is the purpose of homeostasis. If that is so then the greatly altered amounts and concentrations which are characteristic of pregnancy cannot reasonably be assumed to be equally advantageous to the mother's metabolism. The most plausible explanation is that they represent changes which allow maximum efficiency of fetal growth and metabolism.

The fetus, using hormones as manipulators, over-rides and resets the mother's homeostatic mechanism in its own interests; it is the price of viviparity.

Nutritional requirements during pregnancy

Nutritional requirements are specified on the basis of physiological knowledge or, empirically, from the observed dietary habits of healthy people. As knowledge of nutritional physiology has increased, so the requirement standards prepared by various authorities have tended to conform more closely, and distinctions between 'minimum' and 'optimum' requirements have been less used. Table 5.4 summarizes, in a modified form to simplify comparisons, some current recommended allowances for non-pregnant and pregnant women engaged in light activity. The three sets of standards are broadly in agreement. They are all intended to apply to populations; the amounts specified should cover the needs of nearly all healthy individuals in such groups, with an adequate margin of safety. It would be wrong to conclude, without clinical evidence, that because the diet of an individual falls short of a standard it is therefore inadequate.

Table 5.4   Daily recommended allowances for non-pregnant and pregnant women doing light work

	United Nations		USA		United Kingdom	
	Non-pregnant	Pregnant	Non-pregnant	Pregnant	Non-pregnant	Pregnant
Weight, kg	55	—	58	—	55	—
Weight gain, kg	—	10 ± 2	—	11	—	12·5
Energy, kcal	2300	40 000 per pregnancy	2000	2200	2200	2400
Protein, g	56	65	55	65	55	60
Calcium, g	0·4–0·5	1·0–1·2	0·8	1·2	0·5	1·2
Iron, mg	14–28	14–28	18	18	12	15
Vitamin A, IU	2500	2500	5000	6000	2500	2500
Vitamin D, IU	100	400	none	400	100	400
Thiamine, mg	0·9	1·0	1·0	1·1	0·9	1·0
Riboflavin, mg	1·3	1·4	1·5	1·8	1·3	1·6
Nicotinic acid, mg equiv.	15·2	16·5	13	15	15	18
Vitamin B_6, mg	—	—	2·0	2·5	—	—
Folate, μg	200	400	400	800	—	—
Vitamin B_{12}, μg	2·0	3·0	5·0	8·0	—	—
Ascorbic acid, mg	30	50	55	60	30	60

Sources:

UNITED KINGDOM

Recommended intakes of nutrients for the United Kingdom, Department of Health and Social Security, Reports on Public Health and Medical Subjects, No. 120 (HMSO, London 1969).

USA

Recommended dietary allowances. Nat. Acad. Sci., Nat. Res. Counc. Publ. 1964, Washington (1968).

UNITED NATIONS

Calorie requirements. FAO Nutritional Studies, No. 15 (Food and Agriculture Organization of the United Nations, Rome 1957).

Calcium requirements. FAO Nutr. Meetings Rep. Ser., No. 30 (Food and Agriculture Organization of the United Nations, Rome); also WHO Tech. Rep. Ser., No. 230 (World Health Organization, Geneva 1962).

Protein requirements. FAO Nutr. Meetings Rep. Ser., No. 37 (Food and Agriculture Organization of the United Nations, Rome); also WHO Tech. Rep. Ser., No. 301 (World Health Organization, Geneva 1965).

Requirements of vitamin A, thiamine, riboflavin and niacin. WHO Tech. Rep. Ser., No. 362 (World Health Organization, Geneva); also FAO Nutr. Meetings Rep. Ser., No. 41 (Food and Agriculture Organization of the United Nations, Rome 1967).

Requirements of ascorbic acid, vitamin D, vitamin B_{12}, folate and iron. FAO Nutr. Meetings Rep. Ser., No. 47 (Food and Agriculture Organization of the United Nations, Rome); also WHO Tech. Rep. Ser., No. 452 (World Health Organization, Geneva 1970).

The energy cost of pregnancy has already been outlined above and summarized in figure 5.5. Eating to appetite, a woman will gain some 12·5kg in pregnancy, 3·5kg of it depot fat, and her specific energy requirements will total about 70 000kcal; for most of pregnancy, something over 300kcal/day. But because she economizes in her usual activities, the overall energy requirement of the pregnant woman is only about 200kcal above her usual daily non-pregnant needs and that is the recommended allowance by both the United Kingdom and the USA (Table 5.4). There is certainly no basis for the notion that the pregnant woman should 'eat for two'; she should be encouraged to eat sufficient to allow her to gain about 1lb weight per week, a weight gain associated with the best clinical performance.

Pregnancy is not the best time to start slimming, but no harm will be done to the baby by encouraging obese mothers to eat less and gain less than the average 1lb per week. There is no case for restricting diet during pregnancy so severely as to cause discomfort; maternal fat gained during pregnancy is usually lost later without the need to take any dietary measures.

Nutrients. The specific requirement for protein imposed by pregnancy amounts to a maximum, near term, of only some 5 or 6 grams daily. With a varied diet of sufficient energy value, it is difficult to reduce the protein intake to an inadequate level. This holds for most other nutrients, the supply of which tends to be correlated with calorie intake. Danger arises, when, through bad dietary habits, fads, lack of education, or insufficient purchasing power, the dietary mixture is insufficiently varied and especially when important sources of certain nutrients may be omitted almost entirely. It is not uncommon for women, and especially pregnant women, to confess that they never willingly eat fruit or green vegetables, or that they dislike milk or eggs, and aberrations of appetite, occasionally amounting to pica, may distort the dietary pattern. Dietetic inquiry and advice should seek to identify and to remedy such defects and to restore what is recognized to be a good mixed diet. The average nutritive value of a good mixed diet is specified in the recommended allowances (Table 5.4) and under ordinary conditions there is no need for grossly exaggerated intake levels, nor for supplementation of ordinary foods with concentrates.

The role of supplements. It is widely held that the specific needs for iron, calculated as 4–5mg daily, cannot be met by the ordinary diet and that view is reflected by both WHO and the USA in recommended allowances which cannot be met by a normal unsupplemented diet. The recommendations for folate are also based on amounts sufficient to prevent any occurrence of megaloblastic anaemia in a pregnant population; they are not based on the ordinary needs of healthy women.

The recommendations for calcium are also excessively generous and 1200mg daily would certainly require the consumption of above average amounts of milk or milk products. While not wanting to discourage the drinking of milk it should be noted that repeated childbearing by women who consume only about one-third of that allowance does not lead to any depletion of the skeleton.

It has been noted above that some of the physiological adaptations of normal pregnancy masquerade as deficiency signs, but at the same time it must be acknowledged that deficiency states are more common in pregnancy than at other times. It seems most rational, not to prescribe relatively enormous amounts of hypothetically inadequate nutrients, but to observe individual patients carefully so that true deficiencies can be identified and treated appropriately.

Therapeutic dietetics. The dietitian can do much to ease the miseries suffered by some pregnant women from digestive discomforts such as nausea, heartburn, and constipation. It is temptingly easy for the clinician simply to prescribe an appropriate pill and, since most cases improve anyway, to believe he is doing enough. But appropriate dietetic advice can often be equally effective, and offering it gives another channel through which the aims of nutritional education can be pursued. It has been pointed out above (page 95) that oedema during pregnancy should not be regarded as evidence of pathology. Under ordinary conditions no treatment is required and natriuretic drugs are positively dangerous. But in a minority of cases oedema reaches a degree that is uncomfortable and even disabling; and in such cases a low-salt diet (*not* a salt-free diet) may be very helpful.

LACTATION

Preparatory changes in the breasts

Tenderness of the breasts, sensations of tingling or of fullness and sometimes obvious enlargement are early signs of pregnancy. Such early changes during the first two months are probably no more than the result of vascular engorgement, for there is often a reduction of volume between 10 and 14 weeks. Thereafter the breasts enlarge regularly, chiefly or entirely by growth of the gland tissue, but with great individual variation.

The stimulus to growth of the mammary gland is presumed to be hormonal but which hormone or mixture of hormones is unclear. Animal evidence suggests that the major influence is prolactin with ovarian steroids playing no more than a subsidiary role; in human pregnancy chorionic sommatomammotrophin (HCS) may be primarily responsible for breast development.

No direct measurement of the increase of weight of the breasts in pregnancy seems possible for, even if the weight of breasts removed during the puerperium were recorded, the increase could not be estimated without knowledge of the weight of the gland before pregnancy. Growth has therefore been measured as increase of volume by a water displacement method. In primigravidae in early pregnancy (9–12 weeks) the mean volume of one breast, was about 565ml; it rose to about 665ml at 20 weeks and 775ml at term. Multigravidae had a somewhat higher volume at the beginning, about 590ml, and reached a mean of about 780ml at term. There was little change during the last 10 weeks. The increase in primigravidae between the end of the first trimester and term varied from zero to as much as 880ml; with a mean of about 230ml. In multigravidae there was a smaller range about a similar mean. Taking both groups together the increase of volume is estimated at 75ml between 10 and 20 weeks, 100ml between 20 and 30 weeks, and with small allowances for early pregnancy and the last 10 weeks, the total is about 250ml for each breast, 500ml in all.

In primigravidae the increase of breast size declines steeply with age from a mean of about 230ml in those below 20 years of age to a third of that volume in women over 30. The difference with age is less in multigravidae. The

combined estimate of 500ml given above is applicable to young women.

The components of the weight increase have not been precisely described. Since little fat is laid on above the waist line during pregnancy, little of the breast increase will be fat. Clinically the breast appears to be highly vascular and an assumption that 10 per cent of the increase of volume in blood is not likely to be an overestimate. The main component would be expected to be glandular, but the quantity of functional glandular tissues varies as widely as the increase of volume. Autopsy studies of the breasts of recently delivered women have shown variation from the richly glandular structure of the typical textbook illustration, which is almost always found in lower mammals, to breasts composed almost entirely of fibrous tissue. That being so, it is not surprising that the success of lactation may be forecast from the increase in volume of the breasts during pregnancy. The correlation coefficient between milk yield on the 7th day, when the flow is properly established, and the increase of breast volume averaged 0·46 for 77 primiparae or 0·53 when the effect of age was eliminated, the difference suggesting that, for a given increase of breast volume, the younger primiparae produced more milk than the older. Further, the fat content of 7th day milk falls with rising age from 3·25 per cent for primiparae under 20 years of age to 2·83 per cent in primiparae over 30. Since the difference with age is less in multiparae than in primiparae, there appears to be a sort of disuse atrophy of glandular tissue when the breast does not function for many years after sexual maturity. The changes that occur in the menstrual cycle are not sufficient to maintain the functional efficiency of the gland.

But age is not the only, perhaps not even the major, determinant of efficiency in lactation; genetic make-up may be more important. Since substitute mothers and substitute milks have always been available for the human infant, capacity to lactate has seldom or never been of survival value and indeed the overall size of the breast, as distinct from the increase in pregnancy, is but poorly related to milk production. The breast has become more important as a sex symbol than as an organ to provide food for an infant.

The endocrine changes that initiate and control lactation are discussed in Chapter 4. It is not known whether, or to what extent, yield and composition of milk are under hormonal control. General health, physique and state of nutrition appear to have little to do with the inception of lactation and there is no satisfactory evidence that the composition of milk can be much altered by manipulation of the diet except, for instance, for such water soluble components, like the water soluble vitamins, as are stored in only small amounts in the body and appear in milk in close relation to the current supply.

Milk yield

During the first two or three days of lactation there is secretion of only a little, concentrated milk, 'colostrum', after which there is a rapid increase in yield which averages about 400ml at the end of the first week of lactation and about 700ml when lactation is fully established. Individual variation is very wide and within limits the yield adjusts to the demand of the infant.

Yield and fat content are not related and failure of lactation may be due to low yield with a normal or high fat content, or high yield with so low a fat content that the energy supplied will not support growth of the infant. It is estimated that about one-third of women are genuinely incapable of rearing a child on breast milk because of one or other of such abnormalities.

Cost of and requirements for milk production

All the energy-yielding components of breast milk show considerable variation, fat most of all, and the cost will be assessed only on a compromise that may be regarded as average breast milk. It will have about 7 per cent lactose, 1 per cent protein and 3·5 per cent fat, in early lactation, with an energy value of about 65kcal/100ml. The standard infant of 3·3kg weight, if it has only about 400ml milk at first has about 260kcal, or 80kcal/kg body weight. If the usual estimates of requirements of the infant are valid, the yield, or the fat content, or both must rise rapidly to allow normal growth. On the assumption that the infant has reached a weight of about 5·5kg by three months and requires an energy intake to thrive of some 95kcal/kg, then 520kcal, or about 800ml of milk is necessary. With an allowance of between 2100 and 2400kcal for her own use, and an efficiency of 90 per cent in conversion of food to milk energy, the total requirement of the lactating woman by three months of lactation will be something of the order of 2700 to 3000kcal, if the milk is to be produced from current food intake. It is certain that few women are accustomed, or would find it easy, to eat sufficient food to provide 3000kcal and the likelihood is that milk production will be subsidized, energy from the fat accumulated in early pregnancy and calcium from skeletal reserves. The fact that many women find breast feeding exhausting is not surprising.

REFERENCES

Hytten, F. E. & Leitch, I. (1971) *The Physiology of Human Pregnancy*. 2nd ed. London: Blackwell.
Philip, E. E., Barnes, Josephine B. & Newton, M. (1970) Ed. *Scientific Foundation of Obstetrics and Gynaecology*. London: Heinemann.
Shearman, R. P. (1972) Ed. Human Reproductive Physiology. London: Blackwell.

6. Growth and Development of Fetus and Placenta

A detailed knowledge of embryology and of factors influencing fertility, growth and development, can best be obtained in specialist books and journals. It is, however, essential that the obstetrician have some knowledge and understanding of the normal processes and of their complexity. During development the human fetus passes through many phases where the environmental conditions are critical for normal development and at several stages damage may occur which may have obvious and immediate effects or may influence any future development though abnormality is not declared until childhood or adolescence.

Development is customarily divided firstly into an *embryonic phase* which lasts from fertilization for some 60 days (i.e. some 11 weeks from LMP), by which time the fetus has acquired its definitive form, and has built the main outlines of its organs. The first part (some 5–6 days) of the embryonic period from fertilization until implantation has an importance of its own. During the *fetal period* from 60 days until delivery the organs undergo differentiation and maturation at the histological level.

During fetal life the *ova* derived from the original oogonia have undergone a series of changes of meioses and the ovary at birth may contain up to 2×10^6 oocytes with differentiation arrested. Of those, some 200–300 will reach maturity after puberty and become capable of further development. From the birth of the child until each individual ovum is ultimately stimulated to ovulation (i.e. a period ranging from say 13–50 years) meiosis in the ovum is arrested in the metaphase of the premeiotic division and this is a complete resting phase. The chromosomes have already paired awaiting the first maturation division which does not begin until hormonal stimulation causes this individual ovum to prepare for ovulation. Over those years maternal material can be transferred from the granulosa cells to the ovum and it is possible that even **DNA** may pass, suggesting the possibility of maternal or other external influences on the ova. Moreover during the long waiting period chromosomal damage may certainly occur and of course, a very large number of cells atrophy and disappear. The whole period during which an ovum may await ultimate development may last from the third month of fetal life until the mother is fifty.

Under stimulation of ovarian secretion at each menstrual cycle one or more follicles and oocytes begin to mature. The oocyte at this time still has 44 chromosomes plus normally two X chromosomes. Just before ovulation the first maturation division occurs and one daughter cell receives a disproportionately small amount of cytoplasm and becomes the first polar body. Very soon the second division begins and the oocyte with the first polar body enters the Fallopian tube. While the commencement of the second meiotic division is stimulated by release from the follicle the final phase can take place only after fertilization. This phase of second meiotic division is a particularly vulnerable one and the successful fertilization must take place within 12–14 hours. The ovum despite its reserves will die if not fertilized and there is some evidence that trisomy and monosomy and other anomalies are more frequent when the egg at fertilization is close to death (i.e., there has been a longer period of arrest at the second meiotic division).

The *sperm* during passage through the genital tract gradually acquires the ability to penetrate the zonapellucida of the ovum and so fertilize it. This 'capacitation' is due probably to removal of some material from the sperm head and may in fact take place in the endocervix. Following capacitation there is an increase in glucose uptake and lactate production by the sperm.

Passage through the genital tract into the outer end of the Fallopian is very rapid, suggested times varying from 5 minutes to some hours.

Sperm normality is retained for a long period within the male tract but once within the female tract the sperms age rapidly. There is a suggestion that ageing sperms are equally at risk. The sperm may fail to fertilize or the ovum may die soon after fertilization or continue growth to produce abnormal fetuses. In reflex ovulating mammals where coitus occurs only at the time of heat, or where ovulation is stimulated by coitus, relatively fresh ova and sperms are guaranteed. The human does not have this protection.

The capacitated sperm and the ovum in the second meiotic division normally come together in the outer end of the Fallopian tube. Tubal fluids are probably necessary also to aid fertilization by loosening the corona. With penetration of the zonapellucida of the ovum by the whole sperm (head and tail), which enters under influence of hyaluronidase, the second meiotic division is completed and the second polar body formed and extruded. With this division the chromosome number is reduced by half and there are, therefore, within the oocyte 22 autosomes and one X sex chromosome in the female and within the sperm head 22 autosomes and one X or Y sex chromosome. There is in addition the cytoplasm contributed by the sperm tail.

The chromosome of the ovum condenses into a female pronucleus and the sperm head enlarges to form the male pronucleus. Soon the pronuclei membranes break down and the chromosomes are liberated into the cytoplasm and intermix. Fusion is rapid and fertilization is then complete. The two cell stage appears shortly afterwards, this process taking some 36 hours in man.

It is essential that the ovum remain within the tube for 3–5 days. Its passage through the tube is aided by cilia and fluid movement but there is also some contraction of spiral muscles at the uterine end of the tube to retain the ovum in the tube. During this period active metabolism takes place and glucose and other nourishment is contributed by the tubal fluid. Within the ovum even at the 4–8 cell stage there is already mitochrondrial biochemical activity and some differentiation of areas towards ultimate function already within each individual cell. The eight-cell stage is reached in some 60 hours, and the morula stage by the fourth day. Until this time

there is no increase in size of the ovum which is still within the zonapellucida but merely a redistribution of cytoplasm into each of the daughter cells. By the fifth day fluid has appeared within the cell mass. The 'blastocyst' has lost its zonapellucida by the sixth day after fertilization (or the 20–21st day after first day of LMP), and there is clear differentiation of syncytiotrophoblast and cytotrophoblast and inner cell mass.

The ovum by the lytic action of its trophoblast burrows into the endometrium and implantation has taken place. The richly vascularized, oedematous, glycogen rich endometrium is highly favourable to the implantation. In the few days which follow, the endometrium further develops to increase the nutrition available to the implanting embryo. It is two or three days after implantation (i.e. 24th day of cycle) before the full characteristic decidua of pregnancy is developed this being more marked in the area of implantation.

The ovum normally invades the myometrium between a pair of endometrial glands. The actively invading trophoblast, erodes the stroma and breaks into the glands. Slight haemorrhage into the glands in association with the invading trophoblast is seen occasionally externally. This is the placental sign which occurs at the time of the first missed period and may be confusing.

Recognition by the mother

The maternal organism must be aware of the presence of a fertilized egg before implantation so that corpus luteum death is not allowed to occur. The ovum implants on the 20th day and there is full decidual development by the 24th day, by which time HCG can be detected in the urine, i.e. some 10 days after ovulation. HCG can be detected in the plasma certainly 15 days after ovulation and just about the time the period would be missed.

Placental progesterone is also detectable by the time of the first missed period and by the 21st day after ovulation (say 36 days after LMP), the placenta may produce enough progesterone to maintain the pregnancy. It is clear, however, that the timing must be very important and the maternal organism can only become aware of the presence of the fetus a very few days before corpus luteum failure is expected to occur.

DEVELOPMENT OF THE FETUS

Proper development of the trophoblast and inner cell mass require the presence each of the other. The trophoblast some distance from the inner cell mass develops as syncytiotrophoblast and has an invasive lytic character.

The inner cell mass which will ultimately form the fetus has separated from the cells of the trophoblast and has differentiated by the time of implantation. This differentiation into cells with different functions probably begins as early as the 8–16 cell stage.

While the blastocyst is still implanting changes appear in the inner cell mass. The primitive endoderm appears on its inner surface and the remaining cells form the primitive

5 Bronchial buds develop: mesonephros established, metanephros appears, brain vesicles, suprarenal appear.
6 Mullerian duct appears: optic cup well formed: head dominant in size: limb buds seen.
7 Stomach and duodenum and intestine definitive: anal membrane ruptures: cardiac valves: muscle differentiation.
8 Fetal state attained: testes and ovary distinguishable: main blood vessels defined: ossification begins.
10 Pancreatic alveoli present: kidney secreting: enamel organs forming: lymph glands: movement clearly shown.
12–16 Becomes human in appearance: muscle activity: meconium collects: joints appear: body hair appears: sweat glands

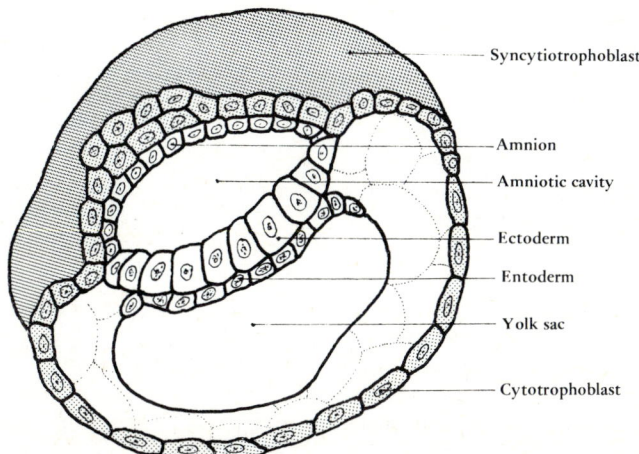

Fig. 6.1 The two-layered ovum at the time of implantation.

ectoderm. The amniotic cavity then appears as a vesicle within the upper part of the inner cell mass.

Following implantation the embryo is a two layer disc within the amniotic cavity (Fig. 6.1).

Developmental landmarks

A very full description can be found in any textbook of human development (*see* Arey, 1966), but certain landmarks can be cited.

Age in weeks (add two weeks for age from LMP)
2–3 Neural groove indicated: Blood islands on yolk sac: Head process present.
4 Neural groove closes: eye vesicles appear: heartbeat: thyroid and liver buds detectable.

develop: sense organ differentiation is completed: brain well developed; etc.

After this period the chief changes are growth and further histological differentiation, the cells gradually coming to assume their final form under the gene influence in their nuclei.

Determination and differentiation of sex

The ultimate sex of the individual is determined by a series of complicated manoeuvres not yet fully understood. The reader is referred to Short (1972) for an extensive discussion.

Genetic sex is determined largely by the sex chromosomes. The cells of the normal human female have two X chromosomes and all ova contain two such chromosomes. Each X chromosome carries at least sixty genes for characters such as colour vision, blood clotting and certain diseases such as muscular dystrophy. The male has an XY chromosome system and some of his sperms carry an X chromosome and the others a Y. Genetic sex of the offspring is determined by the male sperm in the human. The normal female inactivates one of her X chromosomes about the 12–16th day. Females with more than one X chromosome randomly inactivate all but one. The inactivated X chromosomes replicate and are, in the adult seen as inclusion (Barr Bodies) in the female cells or as the drum sticks in the leucocytes. A male similarly with two X chromosomes, e.g. XXY (Klinefelter) will inactivate one and show an inclusion body. Inactivation of the X from mother or father is random, 50 per cent being maternal and 50 per cent paternal in origin. Any abnormal X is selectively inactivated. The germ cells do not take part in inactivation.

Once the genetic balance of the fetus is restored by making only one X chromosome functional, sexual differentiation of the gonads begins, by differentiation of the genital ridge. The basic pattern of development is female but *the presence of a Y chromosome in the male fetus* forces differentiation along male lines with the persistence of the medullary sex cords which develop the seminiferous tubules. The Mullerian duct system is locally inhibited by the presence of a Y chromosome and conversely the Wolffian duct system is actively stimulated so that gonadal sex is established.

Differentiation of the *external genitalia* occurs later under the *direct influence of the hormones secreted* by the ovary or testis. Variations or anomalies of such hormones may alter the appearance at almost any stage of development, varying from intra-uterine virilization due to the exhibition of norethisterone to the mother, to the hair growth and voice changes secondary to virilizing ovarian tumours in the adult.

The *hypothalamus*, which controls sexual function, appears at birth to be sexually undifferentiated. Certainly in the rat an injection of androgen to a newborn female rat within the first five days of life results in a permanent lack of oestrous, no ovulation, and loss of female sexual behaviour when the rat reaches adulthood.

Similarly, male rats treated with anti-androgen preparations will develop the cyclical pattern of the female. It would appear, therefore, that at birth the hypothalamus is largely undifferentiated in its functions but that masculinity is impressed upon the hypothalamic behaviour by a surge of androgen from the gonad, round about, or within the first few weeks of the time of birth. The details of determination of hypothalamic sex is, however, not fully known in the human.

Aberrations of sexual differentiation, sexual determination and sexual behaviour are relatively common and of interest; these are described later.

The main hormones which appear to affect sexual differentiation of the brain are the androstenedione and testosterone which can be converted to oestrogen.

Breast development

The primitive mammary bud at the cranial end of the milk line appears in the third or fourth week of fetal life. By the fifth month the deeper layers proliferate and produce secondary epithelial buds which pass deep into the subcutaneous cellular tissues. The cords branch further and develop a lumen and there is further growth and branching up until term. Breast tissue at term may respond to maternal hormones and the breast of the newborn may be swollen and lactate.

Development of the lung

The fetal lung develops from endoderm and mesoderm. The first sign of lung development is at about the third to the fourth week. Glycogen stored within the tissue provides energy for growth by dichotonous branching and by the *24th week* at the latest 75 per cent of all branching has taken place, the bronchi are ciliated and patent, and there are terminal bronchioles lined with cuboidal epithelium which is later shed to produce large terminal air spaces. True alveoli with elastic tissue are a very much later development which may not be completed until after birth. Capillaries associated with air spaces develop rapidly from the *20th week* and the capillary alveolar relationship necessary may be developed earlier or later and is not complete often until adequate respiration is fully begun. Surface tension within the alveoli at first breath resists expansion and makes the establishment of adequate residual capacity difficult. It is the action of *surfactant* which appears first at *23-24 weeks* to permit this loss of tension and allow residual capacity which makes it of vital importance. Surfactant is associated with the appearance of a methyl transferase system and such development is adversely affected by acidosis, hypothermia and hypoxia. Viability is just possible by 24 weeks in the most well developed lungs.

Respiratory movement *in utero* allows some flow of fluid from the lung passages to and from the amniotic cavity. Surfactant is therefore detectable in the amniotic fluid. Fetal respiratory movement recorded by ultrasound may be useful as a sign of fetal wellbeing (*see* Chapter 18).

During fetal life the lung fills the whole of the chest cavity, the passages being full of fluid which is later expelled at the time of birth and what remains absorbed by the pulmonary lymphatics. Independent pulmonary expansion at birth (Davis, 1970) requires clear airways, adequate alveolar area, stable expanded alveoli, adequate pulmonary perfusion, adequate oxygen carrying capacity, satisfactory fetal lymphatic drainage and normal carbohydrate activity and rhythmic respiration.

Fetal circulation

The first fetal circulation begins at a vitelline stage when the fetus is living only on its reserves, and lasts until the 5th week. From then on the placental circulation develops. The heart becomes a four chamber organ by the 7th week. In late pregnancy fetal blood reaches the placenta via the umbilical arteries; from the placenta it reaches the fetus via the umbilical vein. Blood from the umbilical vein (some 70-80 per cent saturated with oxygen) passes to the left lobe of the liver which therefore, receives the most highly oxygenated and nutrition carrying blood from the placenta. A major amount of the flow is bypassed through the ductus venosus to the inferior vena cava where it joins the blood flow from the lower extremity and is somewhat diluted (some 70 per cent saturated). Reaching the right heart most of the blood is immediately directed to the left heart via the foram ovale. It is again somewhat diluted by the minimal pulmonary coronary and other outflow and then passes to the aorta (60 per cent saturated) and so to the coronary vessels, brain and upper part of the body. The remainder of the blood after mixing with the blood in the ductus arteriosus passes to the abdominal aorta and the rest of the body below that point.

Blood returning from the superior vena cava passes to the right heart and is then directed largely via the ductus arteriosus from the pulmonary vessels to the aortic arch.

The freshest (oxygen plus nutrition) blood goes therefore, to the left lobe of liver, brain and coronary vessels. The right lobe of liver receives poorly oxygenated blood (less than 30 per cent saturated) via the portal circulation and the hepatic arteries and in conditions of severe anoxia when that blood contains virtually no oxygen may suffer necrotic change.

At birth, with removal of the placenta and cessation of umbilical flow there is reduction of pressure in the (R) heart and the foramen ovale (fails to open and) is held loosely closed by pressures in the (L) heart being a little higher. Closure by adhesion is later and sometimes incomplete. The ductus arteriosus closes partially quite quickly and finally slowly over many days largely as a result of contraction of the muscle in its wall under the influence of increasing pO_2 in the contained blood. In conditions of anoxia the ductus may remain open thus contributing further to the problem of the anoxia. At birth the muscle walls of the ventricles are equal in thickness but rapidly the left ventricular wall grows much thicker as the fetus grows, and the blood pressure rises with increasing resistance to outflow.

DEVELOPMENT OF THE FEMALE GENITALIA

At the 5th week the primordial germ cells migrate within the dorsal mesentery from their original site near the yolk sac to reach the previously undifferentiated gonad. In the genital ridges the primitive sex cords proliferate and those cords become ultimately seminiferous tubules in the male and medullary cords in the female. Those cords make junction with a duct of the primitive mesonephros thus uniting the gonad with the mesonephritic duct system. The Wolffian duct is probably formed from one of the tubules of the mesonephric duct gradually establishing itself separate from the mesonephric duct itself along almost its whole length, although it has been suggested that the Wolffian duct is the original pronephric duct which persists and is part of the mesone-phric collecting system.

The Mullerian ducts are formed by in-vagination of the epithelium of the coelome over the genital ridge at the cranial end. Beginning as an epithelial bud the duct penetrates the mesenchyme of the ridge as it grows downwards.

Up until the 7th week of development the genital tracts have the same appearance in both male and female embryos, i.e. there are two Wolffian and two Mullerian ducts. Gradu-ally, however, in the absence of the Y chromo-some the Wolffian duct degenerates and the Mullerian ducts develop and move caudally. The Mullerian ducts ultimately cross the mid-line and the terminal parts of the ducts fuse to form a single median duct which ultimately is the primitive uterus and cervix. The vagina is then formed below that as a budding downwards from the end of the fused Mullerian ducts and this downward budding passes close to and alongside the terminal part of the mesonephric duct. The downward developing vagina meets and fuses with the lateral aspect of the urogenital sinus, part of which proliferates to meet the downward descending vaginal bud which arises from the Mullerian epithelium. The vagina is, there-fore, formed in its upper two-thirds (at least) by epithelium of Mullerian origin and in its lower third by epithelium of origin from endoderm of the urogenital sinus.

By the 4th month the uterus and vaginal areas are definitive, and capable at this time of responding to maternal hormones. All the enzyme systems and the endometrium are intact and function in late fetal life. Glands appear by the 5th month and by term may be almost pre-menstrual in appearance with secretory granules. The uterus and cervix grow throughout pregnancy continuously although at term the cervix is larger than the uterus itself.

Normal female development occurs only in the absence of androgen. Undue androgenic stimulation for example in the female between the 8th and 16th week may prevent normal down growth and development of the vaginal bud and allow the vagina to open into the urethra.

Gradually as development proceeds the perineal portion of the urogenital sinus flattens out so that the urethra and the vaginal orifices reach the surface of the vestibule. By seven weeks the urogenital and anal areas of the cloacal membrane are separated by the peri-neum and by the 9th week the membrane disappears. Further differentiation of the female external genitalia develops during the third month.

Failure of fusion of the terminal portion of the Mullerian ducts results in complete or partial doubling (with a septum) of the uterus, cervix and perhaps of the upper two-thirds of the vagina.

Failure of development of the tissues of the genital ridge on one side will result in a single horn uterus with often the absence of or an abnormal renal or collecting system on the same side.

Lipid metabolism

Synthesis of long chain fatty acids and tri-glycerides takes place in fetal liver, brain and other tissues early in fetal development. Long chain fatty acids also reach the fetus from the mother.

The human fetus synthesizes fat primarily from carbohydrate and the levels, especially of palmitic acid, are high in the normal fetus at birth after the 34th week, but not in the premature where they have not yet been laid down or in the post-mature where they have been used up. At term of course, there is in the posterior triangle of the neck and below the scapulae areas of *brown adipose tissue* able to produce heat in conditions of cold or in aerobic conditions, without shivering. This fat is not useful in hypoxic conditions. The fats of this tissue are mainly triglycerides and exist in many tiny vacuoles within the cytoplasm. The cells have large mitochrondria and a central nucleus.

Cholesterol and several of the complex lipids are of special importance in the forma-tion of myelin in brain development. Brain development can be permanently retarded by under nutrition at certain stages sufficient to limit the supply of precursors for the syn-thesis of lipids and other substances. This is particularly true from the seventh month of fetal life to the first few months of post-natal life. It is unlikely that, except in severe condi-tions of malnutrition in the mother, a child *in utero* could be severely affected. The risk is mainly to those infants born prematurely.

The classical diabetic baby is fat due prob-ably to the effect of excess insulin from the fetal pancreas as a response to a high glucose load from the mother or in response to insulin antagonists of maternal origin.

Serum proteins

In the maternal serum as pregnancy progresses the concentrations of albumin and pre-albumin and of α_1 acid glycoprotein falls, but there is no fall in the total circulating albumin or pre-albumin mass. The fall is due to dilution. *Alpha one* acid glycoprotein would appear to be the only globulin which shows an absolute fall. Several globulins remain unchanged in concentration but in others the concentration actually rises. The total effect is to raise the level of globulin and the A/G ratio may reverse.

In pre-eclampsia there is a loss of proteins of intermediate molecular weight and some globulins show low levels (Studd *et al.*, 1970).

Walker and Wahab (1956) have shown at term the fetal umbilical vein and artery levels in relation to the maternal arm vein levels at rest following spontaneous and easy labour. The fetal total protein level is some 90 per cent of the mother. The albumin is some 105 per cent of the mothers, the α_1 globulin some 60 per cent, the α_2 some 70 per cent, the β 40 per cent, and the γ being 120 per cent of the mothers (by paper electrophoresis). They have also shown that where labour is not allowed to occur and an elective Caesarean section has been done, the levels of all fetal proteins are somewhat lower, especially the γ globulins which are then lower than the mothers. After prolonged labour or in conditions of fetal stress, the β proteins in the baby were clearly elevated. The immunoglobulins would appear to be enhanced in transfer by labour and the fetal response to labour would appear to alter the globulin levels.

There is no clear effect on the cord blood of most pregnancy anomalies even of maternal malnutrition. There is a relative deficiency in fetal blood of fibrinogen.

These earlier techniques of the use of paper electrophoresis have, however, been completely superseded by modern techniques (Stimson, 1972), (Studd *et al.*, 1970) but full studies of the maternal and fetal relationships are not yet available.

In the fetus myoglobin acts as a short term oxygen store to the mitochondria of the fetal heart and facilitates oxygen diffusion in fetal cardiac muscle. It is probably not of any particular value in the skeletal muscle of the fetus.

Amino acids

These are essential building materials for protein and they have been studied in maternal and fetal blood by Young and Prenton (1969), Cockburn, Giles, Robins and Forfar (1973), and by Patel (1972) whose original papers should be studied.

In the mother the free amino acid concentration is reduced from about the 8th week and does not change much after that time. The reduction is more marked in the essential amino acids. At delivery the umbilical cord vein and artery levels are some 80 per cent higher than the levels in the maternal cubital veins.

In the *small for dates* baby with or without pre-eclampsia, the maternal venous concentrations are higher than in the normal pregnant mother, suggesting some degree of transfer failure, but this could also be caused by low maternal plasma volume.

Amino nitrogen uptake is not related to uterine blood flow but more to the metabolic activity of the fetus. The actual uptake would seem to be much greater than necessary for growth. The excess is converted to urea and returned to the mother.

Fetal blood

Angioblastic cells separate early from the wall of the blastocyst and by the 3rd week blood islands exist in the wall of the yolk sac. Haemopoetic function is however, taken over by the fetal liver by the 6th week, and is maximum there by the 3rd month. Liver haemopoesis normally becomes minimal by late pregnancy when marrow haemopoesis is fully developed. The capacity of the liver for haemopoesis is still present however, and it becomes an active source of red cells in conditions of fetal anaemia or hypoxia.

There are three generations of red cells—a primitive group which disappears by about 12 weeks; a fetal group arising early and still present in large numbers at term (and mostly disappearing in early neonatal life); and an adult type detectable by the 12th week and by term composing the majority of the cells in the normal state.

THE RED CELLS

The red cell count rises from 1 500 000 per cmm at the 10th week to 3×10^6 by the 24th week and then slowly until term by which time in the well oxygenated fetus it is 4×10^6. The range at term is from $4-5 \times 10^6$. The packed cell volume at term is 45 per cent but higher when the haemoglobin and red cell count are high. The red cell diameter falls from a mean at 10 weeks of 10.5μ, (the range is from $6-17.5\mu$ but at least 90 per cent are more than 9μ in diameter) to 8·3 at term with still a very wide range ($5-11.5\mu$) in cell size (Turnbull and Walker, 1955).

HAEMOGLOBIN

The total haemoglobin level rises steadily from 9g/100ml at the 10th week (all fetal) to reach 14–15g by the 22nd–24th week and it is likely to remain at or about that level in the normal well oxygenated healthy fetus. At birth however, the reading in cord vein blood may vary from 12–20g/100ml with a mean of 16·5g/100ml (Walker and Turnbull, 1953).

Human fetal blood contains haemoglobin F and haemoglobin A. These are distinguished by their globins. There would seem little obvious virtue to the fetus of having haemoglobin F since the oxygen affinity of the haemoglobin in solution is identical. The fetal red cell differs from the adult in its membrane structure and composition, in its metabolic and enzymatic constitution as well as in its contained haemoglobin. 2·3 diphosphoglycerate (DPG) present in high concentration is largely responsible for influencing the oxygen affinity of the haemoglobin contained in the fetal cell.

The affinity of fetal blood for oxygen is determined largely by the 2·3 DPG content of the fetal cells but is also influenced by the actual content of fetal haemoglobin and each is influenced by the other. Oxygen affinity and the characteristic loading or offloading of oxygen by the haemoglobin in various tensions, pH and temperatures is shown by the shape and position of the disassociation curve.

In the fetal mammal the curve of the fetus is (under standard conditions of pH and temperature) to the left of the mother's and somewhat more vertical in shape. Typical curves and relationships are shown in figure 6.2. Only those parts of the curve below 90 per cent saturation are shown as it is at and below those levels the materno-fetal transfers take

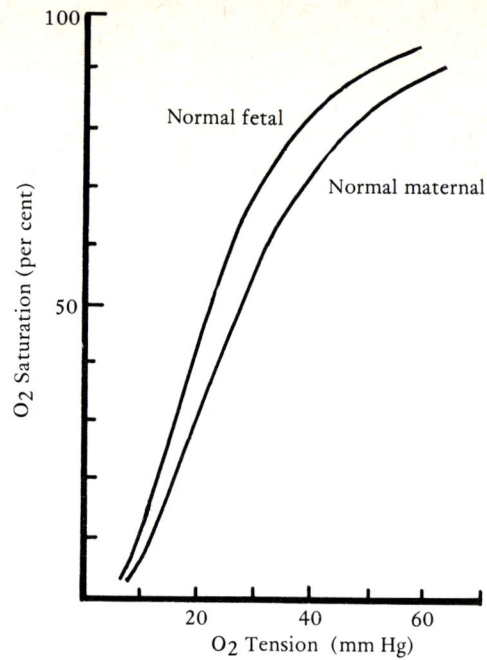

Fig. 6.2   The disassociation curve for oxygen of the arterial blood of human mother and fetus under standard conditions.

place. This is in the vertical part of the curve where even at very low saturation with oxygen the fetal blood can maintain relatively high tension to provide oxygen to its tissues. A fall in saturation in the umbilical vein from 70 per cent to 40 per cent in association say with maternal hypoxia or in prolonged pregnancy is reflected by a tension drop of only 10–12mm Hg.

The fetus picks up oxygen from the maternal intervillous space but there is a clear placental (villus) need for oxygen before the fetal blood is supplied. However, the position of the fetal curve to the left of his mother clearly increases the gradient between and facilitates the transfer of oxygen.

Mathers et al. (1970) have, however, shown that the presence of fetal blood with fetal haemoglobin in the fetus is not necessary for survival as fetuses whose blood has been totally replaced by adult blood by intra-uterine transfusion have then a disassociation curve for oxygen which has a normal adult situation and characteristic and may in fact, at in vivo levels of pH, lie to the right of the mother's. It may, therefore, have a somewhat lesser affinity for oxygen. Those babies grow and develop normally.

FACTORS INFLUENCING THE FETAL BLOOD

Certain of the changes seen in late pregnancy are those of growth and maturation. These are the changing size of cells, the increase in adult haemoglobin levels and the appearance of adult cells with adult characteristics. Other changes in levels of total, fetal and adult haemoglobin and the haematocrit and cell volume are influenced by the environment in which the fetus is forced to live.

Blood gases

The special features of the fetal circulation allow highly oxygenated blood to go to the liver, brain and coronary vessels. It is not possible to give absolute values for the blood gas levels in the various vessels in the human fetus in late pregnancy, but it is likely that those will be close to those reported in the sheep and monkey in the steady state situation (Comline and Silver, 1970), (Meschia *et al.*, 1965).

Comline and Silver have shown that from mid-pregnancy in the ewe, fetal blood gas tensions remained fairly static at a pO^2 in the umbilical vein of 50mm and in the artery of 30mm. The pH, PCV, lactate and glucose levels also remain static. With increasing age, after 110 days or so, there is a tendency of the pO_2 in the umbilical vein to fall to 40–34mm, suggesting some defect in the supply system. There is however, no evidence of a rise in the fetal blood haematocrit despite the fall in pO_2.

In the human in normal late pregnancy it is likely that a situation similar to that in the sheep may well exist. In the fetal vessels there would be before term no rise in haemoglobin and no fall in pO_2 or oxygen saturation or a rise in lactate. However, in the human situation many pregnancies are abnormal. Walker (1954) who investigated conditions of this kind suggested that in the human, haemoglobin levels close to the normal adult level and a relatively high umbilical vein and artery pO_2 were normal for late pregnancy. Where at delivery the fetal blood had a high oxygen capacity and the oxygen saturation was low, the situations were usually clinically abnormal and associated with conditions causing intra-uterine anoxia. There is still some doubt about accepting the simplicity of this arrangement as the definitive studies have not yet been done. However, it is clear that in the premature fetus, especially in pregnancy associated with anoxia producing conditions and in many 'light for dates' babies

(Haworth, Dilling and Younaszai, 1967), haematocrit levels are very high and this is not due to dehydration. Moreover, in prolonged pregnancy where the fetus has signs of dysmaturity the blood shows markedly elevated levels of erythropoetin (Finne, 1966), and a similar feature was seen in other anoxic producing conditions *viz.* pre-eclampsia and occasionally diabetes. Those conditions have been previously shown to be associated with fetuses which have high red cell levels, high haemoglobin levels and low oxygen levels in the umbilical vein (Walker, 1953).

The premature and the 'light for dates' baby from seriously abnormal pregnancy may, therefore, be born with blood with a very high haematocrit, a high viscosity and low oxygen. A very few hours after birth the blood will become highly concentrated and produce a further fetal risk.

In summary, it appears that the actual haemoglobin level in the cord blood at birth may vary with the degree of intra-uterine anoxia. Intra-uterine anaemia will be present when very low levels are to be found. The fetus *in utero* appears to live and mature in an oxygen environment well below that expected by adult standards. This is achieved partly by a relatively large cardiac output and partly because the fetus is geared to live at this level. There are many mechanisms which protect against temporary deficiencies in supply but occasionally a level is reached at which compensation is impossible and then the damage of hypoxia occurs.

For a full description of the physiopathology the reader should study the relevant reviews.

GROWTH

Glucose is the main source of fetal energy and the body fats are built mainly from carbohydrate. Cholesterol metabolism is dependent on glucose. The requirement of glucose crosses the placenta by facilitated diffusion. In the very early fetus and placenta the pentose phosphate pathway is extremely important since it facilitates nucleic acid, lipid and steroid synthesis. Later the pattern is more adult.

Metabolic protection of the brain during intra-uterine anoxia may be produced by the ability of the tissues to metabolize substrates like pyruvate and lactate. There is said to be limited ability of the fetus to metabolize liver glycogen in anoxia, but some workers see this glyconeolysis as rather more common than often reported.

The citric acid cycle may take place in a limited oxygen situation and a complicated system requiring oxidized co-enzymes may enable pyruvate produced by glycolysis to be metabolized to release energy.

While glucose is the main source of energy, the fetus also needs amino acids, fatty acids and vitamins, salts and metals for growth. The amounts of glucose available to the fetus are associated with the concentrations in the maternal blood and the rates of flow of maternal and fetal blood. Poor concentrations or poor flow can cause fetal growth retardation. Fetal glucose utilization is tied to fetal insulin production.

The cells of the early embryo have a strong drive to multiply and regenerate and retarded somatic growth due to reduction in cell numbers is rare. This may occur however, later in the brain in serious conditions of deficiency. Control of such division and differentiation is a function of the genetic information contained within the cell nuclei and also by the inductive effects of associated tissues.

In the premature child the outstanding deficiency is one of fat, but most mammalian fetuses carry very little fat and the human child is an exception. The concentration of protein potassium, magnesium and iron are roughly the same in the 1500g or 3500g fetus (Widdowson and Spray, 1951).

General organ weight

Growth of the fetus depends on the food available and the efficacy of the supply system. It is generally stated that there are three phases of cell growth, increase in number, increase in number and size and later, increase in size alone. Increase in numbers depends on maintained DNA synthesis. Winick (1969) has shown that while this pattern affects cell tissues at different times, there is a particular pattern for the brain. Malnutrition to the brain late in pregnancy can interfere with cell division and therefore, cell numbers, at or about birth may interfere both with numbers and size and after about one month of life with size only. Deficiency in size is recoverable, lack of numbers cannot be improved. Each area of the brain has its own timing and pattern, the cerebellum is more sensitive than the cortex.

Prenatal malnutrition renders an animal unduly sensitive to the growth retarding effect of neonatal malnutrition.

Once the period of embryogenesis and organogenesis are past future differentiation follows defined lines and growth in cell numbers continues. Anomalies of development can still however, appear, many due to previous interference or damage, but some arising due to direct damage to developing tissues at this time, e.g. thalidomide or X-ray.

It is customary to decide the quality of fetal growth by fetal weight at birth when that weight is compared to some standard selected as representative of the group in question. Length, more difficult to ascertain with accuracy, is rarely used. Mean birth weight in populations is inevitably a mixture of mean fetal growth and of mean maturity at birth. Poorly nourished communities have poorly grown babies and a large number of prematurely born babies, and therefore, an artificially low mean birth weight. Birth weight obviously is also related to the size of the maternal uterus and the efficiency of its supply system—small women, therefore, tend to have smaller babies. Babies born at altitude (e.g. Denver, Colorado) have a lower birth weight than those born in similar communities at sea level.

Those, and other subtle variations in birth weight, are discussed by Ounsted and Ounsted (1973). In practice however, within the United Kingdom birth weight is related to:

1. Maternal height—Tall mothers have bigger babies.
2. Maternal weight—Heavier mothers have heavier babies.
3. Parity—First babies tend to be smaller than subsequent ones.
4. Maternal cigarette smoking—heavy smokers have smaller babies.
5. Baby sex—Female babies are smaller than male babies.

In the Perinatal Mortality Survey, 1958 (Boulter and Alderman, 1969), a clear social class difference was seen in the weights of babies born between 35 to 43 weeks. Variations within social classes can, however, be largely explained on the basis of one or other of the above factors.

Recently there is increasing evidence that women who are small because of poor nourishment in childhood or at puberty, and are much better nourished after that time tend to grow bigger babies than would be expected. This, of course, increases the risk of difficult labour since being poorly grown they often have contracted pelves.

Effect of multiple birth

The human uterus has a limited capacity to grow fetal tissues. In general the weight of multiple babies is the same as single ones up until about 26–30 weeks' gestation. After that time a total weight of baby of some 12–16 pounds is the best the average uterus can achieve. This is true for the multigravid uterus which has already grown and produced one or more well grown babies. The primigravid uterus cannot stretch to that extent and premature delivery is one of the serious problems of multiple pregnancy in the primigravida (*see* Chapter 22).

Growth curves

Strictly those are not curves of growth known to have been followed by individual babies but are composite curves of baby weights at birth. Many such curves have been produced and it is essential (Walker, 1967) that in any discussion of factors influencing birth weight that the actual birth weight curves in the community under study should be known.

Factors responsible for inadequate growth

The normal pattern of growth as discussed by Wong and Scott (1972) in a study in Nova Scotia children, showed that while male babies were slightly heavier and larger and have slightly bigger heads than females, the biological variation was some 13 per cent around the mean at 38–42 weeks' gestation. Males reach 2500g by 34 weeks and females by 35 weeks. At 40 weeks male babies weigh 3600g, becoming slightly larger by 42 weeks (females 3400g and 3500g). The 3rd percentile for 40–42 weeks was 2500g in both sexes. This is an example of a well nourished community and an excellent intra-uterine growth pattern.

The most useful statistics for the United Kingdom are however, the curves published by Thomson, Billewicz and Hytten (1968), and Tanner and Thomson (1970), of 52 004 legitimate single births in the City of Aberdeen from 1948 to 1964. The quality of this material

cannot be faulted. The main 'growth' curve of the average baby in the United Kingdom means that it should be 1000–1100g at 28 completed weeks, 2500g at 35 completed weeks, and 3300g at 40 completed weeks, and should continue to grow at least until 42 completed weeks (3500g), but differences of

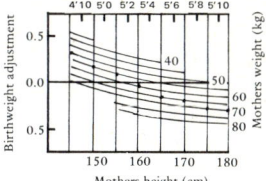

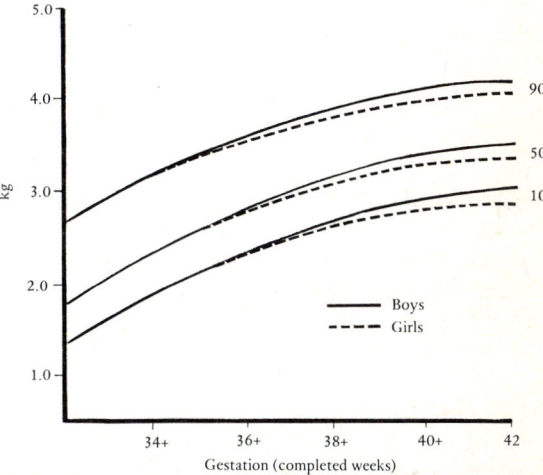

Fig. 6.3 The 10th, 50th and 90th percentile of birth weights of firstborn boys and girls to mothers of a height of 160cm and a mid-pregnancy weight of 50kg. The small chart above shows the adjustment to be made for expected weights for mothers of different height and mid-pregnancy weight. Drawn from Tanner and Thomson (1970).

±500g mean at 40 weeks occur between very tall, heavy mothers, and those who are small and light (Fig. 6.3).

Poor fetal growth—(The 'light for dates' fetus)

Inadequate fetal growth *in utero* as a clear explanation for small babies born at 'term' was suggested by McBurney (1947), and the long term functional inadequacy of these babies was described by Baird in 1959. Since then of course, a vast complicated and somewhat confused literature has developed (Warkany, Monroe and Sutherland, 1961).

Inadequate growth of the fetus is assumed when at birth the weight is below a level selected against a mean for that period of gestation for babies of that community. Obviously as many babies are below the mean as above, but the level at which poor growth or 'light for dates' is to be determined is taken usually as the weight below the *10th percentile* (Fig. 6.3). Occasionally in some series statistical use is made of the somewhat more easily calculated 'Standard Deviation from the Mean' and one or two 'SD below the mean' is selected to define the 'light for dates' baby. However, in practice, for follow-up and other studies the '2 SD below the mean' criteria is too low and selects out a biologically inferior and possibly congenitally abnormal group, rather than selecting those otherwise normal babies who have suffered inadequate intra-uterine nutrition. The group is best selected by the 10th percentile.

Organ weights

Where the fetus is poorly grown for gestational age, and especially when there is considered to be an element of malnutrition some body organs appear to have a lower relative weight than others (Grunewald, 1965, and Wigglesworth, 1968). There is a lack of subcutaneous white fat, a relatively larger heart and brain, and a liver small with depleted glycogen. The thymus with depleted lymphocytes is also small, the lungs are smaller because of small cell size, and the adrenals relatively smaller with a poorer stress response. Brown adipose tissue is also depleted of fat. In a long standing 'malnutrition' situation fetal length is also reduced.

Dobbing (1970 a & b) has with others shown that in such cases the brain, even though apparently escaping the effect of malnutrition, may well have suffered because the main period of cell division extends from the 30th week of gestation until 18 months of age. Inadequate availability of lipid precursor and of long chain fatty acids from an undernourished mother may limit the total cell mass (Winnock and Rosso, 1969). They have shown that brains from severely malnourished children have very many fewer brain cells than would have been expected with adequate nutrition.

The child suffering brain malnutrition and inadequacy grows into an adult with poor functional efficiency. The inadequate physical and mental development of this adult does not allow him by his own effort to extricate himself from poor social conditions and inadequate

employment opportunity in time to prevent his children suffering similarly. This type of long-term sequelae explains simply most of the perpetuation of poor quality children in the poor social groups of the community much better and much more accurately than any need to find any special genetic constitutional pattern. This problem can be handled only by the most skilled obstetric and paediatric care and an improvement in the social conditions into which those children are born.

Effects of malnutrition

Where the cause of poor fetal growth is essentially that of undernourishment of the mother and only that, lack of physical growth of the conceptus is said not to become obvious until after the 30th week.

Clinically poor growth of the uterus and contents in the abnormal situation may be obvious before that time. It is also suggested that the maternal fat gain in early pregnancy is an energy source for the fetus in late pregnancy and that when the mother has a poor early pregnancy nutritional state she cannot nourish her child adequately later in the pregnancy, but this should be overcome by good late pregnancy nutrition.

Trophoblast cells have priority over maternal tissues early in gestation and up until about mid-pregnancy fetal weight is probably unaffected by maternal malnutrition, but the area attained by the placenta and clearly established will limit the ultimate nourishment it can transfer to the baby. Probably the best known study is that of Smith (1947). On September 17, 1944, the Dutch underground movement initiated a transport strike and held this until liberation in May, 1945. Little or no food or coal was allowed into the major cities and the calories available to the civilian population dropped in some instances to less than 730 for pregnant women with only 33g of protein of which 9g was animal. Starvation increased infertility (and amenorrhoea). If in the first trimester it was followed by a high incidence of premature labour with babies of low birth weight. Starvation in the third trimester was followed by a fall in the mean birth weight and an increased infant mortality (Zusser and Stein, 1975).

Similar studies in India and South Africa have shown that the small poorly nourished mother with low pregnancy weight gain has a high incidence of premature birth, poor fetal growth, poor baby weight at term, and 30 per cent of the babies at term weighing less than 2500g. For a study of the effects of nutrition on fertility *see* Gopalon and Naidu (1972) and Gopalon (1970).

Even in the United Kingdom, the situation is similar. Thomson, Billewicz and Hytten (1968) made a full assessment of birth weight in a large series. They reported the expected weights and percentiles of Aberdeen children who are on the whole larger than most American series, but smaller than the Swedish. They show, for example, that if the mother weighs 50kg at 20 weeks' gestation and measures 160cm (5′ 3″) in height (mean)—first born children ought to weigh 3200g-3300g at 39–42 weeks, and the 5th percentile should be well over 2800g. If the mother is under 150cm (5′) in height then the child weighs 0·2–0·3kg less. This reduced the 5th percentile level to 2300g at the 39th week but still 2500g by 41 weeks. In heavier and taller primigravidae the 5th percentile at 40+ weeks may be as high as 3000g. Discussion of poor growth syndrome starts from a different level in different situations. Is it correct therefore, to compare the 3000g baby of a tall fit mother (5th percentile at term) in its behaviour with the 2400g (5th percentile) baby of the smaller height mother and would such comparisons be meaningful. It is better to use the best as the standard and examine and study those children who fall below the levels of the best, but who are, of course, often apparently normal. Study of well nourished pre-school children of different ethnic groups shows little variation between groups, but if there is poverty and malnourishment the difference is great. It is likely in the fetus that almost all ethnic weight difference is associated with varying capacity of the uterine supply system to grow the child and is not associated with ethnic group as such.

Poor fetal growth has been achieved artificially in the sheep and in the monkey by limiting the total arterial flow to the uterus or alternatively by limiting the total placental area available to the fetus and weight deficiency up to 30 per cent can be achieved.

However, abnormal growth in the human fetus, the truly 'low birth weight child', arises often from very different situations. Frequently the mother appears to be well nourished. We have, therefore, two main groups together, with several sub-groups; the child light at birth because the mother is malnourished, or small, or both, and the child light at birth because of some process interfering with his growth but not a general maternal malnutrition state. Frequently general and specific malnourishment co-exist.

CONDITIONS ASSOCIATED WITH POOR FETAL GROWTH

The fetus poorly grown because of maternal malnutrition is probably poorly grown only in the latter 12 weeks. The fetus poorly grown because of poor maternal supply system, i.e. small uterus and poor vascular supply may be poorly grown throughout or also only in the later weeks—e.g. in twins. The fetus poorly grown because of a disease situation may have his growth halted at any stage.

Walker (1967) discussing the 'light for dates' baby' from the viewpoint of oestrogen excretion in maternal urine suggested, following the work of Coyle and Brown (1963) that steadily rising maternal urinary oestrogen readings even at a level below the normal mean, suggested progressive though slow fetal growth, but that oestrogen levels halting or in fact falling after 30 weeks suggested slowing or cessation of growth and were more serious for immediate outcome.

Low grade essential hypertension, mild to moderate pre-eclampsia and chronic nephritis seem to have in general little or no serious effect on fetal growth. Severe pre-eclampsia, the heavy albuminuria of the nephrotic syndrome and long standing hypertension however, have a depressing effect. There is one syndrome as yet little described where the poor weight gain precedes the hypertension and albuminuria which often gets the credit.

Reid (1961) and Walker (1967) pointed out clearly that women who deliver one low weight baby had at least a 30 per cent chance of repeating this and some women could not grow a normal sized child. Many of these women have abnormal uteri (septate etc.) or have abnormal vasculature. Ounsted and Ounsted suggest the possibility of a more subtle genetic effect.

Poor ultimate fetal weight is seen also in mothers with congenital heart disease or chronic chest conditions, thyrotoxicosis and chronic disease of any kind. Low weight at birth is often associated with threatened abortion early in the pregnancy but *not* as a general rule in late pregnancy bleeding.

Deformed fetuses are usually poorly grown except for some hydrocephalics.

Chronic maternal malaria is responsible for suppression of fetal growth and where malaria eradication programmes are adequate, fetal birth weight rises dramatically (Macgregor and Avery, 1974).

Excessive weight

Excessive weight at birth is, however, a function classically of the hyperglycaemia of the diabetic mother. Here the excessive growth of the child may be related to his insulin response to the high sugar transferred to him, or to transplacental maternal insulin antagonists.

Babies high in the 90th percentile are seen in the healthy multigravidae already with four or five children and some women in this group can grow fifteen, or more, pounds of multiple pregnancy. This is a question of uterine growth, size, and supply system.

GROWTH AND DEVELOPMENT OF PLACENTA AND CORD

When conception has occurred the hormones of the corpus luteum, and perhaps also chorionic gonadotrophin derived from the trophoblast modify the endometrium to form the decidua. There is swelling of the stromal cells which become oval in shape, with large pale nuclei, and faintly-staining cytoplasm. The superficial layers contain tightly packed cells, with small glands having long thin necks (decidua compacta), while the deeper layers

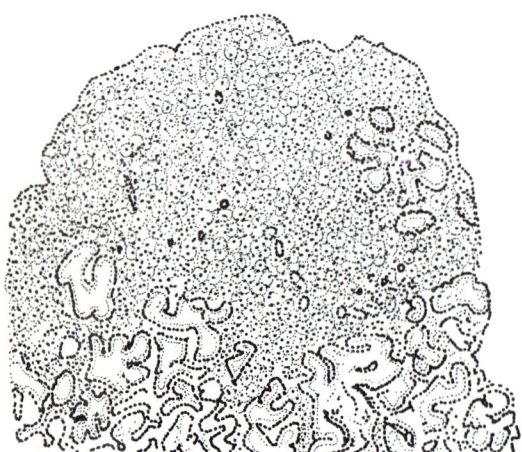

Fig. 6.4   Decidual change in the endometrium. (Compare with Fig. 4.18a & b.) Menstrual cycle.

have a more open appearance due to the distended gland bodies (decidua spongiosa) (Fig. 6.4). The columnar epithelium of the endometrial glands atrophies after implantation, but those parts of the glands embedded in the myometrium persist, and form the origin of the new endometrium which regenerates after delivery. Shortly after implantation the decidua is described as having three components. The decidua capsularis covers the surface of the ovum. The decidua basalis lies between the ovum and the uterine wall. The decidua parietalis lines the rest of the uterine cavity (Fig. 6.5). In later development the decidua basalis will form the placenta, and the other two parts fuse as the ovum increases in size.

At implantation (day 6) the cells of the trophoblast erode the superficial cells of the decidua, and within the next few days the ovum becomes completely surrounded by trophoblast (Fig. 6.6). Its nourishment is obtained initially by lysis of the decidual cells.

Before the 13th day, the outer layer of trophoblast (syncitiotrophoblast) begins to form finger-shaped projections which will develop into villi (Fig. 6.7a). Two days later the inner layer of trophoblast (cytotrophoblast) invades the villi to form a central core, and erosion of maternal vessels occurs so that the villi are bathed in maternal blood (Fig. 6.7b). About day 18 a projection of mesenchyme enters each villus, and vascular islets, the future circulation of the fetal side of the placenta, appear (Fig. 6.8). On day 21 the intravillous vascular network meets the umbilical vessels to establish the fetal circulation. A proportion of the villi fuse with the decidua and remain avascular (Fig. 6.9). Their function is to anchor the placenta to the uterine wall.

Towards the end of the 8th week, the villi begin to group together in the region of the decidua basalis and disappear from the remainder of the surface of the ovum. At 12 weeks the placenta is clearly defined.

The placenta weighs about 20g at 10 weeks, 170g at 20 weeks, 430g at 30 weeks and 650g at term (mean figures with considerable variation). There is some correlation between fetal weight and placental weight at term. The fetal placenta is divided into cotyledons each of which is a separate fetal vascular system, supplied by one artery and drained by one or

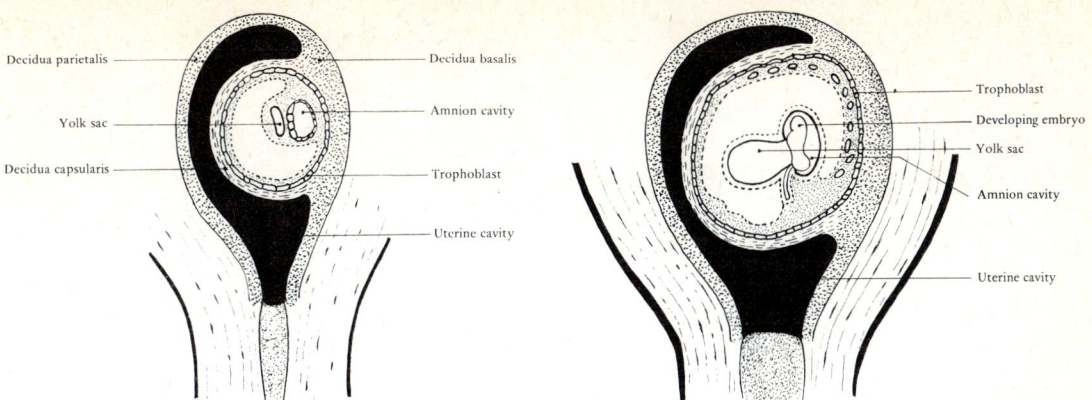

Fig. 6.5 Differentiation of decidua.

Fig. 6.6 Day 8.

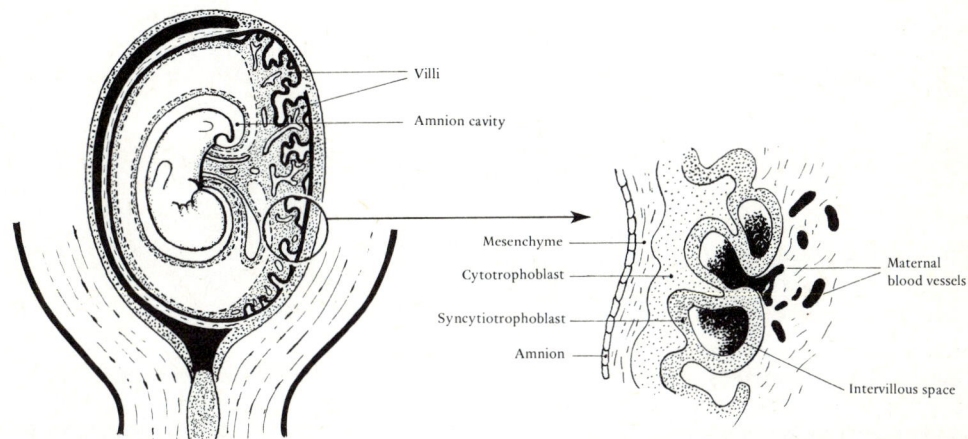

Fig. 6.7a Day 12.

Fig. 6.7b Day 12.

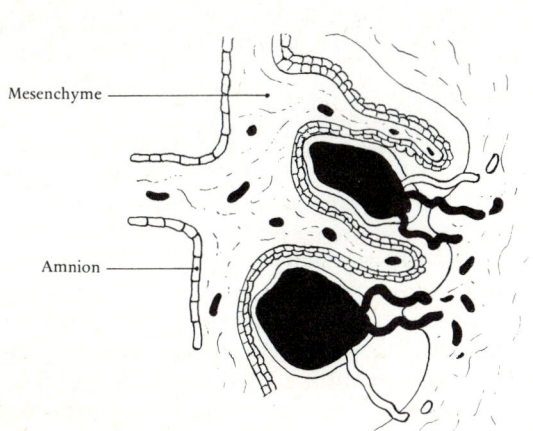

Fig. 6.8 Day 18.

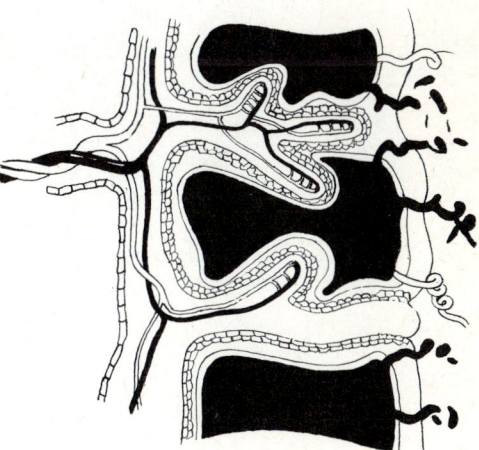

Fig. 6.9 Day 21.

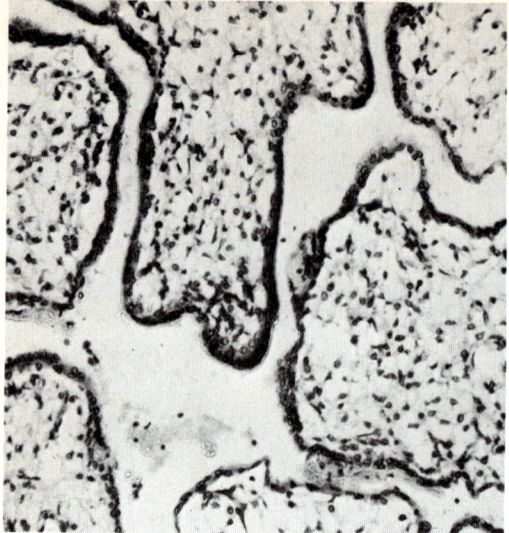

Fig. 6.10   Sections of villi at 12th week.

more veins (Fig. 6.14). The number of fetal cotyledons (60–200) does not increase after 12 weeks, but growth occurs by continuing proliferation of peripheral villi right up to term. The villi themselves change considerably. At 12 weeks they are large (up to 0·3 mm in diameter) with two well-defined layers of trophoblast. Capillaries are small and located centrally in the connective tissue core (Fig. 6.10). At term the villi are much smaller (0·05–0·1 mm), the capillaries are larger and near the surface, and the cytotrophoblast cells are few. Fibrin deposits on the surface of villi are commonly seen (Fig. 6.11).

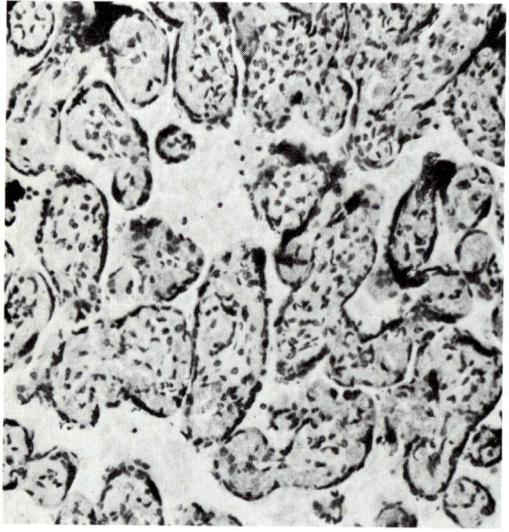

Fig. 6.11   Sections of villi at term.

The placenta at term

The placenta is disc-shaped, about 20cm in diameter, 2·5cm thick in the middle and tapering towards the edges. The fetal surface is covered by amnion, which is easily stripped off except at its close attachment to the umbilical cord. Beneath the amnion lies the chorion within which run the fetal vessels before dipping down into the depths of the placenta. Arteries cross superficial to veins (Fig. 6.12). The maternal surface is lobulated

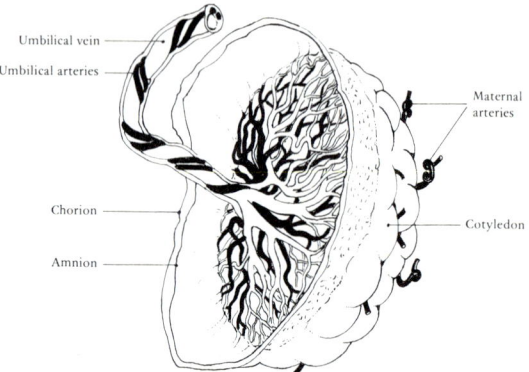

Fig. 6.12   Placenta at term.

in appearance. These maternal 'cotyledons' correspond to one, or more usually several, fetal cotyledons. A spiral artery enters the middle of each, and several peripheral veins return blood to the maternal circulation. The umbilical cord normally contains two arteries and one vein in a jelly-like substance (Wharton's jelly) and is covered with amnion. It is usually inserted near the centre of the placenta. Its length is usually between 50 and 100cm but figures of 2–250cm have been recorded.

Placental circulation

The uterus is supplied by the uterine and ovarian arteries which anastomose along the lateral border and give off branches which penetrate the myometrium (Fig. 6.13). As many as 100 arterioles supply blood directly to the intervillous space under high pressure. It has been shown in non-human primates that the blood enters the placenta in spurts, not all arterioles delivering blood at the same time. It is likely that a similar process occurs in the human. As the blood encounters the villi it is slowed and dispersed laterally, bathing the

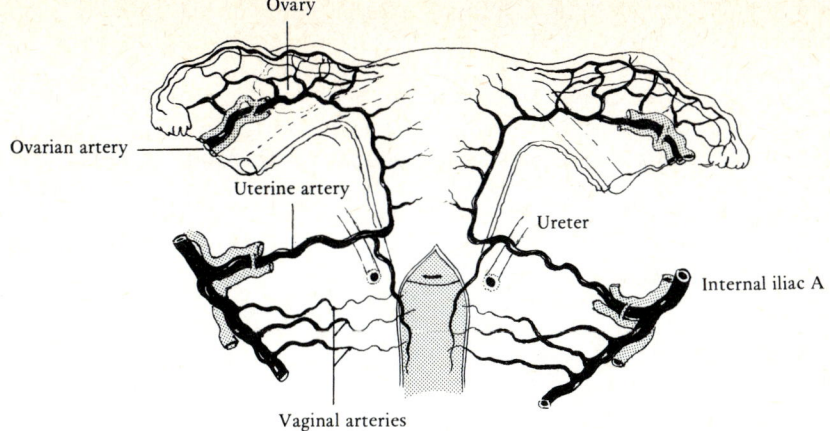

Fig. 6.13   Maternal circulation.

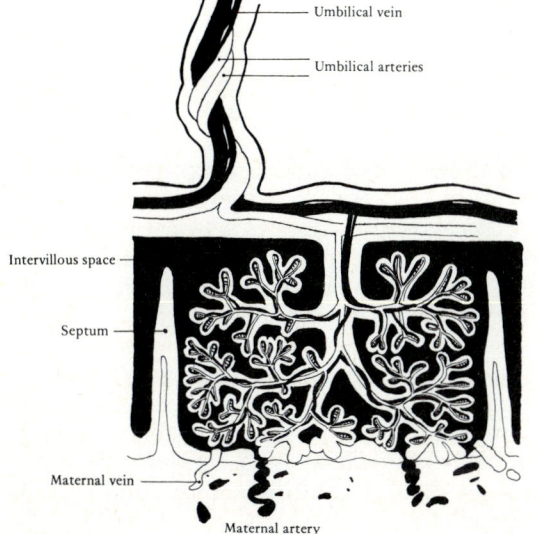

Fig. 6.14   Diagram of placental vasculature.

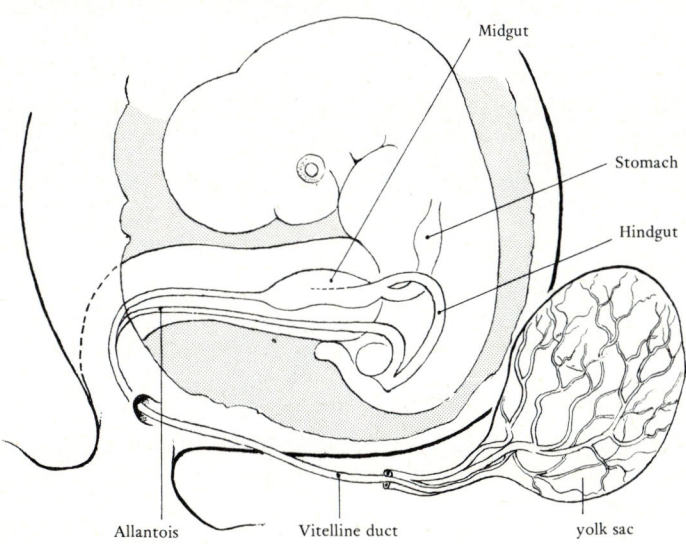

Fig. 6.15   Formation of umbilical cord.

villi and eventually collecting in the maternal veins. About 500ml of blood passes through the intervillous space each minute.

The fetal circulation arises as two branches of the internal iliac arteries which convey about 50 per cent of the cardiac output to the placenta. There is a constant anastomosis between these arteries about 1cm from the placental surface. Branches of the arteries spread to all parts of the placenta, entering the cotyledons vertically and dividing progressively into the villous capillaries (Fig. 6.14). There are no valves in the placental vessels, and they almost certainly have no nerve supply.

DEVELOPMENT OF THE UMBILICAL CORD

As the embryonic plate grows and there is an increased growth of ectoderm the ventral area of the embryo becomes enfolded by ectoderm and the amnion increases in size to envelope the developing embryo.

The yolk sac becomes partly enclosed to form the gut and a portion is nipped off leaving the residual yolk sac connected by the vitelline duct to the gut (Fig. 6.15). An area of hind gut (the allantois) has protruded into the extra-embryonic coelom and has acquired mesoderm associating it with the primitive body stalk. The original yolk sac blood vessels gradually disappear and definitive blood vessels connecting the fetus to its developing placenta arise in the mesoderm of the allantoic duct. As the amnion envelopes the fetus at about the 6th week and covers the developing placenta it includes within its folds: The stalk of the yolk sac (vitelline duct); the allantois and its vessels and the primitive mesodern of the original body stalk and for a little time part of the extra embryonic coelom (Fig. 6.16).

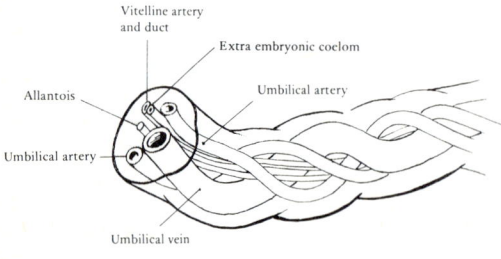

Fig. 6.16   Elements of the umbilical cord.

The adult umbilical cord contains, therefore, remains of vitelline duct and allantois but mainly three blood vessels, a large central umbilical vein (the right vein having disappeared early) and (except rarely) two arteries which spiral round the vein. The ground substance (Wharton's jelly) is rich in mucoid, poor in fibres, contains neither intrinsic vessels nor nerves. It varies greatly in amount.

Abnormalities of placenta and cord

The cord varies greatly in length from a few inches to several feet and excessively short or long cords prove dangerous to the child.

The cord may be inserted into the placenta in several ways. Normally it is inserted in mid-placenta and the vessels fan out equally in all directions. The cord may reach the placental edge (battledore insertion). Occasionally the cord is inserted into the membranes, and vessels run free in the membranes spreading as they go to the placenta (membraneous insertion).—Very occasionally those vessels run across the membranes in front of the baby's head and are ruptured during labour or at rupture of membranes (vasa praevia). Other rare anomalies are discussed later.

Rarely the extra embryonic coelom persists into the cord close to the fetus with failure of proper closure at the umbilicus. This allows herniation of gut or liver into the cord. The distended herniation is an omphalocele which may be damaged during delivery and may be difficult to repair.

The placenta is usually implanted on the anterior or posterior region of the upper part of the uterus. Fundal insertion may predispose to uterine inversion. Insertion into the lower part of the uterus (placenta praevia) is an important clinical complication of pregnancy.

Occasionally the placenta is in two parts (placenta duplex) with vascular connections in the membranes. If one part is much smaller than the other it is termed a succenturiate lobe, and may be left *in utero* after delivery of the placenta, causing post-partum haemorrhage (Fig. 6.17).

In the circumvallate placenta, the membranes are attached, not to the edge of the placenta, but some distance within (Fig. 6.18). The margin of the placenta is much thicker than usual, and undermines the decidua. The cause of this condition is not known for certain. It has been suggested that the fertilized ovum

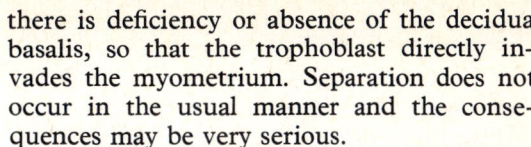

Succenturiate

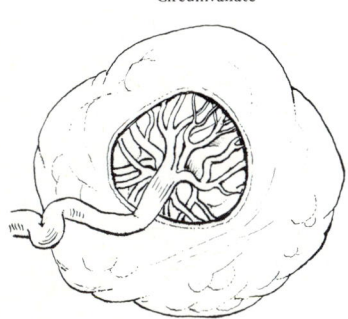

Fig. 6.17   Placenta with succenturiate lobe.

Circumvallate

Fig. 6.18   Circumvallate placenta.

there is deficiency or absence of the decidua basalis, so that the trophoblast directly invades the myometrium. Separation does not occur in the usual manner and the consequences may be very serious.

The placenta may be unduly large in severe Rhesus haemolytic disease and in diabetes.

PLACENTAL INFARCTS

These result from local interference with part of the maternal circulation to the placenta. They appear as white, yellow or brown areas, smooth and uniform, usually close to the decidual surface (Fig. 6.19). It is unusual to find a term placenta free from infarcts, but the amount of tissue destroyed varies greatly. There is conflicting evidence of an increased incidence of infarction in those conditions of pregnancy known to interfere with fetal growth, e.g. hypertension, renal disease.

'PLACENTAL INSUFFICIENCY'

This is a diagnosis often made retrospectively as a cause of fetal death, fetal distress in labour, or poor fetal growth. It is also suspected antenatally when maternal hormone levels are found to be low, or there is other evidence of growth retardation. As has been stated earlier, there is a close relationship between fetal and placental size, and it is most likely that the

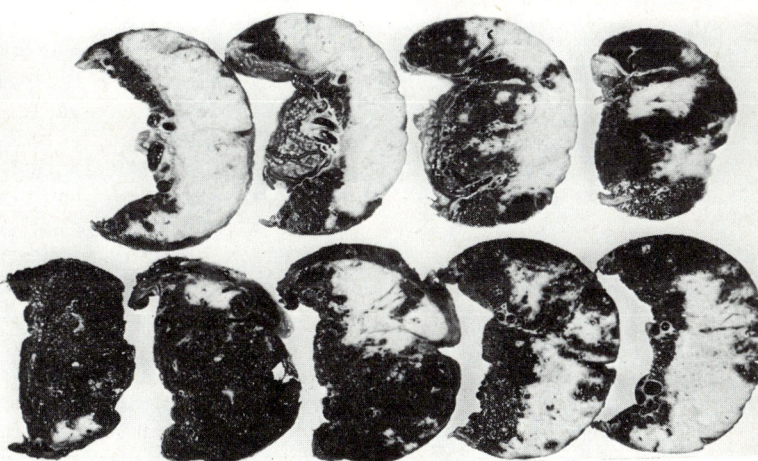

Fig. 6.19   A grossly infarcted placenta (white areas are infarcts).

has implanted more superficially than usual, or that there has been continuing proliferation of villi after the original limits of the placenta have been determined. It is alleged that spontaneous abortion is more common in the presence of this variation in placental form.

Placenta accreta is a rare condition in which

abnormality in these cases is in the maternal blood supply to both placenta and fetus, and in the original area of placenta insertion. Examination of the delivered placenta will not reveal the basic abnormality which most probably involves the arterioles as they pass through the myometrium.

Placental transfer

The placenta has often been referred to as the fetal lung. While its respiratory functions are of course, vital to the developing fetus, there are many other essential functions which are increasingly being recognized as important in clinical obstetrics.

Every substance which passes from the maternal to the fetal circulation does so by way of the placenta. The maternal circulation in the intervillous space is in direct contact with the trophoblast, but the two layers of this structure and the capillary endothelium normally remain intact. Transfer between the two circulations may occur by simple diffusion, by active transport, or by an intermediate procedure referred to as facilitated transfer.

Simple diffusion

The transfer of the respiratory gases, oxygen and carbon dioxide, is a good example. The rate of diffusion is dependent upon the relative flow rates of maternal and fetal bloods, difference in concentration on the two sides of the membrane, the surface area of the membrane and the thickness of the membrane. The greater oxygen affinity of fetal haemoglobin is of assistance, although not essential to normal fetal development (Fig. 6.2).

The maternal blood supply to the placenta

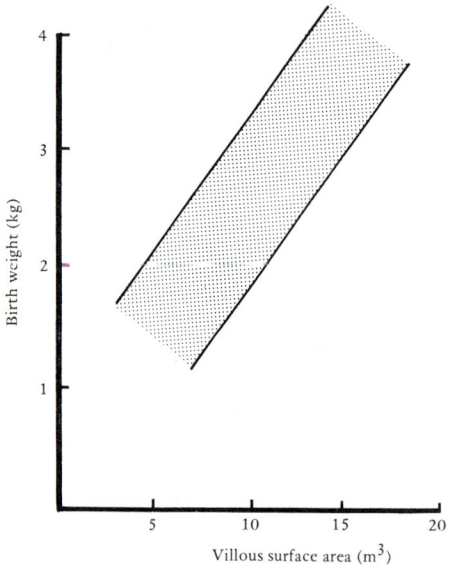

Fig. 6.20   Relation between fetal weight and total villous surface area (normal range).

is liberal—estimates suggest a figure in the region of 500ml per minute in the normal term pregnancy. The area of interchange between the two circulations is in the region of 11 sq metres, and it has been shown that this area is directly proportional to the weight of the fetus (Fig. 6.20).

The thickness of the tissues interposed between the two circulations cannot be measured accurately as it may vary. It is probable that simple diffusion occurs preferentially across the region of cytoplasm away from the nuclei, and it has been suggested that in situations in which the fetus is short of oxygen there is migration or clumping of the nuclei of the trophoblast to increase the area available for diffusion.

The oxygen tension of the maternal blood supplied to the placenta is high—slightly higher than in the non-pregnant state due to the effect of progesterone on respiration. Likewise the maternal carbon dioxide tension is lowered. Fetal blood returning to the placenta has a low oxygen pressure, and a higher level of carbon dioxide, thus facilitating transfer of these two substances.

The higher oxygen affinity of fetal haemoglobin means that it can take up oxygen to a greater degree at lower oxygen tensions than could adult haemoglobin. The slightly higher concentration of haemoglobin in fetal blood also acts to the advantage of the fetus. Carbon dioxide is able to cross the placenta at about 40 times the rate of oxygen, for the same pressure gradient between the two circulations. It is therefore most unlikely that CO_2 retention should become a problem, rather than O_2 lack. In the clinical situation of fetal distress there is a build-up of fixed acids in the fetal circulation, the pH is lowered shifting the oxygen dissociation curve to the right which leads to a decrease in the oxygen affinity of the fetal blood.

It must be remembered that the placenta itself requires an oxygen supply, some 25 per cent of that used by the fetus.

Carbohydrates

Glucose is the principal source of energy for the human fetus, crossing the placenta by facilitated transport. The level in the fetal blood varies in accordance with the maternal level, but is always lower. There is normally a considerable excess of glucose over the supply of oxygen required for its metabolism. The fetus is able to store glycogen, particularly in the liver, in higher concentration than the adult.

Proteins

The essential amino acids are readily transported across the placenta. Active transport results, in some cases, in higher concentrations in fetal than in maternal blood. There are also differences in transfer rate between L and D-isomers of some substances.

Large molecular weight proteins can also cross the placenta, γ-G immunoglobulin being one of the most important transferred in large amount. Size alone is not the only determinant of the rate of transfer, as only small amounts of albumen (molecular weight 70 000—half that of IgG) cross the placenta. There is some evidence from animals that pinocytosisis may be involved.

Electrolytes

Sodium, potassium and chloride probably cross by simple diffusion. Calcium, iron and phosphorous are present in higher levels in fetal than maternal blood suggesting active transport. Unbound iodine crosses very readily, and is taken up in the fetal thyroid more readily than in the maternal.

Vitamins

The water soluble vitamins are found in higher concentrations in fetal blood, while the fat soluble ones are in lower concentration.

Lipids

Phospholipids and cholesterol do not cross intact, but the placenta is readily permeable to acetate and many free fatty acids.

REFERENCES

Butler, N. R. & Alberman, Eva D. (1969) *Perinatal Problems* (Survey 1958). Edinburgh: Livingstone.

Cockburn, F., Giles, N., Robins, S. P. & Forfar, J. O. (1973) Free Amino Acid Composition of Human Amniotic Fluid at Term. *J. Obstet. Gynaec. Brit. Cwlth*, **80**, 10.

Comline, R. S. & Silver, M. (1970) pO$_2$, pCO$_2$ and pH Levels in the umbilical and uterine blood of the mare and ewe. *J. Physiol*, **209**, 587–608.

Comline, R. S. & Silver, M. (1970) Daily changes in foetal and maternal blood of conscious pregnant ewes, with catheters in umbilical and uterine vessels. *J. Physiol*, **209**, 567.

Coyle, M. G. & Brown, J. B. (1963) Urinary excretion of oestriol during pregnancy—results in normal and abnormal pregnancy. *J. Obstet. Gynaec. Brit. Cwlth*, **70**, 225.

Davis, J. (1970) The first breath and development of the lung. In *Scientific Foundations of Obstet. & Gynaec*. Edited by E. E. Philipp, Josephine Barnes & A. Newton. London: Heinemann.

Dobbing, J. (1970) The effects of early growth retardation on the human brain. *J. Path*, **101**, 13.

Finne, P. H. (1966) Erythropoitin levels in cord blood as evidence in intrauterine asphyxia. *Acta paediat. scand*, **55**, 478.

Gopalan, C., Naidu, A. & Nadamuni (1972) Nutrition and Fertility. *Lancet* **ii**, 1077.

Gopalan, C. (1970) Nutrition—in *Scientific Foundations of Obstet. & Gynaec*. Edited by E. E. Philipp, Josephine Barnes & A. Newton. London: Heinemann.

Grunewald, P. (1965) *Some aspects of foetal distress—in Gestational Age, Size and maturity*. Edited by Dawkins & MacGregor. London: Spastics Soc.

Haworth, J. C., Dilling, Louise & Younoszai, M. K. (1967) Relation of blood-glucose to haematocrit, birthweight, and other body measurements in normal and growth-retarded newborn infants. *Lancet*, **ii**, 901.

Macgregor, J. D. & Avery, J. G. (1974) Malaria Transmission and fetal growth. *Brit. med. J.*, **ii**, 437.

Mathers, N. P., James, G. B. & Walker, J. (1970) The oxygen affinity of the blood of infants treated by intrauterine transfusion. *J. Obstet. Gynaec. Brit. Cwlth*, **77**, 648.

Meschia, G., Cotter, J. R., Breathnach, C. S. & Barron, D. (1965) The hemoglobin, oxygen, carbon dioxide and hydrogen ion concentrations in the umbilical bloods of sheep and goats as sampled via indwelling plastic catheters. *Quart. F. Exp. Physiology*, Vol. **50**, 185.

Patel, N. (1972) Amino acid concentrations in normal and abnormal pregnancies. *Proceedings of the Third European Congress of Perinatal Medicine*. Vienna: Hans Huber.

Reid, S. M. (1961) Unexplained prematurity: Investigation of possible causes. *J. Obstet. & Gynaec. Brit. Cwlth*, Vol. **68**, p. 796.

Short, R. V. (1972) *Sex determination and differentiation in embryonic and foetal development*. Edited by C. R. Austin & R. V. Short. Cambridge Univ. Press.

Smith, C. A. (1947) *Effects of the hunger winter (1944–45) in Holland upon pregnancy and the newborn infant*. Maandschr. v. Kindergeneesk, **15**, 121–141 (April 1947).

Stimson, W. H. (1972) Studies in the changes in the concentrations and total mass of individual serum proteins during late pregnancy. *J. Clin. Biochem*, **5**, 3.

Studd, J. W. W., Starkie, C. M. & Blainey, J. D. (1970) Serum protein changes in the parturient mother, fetus and newborn infant. *J. Obstet. Gynaec. Brit. Cwlth*, **77**, 511.

Tanner, J. M. & Thomson, A. N. (1970) Standards for birthweight at gestation periods from 32 to 42 weeks allowing for maternal height and weight. *Archs. Dis. Childh*, **45**, 566.

Thomson, A. N., Billewica, W. Z. & Hytten, F. E. (1968) The assessment of fetal growth. *J. Obstet. Gynaec. Brit. Cwlth*, **75**, 903.

Turnbull, E. & Walker, J. (1955) Haemoglobin and red cells in the human fetus. II. The Red Cells. *Archs. Dis. Childh*, **30**, 102.

Walker, J. & Turnbull, E. P. N. (1953) Haemoglobin and red cells in the human foetus. *Lancet*, **ii**, 312.

Walker, J. (1954) Foetal Anoxia. *J. Obstet. & Gynaec. Brit. Emp.*, **61**, 162.

Walker, J. & Wahab, A. (1956) *Personal Communication.*

Walker, J. (1967) The 'Small for Dates' Baby. *Proc. R. Soc. Med.*, Vol. **60**, 877.

Warkany, J., Monroe, B. B. & Sutherland, B. S. (1961) Intrauterine growth retardation. *Amer. J. Dis. Child.*, **102**, 249.

Widdowson, E. M. & Spray, C. M. (1951) Chemical development in utero. *Archs. Dis. Childh.*, **26**, 205.

Wigglesworth, J. S. (1969) Pathological and experimental studies in intrauterine malnutrition. *Proc. Nutrit. Soc.*, **28**, 31.

Winick, M. (1969) Malnutrition and brain development. *J. Paediat*, **74**, 667.

Winick, M. & Rosso, P. (1969) Head circumference and cellular growth of brain in normal and marasmic children. *J. Paediat*, **74**, 774.

Wong, K. S. & Scott, K. E. (1972) Fetal growth at sea level. *Biol. Neonate*, **20**, 175.

Young, M. & Prenton, M. A. (1969) Maternal and fetal plasma amino acid concentrations during gestation and in retarded fetal growth. *J. Obstet. Gynaec. Brit. Cwlth*, Vol. **76**, 333–344.

FURTHER READING

Austin, C. R. & Short, R. V. (Ed.) Reproduction in Mammals. *Embryonic and Foetal Development* (1972) Cambridge Univ. Press.

Ayre, L. B. (1965) *Developmental Anatomy*. London: Saunders.

Comline, K. S., Cross, K. W., Dawes, G. S. & Nathanielsz, P. W. (Ed.) *Foetal and Neonatal Physiology* (1972) Barcroft Symposium. Cambridge Univ. Press.

Dawes, G. S. (1968) *Foetal and Neonatal Physiology*. London: Year Book Publishers.

Hodari, A. A. & Morcina, F. G. (Ed.) *Physiological Biochemistry of the Foetus* (1972) London: Thames.

Horsky, J. & Stenkra, Z. K. (Ed.) *Intrauterine Dangers to the Foetus* (1967) (Symposium) Excerpta Med. Found.

Ounsted, N. & Ounsted, C. (1973) On Foetal Growth Rate. *Clinics in Dev. Med*, No. **4**. Spastic Med. Pub. London: Heinemann.

Tuchman-Duplessis, H. & Haegel, P. (1972) *Illustrated Human Embryology*. Vol. **1** Embryogenesis. Vol. **2** Organogenesis. London: Chapman and Hall.

Wolstenholme, G. E. W. & O'Connor, N. (Ed.) *Somatic Stability in the Newlyborn* (1961) London: Churchill.

Wolstenholme, G. E. W. & O'Connor, N. *Foetal Autonomy* (1969) London: Churchill.

Zusser, M. & Stein, Z. (1975) Maternal nutrition and low birth weight. *Lancet*, **ii**, 664.

7. Genetics in Relation to the Practice of Obstetrics and Gynaecology

INTRODUCTION

In recent years, because of advances in medicine and surgery, the incidence of diseases due to infections and nutritional deficiencies has gradually declined. The result has been an increase in the proportion of disorders which are largely or even entirely genetically determined.

In a recent survey of the causes of childhood deaths in a large industrial area of Britain, it was found that over 40 per cent were due largely or entirely to genetic factors (Roberts *et al.*, 1970). Problems presented by genetic disease are therefore not uncommon, and the physician is being asked more and more often to give advice on such problems.

The most important genetic problems in the practice of Obstetrics and Gynaecology involve delayed or abnormal sexual development, recurrent abortion, genetic counselling in families with genetic disease and antenatal diagnosis. More detailed treatment of these subjects can be found in Yunis (1974) and Emery (1975).

SEX CHROMOSOMAL ABNORMALITIES

Sexuality may be defined in terms of genetic, chromosomal, gonadal, hormonal and psychological factors. Any discrepancy between the latter and any of the former factors may result in psycho-sexual behaviour problems such as homosexuality, transexuality and transvestism. In this chapter, however, we shall only be concerned with intersex conditions in which genetic factors are of predominant importance. Many such disorders are associated with abnormalities of the sex chromosomes.

Diagnosis

Man has 46 chromosomes comprising 22 pairs of non-sex chromosomes (*autosomes*) and a pair of sex chromosomes: XX in the female and XY in the male. There are several cytogenetic techniques available for studying a patient's sex chromosome constitution. These techniques include sex-chromatin and fluorescent studies of cells obtained with a buccal smear, examination of 'drumsticks' in polymorphonuclear leucocytes in blood smears, and chromosome studies on peripheral blood leucocytes. Dermatoglyphics or the study of dermal ridge patterns may also be of some value but has limited clinical application.

Sex chromatin studies are carried out on cells obtained with a buccal smear and are then stained with an appropriate stain such as cresyl violet. In normal women there is a small dark staining body at the periphery of the nucleus in about half the cells examined. A similar body is not found in normal males. This is the sex-chromatin body and represents an X chromosome which is inactive and contracted down. The number of sex-chromatin bodies is one less than the number of X chromosomes. Thus the normal female has one sex-chromatin body, a female with three X chromosomes has 2 sex-chromatin bodies and a female with an XO sex chromosome constitution resembles the male in having no sex-chromatin bodies.

The Y chromosome can also be identified in buccal smears because the Y chromosome fluoresces when stained with certain quinacrine dyes. By a combination of staining for the sex-chromatin body and for the fluorescent Y chromosome it is possible from examination of a buccal smear to determine a person's sex chromosome constitution.

Another way in which the number of X chromosomes can be determined is by examination of the nuclei of polymorphs in stained peripheral blood smears. About 3 per cent of polymorphs of females have a small accessory nuclear lobule resembling a drumstick which projects from the main mass of the nuclear lobes. This is not seen in polymorphs from males, or females with an XO chromosome constitution. Unfortunately the number of drumsticks is not directly related to the number of X chromosomes when there are more than two.

Finally, when the morphology and characteristics of all the chromosomes are to be studied, then resort must be made to studying chromosomes in cultures of peripheral blood leucocytes or skin fibroblasts. In this way the number, size and shape of all the chromosomes (*karyotype*) can be studied (Fig. 7.1). This is a

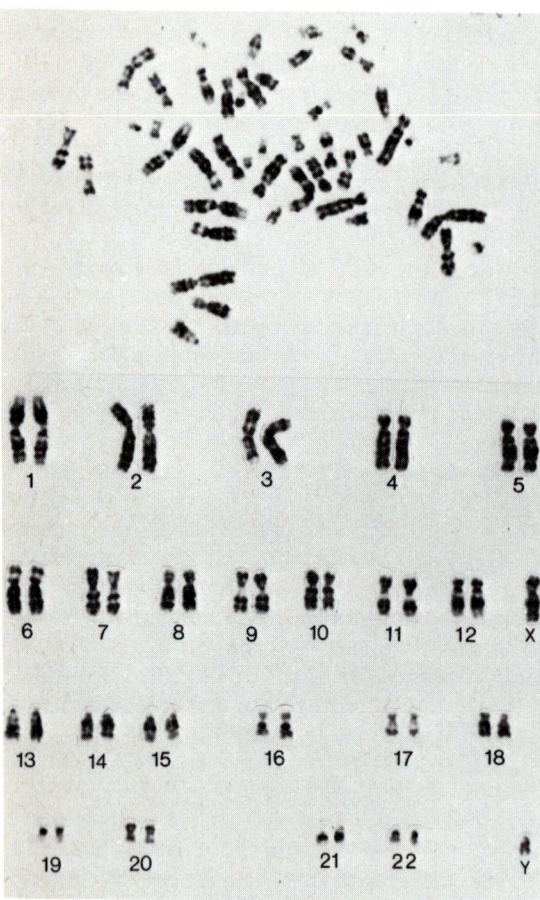

Fig. 7.1   Karyotype of a normal male.
(kind permission of Professor H. J. Evans)

task for the specialist cytogenetic laboratory. By fluorescent staining techniques it is now possible to identify each of the individual chromosomes.

Aetiology

A variety of sex chromosome abnormalities have been reported. In each case there is loss or gain of whole or part of one of the sex chromosomes.

Sex chromosome abnormalities may be divided into those which result from an error in cell division (*non-disjunction*), so that a whole sex chromosome is gained or lost, or from loss of part of a chromosome (a *deletion*). Non-disjunction usually occurs during gametogenesis and is illustrated in figure 7.2. If non-disjunction occurred during oogenesis and the ovum containing no sex chromosomes was fertilized by an X-bearing sperm the result would be a zygote with an XO sex chromosome constitution. If the ovum was fertilized by a Y-bearing sperm then the result would be a zygote with a YO sex chromosome constitution. Since no individual with this sex chromosome constitution has been found it is presumably lethal. Cases with four or more sex chromosomes cannot be explained by a single non-disjunctional event and we have to presume that two such events have occurred, one during meiosis I and the other during meiosis II. XYY individuals can only result during spermatogenesis if non-disjunction occurs at meiosis II. The cause of non-disjunction is not known. In the case of Down's syndrome (mongolism) and Klinefelter's syndrome it appears to be related to maternal age but this is not so in Turner's syndrome. The mothers of patients with Down's syndrome and Turner's syndrome have an increased frequency of thyroid antibodies, but how this is related to the cause of non-disjunction is not clear. In the case of Down's syndrome X-radiation has also been implicated but the evidence is far from being conclusive.

A shorthand notation is often used in describing chromosome abnormalities. Some of the abbreviations now being used include *p* and *q* for the short and long arms of chromosomes respectively, *t* for a translocation, *i* for an isochromosome and *r* for a ring. Addition of all or part of a chromosome is represented by a + sign and loss by a − sign after the chromosome to which they refer. It is customary to state first the number of chromosomes, followed by the sex chromosome constitution and then a note of any chromosomal abnormalities. Thus a normal female is represented as 46,XX and a normal male as 46,XY and a boy

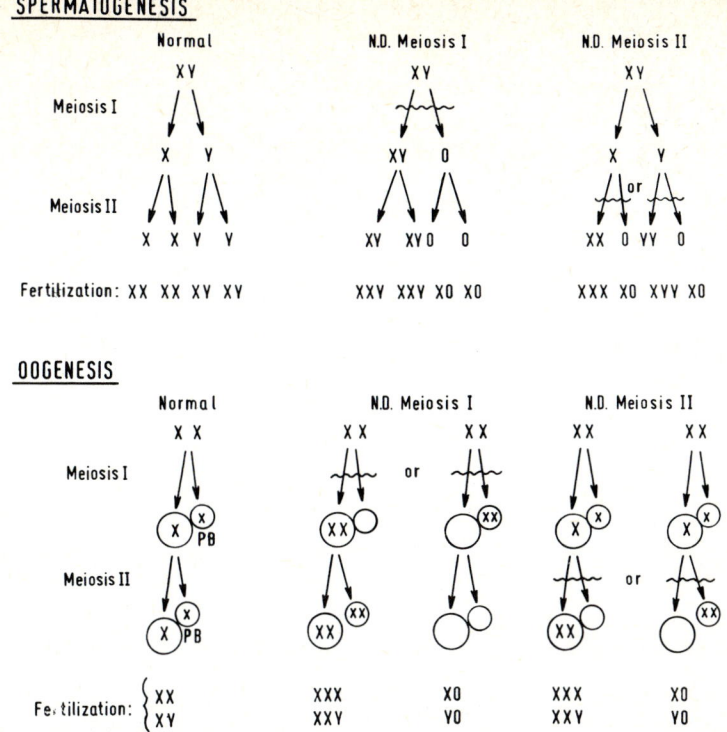

SPERMATOGENESIS

Fig. 7.2   The results of non-disjunction (ND) occurring at the first or second meiotic division in spermatogenesis and oogenesis.

with Down's syndrome with 47 chromosomes and an extra number 21 as 47,XY,21 +. Other variations will be described as they are encountered.

Ovarian dysgenesis (Turner's syndrome)

The term ovarian dysgenesis refers to the condition in which the ovaries are reduced to streaks of connective tissue ('streak gonads') with few if any Graafian follicles. The result is that such individuals rarely ovulate and therefore have primary amenorrhoea and are sterile. The breasts are usually undeveloped. This condition occurs if there is loss (deletion) of a long arm of one of the X chromosomes (46,XXq−).

Ovarian dysgenesis, however, is usually associated with various other congenital abnormalities when it is then referred to as Turner's syndrome (Fig. 7.3). Such individuals are rarely more than 5 feet in height, often have pigmented naevi, webbing of the neck, low posterior hairline, shield-like chest with widely spaced nipples, cubitus valgus (increased carrying angle), short fourth metacarpal and

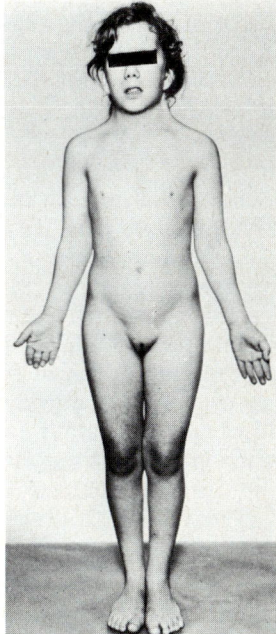

Fig. 7.3   Patient with Turner's syndrome with an XO sex chromosome constitution.

metatarsal bones, and coarctation of the aorta. Intellectual development is usually normal. In Turner's syndrome there is always loss of the *short* arm of one of the X chromosomes which very rarely may occur alone (46,XXp −), or more commonly is associated with the loss of an entire X chromosome (45,XO). Occasionally a female with Turner's syndrome has two X chromosomes but one is greatly enlarged due to duplication of the long arm and loss of the short arm. This abnormal chromosome is called an isochromosome and is believed to result from the centromere having divided transversely instead of longitudinally during cell division. This is represented as 46,XXqi. The relevant findings in patients with ovarian

testes and include small size (less than $\frac{1}{2}$ inch in diameter) and almost complete obliteration of the seminiferous tubules which are converted to hyaline masses. The Leydig (testosterone-producing) cells are unaffected and occupy the spaces between the shrunken tubules. As a consequence of these changes, individuals with this syndrome often have normal secondary sexual characteristics with a normal sized penis but there may be some gynaecomastia (Fig. 7.4). In all males with this syndrome however, spermatogenesis is usually entirely absent and they present as infertility. About 1 in 4 is mentally retarded.

Most patients with Klinefelter's syndrome have an XXY sex chromosome constitution

Table 7.1   Findings in female patients with ovarian dysgenesis and Turner's syndrome

Karyotype	Sex chromatin	Ovarian dysgenesis	Turner's syndrome (including short stature)
45,XO	−	+	+
46,XXp −	+	+	+
46,XXqi	+ (large)	+	+
46,XXq −	+ (small)	+	−

dysgenesis and Turner's syndrome are summarized in Table 7.1.

It is clear from these findings that full chromosome studies with karyotype analysis may be necessary to establish the correct chromosome constitution in some cases of ovarian dysgenesis.

The occurrence of short stature, webbing of the neck, cubitus valgus and certain other congenital abnormalities has been described in both males and females with apparently normal karyotypes. This syndrome has been variously described as 'male Turner syndrome' or 'female pseudo-Turner syndrome'. More recently such cases have come to be referred to as Noonan's syndrome after Dr Jacqueline Noonan who first drew attention to the syndrome in 1963. It appears to be inherited but the precise mode of inheritance is not clear: it may be an X-linked or autosomal dominant trait.

Seminiferous tubule dysgenesis (Klinefelter's syndrome)

The cardinal pathological features of Klinefelter's syndrome are seen in the postpubertal

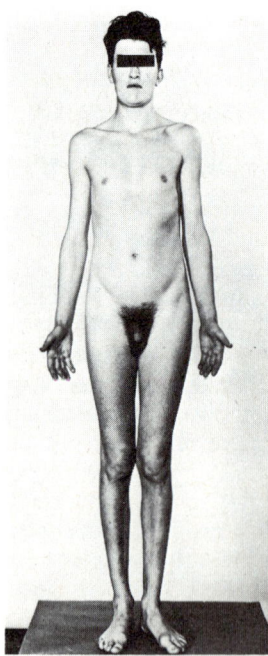

Fig. 7.4   Patient with Klinefelter's syndrome with an XXY sex chromosome constitution.

(47,XXY) and can be easily detected because they are sex-chromatin positive. However, patients have been described with this syndrome who are 48,XXXY and even 49,XXXXY. These individuals have 2 and 3 sex-chromatin bodies respectively, are always mentally retarded and often have congenital abnormalities not usually seen in XXY cases.

Mosaics

A mosaic is an individual with two or more distinct cell populations with different karyotypes which are usually distributed throughout the body in a random manner. A great variety of mosaics have been described in man. For example, patients with Turner's syndrome may be 45,XO/46,XX, or 45,XO/47,XXX, or 45,XO/46,XX/47,XXX (3 cell lines) etc. The patient will appear more normal the greater the proportion of cells with a normal female XX sex chromosome constitution. Mosaicism has not only been described in Turner's syndrome but also in other chromosomal abnormalities including Klinefelter's syndrome (46,XY/47,XXY, or 46,XY/48,-XXXY, or 46,XY/47,XXY/48,XXXY etc). More than one cell line may be detected in a single tissue (e.g. blood) or mosaicism may only be evident when different tissues have been examined; for example, skin fibroblasts and peripheral blood leucocytes.

Mosaicism can arise in two ways. It may be the result of non-disjunction in early embryogenesis with the persistence of more than one cell line. Thus if a zygote has two X chromosomes and non-disjunction occurs so that one daughter cell receives three X chromosomes (XXX) while the other receives only one X chromosome (XO) this will result in an XO/XXX mosaic. This appears to be the way in which many mosaics arise. However, another possible cause of an XX/XY mosaic is double fertilization, that is by fertilization of two eggs or an egg and a polar body by two spermatozoa—the resulting two diploid nuclei then both contribute to the formation of an individual. This appears to be a rare event but evidence that it can occur in man has been obtained from blood group and other studies of the parents of certain patients who are known to be mosaics.

The diagnosis of mosaicism is not always easy because though most of the cells of a normal person will have the modal number of 46 chromosomes, some cells may have lost or gained a chromosome as a consequence of technical factors. If mosaicism is suspected it must be established that in the hypomodal and hypermodal cells it is always the same chromosome which is missing or is in excess.

Hermaphroditism

True hermaphrodites have both ovarian and testicular tissue. All degrees have been described from those who appear to be almost like a normal male to those who appear to be almost like a normal female. There are varying degrees of bisexuality in the genitalia as well as in the general physique (Fig. 7.5). At laparotomy an

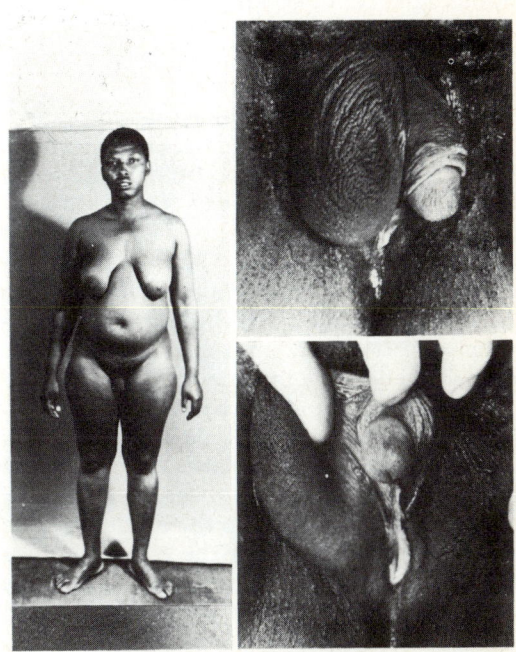

Fig. 7.5 Patient with true hermaphroditism, sex chromatin positive and an XX sex chromosome constitution.

(kind permission of Dr E. Wilton)

ovary may be found on one side and a testis on the other, or there is a mixture of ovarian and testicular tissues (ovo-testes) on both sides or sometimes only on one side, the gonad on the other side being an ovary or a testis.

It would be expected that true hermaphrodites might be XX/XY mosaics. Some are, but the majority have an ostensibly normal XX sex chromosome constitution. The reason for this is not clear. There is always the possibility that if studies have been limited to a single tissue, usually peripheral blood, mosaicism of the XX/XY type might not have been excluded. However, many XX cases have been subjected to thorough cytogenetic investigation but no evidence of mosaicism has been obtained. It has been suggested that in these cases the paternal X chromosome may carry male-determining genes as a result of crossing-over between the X and Y chromosomes during meiosis in spermatogenesis.

Pseudohermaphroditism

In pseudohermaphrodites there is a discordance between the external genitalia and the true gonadal sex. Thus, a male pseudohermaphrodite has testes but female external genitalia and breast tissue, whereas a female pseudohermaphrodite has ovaries but masculinized genitalia.

An example of male pseudohermaphroditism is the Testicular Feminization Syndrome. Affected persons appear to be perfectly normal females with breasts and female external genitalia but they have no uterus, do not menstruate and are sterile. Chromosome studies of patients with this syndrome have shown that they have an XY sex chromosome constitution and do in fact have testes which are often located in the inguinal canal and sometimes mistaken for a hernia. The reasons why these individuals appear to be normal females and do not have any outward manifestations of masculinity is believed to be because their tissues are unresponsive to the effects of male hormones synthesized by the testes. This is an inherited disorder but whether it is an autosomal dominant trait with male limitation or an X-linked recessive trait is not clear.

Female pseudohermaphrodites have normal ovaries and female internal genitalia and an XX sex chromosome constitution but with masculinized external genitalia. This may be iatrogenic, induced in a female fetus by the ingestion of androgens by the pregnant mother. Alternatively it may be due to the adrenogenital syndrome, an inborn error of metabolism associated with a defect of a specific enzyme necessary for the synthesis of cortisol. The pituitary gland compensates by secreting excessive amounts of ACTH which stimulates the adrenal cortex with the resultant excess production of androgens and cortisol-precursors. This condition is inherited as an autosomal recessive trait and affects both sexes. In the female the earliest signs of masculinization are present at birth with enlargement of the clitoris and varying degrees of fusion of the genital folds. In the male, within a short time of birth, the penis starts to enlarge and later features of precocious pseudo-puberty appear.

Other sex chromosome abnormalities

Two other sex chromosome abnormalities remain to be discussed: the XXX female and the XYY male. Females with three or even four X chromosomes have been described. They are sometimes mentally retarded though in all other respects they appear to be perfectly normal females. The XYY male has received considerable publicity in recent times. This chromosomal abnormality was first thought to be associated with mental subnormality and aggressive antisocial behaviour. However, in recent studies such individuals have been found in the general population by chance and though often tall are not necessarily delinquent or mentally retarded. So far all the children of XXX females and XYY males have been normal in contrast to the offspring of women with Down's syndrome, half of whose children are similarly affected. The reason why XXX females and XYY males do not have children with extra sex chromosomes is not known.

Meiotic studies

So far we have been concerned only with *somatic* chromosomes derived from peripheral blood leucocytes or skin fibroblasts. It is possible, however, to study chromosomes undergoing meiosis from biopsied testicular or even ovarian tissues. In this way the morphology and pairing behaviour of chromosomes in spermatocytes and oocytes may be studied. Certain chromosomal rearrangements (which may be the cause of fetal abnormality) may be clearly recognized in meiotic material from the configuration of pairing homologous chromosomes (bivalents). For example, a chromosome *inversion*, whereby a segment of a chromosome is inverted, may be recognizable from its abnormal pairing behaviour and configuration in meiotic material. Meiotic studies in testicular tissue may also be helpful in understanding the cause of certain forms of male sterility.

However, the introduction of the new banding techniques whereby parts of individual somatic chromosomes can be clearly identified may in fact make the need for meiotic studies not quite so important in the future.

AUTOSOMAL ABNORMALITIES

Abnormalities of the non-sex chromosomes (autosomes) may be subdivided into numerical and structural abnormalities. Numerical abnormalities involve the loss or gain of one or two chromosomes (*aneuploidy*) or even the gain of a whole chromosome set. The latter condition is referred to as *triploidy* (69 chromosomes). Survival after birth with triploid cells in every tissue of the body is extremely rare and all reported cases have died shortly after birth. *Monosomy* or the loss of an autosome is also lethal. However, *trisomy*, or the addition of an extra autosome has been described in several disorders in man. The commonest of these is Down's syndrome with 47 chromosomes, the extra chromosome being a number 21.

Structural abnormalities of the autosomes include *translocations*, in which there is an exchange of genetic material between non-homologous chromosomes, and *deletions* in which a segment of a chromosome has been lost. Though the majority of children with Down's syndrome are trisomic for chromosome 21, a few (about 3 per cent) have the normal number of 46 chromosomes. In these cases the extra chromosome 21 is present but has been translocated either to another chromosome 21, to a chromosome 22 or more usually to chromosome 14 or 15. In such cases one of the parents may carry the chromosome translocation but has only 45 chromosomes. These individuals appear perfectly normal because they have only two chromosomes 21. However, their recognition is important as they run a comparatively high risk of having a child with Down's syndrome (*see below*).

Apart from Down's syndrome, most autosomal abnormalities are rare. Some of the salient clinical features of recognized autosomal abnormalities are summarized in Table 7.2.

Table 7.2   Autosomal abnormalities associated with recognized clinical syndromes (*From* Emery, 1975)

Chromosome abnormality	Syndrome	Clinical features
trisomy-21 translocation 14 or 15/21 translocation 22/21 translocation 21/21	Down's	characteristic facies mental retardation hypotonia congenital heart disease Simian palmar crease
trisomy-8	——	moderate mental retardation concomitant strabismus clinodactyly other skeletal defects
trisomy-9	——	abnormal facies skeletal abnormalities hypoplastic genitalia congenital heart disease
trisomy-13	Patau's	motor and mental retardation microcephaly microphthalmia cleft palate/hare lip polydactyly congenital heart disease
trisomy-18	Edwards'	motor and mental retardation flexion deformities of fingers micrognathia 'rocker-bottom' feet congenital heart disease
trisomy-22	——	mental and motor retardation microcephaly abnormal facies and ears
trisomy-4p	——	abnormal facies digital anomalies foot deformities

Table 7.2   Autosomal abnormalities associated with recognized clinical
syndromes—*continued*

Chromosome abnormality	Syndrome	Clinical features
trisomy-9p	——	abnormal facies
		large, low-set ears
		mental retardation
		incurred and short V digit
4p–	——	mental retardation
		abnormal facies
		cleft plate
		coloboma
		epilepsy
		hypospadias
		scalp defects
5p–	Cri du chat	mental retardation
		microcephaly
		hypertelorism
		characteristic cry
13q–	——	mental and motor retardation
13r		abnormal facies
		microcephaly
		abnormal thumbs
		abnormal ears
18q–	De Grouchy's	mental retardation
		'carp mouth'
		abnormal ears
		tapering fingers
18p–	De Grouchy's	mental retardation
		ocular abnormalities
		abnormal ears
		dental decay
		CNS abnormalities
18r	——	combination of 18p– and 18q– features
21q– (G deletion syndrome I)	'anti-mongolism'	antimongoloid slant of eyes
		hypertonia
		micrognathia
		growth retardation
		skeletal malformations
22q– (G deletion syndrome II)	——	epicanthic folds
		hypotonia
		syndactyly
		retarded development

RECURRENT ABORTION

About 15 per cent of all conceptions terminate in either a spontaneous abortion or a still birth; and more than 30 per cent of spontaneous abortions have a chromosome abnormality. Many of these chromosomal abnormalities, which include autosomal monosomy (loss of an autosome) and triploidy (an extra set of chromosomes, i.e. 69 rather than 46), have not been found in live-born babies and are therefore presumably lethal. Others, such as XO, can be compatible with survival. The risk of recurrence in these types of abnormalities is small. Occasionally in cases of recurrent abortion one of the parents carries a trans-location which in the unbalanced state in the fetus is lethal. The parent who carries the translocation has the normal amount of genetic material and is therefore perfectly healthy. Depending on the particular type of chromosomal rearrangement found in the carrier parent the risks of further abortions may be very high. In some instances it might be predicted that no live birth would be possible. In cases of recurrent abortion where the cause is not obvious, chromosome studies on both parents may therefore be helpful. Evidence suggests however, that a chromosome rearrangement is a rare cause of recurrent abortion.

Almost 50 per cent of abortions from women

who have conceived after discontinuing oral contraceptives have a chromosomal abnormality, usually triploidy. The reason for this is not known but the investigation of this phenomenon may throw more light on the cause of spontaneous abortions and chromosomal abnormalities in general.

GENETIC COUNSELLING

The genetic counsellor is concerned with such problems as the advisability of cousin marriages, child adoption and because of his

gene on an autosome is said to be inherited as an autosomal trait and may be dominant or recessive. A trait which is determined by a gene on one of the sex chromosomes is said to be sex-linked and may also be either dominant or recessive. However, apart from the possible exception of hairy ears, there appear to be no Mendelizing genes on the Y chromosome and therefore sex-linkage is synonymous with X-linkage. X-linked dominant traits, apart from the Xg blood group, are rare and will not be dealt with. A list of some of the more common unifactorial disorders and their modes of inheritance are given in Table 7.3. These

Table 7.3   Modes of inheritance of some genetic (unifactorial) disorders

Autosomal dominant	Autosomal recessive	X-linked recessive
Achondroplasia	Albinism	Aldrich syndrome
Facio–scapulo–humeral muscular dystrophy	Alkaptonuria	Choroideremia
Haemoglobin variants	Fibrocystic disease	Deutan & Protan colour blindness
Holt–Oram syndrome	Friedreich's ataxia	Duchenne muscular dystrophy
Huntington's chorea	Galactosaemia	G-6-PD deficiency
Marfan's syndrome	Hartnup's disease	Fabry's disease
Neurofibromatosis	Homocystinuria	Haemophilia A & B
Polyposis coli	Hurler's syndrome	Hunter's syndrome
Porphyria variegata	Laurence-Moon-Biedl syndrome	Lesch-Nyhan syndrome
Tuberose sclerosis	Limb girdle muscular dystrophy	Nephrogenic diabetes insipidus
Waardenburg's syndrome	Maple syrup urine disease	Ocular albinism
	Niemann–Pick's disease	Oculo-cerebro-renal syndrome
	Phenylketonuria	
	Pseudoxanthoma	
	Refsum's syndrome	
	Tay–Sachs disease	
	Werdnig-Hoffmann's disease	
	Wilson's disease	

knowledge of cytogenetics, delayed or abnormal sexual development, infertility, and recurrent abortion where there is no obvious gynaecological cause. The primary concern of the genetic counsellor however, is with calculating and explaining the risks of recurrence of genetic disease.

In discussing recurrence risks it is convenient to divide genetic disease into three groups: unifactorial, multifactorial and chromosomal disorders.

Unifactorial disorders

These are so-called Mendelian traits or single gene defects. A trait which is determined by a

disorders, though individually rare, are important because they are often serious and the chances of recurrence in other members of a family may be very high.

Autosomal dominant traits affect both males and females, and if they have little effect on survival can often be traced back through several generations (Fig. 7.6). If however, the disorder significantly reduces the chances of an affected person having children then only a few instances of an affected parent and child may occur. With autosomal dominant traits the chance of an affected person having an affected child is 1 in 2. However, if normal parents have an affected child and there is no

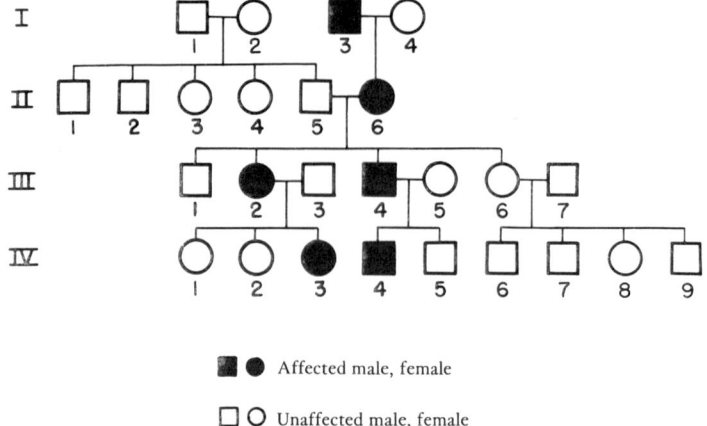

Fig. 7.6   Pedigree pattern of an autosomal dominant trait.

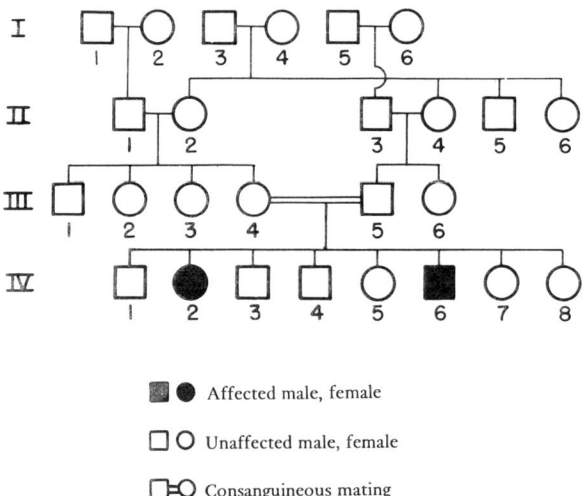

Fig. 7.7   Pedigree pattern of an autosomal recessive trait.

family history of anyone else having been similarly affected, this is presumably the result of a new *mutation* and is therefore most unlikely to recur in any subsequent children. It should be remembered however, that autosomal dominant traits tend to vary considerably in their severity (= *expressivity*). It may be that one of the parents is affected though minimally (= *forme fruste*), the abnormality only being obvious on careful clinical examination. In such circumstances the chances of recurrence are the same as if the parent were severely affected. Very rarely a dominant trait may skip a generation (= *nonpenetrant*).

Autosomal recessive disorders affect brothers and sisters (sibs) but the parents are healthy (Fig. 7.7). With rare recessive disorders

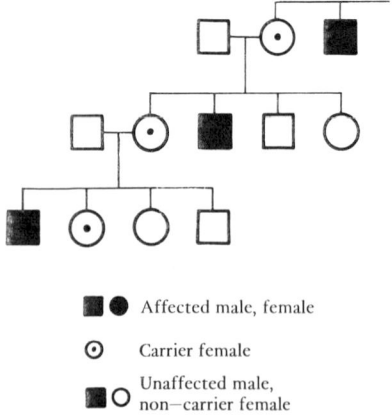

Fig. 7.8   Pedigree pattern of an X-linked recessive trait in which affected males do not reproduce.

the parents are often related but the absence of consanguinity does not mean that a disorder is not a recessive. When parents have had one affected child the chance of recurrence in subsequent children is 1 in 4.

X-linked recessive disorders affect males but very rarely females who are then usually XO. These disorders are transmitted by healthy females (Fig. 7.8) but if the disorder is not so serious, affected males may survive and have children. Since a male transmits his X chromosome to his daughters and his Y chromosome to his sons, all his daughters will be carriers but all his sons will be normal. A woman who is a carrier has a 1 in 2 chance of having a son who is affected and a 1 in 2 chance of having a daughter who is also a carrier. There are now tests available which can detect whether a woman is a carrier of certain X-linked disorders. In this way the sister of an affected boy for example, can be tested and advised regarding her risks of having an affected son.

One very important point to be remembered in genetic counselling is the phenomenon of *genetic heterogeneity*, i.e. that different genes may produce apparently similar disorders. Thus in progressive muscular dystrophy there are X-linked recessive forms (e.g. Duchenne type), autosomal recessive forms (e.g. limb-girdle type), and autosomal dominant forms (e.g. facioscapulohumeral type). The recognition of genetic heterogeneity is essential if reliable genetic advice is to be given. Not only must a precise diagnosis be established but also the mode of inheritance.

A further complication is that a particular disorder may only resemble a genetic disorder and not be inherited at all. Such a disorder which is due to some environmental factor is referred to as a *phenocopy*. Thus various congenital abnormalities can occur following the ingestion of certain drugs during pregnancy (e.g. thalidomide, antifolates, progestins), exposure to radiation and rubella infection. Once such a causative agent has been identified then the disorder is unlikely to recur again in a subsequent pregnancy and the parents can be reassured.

Multifactorial disorders

There are many fairly common disorders where there is a definite familial tendency, the proportion of affected relatives being greater than in the general population. However, the proportion of affected relatives is often of the order of 1 in 20 (5 per cent) and therefore much less than would be expected for a unifactorial trait. It seems likely that such conditions are caused by many genes plus the effects of environment, so-called multifactorial inheritance.

It is assumed that in multifactorial inheritance an individual has a *liability* to developing a particular disorder. This liability includes not only his genetic predisposition but also the environmental circumstances which render him more or less likely to develop the disease. It is assumed that in the general population and in relatives of affected individuals, liability to a particular disorder is normally distributed but the curve for relatives is shifted to the right (Fig. 7.9). The points on the curves

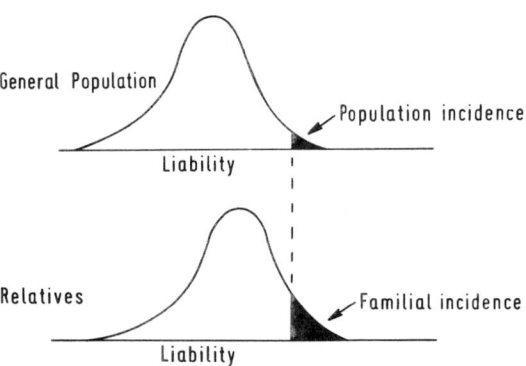

Fig. 7.9 Hypothetical curve of liability in the general population and in relatives for an hereditary disorder in which the genetic predisposition is multifactorial.

above which all individuals are affected is the threshold. In the general population the proportion above the threshold is the population incidence and among relatives the proportion above the threshold is the familial incidence. This model has been applied to measurable characters (such as stature and intelligence) and also to explain the familial incidence of such conditions as diabetes mellitus, various congenital abnormalities (anencephaly and spina bifida, club foot, congenital pyloric stenosis etc.), schizophrenia, ischaemic heart disease, hypertension and peptic ulcer. In such conditions it is not possible to predict recurrence risks based on Mendelian ratios. The risks have to be determined by estimating the frequency of the condition among the relatives of affected individuals, so-called *empiric risks*. Approximate empiric risk figures for some

Table 7.4   Empiric risks for some common disorders (in per cent)
(*From* Emery, 1975)

Disorder	Incidence	Sex ratio M:F	Normal parents having a second affected child	Affected parent having an affected child	Affected parent having a second affected child
Anencephaly	0·20	1:2	2	—	—
Cleft palate only	0·04	2:3	2	7	15
Cleft lip ± cleft palate	0·10	3:2	4	4	10
Club foot	0·10	2:1	3	3	10
Cong. heart disease (all types)	0·50	—	1–4	1–4	—
Diabetes mellitus (early onset)	0·20	1:1	8	8	10
Dislocation of hip	0·07	1:6	4	4	10
Epilepsy ('idiopathic')	0·50	1:1	5	5	10
Hirschsprung's disease	0·02	4:1			
male index			2	—	—
female index			8	—	—
Manic-depressive psychoses	0·40	2:3	—	10–15	—
Mental retardation ('idiopathic')	0·30 −0·50	1:1	3–5	—	—
Profound childhood deafness	0·10	1:1	10	6	—
Pyloric stenosis	0·30	5:1			
male index			2	4	13
female index			10	17	38
Schizophrenia	1–2	1:1	—	16	—
Scoliosis (idiopathic, adolescent)	0·22	1:6	7	5	—
Spina bifida	0·30	2:3	4	3	—

(Tables 7.2 and 7.4 are reproduced from Emery, A. E. H. (1975) *Elements of Medical Genetics*, 4th edn. Edinburgh: Churchill Livingstone).

common conditions are given in Table 7.4. These risks only apply to conditions which are not inherited in any simple manner. For example, mental retardation due to phenylketonuria is inherited as an autosomal recessive trait and the risk of recurrence to sibs is 1 in 4 (25 per cent). In cases of mental retardation not associated with any particular genetic disorder (i.e. 'idiopathic'), the risk of recurrence to sibs is about 3–5 per cent.

In general recurrence risks for common genetic (multifactorial) disorders are usually low, being of the order of 3–5 per cent. The risks however, may be much higher where:

1. there is more than one affected individual in the family.
2. the index patient is *severely* affected.
3. there is a sex difference in the population incidence, the risks being higher in the relatives of the less frequently affected sex. For example, in pyloric stenosis which is five times

commoner in boys than girls, the proportions of affected relatives of male index patients are 5·5 per cent for sons and 2·4 per cent for daughters, but 19·4 per cent for sons and 7·3 per cent for daughters when the index patient is a female (Carter, 1969). For these reasons empiric risk figures should not be applied in the individual case without some qualification and the possibility must always be excluded that the disorder in question is not a single gene (unifactorial) defect.

Chromosomal abnormalities

Most cases of chromosomal abnormalities whether autosomal or sex-chromosomal, are sporadic. They result from errors in meiosis during gametogenesis (or rarely in early embryogenesis) and the chances of recurrence are small. If, however, one of the parents is a mosaic or carries a translocation the situation is different. When one of the parents is a mosaic, genetic counselling is very difficult because it is impossible to estimate what proportion of the parental gonadal tissue is normal. If one of the parents carries a translocation then empiric risk figures are available. In the case of Down's syndrome with a 14–15/21, or 21/22 translocation, if the mother carries the translocation then the risk of recurrence is about 10 per cent, but if the father carries the translocation the risk is less than 5 per cent. If either of the parents carries a 21/21 translocation it can be predicted that all their children will have Down's syndrome, but fortunately this is very rare.

In giving genetic advice in Down's syndrome it should be remembered that only about 3 per cent of cases have a translocation and half of these arise *de novo* and are not inherited. Most cases of Down's syndrome have trisomy-21 and the chances of recurrence after the birth of an affected child are about 1 in 100. A mother aged 40 or more has a 1 in 50 chance of having an affected child irrespective of whether she has had a previously affected child.

ANTENATAL DIAGNOSIS

Factors which influence the parents' decision as to whether or not they will accept the risk of having an affected child include the severity of the abnormality, whether there is an effective treatment, the actual risk, their religious attitudes and socio-economic status and education. The genetic counsellor does not usually try to influence the parents' decision. If, after consideration, the parents decide that the risks of having an affected child are too great then there are several possibilities open to them. They may decide to practise some form of contraception and possibly adopt a child. Alternatively one of the parents may decide to be sterilized. In situations where both parents are heterozygous for the same rare recessive trait, or the father is affected with a dominant or X-linked disorder, then artificial insemination by donor (AID) is a possibility.

With the liberalization of the Abortion Law, if there is a 'substantial risk' of a serious abnormality in the fetus then termination is possible should the mother become pregnant. In certain disorders *selective* abortion is possible whereby a pregnancy need only be terminated when the fetus is known to be

Table 7.5 Techniques available for the antenatal diagnosis of fetal disorders

A. *Direct* (fetal)
  1. Radiography
    a. Skeletal
    b. Soft tissue (amniography, fetography)
  2. Sonography
  3. Electrocardiography
  4. Fetoscopy
  5. Biopsy
    a. Membranes
    b. Placenta
    c. Fetus
  6. Amniocentesis
B. *Indirect* (maternal)
  1. Blood   e.g. Rh, fetal lymphocytes
  2. Urine   e.g. oestriol excretion

abnormal. This is possible through the techniques of antenatal diagnosis (Emery, 1973).

Techniques available for the antenatal diagnosis of fetal disorders are summarized in Table 7.5. Radiography, sonography, and electrocardiography are of value only in later pregnancy and fetoscopy and the biopsy of placental and fetal tissues is still experimental. The technique used in most laboratories is the examination of the cells and fluid in specimens of liquor obtained by transabdominal amniocentesis. The time when the procedure is carried out is a compromise: the more advanced the pregnancy the easier the technique becomes, yet aspiration must be carried out early enough for termination to be possible should it be indicated. Usually 5–10ml of fluid are obtained between the 14th and 16th weeks of pregnancy. Maternal complications following this procedure are rare, and it seems that risks to the fetus are also likely to be small but these have yet to be fully assessed. There is the theoretical risk of evoking Rhesus sensitization in the mother though this seems unlikely if placental damage is avoided by first locating the placenta by sonography.

The fluid obtained by amniocentesis is centrifuged and the cell-free supernatant used for biochemical studies and the cells for sex-determination, cytogenetic and biochemical investigations. The cells are of fetal origin and largely derived from the fetal skin. Amniotic fluid is contributed to by fetal urine from about the 12th week of gestation.

Sexing the fetus

The fetus may be sexed in early pregnancy by a combination of sex-chromatin and fluorescent

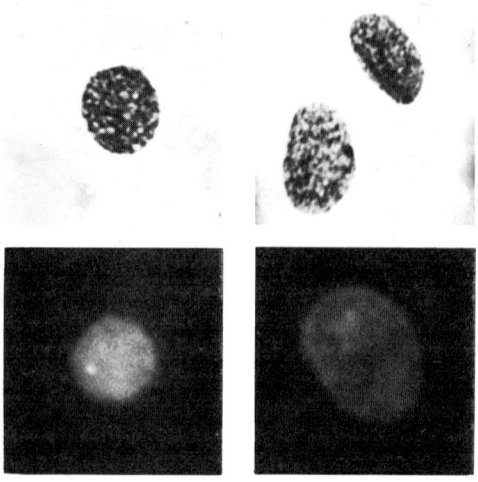

Fig. 7.10   Amniotic fluid cells stained for sex chromatin with cresyl violet (*above*) and for fluorescence with quinacrine hydrochloride (*below*). Cells from a male fetus are sex-chromatin negative and have a fluorescent (Y) body (*left*) whereas cells from a female fetus are sex-chromatin positive and have no fluorescent body (*right*).

(kind permission of Dr M. M. Nelson)

Cytogenetic studies on amniotic fluid cells

Since the cell density is low in amniotic fluid obtained in early pregnancy care is needed in setting up cultures but in experienced laboratories at least 90 per cent of specimens can be successfully cultured. Chromosome analysis of these cultured cells is usually possible within two to three weeks.

These studies are particularly important where one of the parents carries a chromosome translocation which in the unbalanced state produces, for example, Down's syndrome. The technique is also valuable in cases where there is an increased risk of 21-trisomy Down's syndrome. For example, when the mother has already had one such affected child or the mother is over 40 years of age.

studies on amniotic fluid cells (Fig. 7.10). Since these cells are frequently pyknotic not all preparations are found to be satisfactory for these studies and in such cases full karyotype analysis of cultured cells is more reliable for predicting fetal sex. One further complication in all studies of the early fetus by amniocentesis is that it may be a non-identical twin pregnancy and only one sac may be sampled.

One application of fetal sex prediction is in the selective abortion of male fetuses of a known carrier of an X-linked recessive disorder, such as haemophilia or Duchenne muscular dystrophy, which cannot yet be diagnosed *in utero*. In this way the mother can be guaranteed a daughter who will not be affected, but there is a 1 in 2 chance she could be a carrier. Further, in such circumstances on average half the male fetuses aborted will be normal. When it is possible to diagnose the affected male *in utero* then only male fetuses known to be affected need be aborted.

Another application of prenatal sex prediction is in the selective abortion of female fetuses of a father with an X-linked disorder such as haemophilia, since all his daughters must be carriers but all his sons will be normal.

Biochemical studies on amniotic fluid cells

With biochemical studies on cultured amniotic fluid cells it is now possible to diagnose *in utero* a number of inborn errors of metabolism such as galactosaemia, Hurler's syndrome, Tay-Sachs disease and Lesch-Nyhan syndrome. The latter condition, characterized by choreo-athetosis, spasticity, mental retardation and compulsive self-mutilation, is inherited as an X-linked recessive trait. In this disorder both the carrier female and affected male can be diagnosed *in utero*. This of course, is the hope for other X-linked recessive disorders for in this way not only could a mother who is a carrier be guaranteed a healthy son but also a daughter who is not a carrier.

For the antenatal diagnosis of biochemical disorders however, many more cells are required than for cytogenetic investigations and it may be six weeks or more before there are sufficient cells on which to base a reliable diagnosis. This is a serious limitation to the technique but improvements in cell culture techniques will no doubt overcome this problem in the near future.

To avoid the complications of having to culture amniotic fluid cells, another approach to the antenatal diagnosis of metabolic disorders has been the biochemical study of amniotic fluid itself. Here it is assumed that metabolic disorders accompanied by changes in urinary composition might be so detected since fetal urine contributes to the formation of amniotic fluid.

Finally, it is now possible to diagnose anencephaly and most cases of spina bifida in early pregnancy from α-fetoprotein estimations on amniotic fluid and probably maternal serum.

CONCLUSIONS

For families at high risk of having a child with a serious genetic disorder genetic counselling is essential. Not only may this advice prevent the birth of subsequent affected children but it should be designed to dispel feelings of guilt which may accompany the birth of such a child. Through the development of biochemical and other tests it is now possible to detect preclinical cases of certain genetic disorders (such as Duchenne muscular dystrophy) and even healthy carriers of harmful genes. Coupled with the newly developing techniques of antenatal diagnosis and selective abortion, a constructive and helpful approach can be offered to parents at risk of having a child with a serious genetic disorder.

REFERENCES

Carter, C. O. (1969) Genetics of common disorders. *Brit. med. Bull.*, **25**, 52–57.
Emery, A. E. H. (1973) Ed. *Antenatal Diagnosis of Genetic Disease*. Edinburgh: Churchill Livingstone.
Emery, A. E. H. (1975) *Elements of Medical Genetics*. 4th edit. Edinburgh: Churchill Livingstone.
Roberts, D. F., Chavez, J. & Court, S. D. M. (1970) The genetic component in child mortality. *Archs. Dis. Childh.*, **45**, 33–38.
Yunis, J. J. (1974) *Human Chromosome Methodology*, 2nd edit. New York: Academic Press.

8. Bleeding During Pregnancy

Bleeding from the genital tract may occur at any time during pregnancy, and be due to a variety of causes. From a practical point of view, pregnancy bleeding is divided into two main groups—that occurring before 28 weeks of pregnancy and that occurring after 28 weeks of pregnancy.

The first variety is termed early pregnancy bleeding and the latter antepartum haemorrhage.

EARLY PREGNANCY BLEEDING

Bleeding in early pregnancy may be due to:
1. abortion or miscarriage;
2. extra-uterine (ectopic) pregnancy;
3. hydatidiform mole. (*See* Chap. 9.)

Abortion or miscarriage

These terms, which in modern parlance are synonymous, mean the expulsion of the products of conception before the 28th week of pregnancy.

FREQUENCY OF ABORTION

It is difficult, if not impossible, to obtain accurate information about the incidence of abortion. In early abortions, the products of conception may be easily passed with little or no discomfort, and any bleeding may be mistaken for a menstrual period. Frequently, women are not ill, and do not seek medical advice. In some cases, not so many since the introduction of the Abortion Act 1967, there may be deliberate concealment, especially when the abortion has been self-induced. The most comprehensive study performed is that of Stevenson *et al.* (1959) who estimated the incidence of abortion at around 11·8 per cent of all pregnancies, although it seems likely that the figure may, in fact, be higher than this.

THE CAUSES OF ABORTION

The causes of abortion appear to be numerous and much interest has been shown in trying to determine the causes. While advances have been made, much has still to be learned about the fundamental causes for this common condition and there is still much to be done to improve our methods of prevention which are at present somewhat haphazard.

There are two main types of abortion:

a. where uterine contractions occur first and expel the ovum or fetus, and
b. where the ovum or fetus dies first, frequently due to haemorrhage into the decidua and is expelled thereafter.

Aetiological factors leading to abortion may be classified under two main headings:

i. fetal, and
ii. maternal.

i. *Fetal causes*

In many cases, the fetus is not available for detailed examination but where it is, an abnormal conceptus of some type has been found in 40 to 50 per cent of spontaneous abortions. In addition to this, about 6 per cent of specimens which appear normal on external examination and dissection also have a chromosome anomaly. Abortions of less than 120 days' gestation yield the highest number of chromosome anomalies. The commonest disorder is associated with one extra chromosome—trisomy. This disorder may account for nearly half the chromosomaly abnormal abortuses. Monosomy accounts for about 5 per cent, and the third most common type is triploidy, where a whole extra set of chromosomes is present. Some of these abnormalities, e.g. trisomy 21—Down's syndrome—are not necessarily incompatible with extra-uterine life but are usually associated with some form of congenital abnormality. It has also been established that women who have abortions in their childbearing life have a greater incidence of fetal abnormality in their children than women who do not have abortions. It is of interest to note that the incidence of abnormalities in the karyotype of abortuses obtained from therapeutic terminations is only 0·2 per cent. This suggests that these errors in mitosis occur at the very early stages of development. Abnormalities of the chorion are also fetal causes of abortion. The most extreme example of this being hydatidiform mole.

ii *Maternal causes*

Endocrine errors. It is possible that endocrine abnormalities may be a factor associated with abortion but evidence is scanty at present. In a normal pregnancy there is a steady rise in the production of the steroid hormones oestrogen and progesterone and the excretion of their metabolites in the maternal urine. Most of the work on levels of these hormones in abortion has been done from eight weeks of pregnancy onwards, and at this time there is no evidence that a fall in progesterone production either by the corpus luteum of pregnancy or by the trophoblast leads to abortion. Low levels of pregnanediol do occur in a proportion of women who abort but it seems likely that this indicates that the ovum is already dead and hence the trophoblast is producing less hormone. It is probable that the dead ovum is responsible for the low hormone levels and not vice versa.

Evidence is now accumulating with the use of newer and more sensitive methods of hormone assay and the use of ovulation-inducing drugs that at earlier stages of pregnancies, i.e. four to six weeks, there may be abnormalities in the production of hormones by the corpus luteum. How often these lead to abortion is not yet clear but further information on this aspect is awaited with interest. The practical aspects of studying patients other than those on ovulating drugs at the very early stage of pregnancy are not easy.

Other hormones may be implicated in pregnancy failure. Thyroid hormone has been used for the treatment of recurrent abortion but good evidence for a valid effect is lacking.

Nutritional errors. Gross errors of nutrition may lead to sterility and amenorrhoea but it is surprising how poorly nourished women can give birth to normal children. Numerous dietary and vitamin regimes have been used in women who abort but there is little positive evidence to show that minor dietary deficiencies are likely to cause abortion.

Maternal disease. Any severe acute infection of the mother with a high fever is liable to cause fetal death and abortion. In this context, vaccinia may cross the placenta after prophylactic vaccination and infect the fetus causing fetal death and abortion.

Diabetic mothers have a greater tendency to abortion only if the diabetes is poorly controlled. There is no greater incidence of abortion than in normal women if the diabetes is well controlled. In general, severe maternal disease of many types may lead to abortion but it requires to be very severe causing some toxic or anoxic effect on the feto-placental unit before abortion occurs.

Maternal ingestion of certain poisons, e.g. lead, may cause fetal death and abortion.

Abnormalities of the uterus. Developmental abnormalities of the uterus may lead to abortion. The septate or subseptate uterus are the most common varieties encountered. The possibility of a uterine abnormality should always be suspected when the patient has had two or more abortions with no live babies.

Disease of the uterus. The most likely condition to be incompatible with a pregnancy are fibroids of the uterus, especially the submucous variety. Many women, however, with uterine fibroids successfully bear children. In other diseases of the uterus, such as chronic endometritis, the patient usually remains sterile, implantation being prevented by the disease. Cervical lacerations, amputation of the cervix in the course of a repair operation or cone biopsy of the cervix, may result in abortion, due to cervical incompetence. The question of insertion of a cervical suture in these conditions should always be considered.

During history—taking in patients with abortion, emotional upsets, accidents, falls, etc., may all be cited as causal. The evidence for these is variable but in some individuals these causes seem to pertain.

Self-induced abortion. Many so-called spontaneous abortions are, in fact, self-induced although the number is apparently lessening due to the increasing facility of legal termination of pregnancy. Many different methods are used such as abortifacient pills of lead, the introduction of foreign bodies into the uterus and the squirting of water with or without soap or antiseptic into the uterus. These methods are all hazardous in the extreme. Perforation of the uterus or vagina may occur and embolism and sepsis are well known complications.

It is evident then that, in most cases, the cause of the abortion is not known. Attention is now being particularly directed to the very early stages of pregnancy around the time of implantation and early corpus luteum growth. It is hoped that this will lead to a better understanding of the complexity of abortion.

Therapeutic abortion will be discussed in detail in Chapter 43.

Paternal causes

These are more difficult to study, but it is known that male defects are of importance in fertility. Whether abnormalities of the sperm are a factor in causing abortion is not known.

PATHOLOGY OF ABORTION

The immediate cause of spontaneous abortion is a degeneration in the decidua leading to haemorrhage in that site. This haemorrhage usually stimulates uterine contractions which further loosen the ovum and finally it is expelled. In some cases, fetal death may occur first and the ovum be expelled at a later date (Fig. 8.1).

uterus is necessary. Occasionally, the complete sac and placenta are expelled at the same time.

THE CLINICAL PROCESS OF ABORTION (Fig. 8.2)

Threatened abortion

At this stage, haemorrhage is usually slight although a remarkable amount of bleeding may occasionally occur. Pain is usually minimal and is sited usually in the lower abdomen or back. Vaginal examination reveals no or very minimal dilatation of the cervix. Speculum examination should be performed to eliminate local causes of bleeding. Should a retroverted uterus be discovered it should not be replaced at this stage since the stimulation of the uterus at this time is more likely to encourage further bleeding. A watch spring pessary may be inserted after all symptoms have settled.

At this stage, the process is usually reversible and perhaps one-half to two-thirds of cases will settle with treatment.

Treatment should consist of bed rest and

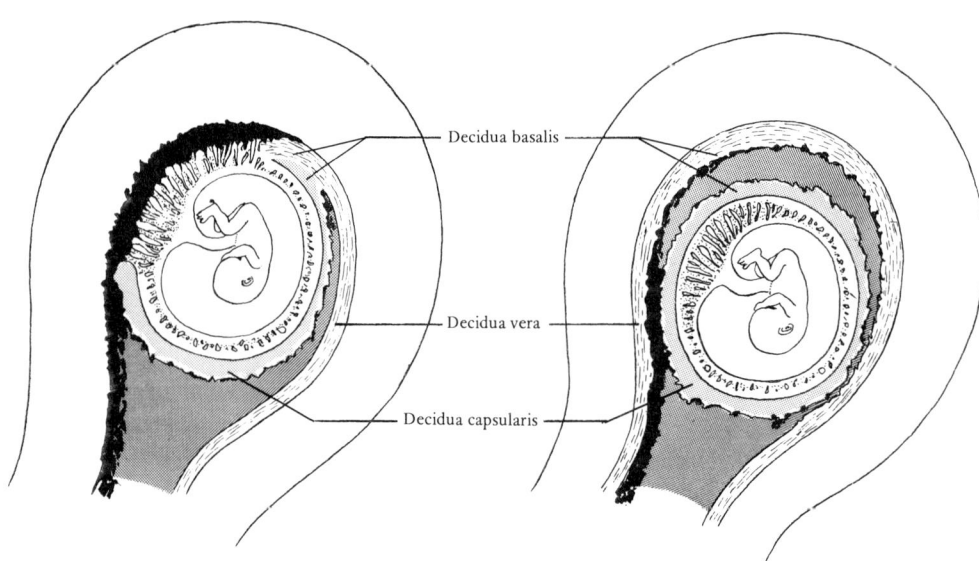

Fig. 8.1   Complete separation of the ovum.

In the early stages of pregnancy the whole ovum may come away complete but more usually portions of trophoblast and decidua are left behind. When the abortion occurs after the placenta is formed at 14 weeks or later, the fetus may be expelled first followed by the placenta, similar to a miniature labour. The placenta, however, may be retained in whole or in part and then evacuation of the

sedation. A barbiturate sedative is usually sufficient and to this might be added an analgesic such as pethidine if pain is troublesome. Morphine derivatives are probably inadvisable owing to their tendency to cause vomiting. There is no evidence that other drugs are beneficial. Various gestagens have been used but their value is not established. The patient should be kept in bed for three to four days

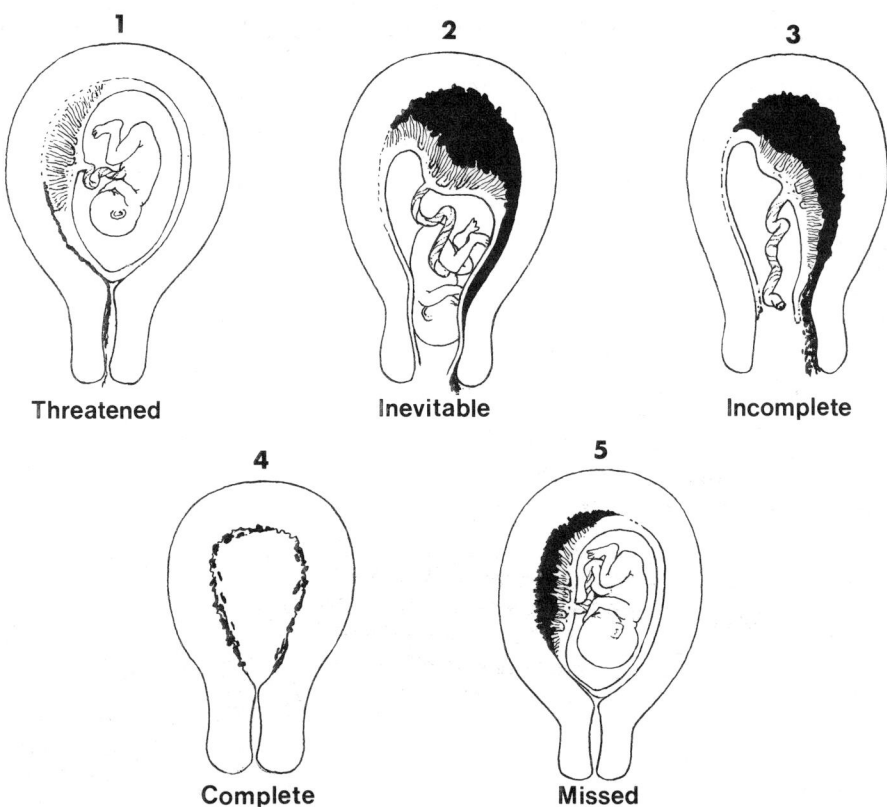

Fig. 8.2   Classification of abortion: 1 Threatened; 2 Inevitable; 3 Incomplete; 4 Complete; 5 Missed.

after the cessation of bleeding, then slowly mobilized. If there is a history of abortion, particularly if the patient has no live children, prolonged bed rest may be advisable. It is not essential to admit a patient with threatened abortion to hospital but if she remains at home she should have adequate help and facilities so that she can obtain the required rest. It is reassuring to the patient at this stage to use a doptone to detect the fetal heart. In this way the viability of the fetus can be ascertained.

If pain and bleeding cease the pregnancy is likely to continue, but in some cases the ovum has died. In the latter patients, the uterus will cease to grow, the signs of pregnancy will disappear and eventually the products of conception will be expelled perhaps in the form of a 'heavy period'. If bleeding continues or uterine contractions increase, the abortion process will progress to the inevitable stage.

Inevitable abortion

At this stage, the abortion process has become irreversible. Pain increases in intensity, bleed-

ing becomes more profuse and the cervix becomes dilated. After a variable period of time, the products of conception are expelled. They may be complete or incomplete. If bleeding stops after passage of the products the likelihood is that the uterus is empty. If bleeding stops after passage of the products, tion is incomplete and evacuation of the remaining products of conception is necessary under general anaesthesia.

If, during the process of abortion, bleeding becomes excessive, blood transfusion may be required and the bleeding can usually be controlled by Ergometrine 0·5mg given intravenously. If there is a likelihood of any material remaining in the uterus, surgical evacuation of the uterine cavity should be performed. If there is evidence of infection this should be controlled by the appropriate antibiotic and then evacuation performed. Should excessive bleeding occur during this waiting period, however, then this takes priority and, even in the presence of infection, it may be necessary to evacuate the uterine cavity.

Septic abortion

The vaginal vault and even the uterine cavity may be invaded by organisms within a few hours of the onset of uterine bleeding. Most of the organisms cause little trouble but if there has been criminal interference or if the vaginal examination is done without due precaution virulent organisms such as coagulase-positive staphylocci, haemolytic streptococci, clostridium welchii or E. coli may be introduced.

The term septic abortion implies an abortion associated with the constitutional signs of infection such as pyrexia, rapid pulse, and malaise. The severity of these signs varies from the very severe picture of Cl. welchii septicaemia to that in which the patient only shows a slight rise in temperature. The patient with a septic abortion must always be regarded as seriously ill. In the majority of cases, septic abortion is probably due to interference and the numbers of septic abortions are, in fact, diminishing as a result of the Abortion Act.

Treatment. The blood of a patient with incomplete abortion should be examined and the degree of leucocytosis estimated. Severe anaemia should be treated by blood transfusion; bacteriological examination must include culture of a vaginal swab, mid-stream specimen of urine and, in serious cases, blood culture.

A gentle vaginal examination should be carried out to determine the degree of dilation of the os and to discover if the ovum is protruding through it. Should the ovum be found to be protruding it should be removed. Tenderness in the fornix or lower abdomen may denote some extra-uterine spread of infection or a pelvic peritonitis.

When a septic abortion is diagnosed the patient should be given a full course of wide-spectrum antibiotic such as ampicillin and when the temperature has settled evacuation of the uterus should be undertaken. If, however, the temperature continues high in spite of antibiotic treatment or if bleeding should occur then it may be necessary to evacuate the uterus forthwith. It is, however, best to try and control the infection first before surgical interference takes place.

Bacterial endotoxic shock. In some patients with septic abortion due to an E. coli or Cl. welchii infection of severe degree, an endotoxic shock may occur. In these cases, the patient is extremely ill. Blood culture should be taken, antibiotics given and intravenous infusion set up. The question of the treatment of shock will be discussed in Chapter 31.

Missed abortion

In this variety of abortion the ovum dies and is retained in the uterus. Sometimes there are signs of threatened abortion at the time of the death of the ovum. Should this occur in early pregnancy the ovum later presents a very typical appearance known as a fleshy, carneous or tubal mole. The embryo is usually absorbed and the liquor amnii disappears. Following the death of the ovum the pregnancy test becomes negative within two or three weeks.

Clinical features. The usual sequence of events is for the patient to say that she thought she was pregnant but now does not feel that the pregnancy is continuing. The breasts may regress, morning sickness disappears and growth of the uterus ceases. If fetal movements have been present these cease and the fetal heart cannot be heard. There may be a history of threatened abortion or a continuous vaginal discharge.

The diagnosis may be difficult. A pregnancy test should be performed but a single negative test should not be considered conclusive. A sonar examination of the uterus (*see* Chapter 28) will show the picture of a non-continuing pregnancy and this test is usually conclusive. A further test which may be carried out from about ten weeks onwards is a 'sonicaid' examination, an ultrasonic examination of the fetal heart which can be detected at this early stage in a normal pregnancy but is absent in a missed abortion. In later pregnancies, X-ray picture may show collapse of the fetal skull.

Treatment. An attempt should be made to empty the uterus as soon as possible. If it is less than twelve weeks' size this can be done by dilatation of the cervix and evacuation of the products of conception. If the uterus is larger than this it may be emptied either by high oxytocin concentration giving the amount required to cause uterine contractions or, in more recent times, by the use of prostaglandins. In the latter case, prostaglandin is given by the so-called 'extra-ovular route' being injected through a Foley catheter into the cervix where it passes between the fetal sac and the uterine wall. Expulsion of the uterine contents usually occurs within 12 hours of the onset of this treatment.

Habitual abortion

It is usually stated that when a woman has had three consecutive abortions she is said to be suffering from the condition of habitual abortion. However, the related complications occur commonly after two consecutive abortions and, therefore, it is more realistic to treat the patient as a 'habitual aborter' once she has had two consecutive abortions. In many cases, the cause of this trouble is not known but various lines of treatment may be considered.

The incidence of habitual abortion is extremely difficult to ascertain and the figures of Malpas (1938) are almost certainly wrong since they are based on unrealistic premises. Goldzieher (1964) has pointed out that Malpas produced no evidence to support his original theory and it should be discarded.

It is evident from more recent work that the chance of abortion increases as the number of the previous abortions increases and the greatest increase occurs between two and three successive abortions. After two consecutive abortions women should be placed in the abortion-prone group since between a half and a third of these women will abort in a third pregnancy. Patients who suffer from habitual abortion have a high incidence of threatened abortion and premature labour in subsequent pregnancies and there is also an increased deformity rate. The perinatal death rate is also greater in these patients in subsequent pregnancies. Particular attention should, therefore, be paid to their antenatal care which should be of a meticulous nature. Chromosomal abnormalities may also be a cause of habitual abortion.

Investigation of a case of habitual abortion. An intensive search for any local uterine cause should be made. The local causes have already been studied and conditions such as chronic pelvic infection, persistent retroversion, congenital uterine abnormalities including incompetent cervix, and uterine hypoplasia should be looked for. In some women, there seems to be a deficiency of the sphincter at the internal cervical os. As pregnancy advances the cervix dilates, the membranes protrude and abortion occurs. The history of these patients is fairly typical in that the original abortion may have been relatively early but subsequent ones usually occur between 14 and 20 weeks. In this sort of patient consideration should be given to the insertion of a cervical suture at an early stage in any subsequent pregnancy. It is also said that other general diseases of the mother cause habitual abortion, but this is only so where they are in an uncon-

trolled state and there is no evidence that diseases such as diabetes, when under good control, cause an increased incidence of abortion.

Treatment of habitual abortion. The treatment of such patients must remain largely empirical and thus a large number of methods or drugs have been used.

Endocrine therapy—gestagens. For many years a deficiency of progesterone from the corpus luteum of pregnancy had been considered to be one of the major causes of abortion and thus many such women were treated with a progesterone in early pregnancy. The natural hormone, progesterone, is not active when given by mouth and is so insoluble, that it is impossible to give a large amount therapeutically. Therefore, progesterone itself, for therapeutic purposes is no longer given. Synthetic gestagens have, therefore, been used. Many of these compounds, although related to progesterone, do not have entirely similar actions and the nor-testosterone derivatives such as norethisterone or norethynodral have been unsuccessful and are potentially dangerous as they have been reported on occasion to cause masculinization of the female fetus. If synthetic gestagens are to be used those more closely related to progesterone itself such as 17 hydroxyprogesterone caproate or the cyclopentyl enol ether of progesterone itself lack such dangers. However, it is apparent from well controlled double blind therapeutic trials conducted by Shearman and Garrett (1963) and by Klopper and Macnaughton (1965) that not even the most carefully selected gestagen is capable of significantly improving the fetal salvage in recurrent abortion. The main cause of early abortion seems to be an inherent defect in the growing conceptus.

Oestrogens. It has been suggested that if uterine hypoplasia is present in a patient suffering from habitual abortion courses of oestrogens before the pregnancy may produce some myometrial hyperplasia. These oestrogens also, however, have the effect of depressing pituitary function and may result in formation of poorer corpora lutea in a subsequent pregnancy.

Thyroid hormone. There seems little value in administering thyroid hormone unless modern methods of investigation show the patient to be hypothyroid.

Diet and vitamins. There is no evidence that any specific avitaminosis is involved in recurrent abortion and vitamin E in the human has not been shown to have any therapeutic value.

General therapy. The most important single factor in the management of patients with habitual abortion is adequate rest and care. It is virtually impossible for this to be obtained at home and, therefore, it is best to admit these patients to hospital for complete physical rest. This should be done before the earliest time at which a previous abortion has occurred and they should be kept in until the sixteenth to twentieth week. By this time placentation is complete and uterine growth can be properly evaluated.

This treatment by itself seems as efficacious as any other form. In the event the patient should have a planned regime of life with ample rest, sound sleep, well-balanced diet and avoidance of sexual intercourse. She should be encouraged psychologically to believe that her pregnancy will go to term and her morale maintained in every possible way. This aspect of management is sometimes referred to by the abbreviated title of 'TLC'—tender loving care—which sums up the need for the closer interest and supervision which such patients require from their medical attendant.

The incompetent cervical os—it has been already stated that some patients suffering from habitual abortion seem to have a deficiency of the sphincter mechanism of the cervix. The classical story is that some time after the 16th week and maybe later, the patient realizes that 'her waters have broken', or may actually see the intact membranes protruding at the vulva. Shortly after, without any significant pain or bleeding, the fetus and placenta are delivered. What has happened is that the cervix has gradually dilated until the membranes protrude through it and abortion occurs.

In many cases, the condition is regarded as 'idiopathic' and no cause can be discovered. In others, there is a history of cervical dilatation for dysmenorrhoea or a dilatation and curettage for menstrual dysfunction. It may be surmised that tearing of the cervical musculature has taken place at operation. In Eastern Europe, a number of patients have this condition as a result of excessive dilatation for termination of pregnancy on a previous occasion. A few patients give a history of a Manchester operation for uterine prolapse when the cervix has been amputated. In other patients, a cone biopsy of the cervix may be recorded and it is certainly worthwhile considering the insertion of a cervical suture in any pregnancy subsequent to amputation of the cervix or cone biopsy.

The condition can be successfully treated by suturing the cervix at an early stage in pregnancy. The diagnosis should be made on the previous history and the cervical suture inserted sometime about the eighth week of pregnancy. There should not be delay until the cervical canal is beginning to open by which time it may be too late and rupture of the membranes may occur either before or during the operation. At operation, the cervix is exposed and a circular purse string suture inserted round it at about the level of the internal os. The suture should be of a material such as mersilk. The cervix should be examined from time to time as pregnancy advances; the purse string suture may be removed at about the 38th week of pregnancy. In some cases, particularly where the patient is elderly and there are no previous live children, delivery may be by Caesarean section. It is probably best to remove the suture after the section to allow free drainage of the uterus in the puerperium. The operation of cervical suture is usually successful in that the pregnancies continue to a viable stage. However, in many patients there are other factors and it is important to watch for 'poor growth syndrome' in the subsequent pregnancy in this type of patient. Should a uterine abnormality such as subseptate uterus be considered to be the main cause of habitual abortion, then a septal operation to remove the septum should be undertaken. The results of this procedure are extremely satisfactory (James, 1970).

MATERNAL MORTALITY FROM ABORTION
Reference is made to this subject in Chapter 2. The most recent confidential inquiry into maternal deaths shows that abortion is still an appreciable cause of maternal mortality and morbidity. Many of these deaths are associated with self-induced abortion and it is to be hoped that as a result of the Abortion Act with the more liberal attitude to abortion, the need for self-induced abortion will diminish and vanish with resultant diminution in mortality from this condition. In the absence of sepsis, morbidity and mortality are very low when treatment is efficiently carried out in optimum circumstances.

Extra-uterine 'ectopic' pregnancy

This refers to a pregnancy occurring outside the uterine cavity. Implantation of the fertilized ovum may occur in the following situations (Fig. 8.3):

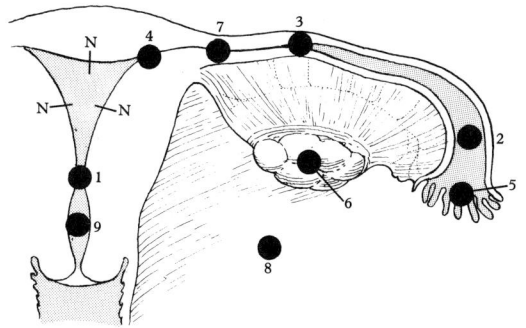

Fig. 8.3   Implantation sites of ovum.
N. Normal. 1. Isthmus of uterus (placenta praevia). 2. Ampulla of tube. 3. Isthmus of tube. 4. Angle of uterus (angular pregnancy). 5. Infundibulum. 6. Ovary. 7. Interstitial portion of tube. 8. Peritoneum. 9. Cervix (cervical pregnancy) – very rare.

1. The ampulla, isthmus, infundibulum and interstitial portion of the tube;
2. The ovary (primary ovarian pregnancy);
3. The broad ligament, bowel, omentum or mesentery (primary abdominal pregnancy).

AETIOLOGY OF ECTOPIC PREGNANCY
Fertilization of the ovum is usually thought to occur in the tubal ampulla and development of the fertilized ovum occurs in this tube so that when it reaches the uterine cavity it is at the correct stage for implantation. It has been suggested that conditions of the tube such as increased tortuosity, adhesions from previous inflammation, obstruction by tumour (rare), deficient peristalsis or diverticulae may delay the passage of the fertilized ovum and lead to tubal implantation. Many cases, however, occur in apparently normal tubes.

The side of embedding of the zygote may be influenced by such conditions as the rapidity of cellular division of the fertilized ovum, the activity of the trophoblast and the amount and composition of the fluid content of the lumen of the tube. It is possible that if the zygote develops beyond a certain point while still in the tube it may imbed in the tubal wall. Developmental anomalies of the tube and the possibility of a well marked decidual reaction in the tube may also favour implantation. Chronic salpingitis is the most common single finding in tubal pregnancy. Women in the older reproductive age-groups, with high parity or a history of abortion, appear to have a greater pre-disposition to ectopic pregnancy (Kleiner and Roberts, 1967).

INCIDENCE OF ECTOPIC PREGNANCY
In Britain, the incidence of ectopic pregnancy is probably about 3 per thousand births and the recurrence rate about 7 per cent. It is higher in areas where there is an increased incidence of tubal inflammation due to causes such as gonorrhoea.

THE PATHOLOGY OF ECTOPIC PREGNANCY
The process of embedding in ectopic pregnancy is similar to that in a normal intra-uterine pregnancy. The zygote buries itself in the wall of the tube through the destructive action of the trophoblast. All the layers of the tube are affected and although the connective tissue cells may take on to a varying extent the appearance of decidual cells, there is no development of true decidua in the tube—this forms in the uterine cavity. The most common site of tubal implantation is in the ampullary portion of the tube and implantation in other parts of the tube is, in fact, rare.

When the ovum is embedded in the ampullary portion, several terminations are possible:

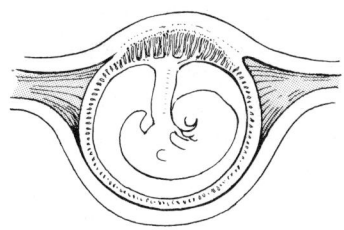

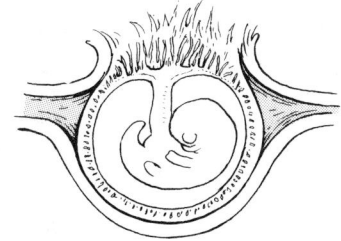

Fig. 8.4   Tubal abortion.

1. tubal abortion;
2. tubal rupture;
3. formation of a tubal mole; and
4. continuation of the pregnancy.

1. *Tubal abortion* (Fig. 8.4)

The ovum is extruded into the peritoneal cavity. When this occurs there is haemorrhage into the peritoneal cavity through the abdominal ostium. This usually stops when the ovum is completely expelled but there is frequently considerable effusion of blood. Bleeding may continue slowly and accumulate in the Pouch of Douglas forming a pelvic haematocele.

2. *Tubal rupture*

This usually occurs before 10 weeks. It may occur suddenly and be accompanied by severe intraperitoneal haemorrhage and collapse of the patient. Gradual rupture is more common due to slow erosion of the tubal wall by the trophoblast and chorionic villi. Should rupture occur in the inferior aspect of the tube between the layers of the broad ligament, haemorrhage is usually limited and a broad ligament haematoma may occur. Growth of the ovum may continue in the broad ligament in a few cases and many examples of extra-uterine pregnancy, which continue to the later months, are of this kind. The broad ligament helps to protect the gestation sac in such cases.

3. *Formation of a tubal mole*

In this case, haemorrhage has occurred around the ovum but has been limited. Usually the mole disintegrates slowly, and a haematosalpinx forms. Occasionally, infection occurs and a pyosalpinx results.

4. *Continuation of the pregnancy*

This is rare and occurs mainly in countries where patients do not so regularly report minor symptoms which may occur in these cases in early pregnancy.

Implantation in the isthmus and infundibulum are rare and early rupture usually occurs in these situations. If implantation occurs in the interstitial portion of the tube, the uterus is found to be enlarged at one corner. Here the diagnosis may be very difficult since the findings resemble lateral flexion of a gravid uterus, angular pregnancy, pregnancy in a rudimentary horn, or pregnancy in a uterus bicornis. Rupture is the usual outcome but not until after 12 weeks.

Haemorrhage is usually severe due to a tearing of the large vessels at the cornu.

OVARIAN PREGNANCY

This is rare and for certain diagnosis it is necessary to demonstrate an intact tube and ovarian tissue in the wall of the gestation sac. Rupture generally occurs in ovarian pregnancy.

PRIMARY ABDOMINAL PREGNANCY

This does occur, the most common site being the Pouch of Douglas. Embedding may also occur in the broad ligament, mesentery and omentum.

UTERINE CHANGES IN ECTOPIC PREGNANCY

The uterus increases in size to that of an 8–10 weeks' gestation. The endometrium is altered to become a decidua, a fact first described by William Hunter. The decidua resembles that of an intra-uterine pregnancy and is generally shed, either whole or in part, after the death of the ovum. This may lead to a mistaken diagnosis of intra-uterine pregnancy but histological examination will show the absence of chorionic villi—a very important diagnostic point.

CLINICAL FEATURES OF ECTOPIC PREGNANCY

The symptoms of ectopic pregnancy are very variable and depend upon the course and outcome of the pregnancy. It is convenient to discuss the clinical features under three headings—before disturbance, after disturbance and continuation of the pregnancy.

Before disturbance

The early symptoms of pregnancy occur, namely, amenorrhoea, breast changes, early morning sickness and frequency of micturition. Amenorrhoea is not always present and a clear history of this is absent in some 30 per cent of cases. This is an important factor as it is often assumed that amenorrhoea is essential before a diagnosis of ectopic pregnancy can be made. There are few symptoms directly attributable to the extra-uterine pregnancy at this stage. Such symptoms may be very mild and amount to only spasmodic abdominal pain related to one or other iliac fossa. Depending on the patient's pain threshold she may or may not seek medical advice at this stage. Pelvic examination reveals the early signs associated with a uterine pregnancy. There is softening of the cervix and globular enlargement of a softened uterus, related to the formation of the decidua. At this stage, careful palpation of the adnexa may reveal the presence of the swollen tube but this is not always easy to recognize. The differential diagnosis includes the tubo-ovarian swelling associated with a uterine pregnancy and cystic enlargement of the ovary causing short term amenorrhoea. If an undisturbed ectopic pregnancy is suspected the patient should be admitted to hospital. A pregnancy test may be helpful but a negative test does not rule out the possibility of ectopic pregnancy at this stage. The optimum method of diagnosis is laparoscopy when the ectopic pregnancy may be visualized directly. Laparoscopy should always be performed when ectopic pregnancy is possible.

After disturbance

If disturbance of a tubal gestation occurs it is accompanied by intra-abdominal bleeding. The amount of bleeding varies from case to case and thus alters the clinical picture. If the haemorrhage is rapid and severe, the signs and symptoms assume an acute form and an acute abdominal emergency results. If the bleeding is slight or slow and clot formation occurs the signs and symptoms will be more chronic.

Acute—50 per cent of all cases of a tubal gestation give rise to acute abdominal symptoms. Rapid and severe haemorrhage is associated with sudden rupture of the tube on its peritoneal aspect. A similar result may less frequently arise from tubal abortion. If the haemorrhage takes place into the peritoneal cavity and is severe the classical features are of severe intra-abdominal haemorrhage. The onset of symptoms is dramatic and the patient is suddenly seized by severe abdominal pain at first localized but quickly spreading throughout the lower abdomen. She may feel as if something has given way and the initial attack of pain may be associated with nausea or vomiting. The pain continues and evidence of shock and blood loss accumulate. Pallor, rapid and feeble pulse, falling blood pressure and sighing respiration all follow. Death of the ovum and vaginal bleeding occur sooner or later as a result of separation of the uterine decidua which is usually expelled in fragments, but, on occasion, may be expelled intact as a decidual cast. This may cause confusion and result in a diagnosis of intra-uterine pregnancy being made. Typically, the patient may complain of shoulder pain, a reflex symptom due to irritation of the diaphragm by blood irritating the lower surface. The side affected by this pain does not necessarily indicate the side of the ectopic pregnancy. It may be helpful in the diagnosis of ectopic pregnancy to raise the foot of the bed in order to encourage tracking of blood upwards to irritate the diaphragm. This is quite a useful aid to diagnosis in some cases.

On abdominal examination, there is distention and resistance to palpation and generalized tenderness. The presence of free fluid in the peritoneal cavity may be indicated by a shifting dullness. The cervix is softened; and the uterus, if felt, will be slightly enlarged; there is a doughy fullness in the fornices and marked tenderness on moving the cervix. There may also be uterine bleeding. The clinical features are all indicative of massive intra-peritoneal haemorrhage. In a married woman of childbearing age the most likely cause of such bleeding is rupture or abortion of a tubal pregnancy and, in the classical case, there is usually little difficulty in arriving at a rapid correct diagnosis. In the less obvious case, the differential diagnosis includes other acute abdominal emergencies such as perforation of a peptic ulcer or acute torsion of an ovarian tumour. Occasionally, massive intra-abdominal bleeding may result from rupture of a small luteal or follicle cyst but, as a rule, this diagnosis is only reached after laparoscopy is performed for the provisional diagnosis of disturbed tubal gestation.

Treatment consists of blood transfusion so that the patient is resuscitated to a reasonable degree before operation. It may, however, be difficult to raise the blood pressure much above 100 systolic. It may, therefore be necessary to operate on a patient in this condition because as soon as the intra-peritoneal haemorrhage is stopped the general condition of the patient immediately begins to improve. Therefore, operation should not long be delayed and, in an extreme emergency, immediate operation is mandatory. Failure to operate as soon as the diagnosis is made is the main avoidable factor leading to death (Confidential Enquiries into Maternal Deaths in England and Wales 1967–69). At operation, the affected tube should be removed but the ovary should be left if possible. Recovery after this operation is rapid and complete.

Chronic—In about half the cases of disturbed tubal pregnancy the signs and symptoms are of a more chronic variety. This may be the result of either a gradual rupture of the tubal wall or an abortion where the bleeding is relatively slight or slow or to extra-peritoneal rupture when the extent of the bleeding is limited by clot formation within the broad ligament. Intra-peritoneal bleeding of this type will lead to the formation of a peritubal haematocele, a peritubal haematocele around the abdominal ostium, or a pelvic haematocele, which is a collection of blood in the Pouch of Douglas. An intra-ligamentary haematocele may follow extra-peritoneal bleeding between the layers of the broad ligament. In these circumstances, the patient does not usually present as an emergency but her complaint is of persistent lower abdominal pain associated with irregular uterine bleeding and sometimes attacks of fainting and vomiting. The attacks of fainting are of particular significance in this type of case. Abdominal examination may show a moderate distension and tenderness and, if the haematocele is of sufficient size, it may be palpated as a firm tender swelling arising from the pelvis and extending upwards for a varying distance into the lower abdomen. Pelvic examination reveals uterine bleeding, a uterus enlarged to the size of about eight weeks' gestation and a tender firm swelling either in the site of one or other of the appendages or behind and below the uterus in the Pouch of Douglas. The pulse rate may be moderately increased, the temperature slightly raised and there may be an increase in white count and a rise in ESR. The diagnosis in these cases may be very difficult and the pregnancy diagnosis test is unreliable in that it is positive in only about half of the cases. The differential diagnosis is from uterine abortion, ovarian tumours with or without pregnancy and inflammatory conditions such as pyosalpinx or appendix abscess. In this type of case, laparoscopy should be performed and the pelvic organs inspected. This is a better method of diagnosis than any pregnancy test although a pregnancy test may be done as an additional diagnostic measure. The old method of puncture of the Pouch of Douglas with a needle is not particularly helpful since very frequently blood is obtained even though there is no pelvic haematocele.

Treatment is by operation if the diagnosis is clinched by laparoscopy and salpingectomy should be performed.

Continuation of the pregnancy

Pregnancy may continue to the later months or even to term either within the tube or as a secondary tubo-ovarian pregnancy. This is extremely rare but depends, to some extent, on the country and the pain threshold of the patient. Where medical services are easily obtained and the threshold of pain is low, continuation is rare. In other circumstances such as developing areas continuation of extra-uterine pregnancies is much more common. The main features to be looked for are the abnormal situation and lie of the fetus and the ease of palpation of fetal parts with the absence of an intervening uterine wall. A lateral X-ray of the patient lying on her back shows that some of the fetal parts are posterior to the maternal spine, a condition which never occurs in a patient with an intra-uterine pregnancy. This is something sufficient to clinch the diagnosis.

Treatment consists of delivery of the fetus by abdominal operation.

In the case of continuation of a tubal pregnancy the placenta and tube may be removed but in secondary abdominal pregnancy it may be impossible to do this without causing excessive haemorrhage and, therefore, the placenta in these circumstances should be left since it will be gradually absorbed and disappear. The modern mortality from ectopic gestation, although present, is very low mainly due to adequate treatment of haemorrhage and shock and rapid operation.

There is an increased likelihood of ectopic pregnancy in the other tube in a patient who has already had one due to the possibility of adhesions being present in that tube either before or after the operation.

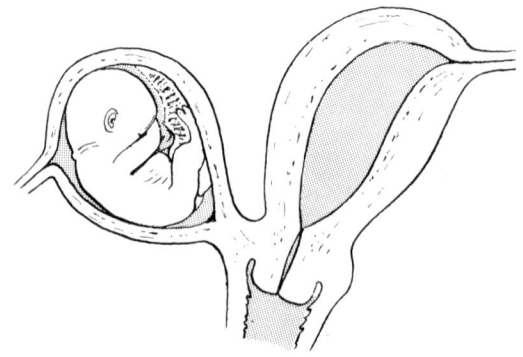

Fig. 8.5   Pregnancy in Rudimentary Horn.

PREGNANCY IN A RUDIMENTARY HORN

This malformation and some of the disturbances it may produce have been referred to already but here reference must be made to the gravid rudimentary horn which clinically resembles ectopic pregnancy in many details. The connection between the two horns of the uterus in these cases is by a fibromuscular band somewhere between 2–5cm in length (Fig. 8.5). This band may be attached to the normal horn about the level of the internal os, although its lower margin may be as low as the external os. Usually no canal is present and if one exists it is incomplete. Impregnation may, therefore, occur by the spermatozoa passing through the normal half of the uterus and tube and impregnating an ovum which·has been shed from the ovary connected with the rudimentary horn. In a few instances, however, the ovum may have come from the other ovary as the corpus luteum has been observed in the ovary connected with the normal horn. The fertilized ovum passes into the rudimentary horn and there develops.

The course of pregnancy in a rudimentary horn is variable. In a proportion of cases rupture occurs due to the poorly developed musculature. The time of rupture depends largely on the state of development of the rudimentary horn. It frequently occurs between the 16th and 20th week but, in some cases, it takes place earlier or, in others, even later. Cases have been recorded where pregnancy advanced to term.

The clinical features of rupture include recurrent attacks of abdominal pain, tenderness, fainting, vaginal bleeding and expulsion of a decidua from the normal uterine horn. Rupture and collapse may occur suddenly without premonitory symptoms. When the pregnancy continues to term spurious labour occurs, and fetal death results.

A gravid rudimentary horn is seldom diagnosed before laparoscopy. Tubal pregnancy is the usual diagnosis in the first instance. The relative position of the two round ligaments and the separation of the tumour from the uterus are important features, particularly in the early months; as pregnancy advances the sac becomes so large that these landmarks are obscured. In late pregnancy the gravid horn may be mistaken for a normal uterus and the non-gravid normal horn for a fibroid or an ovarian tumour.

The treatment is to remove the gravid rudimentary horn, but occasionally the association of the sac and the other horn of the uterus is so intimate that hysterectomy of both horns is advisable.

ANGULAR PREGNANCY

'Angular' pregnancy is a definite clinical entity and occurs when the zygote becomes implanted in the angle or cornua of the uterus. The implantation site appears to be either directly over the tubal opening or just external to it in the interstitial portion of the tube. The condition is quite distinct from the typical interstitial variety of ectopic pregnancy, for the ovum develops not into the wall of the uterus but towards the uterine cavity.

The clinical features of this condition are:

1. severe pain;
2. lateral distension of the uterus on the affected side;
3. tendency to abortion.

In a number of cases the placenta is retained and difficult to remove as it is held up in the sacculation at the uterine angle.

BLEEDING IN THE LATER MONTHS OF PREGNANCY

Bleeding which occurs from the genital tract after the 28th week of pregnancy and before delivery is called antepartum haemorrhage. This is a sign of the utmost importance because irrespective of its cause, antepartum haemorrhage is associated with increased risks to both mother and fetus.

The causes of antepartum haemorrhage can be classified as follows:

1. bleeding from an abnormally situated placenta (placenta praevia; unavoidable haemorrhage)
2. bleeding from a normally situated placenta (abruptio placentae; accidental haemorrhage)
3. bleeding from cervical and vaginal lesions.

The incidence of the various varieties of antepartum bleeding is given in Table 8.1.

Placenta praevia

In placenta praevia, part of the placenta is attached to that area of the uterine wall which forms the lower segment. The lower segment of the uterus forms from the isthmus in the non-pregnant organ and is defined as that

Table 8.1   Antepartum haemorrhage, 1949–58. All Aberdeen City cases—30 195 single pregnancies (overall perinatal mortality, 31 per 1000 births)

Type of A.P.H.	Pregnancies with A.P.H.	Incidence (per cent)	Perinatal Fetal Loss (per cent)	Perinatal Mortality (per 1000) births).
Placenta praevia	126	0·42	13	0·53
Accidental haemorrhage (Concealed and Mixed)	223	0·74	51	3·7
Accidental haemorrhage (External or Revealed)	521	1·73	7·7	1·3
Haemorrhage from Cervix or Vagina	8	0·03	—	—
All A.P.H.	878	2·91	19·7	5·53

portion of the uterine wall which lies below the level of the peritoneal reflection from the anterior surface of the uterus on to the bladder. The lower segment stretches and thins out in later pregnancy and especially in labour so that at term it extends to about 3 inches (6·6cm) from the internal os. If the less expandable placenta is situated in this area it will become separated from its uterine attachment either before or during labour. This provokes bleeding from the placental sinuses which is usually maternal in origin although fetal loss may also occur from vessels in torn placental villi. The old name for placenta praevia was 'unavoidable haemorrhage' which accurately described the inevitable nature of the bleeding which occurs in this condition. The more extensive the area of attachment of the placenta to the lower segment the greater the risk of severe haemorrhage.

AETIOLOGY
Little is known about the cause of placenta praevia but the incidence increases with age. The condition is also associated with twin pregnancy possibly due to the larger area of the placental site in these cases.

There are other possible aetiological factors. (1) The ovum may become implanted by chance in the decidua of the lower part of the uterus and thus placental development will occur in the lower segment. (2) Alternatively defective vascularization of the decidua following inflammatory or other changes may result in a limited blood supply to a placenta which implants in such an area. The placenta, therefore, may attempt to compensate by spreading over a larger area of the uterine wall and come to lie in the lower segment. Such theories are, however, rather speculative and it is difficult to provide conclusive proof of the mechanisms for placenta praevia.

CLASSIFICATION OF PLACENTA PRAEVIA
There are classically four main types of placenta praevia:

1. The placenta is mainly in the upper segment but its lower margin dips into the lower segment.

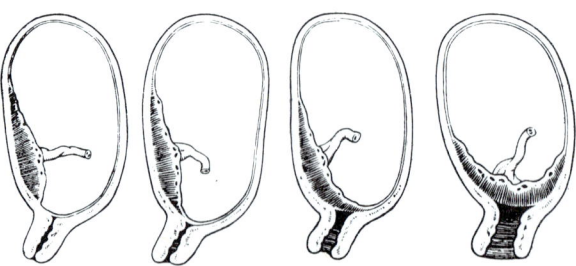

Fig. 8.6   Varieties of placenta praevia: 1. Placenta just dipping on to lower segment; 2. Placenta at margin of internal os; 3. Placenta covers internal os when closed or partly open; 4. Placenta covers lower segment so that it overlies the os even when fully open.

2. The placenta reaches the margin of the internal os.

3. The placenta covers the internal os when closed or partly open.

4. The placenta is so situated in the lower segment that it still covers the os even when the latter is fully dilated.

The classification, which was helpful when older methods of treatment were used, is probably outmoded and it is now more practical to refer to major and minor degrees of placenta praevia. A minor degree of placenta praevia corresponds to type 1 in the old classification and all the other types should be regarded as major degrees. This classification is more relevant to present day practice because major degrees of placenta praevia are now treated by Caesarean section and only in minor degrees should vaginal delivery be contemplated.

SIGNS AND SYMPTOMS

Painless vaginal bleeding is the most characteristic event in placenta praevia. It usually occurs after 30 weeks for the first time but there may be a history of bleeding occurring before this. The severity of the bleeding varies greatly but, on the first occasion, it is frequently slight and stops spontaneously. This is known as a 'warning' haemorrhage. The greater the degree of placenta praevia, the more likely it is that severe haemorrhage will occur later in the pregnancy, although in some patients there may be no bleeding at all until labour begins. In some cases severe haemorrhage will lead to shock or collapse which is directly proportional to the amount of blood lost. Where there has been a pre-existing anaemia, as in some women with large families, this factor will aggravate the degree of shock caused by the heavy blood loss. It must never be forgotten that patients with placenta praevia face a small but real risk of life-endangering haemorrhage.

Although the absence of pain is said to be characteristic of placenta praevia abdominal pain may occur where there is also some separation of the placenta situated in the upper segment of the uterus. The combination of placenta praevia and abruptio is uncommon and there is no connection between pre-eclampsia and placenta praevia although the two conditions may occur quite fortuitously in the same patient.

On abdominal palpation in cases of placenta praevia, the uterus is soft and the presenting part is frequently high above the pelvic brim or deviated into one or other iliac fossa. The possibility of placenta praevia should always be considered in cases of malpresentation even in the absence of antepartum haemorrhage.

DIAGNOSIS OF PLACENTA PRAEVIA

The diagnosis of placenta praevia should be suspected in every case of antepartum vaginal bleeding. The only sure way of making a diagnosis is by digital examination and this should never be performed unless in the operating theatre with full facilities for rapid Caesarean section immediately available. Many sophisticated methods of localizing the placenta have been described and their relative merits will now be discussed.

TECHNICAL DIAGNOSTIC METHODS

Ultrasound—This is nowadays the most satisfactory method of diagnosing placental position and is described in detail in Chapter 28. It can be difficult even with this technique to know the exact type of placenta praevia which is present but if the placenta is clearly seen in the upper segment then the possibility of placenta praevia can be eliminated almost with certainty.

The soft tissue method—This causes minimum disturbance to the mother and fetus and, in experienced hands, the diagnostic accuracy of this technique is 95 per cent or over. The majority of placentae are wholly implanted either on the anterior or posterior uterine walls and may be easily seen on a single erect lateral film.

Other radiological diagnostic methods—These are fully described in textbooks of X-ray diagnosis and only short summaries of the main points will be given here (*see A Textbook of X-ray Diagnosis* vol. 5, 4th Edition, p. 113). The placenta, the amniotic fluid and the uterine wall all cast a similar density on the film. The placenta, however, occupies space, casting a discoid shadow and thereby causing a local increase in the width of the combined shadows up to 9cm at its widest. The outline of the fetus is determined by the translucency caused by subcutaneous fat. In the later weeks of pregnancy, calcification of the placenta is sometimes observed and this identifies the placental site beyond doubt. The accuracy of localization of the placental site increases with the period of gestation and soft tissue radiography should, if possible, be carried out in the last six weeks of gestation, preferably near term. During the later part of pregnancy, the lower uterine segment is considered to lie at the level of the promontory of the sacrum posteriorly and just above the upper margin of the symphysis anteriorly, the transition zone between upper and lower segments being 4–5cm in length. The presence of a low lying placenta will result in displacement of the presenting part from its normal symmetrical position in the pelvic brim. The use of the semi-recumbent position facilitates the recognition especially of the posterior placenta which overlaps the sacral promontory. The technique of this examination is described in Chapter 28.

Amniography—This method involves the injection of a water-soluble contrast medium into the liquor amnii. The placenta is identified as a localized area of flattening in the contour of the opacified amniotic sac associated with an apparent soft tissue thickening between the outline of the amniotic sac and the external contour of the uterine wall.

Outlining the bladder and rectum by contrast medium—This method is no longer in use due to the frequent errors which occurred in interpretation.

Vascular techniques

1. Pelvic Arteriography
2. Intravenous Placentography.

These methods are helpful when localization is required prior to 34 weeks but have really been superseded by sonar.

Pelvic arteriography is performed by percutaneous retrograde injection via the femoral artery using the technique described by Seldinger in 1953. Since it is important to show the uterine arteries, the catheter has to be introduced as far as the bifurcation of the aorta. The ovarian arteries should also be outlined since they may take part in the blood supply to the uterus during pregnancy.

Those interested in this technique should consult the monogram by Fernstrom (1955). The technique is not without morbidity, haematoma formation being a particularly troublesome complication.

Radioisotopes—This method was introduced by Browne and Veall in 1950 using Na^{24}. The isotope accumulates in the placental pool and the placenta can be localized by an isotope counter over the abdominal wall. Other suitable are I^{131} tagged serum albumin, Cr^{51} tagged erythrocytes and Tc^{99} labelled serum albumin.

Definition by this method is not as good as by sonar but it is used in some centres.

Thermography—This method involves the sensing and recording of the longer wavelength infra-red emission from the body. The amount of emission depends mainly upon the temperature of surface. Skin temperature is proportional to the blood flow to the placenta and allows it to be identified on a thermogram, although considerable difficulties can be encountered in the interpretation of results.

The technique of placental localization used will depend on the facilities available. The modern sonar apparatus is very effective and can be used at all stages of gestation. The lower segment does not, however, form fully until after 28 weeks so that a placenta which appears to be low lying before this maturity, may prove to be lying in the upper segment when a repeat picture is taken some weeks later. It is, nevertheless, the best method now available and in competent hands should enable the placenta to be localized with accuracy in 98 per cent of patients.

TREATMENT OF PLACENTA PRAEVIA

Even with modern methods of placental localization, the diagnosis of placenta praevia is not made with certainty until the placenta is felt or visualized in the lower segment. This can be done either at the time of vaginal examination under anaesthesia in the operating theatre or during Caesarean section. The problem that confronts the clinician, therefore, is the management of antepartum haemorrhage where the diagnosis is not known but placenta praevia must be suspected. The management of antepartum haemorrhage will be discussed below, after considering the other causes of vaginal bleeding in the later months of pregnancy.

Abruptio placentae

Abruptio placentae denotes haemorrhage after the 28th week of pregnancy due to separation of a normally situated placenta, i.e. one placed entirely in the upper uterine segment. The alternative term, accidental haemorrhage, arose from the old and mistaken belief that haemorrhage from a normally situated placenta was the result of an 'accident'. It is suggested, therefore, that 'abruptio placentae', which simply describes the event of placental separation, should be used as the more satisfactory term.

TYPES OF ABRUPTIO PLACENTAE

Patients with abruptio placenta can be divided into three main clinical types, as follows:

1. Abruptio placentae with concealed haemorrhage. This includes all cases where retroplacental clot is found at delivery, and external blood loss is absent.

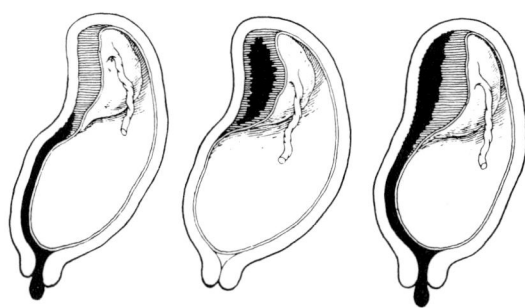

Fig. 8.7   Varieties of accidental haemorrhage.

2. Abruptio placentae with revealed haemorrhage. This is where bleeding occurs from the lower margin of a normally situated placenta. The blood escapes vaginally and especially when the blood loss has been small, the clinical features may closely resemble those of placental praevia.

3. Abruptio placentae with mixed haemorrhage. In this type, the features of concealed and revealed haemorrhage are both present, some blood being retained in the uterus and some escaping vaginally.

EPIDEMIOLOGY

The reported incidence ranges between 1 in 55 deliveries and 1 in 50, depending on the diagnostic criteria. An epidemiological study from Aberdeen demonstrated that the groups at highest risk of developing concealed abruptio were young primigravidae aged 19 years or less and women of high parity above the age of 35 years. Many of the primigravidae who developed concealed abruptio placentae had pre-existing pre-eclampsia but in multiparae, the association between pre-eclampsia and abruptio was less obvious.

In revealed abruptio placentae, the highest incidence was found in very young women of high parity. When revealed abruptio occurred

in primigravidae, the risks were greatest in the younger and the older age-groups. In contrast to the concealed variety there was less evidence to link pre-eclampsia with revealed abruptio placentae.

AETIOLOGY OF ABRUPTIO PLACENTAE

1. As has been discussed above, there is a statistical association between abruptio placentae and pre-eclampsia and chronic hypertension has also been suggested as a predisposing factor in the aetiology of abruptio. In some cases, however, hypertension and proteinuria may develop as a compensatory response to abruptio so that the statistical association between pre-eclampsia and abruptio does not by itself establish a causal relationship. Placental abruption, however, frequently occurs in cases of eclampsia so that it is probable that high blood pressure plays an important part in the aetiology of at least some cases of abruptio.

2. External cephalic version can result in placental separation and this is particularly likely to happen when external version is carried out under general anaesthesia, when the operator may yield to the temptation to use excessive force.

3. Decompression of an overdistended uterus can precipitate abruptio placentae following spontaneous or artificial rupture of the membranes.

4. Dietary factors may play an important part in abruptio placentae. Attempts were made to relate abruptio placentae to folic acid deficiency (Hibbard, 1964) but this has not been confirmed. There is no doubt, however, that the worst cases of abruptio placentae seem to occur in women who lack adequate antenatal care. It is likely that such women will also have a generally poor standard of nutrition and any folic acid deficiency in these cases may not be the specific factor responsible for the abruptio but simply a reflection of their general nutritional state. Since abruptio placentae is a recurring condition, it is important that women who suffer an abruptio should have any anaemia corrected and be given useful dietary advice.

CLINICAL FEATURES OF ABRUPTIO PLACENTAE

1. Revealed abruptio placentae

This group contains cases where the clinical features may be indistinguishable from those of a minor degree of placenta praevia. Bleeding may begin after some sudden physical effort but frequently commences at rest without any obvious cause. Bleeding at first is bright red and this may change to a dark brown discharge. In the mild case, the patient frequently feels well, the uterus is of normal size and the fetus is readily palpable with a normal heart rate. There may be slight abdominal pain but frequently no pain is complained of and the uterus is quite soft. In other cases, there may be local tenderness over the uterine wall where separation of the placenta has occurred.

2. Concealed abruptio placentae

In this, the severest type of abruptio, abdominal pain is severe and the patient rapidly becomes shocked. The pain is constant. The pulse is fast and feeble and the blood pressure is usually low. One can, however, be mis-led by the blood pressure which may, in some cases be quite normal or even elevated. This usually occurs when pre-existing hypertension has been present. In spite of the blood loss, the blood pressure does not fall to what are normally considered hypotensive levels but the patient is clinically shocked. These women, however, usually have a rapid pulse, though on occasion it may be slow in the initial stages. Abdominal examination reveals a very hard, tender uterus with difficulty in palpating the fetal parts; the term 'woody' is used to describe this uterus. In concealed abruptio placentae the fetal heart is usually inaudible because fetal death occurs rapidly. Initially there may be no vaginal bleeding but usually a slight trickle starts as the blood seeps down between the membranes and the uterine wall. It is important to realize that the external blood loss may be very slight compared with the internal and is usually quite out of proportion to the degree of collapse which is present. Catheterization of the bladder reveals scanty secretion of urine.

The uterus may continue to enlarge from haemorrhage so that it becomes more distended—an important sign since it may indicate that paralysis of the uterine muscle has occurred and rhythmic contractions may not begin. The blood, therefore, is not expelled from the uterus and it is usually some time before labour occurs. If abdominal section is performed, the uterus is found to be darkly coloured in many areas and occasionally the peritoneal covering is split by the haemor-

rhage leading into the peritoneal cavity. This mottled appearance following concealed abruptio placentae was first described by Couvelaire in 1912. If the uterus is incised, the placenta will be found almost completely separated with a large retroplacental clot.

If no treatment is given, the patient may die in shock but with adequate treatment improvement generally occurs and is followed by the onset of labour. Progress is frequently rapid once the membranes are ruptured and the placenta, blood clot and fetus are usually expelled rapidly. Severe post-partum haemorrhage may occur due to hypofibrinogenaemia and even a small loss will be serious if the patients are in an exsanguinated condition.

3. Mixed abruptio placentae

A mixed variety of abruptio placenta may also occur when both 1 and 2 are present. In this type of case, both internal and external bleeding occur from the beginning. The condition may not, at first, seem serious as the external blood loss may be relatively slight but the amount of abdominal pain and degree of collapse indicates that there is considerable internal haemorrhage as well. In the mixed variety of abruptio placentae, premature labour may follow the placental separation and this accounts for an important part of the perinatal loss associated with abruptio.

Differential diagnosis

In concealed haemorrhage, the diagnosis is seldom difficult since shock, abdominal pain, a hard, tender uterus, the absence of fetal heart sounds and the difficulty in palpating fetal parts add up to a typical picture. Two other conditions, however, may cause similar symptoms—rupture of the uterus and acute hydramnios. Rupture of the uterus is more likely in patients with a previous uterine scar and it is also more likely to occur in multiparous patients. If the uterus has ruptured, the fetus may be expelled into the abdomen and may be unusually easy to palpate, the uterus being a palpable mass separate from the fetus. If rupture is incomplete, with the fetus still in utero, the pain is generally less severe than with concealed haemorrhage and the uterus is not so hard. The degree of shock present in rupture depends on the amount of blood lost.

In acute hydramnios there may have been a history of increasing size of the uterus over a period of weeks. The uterus may be very tender but the patient is not usually shocked.

The fetal heart is usually audible and the uterus is not very tender. In most cases, the differential diagnosis is fairly simple, but on occasion it can be extremely difficult.

Other acute conditions of the abdomen, such as acute surgical conditions, must always be kept in mind and degeneration of a fibroid may also give rise to similar acute abdominal symptoms.

Local causes of antepartum haemorrhage

Localized abnormalities of the vagina or cervix may be the cause of antepartum vaginal bleeding. The commonest of these are simple lesions such as cervical erosion, cervical polyp or vaginitis. Carcinoma of the cervix, although an uncommon cause of antepartum haemorrhage, should never be forgotten because it is important that it should be diagnosed with the least possible delay. Such extra placental lesions are only discovered on speculum examination but bleeding may still have originated from the placental site, even in the presence of some local cause of antepartum haemorrhage.

TREATMENT OF ANTEPARTUM HAEMORRHAGE
When painless bleeding occurs in the latter half of pregnancy, the patient should be transferred to hospital at once without either vaginal or rectal examination being performed. Any examination may be sufficient to disturb the placental site and if it should be low-lying this could cause torrential bleeding. No vaginal examination should be performed in the patient's home. If the bleeding is severe it will be necessary to call the Obstetric Flying Squad and it is good policy to use this service if there is any doubt about the amount of blood lost or where further haemorrhage may occur during transport to hospital.

If the patient has lost much blood and her pulse and blood pressure are affected, immediate transfusion is required. Vaginal packing is dangerous since it may precipitate further bleeding and produce infection. Fluids by mouth are contra-indicated since an anaesthetic may presently be required.

Treatment of antepartum haemorrhage in hospital
For practical purposes the treatment of antepartum haemorrhage can be discussed under three categories:

1. Slight antepartum haemorrhage without abdominal pain.

2. Antepartum haemorrhage with abdominal pain.
3. Heavy antepartum haemorrhage.

1. *Slight antepartum haemorrhage without abdominal pain*
This is the commonest way in which the problem of antepartum haemorrhage presents to the clinician. The patient is admitted to hospital at once and kept in bed until the bleeding has been stopped for a few days. The objective in management is to allow the pregnancy to continue in the fetal interest until 38 weeks when delivery of the patient is undertaken. This policy of expectant treatment was popularized by Macafee (1945) and has reduced the high fetal mortality due to prematurity which was present when a policy of early intervention was fashionable. This management is suitable when painless haemorrhage has been slight and the pregnancy has not reached 38 weeks. Treatment can only be performed in hospital where the patient is under constant supervision and where immediate active measures can be adopted if, and when, they are necessary. During expectant treatment, the patient's general condition should be investigated, any anaemia corrected and the blood group and Rhesus factor determined. Two pints of blood should be constantly available for use in the event of sudden and serious haemorrhage.

During the stay in hospital, the fetal presentation should be determined and the duration of the pregnancy established. Radiological and ultrasonic examination are carried out to locate the site of the placenta and to determine any gross fetal abnormality.

On admission to hospital, when the bleeding has been slight, the patient should be examined with a vaginal speculum to see if blood is coming from the region of the vagina or cervix. If bleeding has been more than 20ml, this examination should be postponed until bleeding has settled. In this way, unsuspected lesions, such as carcinoma of the cervix, will be found. On no account should any attempt be made to pass a finger through the cervix.

If the placenta is localized in the upper segment and the patient has had a single minor episode of antepartum haemorrhage about 30 weeks, she may be allowed home, but should be re-admitted at 38 weeks for examination or if any further bleeding should occur. Since antepartum haemorrhage may be associated with placental failure, fetal monitoring by measurement of urinary oestriols and bi-parietal cephalometry should be started.

In some cases of antepartum haemorrhage, fetal blood loss may be suspected, particularly when the fetal heart is rapid. In these circumstances, some of the external vaginal blood loss should be examined for fetal cells by the Kleihaur test. If this confirms fetal bleeding, immediate delivery in the interests of the child may be indicated. Where there is doubt about the fetal maturity, estimation of fetal lung maturity may be carried out by measuring the liquor sphingomyelin/lecithin ratio. In many cases the test has proved very useful in indicating the optimum time for delivery. Since the test involves amniocentesis, however, it is not recommended as a routine, because the passage of a needle into the uterus might precipitate further bleeding in a patient with a history of antepartum haemorrhage.

In the majority of cases, the pregnancy can be allowed to continue until 38 weeks when examination under anaesthesia is carried out. If the patient has her first episode of antepartum haemorrhage after 38 weeks, this examination should be carried out without delay.

Examination under anaesthesia. Vaginal examination in a case of antepartum haemorrhage can only be performed in theatre with the following precautions:

a. The patient should be anaesthetized before examination is carried out. This is important because if heavy bleeding is provoked at the time of examination, the patient becomes restless and shocked and this is an unsuitable situation in which to induce anaesthesia. It has become an increasingly common practice to examine patients in theatre without anaesthesia, intending to anaesthetize them quickly if bleeding occurs. The argument in favour of this is the risk associated with the induction of anaesthesia. For the reason stated above, however, examination without anaesthesia can be dangerous and it is doubtful if a really satisfactory exploration of the lower segment to exclude placenta praevia can be performed on the conscious patient. If examination without anaesthesia has a place, it is restricted to parous women in whom the fetal head is deeply engaged.

b. All instruments should be set for immediate Caesarean section.

c. The patient should be catheterized, should be in the dorsal position (not the lithotomy) and should have her abdomen prepared and covered with a theatre towel.

d. An intravenous infusion should be running and two pints of blood should be present in theatre.

e. There should be an assistant scrubbed ready to proceed with immediate section.

These precautions enable immediate section to proceed if heavy bleeding is provoked.

The subsequent action taken depends on the findings at the time of examination under anaesthesia. If the placenta is felt to be coming to within 2–3cm of the internal os by the finger being inserted through the cervix, then delivery by Caesarean section is mandatory.

As placenta praevia is a non-recurring condition, it is advisable to perform lower segment Caesarean section whenever possible. With the adequate availability of blood for transfusion, even when there are large veins over the anterior aspect of the lower uterine segment, a lower uterine segment section can be performed with minimum risk. Some, however, would prefer to perform the classical operation but this is much more likely to give rise to trouble in a subsequent pregnancy and the convalescence may be more complicated than that of a lower segment operation.

If the placenta can be felt to be dipping into the lower segment with the head well into the lower pole of the uterus, it is reasonable to rupture the membranes. If bleeding is not provoked and the fetal heart remains satisfactory, labour can be allowed to continue. If, during the labour, bleeding is provoked by contractions, Caesarean section should be performed without delay. Where there is any doubt about the need for section, it is wiser to err on the side of safety and proceed to abdominal delivery. By this management over 80 per cent of placenta praevias will be delivered by Caesarean section.

If placenta praevia is not present, some authors have recommended that the pregnancy can be allowed to continue and spontaneous labour awaited. The alternative and probably better policy is to proceed to rupture of the membranes and immediate syntocinon stimulation. When antepartum haemorrhage has occurred which is not due to placenta praevia, there is increased perinatal mortality. Oestriol levels are lower following antepartum haemorrhage and further haemorrhage could occur to endanger fetal wellbeing. In view of the efficiency of modern methods of induction of labour, there seems little to gain and much to lose by allowing the pregnancy to continue after 38 weeks when there has been a history of antepartum haemorrhage.

2. *Antepartum haemorrhage with abdominal pain*

When antepartum haemorrhage is complicated by abdominal pain, this usually indicates the diagnosis of abruptio with at least some of the blood concealed within the uterus. The subsequent management depends on whether the fetal heart is still present or not.

In severe internal cases of abruptio placentae the fetal heart is usually absent and treatment should be directed to combating shock, correcting any coagulation defect and then expediting delivery. In all cases of severe abruption blood transfusion is essential and two pints of whole blood should be transfused immediately. The best way to monitor the transfusion requirements is to set up a central venous pressure line. This is probably best done via an antecubital vein and if the pressure exceeds 20cm of water, it usually indicates over-transfusion. The CVP line is an excellent way of controlling the amount of blood required. When the fetus has succumbed due to abruptio placentae, even though no external bleeding is evident, it can be reckoned that at least $2\frac{1}{2}$ pints of blood have been lost.

One of the major complications of abruptio placentae is hypofibrinogenaemia and the presence of this has to be constantly assessed. The use of fresh blood in the treatment of abruptio has great advantages over banked blood because it contains platelets and the labile clotting factors which may help to restore normal blood clotting. Laboratory methods of measuring fibrinogen take time and it is therefore necessary to use a simple and rapid test to determine the plasma fibrinogen level. A clot observation test of Weiner is suitable for this. About 5ml of blood are withdrawn into a test tube and if the fibrinogen in the blood is decreased to a critical level, no coagulation may occur at all. In other cases, there will be delayed clotting beyond the normal time of 10 minutes, the clot will be smaller than normal and will fragment readily throughout the next hour. It is advisable to repeat this test hourly until delivery. The level of fibrino-

gen can be determined in the laboratory and this should be done as rapidly as possible. The normal value for pregnancy is in the region of 450mg per centage. This may fall to 100mg or less in cases of abruptio when clotting failure is present. Details of clotting mechanisms and the cause of hypofibrinogenaemia are fully discussed in the chapter on blood coagulation but the hypofibrinogenaemia is probably due in part to widespread intravascular coagulation and the use of heparin has been suggested on theoretical grounds to combat this. However, heparinization in a patient with severe haemorrhage is potentially dangerous and could lead to further bleeding. This mode of treatment has not been established as helpful at the present time.

In abruptio placentae it is important to get the patient delivered as soon as possible. Prolongation of the period of abruptio placentae is dangerous. During this time the extent of the detachment of the placenta may increase, the bleeding may persist and the complications of hypofibrinogenaemia and acute renal failure may supervene. The aim should be to try to deliver the patient within six hours or so. Once blood transfusion has been commenced and the shock has been treated, the membranes should be ruptured and syntocinon infusion commenced. Labour is usually rapid and the induction to delivery interval relatively short. If labour does not commence with this treatment then Caesarean section may become necessary.

In cases in which abruptio is moderate and the fetal heart is still present, consideration should be given to immediate Caesarean section in the interests of fetal salvage. It was often argued that babies delivered by section after abruptio usually died of respiratory distress. In a study by Lunan (1973), however, it was found that this was not so and he suggested that the prompt use of Caesarean section would save a small number of babies who would otherwise have been lost due to further separation of the placenta in labour.

At delivery, fetus, placenta and retroplacental clot may be rapidly expelled together or shortly after each other. This is a danger period, since serious post-partum haemorrhage may occur due to uterine atony and hypofibrinogenaemia. Careful watch on the uterus at this time is therefore necessary and oxytocics should be held ready for administration.

A catheter should be inserted to the bladder

as soon as the patient is admitted to hospital so that urinary output can be carefully measured. If there has been suppression of urine due to the acute shock, this can be treated by an infusion of Mannitol. If, after treatment of the shock, anuria or oliguria persist, 20gm of Mannitol should be given intravenously over a period of five to ten minutes. The objective should be to maintain a urinary flow of at least 100ml per hour.

Acute renal failure is a complication of abruptio placentae which usually is only seen following the severe forms. Proteinuria of some degree is almost always present. If energetic treatment of the shock and oliguria are instituted early, the likelihood of acute renal failure is greatly diminished. The cause of the renal tubular damage is probably related to blood loss and vasospasm. Cortical ischaemia also may occur and result in focal cortical necrosis. If renal failure does supervene, then haemodialysis may be required until the kidney recovers its function.

3. Antepartum haemorrhage with severe haemorrhage

In some cases, patients may be admitted with severe vaginal haemorrhage. Particularly when there is a high presenting part or transverse lie, examination under anaesthesia may waste valuable time and provoke further bleeding. In these circumstances, it is advisable to proceed immediately to Caesarean section. Even when the fetus is dead, it is safer to deliver the patient by Caesarean section when there is severe haemorrhage, than to resort to the older methods of vaginal manipulation.

PROGNOSIS OF MOTHER AND CHILD FOLLOWING PLACENTA PRAEVIA

Maternal death should now be a rarity in cases of placenta praevia. The great improvement, over the years, in the results in placenta praevia has been due mainly to three factors:

1. earlier hospitalization without vaginal examination;
2. liberal use of blood transfusion;
3. more frequent employment of Caesarean section.

Antibiotics too have played their part. Fetal mortality, stillbirth and neonatal death are mainly due to respiratory distress syndrome, prematurity and to a higher incidence of fetal abnormality.

Expectant treatment has reduced the loss due to prematurity, whilst Caesarean section has lessened the loss from anoxia resulting from placental separation, compression of the placental site and compression of the cord. The better management of premature babies has also played its part in improving the results. The technique of assessing fetal lung maturity by measuring the sphyngomyelin/lecethin ratio has proved very satisfactory in assessing the maturity of the fetal lung in cases with doubtful maturity thus helping to prevent fetal respiratory distress syndrome. The steady improvement in results is probably due to this combination of factors rather than to any one of them in isolation

PROGNOSIS OF MOTHER AND CHILD FOLLOWING ABRUPTIO PLACENTAE

Maternal mortality—This was formerly very high, but with more active measurements of management it has now been reduced to 1 per cent or less and, indeed, few patients should now die from abruptio placentae. The maternal prognosis is dependent upon the degree of severity of the abruptio and whether complications such as coagulation defects and renal complications develop, although both of these may be prevented by energetic treatment.

Fetal mortality—In severe cases, the fetal mortality is 100 per cent. In mild or moderate cases, the stage of gestation is an important factor in the mortality rate. When separation of the placenta has caused the loss of over 2 litres of blood, fetal death is almost invariable.

Table 8.2   Survival related to clot size (Lunan, 1973)

Size of clot	Number of cases	Number of babies	Perinatal loss	Percentage loss
Small	125	128	17**	13·3
Medium	103	105	21	20·0
Large	151	151	108	71·5
Total	379	384	146**	38·0

* Each asterisk signifies a twin pregnancy.
(Courtesy of the Editor, Journal of Obstetrics & Gynaecology of the British Commonwealth.)

Table 8.2 shows the survival related to the severity of the disease.

Late prognosis—Women who have suffered from severe abruptio placentae usually make a complete recovery and many have no trouble in future pregnancies. A proportion do, however, have recurrent abruptions so that careful attention is required during subsequent antenatal care.

REFERENCES

Browne, J. C. M. & Veall, N. (1950) *J. Obstet. Gynaec. Brit. Emp.*, **57**, 566.

Fernström, I. (1955) *Acta Radiol. (Stockh.)*, Suppl., 122.

Goldzieher, J. W. (1964) *J. Amer. med. Ass.*, **188**, 132.

Hibbard, B. M. (1964) *J. Obstet. Gynaec. Brit. Cwlth.*, **69**, 282.

James, G. B. (1970) *Proc. roy. Soc. Med.*, **63**, 1045.

Kleiner, G. J. & Roberts, T. W. (1967) *Amer. J. Obstet. Gynec.*, **99**, 21.

Klopper, A. & Macnaughton, I. (1965) *J. Obstet. Gynaec. Brit. Cwlth.*, **72**, 1022.

Lunan, C. B. (1973) *J. Obstet. Gynaec. Brit. Cwlth.*, **80**, 120.

Macafee, C. H. G. (1945) *J. Obstet. Gynaec. Brit. Emp.*, **59**, 786.

Malpas, P. (1938) *J. Obstet. Gynaec. Brit. Emp.*, **45**, 932.

Shearman, R. P. & Garrett, W. S. (1963) *Brit. med. J.*, **1**, 292.

Stevenson, A. C., Dudgeon, M. Y. & McClure, H. I. (1959) *A. num. genet.*, **23**, 395.

9. The Trophoblast, the Membranes and the Amniotic Fluid

CLASSIFICATION

There are many classifications of Trophoblastic Disease but one of the simplest based on the clinical behaviour of the disease is:

> Hydatidiform Mole.
> Invasive Mole.
> Choriocarcinoma.

Hydatidiform mole

The characteristic vesicles were, at one time, thought to contain worms hence the name which is deeply entrenched in the literature and it will be difficult to get the more descriptive term *vesicular mole* accepted. The aetiology of the condition is obscure but if it is postulated that there is some abnormality of the trophoblast itself which allows accumulation of fluid to occur within the villi which in turn become distended and the blood supply becomes cut off by the consequent pressure then a reasonable explanation of the appearance of hydatidiform mole is possible. The macroscopic appearance is striking: villi become very swollen and translucent attaining sizes of 5mm or even more. The villi often exist in clusters like grapes and a very large number may be present in any one pregnancy. In almost all cases there is no trace of a fetus.

MICROSCOPIC APPEARANCE
The villi are swollen, the stroma may show only mild oedema or may be totally liquefied. Blood vessels are usually absent. The trophoblast surrounding the villus is often stretched but in other areas there may be mild or marked overgrowth (Fig. 9.1). There is wide variation in the proportions of syncytiotrophoblast to cytotrophoblast and in the occurrence of abnormal cells.

CLINICAL FEATURES
It is not surprising (*see above*) that a hydatidiform mole not infrequently grows faster than a pregnancy. Unfortunately this is not always the case, presumably because the villi die from pressure on the blood supply and, therefore, though 'larger than dates' is the rule, it does not automatically follow. Sooner or later the mole pregnancy will bleed and finally vesicles will be passed which are pathognomonic of the condition. Patients are often unwell, multiparous patients will state that the mole pregnancy was unlike previous normal pregnancies. Nausea and vomiting even to the extent of the clinical syndrome of hyperemesis gravidarum occur frequently. Very occasionally hypertension with albuminuria and oedema (pre-eclampsia) will occur. Since the fetus is almost always absent the feto-placental unit production of oestriol is usually reduced to that of maternal origin and this has been used in the differential diagnosis (Macnaughton, 1965). The level of human chorionic gonadotrophin (HCG) is usually greatly raised and ordinary pregnancy tests have been used in the diagnosis. The urine is diluted 1:10, 1:100 and 1:1000. A positive 'pregnancy' test in urine diluted 1:100 is strongly suggestive of mole

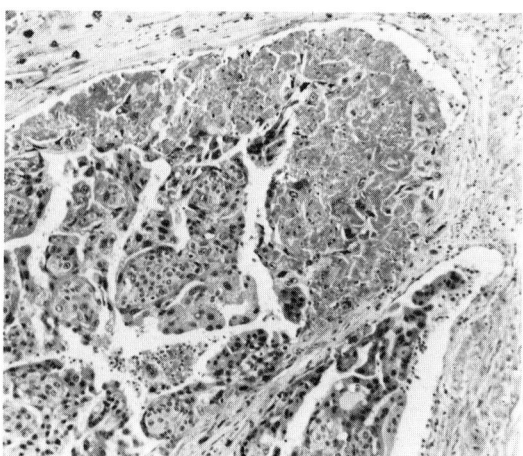

Fig. 9.1 The histology of hydatidiform mole reflects the vesicular macroscopic appearance. However in all moles there are areas of chorionic tissue overgrowth as is illustrated here.

but a negative test at this dilution by no means excludes the diagnosis. Moreover moderately high levels are not completely reliable. A twin pregnancy may give levels of HCG which overlap the levels found in hydatidiform mole. The differential diagnosis usually includes mistaken dates and twin pregnancy because of the size, and threatened abortion of a 'normal' pregnancy because of the bleeding. X-rays can be helpful in that the fetus is absent but at such an early stage in pregnancy when the diagnosis is required their quality must be high. Much the best method of diagnosis is by ultrasound. The appearance is usually characteristic of the condition—see Chapter 28. The association of a soft enlarged uterus and the bilateral granulosa lutein cysts which may accompany the condition make a typical though unusual clinical picture.

TREATMENT

Once the diagnosis has been confirmed the uterus should be evacuated. In the past hysterotomy was often the method of choice but the advent of suction termination has increased the safety of vaginal evacuation. Care is needed because of the softness of the uterus and the ease with which it can be perforated and patience is needed because of the time taken to evacuate such a large mass of tissue.

Some authors have advocated the use of prophylactic hysterectomy in older patients not wishing further family. Prophylactic chemotherapy has also been suggested. If the abdomen should be opened, the lutein cysts commonly present in the ovaries from the effect of the high level of HCG should not be touched since they will return to normal as the hormone level falls. Since some part of the molar tissue was almost always left behind it was common practice that curettage be performed a week after first evacuation when the uterus is considerably involuted but this may be less necessary when successful suction evacuation has been carried out.

Follow up. Since choriocarcinoma is much the most feared complication of hydatidiform mole (occurring after one mole in thirty) and being uniformly fatal if not treated (while being uniformly curable if treated early) it is encumbent on all doctors caring for patients recently delivered of a hydatidiform mole to ensure an adequate and thorough follow-up. The previous practice of seeing patients at three monthly intervals is totally inadequate and a normal 'pregnancy test' is not sensitive enough to ensure the safety of the patient. In the early stages after delivery of a mole it is necessary for the patient to be followed up at least fortnightly, and preferably weekly with measurement of urinary output of HCG by radioimmunoassay. If the titres of HCG remain low at the end of six months then monthly assay is acceptable and should be continued for two years. Such intensive follow-up of patients requires considerable organization. Three centres in the United Kingdom, London, Sheffield and Dundee have developed just such an organization to collect, by post, aliquots of urine directly from patients and send the results (radioimmunoassay of HCG levels) to their supervising doctors. While this organization is designed to relieve the doctor of the administrative chore of checking on defaulters the centres will also do assays for doctors on request.

With regard to *clinical* aftercare, after discharge from hospital the patient should be seen in one month. Further clinical examination subsequent to this may be necessary to reassure the patient, or the doctor, but it is in no way necessary nor often helpful in the early diagnosis of persistent mole, invasive mole or choriocarcinoma.

Invasive mole

Since, as part of its normal physiological role, trophoblast is required to invade the decidua it is not entirely surprising that trophoblast from a mole may also be invasive. On occasion this invasion goes well beyond decidua into uterine muscle and even beyond. There may be deposits of molar tissue elsewhere in the body (normal trophoblast can often be found in the lungs of women dying suddenly in pregnancy). Secondaries in the vagina and the vulva have been found in association with a mole. Sometimes there may be massive intraperitoneal bleeding from the perforation of an invasive mole through the serosa of the uterine wall and bleeding may also occur from secondary deposits on the vulva and in the vagina. Very often the presence of an invasive mole has been diagnosed by noting a persisting or rising titre of HCG in the presence of negative curettings of the uterine cavity. When this occurs arteriography is often instructive and will show a widespread intra mural blood supply often amounting to an arteriovenous anastomosis. (Borell and Fernstrom, 1961.)

TREATMENT

There are many examples in the literature of even advanced forms of invasive mole regressing satisfactorily but few, today, would await this event when chemotherapy is so successful. If the condition were invasive mole one would expect a rapid response to chemotherapy (cf. choriocarcinoma *below*). Surgery should be confined to controlling emergency situations such as haemorrhage and where excision is necessary this means hysterectomy in the case of internal bleeding and local excision in the case of vulval or vaginal haemorrhage.

Choriocarcinoma

Gestational choriocarcinoma is a unique neoplasm. In 1971 Park so described it because it was the first and still the only malignant neoplasm generally accepted as curable after systemic spread had occurred. Since then some other forms of cancer may qualify for cure but choriocarcinoma is unique in still other ways. As described above, it is composed of elements which, by their nature, are physiologically capable of invasion and even metastases. It is immunologically distinct from the host (the fetus, a mole and choriocarcinoma can all be considered allografts) and this may not be unconnected with the success of treatment. Again as has been described above, choriocarcinoma is a relatively frequent occurrence after hydatidiform mole. Its occurrence, after normal pregnancy and abortion, is much less likely (1:50 000 UK). Choriocarcinoma can, very rarely, appear to arise spontaneously from the ovary and certainly arises spontaneously from the testis. Such choriocarcinoma tissue, although sufficient in many cases to give positive pregnancy tests is not usually a pure growth. It is associated with other neoplastic tissues usually from a teratoma and the response to treatment is markedly poorer (*see* Chapter 38).

Diagnosis of choriocarcinoma can be extremely difficult. If it follows a mole it should not be missed if adequate follow-up with radioimmunoassay assessment of urine and/ or plasma is undertaken. In such cases treatment can be started early in the history of the condition and a very high success rate assured (Bagshawe *et al.*, 1973). If, however, choriocarcinoma follows normal pregnancy it may not be suspected and it may cause symptoms so varied as to present itself to almost all the specialists in medicine. Among the common possibilities are presentation to the physician as a lung secondary, to the neuro-surgeon as a brain secondary, to the ophthalmologist as an eye secondary, to the physician as a pyrexia of unknown origin; the list is almost endless. Whenever the condition is suspected estimation of HCG in urine and plasma by radioimmunoassay is always indicated.

TREATMENT

The treatment of choice is chemotherapy and the drug of choice is Methotrexate an antifolic acid agent. Other chemotherapeutic agents are used in cases where resistance to Methotrexate develops but this is unusual. Response of the choriocarcinoma can be accurately monitored by daily estimations of HCG during treatment. The toxic effect to the patient can be monitored by daily white counts. With two such precise monitors of disease response and patient response to treatment it is possible to treat the condition vigorously with minimum risk to the patient. At the end of a course of treatment daily HCG estimation is continued and persistence of the growth can be recognized at a much earlier stage than would be clinically possible. A further course of treatment is then indicated. This cycle is repeated until no further evidence of persistence of growth occurs.

From the patients point of view Methotrexate treatment can have distressing local effects, in particular stomatitis, and glossitis which can be extremely painful. The use of an intra-muscular injection of folinic acid greatly reduces and often eliminates this problem by preventing the effects of local folic acid deficiency on the gastrointestinal epithelium without interfering with the systemic action to any significant extent.

Surgery is inappropriate in the acute stage of the disease apart from symptomatic treatment, e.g. to control haemorrhage. In certain cases after chemotherapy has been used surgery may be indicated to eradicate a small persistent focus of growth which occasionally persists in the uterus. Metastases respond well to chemotherapy although care must be exercised in the case of cerebral metastases since too vigorous treatment may cause widespread tumour necrosis and cerebral haemorrhage.

Methotrexate may need to be given intrathecally. Since it is usual for repeated treatments with intervals between to be required, the treatment is prolonged and since the white count is often depressed the safety of the patient is greatly increased if they can be isolated from infection. The patient should therefore be treated only *in special* units equipped with facilities for isolation and for rapid and reliable radioimmunoassay assays of HCG on a daily basis. Special centres concentrating therapy also ensure an expert staff with adequate experience.

If the condition is diagnosed within three months of the precipitating cause, the results are uniformly good and if within six months then more than 80 per cent of the patients will make a complete recovery. If diagnosis and treatment is delayed beyond six months the success rate falls off. The majority of patients, if they wish, are able subsequently to become pregnant but it is preferable to delay pregnancy for two years and ensure that there is no recurrence of choriocarcinoma by repeated HCG estimations. Obviously a pregnancy during this time may cause confusion in diagnosis and during this time effective contraception should be prescribed. There is a further theoretical reason for delay to allow the death of any oocytes perhaps damaged at a developing stage by the chemotherapy (*see* Chapter 38).

If after this time a pregnancy does occur, check for HCG levels should be carried out at three weeks' postpartum and this should be repeated in each subsequent pregnancy since choriocarcinoma may apparently recur after later pregnancy.

AMNIOTIC FLUID

Introduction

Amniotic fluid plays an important part in the physical development of the fetus because the fluid protects the fetus from mechanical shock and provides a weightless and constant temperature environment. There has been a great increase in interest in amniotic fluid since the realization that the fluid is a useful diagnostic aid in many fields and further advances of knowledge in both the diagnostic and physiological fields are likely.

Physiological background

AMNIOTIC FLUID VOLUME IN NORMAL PREGNANCIES

Amniotic fluid is present in pregnancies of 8 weeks' gestation. The average volume of fluid present at 10 weeks' gestation is 34ml and it increases steadily to nearly 400ml at 19 weeks (Abramovich, 1968) (Table 9.1).

Table 9.1   Amniotic fluid volume in early and mid-pregnancy

Gestational age (weeks)	Amniotic fluid volume (ml)
10	34
14	100
19	383

Between 20 weeks and 37 weeks several investigators have shown that the amount of fluid increases to a peak at about 37–38 weeks' gestation, the volume ranging between 500ml and 1100ml. There then appears to be a steady decrease as only small volumes are present in prolonged pregnancy (Table 9.2).

Table 9.2   Amniotic fluid volume from term to 44 weeks

Gestational age (weeks)	Volume amniotic fluid (ml)	
	Elliott & Inman (1961)	Beischer et al. (1969)
40	791	—
41	636	—
42	324	484
43	—	332
44	—	162

It should be realized that not all pregnancies behave in this way as Queenan *et al.* (1972) have shown with serial determinations that variations in the upward or downward trends of fluid volume can occur at any stage of gestation.

Methods of estimation of amniotic fluid volume
In early pregnancy the most accurate method of measurement is the removal of the intact sac at hysterotomy or after pregnant hysterectomy. If there is a continuing pregnancy or the length of gestation is greater than 20 weeks then the only accurate method is that using the principle of dye dilution. Clinical examination of the pregnant uterus will often suggest that abnormalities of volume exist but give no

information on the volume present. Ultrasonic methods do likewise. In dye dilution tests, a known volume or weight of substance is injected into the amniotic fluid and after suitable mixing has occurred, a sample of fluid is obtained and the concentration of the injected substances determined. Many substances have been used including Congo Red and Coumassie Blue but sodium aminohippurate (PAH) is most commonly used at the moment.

Constituents

Osmolality
Up to 16 weeks' gestation the osmolality of amniotic fluid is similar to that of maternal plasma (average 278mosmol/kg) but as the fetus matures the fluid osmolality drops till at term it averages 250mosmol/kg (Gillibrand, 1969), with a range of 230–260mosmol/kg.

Electrolytes
Amniotic sodium and potassium concentrations are similar to those of maternal plasma till mid-pregnancy while chloride concentrations are higher than plasma. In the second half of pregnancy the concentration of potassium remains steady while that of sodium and chloride fall, the average sodium level being 128mEq/1 (range 117–138mEq/1) and the chloride level 99mEq/1 (95–104mEq/1) (Gillibrand, 1969).

The fall in osmolality and electrolyte values towards term are not definite enough to be of clinical use and the underlying physiological reason has not yet been explained.

Non-protein Nitrogen
Urea, uric acid and creatinine. The concentration of urea remains unchanged till 20 weeks' gestation when it rises slowly to about 25mg per cent at term (Lind *et al.*, 1969) while uric acid and creatinine values rise steadily throughout pregnancy. Creatinine levels have been used for assessing fetal maturity, with the fetus at 37 weeks having a fluid creatinine concentration of 2·0mg/100ml or more (Pitkin and Zwirek, 1967). However, controversy exists about its use as there are some undoubtedly mature fetuses with low amniotic fluid levels. Some of the urea, creatinine and uric acid in amniotic fluid comes from fetal urine but it has also been shown that urea and creatinine are capable of being absorbed and excreted via fetal skin and fetal surface of

the placenta in mid-pregnancy. The fetal surface of the placenta remains a pathway of transfer between fluid and fetal circulation at term (Abramovich, unpublished).

Amino acids
The levels of amino acids in amniotic fluid have been well documented. Emery *et al.* (1970) noted three patterns of change. The first group acids remained steady throughout pregnancy (e.g. proline), in the second group there was a steady fall from the first trimester to term (e.g. glycine) while in the third group the levels rose till 16 weeks, fell steadily till 36 weeks and then rose till term (e.g. valine). Fetal urine is one source of amniotic amino acids but other routes of entry (e.g. fetal surface of the placenta or fetal skin) are likely to be operative, at least up to mid-pregnancy.

It is as yet unclear whether the amino acid concentration of amniotic fluid can be used in the ante-natal diagnosis of inborn errors in metabolism, there being conflicting reports in the literature on this subject.

Glucose, pyruvate and lactic acid
There is conflicting evidence on the clinical importance of the levels of these substances in amniotic fluid. Wood *et al.* (1963) found that the glucose and lactic acid levels at term were 13mg/100ml and 38·7mg/100ml (mean values) and that if the glucose level fell below 10mg/100ml or the lactic acid level rose above 40mg/100ml there was often delay in the onset of respiration. Schreiner and Schmid (1969) found that amniotic glucose at 10–11 weeks was 53·7mg/100ml falling to 22mg/100ml at term. Cohen (1970), however, found no correlation between the levels of glucose, lactate or pyruvate and fetal distress or condition of the infant at birth.

Acid-base Balance
There appears to be no correlation between the fetal state and amniotic fluid acid-base balance. Seeds and Helligers (1968) showed that the fluid becomes more acid as pregnancy progresses, the pH falling from 7·3 at 10–20 weeks to 7·1 at term. Carbon dioxide tension rose from 41mmHg in early pregnancy to 51mmHg at term and the bicarbonate concentration fell from 16·6mm/1 in early pregnancy to 14·8mm/1 at term.

Bilirubin
The amount of bilirubin and bilirubin-like pigment, as measured chemically or spectro-

photometrically is used clinically to assess the degree of severity of rhesus haemolytic disease of the newborn. A sample of fluid is obtained by amniocentesis at about 28 weeks' gestation with minimal light exposure. After centrifugation and/or filtration to remove particulate matter it is examined in a spectrophotometer over a range of wavelengths. If the fluid contains bilirubin there will be an absorption band at 450nm, but contamination with blood or blood pigment causes technical difficulties. One method of interpretation of the results uses the difference in optical density between the height at the 450nm band and the vertical distance from a line joining the points of the curve at 365 and 550nm (Liley, 1963). The tap is commonly repeated after 2–3 weeks with a decision on timing of induction being made on amount of bilirubin relative to stage of gestation, past rhesus obstetric history, maternal antibody titre and paternal genotype.

It should be realized that bilirubin is found in normal (i.e. rhesus unaffected) amniotic fluid from 10 weeks' gestation, the level rising till 18 weeks, levelling off till 25–26 weeks and then falling till its disappearance at 36 weeks. The major pigment present is unconjugated bilirubin which is not excreted by the kidney. The pathway by which the bilirubin enters amniotic fluid is thus likely to be via umbilical cord, fetal surface of the placenta and up to 20 weeks' gestation, through fetal skin. It has been suggested that there is also a pulmonary origin but the amounts originating from the lungs would be small.

Proteins

Total protein concentration in amniotic fluid varies widely in different cases. In early pregnancy the amounts range from 0·1 to 0·6g/100ml but tend to rise till at 24 weeks' gestation the mean level is 0·64g/100ml. From then till term the concentration drops, averaging about 0·28g/100ml at term (Queenan et al., 1970). The difficulty in discussing protein concentration is that each different technique used in measurement gives a different value.

It is generally believed that amniotic fluid proteins are of maternal origin with a likely site of entry being via the amniochorion. Recently, however, the fetal origin or some of the proteins has been suggested with the description of α-feto-protein, the concentration of which in the second trimester ranged

from 280 to 2600ug/100ml and fell at term to 1·5–53·5ug/100ml. This protein originates in part in the fetal liver, is found in fetal urine and can also be detected in maternal plasma (Seppala and Ruoslahti, 1972). Its importance lies in the elevated levels found in amniotic fluid in early pregnancy in cases of anencephaly and spina bifida, thus enabling early diagnosis in these cases (Brock and Sutcliffe, 1972). Care should be taken, however, as elevated levels have been described in cases of fetal distress and intra-uterine death.

Cells

Various authors have examined the cells found in amniotic fluid but they used different staining methods and differing modes of cell classification. Thus any comparison of their findings is difficult. The number of cells found in the fluid in early pregnancy is small with the numbers increasing towards term. The origin of the cells is multiple: from the amnion, the umbilical cord, the fetal mouth and respiratory tree, the bladder and vagina and from the skin. Using the Harris-Storr stain, Huisjes (1970) described nucleated and anuclear eosinophilic cells, small and large cyanophilic cells and polygonal cells with orange staining cytoplasm mainly appearing after 38 weeks and originating from the skin. Lind et al. (1971) using the terminology of cervical cytology, described basal, precornified and cornified cells.

A much used method of assessing fetal maturity has been the staining of cells with 0·1 per cent Nile blue sulphate. When greater than 10 per cent stain orange it is thought that the fetus is mature. The orange staining is caused by the adherence to the cell surface of neutral lipids. The method is reliable but should not be used as the only indicator in assessing fetal maturity.

Hormones

At one stage it appeared that the levels of some steroids in amniotic fluid would provide information on the performance of the feto-placental unit. This hope has not been realized. *Steroids.* The level of total oestriol rises from 28ug/100ml at 20 weeks to 57ug/100ml at 36 weeks and then more than doubles to 135ug/100ml at term (Aleem et al., 1969). The majority of the steroid present is conjugated to glucosiduronic acid. The only clinical correlation known is that the levels of oestriol are suppressed in the presence of severe rhesus iso-immunization.

The levels of other steroids *viz.* testosterone and 17-oxosteroids, cortisol and 17-hydroxy-corticosteroids, progesterone and pregnanediol and C-16 hydroxylated steroids, have been measured in amniotic fluid. At the present time they are only of academic interest. Other hormones *viz.* adrenaline, serotonin, human chorionic gonadotrophin and human placental lactogen, have been found in amniotic fluid but again are, at the moment, only of academic interest.

Prostaglandins

These substances are used clinically in the induction of labour at term and inducing mid-trimester abortions so their presence in amniotic fluid is of interest. Prostaglandin E and F are found in amniotic fluid throughout gestation, increasing in concentration as term approaches. The levels are higher in early labour than before the onset of labour and increase in concentration in proportion to cervical dilatation. It is possible that the accumulation of the prostaglandins in amniotic fluid near term is related to the increased uterine activity at this time (Keirse *et al.*, 1974).

Lipids and Phospholipids

The importance of lipids and phospholipids in amniotic fluid lies not in the presence of varying levels of mono-, di- and triglycerides but in the presence of lecithin, a phospholipid which is thought to be a major chemical component of surfactant. This substance lowers surface tension in the lung alveoli and if its synthesis is inadequate in the newborn then secondary changes in the lungs occur with the infant developing the respiratory distress syndrome (RDS). It is believed that surfactant, produced by the β cells of the alveolae is found in amniotic fluid and on this basis, several tests have been developed to measure its level and thus predict the maturity of the fetal lung. It is hoped that in this way the development of RDS can be predicted and indeed prevented, either by *in utero* treatment (corticoids given to the mother) or by delay in induction of labour.

At the present moment, the main tests used are lecithin/sphingomyelin ratio (L.S. ratio), lecithin concentration and the 'shake' or 'foam' test. The L.S. ratio test depends on the fact that before 30 weeks' gestation the concentration of sphingomyelin exceeds that of lecithin but that after this time, the lecithin concentration is greater, rising sharply at about 35 weeks when biochemical (surfactant) maturation of the lung occurs. When the lung is mature the L/S ratio (as measured in a densitometer) is greater than 2 and the infant will not show evidence of respiratory distress as caused by lack of surfactant. It is suggested that fetal lung maturity is advanced when the fetus is stressed (e.g. maternal toxaemia or ruptured membranes) and delayed in the presence of diabetes mellitus.

This test has aroused controversy in that there are many cases where the ratio lies between 1·5 to 2·0, the so-called 'grey area'. The ratio is not of much help in these cases as the infant may or may not develop respiratory distress. Generally speaking the gestation of these infants lies between 32 and 37 weeks, just the time when it is well-known that RDS is more likely. Further argument has been aroused by differing technical procedures used. Thus a final conclusion of the validity of the L/S ratio is impossible at present.

Similar controversy surrounds the use of lecithin concentration, the arguments against its use being that the concentration is dependent on the volume of amniotic fluid and it shows general overall maturity rather than a specific lung maturity.

The 'shake' or 'foam' test, where increasing dilutions of uncentrifuged liquor are shaken with 95 per cent ethanol to give a circle of stable bubbles visible at the meniscus when surfactant is present is a good non-specific screening test, far simpler than the complex laboratory tests discussed above. Where it is negative, further investigations are then necessary. In the future it is likely that far more specific and non-controversial tests for the measurement of lung alveolar fluid will be developed, giving a more clear-cut clinical answer.

Origin

The origin of amniotic fluid in early pregnancy is unknown. The similarity of composition between maternal plasma and amniotic fluid in early pregnancy together with some experimental evidence from rhesus monkeys suggests that it is a transudate from maternal plasma. Equally it can be suggested that the fluid is a transudate from fetal plasma as there is a close correlation between fetal length and weight and the fluid volume as well as a similarity of composition between the fluid and fetal plasma. It has also been shown that water, electrolytes, creatinine and urea can cross between the fetal circulation and the fluid via fetal skin (up to 20 weeks—till keratinization of skin occurs), umbilical cord and fetal surface of the placenta (Abramovich and Page, 1973). It is not thought that fetal urine is an important source of amniotic fluid in early pregnancy.

Fetal swallowing

The fetus begins to swallow amniotic fluid early in pregnancy and by 10–12 weeks' gestational age is swallowing definite but minute amounts. By 18 weeks of age the fetus swallows (depending on its size) between 4 and 11ml in 24 hours while at term the amount is about 300–400ml in 24 hours (Abramovich, 1970). Though it is widely believed that the inability of the fetus to swallow in cases of tracheo-oesophageal fistula, oesophageal atresia and anencephaly produces polyhydramnios and further that fetal swallowing controls the amniotic fluid volume, there is evidence to the contrary. There are many reports of normal volumes of fluid in these cases; it has been shown that some anencephalics swallow and that the volume of fluid does not appear to be influenced by the presence or absence of swallowing. Furthermore, recent investigations on normal infants with hydramnios suggests that the volume of fluid swallowed is little different from those infants with normal amniotic fluid volumes.

Fetal voiding

The fetus voids *in utero* throughout pregnancy, urine having been found in the bladder of fetuses aged 11 weeks. The amounts passed in early pregnancy are small, perhaps rising to 10ml/24 hours at 18 weeks' gestation. This urine is hypotonic with an osmolality of 144mosmol/kg and remains hypotonic throughout pregnancy (Abramovich, 1970). The fetus voids intermittently throughout the day, apparently has no diurnal variation in output and voids a mean of 590ml/24 hours at 39 weeks (Campbell *et al.*, 1973). Further work suggests that this figure is too high with levels of 300–400ml/24 hours being more common.

Where the amniotic fluid volume is within normal limits, fetal urine provides an important source of the water of amniotic fluid but it appears likely that an equivalent volume of fluid is swallowed daily by the fetus. Where polyhydramnios is present, fetal voiding is less likely to be important in the fluid dynamics.

Respiratory tract

The importance of the lungs as a source of amniotic fluid is uncertain though there is no doubt that fluid is secreted by the respiratory tract. Some fluid from the trachea enters the amniotic cavity as shown by measurements of lecithin concentrations in tracheal and amniotic fluid but it is believed that the bulk of the lung fluid production is swallowed by the fetus. The fetus breathes spontaneously *in utero* both in the lamb and the human but in the lamb, the respiratory movements do not give rise to sufficient trachael flow to clear the respiratory dead-space (Boddy and Mantell, 1972). The position in the human is unknown, but in the normal fetus it is unlikely that amniotic fluid volume is much influenced by fetal lung fluid production.

CONTROL OF AMNIOTIC FLUID VOLUME

What controls amniotic fluid volume is unknown but recent work has enabled a clearer picture of the situation to emerge. As discussed above there are many pathways available for the passage of water, electrolytes, urea and creatinine in both directions between the fetal circulation and amniotic fluid. At term these exchange pathways include the umbilical cord, and as a major site, the fetal surface of the placenta. The fetal skin, an important site in mid-pregnancy, ceases to act as a pathway as soon as keratinization occurs (i.e. after 20 weeks' gestation). Though exchange takes place across these sites, undoubtedly actual transfer of water, electrolytes etc. can occur with an increase or decrease in their concentration on the appropriate side of the membrane. The site of fluid transfer between fetal and maternal circulations is across the placenta and between amniotic fluid and mother across the amniochorion. This latter site is of little importance when actual flows of fluid are taken into account as no more than 20–30ml of water/day pass out from the amniotic cavity across the fetal membranes to the maternal circulation.

Previous workers (Hutchinson *et al.*, 1959) using isotopes of water have suggested that there were large exchanges of water between maternal circulation, fetal circulation and amniotic fluid but it has now been realized that these figures were in fact showing only that the membrane surfaces were permeable to water as there is in fact a 1 for 1 exchange of water molecules i.e. a molecular exchange and not a bulk flow (as in urine production) of water. It should be realized that it is being suggested that a bulk flow of water can occur across the umbilical cord or fetal surface of the placenta and that isotope experiments are not the method that should be used to demonstrate these bulk flows.

Though there is no doubt that fetal swallowing and voiding are important factors in the control of the fluid volume there are many cases where the fetus is not or cannot swallow fluid or is unable to pass urine *in utero* yet the amniotic fluid volume is within normal limits. Thus where one pathway of bulk fluid flow (e.g. swallowing or voiding) is inoperative, bulk flow must be occurring across one or all of the pathways described above. What controls flow across these pathways is unknown but it can be suggested that the factors that control the osmotic tonicity of the fetal plasma (and perhaps of maternal plasma) play some part in the control of amniotic fluid volume.

Clinical factors

Appearance

Amniotic fluid in early pregnancy contains bilirubin, the colour ranging from pale straw to deep yellow. After mid-pregnancy (in absence of rhesus haemolytic disease) the concentration of bilirubin decreases and usually by 36 weeks the fluid is colourless. During the last few weeks of pregnancy the fluid becomes cloudy with vernix caseosa (clumps of desquamated fetal skin cells and free lipid material) being seen in most cases. Abnormal coloration may be seen from contamination with blood, bilirubin or in cases of fetal distress, meconium.

Polyhydramnios

This is a condition where the volume of amniotic fluid is increased to greater than 1500ml. It may be acute or chronic. In acute hydramnios, a very rare condition (the incidence is about 1 in 10 000 to 1 in 20 000), the uterus becomes grossly distended over a very short period (a matter of days). The patient may complain of pain, becomes dyspnoeic and a diagnosis of placental abruption may be made. This condition usually occurs around the 6th month of pregnancy. There is no effective method of treatment apart from rupture of membranes or amniocentesis. The amniotic fluid does not vary from normal in its composition.

Chronic hydramnios, usually referred to as hydramnios, is more common than the acute variety with an incidence of about 1 in 150, the recorded incidence rising with the amount of interest taken in the subject. Clinically the diagnosis is made by finding a uterus larger than dates with difficulty in palpating fetal parts. The fetus may be more easily ballotable and a fluid thrill will be elicited. Normally hydramnios is diagnosed in the last trimester but the fluid accumulates slowly from earlier in pregnancy. The patient may complain of abdominal pain or discomfort, she may be dyspnoeic and have oedema of the lower limbs and abdominal wall. The common clinical associations of hydramnios are:

1. Anencephaly.
2. Oesophageal and duodenal atresia.
3. Maternal diabetes mellitus.
4. Hydrops fetalis (rhesus iso-immunization).
5. Multiple pregnancy.
6. Idiopathic.

There is no scientific evidence to confirm the association of polyhydramnios and pre-eclampsia. In fact there appears to be a diminution of the fluid volume in both pre-eclampsia and essential hypertension (Elliot and Inman, 1961).

In most reported series of hydramnios by far the greatest percentage of cases was associated with a normal fetus while the next largest group consisted of fetal abnormalities. Where multiple pregnancy is concerned, the clinician must be aware of pseudo-hydramnios where a normal volume of fluid surrounds each fetus yet the total volume in the uterus exceeds 1500ml.

When a diagnosis of hydramnios is made, a plain X-ray of the abdomen should be performed to exclude fetal bony abnormality and multiple pregnancy, while the maternal carbohydrate tolerance should be investigated using a glucose tolerance test. Rhesus iso-immunization will have been previously excluded by the examination of the mother's rhesus blood group and presence or absence of rhesus antibodies.

The treatment of hydramnios is difficult in that the only method known to reduce the volume of the fluid is mechanical i.e. by amniocentesis to remove the fluid abdominally or of course by artificial rupture of the membranes. In performing amniocentesis the clinician runs the risk of inducing premature labour in certain cases. If a large amount of fluid (500–1000ml) is being removed this should be done slowly and may need to be repeated at regular intervals. The maternal and fetal dangers of hydramnios include premature labour, cord prolapse, malpresentation, premature placental separation (presumably because of the escape of the excess fluid causing a decrease in the area of uterine wall beneath the placenta) uterine dysfunction and post-partum haemorrhage. These last two complications are associations of uterine atony consequent upon uterine overdistension though the judicious use of oxytocic drugs can control this problem.

Oligohydramnios
This condition may be diagnosed when the amniotic fluid volume is greatly reduced. An arbitrary limit of 300ml at term may be set. Conditions in which oligohydramnios occurs where the fetus is normal include retarded fetal growth with or without pre-eclampsia, and prolonged pregnancy. The classical clinical association of oligohydramnios is renal agenesis. In these cases the fetus also has abnormal (Potter) facies and hypoplastic lungs but cases of renal agenesis with normal fluid volumes have also been described.

When oligohydramnios occurs early in pregnancy there can be fetal dangers where adhesions between the amnion and parts of the fetus can cause serious deformity even including amputation. It has also been suggested that club foot is associated with oligohydramnios.

Amniocentesis
In this procedure amniotic fluid for diagnostic purposes is obtained by transabdominal puncture. It may be performed with safety from about 12–14 weeks' gestation, the indications being discussed below. The technique is relatively simple involving the passing of a lumbar-puncture type needle through the skin into the amniotic cavity and withdrawing a small aliquot of fluid. The procedure is explained in detail to the patient, who may nevertheless require sedation. An ultrasonic scan to define the site of the placenta should have been performed. The patient must have emptied her bladder. The procedure is performed with the usual sterile precautions as infection must be prevented. In early pregnancy a mid-line site is used, local anaesthetic having been injected into the layers of skin and subcutaneous tissues. Later in pregnancy the site of puncture is usually over the nape of the fetal neck though avoiding the placenta takes precedence. Usually it is sufficient to withdraw 10–15ml of fluid which should be protected from the light if the bilirubin concentration is being measured.

The difficulties of amniocentesis include a dry tap (no fluid being obtained) or a 'bloody' tap, though prompt centrifugation of the fluid may avoid the necessity of repeating the procedure in 1–2 weeks. The dangers of the test are mainly theoretical as the complication rate is low. Complications include spontaneous rupture of membranes, premature labour, premature separation of the placenta, intra-uterine infection, fetal organ puncture, and maternal damage (bladder, bowel, abdominal wall haematoma). Some authorities recommend the injection of anti-D if an Rh-negative woman without antibodies undergoes the procedure.

DIAGNOSTIC USES OF AMNIOTIC FLUID
The use of amniotic fluid for diagnostic purposes is a rapidly expanding field. Fluid obtained early in pregnancy (12–20 weeks) is used in the diagnosis of:
a. genetic enzyme defects.
b. fetal sex and chromosome defects (including sex-linked diseases).
   This topic is discussed in Chapter 7.
c. anencephaly and open spinal defects, where α-fetoprotein levels are measured (*see above*).

Between 24 and 34 weeks, the main diagnostic use of amniotic fluid lies in the field of Rhesus iso-immunization. From 32–34 weeks to term the timing of fetal lung maturity may be diagnosed using the 'shake test', L/S ratio or the lecithin concentration. Likewise use of amniotic fluid characteristics is helpful in assessing general fetal maturity. Tests used include Nile blue staining of amniotic cells, creatinine levels and in some laboratories, lecithin concentration.

It must be remembered in any discussion on amniotic fluid that the field is rapidly expanding with new information becoming constantly available so that some of the opinions expressed above must be re-interpreted in this light.

REFERENCES

Abramovich, D. R. (1968) The volume of amniotic fluid in early pregnancy. *J. Obstet. Gynaec. Brit. Cwlth.*, **75**, 728.

Abramovich, D. R. (1970) Fetal Factors Influencing the Volume and Composition of Liquor Amnii. *J. Obstet. Gynaec. Brit. Cwlth*, **77**, 865.

Abramovich, D. R. & Page, K. R. (1973) Pathways of Water Transfer between Liquor Amnii and the Fetoplacental Unit at Term. *Euro. J. Obstet. Gynaec.*, **3/5**, 155.

Aleem, F. A., Pinkerton, J. H. & Neill, D. W. (1969) Clinical Significance of the Amniotic Fluid Oestriol Level. *J. Obstet. Gynaec.*, **76**, 200.

Bagshawe, K. D., Wilson, H., Dublon, P., Smith, A., Baldwin, M. (1973) Follow-up after Hydatidiform Mole: Studies using Radioimmunoassay for Urinary Human Chorionic Gonadotrophin (H.C.G.) *J. Obstet. Gynaec. Brit. Cwlth.*, **80**, 461.

Beischer, N. A., Brown, J. B. & Townsend, L. (1969) Studies in Prolonged Pregnancy III. *Amer. J. Obstet. Gynec.*, **103**, 496.

Boddy, K. & Mantell, C. D. (1972) Observations of Fetal Breathing Movements Transmitted through Maternal Abdominal Wall. *Lancet*, **ii**, 1219.

Borell, J. & Fernstrom, I. (1961) Hydatidiform mole diagnosed by Pelvic Angiography. *Acta Radiol.*, **56**, 113.

Brock, D. J. H. & Sutcliffe, R. C. (1972) Alpha-fetoprotein in the Antenatal Diagnosis of Anencephaly and Spina Bifida. *Lancet*, **ii**, 197.

Campbell, S., Wladimiroff, J. W. & Dewhurst, C. J. (1973) The Antenatal Measurement of Fetal Urine Production. *J. Obstet. Gynaec. Brit. Cwlth.*, **80**, 680.

Cohen, B. M. (1970) The Relationship between the Fetal Condition and the Biochemical Analysis of Amniotic Fluid at Induction of Labour. *J. Obstet. Gynaec. Brit. Cwlth.*, **77**, 496.

Elliot, P. M. & Inman, W. H. W. (1961) Volume of Liquor Amnii in Normal and Abnormal Pregnancy. *Lancet*, **ii**, 835.

Emery, A. E. H., Burt, D., Nelson, M. M. & Scrimgeour, J. B. (1970) Antenatal Diagnosis and Amino-acid Composition of Amniotic Fluid. *Lancet*, **i**, 1307.

Gillibrand, P. N. (1969) Changes in the Electrolytes, Urea and Osmolality of the Amniotic Fluid with Advancing Pregnancy. *J. Obstet. Gynaec. Brit. Cwlth.*, **76**, 893.

Huisjes, H. J. (1970) Origin of the Cells in the Liquor Amnii. *Amer. J. Obstet. Gynec.*, **106**, 1222.

Hutchinson, D. L., Gray, M. J., Plentl, A. A., Alvarez, H., Caldeyro-Barcia, R., Kaplan, B. & Lind, J. (1959) The role of the Fetus in the Water Exchange of Amniotic Fluid of Normal and Hydramniotic Patients. *J. Clin. Invs.*, **38**, 971.

Keirse, M., Flint, A. & Turnbull, A. C. (1974) F prostaglandins in Amniotic Fluid during Pregnancy and Labour. *J. Obstet. Gynaec. Brit. Cwlth.*, **81**, 131.

Liley, A. W. (1961) Liquor Amnii in the Management of Pregnancy Complicated by Rhesus Sensitization. *Amer. J. Obstet. Gynec.*, **82**, 1359.

Lind, T., Parkin, F. M. & Cheyne, G. A. (1969) Biochemical and Cytological Changes in Liquor Amnii with Advancing Gestation. *J. Obstet. Gynaec. Brit. Cwlth.*, **76**, 673.

Lind, T., Billiewicz, W. Z. & Cheyne, G. A. (1971) Composition of Amniotic Fluid and Maternal Blood Through Pregnancy. *J. Obstet. Gynaec. Brit. Cwlth.*, **78**, 505.

Macnaughton, M. C. (1965) Urinary excretion of oestrogen and pregrandiol in Hydatidiform Mole. *J. Obstet. Gynaec. Brit. Cwlth.*, **72**, 249.

Pitkin, R. M. & Zwirek, S. J. (1967) Amniotic Fluid Creatinine. *Amer. J. Obstet. Gynec.*, **98**, 1135.

Queenan, J. T., Gadow, E. C., Bachner, P. & Kubarych (1970) Amniotic Fluid Proteins in Normal and Rhesus Sensitized Pregnancy. *Amer. J. Obstet. Gynec.*, **108**, 406.

Queenan, J. T., Thompson, W., Whitfield, C. R. & Shah, S. I. (1972) Amniotic Fluid Volumes in Normal Pregnancies. *Amer. J. Obstet. Gynec.*, **114**, 34–38.

Schreiner, W. E. & Schmid, J. (1969) The Clinical Significance of Biochemical Tests on the Amniotic Fluid. *Perinatal Medicine*—edited by P. J. Huntingford, K. A. Huter & E. Saling. New York and London: Academic Press.

Seeds, A. E. & Helligers, A. E. (1968) Acid-base Determinations in Human Amniotic Fluid Throughout Pregnancy. *Amer. J. Obstet. Gynec.*, **101**, 257.

Seppala, M. & Ruoslahti, E. (1972) Alpha Fetoprotein in Amniotic Fluid. *Amer. J. Ostet. Gynec.*, **114**, 595.

Wood, C., Acharya, P. T., Cornwell, E. & Pinkerton, J. H. M. (1963) The Significance of Glucose and Lactic Acid Concentration in the Amniotic Fluid. *J. Obstet. Gynaec. Brit. Cwlth.*, **70**, 274.

FURTHER READING

British Medical Journal (1974) Ed. Better results with choriocarcinoma, **ii**, 543.

Coutts, J. R. T., Macnaughton, M. C., Ross, P. E., Walker, J. (1969) Steroidogenesis in a Case of Hydatidiform Mole. *J. Endocr.*, **44**, 335.

10. Hypertensive Disorders of Pregnancy

A raised level of blood pressure found during pregnancy may be due to a hypertensive condition antedating the condition: to a latent hypertensive condition becoming manifest, or to a condition arising for the first time during the pregnancy. It is sometimes extremely difficult to tell during the pregnancy or even afterwards which of these has caused the rise in blood pressure during the pregnancy. This is particularly true if hypertension persists after the pregnancy. One woman in four has a rise of blood pressure above normal in her first pregnancy (MacGillivray, 1961). The commonest cause of hypertension in pregnancy appears to be a condition which is specific to pregnancy, and this will be dealt with first.

HYPERTENSION OF PREGNANCY

It has been recognized from ancient times that convulsions could occur during pregnancy towards the end, during labour or after delivery. This condition is called eclampsia, which means a sudden flash of light, and the name was given presumably because the condition occurred without warning like a flash of lightning. When it became customary for doctors to test the urine it was found that some of those women having a grand mal type of convulsion occurring for the first time during pregnancy had albuminuria. Many of them also had oedema. Later when the sphygmomanometer was invented it was found that such women also had hypertension. It is now recognized that hypertension is the basis of this condition, but not all pregnant women who develop hypertension, no matter how severe, will develop convulsions. Many terms have been used to describe this condition. Although there is no dispute about the use of the term eclampsia where fits occur the syndrome without convulsions has been variously named albuminuria of pregnancy, pre-eclampsia, toxaemia of pregnancy (because it

was thought that a toxin from the placenta might be causing the condition) or pre-eclamptic toxaemia. Continental obstetricians are keen on the term 'gestosis', but this is not a term favoured by English speaking obstetricians. Obstetricians are agreed that hypertension is the one essential part of the syndrome and attempts have been made to agree on a suitable term incorporating the word hypertension; for example, 'specific hypertensive disease of pregnancy' has been suggested by Pickering, but even though it is technically preferable this is rather a long term. In the UK the name generally used is pre-eclampsia and until another term is adopted by international agreement we will use that term in the text. It is generally conceded that proteinuria is a manifestation of a more severe form of the disease. The other part of the triad, oedema, is less readily acceptable as many otherwise normal pregnant women have oedema. About 40 per cent of Aberdeen primigravidae develop oedema (Thomson, Hytten and Billewicz, 1967). Oedema was present in 35 per cent of those who remained normotensive, in 60 per cent of those who develop hypertension and in about 85 per cent of patients who had both hypertension and proteinuria. It is sufficient to recognize that patients with oedema are more liable to develop pregnancy hypertension and should be observed more closely, but there is no need to include oedema in the classification.

Measurement of blood pressure
It would seem to be a relatively easy matter to determine the normal levels of blood pressure throughout pregnancy, but there has been difficulty in doing this because of the need to study sufficiently large numbers of women throughout pregnancy by standard techniques, because of the difficulty of determining what is a normal pregnancy and also because of the difficulties in methodology of recording the blood pressure. The American Heart Associa-

tion concluded, 'It should be clearly recognized that arterial pressure cannot be measured with precision by means of sphygmomanometers'. Many factors cause variation in the blood pressure and it is difficult to standardize for them all. As it appears that the hypertension of pregnancy is due to vasoconstriction it is of more importance to measure the *diastolic* pressure accurately than the systolic pressure, and there is much debate about whether the diastolic pressure should be measured at phase 5 (disappearance) or at phase 4 (muffling). In hyperkinetic states such as pregnancy there is particular difficulty as the sounds may still be present at zero pressure on the cuff. It is, therefore, recommended *that the diastolic pressure should be taken at phase 4 (muffling)*.

The systolic pressure is affected by posture but the diastolic is not. The blood pressure tends to fall late in the first and in the second trimester of pregnancy and rises again in the third trimester, and is still up at the post-natal visit six weeks after delivery (Fig. 10.1). If the

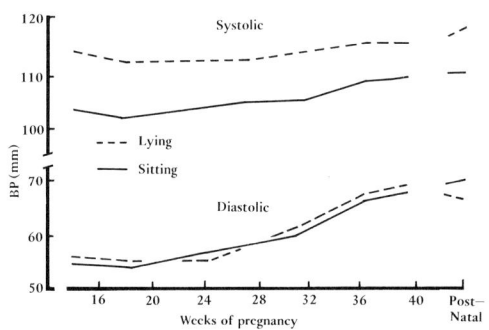

Fig. 10.1 The systolic and diastolic pressures recorded sitting and lying, during pregnancy and at the post-natal visit six weeks after delivery.

blood pressure has been high before pregnancy it may appear to be normal during the first and second trimesters and will then rise again in the third trimester. It is impossible without prior knowledge of the pre-pregnancy or very early pregnancy blood pressure to determine whether this late rise is due to essential hypertension which antedated pregnancy or to pregnancy hypertension. In the American classification of this condition a rise of blood pressure of 15mm or more during pregnancy is diagnostic, but in the United Kingdom it is generally accepted that the critical level of blood pressure is 90mm mercury diastolic blood pressure irrespective of the amount by

which the blood pressure has risen because proteinuria is very unlikely to appear before the diastolic pressure reaches 90mm mercury. The rise to this level must be maintained or recur in 24 hours however. The 15 point rise in diastolic pressure may however be a useful guide in women with a low normal level.

The severity of the condition is sometimes judged by the level which the blood pressure reaches, but generally in British obstetrics the severity is judged by the presence or degree of proteinuria. A trace of protein is usually ignored. Oedema occurs in 40 per cent of primigravidae, and it is not usually taken into account in the classification of the disease or in judging the severity of the condition.

INCIDENCE OF PRE-ECLAMPSIA

It is very difficult to obtain any precise knowledge of the incidence of the condition in various parts of the world largely due to these problems of definition and the absence of knowledge of the pre-pregnancy or early pregnancy blood pressure. An international survey of the disease was carried out in 1958–59 on primigravidae under the age of 30 from 10 countries (Roulet, 1961). The blood pressure was recorded at the 20th week and again later in pregnancy. The results although not justifying firm conclusions allowed some tentative hypotheses to be made. First that the response of the cardiovascular system to pregnancy does vary from one country to another. Secondly that the extent of the response is unrelated to the initial level of blood pressure, so that presumably the factors responsible for it are by and large different from those that determine the normal level of blood pressure, and thirdly the response has no obvious relation to diet, and in particular to protein content. Countries with a high protein diet in which may be included Switzerland and Australia show small response, whereas Nigeria and Japan where the content of animal protein in the diet is certainly lower show an appreciably greater change. The blood pressure in both early and late pregnancy was higher in Eire and Scotland, and lowest in London, in the more detailed study carried out in the British Isles and Eire. The percentages of primigravidae having a blood pressure of 145/95mm of mercury or more in the second half of pregnancy in Ireland, Scotland and England were 23·5, 18·6 and 17·5 respectively. The percentages developing proteinuria were London 2·9 per cent, rest of

England 3 per cent, Eire 3·5 per cent and Scotland 4·1 per cent. Proteinuria seldom developed until the diastolic pressure rose to 85–90mm of mercury. There were strong indications from Israel, Nigeria and Jamaica that blood pressures there are lower than in Western Europe. Differences have been found in the incidence of pre-eclampsia in various Israeli immigrant and indigenous populations, European or American groups and local inhabitants having an incidence more than twice that of oriental groups. In Trinidad there is a higher incidence of the condition in East Indians than in Negroes, and in Fiji a higher incidence in those of Indian descent than in native Fijians. There are variations not only between different countries but also between the racial groups within a country. The incidence of *eclampsia* also varies throughout the world, but it is almost certainly due to different standards of antenatal care.

One of the most striking features of pre-eclampsia is that it is mainly a disease of primigravidae. This is particularly true of proteinuric pre-eclampsia in which the incidence in second and subsequent pregnancies is about one-fifth of that in first pregnancies. The incidence of mild pre-eclampsia (late hypertension only) is halved in second and subsequent pregnancies. Women who have had a previous abortion of a 12 or more weeks' pregnancy are less liable in their first viable pregnancy to develop pre-eclampsia than in a woman who has not had a previous pregnancy, so that a pregnancy of relatively short duration reduces the chance of developing pre-eclampsia but not to such a degree as a previous full-time pregnancy.

A study by Hall (1967) in Aberdeen showed that there has been a drop in the incidence of pre-eclampsia between 1950 and 1963. The incidence of proteinuric hypertension fell from 6·7 per cent in 1950–53 to 3·7 per cent in 1960–63, although that of mild pre-eclampsia with hypertension alone remained about the same, 21·2 per cent and 19·1 per cent respectively for the two periods. The reduced incidence was not due to a lower weight gain in the later years or to a difference in the gestation at delivery.

WEIGHT AND WEIGHT GAIN
There is a high incidence of low birth weight babies when the maternal weight gain is less than $\frac{3}{4}$ of a pound (0·34kg) per week. On the

other hand when the weight gain is high, i.e. $1\frac{1}{4}$ pounds (0·57kg) per week or more between the 20th and 30th weeks, the incidence of hypertension of pregnancy and proteinuric hypertension is increased (Fig. 10.2). It is

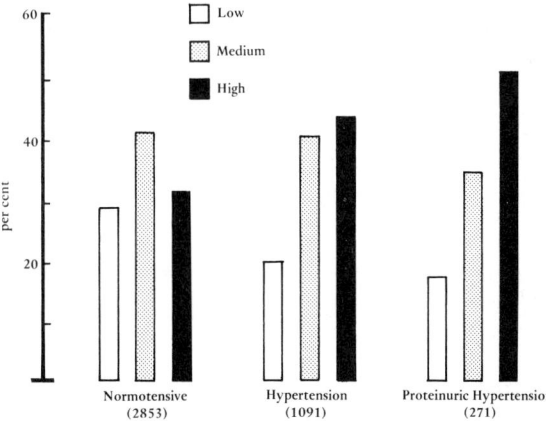

Fig. 10.2   The effect of weight gain on the incidence of hypertension of pregnancy and proteinuric hypertension.

noteworthy too that some women with a low weight gain can develop hypertension and proteinuria in late pregnancy, so that although retention of fluid is associated with pre-eclampsia it is not an essential part of the picture. The higher the weight gain the greater the weight of the baby provided that severe pre-eclampsia does not occur. When the total body water is measured it is found that there is a direct relationship between total body water and the weight of the baby in primigravidae (Duffus, MacGillivray and Dennis, 1970). The total body water is usually increased in pre-eclamptic toxaemia but this depends on whether there is oedema present or not. Similarly the sodium space is increased in pre-eclampsia with oedema, but not if there is no oedema. It seems from this and also from bromide space measurements that neither water retention or sodium retention are essential parts of the pre-eclamptic picture.

OTHER FACTORS INFLUENCING INCIDENCE
Although there have been many suggestions that this condition occurs more frequently in poor socio-economic groups, it seems that the wives of men in the middle social classes have a higher incidence than those of the lower or upper social class (Table 10.1). Cigarette smoking is associated with a lower incidence of proteinuric hypertension (Fig. 10.3). There is a

Table 10.1   The incidence of proteinuric pre-eclampsia by social class
(1723 primigravidae) 1960, 1964

Social class	Incidence of proteinuric pre-eclampsia
I and II	2·4%
III	5·2%
IV and V	3·4%

Table 10.2   City of Aberdeen: Primigravid twin pregnancies
(number of cases in parentheses)

	Monozygotic	Dizygotic
Normotensive	44·3%	52·1%
Late pregnancy hypertension	28·6%	25·2%
Proteinuric hypertension	27·1%	21·1%
	100% (70)	100% (142)

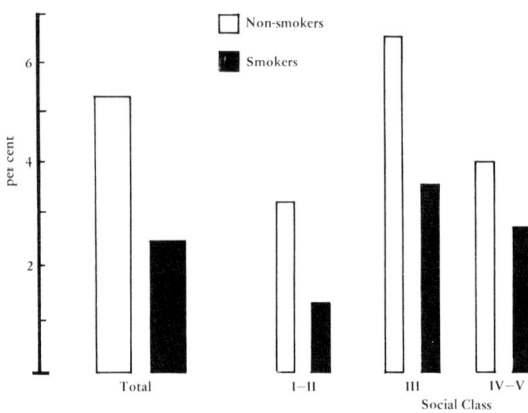

Fig. 10.3   The influence of cigarette smoking and social class on the incidence of proteinuric hypertension.

much higher incidence in twin pregnancies but there is no difference between the incidence in monozygotic and dizygotic twin pregnancies (Table 10.2). The zygosity was determined accurately by blood grouping and enzyme typing. The condition is also more common in conditions with large placentas—the so called hyperplacentosis found in diabetes, hydatidiform mole and hydrops fetalis. There is also a familial tendency to late hypertension (mild pre-eclampsia) and proteinuric hypertension in women whose sisters or mothers have had the condition. In Aberdeen it was found that sisters of primigravidas who developed pre-eclampsia or some degree of hypertension had a higher incidence of pre-eclampsia or hypertension in their first pregnancy than did the sisters of primigravidas who had not suffered from either condition. The

incidence of 'toxaemia' in pregnancy approaches 40 per cent in both the sisters and daughters of women who had eclampsia (Chesley, Cosgrove and Annitto, 1962).

CLINICAL FEATURES

One of the great dangers of this condition is that symptoms do not usually occur until the disease is at an advanced stage. It is essential, therefore, that the blood pressure is checked regularly and more frequently towards the end of pregnancy in primigravidae (see Chapter 16). The urine must also be tested and excessive weight gain and oedema looked for. The symptoms which may occur are headache, which is typically frontal in distribution, visual disturbances, such as dimness of vision, spots floating in front of the eyes, flashes of light and diplopia signify a constriction of the retinal vessels. Opthalmoscopic examination may reveal nipping of the vessels, narrowing, silver wire appearance and in very severe cases haemorrhages and exudates and retinal detachment. In very severe cases blindness, which is fortunately usually temporary, can occur either due to the severe vasoconstriction or to retinal detachment. Vomiting and epigastric pain are also late features and indicate that convulsions are imminent. The epigastric pain is thought to be due to haemorrhage occurring under the capsule of the liver and this may also cause the vomiting, but it might possibly be due to cerebral oedema. As the condition progresses the output of urine is reduced and in very severe cases anuria may develop.

The development of frontal headache, epigastric pain, severe vomiting, visual disturbances or oliguria is of very serious import and can herald the onset of eclampsia.

DIFFERENTIAL DIAGNOSIS

When the blood pressure has been known to be normal in early pregnancy a diagnosis of specific hypertensive disease of pregnancy or mild pre-eclampsia can be made with a fair degree of certainty if the blood pressure rises to 90 diastolic or above and is maintained at this level in the third trimester. Whether this hypertension of pregnancy is a mild form of the condition which is associated with proteinuria in pregnancy, or a manifestation of a latent tendency to essential hypertension is much more difficult to determine, but there is no difference in the management or the treatment of these two causes of hypertension of late pregnancy. If it is not known whether the blood pressure was normal or not in early pregnancy then the hypertension may be due to an essential hypertension, a chronic pyelonephritis, very rarely a renal artery stenosis or a coarctation of the aorta or even a phaeochromocytoma. A coarctation can be detected by palpating the femoral and radial pulses and a phaeochromocytoma may be detected if the blood pressure is very labile and a rise in blood pressure is associated with a severe headache. Estimation of catecholamines may be helpful if a phaeochromocytoma is suspected.

If in addition to the hypertension there is also proteinuria then chronic glomerulonephritis and chronic pyelonephritis might be the cause. If it is due to chronic glomerulonephritis there may be a history of a previous attack of acute nephritis, and the hypertension and proteinuria would be found before 24 weeks. The specific gravity of the urine may be low and haematuria may be present with casts. The blood urea is usually raised more than in severe pre-eclampsia. In chronic pyelonephritis a rather similar picture occurs, but culture of the urine may reveal organisms.

COMPLICATIONS

Eclampsia

With proper antenatal care it is now considered that eclampsia should rarely occur, but occasionally it can occur without severe premonitory symptoms and there may be a very rapid onset of the signs. The convulsions are epileptiform in type. There is usually a premonitory twitching of the face followed by a tonic phase lasting for one or two minutes, and then a clonic phase in which the woman may be very violent and may injure herself. This again lasts for about two minutes and is followed by a phase of coma which can last for some hours, but usually only for a matter of minutes. During the tonic stage the jaws are tightly closed and the tongue may be severely bitten. During the convulsions the breathing is stertorous and the woman becomes cyanosed and her face is congested. The temperature may rise to 104 or 105°F (40 or 41°C), during the attack and this is regarded as a serious sign.

Convulsions can occur either before labour, during labour or up to 48 hours after delivery. There may be only one post-partum convulsion, but in some cases there may be repeated fits with or without brief spells of consciousness between. Rapidly recurring fits are considered to be a poor prognostic sign, but usually nowadays there should be no difficulty in controlling fits with anticonvulsant therapy. Cases have been described in which coma and death have occurred without any preceding convulsions and at post-mortem the organs have shown the characteristic lesions of eclampsia. The presence of the signs of pre-eclampsia usually makes the diagnosis of eclampsia straightforward, but when convulsions occur without hypertension or proteinuria, a simple faint, epilepsy, cerebral-vascular accidents or even amniotic fluid embolism have to be considered.

Placental abruption

This is usually considered to be a complication of pregnancy hypertension, but in many cases it is not known whether the hypertension and proteinuria preceded the abruption of the placenta or not. In most cases the hypertension and proteinuria are noted after the abruption has occurred and it is difficult if not impossible to know if there was a rapid onset of hypertension and proteinuria just prior to the abruption. Occasionally abruption of the placenta may occur during or after eclamptic convulsions. Coagulation failure usually occurs in cases where there is abruption with eclampsia but rarely the failure can occur where there is eclampsia without abruption of the placenta. When eclampsia with antepartum or post-partum haemorrhage occur then there is a serious risk of acute renal failure occurring.

Intra-uterine death of the fetus can occur

due to placental separation or to placental failure.

Retinal detachment

Fortunately this is rare and permanent damage is not usual. Temporary blindness is more commonly due to severe vasoconstriction and oedema, and permanent blindness has usually been ascribed to a lesion in the optic tract or the optic centre in the brain.

Jaundice

This is also a rare complication and indicates severe hepatic involvement.

LATE EFFECTS

The late effects of severe hypertensive disease of pregnancy or of eclampsia seem to be very rare if they occur at all. At one time it was thought that chronic nephritis was a sequel of pre-eclampsia or eclampsia, but it is probable that such cases were in fact due to pre-existing chronic glomerulo-nephritis or pyelonephritis. It seems too that hypertension is not caused by the specific hypertensive disease of pregnancy, but that women who were predisposed to

Chesley (1956) originally taught that prolonged pre-eclampsia often caused chronic hypertension but now believes that pre-eclamptic women who are found to have hypertension at follow up probably had this predisposition before pregnancy.

PROGNOSIS FOR BABY

The perinatal death rate from pre-eclampsia or 'toxaemia' has been presented in 'Perinatal Problems', the second report of the British Perinatal Mortality Survey. The perinatal mortality rate in primigravida was 6·2 for toxaemia. The only other cause which was greater than this was deformities at 6·5 in second pregnancies. The overall 'toxaemia' perinatal mortality rate was 2·2 whereas the deformity perinatal mortality rate was 4·6, and the prematurity perinatal mortality rate was 4·7. The toxaemia perinatal mortality rate was 3·9 in those aged under 20, 3·4 in those aged 20–24, 3·2 in those aged 25–29, 4·4 in those aged 30–34 and 6·9 in those aged 35 and over. Within parity groups the rates rose with age. The perinatal mortality in relation to the amount of proteinuria is shown in Table 10.3.

Table 10.3   Perinatal mortality in relation to the amount of proteinuria

Proteinuria	Perinatal mortality
Nil or trace	23·2%
Under 1g/litre	55·6%
1–2g/litre	75·6%
2g/litre or more	300·2%

hypertension in later life manifest a rise in blood pressure during pregnancy. Those who develop proteinuria as well as hypertension in late pregnancy do not have any more tendency to hypertension in later life than do nulliparous women. (Adams and MacGillivray, 1961.)

There is no correlation between the duration of pre-eclamptic signs and the incidence of residual hypertension in the mother. (Gibson, 1956.) Dieckmann, Smitter and Rynkiewicz (1952) concluded that pre-eclampsia does not produce residual hypertension, but that the 30 per cent of cases who do have an elevated blood pressure in later life represent cases of mild or latent hypertension which have progressed with age to the same extent as they would have done had they not become pregnant. Platt (1958) found in a study of identical twins that the nulliparous twin frequently has the same level of blood pressure as her sister who has had 'toxaemia'.

There is no greater perinatal mortality in those with no proteinuria or a trace than in the normotensives. Perinatal deaths from toxaemia are most difficult to prevent in those cases where the onset of the condition is fulminating and occurs early in the third trimester while the fetus is still small and immature. When proteinuria is present there is frequently growth retardation. In recent years there has been a fall in perinatal mortality from pre-eclampsia probably associated with modern intensive monitoring methods.

PATHOLOGY

Most of the changes which have been described in the organs have been found at post-mortem in women dying of eclampsia, but there is also now information from renal, liver and placental bed biopsies from women with pre-eclampsia or proteinuric hypertension (Robertson, Brosens and Dixon, 1967). The earliest lesion appears to be a fibrinoid necrosis of the arterial walls, and later the damaged vessel is

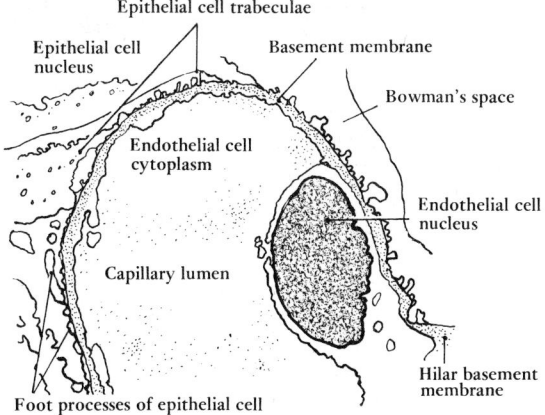

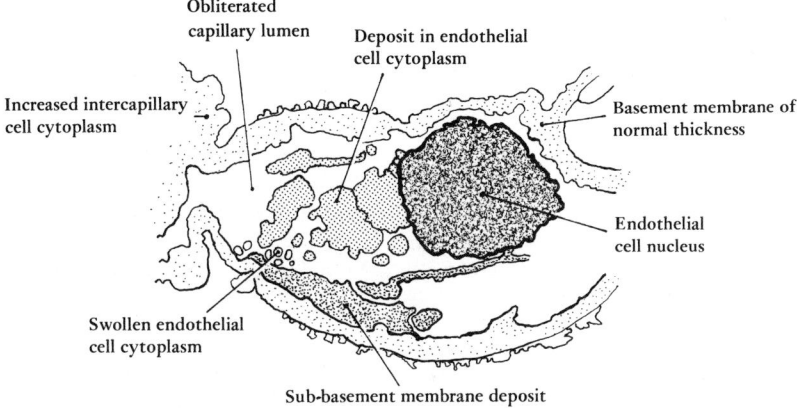

Fig. 10.4A Diagrammatic representation of an electron microscopic picture of the capillary loop of the renal glomerulus showing the protrusion of the endothelial cell nucleus into the wide open capillary lumen. The endothelial cytoplasm is thin and the basement membrane becomes thickened near the hilar area.
B Diagrammatic representation of an electron microscope picture of the capillary loop of the renal glomerulus in pre-eclampsia showing the obliteration of the capillary lumen. There are deposits in the cytoplasm of the swollen endothelial cells and in the sub-basement membrane. The basement membrane is of normal thickness.

infiltrated by lipophages, fibrinoid vasculosis or acute atherosis.

Govan (1961) found changes in fatal eclampsia varying in degree from fibrinoid vasculosis to complete necrosis of the vessels in the brains, livers and kidneys. He considered that the lesions in these organs were of a similar nature and due to a common vascular reaction.

Fibrinoid vasculosis is found in hypertension, hyperergy and vascular stasis. It seems unlikely that there is any excessive allergic reaction in pre-eclampsia. Vascular spasm causing the hypertension could give rise to damage of the vessel walls and this together with the local hypoxia could lead to deposition of fibrin. On the other hand coagulation defects could cause fibrin deposits which in turn would lead to hypertension. The renal glomerular changes found in this condition are unique to the disease on both light and electron microscopy. The

most important feature is the striking swelling of the endothelial cytoplasm of glomerular capillaries (Pollak and Nettles, 1960) (Fig. 10.4). Epithelial cytoplasmic swelling and vacuolation contribute to the narrowing of the capillary lumen. The basement membrane is not significantly thickened or otherwise altered in the great majority of cases, and this disease cannot, therefore, be classified as a type of membranous glomerulo-nephritis.

The causes of these renal changes remain obscure and it is doubtful whether they are primary or secondary to some generalized effect, but the latter is almost certainly the case. The same can be said of the changes in the placental bed, which are the same in pregnancies complicated by essential hypertension, pre-eclampsia or both of these conditions.

Robertson and co-workers (1967) compared the acute atherosis of pre-eclampsia with the renal artery lesions found in rejected human kidney transplants and considered that there was a striking similarity in the patchy fibrinoid necrosis of muscle, the intimal hyperplasia and the infiltrates of lipophages and mononuclear cells. They suggest that there may be an immunological component in the vascular lesions of pre-eclamptic toxaemia because of the morphological similarities of acute atherosis to arterial lesions in other diseases known or suspected to be associated with antigen–antibody reactions. The lesion in the liver is a generalized haemorrhagic necrosis and fibrin can be identified in the liver as well as in the kidneys and lungs of women dying of eclampsia. If the haemorrhages have occurred in the pontine areas this causes a hyperpyrexia. The lungs from fatal cases of eclampsia show oedema and congestion and in some there may be evidence of bronchial pneumonia. Any changes such as dilatation of the left ventricle found in the heart are probably secondary to the lung changes.

In the placenta in pre-eclampsia the Langhan's cells proliferate and show a greater degree of variation in size than in normal and there is degeneration of the syncytium.

Functional pathology

The rise in blood pressure which occurs in toxaemia could be the result of an increase in blood volume or in cardiac output greater than that seen in normal pregnancy or of a higher peripheral vascular resistance or of an increased viscosity of the blood. The cardiac output is either normal or only slightly increased. There is a reduction in plasma volume in severe cases. The viscosity of the blood is not increased. This leaves peripheral vascular resistance as the probable cause of the hypertension. An increase in peripheral resistance in late pregnancy occurs in both pre-eclamptic and hypertensive women, but in pre-eclampsia the vascular resistance returns to normal earlier in the puerperium than in hypertensive subjects (Ginsburg and Duncan, 1967).

Various measurements of blood flows have been made in hypertension of pregnancy, and the conclusions in general are that cerebral, cardiac and hepatic blood flows are normal, *while renal and uterine blood flows are decreased*. It is of interest to note that the same results are found in essential hypertension in pregnancy.

There is a reduced peripheral blood flow in pre-eclampsia and probably this reduction in most cases takes place mainly in the skin, but there is possibly also a decreased muscle blood flow as well (Spetz, 1965).

Clearance studies have definitely established that renal plasma flow and glomerular filtration rate are reduced in pre-eclampsia as compared with a normal pregnancy of the same gestation. There has been a great deal of controversy over the role of salt in pregnancy hypertension. Some workers maintain that sodium retention is an essential feature of the condition (Chesley, 1966), but others maintain that

there is no more retention of sodium and water in the pre-eclamptics without oedema than there is in normal pregnancy (MacGillivray, 1967). It seems then that oedema and water and salt retention are not an essential part of pre-eclampsia.

The water and salt retention which occurs in normal pregnancy is probably due to oestrogens or aldosterone, but both of these are either at normal or below normal levels in pre-eclampsia. The cause of the oedema in pre-eclampsia cannot as yet be satisfactorily explained, but the lowered plasma proteins and increased capillary permeability play a part. Generalized oedema may be due to the binding of water by depolymerized mucopolysaccharides in the skin. There is a marked haemoconcentration in cases of pre-eclampsia and the plasma volume is reduced from around 4000ml to less than 3500ml. There is a fall in the plasma proteins and there is a reduction in the albumin/globulin ratio.

Earlier studies of serum proteins using paper electrophoresis (MacGillivray and Tovey, 1957) showed that in pre-eclampsia there is a further depression in serum albumin and an elevation of the α-2-globulin and β-globulin fractions compared to normal pregnant women. The γ-globulin was decreased. Recent studies using immunoelectrophoresis (Studd, Blainey and Bailey, 1970) showed a decrease in the concentration of serum albumin, transferrin and haemopexin and increased concentrations of α-1-glycoprotein, α-2-macroglobulin and β-lipoprotein in cases of severe pre-eclampsia. These workers considered that the pattern was similar to that found in the nephrotic syndrome. Honger (1967 and 1968) has shown that the intravascular mass of albumin is unchanged in normal pregnancy and that the hypoalbuminaemia is due to haemodilution and to suppression of the synthesis of albumin in the liver by oestrogen. Honger (1968b) claimed that albumin synthesis is significantly greater in pre-eclampsia than in normal pregnancy and that the lower concentration of serum albumin is the result of loss of protein in the urine.

There is a marked increase in uric acid concentration due either to the inability of the kidney to excrete uric acid or to an increased tubular reabsorption. Unlike the kidney, hepatic blood flow is unchanged in pregnancy in spite of the increased cardiac output and blood volume. The liver function tests in pre-eclampsia may show a rise in serum glutamic oxalacetic transaminase and lactic dehydrogenase and impairment of the bromsulphthalein excretion.

AETIOLOGY

It seems that as each new discovery has been made in medicine it has been used to formulate a new theory to explain the cause of eclampsia and pre-eclampsia and various forms of therapy ranging from mastectomy and colonic lavage to antibiotics and hormones have been used. It is only possible to give a very brief outline of some of the more important theories which have been advanced.

Placental

As placental tissue must be present before this disease occurs it is not surprising that the placenta has often been blamed, and it was thought that a toxin was produced from the placenta hence the name toxaemia for this disease. It was also suggested that the infarcts of the placenta were the cause. Infarcts are probably more frequent and extensive in pre-eclampsia but they also occur in normal pregnancies. More recent work has shown that there is no correlation between infarcts and pre-eclampsia, and it is probable that any increase in the incidence of infarction is due to the disease and is not the cause of it. In hydatidiform mole which is associated with a high incidence of pre-eclampsia no typical placental infarcts occur. It was also thought that placental damage caused a fall in monoamine-oxidase which is an inhibitor of sympathomimetic amines and that one of these, in particular, tryptamine was produced in excess and as this is a pressor substance this could account for the disease. It has not been confirmed that tryptamine is found in excess in pre-eclampsia, nor indeed has any pressor substance.

Increased abdominal pressure

This was one of the earliest theories about the aetiology of pre-eclampsia but it has never been found in women with other abdominal tumours.

Renal factors

It was suggested that renin might be the cause but it has been found by Brown and co-workers (1966) that the levels of renin are lower in severe pre-eclampsia than in normal pregnancy.

Sophian (1955) has for many years been the champion of the utero-renal vascular reflex theory which is supposed to be due to overdistension of the uterus. The objection to his theory is that pre-eclampsia and eclampsia can occur in association with extra-uterine pregnancies.

Immune response

The suggestion has been made that there is maternal-fetal incompatability in pre-eclampsia giving rise to an antigen-antibody reaction. The hypothesis postulated by Platt, Stewart and Emery (1958) does not agree fully with immunological principles nor with the natural history of pre-eclampsia.

No satisfactory hypothesis has yet been advanced to explain the immune response and the renal lesions of pre-eclampsia are not associated with the deposition of complement of antigen-antibody complexes. Some workers have demonstrated antibodies against the placenta in greater numbers of women with pre-eclampsia than in normal pregnant women, but this has not been confirmed by other workers. Several workers have suggested that there is evidence of an antigen reaction in pre-eclampsia and have claimed to demonstrate antibodies. The lesions seen in the placental bed are also similar to those that might be found on an immunological basis, but workers who have studied electronmicroscopic sections of the kidneys suggest that the renal lesion is not the same as that found in glomerular nephritis.

Hormonal disturbances

Attempts have been made to show that there is an increased amount of pituitary antidiuretic and vasopressor hormone, but so far the evidence has not been accepted by other workers. The findings of pre-eclampsia in women with diabetes insipidus makes it unlikely that the posterior pituitary is at fault. It has also been suggested that excessive chorionic gonadotrophin caused a hypersensitivity to normal amounts of circulating vasopressor substances. A deficiency of progesterone and oestrogen has been postulated, but there is no evidence to show that this occurs nor that this would cause the syndrome.

Browne (1958) suggested that the hypertrophic anterior pituitary gland produced an excess of corticotrophin which causes an overstimulation of the adrenal cortex. This produces an excess of gluco-and-mineralocorticoids. A Cushingoid syndrome would, therefore, develop in every pregnant woman if the monoaminoxidase from the placenta did not inactivate the adrenal pressor and salt retaining hormones. If there is reduced oxygen tension resulting from uterine ischaemia the placental protective activity decreases. Uterine ischaemia tends to develop when there is overdistension of the uterus as with twin pregnancy and hydramnios, with increased uterine tension as in the primigravida or with constricted blood vessels as in pre-existing hypertension.

Diet

It has been suggested that both excess and deficiencies of diet and of certain articles of diet, particularly, vitamins might be the cause but the World Health Organization Expert Committee (1965) concluded that there seems to be no scientific basis for believing that deficiency or excess of any essential nutrient predisposes to pre-eclampsia and eclampsia.

Salt retention

There has been a great deal of controversy over the role of salt in pre-eclampsia. Some workers maintain that sodium retention is an essential feature of pre-eclampsia (Chesley, 1966; Plentl and Gray, 1959) while others have maintained that there is a greater water than salt retention (MacGillivray and Buchanan, 1958; Davey, O'Sullivan and Browne, 1961). The probable explanation for the different findings is that the results depend on the selection of cases and is dependant on whether the pre-eclamptic patients have oedema or whether the normal control patients have oedema. The adverse effects of sodium chloride was postulated by Harding and Van Wyck (1930) when they caused eclampsia in women with pre-eclampsia by giving intravenous injections of 300ml of a 6 per cent solution of sodium chloride.

This does not prove that ingestion of salt is harmful but probably in women with oliguria it would be prudent not to give too much salt. This in no way suggests, however, that salt retention is the cause of pre-eclampsia.

The possible cause of the sodium retention in pregnancy and in particular in pre-eclampsia could be related to the renin-angiotensin-aldosterone mechanism. In normal pregnancy there are raised levels of renin and aldosterone. It is known that progestational steroids have a natriuretic effect and this might cause the rise in aldosterone excretion because the rate of progesterone excretion is high in normal pregnancy. The urinary excretion is increased when progesterone is given to non-pregnant subjects in doses comparable to the rate of secretion of this hormone in pregnancy (Landau, Bergenstal, Lugibihl and Kascht, 1955). The increased renin levels reported by Brown, Davies, Doak, Lever and Robertson (1963) would initiate this compensatory increase in aldosterone production.

Brown and co-workers (1966) found that renin values for hypertensive pregnant women did not differ markedly from normal pregnant women, but the most severely hypertensive group had a mean renin concentration lower than normotensive pregnant women. The concentration of renin substrate has been found to be lower in pre-eclampsia and this may reduce apparent renal activity. However, the sensitivity to an infusion of angiotensin is greatly increased in pre-eclamptic pregnancies compared with normotensive pregnant women (Talledo, Chesley and Zuspan, 1968), so that it may be that the net effect is greatly increased.

Uteroplacental ischaemia

Bastiaanse and Mastboom (1949) believe that uterine ischaemia with poor intervillous circulation is the cause of pre-eclampsia. They noted that the vascularization of the uterus is much less in a primigravida than in a multigravida which accentuates the ischaemia and which explains the frequency in first pregnancies, but not in subsequent ones, as the improved blood supply remains after pregnancy.

There is an atherosis of the blood vessels of the placental bed and probably a reduction in uterine blood flow, but it is not known whether this is cause or effect.

Browne and Veall (1953) showed with radioactive sodium that the placental blood flow is reduced by more than 50 per cent in pre-eclampsia.

Disorders of blood coagulation

In some fatal cases of eclampsia a widespread fibrin deposition has been a prominent finding. Examination of renal biopsies from cases of pre-eclampsia by immuno-fluorescent techniques has also shown that the material in the glomerular deposits is fibrin. In normal pregnancy there is a trend towards intravascular coagulation and when the homeostatic balance between coagulation and fibrinolytic activity is disturbed, imbalance occurs locally and fibrin is deposited in the placental circulation causing placental ischaemia and insufficiency, and also in the renal vascular system causing proteinuria and hypertension. The eclamptic seizures may be due to microemboli or thrombi composed of platelet aggregates and fibrin temporarily obstructing the cerebral micro-circulation.

The placenta is a very rich source of thromboplastin and it is thought that damage to the trophoblast, possibly the result of ischaemia or hypoxia, might allow the passage of thromboplastin from the placenta into the maternal circulation. There is then a disseminated intravascular coagulation. Mackay, Merrill, Weiner, Hertig and Reid (1953) suggested that thromboplastin liberated from the placenta produced a generalized Schwartzman reaction.

More recently it has been observed that the pulmonary vessels can also be involved in this localized intravascular coagulation process in both pre-eclampsia and eclampsia. It is not yet clear, however, whether the hypertension and vasoconstriction of pre-eclampsia causes placental damage resulting in the release of thromboplastin or whether it is the coagulation process produced by the thromboplastin which gives rise to the hypertension.

Plasminogen activator seems to be the substance which keeps blood vessels free of fibrin deposits and thus allows a free blood flow and to some extent control of the blood pressure. When there is impairment of production of plasminogen activator deposition of fibrin is likely and a compensatory hypertension could develop to overcome the peripheral vascular resistance caused by the intravascular fibrin. Significantly higher levels of fibrin breakdown products were found in cases of severe pre-eclampsia than in normal pregnancy and following eclamptic seizures the level of the breakdown products sharply increased (Bonnar, MacNicol and Douglas, 1971).

Pressor substances

Monoamine oxidase catalyses the oxidative deamination of many sympathomimetic amines (e.g. adrenaline oxytyramine and tyramine) and thereby abolishes their vasopressor effect. If there was a deficiency of monoamine oxidase this would allow a build up of amines, in particular, 5-hydroxytryptamine which would cause vasoconstriction of the blood vessels of the placenta. Several workers have found that monoamine oxidase is deficient in toxaemic placentas, but the blood levels of 5-hydroxytryptamine were not significantly different between pre-eclamptics and normals (Senior, Fahim, Sullivan and Robson, 1963). This has been confirmed by Krupp and Krupp (1960). In spite of prolonged searching by many workers for a toxic or pressor substance in pre-eclampsia none have yet been identified.

Vascular hypersensitivity

Although no excess of pressor substance has yet been

identified in pre-eclampsia an increased sensitivity has been demonstrated in pre-eclamptic women to noradrenaline, adrenaline, vasopressin and angiotensin compared to normal pregnancy. Apart from the fact that no one has with certainty identified an excess of pressor substance the experiments of Page (1938) seem to exclude the possibility of an excess of pressor substance. He transfused 400ml of blood from patients with eclampsia or severe pre-eclampsia into normal pregnant women without causing any increase in blood pressure. It is unlikely that anyone would be willing to repeat such experiments nowadays on ethical grounds but in the study of Tatum and Mule (1962) patients were retransfused in the puerperium with their own blood, which had been collected while they had severe pre-eclampsia and a transient but significant increase both in systolic and diastolic pressure was produced. We (Pirani and MacGillivray, 1973) have confirmed this work but instead of using whole blood the serum from patients was taken and stored while they had severe pre-

eclampsia and the red cells were replaced. Either the patients have in their blood a pressor substance which causes a rise in the puerperium, but this was not found in normal pregnant women after they were delivered, or alternatively these pre-eclamptic women have a hypersensitivity to normal amounts of circulating pressor substances. If Page's work is correct and can be taken as indicative of an absence of any excess of pressor substance then this experiment is suggestive of hypersensitivity as the cause. The fact that the babies of mothers who have had pre-eclampsia do not show any rise in blood pressure indicates that any pressor substance does not pass through the placenta, or that the baby's cardiovascular system is not sensitized to pressor substances.

When a ganglion blocking agent is injected into normal pregnant women there is a fall in blood pressure probably because the autonomic nervous system is correcting the effect of a vasodilator substance. When it is injected into patients with

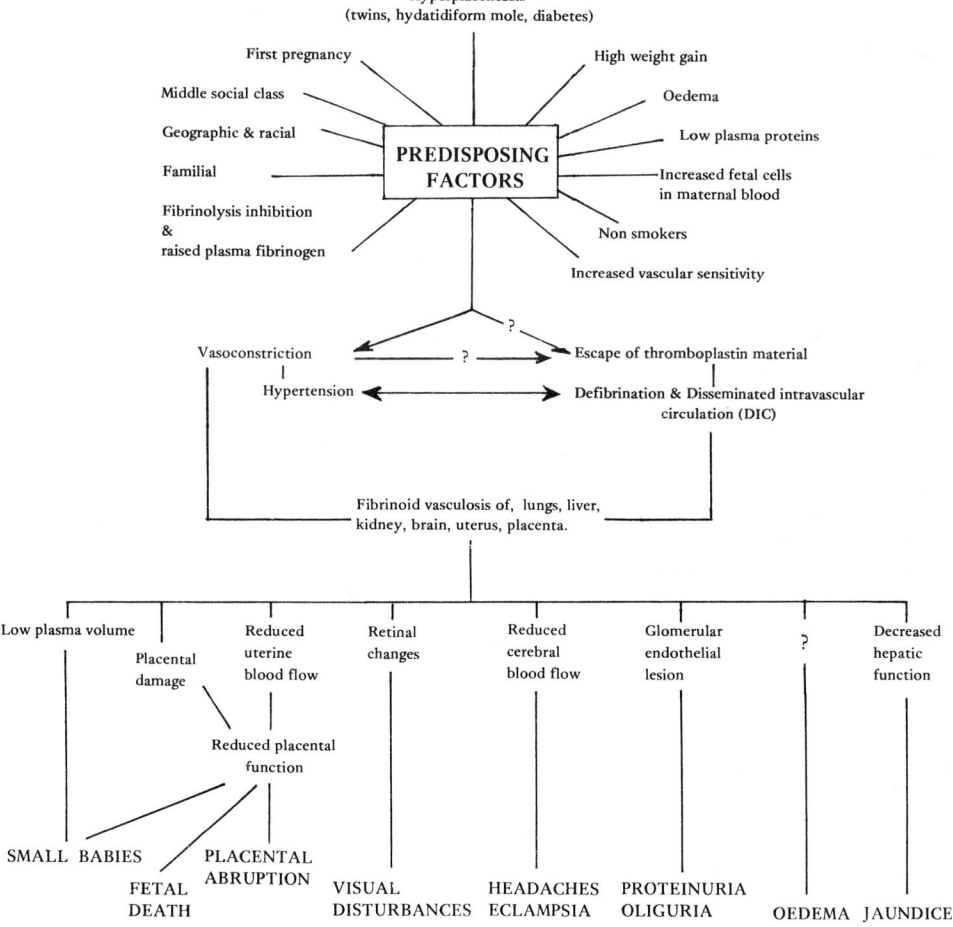

Fig. 10.5   A schematic representation of the factors which predispose to the development of pre-eclampsia and the mechanism of the production of pre-eclampsia.

pre-eclampsia there is very little effect suggesting that there is a lack of vasodilator substance in this condition.

The factors predisposing to the development of pre-eclampsia and the mechanism of production of the lesions are summarized in figure 10.5.

Methods of therapy in hypertension of pregnancy

The best treatment would be prevention, but as we do not know the cause we therefore do not know how to prevent this condition. The next best line, therefore, is early detection of the condition and this requires careful observation of the weight gain, the early detection of oedema, careful recording of the blood pressure and testing of urine for protein. In early cases when there is high weight gain the patient should be seen frequently, so that any rise in blood pressure can be detected. The same applies to women with oedema. Various tests such as the cold pressor test and the flicker fusion test have been tried to detect the very early changes of pre-eclampsia, but they have not been found to be of practical value.

Bed rest
Bed rest is probably one of the most effective methods of treating the condition, although we do not know exactly how it is effective. It has been shown by Morris, Osborne, Payling-Wright and Hart (1965) that bed rest increases the placental blood flow. It also reduces the venous pressure in the lower extremities and allows a reabsorption of a considerable quantity of fluid from these areas.

Salt restriction and Diuretics
A normal pregnant woman when given a water loading test will excrete 100 per cent of the test dose in three hours provided she lies on her side. The percentage output falls to about 30 per cent when the patient is in the dorsal position, and to 30 per cent or less if she stands or moves about. In a pre-eclamptic subject the output of water is reduced to 20 per cent if the test dose is done in the supine position, but with the patient lying on her side it may increase above 50 per cent (Govan, 1962). The amount of salt in an ordinary diet has no effect on the clinical course of pre-eclamptic patients (Bower, 1964; Mengert and Tacchi, 1961). Diuretics may be used to increase the disappearance of oedema but there is some evidence to indicate that they decrease placen-

tal function (Gant, 1973). Thiazides do not significantly lower the blood pressure in toxaemia (MacGillivray et al., 1962; Menzies, 1964) and have indeed proved dangerous by induction of severe hyponatraemia (Brewer, 1962).

A double blind investigation on the continuous prophylactic use of Hydrochlorothiazide, 50mg daily, in 1030 obstetrical patients was carried out by Kraus, Marchise and Yen (1966). They demonstrated that there was no alteration in the incidence of pre-eclampsia, hypertension, prematurity, congenital anomalies or perinatal mortality.

A rise in blood urea and uric acid can be produced by the excessive use of thiazide diuretics and hyperglycaemia and glycosuria in diabetic or pre-diabetic patients may be aggravated.

Some obstetricians advocate the use of a low calorie diet or diuretics to prevent or to treat pre-eclampsia but a recent controlled trial (Campbell and MacGillivray, 1973) has shown that there is no difference in the incidence of proteinuric pre-eclampsia in primigravidae given a thiazide diuretic or a low calorie diet compared with matched controls but the weight of the babies were reduced. There is *no evidence to suggest that diuretics or diets reduced the incidence of pre-eclampsia or improve the condition once it is established.*

Sedation
Magnesium sulphate was popular as part of the Stroganoff treatment which originated from Russia in the early part of the century and its use has continued mainly in North America, in the treatment of eclamptic convulsions or as a sedative in the severe form of pre-convulsive state. Large doses of magnesium sulphate may produce depression of the vital centres. The margin of safety is less than that of barbiturates or Paraldehyde and its use has largely been replaced by barbiturates even in North America.

The so-called 'lytic cocktail' was extensively used in the treatment of eclampsia by Menon (1961) in Madras. The cocktail is composed of 25mg of Chlorpromazine, 100mg of Pethidine and 50mg of Promethazine. Although it is a good anticonvulsant respiratory depression is liable to occur in the babies.

At one time *Morphia* was used extensively in the treatment of fulminating pre-eclampsia and eclampsia, but its use is now considered to be for first aid measure only. *Amylobarbitone Sodium (Sodium Amytal)* is a popular sedative and anticonvulsant. It is usually given in a dose of 200mg nightly or four- to six-hourly depending on the severity of the condition. *Paraldehyde* is still popular in some places but it is usually given rectally and is not a very efficient anticonvulsant. *Diazepam* (Valium) is an efficient anticonvulsant and has some hypotensive effect, particularly if used with Phenobarbitone, but overdosage is relatively easy and respiratory depression may be encountered particularly if the Diazepam is given in conjunction with barbiturates. It is given in an initial dose of 20mg intravenously and a further four injections of 20mg are given intramuscularly over a period of four to six hours. Alternatively an intravenous infusion can be used.

Chlormethiazole (Heminevrin) given in a strength of 0·8 per cent as a continuous intravenous infusion is a very useful anticonvulsant. Initially it is administered at 60 drops a minute for five to ten minutes until the patient is well under sedation. The drip is then maintained at 15 drops a minute, but it is increased if the patient becomes restless and is reduced if she is too well under sedation. The patient sleeps quite soundly but is easily roused and remains rational and co-operative. The perinatal mortality with Chlormethiazole was only half that found with Bromethol or Paraldehyde (Duffus, Tunstall and MacGillivray, 1968). Epidural anaesthesia can be used in conjunction with sedatives when the patient is in labour.

Hypotensive therapy
Hypotensive therapy is useful only in severe pre-eclampsia to control the blood pressure while labour is being induced and during the course of labour and in the early post-partum period. There is no evidence that hypotensive therapy reduces the perinatal mortality. Some believe that hypotensive therapy should be used in the treatment of pre-eclampsia, but it is important to remember that there is no evidence that there is any improvement in uterine blood flow, that although the blood pressure is reduced the amount of protein in the urine is not decreased. There is a danger that the fall in blood pressure may be taken as an indication of improvement in the pre-eclamptic condition and that the pregnancy may be continued for an unduly long time. In the acute treatment of hypertension in

severe pre-eclampsia or eclampsia an intravenous infusion is necessary. A drug commonly used is *Puroverine*. This is given at a rate of 40 drops/minute of a solution of 1mg of Puroverine in 5 per cent glucose solution until the blood pressure starts to fall. It is preferable, if possible, to administer the Puroverine through a slow infusion pump. Puroverine which is an alkaloid of Veratrum Viride can cause bradycardia. In such cases the dosage is reduced.

Hydrallazine (Apresoline) produces its hypertensive effect by acting directly on the wall of the blood vessel and acts best with the patient lying flat in bed. The initial intravenous dose is 20mg given intravenously. Tachycardia which is one of the side effects can be controlled by giving Practolol. The Hydrallazine can be given by a slow infusion pump delivering a solution containing 400mg of Hydrallazine in 300ml of 5 per cent dextrose. The rate is regulated so that 20mg of Apresoline are delivered in 20 minutes initially, and then the rate is slowed to maintain the blood pressure at the required level. If the maternal pulse rate rises to 120 beats/minute, 5mg of Practolol (Eraldin) are given by slow intravenous injection. This can be repeated up to a total of 20mg.

Methyldopa (Aldomet) in an infusion containing 1mg in 100ml of 5 per cent dextrose is given over a period of about an hour to achieve the reduction in the blood pressure required and a maintenance dose can be continued thereafter. There is no place for oral hypotensive agents in the treatment of pre-eclampsia, because by the time there is an efficient hypotensive effect the condition has usually progressed so far that termination of the pregnancy has to be considered. If the condition is less severe there is probably no need for hypotensive therapy anyway, and the use of sedatives is sufficient.

Anticoagulant therapy
As disseminated intravascular coagulation is thought to occur commonly in pre-eclampsia there have been several attempts to treat the condition with heparin. Although some have claimed successes others have not been able to show any benefit in cases of pre-eclampsia. Anticoagulant therapy with heparin is used in the treatment of micrangiopathic anaemia which is a rare complication of severe pre-eclampsia.

In an effort to raise the plasma osmotic pressure various substances such as Dextran, Sucrose or plasma have been administered. These diffuse through the capillary walls less readily than glucose, but only the larger Dextran molecules stay in the plasma for any length of time. When the plasma osmotic pressure increases, there is a reduction in glomerular filtration so that this tends to inhibit the loss of the oedema fluid. It is doubtful if such measures to increase the osmotic pressure are of practical value, but it may be that Dextran could be beneficial, not only by causing a diuresis, but also by tending to prevent intravascular coagulation.

MANAGEMENT ROUTINES

Antenatal care

A large part of antenatal care is concerned with the early detection of pre-eclampsia (Chapter 16). The routine taking of blood pressure, recording of weight gain, testing of the urine for protein and inspection for evidence of oedema are all part of this early detection. The weight gain, of course, may be below average in which case the condition which must be suspected is retarded intra-uterine growth of the fetus, but where the weight gain is considered to be excessive, that is more than $1\frac{1}{4}$lb (0·57kg) per week, then it must be considered that the patient is at risk of developing pre-eclampsia. Similarly if oedema is detected, this also indicates a potential tendency to the development of pre-eclampsia. Oedema is looked for in the feet, in front of the tibia, in the sacral region, abdominal wall, fingers and the face. If oedema of the fingers develops the rings become tight.

It is not necessary to undertake any active treatment if there is oedema or high weight gain except that in general terms it is preferable that a woman should not deposit too much additional fat early in pregnancy. As diuretics do not reduce the chance of pre-eclampsia developing there is no advantage in putting these women on to a reduced salt intake. At each attendance at the clinic the woman should be asked about her symptoms and in particular about headache or visual disturbances. It is essential that women with a high weight gain or oedema should be seen frequently as they are at somewhat greater risk of developing hypertension and proteinuria, particularly in a first pregnancy. If the blood pressure is found to be raised to a diastolic pressure of 90 or more after rest she should be admitted to

hospital. This should also happen if there is protein in more than trace amounts in a midstream specimen of urine. If the blood pressure is just below 90mm or falls below 90mm on resting the patient should be asked to rest at home, mild evening sedation should be prescribed, e.g. Sodium Amytal, 200mg, and to return to the antenatal clinic in a few days' time, when the blood pressure can be checked again after resting.

On admission to hospital a careful assessment is made of the patient, and in all but the mildest cases the urinary output is charted. The blood pressure is recorded twice daily and the patient is weighed daily. Where more than a small amount of protein is present, the amount in 24-hour specimens of urine is estimated by the Biuret method or the Esbach method, although this is not so accurate. Blood may be taken for estimation of sodium, potassium, urea and plasma proteins. If the facilities are available estimations are made of plasma or urinary oestriol, human placental lactogen, heat stable alkaline phosphatase or other indicators of the fetal and placental functions. The rate of growth of the fetus is estimated by ultrasonic measurement of the biparietal diameter. If the condition is mild the only treatment required is bed rest and mild sedation with either Amylobarbitone Sodium (Sodium Amytal), 60mg, Chlormethiazole (Heminevrin), 500mg, or Diazepam (Valium), 5mg, eight-hourly. In most cases, particularly if the blood pressure has risen late in pregnancy there will be a fall in the blood pressure soon after admission to hospital. The patient may then be gradually mobilized and after she has been ambulant for a day she may be allowed home to attend the antenatal clinic as an outpatient provided tests of fetal growth and placental function are satisfactory.

If the blood pressure remains up and particularly if proteinuria is present the patient must stay in hospital and the sedation may have to be increased. She may be allowed up to the toilet but otherwise bed rest should be complete. The progress of the mother and the fetus must be monitored carefully.

The main problem is to decide when the baby should be delivered. If the condition has come on early and is progressing rapidly, heavy sedation is required and this may have to be given intravenously. The treatment is then very similar to that for eclampsia (*see* page 188). A decision has to be made on whether there is a continuing growth of the fetus or whether growth has ceased and that further continuation of the pregnancy will only hazard the fetus and the mother. If the condition is severe at about 30 weeks it is unlikely that it will be possible or desirable to try to continue the pregnancy beyond 34 weeks unless there is clear evidence from the fetal monitoring that the feto-placental unit is not being unduly depressed. If the condition is very severe before 30 weeks then it will be, in general, hopeless to carry on the pregnancy, but it is worth trying heavy sedation and bed rest for a day or two to see if there is any response, because otherwise labour has to be induced or even a Caesarean section performed with very little hope of producing a baby which will survive.

The mother's condition has also to be watched carefully and if there is any evidence that there is impending renal failure as evidenced by a falling urinary output, and increasing proteinuria then this indicates that the pregnancy should be terminated. If the pregnancy is carried on too long then the fetus is at considerable risk and death *in utero* will occur. When this does occur the blood pressure will gradually fall and the oedema, if it is present, will disappear and the proteinuria

will also diminish. There will be, in other words, a general improvement in the patient's condition. Once the decision has been made that there is nothing more to be achieved and that there is an imminent risk of the baby dying *in utero*, or alternatively that the pregnancy has continued sufficiently near to term to give the baby a good chance of survival a decision is made to terminate the pregnancy. In some cases it may be helpful to estimate the chance of fetal survival by examination of the liquor (*see* Chapter 18). A decision is then made regarding the type of delivery.

When labour is induced the severe pre-eclamptic patient delivers rather readily as it is known that there is increased uterine activity in the toxaemic patient (Cobo, 1964). If it is anticipated that labour might be prolonged because of uterine dysfunction or fetal malposition or if after a short trial a rapid easy labour is not occurring, Caesarean section should be performed. Monitoring of those high risk babies is essential in labour as described in Chapter 19 (the management is summarized in Table 10.4).

Management of eclampsia
Eclampsia may occur in the patient's home but it is more likely nowadays that it will occur

Table 10.4 Management of pre-eclampsia

At Antenatal Clinic	BP ≥ 90mmHg	– Either admit to hospital or rest at home and see in three or four days. Give sedative. Advise to contact doctor immediately if symptoms develop.
	Weight gain	– ≥ 1·25 lb (0·57kg) per week—see weekly to check BP. Do *not* give diuretic.
	Oedema	– See weekly to check BP—do *not* give diuretic.
	Proteinuria	– ≥0·25gm/litre—ADMIT FORTHWITH.

IN HOSPITAL	Bed rest and sedation. High protein diet. CHART – Weight; BP; oedema; fluid intake; urinary output: Protein in 24 hours' urine, plasma electrolytes, urea, proteins. MONITOR FETO-PLACENTAL FUNCTION BY ALL AVAILABLE MEANS.
	EARLY MILD CASE <37 weeks: nil or trace proteinuria — If BP returns to normal allow home and see frequently at clinic thereafter. If BP static observe in hospital. If BP rises and proteinuria develops treat as EARLY SEVERE.
	EARLY SEVERE CASE <37 weeks: 0·25gm protein per litre urine — INTENSIVE CARE. If there is deterioration as signified by clinical condition and feto-placental function tests then deliver but continue to 34 weeks if possible. Estimate Lecithin/Sphingomyelin ratio in liquor and ? give betamethasone before delivery. If there is rapid deterioration treat as eclampsia.
	LATE MILD CASE ≥37 weeks: no proteinuria — If BP returns to normal allow home and see twice weekly at clinic. If BP static induce labour at term. If proteinuria develops induce labour.
	LATE SEVERE CASE ≥37 weeks: significant proteinuria — If condition does not improve after a few days' treatment induce labour or deliver by Caesarean Section.

when she is in a maternity hospital and in such circumstances she should be nursed in the intensive care area of the hospital. Should convulsions occur outside of hospital adequate sedation must be given before she is transferred. The maternity emergency service or 'Flying Squad' must be summonsed and a suitable form of sedation given, usually intravenously before the patient is transferred.

Many sedatives have been used in the treatment of severe pre-eclampsia and eclampsia. The best sedative would be one which would effectively control the convulsions without depressing the respirations of the baby when it was born and it should also be easy to administer. As a first aid measure in the patient's home morphine sulphate grain 15 intravenously is very useful but it is preferable to use one of the anticonvulsants in common use described on page 184. During transfer oxygen should be given and an adequate airway must be maintained.

The routine care is that for any patient under heavy sedation. She should be moved from one side to the other about every two hours. In an emergency situation oxygen should be forced in by squeezing the re-breathing bag. A suitable rubber gag should be available and should be inserted between the teeth to prevent the patient biting her tongue. *It is preferable not to darken the room as it is important that the patient's colour should be observed closely so that any evidence of cyanosis can be detected early.* The sedation should be sufficient to prevent any stimulation from light but excessive noise is best avoided. The patient should be protected from injuring herself during a convulsion. Such patients are liable to fall out of bed or to strike their heads against the bed, and therefore may require to be restrained. After suitable sedation has been given a catheter should be passed and left in the bladder.

An alternative or an adjuvant to the use of sedatives are the hypotensive drugs. Puroverine or hydrallizine (Apresoline) can be given as an intravenous infusion to control the blood pressure, for example, *puroverine and chlormethiazole* or *hydrallizine and diazepam* are quite often used together. In addition, epidural anaesthesia is particularly useful when the patient is in labour. Often only one convulsion occurs and the condition is rapidly brought under control by using intravenous therapy. There are occasional

cases where several convulsions occur, but these can usually be brought under control by increasing the intravenous sedation and also using an antihypertensive drug. Occasionally the patient may need to be curarized and treated by intensive respiratory support therapy. Once the convulsions are under control labour is induced if the patient is not already in labour or delivered. This is done by artificial rupture of the membranes combined with syntocinon infusion. If it is antici-pated that

ERRATUM

On page 188, seventeen lines down in the left-hand column, "grain 15" should read "15 mg".

difficult l section is c that ergon delivery of or eclamps pressure. T creased or an intramuscular injection of syntocinon can be given if no infusion is being given. It has been observed that the uterus in eclampsia or severe pre-eclampsia is more active and sensitive to oxytocin.

After delivery it is essential that adequate sedation is maintained as many convulsions occur post-partum. Post-partum eclampsia can occur up to 48 hours after delivery, but there are other cases where convulsions occur later than this without any other explanation and these usually have to be considered as cases of eclampsia after all other causes have been excluded. Intravenous therapy should be continued and thereafter sedation is maintained with oral dosage. A diuresis occurs spontaneously usually about 48 hours after delivery, but this may require to be stimulated by giving a mannitol infusion. The protein gradually disappears from the urine but it usually takes several days or even weeks before the blood pressure returns to normal levels.

The patient is seen for follow-up six weeks after delivery and the blood pressure and urine are checked. If there is residual hypertension and particularly if there is proteinuria, full renal investigations are carried out. It is usually considered that pre-eclampsia does not cause permanent renal damage and if any lesion is found it is more likely to have been a pre-existing condition. If the blood pressure has returned to normal the patient can be reassured that she is unlikely to have recurrence of pre-eclampsia in a subsequent pregnancy. If she is put on to an oral contraceptive, particular attention should be paid to monitoring the blood pressure.

ESSENTIAL HYPERTENSION IN PREGNANCY

As already indicated many of the women developing hypertension in late pregnancy are probably revealing a latent tendency to essential hypertension and it is very difficult, if not impossible to differentiate between essential hypertension and hypertension of pregnancy. There is usually a strong family history of hypertension amongst relatives and hypertension in late pregnancy is frequently found among the sisters of women who developed a raised blood pressure in late pregnancy without proteinuria. These women are also very liable to develop hypertension in later life. Although it is usually stated that essential hypertension is uncommon under the age of 30 it is probable that the latent hypertension is revealed by pregnancy at a much earlier age. Severe essential hypertension, however, is uncommon under the age of 30 even in pregnant women.

If the blood pressure is noted to be raised before the third trimester it is probable that the patient is suffering from essential hypertension and should be treated accordingly. It has to be remembered too that the blood pressure falls in the first and second trimesters of pregnancy, so that a diastolic pressure above 80mm of mercury in the early weeks of pregnancy is suspicious if not diagnostic of essential hypertension. Many of the women who have essential hypertension at the beginning of pregnancy have a further rise in pressure in the third trimester and about half of these will also develop proteinuria. *This is considered to be a superimposed pre-eclampsia.*

The incidence of proteinuric pre-eclampsia in primigravida was found to be 9 per cent in women with a blood pressure of 80mm or more at the 20th week of pregnancy compared to 3 per cent in women with blood pressure below this level (MacGillivray, 1961).

The risk to the baby is always considered to be greater in women with essential hypertension. This is largely due to the development of superimposed pre-eclampsia. The proteinuria is probably the best guide to the fetal prognosis and there is little greater risk to the baby of the mother who had hypertension only, unless the pressure is very high. The prognosis for the mother is dependant on the severity of the hypertension and the duration of the hypertension. There is no evidence that any permanent deterioration occurs in the essential hypertension following pregnancy, but if there is superimposed pre-eclampsia the essential hypertension tends to worsen. Occasionally malignant hypertension develops on an essential hypertension during pregnancy with the development of headache, papilloedema and albuminuria. This, of course, is very difficult to distinguish from proteinuric pre-eclampsia.

Treatment

If the condition is severe and of long standing then termination of pregnancy must be considered, but the decision must be balanced against the number of children the woman has had. If it is her first pregnancy and she is very anxious to have the baby then the risks have to be explained to the mother and rest and therapy are carried out during the pregnancy to try to achieve a live birth without unduly endangering the mother. Modern hypotensive therapy can be helpful but if there is severe long standing hypertension the risks of severe pre-eclampsia and of cerebral haemorrhage and heart failure during pregnancy are still considerable. It is sufficient in mild cases of essential hypertension to advise rest and she should be seen frequently to determine whether the blood pressure is rising and whether albuminuria is developing. If the hypertension is more severe the patient is put on to a hypotensive agent, for example Methyldopa, 250mg tds with an increase by 250mg every third or fourth day until a satisfactory level of blood pressure is achieved. Another commonly used hypotensive drug is Reserpine in a dose of 0·25mg bd but this may cause depression in the mother.

Results of hypotensive therapy for essential hypertension in pregnancy have not proved to be very encouraging so far as the fetal survival rate is concerned, but no large series of cases with a controlled study have so far been reported. A group of 32 women with severe hypertension in early pregnancy treated with Methyldopa had a perinatal mortality of 9·3 per cent (Kincaid-Smith, 1966). In two of the three cases with perinatal deaths proteinuria developed before the 30th week. Townsend (1958) found a perinatal mortality of 16 per cent when mothers had an initial diastolic pressure of 110mm Hg and this rose to 50 per cent when proteinuria occurred.

RENAL DISEASE AND HYPERTENSION

In this chapter the conditions which will be considered are proteinuria in early pregnancy, proteinuria in later pregnancy, Bright's disease, acute nephritis, polyarteritis, systemic lupus erythematosus, nephrotic nephritis, chronic nephritis, polycystic disease of the kidneys, renal tuberculosis and chronic pyelonephritis.

ACUTE GLOMERULO NEPHRITIS

This is a condition found mostly in children and adolescents so that it is rarely seen in pregnancy.

Oedema, hypertension and albuminuria occur but in addition there is loin pain and haematuria. The condition should be readily differentiated from pre-eclampsia because of the many casts and red cells in the urine. If the condition is treated promptly the oedema subsides quite quickly and the pregnancy is not likely to be interfered with. If, however, treatment is delayed the blood pressure will tend to rise and there is a risk of intra-uterine death of the fetus or abortion. In very severe cases patients do not respond to treatment and die of renal failure. The treatment of acute nephritis is with Penicillin for the infection and fluids only in limited amounts until a diuresis begins and the blood pressure falls. Should the condition not respond to this treatment termination of pregnancy is usually indicated and the treatment for acute renal failure initiated.

SYSTEMIC LUPUS ERYTHEMATOSUS

This relatively rare auto immune disease occurs most commonly in the childbearing years. There are periods of remission during the disease, and it is thought that pregnancy does not alter the course of the disease in the majority of patients. There is usually proteinuria, haematuria and oedema present and in addition many generalized manifestations such as joint pains, pleurisy and pericarditis. Active disease may be exacerbated by pregnancy. The treatment of the condition is with corticosteroids but the abortion rate and still-birth rates are still high. Babies are not affected by the disease when they are born alive.

POLYARTERITIS NODOSA

This condition very rarely complicates pregnancy. It is another collagen disease and is treated with cortisone, but the prognosis for the mother is poor. In addition to the renal manifestation and hypertension there are gastro-intestinal, neurological and joint disturbances.

NEPHROTIC NEPHRITIS

This is a rare condition in pregnancy and there is usually no hypertension. There is, however, marked oedema and proteinuria and the plasma proteins fall markedly. A similar picture is produced by other disorders such as diabetes, renal vein thrombosis, systemic lupus erythematosus and malaria (Marcus, 1963). The prognosis for the mother and baby is good in this condition but the baby may be poorly grown.

Treatment is by giving a high protein diet and a thiazide diuretic. Alternatively diuresis may be obtained in such cases by giving Spironolactone, 25mg four times a day. This blocks the increased secretion of aldosterone which occurs in the nephrotic system. There is a serious risk of thrombo-embolism and infection if cortisone is used in therapy.

CHRONIC NEPHRITIS

Probably this occurs less commonly in pregnancy than has been suggested and many of the cases diagnosed as chronic Bright's disease have been due to chronic pyelonephritis. The diagnosis is difficult to make without renal biopsy which is in general contraindicated during pregnancy. A large number of granular and cellular casts are found in the urine of patients with chronic nephritis and a past history of haematuria or oedema may be present. It is often impossible without renal biopsy to tell whether the condition is chronic Bright's disease, chronic pyelonephritis or pre-eclampsia. However, if chronic nephritis is associated with proteinuria and urinary casts and is found in early pregnancy without hypertension the diagnosis is clear. In such cases the outlook for the pregnancy is good. The condition does not seem to be adversely affected by pregnancy provided that pre-eclampsia does not occur. If there is hypertension present as well in early pregnancy then the prognosis is much worse. Abortion and abruption of the placenta are likely to occur. Superimposed pre-eclampsia is common and a fetal mortality between 30 and 40 per cent is to be expected.

If there is proteinuria alone and hypertension does not supervene then the management of pregnancy differs little from normal apart from closer observation. If there is hypertension as well as albuminuria the renal function should be assessed as carefully as possible and termination of pregnancy might be necessary, but in women who have insisted on continuing with the pregnancy with marked hypertension and proteinuria a few have been able to produce live babies. Anaemia is common in cases of chronic nephritis and has to be treated sometimes with transfusion of packed cells. The management in the later weeks of pregnancy is similar to that for severe pre-eclampsia.

POLYCYSTIC DISEASE OF THE KIDNEYS

This is rarely found in pregnancy. It is a strongly hereditary disease. If renal failure has not developed then the condition has little effect on the course of the pregnancy. If hypertension is present the prognosis is worsened, particularly if the blood urea is raised. The outlook for both mother and baby becomes much more serious and termination of the pregnancy should be performed. The diagnosis is made on the basis of the enlargement of one or both kidneys, the family history and the recurrent proteinuria and haematuria.

PROTEINURIA IN EARLY PREGNANCY

This should be investigated by taking a careful history, both obstetrical, medical and family. The presence of postural or orthostatic proteinuria should be excluded by testing the first specimen passed in the morning. If this is free of protein the condition may be orthostatic. A mid-stream specimen of urine should be examined for casts and red cells and also cultured for organisms. Three early morning specimens of urine should be cultured to exclude the possibility of tuberculosis. A simple urine concentration test should be carried out. The specific gravity of the first morning specimen or urine is tested after the patient has had no fluids from the previous evening. If the specific gravity is greater than 1024 this indicates good renal function. If the concentration is less than this then blood urea and inulin clearance should be performed. A creatinine clearance test is less reliable than the inulin clearance.

If the proteinuria develops in later pregnancy the same careful elimination of other causes such as anaemia, contamination of the urine and posture should be excluded. Generally speaking it is not possible to differentiate between cases developing proteinuria in late pregnancy and it is necessary to wait until after the baby is delivered before full investigations can be carried out. It is sometimes helpful to estimate the uric acid in the blood as the levels are raised in pre-eclampsia but not in essential hypertension.

REFERENCES

Adams, E. M. & MacGillivray, I. (1961) Long term effect of pre-eclampsia on blood pressure. *Lancet*, **ii**, 1373.

Bastiannse, M. A. & Mastboom, J. L. (1949) Etiology of eclampsia. *Belg. Tijdschr. Geneesk.*, **5**, 637.

Bonnar, J., McNicol, G. P. & Douglas, A. S. (1971) Coagulation and Fibrinolytic Systems in Pre-eclampsia and Eclampsia. *Brit. med. J.*, **ii**, 12.

Bower, D. (1964) The influence of dietary salt intake on pre-eclampsia. *J. Obstet. Gynaec. Brit. Cwlth.*, **71**, 12.

Brown, J. J., Davies, D. L., Doak, P. B., Lever, A. F. & Robertson, J. I. S. (1963) Plasma renin in normal pregnancy. *Lancet*, **ii**, 900.

Brown, J. J., Davies, D. L., Doak, P. B., Lever, A. F. & Robertson, J. I. S. (1966) Plasma renin concentration in the hypertensive diseases of pregnancy. *J. Obstet. Gynaec. Brit. Cwlth.*, **73**, 410.

Browne, F. J. (1958) Etiology of pre-eclamptic toxaemia and eclampsia. Fact and theory. *Lancet*, **i**, 115.

Browne, J. C. M. & Veall, N. (1953) The maternal placental blood flow in normotensive and hypertensive women. *J. Obstet. Gynaec. Brit. Emp.*, **60**, 141.

Chesley, L. C. (1956) Toxaemia of pregnancy in relation to chronic hypertension. *West. J. Surg. Obstet. Gynaec.*, **64**, 284.

Chesley, L. C., Cosgrove, R. A. & Annitto, J. E. (1962) A follow up of eclamptic women. *Amer. J. Obstet. Gynec.*, **83**, 1360.

Chesley, L. C. (1966) Sodium retention and pre-eclampsia. *Amer. J. Obstet. Gynec.*, **95**, 127.

Cobo, E. (1965) Uterine hypercontractility in toxaemia of pregnancy. *Amer. J. Obstet. Gynec.*, **90**, 505.

Davey, D. A., O'Sullivan, W. J. & Browne, J. C. M. (1961) Total exchangeable sodium in normal pregnancy and in pre-eclampsia. *Lancet*, **i**, 159.

Dieckmann, W. J., Smitter, R. C. & Rynkiewicz, L. (1952) Pre-eclampsia—eclampsia does not cause permanent vascular-renal disease. *Amer. J. Obstet. Gynec.*, **64**, 850.

Duffus, G. M., Tunstall, M. E. & MacGillivray, I. (1968) Intravenous chlormethiazole in pre-eclamptic toxaemia in labour. *Lancet*, **i**, 335.

Duffus, G. M., MacGillivray, I. & Dennis, K. J. (1971) The relationship between baby weight and changes in maternal weight, total body water, plasma volume, electrolytes and proteins and urinary oestriol excretion. *J. Obstet. Gynaec. Brit. Cwlth.*, **78**, 2, 97.

Gibson, G. B. (1956) Further observations on the progress in toxaemia of late pregnancy. *J. Obstet. Gynaec. Brit. Emp.*, **63**, 833.

Ginsburg, J. & Duncan, S. L. B. (1967) Peripheral blood flow in normal pregnancy. *Circulation Review*, **1**, 356.

Govan, A. D. T. (1962) Renal function, water, electrolytes and oedema in pregnancy. *Postgrad. med. J.*, **38**, 214.

Griess, F. C. (1963) The uterine vascular bed effect of adrenerjic stimulation. *Obstet. Gynaec.*, **21**, 295.

Hall, M. H. (1967) Changes in pre-eclampsia in Aberdeen from 1950–1963. *Paper presented at the Northern Obstetrical Society Meeting in May, 1967.*

Harding, V. J. & Van Wyck, H. B. (1930) Effects of hypertonic saline in toxaemia of later pregnancy. *Brit. med. J.*, **ii**, 589.

Honger, P. E. (1967) Intravascular mass of albumin in pre-eclampsia in normal pregnancy. *Scand. J. Clin. Lab. Invest.*, **19**, 283

Honger, P. E. (1968a) Albumin metabolism in normal pregnancy. *Scand. J. Clin. Lab. Invest.*, **21**, 3.

Honger, P. E. (1968b) Albumin metabolism in pre-eclampsia. *Scand. J. Clin. Lab. Invest.*, **22**, 177.

Kincaid-Smith, P., Bullen, M. and Mills, J. (1966) Prolonged use of methyldopa in severe hypertension in pregnancy. *Brit. med. J.*, **i**, 274.

Kraus, G. W., Marchese, J. R. & Yen, S. S. C. (1966) Prophylactic use of hydrochlorothiazide in pregnancy. *J. Amer. Med. Assoc.*, **198**, 1150.

Krupp, P. & Krupp, I. (1960) Serotonin and toxaemia of pregnancy. *Obstet. Gynaec.*, **15**, 237.

Landau, R. L., Bergenstal, D. M., Lugibihl, K. & Kascht, M. E. (1955) The metabolic effects of progesterone in man. *J. Clin. Endocr.*, **15**, 1194.

Lee, M. R. (1969) Renin and hypertension. London: Lloyd Luke Medical Books Ltd.

MacGillivray, I. & Buchanan, T. L. (1958) Total exchangeable sodium and potassium in non-pregnant women and in normal and pre-eclamptic pregnancy. *Lancet*, **i**, 1090.

MacGillivray, I. (1961) Hypertension in pregnancy and its consequences. *J. Obstet. Gynaec. Brit. Cwlth.*, **68**, 4, 557.

Mackay, D. G., Merrill, S. J., Weiner, A. E., Hertig, A. T. & Reid, D. E. (1953) Pathological anatomy of eclampsia, bilateral renal corticonecrosis, pituitary necrosis and other acute fetal complications of pregnancy and their possible relationship to generalized schwartsman phenomena. *Amer. J. Obstet. Gynec.*, **66**, 507.

Marcus, S. L. (1963) The nephrotic syndrome during pregnancy. *Obstet. Gynaec. Sur.*, **18**, 511.

Mastboom, S. L. (1956) A hypothesis of the etiology of toxaemia with late pregnancy. *Mod. Trends Obstet. Gynaec.*, 179–190. Edited by K. Bowes. New York: Paul B. Hoeber Inc.

Mengert, W. F. & Tacchi, D. A. (1961) Pregnancy toxaemia and sodium chloride. Preliminary Report. *Amer. J. Obstet. Gynec.*, **81**, 601.

Menon, M. K. K. (1961) The evolution of the treatment of eclampsia. *J. Obstet. Gynaec. Brit. Emp.*, **68**, 417.

Morris, N., Osborne, S. B., Wright, H. P. & Hart, A. (1965) Effective uterine blood flow during exercise in normal and pre-eclamptic pregnancy. *Lancet*, **ii**, 481.

Page, E. W. (1953) *The hypertensive disorders of pregnancy.* Springfield, Illinois: Charles C. Thomas.

Paterson, M. L. (1960) The role of the posterior pituitary antidiuretic hormone in toxaemia of pregnancy. *J. Obstet. Gynaec. Brit. Emp.*, **67**, 883.

Perinatal Problems. *The Second Report of the British Mortality Survey* (1858). Edited by N. R. Butler. London: E. & S. Livingstone.

Pirani, B. B. K. & MacGillivray, I. (1973) In preparation.

Platt, R. (1958) Chronic hypertension following pre-eclamptic toxaemia: the influences of familial hypertension on its causation. *J. Obstet. Gynaec. Brit. Emp.*, **65**, 385.

Plentl, A. A. & Gray, M. J. (1959) Total body water, sodium space and total exchangeable sodium in normal and toxaemic pregnant women. *Amer. J. Obstet. Gynec.*, **78**, 472.

Pollak, V. E. & Nettles, J. B. (1960) Preliminary observations on the differential diagnosis of toxaemias of pregnancy by means of renal biopsy. *Amer. J. Obstet. Gynec.*, **79**, 866.

Robertson, W. B., Brosens, I. & Dixon, H. G. (1967) The pathological response of the vessels of the placental bed to hypertensive pregnancy. *J. Path. Bact.*, **93**, 581.

Roulet, F. (1961) Pre-eclampsia and eclampsia in pregnancy. 7th Conference of the International Society of Geographical Pathology, London (1960) *Pathologia Microbiol.*, **24**.

Senior, J. B., Fahim, I., Sullivan, F. M. & Robson, J. M. (1963) Possible role of 5-hydroxytryptamine in toxaemia of pregnancy. *Lancet*, **ii**, 553.

Sophian, J. (1955) Myometrial resistance to stretch the cause of pre-eclampsia. *J. Obstet. Gynaec. Brit. Emp.*, **62**, 37.

Spetz, S. (1965) Peripheral circulation in pregnancy complicated by toxaemia. *Acta Obstet. Gynec. Scand.*, **44**, 243.

Studd, J. W. W., Blainey, J. D. & Bailey, D. E. (1970) Serum protein changes in the pre-eclampsia/eclampsia syndrome. *J. Obstet. Gynaec. Brit. Cwlth.*, **77**, 796.

Talledo, O. E., Chesley, L. C. & Zuspan, F. P. (1966) Spontaneous uterine hypercontractility in eclampsia. Symposium on Toxaemia of Pregnancy. Edited by F. P. Zuspan. *Clin. Obstet. Gynaec.*, **9**, 910.

Tatum, H. J. & Mule, J. G. (1962) The hypertensive action of blood from patients with pre-eclampsia. *Amer. J. Obstet. Gynec.*, **83**, 1028.

Thomson, A. M., Hytten, F. E. & Billewicz, W. Z. (1967) The epidemiology of oedema during pregnancy. *J. Obstet. Gynaec. Brit. Cwlth.*, **74**, 1.

Townsend, S. L. (1958) *Thesis for Doctor of Medicine.* Australia: University of Melbourne.

World Health Organization Expert Committee (1965) Expert Committee on pregnancy and lactation. *Wld. Hlth. Org. tech. Rep. Ser.* **302**.

11. Other Specific Diseases of Pregnancy

VOMITING IN PREGNANCY

Nausea and vomiting are common in the early months of pregnancy, but it is only rarely nowadays that the vomiting becomes severe. Nausea and vomiting are sometimes the first indications that the woman is pregnant and can occur before a menstrual period is missed. The vomiting typically occurs in the mornings and usually clears up by the fourth month of pregnancy.

HYPEREMESIS GRAVIDARUM

Occasionally the nausea and sickness experienced in the mornings becomes worse and extends over the whole day. There is no clear cut division between what is morning sickness and what is excessive vomiting of pregnancy. It is only a matter of degree and both conditions should be treated, although morning sickness often requires little in the way of treatment apart from advice about diet.

The onset of hyperemesis is usually insidious and there is a gradual deterioration in the patient's condition. As vomiting is so common in pregnancy the woman will often not seek any advice until she is quite ill.

At one time it was thought that an excess of chorionic gonadotrophin was responsible for hyperemesis because it is known that in cases of hydatidiform mole there is very often excessive vomiting. It is now known that there is no excess of chorionic gonadotrophin in the great majority of cases. There is, however, apparently a neurotic element in many of these women and it is probable that hyperemesis gravidarum is not a distinct entity from morning sickness of pregnancy. The woman starts off with morning sickness and because of a combination of emotional and metabolic factors the vomiting worsens and a vicious cycle develops. It is known that starvation causes a much more intense ketonaemia and

ketonuria than in the non-pregnant. Thus the woman with hyperemesis becomes starved and dehydrated and there is a strong smell of acetone in the breath. The vomiting becomes worse so that she cannot even take fluids. Weight loss becomes marked and the skin becomes pale and dry and in very severe cases jaundiced. The pulse becomes rapid and there is a fall in blood pressure. Nystagmus may be present. There is marked haemoconcentration and a rise in blood urea, uric acid and non-protein nitrogen. The plasma sodium and chloride fall and in severe cases so does the potassium. The urine is scanty in amount and the chloride content may be low or absent. Specific gravity of the urine is high and ketones are present. In severe cases protein and bile may appear in the urine. In very severe untreated cases drowsiness, coma and death can occur.

Pathology

The liver shows the changes of starvation with gross fatty infiltration. This occurs because the liver is unable to cope with the fat, which is transported to it for use as energy. The kidneys may show fatty degeneration of the convoluted tubules and the heart is small and atrophic with subendocardial haemorrhages. There is a condition associated with severe starvation called Wernicke's encephalopathy in which there are petechial haemorrhages in the brain stem, particularly in the corpora mammillaria and in the floor of the fourth ventricle. These changes are found in cases dying of hyperemesis gravidarum.

Diagnosis of hyperemesis gravidarum

It is extremely important to remember that because a woman is pregnant and is vomiting the condition is not necessarily hyperemesis gravidarum. It is important to exclude conditions such as gastro-enteritis, cholecystitis, hepatitis, peptic ulceration, pyelonephritis, pyloric stenosis and even carcinoma of the stomach or cerebral tumour. The history, the type of vomiting and the presence or absence of pain are the most useful points in differential diagnosis.

Treatment

It is very often found that the morning sickness is aggravated by certain foods, by heavy fatty meals and also by smells such as cigarette smoke or food cooking. It is important, therefore, to advise the woman to avoid spiced or fancy foods, and also to take small meals frequently and to avoid smells which upset her. A high carbohydrate diet with plenty of fluids should be taken, and it is usually advisable for the woman to take a sweetened drink before rising in the morning. If possible she should have her food cooked for her so that she avoids the smell of cooking. As well as giving reassurance it is sometimes desirable to give a mild sedative or tranquillizer such as phenobarbitone, 30mg or diazepam (Valium), 5mg three times a day, promazine hydrochloride (Sparine), 25mg twice daily and an antiemetic such as prochlorperazine (Stemetil) 5mg twice daily or tablets containing pyridoxine such as Debendox and Nidoxital or promethazine (Avomine). A good guide to progress is given by the patient's weight.

The severe case

Continuing vomiting and loss of weight are indications for hospitalization. It is very often found that when the woman is admitted to hospital the vomiting ceases dramatically. In such cases a fluid diet can be given and gradually an ordinary diet is introduced and in a few days it is possible to allow the patient home, but it is important that the patient should be sufficiently reassured and any underlying emotional cause established and corrected before allowing the patient home.

Severe cases are assessed to determine how much fluid, glucose and electrolytes are required to correct the biochemical imbalance. A useful indication can be obtained from examination of the urine. The volume, specific gravity, acetone content, and amount of chlorides can be used to assess how much sodium chloride and dextrose solutions should be given. Bottles containing 4·3 per cent dextrose in 0·18 per cent sodium chloride solution are used and the amount to be given assessed by the urinary output. Plasma electrolytes are measured and if the potassium is low, 1gm is added to each bottle of saline. Aneurine should be given to all cases of hyperemesis in a dose of 100mgs daily. Sparine, Stemetil and Largactil (Chlorpromazine) can also be given. In the majority of cases there is rapid improvement on this regime and small amounts of fluid can be given by mouth and gradually increased. In the past termination of pregnancy was sometimes required because of hyperemesis but this must be very rare indeed nowadays, and correction of fluid and electrolyte imbalance and control of emotional factors ensures recovery from the condition.

LATE VOMITING OF PREGNANCY

It is doubtful if there is a separate disease entity directly due to pregnancy which causes excessive vomiting in the later months. Such excessive vomiting is almost always due to some underlying condition such as pyelonephritis, pre-eclampsia or occasionally fatty liver. Multiple pregnancy and hydramnios may also cause such distension that vomiting results. In some cases of hiatus hernia resulting from pregnancy there can be excessive vomiting associated with heartburn. In some cases of hyperemesis gravidarum vomiting continues intermittently right on towards the end of pregnancy. In cases of vomiting starting in late pregnancy it is necessary to make a very careful assessment to determine the cause, but if none is found then the case is treated along the same lines as that of hyperemesis gravidarum, but termination of the pregnancy by induction of premature labour can be resorted to more readily than induction of abortion in cases of hyperemesis gravidarum.

JAUNDICE IN PREGNANCY

Hepatic disease is fortunately rare in pregnancy because when it does occur it is very serious. Hepatic function is not altered by normal pregnancy, so far as can be judged by routine hepatic function tests; for example, the turbidity tests, serum bilirubin and transaminases are normal throughout pregnancy. The bromsulphthalein excretion is normal in early pregnancy but may be slightly impaired towards the end of pregnancy because of the slowing of the conjugation of the dye in the liver. The alkaline phosphatase levels rise in pregnancy, but the increase is due to the heat stable fraction which is derived from the placenta. The level of albumin falls progressively during pregnancy. This is not due to haemodilution as the globulin fractions rise. Serum cholesterol levels rise markedly during pregnancy and may exceed 250mg/100ml. Spider naevi and palmar erythema are common in pregnancy but this is due to the high levels of circulating oestrogens and not to hepatic failure.

Jaundice may be caused by (1) conditions arising due to pregnancy, (2) intercurrent conditions, (3) hepatotoxic drugs and (4) pre-existing liver disease, not directly related to pregnancy. In the first group jaundice may be due to obstetric acute yellow atrophy, hyperemesis gravidarum or eclampsia. In the second group jaundice may be due to viral hepatitis, blood transfusion, infection with Clostridium or in the third drugs such as promazine and in the fourth cholecystitis.

1. Jaundice due to conditions of pregnancy

a. ACUTE FATTY LIVER
This was originally called 'obstetric acute yellow atrophy of the liver' by Sheehan (1940). This is a rare and usually fatal disease and its cause is unknown, but it has been suggested that it might be related to marked protein malnutrition as the morphological appearances in the liver resemble experimental lesions produced in animals by protein anabolic depressants. It is also suggested that large doses of Tetracycline can cause the lesions. The characteristic histological appearances of the liver are the many small intracytoplasmic lipid-laden vacuoles arranged around the centrally placed normal nuclei. This occurs in the central portions of the lobules and the periportal liver cells are normal. There is no evidence of necrosis of the liver cells, which is a characteristic feature of acute hepatic necrosis. The condition usually arises in the latter weeks of pregnancy and jaundice develops after vomiting and epigastric pain have been present for a few days. The condition progresses to hepatic failure with mental confusion, deepening jaundice and haemorrhages in the skin and mucous membranes. The liver function tests show only a slight increase in the turbidity tests and transaminases. This differentiates the condition from acute viral hepatitis with which it is otherwise readily confused. The baby is usually stillborn. No treatment is effective, but blood transfusions may be helpful if haemorrhages occur.

b. HYPEREMESIS AND LATE VOMITING OF PREGNANCY
In these conditions the severe vomiting may produce a deficiency of lipotropic factors such as choline and methionine. This results in a mobilization of fat from the mother's depots which is deposited as droplets of neutral fat in the liver cells. The infiltration of the liver cells with large droplets of fat can be seen histologically in cases dying of severe hyperemesis or late vomiting of pregnancy. There may be also some necrosis of the cells in the centres of the lobules. Pregnancy predisposes to this fatty infiltration of the liver because the growing fetus requires large amounts of lipotropic substances. Jaundice developing in cases of hyperemesis or late vomiting of pregnancy is of grave prognostic importance.

c. PRE-ECLAMPSIA AND ECLAMPSIA
This is a rare complication and can occur both in severe pre-eclampsia as well as in eclampsia. The jaundice is haemolytic in type. Apart from termination of the pregnancy there is no known treatment other than the control of the eclampsia.

d. RECURRENT INTRAHEPATIC CHOLESTATIC JAUNDICE
This type of obstructive (cholestatic) jaundice appears in the last trimester of pregnancy. In the mildest form jaundice is absent and the only abnormality is pruritus. Jaundice is rarely deep, the urine is dark and the stools are pale. There is no pain and no upset apart from the pruritus. The jaundice disappears within one or two weeks of delivery and the prognosis is excellent. The condition recurs in subsequent pregnancies. Serum transaminases are usually normal or slightly increased. Histological examination shows bile stasis. The cause of the condition is unknown, but may be due to a cholestatic reaction caused by a steriod. There is an association between jaundice following the administration of oral contraceptive pills and intrahepatic cholestasis of pregnancy. Oral contraceptives should not be given to patients who have previously suffered pruritus in pregnancy.

2. Intercurrent jaundice of pregnancy

a. VIRAL HEPATITIS
Hepatitis is most frequent between the ages of three and ten, so that family contact exposes mothers to the risk of infective hepatitis.

Pregnant women are not more susceptible to hepatitis whether of the infective or serum variety than the general population. Viral hepatitis is not any more lethal to pregnant women unless they are undernourished, and a favourable outcome can usually be expected for the mother with hepatitis. The clinical course, results of liver function tests and histological appearance of the liver are the same as in the non-pregnant. The course of severe hepatitis is not influenced by termination of pregnancy, and this should be avoided. There is no positive evidence that hepatitis causes fetal abnormalities. Viral hepatitis is the commonest cause of jaundice in pregnancy.

b. GALL STONES

Gall stones are associated with obesity and parity and jaundice can be caused in pregnancy by stones in the common bile duct, but this is surprisingly rare. The management is the same as for the non-pregnant.

3. Hepatotoxic drugs

Any drug which decreases hepatic synthetic processes such as Tetracycline can cause jaundice. Sensitivity to Chlorpromazine is infrequent. Halothane can cause jaundice if given repeatedly.

4. Pre-existing liver disease

It is very rare for a woman with hepatic cirrhosis to conceive and abortion is likely to occur. Active chronic hepatitis (lupoid hepatitis) is an uncommon condition affecting young women. Amenorrhoea is usual but some patients have borne children.

The coincidence of a co-existence of a liver disease and pregnancy is not in itself an indication for termination, but special care has to be taken during the pregnancy.

SKIN DISEASES IN PREGNANCY

The incidence of skin diseases in pregnancy is low and serious skin diseases are very rare in pregnancy, but there are a few skin conditions which are peculiar to pregnancy.

During pregnancy there are many skin changes which are physiological. Pigmentation with melanin is common on the face and forehead (chloasma) and on the abdomen (linea nigra). This is thought to be due to the direct stimulant effect of progesterone on the melanocytes and pigmentation can occur in women on oestrogen/progestagen contraceptive pills. Pigmentation also commonly occurs around the nipples and umbilicus.

PALMAR ERYTHEMA

Palmer erythema particularly over the thenar and hypothenar eminences is very common and is thought to be due to the increase in oestrogen production.

Spider naevi are also thought to be due to the increased oestrogen, but are less common. They are distributed on the face, neck, upper arms and chest.

Striae gravidarum are very common particularly towards the end of pregnancy. They are found on the abdomen, breasts, flanks, buttocks and thighs. The elastic fibres in the dermis disappear and the epidermis is thin and atrophic. Striae are at first purplish-pink, but later become white. They are sometimes associated with pruritus.

Hypertrichosis is common but usually slight in pregnancy. Occasionally it can be excessive, but fortunately it tends to disappear after delivery.

Skin disease peculiar to pregnancy

PRURIGO GESTATIONIS

This is a papular eruption usually found on the abdomen, thighs and buttocks, and on the dorsal surfaces of the hands or feet. It usually begins in the middle trimester and causes intense itching. The cause is unknown and the treatment is empirical with antipruritic lotions and antihistamines.

HERPES GESTATIONIS

There is at first erythematous patches on the extremities or trunk. These are followed by vesicles rather like herpes and occur in rings. Bullae are formed and may become pustular or haemorrhagic. The rash may spread to the whole body. Eosinophilia is a striking feature. The prognosis for the mother is usually good although a few fatal cases have been reported, but the prognosis for the fetus is poor. The perinatal death rate is high and there is a higher incidence than normal of fetal abnormality. Treatment is aimed at avoiding secondary infection and corticosteroid therapy is given. If infection should occur a broad spectrum antibiotic is given.

IMPETIGO HERPETIFORMIS

This is another skin condition occurring in

pregnancy in which the prognosis for the baby is poor. The lesion is composed of pustules arranged in rings or groups, and there are no vesicles. It causes less itching than herpes gestationis and there is less eosinophilia. The mother becomes severely ill with pyrexia, rigors and vomiting. There is no specific treatment for the condition.

PAPULAR DERMATITIS OF PREGNANCY

Again there is a high fetal mortality in this condition, which is characterized by a generalized papular eruption which is intensely itchy. The rash is spread over the trunk, arms and legs. The condition is treated with prednisolone.

Skin conditions commonly occurring in pregnancy

Skin disorders of the vulva and thighs are common in pregnancy and are due to trichomoniasis, moniliasis or intertrigo. Examination of the vaginal discharge will reveal either trichomonas vaginalis or candida albicans. The former is treated with Metranidazole (Flagyl) 200 mgs t.d.s. for seven days. Moniliasis is treated with Nystatin pessaries. Intertrigo usually occurs in other situations than the vulvar region, such as the axillary folds, intergluteal cleft or submammary folds. The areas are treated by washing and powdering, but if a secondary infection has occurred steroid ointments and broad spectrum antibiotics may be necessary.

PSORIASIS

There is a difference of opinion about whether psoriasis is more common in pregnancy or not, but it seems unlikely that psoriasis is precipitated by pregnancy. The condition may be worsened in pregnancy because of the increased perspiration and increased weight. Treatment follows the usual lines with baths, steroid creams and other conventional remedies.

ECZEMA

This is commonly found on the areola and nipple in pregnant women.

PITYRIASIS

This common fungus disease is often seen in pregnant women. The condition seems to be difficult to cure during pregnancy and is treated along the conventional lines with hot baths, application of 10 per cent solution of sodium thiosulphate and salicylic acid and benzoic acid ointments.

PRURITUS IN PREGNANCY

Itching is quite common during pregnancy but is usually mild. Localized pruritus often occurs around the vulva or anus and is usually due to intertrigo or trichomoniasis or moniliasis. Any skin disorders of the area may cause itching. Dermatitis may be caused by clothing or other substances causing sensitization. Pediculosis pubis may also cause itching. Treatment of localized pruritus is of the underlying cause.

Generalized pruritus may be due to any of the dermatoses of pregnancy, which have already been discussed. Metabolic disorders such as diabetes, jaundice and uraemia can cause itching as can blood diseases such as leukaemia and reticulo-endothelial diseases such as Hodgkin's disease. Generalized itching can also be caused by the toxic effects from drugs. Both localized and generalized pruritus may be due to psychogenic causes.

POLIOMYELITIS

Pregnant women are more likely to contract poliomyelitis than women of similar age who are not pregnant. The World Health Organization's Expert Committee (1954) on poliomyelitis stated that poliomyelitis ran a more severe course in pregnancy than in the non-pregnant. Possibly this is due to an increase in hormones, particularly cortisol in pregnancy aggravating the condition as it has been shown that cortisone increases the susceptibility of experimental animals. The spinal type of the disease seems to be commoner than the bulbar type in pregnancy, so that the death rate is not so high. In many countries including Britain, vaccination of pregnant women with poliomyelitis vaccine is a standard procedure. Oral vaccine is used and given in three doses. It is well known that women who develop poliomyelitis in pregnancy or who have had poliomyelitis of the paralytic form can have a painless normal first stage of labour, but a forceps delivery is usually required for the second stage.

RHEUMATOID ARTHRITIS

Pregnancy occurring in women with rheumatoid arthritis is of particular interest because of the frequent spontaneous remissions of the disease which occur during pregnancy. This is usually thought to be due to the increase in the level of hydroxycorticoids in the plasma.

RHEUMATIC FEVER

Although this is a disease of young adults it appears to be very rare in pregnancy. It may manifest itself either as a carditis or an arthritis.

SYSTEMIC LUPUS ERYTHEMATOSUS

The course of this disease is not altered by pregnancy, but there are spontaneous periods of remission, which may coincide with pregnancy. The condition is of particular importance when there is renal involvement or hypertension, and in such cases there is an increased maternal risk and a markedly increased fetal risk. The condition is of importance in the differential diagnosis of hypertension and proteinuria in pregnancy (*see* Chapter 10). The women may fall pregnant while they are on treatment with corticosteroids and immunosuppressive drugs, which may have a teratogenetic effect on the fetus and this may be an indication for termination of pregnancy in addition to the disease itself.

VIRAL AND BACTERIAL INFECTIONS IN PREGNANCY

The importance of viral infection to the mother in pregnancy is largely the risk of infection to the child. Chapter 12 should be read in relation to all infectious conditions in pregnancy.

Rubella (German measles)

In view of the risk of this disease in pregnant women to their fetus, routine vaccination is now offered to all female children at or about puberty unless they are already shown to be immune. Nurses, female medical students and other young females likely to be exposed to rubella or likely to be in contact with women in early pregnancy are similarly offered protection.

In early pregnancy routine screen will disclose non-protected mothers but no action can be taken until after delivery when routine protection should be offered. When a woman in early pregnancy reports that she has been exposed to rubella, blood should be taken immediately for HAI titre estimation. A rise in titre due to new infection does not take place until the time of the appearance of the rash 12–14 days after exposure so that early estimation will allow assessment of the previously protected state. A second blood should be taken 14 days after the first and a four-fold rise will be clear evidence that infection has occurred, and a third may be necessary. It should be possible then to decide whether the mother was previously immune or whether she has been infected by the current exposure. If she has been infected then the risk to the child is very great (see Chapter 23).

It is a good idea to obtain, if possible, a sample of the blood of the source child or adult since many of the infections said to be rubella are not, e.g. echo virus can cause a similar rash and is *not* a risk to the fetus. Occasionally it is worthwhile estimating the specific IGA antibody in the mother as proof of infection or re-infection.

Non specific gamma globulin is of no value and should not be offered.

Therapeutic abortion should be offered if proven infection occurs in the first 12 weeks of pregnancy and should be considered even up to 16 weeks.

Toxoplasmosis in the mother is common in the hot and humid areas of the world where up to 30 per cent may be infected by T. Gondi. The fetus is infected only when the mother is first infected during the actual pregnancy. The condition may be characterized in the mother by fever, fatigue and lymphadenopathy. Serial serological tests are necessary for diagnosis. If there is clear evidence of maternal infection, the child cannot be protected.

Other infections are discussed in Chapter 12 and the effects on the fetus in Chapter 13.

REFERENCES

Sheehan, H. L. (1940) The Pathology of Acute Yellow Atrophy and Delayed Chloroform Poisoning. *J. Obstet. Gynaec. Brit. Emp.*, **47**, 49.
Wld. Hlth. Org. Tech. Rep. Ser. (1954) No. **81**, 10 (Geneva).

FURTHER READING

Barnes, C. G. (1970) *Medical Disorders in Obstetric Practice*. Oxford and Edinburgh: Blackwell.
Campbell, M. (1961) Place of Maternal Rubella in the Aetiology of Congenital Heart Disease. *Brit. med. J.*, **i**, 691.
Fairweather, D. (1968) Nausea and Vomiting in Pregnancy. *Amer. J. Obstet. Gynec.*, **102**, 135.
Gregg, N. M. (1941) Congenital Cataract Following German Measles in the Mother. *Transaction of the Opthalmological Society of Australia*, **3**, 35.
Leading Article: (1957) *Brit. Med. J.*, **i**, 1352.
Sherlock, S. (1968) Jaundice in Pregnancy. *Brit. Med. Bull.*, **24**, 39.

12. Medical Disorders

SECTION 1: CARDIOVASCULAR SYSTEM

Introduction and background

Since earlier editions of this textbook were published, certain trends in the prevalence of the types of heart disease likely to affect women of child-bearing age have reached such a stage that it has become necessary to reconsider the whole subject of heart disease in pregnancy in the light of its relevance to every day obstetric practice in this and similar countries.

By far and away the most important of these trends has been the dramatic reduction in rheumatic fever and consequent rheumatic heart disease (Fig. 12.1) which, in the past, accounted for the vast majority of cases. So much so, that for many years, the care of women with heart disease during pregnancy depended largely upon the knowledge of how those with rheumatic lesions of the mitral valve reacted at various stages, in the natural history of their disease, to the circulatory burden imposed by pregnancy upon the cardiovascular system. Although this changing incidence is not yet too obvious in adult medical wards, where one still sees many patients in middle and late middle life with severely damaged valves that require surgical treatment, acute rheumatism has all but disappeared from paediatric practice. The question for a number of years has more often been: is the heart affected, rather than, how seriously has it been damaged. The inevitable result of such a change is now becoming evident at cardiac antenatal clinics in the decreasing number of young women with heart disease and the lessened severity of their lesions. Along with this decrease in rheumatic heart disease has come a small but steady increase in the number of patients with congenital heart disease whose improved prognosis following successful surgical treatment

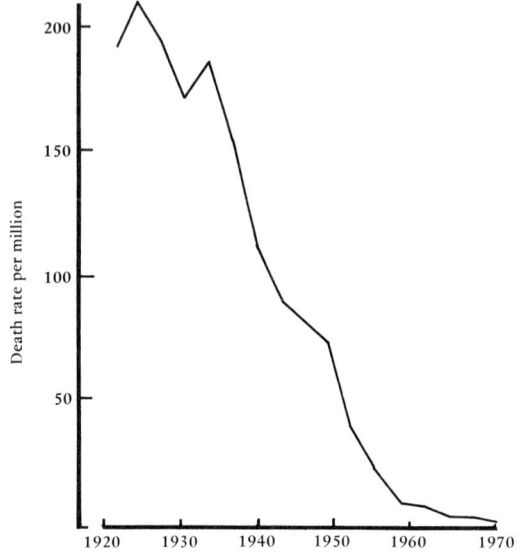

Fig. 12.1   UK deaths from rheumatic fever (1921–71) age 0-14 years.

has brought them to marriagable age; a trend that seems likely to continue. In fact, the number of new patients with rheumatic heart disease has now fallen to such a low level that during the years 1967–69, the last for which

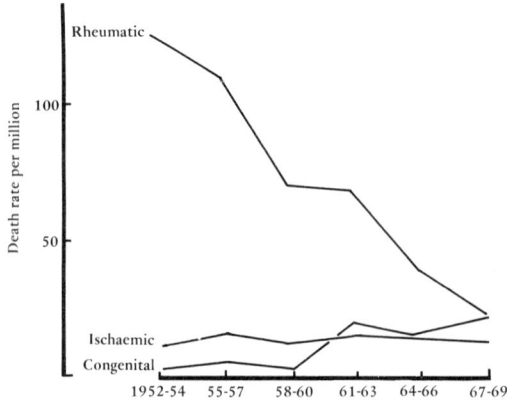

Fig. 12.2   The changing pattern of maternal deaths from disease (Scotland, England and Wales, 1952–69).

official statistics are available, rheumatism was for the first time less important than congenital and ischaemic heart disease as a cause of maternal mortality in the United Kingdom (Fig. 12.2). In England and Wales congenital cardiac malformations are now actually responsible for more maternal deaths than acquired valvar lesions.

These great changes in the pattern of heart disease have occurred during a time of great therapeutic change. Present day antibiotics, anaesthetics, diuretics, surgery and intensive care facilities, together with current social attitudes concerning contraception, sterilization and abortion, allow for a much more rational approach towards pregnancy and childbearing, and for intelligent family planning. *Future emphasis should be upon prophylaxias.* Young women known to have heart disease should be encouraged to seek cardiological advice, if possible before marriage and certainly before pregnancy, so that the risks can be assessed and necessary measures taken to anticipate or avoid them. In general they should be advised to have two well spaced pregnancies when still young and no more.

With the exception of some congenital cardiac malformations, successful surgical treatment will not alter this advice because even when it is necessary and possible it is usually palliative rather than curative. At best it improves the cardiovascular system seldom restoring it to normal. It is important also to remember that women with significant heart disease and severe symptoms run a serious risk of spontaneous abortion, premature labour, stillbirth and neonatal death.

A careful routine clinical examination of the cardiovascular system early in pregnancy is extremely important and should be carried out at the first antenatal visit, which is often early in pregnancy before the hyperkinetic circulatory state has become fully established and has modified the signs of heart disease. Centres of any size should always have antenatal cardiac clinics to which all patients suspected of having heart disease should be referred to be cared for by physicians and obstetricians with a special knowledge of heart disease in pregnancy. Although a high index of suspicion inevitably entails the reference of many women without organic heart disease,

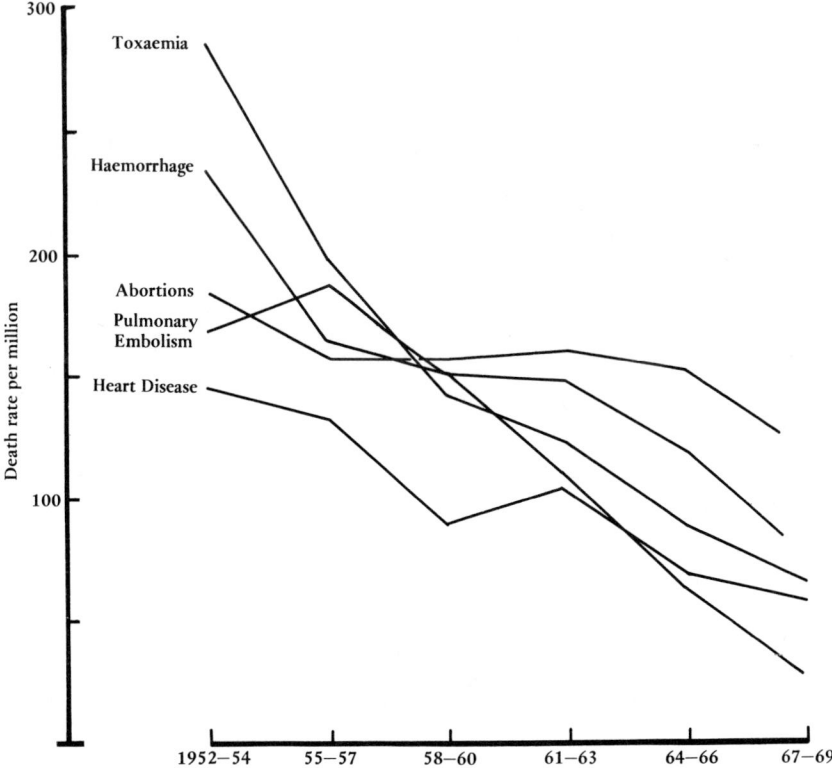

Fig. 12.3   The changing pattern of maternal deaths (Scotland, England and Wales, 1952–69).

it is rewarded by the timely detection of some previously unsuspected, but potentially dangerous cardiac lesions.

It is therefore against this background that we must approach the problems presented by heart disease in pregnancy, realizing that although like the other major causes of maternal mortality (Fig. 12.3), it is now responsible for far fewer deaths than it was some years ago, it represents a hard core problem that can only be contained by those with specialist knowledge who are skilled in its management. Having said that, however, we must admit that it is becoming so uncommon that soon few in this country will have much practical experience in the management of severe cases. Fortunately, carefully documented evidence is available from former times (Haig and Gilchrist, 1949; Jones, 1951; Burwell and Metcalf, 1958; Mendelson, 1960; Marquis, 1969), which, if suitably modified in the light of current circumstances, will act as an invaluable guide for future practice.

The effects of pregnancy on the cardiovascular system

The profound circulatory changes that occur during pregnancy are discussed in Chapter 5. Beginning early in the second month, cardiac output increases by so much as 30–50 per cent during the first few months and must be maintained at this level till term. The idea that it fell during the last 8 weeks of pregnancy is now known to be fallacious and arose because early workers underestimated the venous return to the heart by failing to appreciate that when a pregnant woman lay on her back, the gravid uterus obstructed flow through the inferior vena cava. Any lingering sense of false security engendered by the approach of term must therefore be vigorously resisted, especially as the early puerperium, with its sudden circulatory readjustment, is also a time of great hazard.

The clinical signs of this hyperkinetic circulatory state become obvious very early in pregnancy and are in many ways similar to those seen in other conditions causing an increase in cardiac output, such as anaemia, thyrotoxicosis or hepatic failure. The hands are warm with easily felt pulsation in small arteries and distension of small veins. The heart rate is increased to cope with the increased blood volume. The heart itself may become slightly enlarged as a result of its increased stroke volume and feels overactive. Increased flow through it is manifest by a loud third heart sound at the apex and a soft early to mid-systolic murmur along the left sternal edge; physiological signs that are frequently mistaken for evidence of heart disease, especially as increasing body weight and a rising diaphragm so often cause a little simultaneous breathlessness.

To understand how heart disease may affect pregnancy, and be influenced by it, one must be fully conversant with the physiological changes that occur during pregnancy and relate them to the abnormal cardiovascular state. For example, hormonal changes may cause fluid retention and hypervolaemia, which, although well tolerated by normal women, may aggravate what symptoms might reasonably be expected in those with heart disease and which, towards term, may even produce relatively severe disability in women with relatively mild lesions. Changes in the respiratory system require pregnant women to breathe more deeply than normal to compensate for the reduced movement of the diaphragm, thus increasing tidal volume with little or no increase in respiratory rate. These and many other physiological adaptations must be kept in mind when interpreting symptoms or attributing them to heart disease.

It is also essential to appreciate that cardiac signs are notoriously variable during pregnancy. Heart murmurs, especially diastolic ones, may come and go and may vary greatly in intensity. As the hyperkinetic circulatory state begins so soon after conception, it is difficult at times to gauge the true severity of lesions in patients who have not been examined before they become pregnant.

The assessment of risk

With few exceptions, most women with heart disease can survive pregnancy nowadays if they are properly cared for by those with *the necessary experience and resources*. The cardiologist's duty is to assess the likely risks and to explain them in simple terms to the patient, and if necessary to her husband, so that they can make decisions about planning their family. In the now fairly exceptional circumstances where the risk is to life—either of mother or child—this must be clearly stated, as all too often the word *risk* is not taken to include such a serious outcome.

In assessing the risk many factors are taken into account. The nature and severity of the heart disease itself being the first consideration. Severe rheumatic mitral stenosis is obviously of much greater significance than a small congenital defect in the ventricular septum, whereas a large defect with pulmonary hypertension carries a far graver prognosis than a modest degree of mitral regurgitation. The effect of surgical treatment upon the lesion must also be considered. Age is important, because by and large, the younger the patient the better she tolerates pregnancy and its complications. Parity and previous experience are helpful guides because, other things being equal, she will seldom be better, often be the same and frequently be little worse than in previous pregnancies. Signs such as atrial fibrillation and cardiomegaly, which indicate severity of heart disease in a non-specific way, and some specific lesions such as the Eisenmenger syndrome, which experience has shown to carry a high mortality, must also be considered.

With these various points in mind, the patient is examined and if she has heart disease, a decision is made about the desirability of pregnancy and how it should best be managed. The cardiologist then thinks along certain well determined lines:

1. The heart disease is not significant and the patient should, for all practical purposes, be treated as a normal healthy person.
2. The heart disease is significant but not serious and with routine supervision at the antenatal clinic, is not likely to cause trouble during pregnancy, labour or the puerperium.
3. The heart disease is serious. With careful supervision, pregnancy should be successfully concluded with no great risk to the mother or child. She must, however, be prepared to modify her physical activities and take extra rest when advised to do so. She will probably have to come into hospital for a rest late in pregnancy and should have skilled obstetric care at delivery.
4. The heart disease is serious. Pregnancy carries considerable risk with the prospect of prolonged hospital treatment and no guarantee of success. It would be far better to terminate this pregnancy, have the heart improved by surgery if this is feasible and start again.
5. The heart disease is serious. Pregnancy carries grave risks and cardiac surgery has nothing to offer. The pregnancy should be terminated and the patient sterilized. If she is determined to continue with the existing pregnancy, expert medical supervision in hospital should ensure survival and will sometimes result in the birth of a live child.

Advice about these alternatives may be influenced by the age and parity of the patient. The case of the young nullipara desperate for a child is clearly different, from that of the older multipara with live children, because with comparable lesions youth is in her favour and may justify greater risks. When giving advice, each case must first be judged strictly on its *medical* merits. Moral, ethical, sociological or religious beliefs must not influence the initial assessment. Only after the medical situation has been made clear to the patient and her husband can compromise or modification be discussed where the advice given conflicts with their convictions. Fortunately, during the last few years, such conflicts have become increasingly rare.

The management of the patient

During the antenatal period. Once she has embarked upon pregnancy, the care of the patient with heart disease falls into a carefully determined routine. The *cardiac grade* (New York Heart Classification)* is determined and reassessed at each of a series of regular visits to the cardiac antenatal clinic. Following clinical examination, and, if necessary, with the help of electrocardiograms and X-rays, the likely course of events has been predicted and vigilance is maintained to make sure that no unexpected deterioration takes place. The cardiac grade is a rough and ready way of assessing exercise tolerance and functional capacity. Those in Grade I have no disability; those in Grade II are handicapped on fairly strenuous exertion (in this context usually by breathlessness); those in Grade III are incapacitated by ordinary activities; those in Grade IV are breathless at rest and show signs of heart failure. Obviously it is a somewhat crude yard-stick and many physicians subdivide further in their practice (a good II, II/III, etc.), but so long as its limitations are appreciated and symptoms do not take precedence over signs, the regular evaluation of

* The New York Heart Association in 1955 (*Nomenclature and Criteria for Diagnosis of Disease of the Heart and Blood Vessels*. Ed. 5, The New York Heart Association 177).

cardiac grade is of proved value as the basis of out-patient surveillance. Experience has shown (1) that women who have severe symptoms and who are Grade III or IV in early pregnancy are seldom fit for childbearing unless medical or surgical treatment can restore them at least to Grade I or II, and (2) that the risk to both mother and child increases out of all proportion, regardless of the severity of the underlying cardiac lesion, in those who develop severe symptoms and deteriorate to Grades III or IV during pregnancy. For this reason deterioration to Grade III is an indication for hospital admission and active treatment so that the patient may be restored as soon as possible to Grade II and maintained in this state until after delivery, even if this means staying in hospital for the rest of the pregnancy. It is also worth remembering that few healthy women remain in Grade I towards term—especially if they are obese or elderly or both.

This classification takes no account of that most serious of all symptoms, *acute paroxysmal dyspnoea*, which is often nocturnal and may occur in those whose cardiac grade is otherwise good—frequently in young women with tight mitral stenosis who may previously have had little incapacity. When accompanied by pulmonary oedema, it is life threatening and demands immediate bed rest with intensive medical therapy. It is now the commonest cause of cardiac death in pregnancy and is disregarded at the patient's peril.

Acute pulmonary oedema is a grave medical emergency and requires the following vigorous treatment:

1. prop the patient upright in bed or a chair;
2. give 10–20mgm morphine IM or IV;
3. oxygen, if possible under slight positive pressure;
4. 40mgm Frusemide IV.

This should give time to consider the cause or precipitating factor and initiate appropriate therapy, e.g. IV digoxin 0·5–1·0mg if due to rapid paroxysmal dysrhythmia. Other measures that may be used are IV Aminophylline 0·5–1·0g given slowly and reduction of the venous return to the heart by the application of tourniquets to the limbs or as a last resort by venesection. If all else fails positive pressure ventilation may be used.

ROUTINE ADVICE

At their first visit to the cardiac clinic, patients are given a simple explanation of the increased load on the circulatory system in such terms as 'the heart working for two instead of one', and they are advised to take more rest than healthy women; the order of the day being early to bed and late to rise with an hour or two in bed in the afternoon as pregnancy progresses. They should, in addition, be advised to sleep with two, and later on with three or more pillows to compensate for a rising diaphragm and keep the vital capacity of the thorax as large as possible. In this regard too, weight increase should be watched carefully and kept to a minimum.

If all goes well patients in Grades I and II are seen monthly during the first 28 weeks and then every 2 weeks until term. They are warned of the necessity to report symptoms, especially sudden or unexpected breathlessness, which should bring them back at once to the clinic. Any unexpected or unnatural deterioration of the cardiac grade must be investigated and if no obvious cause is found, more rest and possibly a diuretic are prescribed. Each case is judged on its merits, but many will benefit from bed rest in hospital for a week or two before their baby is due.

This regime is suitably modified where the heart disease is causing more disability, and it should be kept in mind that this does not necessarily signify that it is intrinsically more severe. Patients with symptoms whose grade deteriorates should have more frequent observation and often require admission to hospital for investigation and treatment. Sometimes they are allowed to go home again with suitably modified activities; sometimes it is best to keep them under strict medical supervision until they can go home with a baby. Patients who deteriorate to Grade III or IV at any stage in pregnancy should be kept in hospital till safely delivered. Again, each case must be judged on its merits, it being always better to err on the safe side.

Non-cardiac complications of antenatal care must be treated with due regard to the effects upon the heart of both the complication and its treatment. Pre-eclamptic toxaemia, for example, by causing fluid retention, may greatly increase not only the symptoms but also the signs of heart failure in patients with mitral stenosis; thus creating a false impression about the severity of the heart disease and the deteriorating cardiac grade.

During labour

The effects of labour on the cardiovascular system are discussed in Chapter 19. It used to be taught, with good reason, that cardiac patients should be left to go into spontaneous labour and that surgical interference in delivery should be reserved for strictly obstetrical reasons. Low forceps were allowed to shorten the second stage. It is now clear that with modern local or regional anaesthesia, antibiotics, blood replacement, etc., the cardiac condition, though requiring special consideration, need no longer dictate the obstetric action. Even inductions with synthetic oxytocin is safe provided no great volume of fluid is required and violent uterine contractions are avoided (*see* Chapter 19).

Although the factors that require special consideration depend in some measure upon the nature of the heart disease, certain general rules apply in most cases unless it has been judged to be trivial or insignificant, in which case no special consideration is necessary. If it is necessary to induce labour, an effective method that is likely to work quickly should be employed. The patient should be kept propped up, should have an adequate supply of oxygen and should not be given sedatives that are liable to inhibit respiration. Care must be taken to keep the volume of infused fluids to a minimum, and vasopressive substances should be used with caution. Labour should be as short as possible to avoid undue fatigue or pain during the first stage and too much violent bearing down during the second. Forceps should be used to speed delivery where this seems likely to be delayed. *Trials of labour for disproportion or malposition are strictly forbidden.* If there is any question of disproportion or other circumstances suggesting that the natural course of events seems likely to be either prolonged or difficult, a cardiac lesion is an indication for elective Caesarean section. During all labour ward procedures the services of an expert anaesthetist must always be available.

Antibiotics should be used to guard against bacterial endocarditis when there is a definite risk of infection, but their routine use as a prophylactic measure is of doubtful value.

The third stage, a time of profound and rapid circulatory readjustment, is potentially hazardous and requires careful supervision when the cardiac lesion is severe or if the medical preparation for delivery has been inadequate. With the separation of the placenta and contraction of the uterus, a large volume of blood is suddenly injected into the circulation and may cause acute embarrassment, albeit temporary. The principal danger at this time is acute pulmonary oedema, which is now responsible for most of the cardiac deaths that still occur during pregnancy. Analysis of past experience has shown that many of them could have been prevented had the signs of occult peripheral and pulmonary congestion been recognized and treated. All too often digitalis and diuretics were withheld until heart failure was all too obvious. We now know that bed rest by itself, for those who require it, is not sufficient for the stresses of labour and the circulatory readjustments of the puerperium. *Incipient heart failure* demands active therapy and patients whose antenatal supervision has been adequate should have no real difficulty in the puerperium.

The management of the third stage, however, is still important because all patients have not necessarily had the advantage of expert antenatal supervision and unbooked cases may well present as emergencies.

In most cases who have had adequate antenatal supervision, syntometrine may be given with the anterior shoulder and the third stage conducted normally. The patient should be well propped up in bed, with oxygen to hand, and no attempt made to bring about rapid separation of the placenta or sudden contraction of the uterus.

During the puerperium

After their return to the ward, such patients should remain under special care for another 48 hours during which time the heart will usually have come to terms with its changed circumstances. Thereafter, if all goes well, they should gradually rejoin the normal ward routine and most are ready for home in 7 days— provided suitable domestic arrangements can be made. Where the heart has failed, a longer period of intensive medical care and rehabilitation will be necessary.

No woman with significant heart disease should be allowed to go home without advice about contraception, because, although family planning will be discussed in detail after assessment at the postnatal clinic, much marital distress and 'many a slip' results from failure to make arrangements to cover the interval between discharge from hospital and an out-patient appointment some time later.

Postnatal assessment

All patients should be seen again in the cardiac clinic three months after delivery for post-natal cardiac assessment so that the true nature and severity of the heart disease can be determined. This is specially important in patients who were seen for the first time during pregnancy when signs are notoriously variable and the cardiovascular system is under the influence of complex physiological forces.

The various possibilities outlined in the section dealing with the assessment of risk can then be reconsidered with the benefit of hind-sight and decisions taken about the future management of the case. Where the assessment was incorrect, steps should be taken to make certain that mistakes are not repeated, *even if the eventual outcome has been satisfactory.* Surgical treatment may be recommended either to ensure the patient's continued good health or as a prophylactic measure to improve the heart before a further pregnancy. If further pregnancies are neither desired nor desirable, suitable advice about effective contraception should be given or sterilization should be arranged so that nothing is left to chance. Those who are in need of continuing medical care should be transferred to the cardiac clinic for long term follow-up.

Acquired valvar heart disease. This title is now preferred to rheumatic heart disease because many of the patients referred with a history of rheumatic fever have no evidence of heart disease and many of those with acquired lesions, although almost certainly rheumatic, have no history of rheumatism.

With the dramatic reduction in the number of pregnant patients so-classified, and the concomitant decrease in the complexity of what lesions remain, the pattern of heart failure has changed from chronic systemic congestion to acute pulmonary congestion. Fewer older women are now seen and most of the new cases seen nowadays are young asymptomatic women with mitral stenosis who give no history of rheumatic fever. The temptation, in the presence of youth and the absence of symptoms, to reassure them and say they will have no trouble is strong, but must be resisted at all costs because a sense of false security in such circumstances

is responsible for many of today's tragedies. Amongst these women are those with tight stenosis who have not yet developed the pulmonary vascular changes that in some way protect the lungs from sudden exudation of fluid when pressure rises; and for whom any alarming attack of acute paroxysmal dyspnoea may lead rapidly to life-threatening pulmonary oedema. It is therefore worth re-emphasizing the importance of physical signs and X-rays when assessing the risk in such patients whose cardiac grade is I or II.

When considering the place of *surgical treatment* in the management of mitral stenosis during pregnancy, it should be stressed that late pregnancy is not the optimum time for major heart surgery. Ideally, it should be a prophylactic measure before pregnancy com-mences; next best it may be considered very early in pregnancy for those who are thought to be at great risk or whose cardiac grade has shown rapid deterioration; finally, and far less satisfactorily, it may occasionally be necessary later on for those in whom strict medical treatment has failed. Although there are now many reports of pregnancy following valve replacement, pregnancy is no time for by pass surgery. If patients requiring valve replace-ment become pregnant, the pregnancy should be terminated and further pregnancy delayed until surgery has been successfully com-pleted.

Congenital cardiac malformations

Having pointed out that congenital cardiac malformations now rank numerically alongside rheumatic lesions as causes of heart disease seen in pregnancy, it must be re-emphasized that the change in relativity is mainly due to the dramatic reduction in the prevalence of acquired valvar lesions. It is also true, however, that for several reasons, an increasing number of women with congenital malformations are attending antenatal clinics. A highly organized series of medical examinations in neonatal nurseries, child welfare clinics and schools, plus a much better knowledge and under-standing of congenital heart disease amongst the medical examiners, has identified the vast majority of those who are born with malforma-tions long before they reach childbearing age. Many of our present patients in the maternity hospital have been our patients since infancy and they have grown up in a society whose attitudes towards heart disease have changed so much that it is no longer regarded as an impediment to marriage or motherhood.

The majority are of only mild or moderate severity and of no great haemodynamic significance. Most of them tolerate pregnancy well and require no special care or treatment other than that outlined above. The more serious cases have nearly all been either improved or cured by palliative or corrective surgery long before they became pregnant and again cause remarkably little trouble, even those with mild persistent cyanosis. It should be remembered, however, that when the packed cell volume is more than about 60 per cent the chance of producing a live baby is poor, and that residual post-operative malformations, cardiomegaly or disturbances of rhythm may still lead to difficulties during pregnancy in women who so far as exercise tolerance is concerned, regarded themselves as cured before becoming pregnant. Those with severe obstructive lesions or large left to right shunts should have cardiac surgery before pregnancy or, if pregnant, should be terminated and have cardiac surgery before further pregnancy. Those with complex and inoperable lesions, which are often associated with severe cyanosis and gross right ventricular hypertrophy, present considerable problems of management and are best advised against pregnancy. So are those whose pulmonary hypertension is sufficiently severe to result in a right to left shunt through an associated septal defect or ductus arteriosus (the Eisenmenger Syndrome), because this is a particularly lethal combination carrying a maternal mortality in the region of 30–40 per cent. If patients with these severe types of congenital malformations are already pregnant when seen for the first time, termination and sterilization should be advised.

Ischaemic heart disease

This is uncommon in young women of childbearing age and many cases included under this classification are almost certainly not caused by atheroma. The increasing frequency of ischaemic heart disease in young men has been less striking in women and has so far had no impact on the national figures in the Confidential Reports on Maternal Mortality (Fig. 12.2); perhaps because the overall pattern of childbearing in this country has also changed in recent years and most women are having their children at a much younger age than they used to do. However, there is now evidence that the contraceptive pill may be causing an increased prevalence of this type of heart disease in women of childbearing age who were previously thought to be in some way protected until the menopause.

The natural history of pregnancy complicated by ischaemic heart disease is much less well defined than it is in rheumatic and congenital heart disease. As with other types of heart disease, each pregnancy must be judged on its merits taking account of age, parity, heart size, cardiac grade, etc. Successful pregnancies have been recorded in such patients, but as they run a high risk of shortened lives and an unpredictable liability to sudden death, pregnancy should be avoided.

REFERENCES (SECTION 1)

Burwell, C. S. & Metcalfe, J. (1958) *Heart Disease and Pregnancy : Physiology and Management*, London: J. & A. Churchill.
Editorial (1964) *Lancet*, ii, 240.
Haig, D. C. & Gilchrist, A. R. (1949) Heart disease complicated by pregnancy. *Edinb. med. J.*, **101**, 55.
Jones, A. M. (1951) *Heart Disease in Pregnancy*. London: Harvey and Blythe.
Marquis, R. M. (1969) Mitral disease and pregnancy. *J. roy Coll. Physic. Lond.*, **3**, 121.
Mendelson, C. L. (1960) *Cardiac Disease in Pregnancy*. Philadelphia: F. A. Davis.

FURTHER READING

Barnes, C. G. (1970) *Medical Disorders in Obstetric Practice*, 3rd edn. Oxford: Blackwell.
Haynes, D. M. (1969) *Medical Complications During Pregnancy*. New York: McGraw-Hill.
Perkins, R. P. (1971) Inherited disorders of haemoglobin synthesis and pregnancy. *Amer. J. Obstet. Gynec.*, **111**, 120.
Rothman, Doreen (1970) Folic acid in pregnancy. *Amer. J. Obstet. Gynec.*, **108**, 149.
Rovinsky, J. J. & Guttmacher, A. F. (1965) *Medical, Surgical and Gynecologic Complications of Pregnancy*, 2nd edn. Edinburgh: Livingstone.
Steingold, L. (1962) In *Recent Advances in Obstetrics and Gynaecology*, 10th edn., Ch. 8, p. 191. Edited by A. W. Bourne & L. H. Williams. London: Churchill.

SECTION 2: DISEASES OF THE RESPIRATORY SYSTEM

During pregnancy there is increased pulmonary ventilation at rest from early in the first trimester (*see* Chapter 5). During labour, especially in the late first and early second stages, there is a marked increase in inspiratory flow and up to 250 litres per minute may be exceeded. There is therefore a need for free respiratory excursion and the patient in whom gas transfer is embarrassed will need special care.

This is particularly to be remembered when gaseous analgesia or anaesthesia is used and, for example, up to 1500 litres of analgesic gas mixture may be required for a normal primigravid labour (Crawford and Tunstall, 1968).

It has also to be remembered that as a consequence of the hyperventilation there is normally some slight increase in arterial pO_2 and a marked fall in pCO_2 (Andersen and Walker, 1970). Hyperventilation often associated with fear or pain is greatly lessened by the use of epidural anaesthesia.

Upper respiratory infection

Pregnant women are more prone to upper respiratory infection and greater care than usual should be taken—bed rest, warmth and the usual simple measures are adequate if taken early and efficiently. Pneumonia is, however, a more common and relatively serious disease.

Pneumonia

Before the days of active therapy with antibiotics bacterial pneumonia was a frequent cause of maternal death and is still in communities when care is inadequate or absent or during epidemics of influenzal pneumonia. Active and early treatment as in the non-pregnant will prevent serious effects. As with all serious illness, abortion and premature labour may occur in the ill patient and the ill woman with active pneumonia stands labour badly. Pneumonia is a relatively rare complication of the pregnant woman with *varicella* but can be extremely serious (Harris and Rhoades, 1965). Antibiotics should be given routinely and extreme respiratory support may be required especially in the third trimester.

Inhalation pneumonias

Multilobar or segmented pneumonia associated with retention of secretion in the bronchitic or asthmatic patient, or in the ill, or post-operative patient with pulmonary collapse or inadequate respiratory excursion may be severe and prolonged. Therapy will be as in the non-pregnant but should be active. In post-operative pulmonary collapse active physiotherapy is indicated and occasionally bronchoscopy is necessary. The classical inhalation pneumonia of the pregnant woman *Mendelson's syndrome* is that associated with inhalation of gastric contents during anaesthesia and, especially before being clearly recognized, was a very serious condition indeed. Multilobar collapse with shock, cyanosis, tachycardia, and dyspnoea immediately follows anaesthesia during which there may (or sometimes not) have been obvious regurgitation or vomiting of stomach contents. Pneumonia with infection of the collapsed areas and abscess may follow. Intensive respiratory support may be necessary for many days but lesser degrees recover with routine therapy. It is believed that the condition follows inhalation of acid stomach contents and that there is a special risk associated with ergometrine used at delivery which may alter pulmonary vascular behaviour. This condition is now very rare with the development of expert obstetric anaesthetic skills and the less frequent use of general anaesthesia but nevertheless is still a risk. Routine use of magnesium trisilicate in labour to lessen the acidity of the stomach contents, intravenous fluid nourishment of the labouring woman who might need anaesthesia, local, pudendal, epidural, or caudal analgesics where possible, and use of an expert practitioner to give general anaesthesia where necessary, have made the incidence very low indeed.

Bronchitis and bronchiectasis

Serious degrees of respiratory embarrassment in the patient with chronic pulmonary disease may rarely make successful pregnancy impossible. Usually, however, there is merely some increase in the discomfort. Special care must be applied to prevent or rapidly treat superadded pneumonic change. Routine therapy as in the non-pregnant, intensified if necessary, is usually sufficient.

Tuberculosis

Pulmonary tuberculosis is a special problem in the tropics and is discussed in Chapter 26. Active tuberculosis in pregnancy in the United Kingdom is a relative rarity. It is generally accepted that pregnancy should not be encouraged within two years of cure of an active pulmonary, renal or other infection—although termination on these grounds is now rarely required. In view largely of the risk to the developing fetus routine radiography of the chest in pregnant woman is now not permitted. Routine check may, however, be necessary in patients with a known or suspicious history or in those recently immigrated from less favoured countries. Active tuberculosis confirmed in pregnancy must be actively treated and hospitalization is probably wise. No special obstetric care is required but the special risk to the baby must be remembered and the baby immediately isolated from the infectious mother until it is obvious that the classical post delivery exacerbation has not occurred and she is cleared to be non-infectious—BCG inoculation helps to protect the infant.

Sarcoidosis

The effects of pregnancy on this relatively rare disease and of the disease on pregnancy are unpredictable. In view of the clinical and pathological resemblance to tuberculosis the necessary investigations are required. Hodgkin's disease and systemic granulomas may require to be excluded. Therapy should be of the disease and isoniazid and corticosteroid may be required. Special care may be required depending on the organs specially involved.

Asthma

Pregnancy often relieves the frequency and severity of attacks but this is by no means always so. Premature labour does not usually follow minor attacks but severe with hypercapnea and hypoxia are often seriously detrimental to the pregnancy. The known asthmatic should always be under the joint care of a respiratory disease physician and the obstetrician. Routine therapy may be salbutamol orally with or without steroids and should be continued although newer therapies with sodium cromoglycate (Imtal) by inhalation may be used to prevent attacks. The moderately acute attack should respond to B_2 stimulants like salbutamol by inhaler. Failure of quick response merits hospital admission where it may be necessary to allow fluid replacement to prevent unduly sticky secretions, oxygen antibiotics, salbutamol by inhaler, aminophylline 250mg IV over 10–20 minutes and occasionally large doses of steroids, e.g. hydrocortisone 100–500mg. In the really serious case expert respiratory support, bronchoscopy and artificial ventilation may be required.

There is no place for the B_1 B_2 stimulants, e.g. adrenaline (epinephrine) in view of the serious cardiac effects and morphine is contraindicated. Therapeutic abortion may be indicated if a previous pregnancy has produced serious risk. Recently asthmatic attacks have been noted on patients during prostaglandin (PGF_2) intravenous therapy for therapeutic abortion. This is due to the broncho restrictive effects of the drug and stops when the drug is discontinued.

REFERENCES (SECTION 2)

Andersen, G. J. & Walker, J. (1970) The effect of labour on the maternal blood gas and acid base status. *J. Obstet. Gynaec. Brit. Cwlth.*, 77, 284.

Crawford, J. S. & Tunstall, M. E. (1968) Notes on respiratory performance during labour. *Brit. J. Anaes.*, 40, 612.

Harris, R. E. & Rhoades, E. R. (1965) Varicella pneumonia complicating pregnancy. *Obstet. & Gynaec.*, 25, 734.

Selikoff, I. J. & Dorfmoun, H. L. (1965) The management of tuberculosis, in *Medical, Surgical and Gynaecological complications of pregnancy*. Edited by Rovinsky & A. F. Guttmacher. Edinburgh: Livingstone.

SECTION 3: ALIMENTARY AND ENDOCRINE SYSTEM

In view of the fact that during the nine months of pregnancy a fetus of about 3400g (7lb 8oz) is formed and nourished it is obvious that the problems of the mother's intake and absorption of food are most important. Usually the intake is increased and there is a corresponding increase in appetite, but disturbances of the digestive system are common. The most frequent is nausea and vomiting early in pregnancy which has been regarded by some as a normal feature of pregnancy. Many of the pathological states peculiar to pregnancy cause vomiting, but the conditions dealt with in this chapter are not discussed elsewhere.

Excessive salivation

Very occasionally, excessive salivation occurs between the second and fifth month of pregnancy. In severe cases up to 1000ml a day may be produced, all of which cannot be swallowed because of nausea. The condition is fairly difficult to treat, but astringent mouthwashes, atropine and sedatives should be tried. Intravenous fluids may occasionally be necessary.

Heartburn

This very common symptom usually appears about the fifth month of pregnancy and often goes away in the last month. It is described as a burning pain and is very similar to that caused by the reflux of gastric contents including bile into the lower end of the oesophagus in patients with hiatus hernia. In pregnancy the reflux is thought to be due to relaxation of the cardia coupled with increase of the intra-abdominal contents. Spasm of the oesophagus may be a factor in some cases. The pain is almost always accentuated by stooping or lying flat. Patients try to obtain relief by continually swallowing saliva, but this may produce vomiting. The patient should as far as possible avoid extreme bending and should sleep propped up by pillows in a semi-recumbent position. Although it is known that the degree of heartburn is not related to the degree of acidity of the gastric contents, temporary relief in most cases is obtained from antacid preparations, such as magnesium trisilicate and aluminium hydro-

xide. Some women suffer a great deal of discomfort despite all forms of treatment and may lose weight and become debilitated. Oesophageal ulceration with ultimate stenosis may follow the very severe case.

Peptic ulceration

Despite the prominence of heartburn and vomiting in the early months there is abundant evidence that pregnancy leads to a remission of symptoms in a very high proportion of women with chronic gastric or duodenal ulceration. Ulcer symptoms often return, however, shortly after delivery. The reason for this beneficial effect of pregnancy is quite unknown. One of the theories suggests that diminished acid secretion may occur during pregnancy, but so far there is no clear evidence that this is the explanation. A hormonal influence has also been postulated and seems to be a very probable explanation, although the mechanism is still obscure. Complications such as haemorrhage and perforation are very rare, and when these require surgery near to term a Caesarean section should be performed first (Jones et al., 1969). In view of the beneficial effect of pregnancy peptic ulceration by itself is seldom an indication for termination of pregnancy.

Ulcerative colitis and regional ileitis (Crohn's disease)

There is little information on the influence of pregnancy on the course of these diseases. They are both subject to remission and relapse and it is impossible to predict the effect of pregnancy on any individual patient. If either disease is inactive initially then pregnancy has little, if any, effect on the symptoms. When these conditions are mild or moderately active the effect of pregnancy is variable. If advice is sought about pregnancy, it is preferable to advise delay until the disease is in an inactive stage. Regardless of symptoms, however, pregnancy is usually taken to term without mishap. When ulcerative colitis develops during pregnancy it is often a very virulent disease and usually it is aggravated after delivery. The main problem of Crohn's disease in relation to child bearing is its significant association with sterility (Fielding and Cooke, 1970).

Jaundice in pregnancy is discussed in Chapter 11.

Acute appendicitis

The diagnosis of acute appendicitis becomes more difficult in the later months of pregnancy so that there is often delay in making a firm diagnosis and performing a laparotomy. It is said that the mortality from acute appendicitis in the later months is ten times as great as that in the early months of pregnancy. Difficulty in making an early clinical diagnosis is due to several causes. Abdominal pain and vomiting may be attributed to the pregnancy. The caecum and appendix may be displaced towards the right flank by the enlarging uterus so that the local signs are in an unusual position and poorly localized while the enlarged uterus obscures rigidity of the abdominal wall.

The differential diagnosis most commonly considered is acute pyelitis. When this condition is severe enough to cause abdominal pain the temperature and pulse rate are usually much higher than with acute appendicitis, and there is commonly a history of rigors. Urine is infected and usually contains numerous pus cells.

The clinical symptomatology of appendicitis is little different from that of the non-pregnant state. The signs may be a little altered but if the possibility is remembered the diagnosis is usually made. Early laparotomy is essential. Peritonitis is usually followed by abortion or premature labour.

Diabetes mellitus

The chief hazard of pregnancy in the diabetic is to the fetus. The combined stillbirth and neonatal mortality rate is about 10 per cent under optimal conditions in specialist centres and greater elsewhere. The fetal risk is relatively high even when the maternal diabetes is still in the asymptomatic (chemical) stage (Karlsson and Kjellmer, 1972).

MATERNAL ASPECT

Improved control of diabetes in children is allowing increasing numbers of young women with relatively long-standing diabetes to marry and become pregnant. The care of such women in pregnancy is a therapeutic challenge to both physician and obstetrician and best exercised in a combined medical-antenatal clinic. The prognosis for the pregnancy depends largely on the duration of the maternal diabetes, for both macro- and more specific microangiopathy increase with time, as do nephropathy and retinopathy. Good diabetic control seems to delay the progress of these complications but not altogether to prevent them. Diabetic *nephropathy* with a raised level of blood urea or severe *retinopathy* with vitreous haemorrhage or of the proliferative type may constitute a *contra-indication to pregnancy*, for both may progress more quickly during pregnancy.

Diagnosis

Women with a diabetic trait tend to show it in pregnancy which therefore represents an opportunity to make the diagnosis much earlier than would otherwise be possible (Drury and Timoney, 1970). Recognition of diabetes at this stage may avert the much later appearance of primary symptoms possibly already associated with complications. The patient who develops overt diabetes in pregnancy will tend to have the typical primary symptoms of diabetes with clearly raised levels of blood sugar, but in milder cases the blood sugar level 2–3 hours after a main meal is much more revealing than the fasting level which is lower than usual in pregnancy (Burt, 1960). If an oral glucose tolerance test is needed, it should be continued for 3 hours, for even in normal pregnancy the rate of fall of the blood sugar tends to be delayed, although the fasting level is typically low. *Chemical diabetes* occurs about six times as frequently in pregnancy as does the overt variety, and, since it is associated with an increased perinatal mortality, it is numerically more important in relation to fetal loss than is overt diabetes. It is important therefore to know which women are worth testing for chemical diabetes and how to treat them, once identified. The intravenous glucose tolerance test seems preferable to the oral one for it has been shown to be more reproducible in pregnancy and is considerably less time-consuming (Hadden *et al.*, 1971; Lind and Hytten, 1969). Furthermore, it avoids the factor of delayed gastrointestinal absorption of glucose which affects the oral test. Glycosuria has long been considered an indication for glucose tolerance testing in pregnancy, but since renal glycosuria is so common, glucose can be found in post-prandial urine specimens with glucose oxidase test strips in about 80 per cent of all pregnant women. It is now known that true fasting glycosuria is much more indicative of diabetes, although it is in fact a reflection of a marked reduction in the renal

revealed hyperplasia of the pancreatic islets of Langerhans, two or more abortions, the presence of a *major congenital fetal anomaly* in a previous pregnancy, the history of having previously produced a *heavy-for-dates* baby (*see* Table 12.1 for 95th percentile weights),

Table 12.1   Smoothed baby weight equivalent to 4082g (ic 95 percentile) at term with maternal height 1·575 metres

Maternal height in metres	1·473	1·499	1·524	1·549	1·575	1·600	1·626	1·651	1·676
34	3·190	3·190	3·290	3·400	3·400	3·515	3·515	3·515	3·630
35	3·290	3·290	3·400	3·515	3·515	3·630	3·745	3·745	3·860
36	3·400	3·400	3·515	3·515	3·630	3·745	3·745	3·860	3·860
37	3·630	3·630	3·630	3·745	3·745	3·860	3·860	3·975	4·090
38	3·745	3·745	3·745	3·745	3·860	3·860	3·975	3·975	4·090
39	3·745	3·860	3·860	3·860	3·860	3·975	4·090	4·090	4·200
40	3·860	3·975	3·975	4·090	4·090	4·090	4·200	4·200	4·315
41	3·975	4·090	4·200	4·200	4·200	4·200	4·315	4·315	4·430
42	3·975	4·090	4·200	4·315	4·315	4·315	4·315	4·430	4·545

(GESTATION IN WEEKS)

threshold for glucose. Thus glycosuria to *Clinistix* (that is true glycosuria) in a *second fasting urine* specimen tested at any time in pregnancy has been found to be associated with an incidence of approximately 20 per cent of chemical diabetes, whereas there is

the presence of an excessive fetal fat outline radiologically in the last four weeks of pregnancy or of unequivocal hydramnios. *Obesity* of the mother, e.g. the top fifteen percentile (*see* Table 12.2) is another indication for glucose tolerance testing, especially when the

Table 12.2   85 percentile weights (kg) (women)
(Without clothing and shoes. Height without shoes)

Height in metres	Age—years					
	15–19	20–24	25–29	30–34	35–39	40–44
1·47	49·0	51·3	53·5	56·7	58·5	61·7
1·50	50·4	52·6	54·9	58·5	59·9	63·5
1·52	51·7	54·4	56·3	59·9	61·2	64·9
1·55	53·5	56·3	58·1	61·2	63·1	66·2
1·58	54·9	57·6	59·4	63·1	64·4	67·6
1·60	56·7	59·0	60·8	64·9	66·2	69·4
1·63	58·5	60·8	62·6	66·7	68·0	71·2
1·65	59·9	62·1	64·0	68·0	69·4	72·6
1·68	61·2	63·5	65·3	69·4	70·8	73·9
1·70	63·1	65·3	67·1	70·8	72·6	75·3
1·73	64·4	66·7	68·5	72·6	73·9	77·1
1·75	65·8	68·5	69·9	73·9	75·2	78·5
1·78	67·6	70·3	71·7	75·3	76·7	80·3

Standard weights during pregnancy should be calculated from the non-pregnant standard weight as follows:

ADD 0·2 kg per week for the first 20 weeks, and then 0·5kg/week up to full term.

no correlation between purely postprandial glycosuria and chemical diabetes (Sutherland *et al.*, 1970). Other good indications for glucose tolerance testing in pregnancy include family history of diabetes in one or more first degree relatives, especially sibling, mother and maternal grandmother, and when the time of onset was before 50 years of age, the history of one or more *stillbirths*, especially if autopsy

mother was herself a heavy-for-dates baby, and so is *multiparity*, defined as five previous pregnancies carried to at least 28 weeks' duration. In circumstances where inadequate facilities for glucose tolerance testing exist, the very presence of these indications warrants special care for the risk to the fetus is increased even where the glucose tolerance is normal.

INFLUENCE OF PREGNANCY ON CARBOHYDRATE TOLERANCE

In normal pregnancy there are a number of changes which affect glucose tolerance. There are increased levels of plasma immunoreactive insulin in spite of active insulinases being in the placenta, increased resistance to injected insulin or sulphonylureas taken by mouth and a smaller Growth Hormone response to hypoglycaemia. Especially in the last trimester, there are high circulating levels of placental lactogen (HPL) which has a relatively weak Growth Hormone-like action on carbohydrate metabolism, and increased levels of cortisol and thyroxine bound to specific carrier proteins. The changes in oral glucose tolerance in normal pregnancy have already been mentioned and both oral and intravenous tests show some progressive reduction of tolerance from the second to the third trimester with a rapid return to higher values post-partum. These changes in normal pregnancy occur within the limits of normal glucose tolerance in the non-pregnant state, but are reflected by the same trends in those who become pregnant when already diabetic. Thus in the first trimester there is an increased incidence of hypoglycaemia associated with the vagaries of appetite and tendency to morning sickness but in the last trimester the insulin requirement rises only to fall quickly postpartum. There is increased lability of levels of glucose and ketones in the blood and this is complicated by the associated renal glycosuria. *Clinitesting* of urine becomes more meaningful in terms of the desirable range of blood sugar levels if only two drops instead of the usual five of urine are tested with thirteen instead of the usual ten drops of water.

EFFECT OF DIABETES ON PREGNANCY

Diabetes is associated with an increased incidence of pre-eclampsia, hydramnios, fetal abnormality and increased weight of the baby and placenta. The same tendency for fetal oversize does not seem to occur when the diabetes is at only the chemical stage, although such individuals may have a history of having previously borne a heavy-for-dates baby. Diabetic mothers with vascular complications also tend to have light-for-dates babies. The baby of a diabetic mother tends to have an increased proportion of fat, to be polycythaemic and to develop hypoglycaemia in the first few days of extra-uterine life.

Among other features positively associated with diabetic pregnancies are abnormal presentations of the fetus, monilial vaginitis, pyelitis and symptomless bacteriuria.

The risk to the fetus

The increased fetal risk in diabetic pregnancies remains the chief problem, for although the baby may be oversize at birth it carries many of the risks of premature babies born to non-diabetic mothers. Of these, the most important is the respiratory distress syndrome, associated with hyaline membrane disease of the lungs, found especially in babies born by Caesarean section. Diabetic pregnancies produce not only an increased proportion of heavy-for-dates babies but also a group who are light-for-dates, and these have a worse prognosis. Congenital anomalies have an increased frequency but do not contribute much to the increased perinatal mortality, which is found largely in association with pre-eclampsia, hydramnios and poor control of the mother's diabetes. Babies of diabetic mothers, like those affected by erythroblastosis fetalis, tend to have hyperplasia of the pancreatic beta cells in the islets of Langerhans. Thus it is not surprising that they should tend to develop hypoglycaemia for a few days postnatally, and, in contrast to their mothers, they have an unusually good tolerance to glucose with relative hyperinsulinism. It seems likely that maternal hyperglycaemia which controls the fetal level of blood sugar, is the main factor of producing hyperinsulinism, although this may occur even when maternal diabetes is very mild. Episodes of maternal hypoglycaemia do not appear to endanger the fetus, but ketosis does and has to be prevented carefully. Thus meticulous control of the maternal diabetes is the main factor which can improve the prognosis for the fetus. A careful balance has to be made between the increased risk of death *in utero* and in the neonatal period. It seems justifiable to allow pregnancy to persist until term only if the maternal control of blood sugar has been excellent, and in most cases delivery between 21 and 14 days before the expected date of delivery is to be preferred. The baby of a diabetic mother should be given the special care of a premature baby even if it appears unusually large. The perinatal fetal loss remains about 10 per cent (about five times normal) even under optimal conditions and to this must be added the increased risk of abortion in diabetic pregnancies.

Management of the pregnant diabetic

Termination of pregnancy with sterilization is advised if the mother already has severe enough nephropathy to be associated with a blood urea level above 50mg/100ml or the haemorrhagic type of retinopathy with seriously impaired vision, even if only in one eye. Where the diabetic has already had several pregnancies and has at least one living child, termination should be considered.

It is important that the pregnant diabetic should be under the combined care of a physician and an obstetrician both with special knowledge of the condition. The principal aim of the antenatal care in the first 28 weeks of pregnancy is to *establish the correct gestational age* by vaginal examinations, repeated clinical assessments and sonar scans from around twenty weeks. Later in pregnancy the early signs of hydramnios, pre-eclampsia and of unduly rapid fetal growth are sought at frequent visits. The physician should see the patient often in order to obtain optimal control of the blood sugar level, for which special instruction of the patient will be required. Weight gain should be carefully supervised and it is not particularly necessary to increase the caloric intake merely because of the pregnancy. Calorie restriction should be used for significantly obese diabetics, so long as the protein content of the diet is not reduced below 1g/kg actual body weight per day. In extreme examples such diets have been associated with overall weight loss during pregnancy and yet with normal birth weight of the baby. Obese diabetics with only chemical diabetes can usually be treated by diet alone. Small doses of sulphonylureas (not more than 100mg of Chlorpropamide a day) have been used successfully for pregnant chemical diabetics of more normal weight and may reverse the maternal diabetes (Sutherland *et al.*, 1973), but larger doses of sulphonylureas seem to increase the perinatal mortality and stimulate hypoglycaemia in the newborn. They do not seem to be teratogenic. If a woman needs a sulphonylurea to control her diabetes before pregnancy, she is best treated with insulin, such as a modest dose of Semitard MC Insulin during pregnancy. This is one of the Monocomponent Insulins which have the theoretical advantage of having little or no antigenicity, for IgG antibodies to Insulin can cross the placenta and may contribute to the development of fetal pancreatic beta cell hyperplasia.

Clinitesting of the urine for sugar should be done before each main meal with only two drops of urine and thirteen of water, as already mentioned, and if the full colour development occurs, ketonuria should be sought using Acetest tablets or Ketostix strips. If either of these tests is strongly positive, the degree of ketosis warrants admitting the patient to hospital for urgent stabilization. Significant ketonuria demands increased dosage of insulin with the use of sucrose containing drinks between meals if there is associated anorexia. In the presence of vomiting intravenous therapy will be needed urgently. The soluble, preferably Actrapid MC, insulin should then be given at a dose of 4–8 units in every hour or by continuous im infusion at a rate of 4–6 units an hour. *Insulin-dependent diabetics* are best treated with the Actrapid MC variety given twice daily, usually about two-thirds of the total dose before breakfast and the remaining one-third before the evening meal. In some patients with an unusually long interval between breakfast and evening meal, a third dose may be needed before lunch. If there is more than minimal glycosuria in a second fasting morning urine specimen, the bedtime snack of carbohydrate should be reduced, and if this proves inadequate, Semitard MC should be given instead of the soluble variety before the evening meal to improve the overnight control. Optimal control of the blood sugar is facilitated by giving the patient a scale of dosage of each insulin based on urine Clinitests. Thus undue glycosuria before breakfast is the signal for increasing the evening dose of insulin, and before the evening meal or lunch the morning dose of insulin. This 'reverse testing technique' tends to reduce the swings of blood sugar level (Stowers, 1972). The overall aim is to achieve as normal levels of blood sugar as possible without disabling hypoglycaemia and to avoid ketosis which will endanger the fetus. If the diabetes is particularly difficult to control during the last trimester of pregnancy, or if there is a history of previous unsuccessful pregnancy it may be advisable to keep the patient closely supervised in hospital with frequent estimations of pre-meal blood sugar levels for weeks or even months. At follow-up visits at a combined medical/antenatal clinic, measurements are made of the patient's weight, blood pressure, urine sugar using Clinistix for the chemical diabetics and both Clinistix and

Clinitest for overt diabetics. Clinitest is effected by lactose and other reducing substances but the non-quantitative Clinistix is specific for glucose. Uristix may be preferred to Clinistix, as measurement should be made also for proteinuria. The obstetrician needs to assess fetal size and presentation, sometimes with the help of a sonar scan and to listen to the fetal heart. Confirmation of fetal maturity may be assessed radiologically after the beginning of the 37th week. Measurements of plasma or urinary oestriol may be of value in assessing the well-being of the pregnancy and deciding when it is best to deliver the patient, especially in the presence of associated hypertension.

DELIVERY

The decision whether to deliver naturally or by Caesarean section is taken primarily on obstetric rather than on medical grounds. The optimum time for delivery will depend largely on freedom from obstetric complications, such as pre-eclampsia and on the assessment of fetal size. In the absence of complications the present tendency is to deliver the mother after 37 completed weeks gestation rather than earlier in order to reduce the neonatal mortality without appreciable risk of increasing the stillbirth rate. Hydramnios, a very large fetus or pre-eclampsia may favour a decision to deliver the mother earlier. Since the commonest cause of neonatal death in diabetic pregnancy is respiratory distress syndrome, associated with hyaline membrane disease of the lungs, efforts have been made to predict the likelihood of this before delivering the patient. The lecithin/sphyomyelin ratio in the amniotic fluid is measured (see Chapter 18) (Bhagwanini et al., 1972; Clements et al., 1972).

The physical exertion of labour in association with anorexia at this time reduces the requirement for insulin and the post-partum insulin dose needed is usually close to that required before the start of the pregnancy. Long labour should be avoided for the sake of the fetus, whose viability may be precarious, and to ease the control of the maternal diabetes. Thus labour is induced surgically at a carefully selected time and controlled with an iv infusion of oxytocin under suitable antibiotic cover. An elective forceps delivery is then done in the second stage and with a paediatrician in attendance to take over the immediate care or resuscitation of the baby. If the baby is a typical 'Cushingoid' progeny of a diabetic mother shoulder girdle dystocia may be a problem.

Before Caesarean section a drip of 10 per cent glucose is run in at a rate of about 500ml in four hours and then Soluble Insulin is given on an eight-hourly basis according to a scale of blood sugar values which may be assessed sufficiently accurately by using Dextrostix. Rather less Soluble Insulin is needed preoperatively than is usually taken before breakfast. If the intravenous drip has to be continued for more than 24 hours, a half litre of 5 per cent Dextrose in physiological saline is included, for there must be a continuous infusion of glucose. When oral feeding is restarted, Soluble Insulin is given shortly before the three main meals, about $\frac{3}{6}$ths of the total daily dose before breakfast, $\frac{1}{6}$th before lunch and $\frac{2}{6}$ths before the evening meal, each dose depending on the result of the Clinitest done on urine passed before that meal. When the insulin-dependent mother is discharged from hospital the level of control of the diabetes should be relaxed sufficiently to reduce the risk of hypoglycaemia which might endanger her handling of the baby. If the diabetes was diagnosed during pregnancy and ketosis never developed, it is likely that insulin or a small dose of sulphonylurea can be discontinued as long as careful observation is made of tests for glycosuria, but a glucose tolerance test should be done four to six weeks after delivery for in about 20–30 per cent of such women diabetes will be found still to be present. In planning contraception it is wise to avoid the use of the standard types of pill which have a definite although fairly weak diabetogenic effect.

It may be reassuring for the diabetic mother to know that even when both parents are diabetic the overall incidence of overt diabetes in their children has not been found in Britain greatly to exceed that in the population as a whole.

Diabetes insipidus

The effect of pregnancy upon the clinical course of diabetes insipidus is variable and unpredictable. The prior existence of diabetes insipidus in a woman does not appear usually to alter her fertility, the course of her pregnancy, the effectiveness of her labour or her ability to lactate (Hendricks, 1954). Before establishing the diagnosis of neurohypophyseal diabetes insipidus it is first necessary to prove that any pregnant woman demonstrating marked polyuria and polydipsia does not have diabetes mellitus, psychogenic polydipsia or nephrogenic diabetes insipidus. Diabetes mellitus is easily identified by the glycosuria and high blood sugar level and a hypertonic saline infusion test (Carter and Robbins, 1947), followed where necessary by an injection of pitressin will differentiate between the other two possibilities. Hypertonic saline will lead to ADH secretion and decreased diuresis in case of psychogenic polydipsia, but not in true neurophypophyseal or nephrogenic diabetes insipidus. While the neurohypophyseal type responds to pitressin by injection, the renal type does not. In cases of incomplete neurohypophyseal failure there will be a partial response to hypertonic saline. In women already known to have diabetes insipidus when they become pregnant it is more common for the symptoms to relapse than to remit during pregnancy. Such relapses may be due to increased enzymatic destruction of ADH in the blood, for inactivation of ADH by blood from pregnant women has been demonstrated *in vitro* (Dieckmann *et al.*, 1950). While severe uterine atony has been reported in some patients with diabetes insipidus, this is rare and labour usually proceeds normally. In such cases it is of course open to doubt the totality of the posterior pituitary deficiency. Normal milk ejection has been reported in cases of diabetes insipidus but suckling stimulates the release of much more oxytocin than ADH (Chau, S. S. *et al.*, 1969).

The main points in the management of pregnant women with diabetes insipidus are to confirm the diagnosis, to deal promptly with urinary retention or infection and to give pitressin tannate in oil or Disipidin snuff to control their symptoms. Some caution is required near to term in the use of such preparations and delivery should not be delayed until after term). There is no contra-indication to using an oxytocin drip, and a watch should be kept for uterine atony post-partum. Lactation usually occurs normally.

Adrenal insufficiency

In normal pregnancy there appears to be an increased formation of cortisol and a decreased rate of its destruction. There is also increased binding of cortisol to its carrier serum protein (transcortin). Thus levels of plasma cortisol rise progressively during pregnancy reaching peak values at the time of labour (Bayliss *et al.*, 1955). Isotopic studies have shown that the daily production of aldosterone is increased in pregnancy to about three times the non-pregnant level (Jones, K. M. *et al.*, 1959).

Patients with untreated Addison's disease seldom become pregnant. Late pregnancy has a favourable effect on Addisonian symptoms but early pregnancy tends to be poorly tolerated due to episodes of severe nausea and vomiting. Hormone studies have shown that most Addisonian pregnant patients have a normal or almost normal rise in the excretion of corticoids, 17-oxosteroids and pregnanediol in the urine (Jailer and Knowlton, 1950). Despite this increase in steroid metabolites in the urine these patients do not respond to the administration of ACTH. The extra steroids of placental origin do not prevent the development of an acute adrenal cortical crisis (Hills *et al.*, 1954). Addison's disease is not an indication for therapeutic abortion but such women need full replacement treatment with Cortisone or Cortisol with increased dosage to cover parturition and the early puerperium when the adrenal crisis would be most likely to occur. Vaginal delivery is in order and the weight and life expectancy of the baby should be nearly or quite normal if the mother's adrenal insufficiency has been well treated.

Porphyria

The most important of the porphyrias found in pregnancy is the acute intermittent type and even this is rare. Its importance is that each case represents a potential maternal death which may be related to the injudicious use of barbiturates, sulphonamides or alcohol. As this form of porphyria presents with hypertension, which may be attributed to pre-eclamptic toxaemia, barbiturates may be prescribed and further exacerbate the condition. The symptoms are protean and in order of frequency include abdominal pain, vomiting, constipation, paresis, psychological disturbance and non-abdominal pain. The commonest signs are tachycardia, hypertension, reduced or absent tendon reflexes, abnormalities of sensation and cranial neuropathies, often with a leucocytosis and mild fever and sometimes with hyponatraemia and hypochloraemia (Goldberg, 1959). Most of the deaths, 27 per cent of 73 patients in one series (Hunter, 1971), were due to failure to recognize the presence of the acute intermittent porphyria and thus to avoid potentially hepatotoxic drugs. The biochemical diagnosis of this type of porphyria depends on finding increased levels of porphyrins and their precursors in the urine, for example d-amino laevulinic acid, porphobilinogen (Watson-Schwartz test) copro- and uroporphyrin.

Pica and craving

Vagaries of appetite are common and may start early in the course of pregnancy. Thus in a study of 600 consecutive pregnant women attending Harlem Hospital, New York, Posner and his colleagues (1957) found that 394 had an urgent and imperative longing, that is a craving, for food, and 10 had Pica which can be defined as a longing to eat substances that are not fit for food, such as coal or clay. Harries and Hughes (1958) found that in their British survey the main craving was for fruit, followed by raw vegetables, confections, pickles and raw cereals. Such attitudes to food are to be contrasted with hyperemesis gravidarium and psychological theories have been constructed to explain them both.

THE THYROID

Physiological changes in pregnancy

It is possible to detect enlargement of the thyroid in pregnancy by clinical means in 25–85 per cent of subjects. Such 'pregnancy goitres' have been regarded as a compensation for the increased renal loss of inorganic iodide in pregnancy (Aboul-Khair et al., 1964), but an important additional factor appears to be a pre-existing iodine deficiency. Thus Crooks and his colleagues (1967) found no increase in goitres in pregnancy in Iceland, whereas an earlier study in the north-east of Scotland by the same group (Aboul-Khair et al., 1964) had shown an increase in the incidence of goitre in women of childbearing age from 37 per cent when non-pregnant, to 76 per cent when pregnant. The difference in the two communities was attributed to the high fish diet in Iceland and was confirmed by measurements of plasma inorganic iodide in the two communities.

The BMR is normal in early pregnancy and then rises from 8 to 25 per cent or more above non-pregnant standards. A number of reasons can be cited to account for such a rise, such as increased cardiac and respiratory work, but it has been suggested that the energy production of a unit mass of maternal tissue remains unchanged if the fetal surface area is added to the maternal surface area. In the puerperium the BMR falls promptly to a nadir several weeks post-partum (Rowe et al., 1931).

The serum protein bound iodine (PBI) rises from early on in pregnancy but the tri-iodothyronine resin uptake falls. The rise in PBI is produced by an increase in thyroxine-binding globulin (Ralli et al., 1964) so that the level of circulating free thyroxine remains normal (Sterling and Brenner, 1966). I^{131} uptake is increased in pregnancy (Ralli et al., 1964) and there is a consistent but variable increase in lipoproteins and cholesterol.

Placental permeability

The 12–24 week old human fetus has levels of thyroxine and PBI which are hypothyroid by adult standards (Osorio and Myant, 1962), but since the protein-binding capacity for thyroxine is also low, free thyroxine levels are similar to those of the mother (Marks et al., 1966). It appears that only free and perhaps weakly bound thyroxine participates in any transplacental flux (French and Van Wyk, 1964). The relevant factors for the transfer rates in each direction are not only the levels in the two circulations, but the size of the two pools of binding globulin. In humans little I^{131} reaches the fetus when radioactive thyroxine is injected into the mother during the early stages of pregnancy (Myant, 1964), but at term there is evidence that relatively large amounts of I^{131}-labelled thyroxine and especially I^{131}-labelled tri-iodothyronine can be transferred from the maternal to the fetal circulation (Grumbach and Werner, 1956; Kearns and Nutson, 1963). Nevertheless it appears that the rate of thyroid hormone transport from the mother is insufficient to support normal skeletal and brain development when the fetus has a primary thyroideal defect. It seems that virtually no thyroid stimulating hormone (TSH) crosses the placenta (Editorial, 1967), but transient neonatal Grave's disease has been attributed to placental transfer of long-acting thyroid stimulator (LATS), since the latter is found in both the maternal and fetal circulations in most cases of maternal Grave's disease (McKenzie, 1964).

Fetal thyroid function

The earliest time when the full adult range of iodinated compounds can be recovered from the fetal thyroid is at about 74 gestational days (68mm stage) (Shepard, 1967) and this corresponds to the time when the thyroid to body weight ratio reaches adult proportions (Shepard et al., 1964) and when the follicles are beginning to accumulate colloid (Shepard, 1967). A normal fetal pituitary-thyroid dependence has been shown to be present in the fifth month of gestation by studies of formation of a fetal goitre by drug-induced hypothyroidism (Davis and Forbes, 1945).

Hyperthyroidism

IN THE NON-PREGNANT
This may well be associated with normal reproductive function, although there appears to be an increased incidence of amenorrhea, oligomenorrhea and menometrorrhagia (Goldsmith et al., 1952). However, studies of the menstrual pattern of fairly small numbers of women with thyrotoxicosis have shown that a significant number are anovulatory with consequent impairment of fertility (Goldsmith et al., 1952). In general, the greater the degree of the hyperthyroidism the greater is the incidence of menstrual irregularities (Benson and Dailey, 1955).

IN THE PREGNANT
Hyperthyroidism has been claimed to have a frequency of about 1 in a 1000 pregnancies (Javert, 1940) and can very rarely be considered to have been precipitated by pregnancy. The course of hyperthyroidism is usually ameliorated in pregnancy (Astwood, 1951), possibly because of the reduced values of plasma inorganic iodide (Aboul-Khair et al., 1964). The perinatal mortality should not be significantly increased (Mussey et al., 1926).

The diagnosis of hyperthyroidism is difficult in pregnancy not only because symptoms such as heat intolerance, dyspnoea and tachypnoea are found in normal pregnancy, wherein the thyroid gland frequently becomes visible and palpable (Aboul-Khair et al., 1964), but most measurements of thyroid function rise normally in pregnancy. Thus an increase in serum PBI can be detected as early as two weeks after conception and normal pregnancy values range from 310–1580nmol/l (mean 700), i.e. 4–20μg/100ml (mean 8·8) compared to 310–630nmol/l (mean 440), i.e. 4–8μg/100ml (mean 5·6) for non-pregnant women (De Mowbray and Tickner, 1952). It is unwise to administer I^{131} in pregnancy (Shepard, 1967) especially after the twelfth week when fetal damage may occur with concentration of the radioactive isotope in the thyroid (Chapman et al., 1948) but I^{132} with its inconveniently short half-life, is relatively safe. Tri-iodothyronine resin uptake tests may be of considerable value in pregnancy (McGoogan et al., 1962), especially as they involve no administration of radio-iodine to the mother or even a need for her to attend a laboratory. More sophisticated tests such as the free thyroxine factor (Goolden et al., 1967) or the T4 free-thyroxine index (Howarth and Ward, 1972), carry the additional advantage that they are unaffected by pregnancy or oestrogen-containing contraceptives, or, in the case of the latter test, by drugs such as iodide or the thiouracils, which may interfere with other tests. In mild cases of possible hyperthyroidism in pregnancy it may be wise to postpone attempts at definitive diagnosis until about six weeks post-partum.

In the treatment of hyperthyroidism in pregnancy it is seldom if ever warranted to perform a therapeutic abortion (Javert, 1940). Such cases are normally managed by using antithyroid drugs, such as Carbimazole, in rather smaller dosage than would be given for non-pregnant patients, because of the danger of producing a cretinous baby (Burrow, 1965). Such treatment should be stopped after 34–36 weeks of gestation for the same reason, although it may need to be resumed post-partum. Subtotal thyroidectomy is reserved for those who fail to follow a medical regime or who have untoward reactions to antithyroid drugs. It is usually contra-indicated by cardiac failure or the initial presentation of the hyperthyroidism in the third trimester of pregnancy.

Hypothyroidism

OVARIAN FUNCTION
Women with hypothyroidism have an abnormally high rate of various menstrual abnormalities, such as amenorrhea or more commonly menorrhagia and metrorrhagia

(Scott and Mussey, 1964). Ovulation may fail to occur and there may be some reduction of oestrogen production from the ovaries (Goldsmith *et al.*, 1952). Furthermore subnormal levels of thyroid hormone have been shown to increase the transformation of oestradiol-17β to oestriol and decrease the formation of 2-hydroxylated metabolites, whereas high levels of thyroid hormone have the reverse effects (Fishman *et al.*, 1965). Such changes in oestrogen levels may be sufficient to disturb the hormonal feedback relationship between the ovary and the pituitary. Progesterone metabolism on the other hand does not appear to be significantly affected by hypothyroidism.

The main effect of oestrogens on thyroid function appears to be to increase levels of serum thyroxine-binding globulin with a secondary rise in PBI but without affecting the levels of free thyroxine (Oliner, 1968). Since most contraceptive drugs contain oestrogens, these also tend to raise levels of serum PBI (Starup and Friis, 1967).

In short, fertility is decreased by hypothyroidism, but even frank myxoedema is compatible with the production of live normal offspring (Osorio and Myant, 1960).

PREGNANCY

The diagnosis of hypothyroidism in pregnancy is difficult and a low level of serum PBI, that is not increased, as normally, in pregnancy, is rather more likely to be due to low oestrogen secretion than to hypothyroidism. When in doubt it is safer to treat such a pregnant woman with full replacement amounts of thyroxine during pregnancy, but to discontinue such treatment in the puerperium when the thyroid status can be more reliably assessed about 6–8 weeks post-partum.

Hypothyroidism is associated in general with an increased tendency to abortion or stillbirth, although their incidence does not correlate well with laboratory evidence of reduced thyroid function (Man *et al.*, 1951). There may be an increased tendency towards congenital anomalies in babies borne by hypothyroid mothers, although the evidence is scanty (Hodges *et al.*, 1952). Some corroborative data were, however, published by Greenman and his colleagues (1962) when they showed a greater incidence of mental and physical abnormalities among children whose mothers had low butanol-extractable iodine levels during pregnancy. It is still unknown whether transport of thyroid hormone across the placenta from mother to fetus can be sufficiently large to prevent hypothyroidism in the fetus by administration of thyroxine (T4) to the mother. Since there is some evidence that tri-iodothyronine (T_3) can cross the placenta more readily (Kearns and Nutson, 1963) it would seem reasonable to treat such mothers with T3 rather than T4 during pregnancy in a dose of 100–200μg/day.

REFERENCES (SECTION 3)

Aboul-Khair, S. A., Crooks, J., Turnbull, A. C. & Hytten, F. E. (1964) The physiological changes in thyroid function during pregnancy. *Clinical Science*, 27, 195.

Astwood, E. B. (1951) Use of antithyroid drugs during pregnancy. *J. of Clin. Endocr.* 11, 1045.

Bayliss, R. I. S., Browne, J. I. McC., Round, B. P. & Steinbeck, A. W. (1955) Plasma 17-hydroxycorticosteroids in pregnancy. *Lancet*, i, 62.

Benson, R. C. & Dailey, M. E. (1955) Menstrual pattern in hyperthyroidism and subsequent post-therapy hypothyroidism. *Surg. Gynec. Obstet.*, 100, 19.

Bhagwanini, S. G., Fahmy, D. & Turnbull, A. C. (1972) Quick determination of amniotic-fluid lecithin concentration for prediction of neonatal respiratory distress. *Lancet*, ii, 66.

Burrow, G. N. (1965) Neonatal goiter after maternal propylthioaracil therapy. *J. Endocr.* 25, 403.

Burt, R. L. (1960) Carbohydrate metabolism in pregnancy. *Clin. Obstet. Gynec.*, 3, 310.

Carter, A. C. & Robbins, J. (1947) Use of hypertonic saline infusions in differential diagnosis of diabetes insipidus and psychogenic polydipsia. *J. Clin. Endocr.* 7, 753.

Chapman, E. M., Corner, G. W., Robinson, D. & Evans, R. D. (1948) Collection of radioactive iodine by human fetal thyroid. *J. Clin. Endocr.*, 8, 717.

Chau, S. S., Fitzpatrick, R. J. & Jamieson, B. (1969) Diabetes insipidus and parturition. *J. Obstet. Gynaec. Brit. Cwlth.*, 76, 444.

Clements, J. A., Platzker, A. C., Tierney, D. F., Creasy, R. K., Hobel, C. J., Margolis, A. J. & Tooley, W. H. (1972) Assessment of the risk of the respiratory-distress syndrome by a rapid test for surfactant in amniotic fluid. *New Engl. J. Med.*, 286, 1077.

Crooks, J., Tulloch, M. I., Turnbull, A. C., Davidson, D. & Skulason, T. (1967) Comparative incidence of goitre in pregnancy in Iceland and Scotland. *Lancet*, **ii**, 625.

Davis, L. J. & Forbes, W. (1945) Thiouracil in pregnancy: effect on fetal thyroid. *Lancet*, **ii**, 740.

De Mowbray, R. R. & Tickner, A. (1952) Diagnostic value of estimations of protein-bound iodine in serum. *Lancet*, **ii**, 511.

Dieckmann, W. J., Egenholf, G. F., Morley, B. & Pottinger, R. E. (1950) Inactivation of antidiuretic hormone of posterior pituitary gland by blood from pregnant patients. *Amer. J. Obstet. Gynec.*, **60**, 1043.

Drury, M. I. & Timoney, F. J. (1970) Latent diabetes in pregnancy. *J. Obstet. Gynaec. Brit. Cwlth.*, **77**, 24.

Editorial (1967) Transplacental passage of thyroid hormones. *New Engl. J. Med.*, **277**, 486.

Fielding, J. F. & Cooke, W. T. (1970) Pregnancy and Crohn's disease. *Brit. Med. J.*, **ii**, 76.

Fishman, J., Hellman, L., Zumoff, B. & Gallagher, T. F. (1965) Effect of thyroid on hydroxylation of estrogen in man. *J. Clin. Endocr.*, **25**, 365.

French, F. S. & Van Wyk, J. (1964) Fetal hypothyroidism. I. Effects of thyroxine on neural development. II. Fetal versus maternal contributions to fetal thyroxine requirements. III. Clinical implications. *J. Pediat.*, **64**, 589.

Gillner, M. D. G., Beard, R. W., Brooke, F. N. & Oakley, N. H. (1975) Carbohydrate metabolism in pregnancy—Parts I and II. *Brit. Med. J.*, **3**, 399, 1402.

Goldberg, A. (1959) Acute intermittent porphyria; a study of 50 cases. *Quart. J. Med.*, **28**, 183.

Goldsmith, R. E., Sturgis, S. N., Lerman, J. & Stanbury, J. B. (1952) Menstrual pattern in thyroid disease. *J. Clin. Endocr.*, **12**, 846.

Goolden, A. W. G., Gartside, J. M. & Sanderson, C. (1967) Thyroid status in pregnancy and in women taking oral contraceptives. *Lancet*, **i**, 12.

Greenman, G. W., Gabrielson, O., Howard-Flanders, J. & Wessel, M. A. (1962) Thyroid dysfunction in pregnancy. Fetal loss and follow-up evaluation of surviving infants. *New Engl. J. Med.*, **267**, 426.

Grumbach, M. M. & Werner, S. C. (1956) Transfer of thyroid hormone across the human placenta at term. *J. Clin. Endocr.*, **16**, 1392.

Hadden, D. R., Harley, J. M., Kajtar, T. J. & Montgomery, D. A. D. (1971) A prospective study of three tests of glucose tolerance in pregnant women selected for potential diabetes with reference to the fetal outcome. *Diabetologia*, **7**, 87.

Harries, J. M. & Hughes, T. F. (1958) Enumeration of the cravings of some pregnant women. *Brit. Med. J.*, **ii**, 39.

Hendricks, C. H. (1954) Neurohypophysis in pregnancy. *Obstet. gynaec. Surv.*, **9**, 323.

Hills, A. G., Venning, E. H., Dohan, F. C., Webster, G. D. Jr. & Richardson, E. M. (1954) Pregnancy and adrenocortical function: endocrine studies of pregnancy occurring in 2 adrenal-deficient women. *J. Clin. Invest.*, **33**, 1466.

Hodges, R. E., Hamilton, H. E. & Keettal, W. C. (1952) Pregnancy in myxedema. *Arch. intern. Med.* (Chicago), **90**, 863.

Howarth, P. J. N. & Ward, R. L. (1972) The T4-free thyroxine index as a test of thyroid function of first choice. *J. Clin. Path.*, **25**, 259.

Hunter, D. J. S. (1971) Acute intermittent porphyria and pregnancy. *J. Obstet. Gynaec. Brit. Cwlth.*, **78**, 746.

Jailer, J. W. & Knowlton, A. I. (1950) Simulated adreno-cortical activity in pregnancy in Addisonian patient. *J. Clin. Invest.*, **29**, 1430.

Javert, C. T. (1940) Hyperthyroidism and pregnancy. *Amer. J. Obstet. Gynec.*, **39**, 954.

Jones, K. M., Lloyd Jones, R., Riondel, A., Tait, J. F., Tait, S. A. S., Bulbrook, R. D. & Greenwood, F. C. (1959) Aldosterone secretion and metabolism in normal men and women and in pregnancy. *Acta Endocrinologica*, Copenhagen, **30**, 321.

Jones, P. F., McEwan, A. B. & Bernard, R. M. (1969) Haemorrhage and perforation complicating peptic ulcer in pregnancy. *Lancet*, **ii**, 350.

Karlsson, K. & Kjellmer, I. (1972) The outcome of diabetic pregnancies in relation to the mother's blood sugar level. *Amer. J. Obstet. Gynec.*, **112**, 213.

Kearns, J. E. & Nutson, W. J. (1963) Tagged isomers and analogues of thyroxine (their transmission across the human placenta and other studies). *Nuclear Medicine*, **4**, 453.

Komins, J. I., Snyder, P. J. & Schwarz (1975) Hyperthyroidism in pregnancy. *Obstet. Gynae. Surv.*, **30**, 522.

Lind, T. & Hytten, F. E. (1969) Blood glucose following oral loads of glucose, maltose and starch during pregnancy. *Proceedings of the Nutrition Society*, **28**, 64A.

Man, E. B., Heineman, M., Johnson, C., Leary, D. C. & Peters, J. P. (1951) The precipitable iodine of serum in normal pregnancy and its relation to abortions. *J. clin. invest.*, **30**, 137.

Marks, J. F., Hamlin, M. & Zack, P. (1966) Neonatal thyroid function. II. Free thyroxine in infancy. *J. Pediat.*, **68**, 559.

McGoogan, L. S., Langdon, R. N., Ogborn, R. E., Copley, J. S. & Burgin, W. W. (1962) Radioactive tri-iodothyronine uptake by red cells in pregnancy. *Amer. J. Obstet. Gynec.*, **83**, 1157.

McKenzie, J. M. (1964) Neonatal Grave's disease. *J. Clin. Endocr.*, **24**, 660.

Mussey, R. D., Plummer, W. A. & Boothby, W. M. (1926) Pregnancy complicating exophthalmic goiter and adenomatous goiter with hyperthyroidism. *J. Amer. med. Ass.*, **87**, 1009.

Myant, N. B. (1964) 'The Thyroid Gland and Reproduction in Mammals' in *The Thyroid Gland*. Edited by Pitt-Rivers, R. H. & Trotter, W. R. London: Butterworth, p. 228.

Oliner, L. (1968) 'Thyroid–Gonadal Interrelationships' in *Gynecologic Endocrinology*. Edited by Gold, J. J. New York: Hoeber, p. 115.

Osorio, C. & Myant, N. B. (1960) The passage of thyroid hormone from mother to foetus and its relation to foetal development. *Brit. med. Bull.*, **16**, 159.

Osorio, C. & Myant, N. B. (1962) The binding of thyroxine by human foetal serum. *Clinical Science*, **23**, 277.

Posner, L. B., McCottry, C. M. & Posner, A. C. (1957) Pregnancy craving and pica. *Obstet. Gynec.*, **9**, 270.

Ralli, J. E., Rubbins, J. & Lewallen, C. G. (1964) 'The Thyroid' in *Hormones V*. Edited by Pincus, G., Thimann, K. & Astwood, E. B. New York: Academic Press, p. 376.

Rowe, A. W., Gallivan, D. E. & Matthews, H. (1931) Metabolism in pregnancy; respiratory metabolism and acid elimination. *Amer. J. Physiol.*, **96**, 101.

Scott, J. C. Jr. & Mussey, E. (1964) Menstrual patterns in myxedema. *Amer. J. Obstet. Gynec.*, **90**, 161.

Shepard, T. H. (1967) Onset of function in the human fetal thyroid: biochemical and radioautographic studies from organ culture. *J. Clin. Endocr.*, **27**, 945.

Shepard, T. H., Andersen, H. U. & Andersen, H. (1964) The human fetal thyroid. I. Its weight in relation to body weight, crown-rump length, foot length and estimated gestation age. *Anatomical Records*, **148**, 123.

Starup, J. & Friis, T. (1967) Thyroid function in oral contraception. *Acta Endocrinologica* (Kobenhavn), **56**, 525.

Sterling, K. & Brenner, M. A. (1966) Free thyroxine in human serum: simplified measurement with the aid of magnesium precipitation. *J. clin Invest.*, **45**, 153.

Stowers, J. M. (1972) A critical appraisal of insulin treatment. *J. roy Coll. Physic.*, London, **7**, 69.

Sutherland, H. W., Stowers, J. M. & MacKenzie, C. (1970) Simplifying the clinical problem of glycosuria in pregnancy. *Lancet*, **i**, 1069.

Sutherland, H. W., Stowers, J. M. Cormack, J. D. & Bewsher, P. D. (1973) Chlorpropamide in chemical diabetes diagnosed during pregnancy. *Brit. med. J.*, **3**, 9.

FURTHER READING

Harris, R. E. & Podolosky, S. (1969) Endocrine complications of pregnancy. 101 cases. *Postgraduate Medicine*, **46**, 123.

Pedersen, J. (1967) *The pregnant diabetic and new newborn.* Copenhagen: Munksgaard.

Prout, T. E. (1966) Thyroid disease in pregnancy. *Amer. J. Obstet. Gynaec.*, **96**, 148.

Rovinsky, J. J. & Guttmacher, A. F. (1965) *Medical, Surgical and Gynaecological Complications of Pregnancy.* Edinburgh: Livingstone.

Sutherland, H. W. & Stowers, J. M. (1975) *Carbohydrate Metabolism in Pregnancy and the Newborn.* Edinburgh: Churchill Livingstone.

White, P. (1965) Pregnancy and diabetes: medical aspects. *Medical Clinics of North America*, **49**, 1015.

SECTION 4: RENAL SYSTEM

The normal physiological changes of pregnancy include retention of sodium, potassium and water, an increase in total blood volume and a rise in cardiac output. Renal perfusion is greatly increased and glomerular filtration rate raised by one-third. During pregnancy the blood urea level is much lower than normal, lying between 2 and 3m.mol/100ml. After the puerperium it returns towards the normal range. In the early months minor orthostatic proteinuria may be found. Glycosuria is a common occurrence.

From about the third month of pregnancy there is increasing dilatation of the ureters and pelvis of the kidneys believed to result from varying concentration of circulating hormones. Later there is compression of the ureters at the pelvic brim, particularly on the right side by the enlarged uterus.

Infection in the urinary tract and kidneys

Four distinct conditions are encountered which are associated with urinary infection. These include frequency, dysuria and occasionally haematuria following sexual activity; symptomless bacteriuria; acute pyelonephritis and clinical features caused by pre-existing renal disease.

The development of semi-quantitative bacteriological methods has facilitated the diagnosis of urinary tract infection. Kass estimated the number of bacteria in urine by counting the number of colonies grown on a plate inoculated with a known quantity of urine. A bacteriological count of 100 000 organisms/ml of urine in properly taken specimens reaching the laboratory within two hours indicated urinary tract infection. Counts below 10 000 organisms/ml urine were due to contamination.

The urine specimen should be collected after swabbing the perineum with soap and water, rinsing with sterile water and drying with a sterile swab. The labia are then held open and the patient asked to empty the bladder. Urine is collected in two containers. The first 30ml or so passed into one container is discarded, the rest is collected in a sterile wide mouthed jar.

Using these methods a number of important points have been established:

The prevalence of urinary tract infection in young females is much greater than in males. At least 5 per cent of girls but only 0·03 per cent of boys acquire bacteriuria during school years. This suggests that anatomical arrangements facilitate the entry of bowel organisms, especially *E. coli*, via the urethra into the bladder. The incidence of asymptomatic bacteriuria which is low in schoolgirls rises after puberty to a peak at the age of 20–30 years. The incidence in married women is ten times as great as in single women. There is little difference between the incidence in married women who have previously been pregnant and those who have not. These findings suggest an aetiological relationship between sexual activity and urinary tract infection.

HONEYMOON CYSTITIS

The group of distressing symptoms which sometimes follows sexual activity in young women has been shown to be frequently associated with infection and has recently received a good deal of publicity. There is no doubt that much misery can be avoided by very simple measures. The recommendations which are often found to be effective include strict local hygiene, a high liquid intake and emptying of the bladder after intercourse. During times of special susceptibility, such as the first two to three weeks after marriage, 50mg of Nitrofurantoin or similar urinary antiseptic may be taken each evening.

ASYMPTOMATIC BACTERIURIA

Since almost three-quarters of all cases of acute pyelonephritis of pregnancy occur in the 7 per cent of women with persistent bacteriuria it is possible to identify those among whom most of the attacks of acute pyelonephritis will occur by culturing the urine of all patients at the beginning of pregnancy. This can readily be done by using dipslides at the antenatal clinic. There is, however, controversy over the question of treatment of these cases with asymptomatic bacteriuria. Some believe that a week's course of Sulphadimidine should be given to abolish the bacteriuria, but in about 15 per cent the urine will remain infected or become re-infected and further treatment with another agent such as Nitrofurantoin 50mg or Nalidixic Acid each evening until the end of pregnancy is given. Other combinations of antibiotics may be required to make the urine sterile. Others, however, believe that many of the cases of asymptomatic bacteriuria will not develop symptoms and that not only is treatment unnecessary, but side effects occur in between 10 and 30 per cent of patients requiring drugs. In a study in Aberdeen, Swapp (1974) found that 86·1 per cent of patients with urinary tract infection had negative bacteriuria at their first antenatal visit. Only 19·6 per cent of patients with asymptomatic bacteriuria at the first antenatal visit developed symptoms of urinary tract infection so that about 80 per cent with asymptomatic bacteriuria would have received an unnecessary course of prophylactic antibiotic therapy. It is thus felt that it is better to await the onset of symptoms and to treat promptly. The problems associated with prophylactic treatment are discussed by Kass (1965) and by Brumfitt and Asscher (1973).

ACUTE PYELENEPHRITIS

Aetiology

1. *Predisposing factors.* It is well recognized that the structural changes which occur in the urinary tract during pregnancy predispose to infection. Dilatation of the upper urinary tract occurs in nearly every pregnant woman although the degree varies from very slight to such marked dilatation that the renal pelvis and ureter may have a capacity of 200ml. On the right side the dilatation is usually more marked affecting the calyces, renal pelvis and ureter down to the level of the pelvic brim where the ureter narrows suddenly. In its pelvic portion the ureter is very slightly dilated. On the left side the calyces and renal pelvis are less frequently involved. On both sides kinks are usually seen but on the right side they are much more pronounced and may be very acute. They are usually situated in the upper third of the ureter and cause definite

narrowing of the lumen. Lateral displacement of the ureters to the outer border of the psoas muscle frequently occurs in the second half of pregnancy. When this happens the ureter escapes compression until it crosses the psoas muscle at the level of the pelvic brim to gain access to the pelvis. Dilatation is more marked in primigravidae than in multiparae. It is found as early as the tenth week of pregnancy. At the end of the fourth month the dilatation is increased by the pressure of the pregnant uterus which is more marked on the right side. To the end of the sixth month dilatation increases but from then to full term it tends to diminish. In conjunction with this dilatation stasis is usually found which begins in the early months, reaching its maximum as a rule at the sixth month and diminishing near full time.

As regards the causal factors it is certain that the uterus can compress the ureters against the psoas muscle at the pelvic brim and for some distance above this point but some dilatation occurs before the uterus is big enough to exert pressure and is due probably to diminished tone of the ureteric muscle. This is possibly caused by progesterone which produces a similar effect on the uterus and the bowel. The tone of the ureter improves from about the sixth month to full term, decreases rapidly again in the first ten days of the puerperium and is restored slowly thereafter. This sudden decrease in the tone of the ureter after delivery corresponds in time to the withdrawal of oestrogens from the circulation and may be due to this factor.

The importance of stasis in the production of pyelonephritis of pregnancy is well shown in the clear relationship between the time of onset of stasis and of infection. Pyelonephritis is more common in primigravidae. It affects the right side more than the left and it usually begins between the fourth and sixth months of pregnancy at the time when the stasis has reached its maximum.

Causal organism. The organism belongs to the coliform group in over 90 per cent of cases and is probably derived from the bowel. It may reach the kidney by the lumen of the ureter or the bloodstream. The recent evidence suggests that in most cases the infection spreads upwards from the bladder along the ureter to the kidney. Reflux of urine from the bladder into the ureter may not be uncommon and in the normally functioning ureter it is probably expelled back into the bladder with little delay so that even if organisms are present in the urine clinical infection of the upper urinary tract will not occur. The result might be very different in a pregnancy, especially one which has reached twenty weeks or more where the urine may be trapped for long periods in the upper urinary tract. This theory would be in keeping with the fact that the incidence of disease agrees very well with the incidence of dilatation and of stasis in the ureters. It is not known whether ureteric reflux is more common in pregnancy nor do we know if symptomless bacteriuria in an early pregnancy is the result of a low grade cystitis or a chronic infection of the kidney. In those women giving a definite history of pyelonephritis in childhood an acute exacerbation is likely to occur very early in pregnancy, certainly before the fifth month, whereas in those women with no previous history of kidney infection pyelonephritis seldom occurs before the end of the fifth month. Another point in favour of ascending infection from a chronic infection of the bladder is that while symptoms of cystitis are relatively common in women soon after marriage symptoms of pyelonephritis are very unusual. Rarely staphylococci or Klebsiella pneumoniae are the causal organisms. Other organisms which include pseudomonas pyocyanea, proteus vulgaris and streptococcus faecalis are found commonly after antibiotic therapy or following catheterization.

Signs and symptoms
Typically the patient is a primigravida in the fifth or sixth month of pregnancy, who develops sudden severe pain in the right costo-vertebral angle. There is great tenderness and high temperature and rapid pulse. Sometimes there is a rigor and the patient vomits. She may have some frequency of micturition with slight dysuria. She looks and feels ill, is flushed, the respiration is rapid and shallow and there is pain on inspiration and a short cough. Usually in a case of this kind the diagnosis is easy after the urine has been examined but pneumonia or pleurisy may be suspected. Localizing features are more marked on the right than on the left side, but often the infection is bilateral.

Diagnosis
The diagnosis is confirmed by examination of the urine. Typically it is strongly acid and

concentrated. It may contain blood cells. Usually there are pus cells and coliform bacilli.

Treatment

Preventative. Patients with asymptomatic bacteriuria during pregnancy should be treated since they are so much more likely to develop acute pyelonephritis. Early studies using Sulphadimidine in a dose of 1g eight-hourly for seven days gave a cure rate for asymptomatic bacteriuria of pregnancy of about 75 per cent. When the patients are followed up until delivery, however, the cure rate fell to 66 per cent. Similar findings have been obtained with Amoxycillin in a dose of 500mg bd for seven days. Recurrent infection has often been shown to be associated with structural deformity due to chronic pre-existing renal disease. These patients have been treated with benefit using Nitrofurantoin 50mg in the evening until the end of pregnancy. Urine samples must be cultured to identify the organisms concerned and to obtain their antibiotic sensitivities.

Curative. In the acute stage abundant fluids are given and usually sulphonamides are administered before the organism responsible for the infection has been identified by culture. A commonly prescribed course is 3g as a loading dose and 1g six-hourly. This should be continued for at least three weeks. If there is evidence of extensive intrarenal infection as shown by biochemical changes in the plasma the course should be continued for two to three months. A specimen of urine should be examined on the fourth day of the course and if pus cells and organisms are still found the antibiotic sensitivity of the organism should be obtained, particularly to Cephalexin, Ampicillin and its derivatives. Despite the excellent immediate response to treatment in acute cases it may be necessary because of reinfection to continue treatment for the rest of the pregnancy. This may be done by giving Sulphadimidine 0·4g, Cephalexin 125mg or Nitrofurantoin 50mg in the evening before retiring. Side effects with these small doses of Nitrofurantoin are very unusual. When reinfection occurs despite the continued use of antibiotic it may be necessary to give larger doses and to vary the antibiotic each week. For example, Nitrofurantoin 100–200mg/day, Cephalexin 500mg three times a day, Nalidixic Acid 2g/day or Ampicillin 250mg four times a day, have been used in this way. Other drugs including Kanamycin and Colistin have also been recommended. These patients are often shown on investigation after delivery to have prominent structural damage, often associated with a history of urinary tract infection.

The drugs now used are so satisfactory that former methods of treatment such as postural drainage, passage or ureteric catheters and nephrostomy are seldom necessary. Occasionally when there is complete blockage of the ureter nephrostomy or even nephrectomy may be necessary. Usually this is associated with pre-existing renal disease.

Renal and ureteric calculi

Although stasis and infection which often occurs in pregnancy should predispose to formation of renal calculi this does not appear to be a frequent occurrence in women of the childbearing age. Even when they form they are unlikely to produce symptoms during pregnancy. The calculi presumably pass easily along the dilated ureters during pregnancy and are not likely to cause symptoms. Calculi are usually found during or after pregnancy in the investigation of persisting pyelonephritis but if the calculus becomes impacted in the ureter severe pain can occur in the loin and may be associated with haematuria. Urethral catheterization may aid in the passage of a ureteric calculus but if there is persisting pain and infection a uretero-lithotomy may have to be performed. Depending on the duration of pregnancy this may be straightforward but in late pregnancy it will be necessary to empty the uterus to gain access.

Polycystic kidney

This hereditary condition is a rare complication of pregnancy and is not usually diagnosed then because of the absence of symptoms and the difficulty of palpating the kidneys due to the enlarged uterus. Hypertension and albuminuria tend to occur in later life but may occur during pregnancy and can give rise to difficulty in differentiating from pre-eclampsia, but the time of onset of the hypertension and proteinuria may be useful in making the diagnosis. Infection is likely to occur in the polycystic kidneys during pregnancy and may cause intractable pyelonephritis. There is marked deterioration of kidney function and an early pregnancy termination may be indicated, but if the condition does not manifest itself until late in pregnancy it should be possible to achieve a live birth without jeopardizing the health of the mother.

Acute renal failure

Oliguria and a transient rise in blood urea usually follow the severe reduction in renal perfusion and glomerular filtration rate caused by acute haemorrhage or dehydration. In this type of oliguria the specific gravity of the urine is high and the urinary concentration of urea greater than 2g/100ml. Diuresis will follow fluid replacement and restoration of blood volume.

Acute pyelonephritis with extensive intrarenal infection occasionally causes severe oliguria. Effective treatment with antibiotics is followed by diuresis.

ACUTE TUBULAR NECROSIS

Acute necrosis of the renal tubular epithelium has several precipitating causes. In obstetrical practice it may be encountered in the early months after septic abortion or the severe dehydration and electrolyte disturbance which may follow persistent vomiting. Later in pregnancy it may result from retroplacental or post-partum haemorrhage, surgical procedures or eclampsia. Transfusion reactions, which were previously a cause, are nowadays uncommon.

Necrosis of the tubular epithelium is scattered along the course of the tubule and not confined to the lower part of the nephron as formerly described. Near the more severely damaged tubules the stroma is often oedematous and shows a cellular reaction. Pigmented casts are seen in the tubular lumen. The glomeruli appear to be structurally normal. Tubular epithelium has very great regenerative ability and if the basement membrane remains intact epithelial regeneration and restoration of tubular continuity are almost complete in 7–10 days.

The main cause of tubular necrosis is now believed to be the severe renal vaso-constriction which follows an extreme fall in systemic blood pressure or a reduction in blood volume after haemorrhage. During pregnancy this is sometimes accompanied by increased intravascular coagulation.

Clinical features

The clinical course of the illness may be divided into the stage of onset, the period of oliguria and the diuretic stage.

The onset is often associated with circulatory failure and overshadowed by the features of the precipitating cause. During this stage there is severe renal ischaemia which determines the degree and extent of the tubular damage. Severe oliguria is by far the most important early sign and the medical staff must be specially alert in charting the urinary output of patients who suffer from any of the recognized precipitating causes of acute tubular necrosis. Symptoms of renal failure may not appear for several days and usually start insidiously. Early symptoms include mental and physical lethargy, apathy, headache, anorexia and nausea. The gradual onset of these features may be ascribed to the precipitating illness and their significance not appreciated. Ultimately they are followed by the progressive development of the full clinical picture of uraemia.

The small amount of urine which is passed is often dark brown in colour, contains albumin, numerous blood cells and casts. There is a gradual rise in the end products of protein catabolism in the blood such as urea, phosphate and potassium. The concentration of these substances increases very rapidly in the presence of extensive tissue trauma. The unusually rapid rise after delivery may be related to involution of the uterus. The electrolyte pattern of the extra-cellular fluid is similar to that in uraemia from any cause. Serum potassium shows a progressive rise and serum calcium usually falls reciprocally with the rise in serum phosphate. The bicarbonate level falls steeply as acidosis develops. The clinical signs of hyperpotassaemia contribute to the features of uraemia as do the retention of nonvolatile products of protein metabolism, alterations in acid base balance, the relative concentration of electrolytes and the osmotic activity of body fluids.

On recovery there is a gradual increase in daily urine volume. Less commonly this is abrupt. This stage may begin at any time from 3–10 days after the onset. Longer periods of oliguria have been reported with ultimate recovery. Although the tubular epithelium is structurally restored return of function takes longer. The large volume of urine passed is mainly the result of an osmotic diuresis produced by the high blood urea. For a short time blood urea levels may continue to rise despite the onset of diuresis. There is also impaired reabsorption of electrolytes and features of sodium and potassium depletion may be found during this stage unless replacement is adequate. Gradually tubular function is restored, the blood urea level falls, the acid base balance is re-established, the body fluids return to their normal chemical pattern and volume.

Treatment

Efforts to prevent or to minimize the extent and severity of the renal lesion include the rapid restoration of blood volume after acute haemorrhage and fluid loss; minimal tissue trauma during surgical procedures and the effective treatment of severe infections. Clinical management of the oliguric stage is designed to minimize the release into the blood of end products of endogenous protein metabolism, especially fixed acids and potassium but above all to avoid over-hydration. In the diuretic stage care must be taken to avoid dehydration and electrolyte depletion.

Water. Increased catabolism in anuric patients causes a rise in total body water. It is now recommended that the water intake should be restricted to 500ml each day in addition to the loss from any other route, including any urine passed. With ideal management there should be a daily weight loss during the oliguric stage of about half a kilogram each day.

Electrolytes. The intake of sodium and potassium should be prevented. Sodium restriction diminishes the tendency to over-hydration which may lead to acute pulmonary oedema and to convulsions. Natural and synthetic fruit juices have an appreciable potassium content and should not be given. The intravenous administration of glucose and insulin causes a transfer of potassium from the extra-cellular fluid to the cells where it is stored with glycogen. It is possible to obtain temporary depression of the potassium level in this way. The plasma potassium may be lowered more effectively by giving resins in the calcium phase either 15g orally two to four times a day or 60g as a retention enema.

The use of sodium bicarbonate or sodium lactate to correct acidosis is a dangerous procedure. Sodium salts given in this way encourage oedema formation. Acidosis is less dangerous than oedema and should be treated only if respiratory distress is severe.

Nutrition. The accumulation of protein end products in extra-cellular fluid is accelerated when the catabolic rate is high and increased when oliguria is prolonged. Protein intake should therefore be restricted and as far as possible daily energy requirements provided by carbohydrate. In the early stage carbohydrate may be given orally in any form the patient can take, provided it is free of electrolytes. 100g of carbohydrate will reduce the breakdown of endogenous protein by about 50 per cent. Highly concentrated solutions of carbohydrate may be given orally such as Hycal (Beecham) containing 400 calories of carbohydrate in 180ml of water. There is some evidence that protein breakdown may also be reduced by giving anabolic steroids, for example Norethandrolone in doses of 30mg by mouth or 50mg by intramuscular injection for five days.

Fats may also be given in combination with carbohydrate either orally or in suitable preparations by intravenous injection. Administration in large amounts by stomach tube is apt to cause diarrhoea. When nausea or gastrointestinal disturbance prevents the oral intake of calories as carbohydrate or fat highly concentrated solutions of glucose or fructose may be given by continuous intravenous infusion. If solutions of glucose above 10 per cent are given into a peripheral vein thrombosis will occur within a few hours. Glucose solutions up to 50 per cent may be given intravenously through an indwelling caval catheter. To each litre of solution 1000 units of Heparin are added to minimize the risk of thrombosis in a central vein. The infusion may be delivered at a rate of about 0·25ml/min.

Infection. These patients are particularly susceptible to infection. It is unnecessary to have an indwelling catheter in the bladder and it is undesirable to give prophylactic antibiotic but frequent routine examination should include a search for foci of infection. When appropriate antibiotics are given it should be remembered that many of them are excreted by the kidney and the dose used should be modified accordingly.

If these measures are introduced at an early stage physico-chemical changes in the internal environment occur slowly. Potassium may not reach the danger level of 7mEq/litre before the tubular epithelium has regenerated and diuresis begins.

Sometimes, however, patients are seen with increased extra-cellular volume with raised effective osmotic pressure, a high potassium level and severe acidosis due to inadequate control in the early stage of anuria or to increased protein catabolism from fever, tissue trauma and involution of the uterus. In these cases peritoneal dialysis or haemodialysis may be life saving.

In the diuretic phase the daily urine volume increases progressively but the blood urea may not begin to fall for several days thereafter. It is important that strict control of water, electrolytes and protein are continued until the levels of urea and potassium fall. Diuresis soon reaches 2–3 litres a day or more partly from the osmotic effect of the high concentrations of urea in the blood and tissues. Should this output continue it may lead to water depletion with excessive loss of salt and potassium. Plasma electrolytes should therefore be measured regularly.

The convalescence of these patients, who have been severely ill, should be gradual. Often they have troublesome though minor symptoms such as muscle weakness, unsteadiness and debility for several weeks after recovery.

SYMMETRICAL RENAL CORTICAL NECROSIS
This is a rare complication of pregnancy. Usually it follows retroplacental haemorrhage and tends to occur in patients who are already anaemic. It cannot be differentiated clinically from acute tubular necrosis which is commoner and is reversible. Patients who may suffer from cortical necrosis must therefore be treated on the lines which have been indicated in the section on acute tubular necrosis. It is rare for tubular necrosis to last longer than 28 days and should oliguria persist after that time specialized investigation is necessary including renal biopsy and consideration of long term treatment by repeated haemodialysis or transplantation.

PRE-EXISTING GLOMERULONEPHRITIS
Patients with chronic glomerulonephritis who become pregnant are likely to show an increase in proteinuria and hypertension. Should this occur in the early months of pregnancy it is extremely unlikely that a viable fetus will be delivered. Deterioration in renal function may occur at any time during the pregnancy.

If renal function is less than half normal, that is if they are known to have a persistent elevation of the blood urea above the accepted upper limit of normal, they should be advised against pregnancy. If, however, despite this advice they do become pregnant or if they are seen for the first time and give a history of previous renal disease when they are already pregnant, it should be terminated when evidence of aggravation of glomerular damage occurs. Those who are able to continue should have the hypertension controlled by Propranolol with a diuretic. They must be seen at very frequent intervals and remain in bed during the later months. The risk of fetal death *in utero* increases as pregnancy advances.

Pregnancy after removal of a kidney

Large numbers of patients have gone through pregnancy after removal of one kidney and provided the remaining one is healthy, there has been no untoward effect from the pregnancy. Successful pregnancies have also been achieved after renal transplant, and even in patients on permanent dialysis.

REFERENCES (SECTION 4)

Brumfitt, W. & Asscher, A. W. (1973) Urinary tract infection. *Proceedings of the Second National Symposium in London,* March, 1972. London: Oxford University Press.
Kass, E. H. (1965) *Progress in pyelonephritis.* Editor E. H. Kass. Philadelphia: Davis.
Swapp, G. H. (1974) Personal communication.

SECTION 5: NERVOUS SYSTEM

Epilepsy

In some patients epileptic seizures occur as a manifestation of local intracranial disease such as a tumour, vascular lesion or infection or present as a feature of a general disturbance such as severe anoxia, extreme hypertension, eclampsia and hypoglycaemia. In a large number of patients, however, the attacks are idiopathic and no primary disease can be found.

Idiopathic epilepsy usually appears before

the age of 20 and may do so during pregnancy. The effect of pregnancy on known epileptic patients is variable as it is in asthma, migraine and some chronic skin disease such as psoriasis. Some patients are improved but often the frequency of attacks is increased.

It is very important to exclude an underlying cause for a convulsive seizure which occurs for the first time during pregnancy. Such patients should be admitted to hospital. The past history and family history should be carefully obtained and a full general and neurological examination conducted. If no cause can be demonstrated by these clinical methods, special investigations should include an X-ray of the skull; the blood Wassermann reaction; the investigation of spontaneous hypoglycaemia by prolonged fasting, by the intravenous tolbutamide test or by estimation of the plasma insulin level; lumbar puncture with chemical, cytological and serological examination of the cerebrospinal fluid. An electro-encephalogram may be helpful by indicating abnormal cerebral rhythms. Depending on the result of these investigations neurosurgical studies may be required. The diagnosis of idiopathic epilepsy is made by exclusion.

The detailed management of epilepsy is described in appropriate textbooks and many anticonvulsant drugs are now available. Phenobarbitone is widely employed. A commonly effective dose is from 90 to 180mg daily in two or three divided doses, but individual dosage is achieved by trial and the smallest amount which will give control is desirable. Phenytoin (epanutin) in an average dose of 100mg three times daily is valuable in major epilepsy. Tridione in a dose of 300mg twice or thrice daily is used in the control of *petit mal* although this disorder is relatively rare in adults. Paraldehyde, 5–10ml intramuscularly, is often effective in controlling status epilepticus and can be repeated safely.

Idiopathic epilepsy is not of itself an indication for terminating a pregnancy. There is an increased incidence of epilepsy in the children of epileptic parents so that it is reasonable to limit the family by sterilization after one or two successful pregnancies. When only one parent is epileptic the risk of a child being affected is only slightly greater than in the average population. If epilepsy in the parents is symptomatic rather than idiopathic (e.g. post-traumatic) there is, of course, no added risk to the children.

Chorea gravidarum

About one in four women who had chorea in childhood can be expected to have a recurrence during pregnancy. The fetus is unaffected by the disease. Control is usually possible with rest and sedation with Chlorpromazine (2·5–5mg thrice daily) and antibiotic for pyrexia.

The disease is rare. Therapeutic termination, formerly advised, is rarely necessary.

Disseminated sclerosis

In the majority of cases the natural course of this disease is one of chronic progression with relapse and remission of symptoms over many years. Foci of demyelination are scattered throughout the central nervous system and clinical signs may be found on examination of the motor and sensory functions of the cranial and spinal nerves.

The majority opinion is that pregnancy aggravates the neurological manifestations but this is difficult to establish and the evidence is not impressive. Termination is very rarely indicated and depends mainly on the severity of the disease and the stage which it has reached in its relentless progress. Patients who are able to continue the pregnancy seldom have difficulty during delivery. Breast feeding is better avoided if there is muscular inco-ordination.

Thrombosis of the intracranial venous sinuses

This complication is not uncommon in the puerperium and it is probable that in patients with minor symptoms the condition is not diagnosed. It is a manifestation of the increased tendency to intravascular thrombosis after delivery and the incidence rises with infection.

Clinical signs vary with the severity of the thrombosis. In many cases headache, giddiness and clouding of consciousness are accompanied by a hemiparesis or weakness of an upper limb and one side of the face; disorders of speech such as motor aphasia or word blindness may occur and, of the cranial nerves, the oculomotor is most commonly affected. In some cases headache and giddiness is followed by an epileptic seizure which may be of Jacksonian type. The cerebrospinal fluid pressure is raised with an increase in protein, erythrocytes and a yellow colour.

In the great majority of cases recovery is complete. Symptoms may, however, remain such as weakness of a limb or intellectual impairment. Occasionally epileptic attacks may follow local cortical damage.

When the diagnosis is established anticoagulants should be used as described in the treatment of phlebothrombosis. Epilepsy is controlled either with phenobarbitone, 90–180 mg daily, in divided dosage or with paraldehyde, 5–10ml intramuscularly. Any infection should be treated with antibiotics.

Maternal birth palsy

This condition is rare and is now thought to result from herniation of the nucleus pulposus involving the lower lumbar intervertebral discs. Backache and pain in the back of the leg or in front of the thigh may be accompanied by signs of a lower motor neurone lesion affecting a group of leg muscles. Most cases recover within a few weeks although the full return of muscle power may take several months.

Treatment is on routine lines with rest in bed until pain disappears, splints to prevent foot drop and physiotherapy to the affected muscle groups. Operative removal of the disc is indicated only in rare cases. Caesarean section might be considered in patients with symptoms before delivery.

Acroparaesthesia

Paraesthesia with 'pins and needles' sensation, numbness, pain and weakness of the muscles of the hands is not uncommon in the later months of pregnancy. Symptoms are worse at night. They disappear within a week or two after delivery. These symptoms are now thought to be due to compression of the median nerve at the wrist in the carpal tunnel. It is probable, from the time of occurrence of symptoms and the rapidity of relief after delivery, that fluid retention and tissue oedema contribute to the nerve compression. Sodium restriction and diuretics may be helpful in those cases which occur shortly before delivery. Considerable relief is often obtained by splinting the hands in flexion during the night. Severe persistent symptoms may be relieved by division of the flexor retinaculum.

Compression of the lateral cutaneous nerve of the thigh gives rise to neuralgia paraesthetica with which there is pain, paraesthesia and sensory loss over the antero-lateral aspect of the thigh. Rest and analgesics are usually sufficient to ease the symptoms but in severe cases it may be necessary to free the nerve from friction by the inguinal ligament.

Spontaneous subarachnoid haemorrhage

This serious condition is seen occasionally in pregnancy. It is not known with certainty whether the rise in blood volume and in cardiac output which occur during pregnancy precipitate vascular rupture in a susceptible patient but it is probably wise to advise against future pregnancies in the case of a patient who gives a history of spontaneous intracranial bleeding.

Haemorrhage may arise from different pathological types of vascular lesion only some of which are accessible to direct neurosurgical attack. In about one-third of the cases haemorrhage is due to rupture of an aneurysm on or about the anterior communicating artery and its junction with the anterior cerebral vessels. The principles underlying the management of this group have recently been clarified. Immediately after the initial haemorrhage there is intense arterial spasm of the adjacent vessels. This not only arrests further bleeding but also causes some of the more serious clinical features. It is largely responsible for the initial coma and for death in some cases; for many of the neurological signs and partly for the severe headache. Since no form of treatment is known to relieve this arterial spasm and since an intracerebral haematoma in this region does not cause cerebral compression, the only contributory treatment is to prevent further haemorrhage. Recurrent haemorrhage after the second day is common.

Although death after the first haemorrhage is relatively rare the mortality rises steeply with successive bleedings. Immediately the diagnosis is made the opinion of a neurosurgeon should be obtained. Angiography and when possible proximal clipping of the involved vessel should be performed in the acute stage provided that the patient is out of coma and showing some signs of recovery. Active treatment of suitable patients will help the mortality compared with those treated conservatively.

Not all pathological types of vascular lesion are suitable for a direct neurosurgical attack and the management of the patient must be guided by a neurosurgeon. It is, however, emphasized that neurosurgical advice should be sought early and investigation initiated as soon as possible after the first haemorrhage.

Myaesthenia gravis

This serious condition with progressive weakness of the muscles is fortunately uncommonly found in pregnancy. Very occasionally the disease may present for the first time in pregnancy. There is no set pattern to the behaviour of these patients during pregnancy as some appear to improve but others deteriorate. The dose of the drugs used for controlling the myaesthenia may have to be altered during pregnancy depending on the response. Particular care must be paid during labour and in the early puerperium to the dosage and it may be necessary to give parenteral treatment during labour and the delivery should be assisted by forceps.

The baby is limp and hypotonic at birth due to transient neonatal myaesthenia. This passes off within the first two weeks but treatment may be required during this time.

Poliomyelitis

The availability of poliomyelitis vaccine has completely altered the picture in pregnancy as pregnant women are more susceptible to develop poliomyelitis. Vaccination against poliomyelitis is now standard procedure in pregnancy and there appears to be no ill-effects on the pregnancy or the fetus.

Although poliomyelitis is more likely to occur in pregnant women the prognosis does not seem to be any worse than in the non-pregnant except when the disease occurs late in pregnancy or in the puerperium. If the disease occurs in early pregnancy abortion is likely to occur possibly because of the high fever. The uterine muscle is not affected so that even in the most severe cases labour can progress normally. Assistance is only required in second stage. Horn (1958) described the management of these cases in detail and recommends Caesarean section only for patients acutely ill with bulbal spinal poliomyelitis. Patients with severe residual disease who require to be kept in a respirator can be delivered vaginally.

The baby is very unlikely to be affected by congenital poliomyelitis. When this occurs the baby is so-called 'rag-doll' and is completely flaccid.

REFERENCES (SECTION 5)

Horn, P. (1958) Obstetric management of poliomyelitis complicating pregnancy. *Clin. Obstet. Gynae.*, **1**, 127.

FURTHER READING

Dovinsky, J. & Guttmacher, A. F. (Eds.) (1965) Medical Surgical & Gynaecological Complications of Pregnancy. Edinburgh: Churchill Livingstone.

SECTION 6: HAEMOPOIETIC SYSTEM

General observations

Anaemia may be defined as a significant reduction of the total, circulating, intracorpuscular haemoglobin. Thus anaemia may be due to a reduction of the total volume of blood from acute haemorrhage (*see* Chapter 31) or to a reduction in the concentration of haemoglobin per unit volume of blood from other causes. Anaemia is frequent in pregnancy and potentially dangerous, and may be of nutritional, infective or hereditary origin or due to a combination of any two or all three of such causes. The first two can usually be prevented or readily treated and the worst effects of the last controlled. The main message of this section must clearly be in the realms of prevention.

In well-nourished communities with competent antenatal care anaemia in pregnancy is uncommon, but in poorly fed communities there is a high incidence of hypochromic and megaloblastic anaemias. Anaemia is especially frequent in the tropics, in conditions of mal-nourishment and with hookworm infestation or sprue. In the tropics too, and to a lesser extent elsewhere, the pandemic heritage of the haemoglobinopathies is potentiated by folate deficiency and infection to constitute a major problem in obstetric management. (The reader is referred to Chapter 26 for a full discussion of the clinical aspects of anaemia in the tropics. The chapters are complementary.)

The normal haematological changes accom-panying pregnancy have been described in Chapter 5. In pregnant women the haemo-globin level, especially in the later months, is usually lower than in the non-pregnant. This fall is accompanied by an absolute rise in plasma volume. In any individual it may not be possible to decide to what extent the fall in haemoglobin is physiological or pathological. Thus a truly scientific basis for the diagnosis of anaemia is not possible and one must adopt an arbitrary standard. The level at which this standard is drawn varies from one community to another. In privileged groups a haemo-globin level of 12g/100ml might be chosen as the level below which the patient could be considered to be anaemic, but usually a level below this must suffice. In Britain a level of 11g/100ml is generally taken, but levels of 10g or even less are not uncommonly used in other countries. The level selected reflects the nutritional state of the community in question.

A classification of the various types of anaemia which may be found in relation to

Table 12.3 Classification of anaemia in relation to pregnancy

1. *Acute posthaemorrhagic anaemia*
2. *Hypochromic anaemias*
   a. sideropenic anaemias—lack of iron;
   b. haemoglobinopathies—defective globin synthesis, either quantitative as in thalassaemia or qualitative as in sickle cell disease—these anaemias are haemolytic as well as hypochromic;
   c. sideroblastic anaemias—defective haem synthesis.
3. *Megaloblastic anaemias*
4. *Anaemias associated with hypertensive toxaemias*
5. *Anaemias associated with infections*
6. *Anaemias uncommon in pregnancy*
   a. haemolytic anaemias apart from the haemolytic aspects of 2(b), 3, 4 and 5;
   b. hypoplastic anaemias;
   c. anaemias due to usurpation of the marrow, especially from leukaemia;
   d. anaemias secondary to splenic disorders.

pregnancy is given in Table 12.3, but, before passing to specific details, a few general points are worth a mention. Haematological classifica-tion does not necessarily imply a real diagnosis, for terms such as hypochromic anaemia and megaloblastic anaemia are merely specific signs which point to a need to find the under-lying cause. Furthermore, in the elucidation of the nutritional anaemias, as indeed of any nutritional disorder, one must remember three important principles, namely that in a *single* malnourished patient there *may* be *multiple deficiencies, multiple sites* of interference with nutrition (food, digestion, absorption, storage and utilization), and *multiple effects* of single deficiencies, e.g. megaloblastic anaemia, epi-thelial changes and abnormal histidine metabolism in folate deficiency.

1. ACUTE POSTHAEMORRHAGIC ANAEMIA

Acute haemorrhage occurs frequently in early pregnancy, especially from abortion and ectopic pregnancy, and, about the time of delivery, from placenta praevia, abruptio placentae and complications of the third stage of labour. Acute haemorrhage is considered in detail in other chapters, but a few general points will now be discussed.

The increased blood volume in pregnancy allows some reserve in late pregnancy for moderate blood loss, but if loss is enough to cause shock, rapid and adequate replacement of blood volume is essential, initially with plasma or a substitute and then with com-patible, cross-matched blood of appropriate ABO and Rhesus groups (*see* Chapters 8 and 20). It is particularly important that full replacement of blood be made in cases of abruptio, for blood loss in that condition may be underestimated and failure to restore blood volume before delivery is an important factor in the occurrence of uncontrollable post-partum haemorrhage in such patients. The depletion of fibrinogen and other clotting factors in this and other haemostatic complica-tions of pregnancy is discussed in Chapter 13.

In assessment of blood loss, only measure-ment of external loss and monitoring of the degree of shock are of value. Immediately after acute haemorrhage the haemoglobin level, red cell count and packed cell volume give no information as to the amount lost; until haemodilution has occurred their values are unaltered. Apart from the risks of radio-activity, serial blood volume estimations are of doubtful value, but in severe cases a record of the central (caval) venous pressure is essential throughout the emergency, to establish whether shock persisting after transfusion is hypovolaemic or not, and to act as a guide to therapy. In this respect it is important to remember in the emergency situation that, apart from the hypovolaemia of blood loss or plasma loss or dehydration, shock may be of cardiac, endocrine, neural or anaphylactoid type, and, particularly in obstetrics, may be due to disseminated intravascular coagulation, as from abruptio, amniotic embolism, intra-uterine death, hydatidiform mole, incompatible transfusion, contaminated transfusion or septicaemia (McKay, 1965).

The blood film after haemorrhage does not give much positive information, with the exception of that characteristic of pre-existing anaemia or thrombocytopenia. Signs of reaction to bleeding (excessive polychromasia of erythrocytes, neutrophil leucocytosis and thrombocytosis) appear later than haemodilution. In relation to massive transfusion with stored blood it should be remembered that such blood contains few platelets and is deficient in chemical clotting factors, that stored erythrocytes assume temporarily a spherical shape, more striking than the slight sphering often seen in apparently normal pregnant women (Chapter 5) and falsely suggestive of a haemolytic process and that impairment of oxygen transport may also occur (Valtis and Kennedy, 1954). Thus blood as fresh as possible should be used for massive transfusion.

2. HYPOCHROMIC ANAEMIAS

a. *Sideropenic or iron deficiency anaemia*

The causes of hypochromic anaemia are so numerous that it is wrong just to equate hypochromia with iron deficiency, treat empirically as such and fail to look for the underlying cause. Iron deficiency may be present at the start of pregnancy, when it may be due to poor diet, gastro-intestinal disorders (including helminth and particularly hookworm infestation), previous menorrhagia, previous abortion, multiparity or previous ante- or post-partum haemorrhage inadequately compensated. Such long-standing iron deficiency, particularly in older multiparous women, may occasionally be part of the Kelly–Paterson (Plummer–Vinson) syndrome of anaemia, glossitis and dysphagia and be accompanied by koilonychia,

cheilitis and gastric achlorhydria. Patients with these symptoms may require vitamins of the B-complex (particularly riboflavin and nicotinic acid) as well as iron. Iron deficiency may develop during the pregnancy because of inadequate stores, inadequate dietary iron, multiple pregnancy, blood loss (as from haemorrhoids) or malabsorption of iron, either alone or as part of a general malabsorption. Folate deficiency is a common accompaniment of such late iron deficiency.

The blood picture in long-standing iron deficiency is usually characteristically hypochromic and microcytic, but, when the anaemia develops rapidly, as with twin pregnancy, only a minority of recently formed erythrocytes may show these features. The typical findings of hypochromic microcytic anaemia are a low mean corpuscular haemoglobin (MCH), a low mean corpuscular haemoglobin concentration (MCHC), a low mean corpuscular volume (MCV), and, in the film, small erythrocytes with pronounced central pallor (ring staining). Leucocytes are usually normal, but neutrophils may show hypersegmentation, especially if there be folate deficiency too. Eosinophilia should be excluded, especially if the patient is from the tropics. Platelets are usually adequate, but thrombocytopenia may occasionally be the underlying cause of a chronic post-haemorrhagic sideropenic anaemia. The reticulocyte count may be slightly raised, particularly if there be blood loss or twin pregnancy, but may be normal, e.g. in patients with chronic infection.

The prevention of sideropenic anaemia will be dealt with later. The treatment of established anaemia is generally accomplished with oral iron and is likely to be more successful if started early. Ferrous sulphate or ferrous gluconate is generally suitable, but may cause gastro-intestinal upsets. Ferrous fumarate or succinate or one of the slow release preparations may be better tolerated, but the writer suspects that some of the upsets may be brought about initially by too high a dosage. The problems of refractory hypochromic anaemia and parenteral therapy will be considered after prophylaxis.

b. *The haemoglobinopathies* (Lehmann and Huntsman, 1974)

The haemoglobinopathies comprise a large number of usually inherited disorders of haemoglobin synthesis, chemically but not always clinically dominant, affecting the formation of globin chains, either quantitatively, as in thalassaemia, or qualitatively, as in sickle cell disease, and commonly causing anaemia which may become more severe in pregnancy. Diagnostic tests will be discussed later—under refractory hypochromic anaemia.

The thalassaemias—(Synonyms: Mediterranean Anaemia, Cooley's Anaemia); (Weatherall and Clegg, 1972). This group of diseases was thought originally to affect only people of Mediterranean origin. β-thalassaemia minor has been described in Scotland (Fig. 12.4A), and any ethnic group may be affected. A full understanding of the thalassaemias requires a knowledge of the chemical structure of normal haemoglobins.

The globin part of the molecule of the predominant haemoglobin of normal adults (HbA) consists of four polypeptide chains, two α and two β. The α chains contain a characteristic sequence of 141 amino-acids; the β contain 146. The normal fetus has a predominant haemoglobin (HbF) which contains two similar α chains, but these are complemented by two other chains, each of 146 amino-acids, the so-called γ chains. There is also another normal adult haemoglobin (HbA$_2$) which contains α chains and δ chains and occurs normally in small amounts—up to about 3 per cent of total Hb.

The thalassaemias are of two main types, classical Mediterranean anaemia, now known as β-thalassaemia, and α-thalassaemia which is particularly common in China and Africa as well as in Greece. In β-*thalassaemia* the total production of HbA is reduced and this leads to hypochromia of the erythrocytes even in the presence of adequate iron. There is a shortened red cell survival and thus a haemolytic element in the anaemia. Another feature of β-thalassaemia is that HbF and HbA$_2$ are usually increased relative to HbA.

From the genetic point of view, the thalassaemias can be divided into the common heterozygous and the rarer homozygous types, and these types are profoundly different clinically. In *homozygous β-thalassaemia (thalassaemia major)* death usually occurs before puberty; thus the obstetrician is highly unlikely to encounter a case. In the *heterozygous form*, β-*thalassaemia* minor, pregnancy may lead to an increase in the severity of the anaemia, particularly if there be folate depletion or infection. If appropriate prophylaxis or therapy of these complications fails to raise the haemoglobin level, the question of transfusion may arise, but it is wise to remember that the patient may be well compensated by vasomotor and chemical changes to a lower level of haemoglobin (Huehns, 1971).

To the obstetrician, however, α-*thalassaemia* is of particular importance, because its most severe homozygous form which occurs in the fetus causes death from haemolytic anaemia, with hydrops and erythroblastosis.

In the heterozygote, α-thalassaemia is usually mild clinically and sometimes difficult to diagnose, because morphological changes in erythrocytes may be slight and there is no excess of HbF or HbA$_2$.

Qualitative abnormalities of the haemoglobin molecule. In these abnormal haemoglobins substitution or deletion of amino-acids has taken place. The effects are protean. Sickle haemoglobin (HbS) causes sickle cell anaemia in the homozygous state or when inherited with other haemoglobinopathies (C, D, thalassaemia or hereditary persistence of fetal Hb). Non-sickling anomalous haemoglobins, e.g. HbC and HbE, may also lead to anaemia in the homozygous state (Giblett, 1969) (Fig. 12.4B).

Sickle cell disease. The sickle cell states comprise the most important group of the haemoglobinopathies, both from the point of view of potential for morbidity and range of geographical and ethnic distribution. Pauling and his associates demonstrated that the sickling phenomenon was due to the presence of an abnormal haemoglobin (HbS) which they separated by electrophoresis. Sickling occurs predominantly in people of African origin, but is also common among Mediterranean and Indian groups. Other foci of high concentration are found in Southern Arabia, and it has been suggested that the anomaly arose there and spread thence to other lands (for precise references *see* Lehmann and Huntsman).

Erythrocytes containing HbS assume a sickle shape when exposed to low oxygen tension or reducing agents (Fig. 12.4C). In *homozygous* sickle cell disease (SS) there is a preponderance of HbS with a slight excess of HbF; in the heterozygous trait (AS) HbS is present in a concentration of 30–45 per cent, the rest being HbA. *Heterozygotes* enjoy relative resistance to falciparum malaria, but paradoxically, homozygotes do not.

The clinical manifestations of haemoglobin SS and SC disease are fully discussed in Chapter 26. The pregnant woman with the trait appears to be more susceptible than normal to urinary tract infection, but otherwise is in no danger unless she becomes severely hypoxic as from a bad anaesthetic. With homozygous SS disease, however, or a combination of sickling with another haemoglobinopathy, especially HbC, i.e. HbSC disease, there is a high risk of morbidity, and, with inadequate antenatal care, appreciable mortality. The pathogenesis of sickle cell anaemia is complex—hypochromia, haemo-

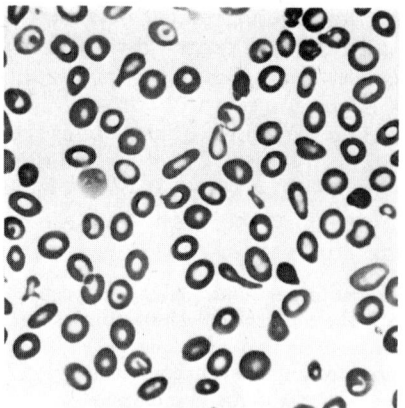

Fig. 12.4a   Blood film (stained Leishman): β-thalassaemia minor in a 20-year-old Scotswoman; mother and mother's sister similarly affected; presented with hypochromic microcytic anaemia associated with menorrhagia, but failed to respond adequately when iron deficiency was corrected; excess of HbF and HbA₂; many more distorted erythrocytes than would be expected with sideropenic anaemia with Hb of 11·5g/100ml, the level when film was made; note also target cells and fragmented forms—schistocytes.

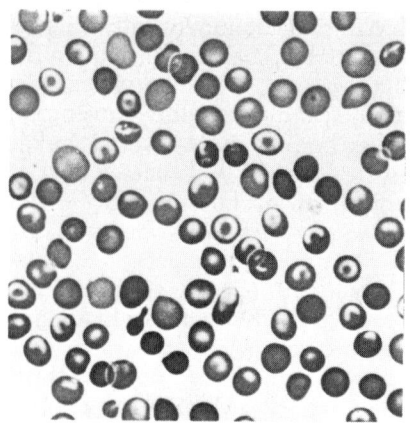

Fig. 12.4b   Blood film (stained Leishman): 32-year-old woman from Singapore, wife of British Serviceman; homozygous haemoglobin E disease; note numerous target cells and small dark, presumably thicker, cells; required transfusion of packed cells for anaemia late in pregnancy after an episode of bronchopneumonia.

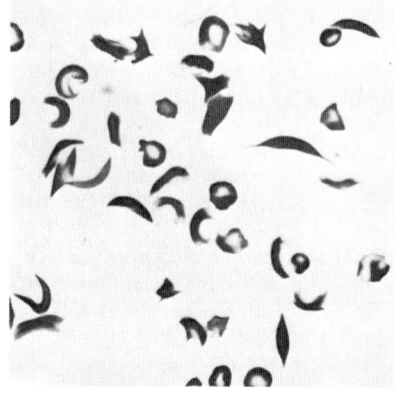

Fig. 12.4c   Positive sickle preparation (incubated with 2 per cent sodium metabisulphite; stained with eosin); primiparous 19-year-old Nigerian housewife; homozygous sickle cell disease, confirmed by electrophoresis, alkali resistance tests and solubility tests—87 per cent HbS, 13 per cent HbF: maintained during pregnancy on 5mg folic acid daily; required two small transfusions of packed red cells after episodes of urinary infection for which intensive antibiotic treatment was given; otherwise remained well with no crises; husband HbAA, infant HbAS.

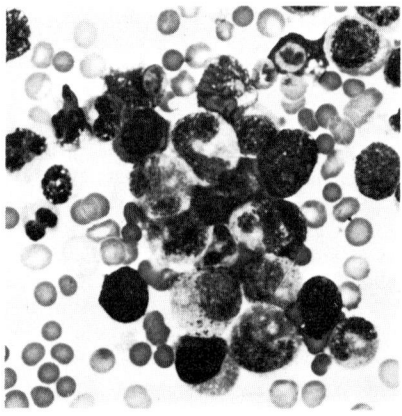

Fig. 12.4d   Sternal marrow smear (stained Leishman): primiparous patient with severe anaemia at mid-term; megaloblast, giant metamyelocyte (near centre) and spherocytes; folate deficiency complicating hereditary spherocyte haemolytic anaemia.

lysis and blockage of small blood vessels all play a part in the outcome, and folate deficiency and infections, especially malaria, respiratory and urinary tract infections, may precipitate crises characterized by pains in bones, joints and abdomen, by fever and sometimes by ischaemic lesions, e.g. necrosis of the head of the femur or of the breast. In HbSS disease, there is often skeletal and sexual immaturity; fertility is relatively low; pregnancy often ends in abortion, stillbirth or prematurity; pre-eclampsia is common; and thromboembolism and cardiac failure may occur. In HbSC disease, on the other hand, sexual maturity and fertility are normal, but in pregnancy dangerous anaemia and thromboembolism are at least as common as in the HbSS patient, possibly because anaemia is initially less severe and the seriousness of the situation is not appreciated (Lewis, 1970).

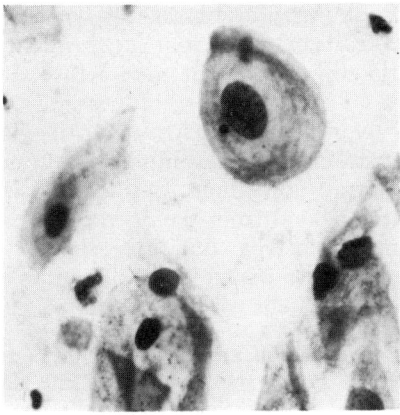

Fig. 12.4e Cervical smear (stained Papanicolaou): epithelial cells showing a wide range of size, one with a giant nucleus; case of megaloblastic anaemia; epithelial cells became normal within 10 days of start of folate therapy.

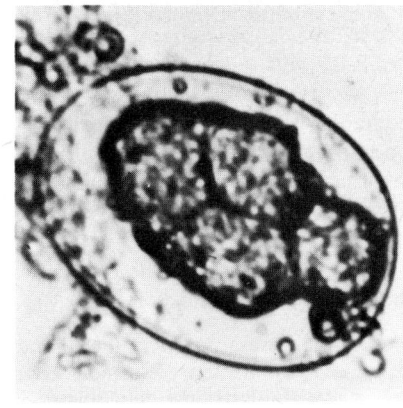

Fig. 12.4f Unstained flotation concentrate from stool; pregnant Pakistani woman with refractory hypochromic anaemia and 20 per cent eosinophilia; characteristic hookworm ovum (ankylostoma duodenale) with scalloped margin inside chitinous envelope.

Prophylactic measures should include oral folic acid, up to 15mg/day, antimalarials where appropriate and antibiotics for incipient bacterial infection. Hypoxia, shock, acidosis and dehydration must be prevented. Analgesics are required for bone pains. Particular care is required with general anaesthesia including the administration of 30–50 per cent oxygen. Regional block is preferable at delivery, but even this has the potential danger of hypotension. There is controversy about the use of blood transfusion, as to the Hb level at which transfusion is indicated, the amount required and how the blood should be given, particularly whether partial exchange and hypertransfusion should be carried out to reduce potential viscosity and reduce the production of sickle cells. Some authorities advise transfusion only when the Hb drops below 6g/100ml and exchange below 4g. A crisis may follow injudicious transfusion, and excessive transfusion in the long term may lead to iron overload (one rather unusual feature of sickle cell disease, however, compared with most other haemolytic anaemias is that sideropenia may occur).

Thus far, various drugs aimed at reducing sickling have been disappointing. Current clinical trials with urea and experiments with cyanate have not been fully assessed and the use of such toxic substances has obvious dangers, particularly in pregnancy.

Splenectomy may occasionally be useful, but in long-standing sickle cell disease the spleen is usually atrophic, fibrotic, siderotic and non-functional and removal of such a spleen is obviously of no value.

c. *Sideroblastic anaemias* (Hoffbrand and Lewis, 1972)

The characteristic morphological change in this group of anaemias is the presence in the bone marrow of ring sideroblasts, erythroblasts containing a perinuclear circle of granules which stain with the Prussian Blue reaction for ferric iron. Sideroblastic anaemias usually present as refractory hypochromic anaemias; they are uncommon generally and rare in pregnancy. Sideroblastic anaemias have a wide range of aetiology and clinical significance as highlighted by the only two cases the writer has seen during pregnancy: one was associated with poor diet and respiratory infection and recovered on pyridoxine; the other was temporarily helped by pyridoxine, but developed Hodgkin's disease which appeared to be the underlying disorder and proved fatal four years after the onset of anaemia. In sideroblastic anaemias, as in the haemoglobinopathies, hypochromia occurs despite a normal or raised serum iron; it is thus important to avoid iron therapy, especially parenteral.

3. MEGALOBLASTIC ANAEMIAS

Megaloblastic anaemia in pregnancy and the puerperium is almost invariably due to folate deficiency and is largely preventable. Even in an apparently normal woman the serum folate level falls as pregnancy advances (Blackledge, 1965) and, especially in poorly nourished communities, if prophylactic folic acid is not given, a variable proportion of pregnant women show haematological changes ranging from florid megaloblastic anaemia to minimal changes in the bone marrow smear without anaemia. In florid cases anaemia may be severe. Morphological changes (hypersegmented neutrophil leucocytes, oval macrocytes, giant metamyelocytes and haemoglobinized or polychromatophilic megaloblasts) are usually demonstrable, if not in ordinary blood films, at least in smears of the *buffy coat from the haematocrit*; the serum folate is usually low (<2mg/ml); thus diagnosis is easy.

In borderline cases, on the other hand, often non-anaemic, identification of minor, transitional changes in erythroblasts and leucoblasts in bone marrow smears is required for diagnosis, but even given such preparations experts differ in their interpretations. Diagnosis is not helped by general haematological data: patients with gestational megaloblastic anaemia may have a normal or low MCHC and a high, normal or low MCV; the leucocyte count is similarly variable; platelets may or may not be reduced. The serum folate level, histidine loading test (FIGLU) and other tests of folate status do not resolve the situation. The red cell folate level may be of some help, but as authorities give such varying ranges of normality, mainly because of variations in techniques of assay, anyone using this parameter must set his own standards.

The rigid scientific approach to the problem implies the need for repeated marrow biopsies from about mid-term on every pregnant woman (Fig. 12.4D). Such a policy is patently impracticable. Buffy coat preparations have served the writer as a useful compromise, but, as they require considerable time and expertise, the only acceptable practical solution is to give prophylactic folic acid (Willoughby and Jewell, 1968) or to give folic acid to anaemic women whose haemoglobin level does not rise on iron therapy.

The protean manifestations of untreated gestational megaloblastic anaemia, however, should not be forgotten. The onset may be rapid, may occur from about mid-term in severe cases, especially in association with iron deficiency, haemolytic anaemia, anticonvulsant drugs, malabsorption syndrome or twin pregnancy, is most frequent in the third trimester but may not be clinically obvious until the puerperium. Indeed the appearance of the patient may be quite deceptive, sometimes pale, but sometimes almost ruddy despite a low haemoglobin. Signs suggestive of pre-eclampsia (oedema, raised blood pressure and proteinuria) are not uncommon (Goodall,

1961b), and may disappear rapidly with folate therapy. Premature labour or intra-uterine death is common in the severe case. Inflammation of mucous membranes may occur, e.g., vulvo-vaginitis, gastro-enteritis, glossitis, stomatitis, cheilitis, respiratory infections and urinary tract infections. Epithelial cells from such lesions and from the cervix, either antepartum or post-partum, may show changes resembling the megaloblastic changes in the haemopoietic cells (*see* Fig. 12.4E).

In a series investigated by the writer and G. D. Blackledge, six of sixteen cases of megaloblastic anaemia diagnosed during pregnancy showed unequivocal evidence of giant hypochromatic nuclei in the cervical smear and six of twelve diagnosed in the puerperium showed similar changes. These abnormalities disappeared after treatment with folic acid. Folate deficiency may predispose to recurrent abortion. Infections may lead to thrombocytopenic purpura, severe neutropenia, haemolysis or disseminated intravascular coagulation. In one such case the writer has observed necrosis of the head of the femur (the patient is not a sickler) (Goodall, 1970).

Cases delivered without treatment may be complicated by intra-partum or post-partum collapse, with or without haemorrhage or by puerperal pyrexia. Haemorrhagic retinopathy may occasionally occur. The blood and bone marrow in either untreated or treated cases may show leukaemoid reactions.

One of the main recent interests in folate deficiency in pregnancy is its possible relationship to abruptio placentae (*see* Chapter 8). The idea has its advocates (Hibbert and Hibbert, 1963) and its opponents (Chanarin, 1969). The precise significance of the relationship is difficult to define, as many of the women in whom folate deficiency and abruptio co-exist are of low income groups, multiparous and possibly also subject to other nutritional disorders.

The pathogenesis of megaloblastic anaemia of pregnancy is likewise complex. The deterioration of folate status which occurs in any pregnancy is no doubt brought about by excessive demands for the synthesis of desoxyribonucleic acid in fetus, placenta, uterus and maternal marrow. Poor diet, malabsorption, multiparity, multiple pregnancy, persistent vomiting, anticonvulsant drugs, pre-existing hypochromic anaemia or haemolytic anaemia may be of importance in particular cases. The only factor common to all would appear to be pregnancy.

However complex the aetiology, prevention is simple (0·3–0·5mg folic acid daily by mouth), and, even when it has been neglected, treatment with oral folic acid (5–10mg tds) is usually successful. As with prophylactic iron therapy, however, there is no guarantee that the woman will take routine therapy. Parenteral folate is seldom required, but may be if there is persistent vomiting or severe malabsorption. Blood transfusion may be required if the anaemia is severe, particularly near term, and, in the presence of cardiac failure, either from the anaemia or co-existing cardiac disease, exchange transfusion or the simultaneous administration of ethnacrynic acid may be required to prevent dangerous overloading of the circulation (*see* Chapter 26).

Response to folic acid is usually assessed on the reticulocyte count and rise in haemoglobin, but specific reaction may be seen in normoblastic change in the buffy coat (usually in about two days—half the time for the reticulocyte rise), a rapid fall in the usually high serum iron and a rise in serum uric acid. Reticulocytosis and rise in haemoglobin may not be optimal during pregnancy and may be inadequate in the presence of infection or iron deficiency.

OTHER TYPES OF MEGALOBLASTIC ANAEMIA

Although the serum vitamin B_{12} level is often slightly reduced in pregnancy, serious depletion is uncommon, and not surprisingly so, as deficiency of that vitamin may lead to infertility (Jackson *et al.*, 1967). Addisonian pernicious anaemia is rare in young women, and, when treated, should not be a problem in relation to pregnancy. Intestinal malabsorption may lead to deficiency of vitamin B_{12} as well as of folic acid. Indeed sideropenia may also occur in such cases and lead to a dimorphic type of anaemia. With severe malabsorption, particularly from gluten enteropathy, the spleen may be shrunken and this is associated with characteristic changes in the blood —'hyposplenism'. Congenital absence of intrinsic factor or failure to absorb cobalamins in the presence of intrinsic factor are exceedingly rare, are due to autosomal recessive genes and thus occur characteristically in children of consanguinous marriages. Dietary deficiency of vitamin B_{12} is uncommon, occurring mainly in strict vegans. Women who smoke cigarettes appear to have low serum vitamin B_{12} levels in pregnancy.

4. ANAEMIAS ASSOCIATED WITH HYPERTENSIVE TOXAEMIAS

Mention has already been made of how megaloblastic anaemia may mimic pre-eclampsia. The two conditions may co-exist, for not infrequently, especially in primiparous patients, one used to see partial response of the 'toxaemia' to folic acid, but, later, a recurrence of oedema, hypertension and proteinuria despite continued folate therapy. Severe sideropenic anaemia may also rarely mimic pre-eclampsia. One interesting feature of the megaloblastic cases with signs of 'toxaemia' is that they do not have fits.

On the other hand, patients with eclampsia may suffer from severe secondary anaemia. This may be of a fulminating type with haemoglobinuria which may be due to the lysis of blood extravasated in the liver (Goodall, 1961a), or when hypertension is severe, may be of micro-angiopathic type, i.e. due to widespread microthrombosis and characterized haematologically by distortion and fragmentation of the erythrocytes and by thrombocytopenia (Brain *et al.*, 1962). Sheehan and Lynch (1973) raise objections to these explanations, but offer no alternative.

Rather paradoxically a rising haemoglobin level is a bad sign in patients with pre-eclampsia, as it denotes rapid extravasation of plasma with increase of blood viscosity and danger of cerebral hypoxia and fits.

5. ANAEMIAS ASSOCIATED WITH INFECTIONS

The presence of any chronic inflammatory process may lead to anaemia. Such anaemia may show a maldistribution of iron: low concentration in the serum; high in the reticulo-endothelial system. Response to oral iron in these cases is often disappointing and the case for parenteral iron doubtful generally and contra-indicated in urinary tract infection (Scott, 1963). Satisfactory response comes usually only after the inflammatory lesion has subsided. The red cells in such cases are usually small and may or may not be hypochromic.

Even today *malaria* is a common cause of anaemia, haemolytic in type, chronic in benign tertian and quartan, acute in the subtertian (falciparum, malignant) form (*see* Chapter 26). Malaria may be transmitted to the fetus. The patient with malignant malaria has fever, haemolytic anaemia and disseminated intravascular coagulation which may affect the brain or other organs. Anyone recently in the tropics is at risk and examination of thick and thin films should be made on the blood of such individuals presenting with any of these signs: fever, headache, acute psychosis, coma, vomiting, diarrhoea or jaundice. The hypersplenism of chronic endemic or latent malaria will be discussed later (*see also* Chapter 26).

Fulminating haemolytic anaemia with haemoglobinuria may also result from *Clostridium welchii septicaemia* particularly after abortion or ignored rupture of the membranes. Pyogenic bacteria (streptococci and staphylococci) may cause less severe grades of haemolysis.

Viral infections of the respiratory tract may cause auto-immune haemolytic anaemia and *viral hepatitis* may be complicated by haemolytic or hypoplastic anaemia. Hypoplasia of the marrow may also be due to *miliary tuberculosis.* Infections of various types, e.g. hepatitis, infectious mononucleosis, brucellosis, may cause transient damage to the marrow with polyploidy of erythroblasts and transient macrocytosis mimicking megaloblastic anaemia.

As already mentioned, infections may cause worsening of anaemias and delay in response to specific therapy, e.g. *E. coli* infections of the urinary tract in megaloblastic anaemia. *E. coli* or salmonella infection may cause crises and bone necrosis in sickle cell disease. Disseminated intravascular coagulation appears to play a part in these acute complicating infections and may be accompanied by cryofibrinogenaemia (presence of cold-precipitable fibrinogen).

6. ANAEMIAS UNCOMMON IN PREGNANCY

a. *Haemolytic anaemias*
Apart from haemolytic aspects of 2(b), 3, 4 and 5 (*see* Table 12.3).

Haemolytic anaemias are characterized by a reduction of the life span of the erythrocyte. They may be inherited or may be due to infections, immune processes, physical factors or chemical agents. Apart from the conditions already discussed they are rare in pregnancy and will only be briefly mentioned. Haemolytic anaemia usually leads to jaundice and the yellow colour of the serum must be differentiated from that of carotenaemia.

Hereditary spherocytic haemolytic anaemia occasionally presents during pregnancy, usually with a megaloblastic crisis due to folate deficiency or a hypoplastic crisis from infection. The anaemia may be very severe in such cases and the reticulocytosis characteristic of most haemolytic anaemias is usually absent. When jaundice is severe, transfusion of packed cells to attain a high level of haemoglobin is required not only to correct the anaemia, but also to reduce the production of bilirubin by substituting normal red cells and to prevent a rapid regeneration of abnormal spherocytes when folic acid or an appropriate antibiotic has been successful in correcting the megaloblastic or hypoplastic process. Splenectomy is indicated, but can usually be delayed until a few months post-partum. Occasionally obstructive jaundice may supervene, because of biliary sludging,

infection or pigment stones, and in these cases of acholuric jaundice which have become choluric, splenectomy must not be delayed. The diagnosis of hereditary spherocytic haemolytic anaemia is usually made by the finding of small, densely eosinophilic erythrocytes (spherocytes) in the blood film and confirmed by increased osmotic fragility in association with a negative direct antiglobulin (Coombs) test.

Hereditary ovalocytic haemolytic anaemia is rare.

Hereditary non-spherocytic haemolytic anaemia is also uncommon, but *genetically determined deficiency of glucose-6-phosphate dehydrogenase* (G-6-PD) is a common basis for haemolytic reactions to drugs, particularly in individuals of Mediterranean or African origin, e.g. primaquine, sulphonamides and nitrofurantoin drugs or favus beans. From the point of view of the obstetrician, however, the G-6-PD problem is important in relation to oxidant drugs used in the treatment of infections in the mother and because deficiency may cause neonatal jaundice in either sex, particularly in infants of Chinese or Mediterranean origin and especially if there is infection or if vitamin K analogues have been given.

Auto-immune haemolytic anaemia varies clinically from acute to chronic, aetiologically from post-infective to neoplastic and serologically as to the types of antibodies. The direct antiglobulin (Coombs) test is positive. Treatment is usually with corticosteroids, but occasionally splenectomy is indicated. Blood transfusion in such cases requires careful cross-matching.

The iso-immune processes responsible for haemolytic disease of the newborn and incompatible transfusion reactions will not be discussed in this chapter, but the danger to the mother of incompatible transfusion must again be stressed, and indeed even in the absence of antibodies Rh-positive blood must *never* be given to an Rh-negative female.

Among *chemicals* toxic to the erythrocyte, *lead* is one which must be kept in mind in relation to obstetrics and gynaecology. Large doses of oxidant drugs may cause haemolysis in a previously normal person, and, as discussed above, G-6-PD deficiency may cause greater susceptibility to such drugs.

b. *Hypoplastic anaemias*
Hypoplastic (aplastic) anaemias are very rare in pregnancy. Industrial hazards, e.g. benzene, or drugs, e.g. chloramphenicol, gold salts or antineoplastic agents may be responsible, as may occupational or therapeutic irradiation, but no apparent cause may be found.

c. *Anaemias due to usurpation of the marrow*
Replacement of the bone marrow by primary or secondary neoplastic disorders, sometimes associated with fibrosis, may cause profound anaemia.

Leukaemia is rare in pregnancy, but Sheehy (1958) published a review of 153 cases (126 granulocytic, 37 acute, 89 chronic; 20 lymphoid, 16 acute, 4 chronic; and 7 acute monocytic; Hoover and Schumacher (1966) analysed 59 acute cases, approximately half granulocytic, a quarter lymphoid and a quarter monocytic. Pregnancy generally has no effect on the leukaemic process, except possibly in relation to its complication by an acute haemorrhagic state with thrombocytopenia and defibrination. Acute leukaemia in the mother causes an appreciable abortion rate (8 per cent) and perinatal mortality (27 per cent). Transmission to the fetus is unlikely to occur; there is only one possible case reported. Management of chronic cases raises the problem of assessing the relative dangers to mother and infant, particularly the danger to the early embryo from steroids, antimetabolites or alkylating agents. In general the leukaemic process is more dangerous than even such potent drugs. The most acute clinical problem occurs with acute myeloblastic, monocytic or myelomonocytic cases complicated by defibrination and by thrombocytopenia from excessive consumption as well as failure of formation. Secondary infection is common. There is no simple approach to the management of leukaemia in pregnancy and each patient must be treated as a unique individual in relation to the complicated pattern of haematological and obstetric problems.

An extensive review of *Hodgkin's disease* associated with pregnancy was published by Barry *et al.* (1962). In 91 pregnancies which were allowed to continue 79 resulted in viable infants and none of these infants had Hodgkin's disease or any other disease patterns. The condition appears to be little affected by pregnancy, except that there may be marginal improvement followed by exacerbations post-partum. As with leukaemia each case must be managed individually and radiotherapy or chemotherapy should not be given in the first trimester. It should also be emphasized that the management of all such cases should be shared with an expert in such treatment.

d. *Anaemias secondary to splenic disorders—hypersplenism*
In pregnant women the problem is mainly found in the tropics (*see* Chapter 26). Latent malaria must be excluded, by therapeutic trial if necessary. Congestive splenomegaly due to portal cirrhosis or hepatic schistosomiasis is also possible. Splenectomy is frequently required, even in infective cases, for specific chemotherapy, though clearing the infection, may not lead to shrinkage of the spleen. These cases of so-called tropical splenomegaly may, like Burkitt's lymphoma, represent exaggerated reaction to repeated infections.

Finally, in relation to splenomegaly, it should be stressed that, apart from the great variation in the size of the spleen from case to case of haemolytic anaemia or leukaemia, the clinical detection of enlargement of the spleen is difficult in late pregnancy. Palpation and percussion are unreliable and radiological examination inadvisable. Ultrasonic scanning may well prove to be the most useful yardstick of splenic size in pregnant women.

Prevention of anaemia in pregnancy

1. ROUTINE BLOOD EXAMINATIONS
Some of the measures required have already been mentioned in relation to the various types of anaemia. Practical aspects of the antenatal care of the blood will now be outlined. The blood of every pregnant woman should be examined at first booking (if possible not later than 8-10 weeks) and thereafter at least at 22-24 weeks, 28-32 weeks and 36-38 weeks. Checks 3-5 days post-partum and at the postnatal clinic are also suggested. Frequent checks are necessary to detect anaemia developing late in pregnancy. Apart from increasing the well-being of the pregnant woman, detection of anaemia at the earliest opportunity may prevent emergencies later in pregnancy and the need for scarce and potentially dangerous blood.

For haematological screening a venous sample in a sequestrenized (EDTA) plastic container is required and clotted samples are also taken at first attendance, one for ABO and Rhesus blood grouping and antibody studies, the other samples for various screening procedures (Chapter 16). Even if only a haemoglobin estimation is required at later checks, *a venous sample should be taken*, as even subclinical oedema in pregnancy may render capillary samples inaccurate from dilution by tissue fluid. It should also be remembered that prolonged stasis with a tourniquet or sphygmomanometer may lead to haemoconcentration of the specimen; so the practice of taking a venous sample immediately after the use of a blood pressure cuff is ill-advised.

The haemoglobin estimation is best done with a photoelectric absorptiometer, measuring the pigment as cyanmethaemoglobin or oxyhaemoglobin (if the latter, standards should be set using the former). A useful, rapid screening test for the presence or absence of anaemia is given by the copper sulphate specific gravity method. Blood results *may be positively misleading if there is delay in transmission of the specimens to the laboratory, particularly if they go through the post.*

Morphological examination of all antenatal specimens of blood, though desirable, may not be possible. It is necessary, however, to examine the blood film, and preferably the buffy coat smear too (Goodall, 1957) from women whose haemoglobin falls below the arbitrary level, say 11g/100ml (9g in the developing countries), taken as indicative of anaemia. Where a satisfactory explanation of anaemia is not given by these screening tests or by the clinical features a marrow biopsy is indicated, but if prophylactic iron and folic acid is taken, such investigations are seldom required. Clotted specimens for serum folate and serum vitamin B_{12} assays should be taken from patients with refractory anaemia.

Patients of African, Mediterranean or Oriental origin and those with refractory anaemia should be screened routinely for abnormal haemoglobins and stools checked for abnormal ova (Fig. 12.4F). Haemoglobin electrophoresis on filter paper at pH 8·6 is the most useful general test. A sickle test (see Fig. 12.4C) using *fresh* 2 per cent sodium meta-bisulphite is also required. Screening tests based on the low solubility of reduced HbS are also advocated. The proprietary 'Sickledex' (Ortho) reagent is useful for the occasional test but expensive for frequent use. A recently published rapid whole blood pre-cipitation test has the advantages of cheapness and of differentiating sickle trait from sickle cell anaemia (Huntsman *et al.*, 1970), but false positive results may occur with anaemia *per se* from excess of plasma or because of the presence of abnormal globulins. For cord blood samples agar gel electrophoresis is the most satisfactory method of demonstrating HbS and HbC (Yawson *et al.*, 1970). The alkali resistance test for HbF and the estimation of HbA_2 by electro-phoresis are required in the investigation of suspected thalassaemia and films should be examined by the acid elution test and periodic acid-Schiff reaction in such cases. Tests for G-6-PD deficiency (Giblett) have already been mentioned.

2. PROPHYLACTIC IRON AND FOLIC ACID

The potentially common hypochromic and megaloblastic anaemias can be prevented in the majority of pregnant women by oral supplements of iron and folic acid. As em-phasized by Bonnar and Goldberg (1969) regular supplements eliminate many so-called physiological anaemias. A daily intake from first attendance of about 50mg of elemental iron and 0·3–0·5mg of folic acid is sufficient in most cases, but larger amounts of both may be required in patients with malabsorption or twin pregnancy. In pregnant women with haemolytic anaemias, especially sickle cell disease, the requirements of folic acid are much larger—5–15mg/day.

Unless the diet is really good, ascorbic acid, 50–100mg daily is a useful additional supple-ment which appears to aid absorption of iron. There is not yet enough evidence to suggest exact requirements for vitamin B complex and vitamin E in pregnancy.

3. REFRACTORY HYPOCHROMIC ANAEMIA

In relation to pregnancy this may be defined in two ways; first, as hypochromic anaemia which is diagnosed at first visit but fails to respond to therapeutic doses of oral iron; second, as hypochromic anaemia developing despite oral prophylaxis with iron and folic acid. In either case the serum iron and iron combining power must be estimated in order to define whether or not there is iron deficiency; the lower limit for serum iron is about 70 microgrammes/100ml, and for saturation of transferrin (siderophilin) about 20 per cent.

If there is sideropenia the following possi-bilities must be considered: failure to take the preparation, malabsorption, chronic bleeding either overt or occult, chronic infection, multiple pregnancy, co-existing vitamin C deficiency.

If the serum iron is high or normal, the possibility of haemoglobinopathy, either thalas-saemia or the presence of haemoglobin variants, must be considered, and, if suitable investiga-tions for these are negative, marrow biopsy should be carried out to exclude sideroblastic anaemia or other lesions of the haemopoietic system and to assess iron stores. Siderocytes and sideroblasts may be found in the ordinary film or buffy coat smear, but usually only in severe cases. Either sternal or iliac crest puncture may be done; the latter is more comfortable for the patient. A general sedative/analgesic should be given as well as local anaesthesia. Smears and sections are required, and bacterial and cytogenetic cultures should be made where indicated.

4. PARENTERAL IRON THERAPY

Parenteral iron therapy may be necessary in patients with proven and serious malabsorption and is seldom justified in other circumstances (*see*, however, Chapter 16). The patient is deficient in iron only if the serum iron level is below 70 microgrammes/100ml and a low degree of iron binding shown by saturation of transferrin below 20 per cent. The serum level fluctuates and is especially difficult to interpret in association with megaloblastic anaemia, falsely high before treatment and falsely low during folic acid therapy. Folate deficiency should be corrected before parenteral iron is given.

Two types of parenteral iron have been used in recent years: 'Imferon' (Fisons), an iron dextran compound, which has been given as a total dose by slow intravenous drip ('TDI'); and 'Jectofer' (Astra Chemicals), an iron sorbital/citric acid complex stabilized with dextrin, which is given in divided intramuscular doses. The dosage and technique of administration are available from the manufacturers and the former should depend on the weight and haemoglobin deficit of the patient.

Initially 'Imferon' by 'TDI' seemed to be the answer to the problem of parenteral iron therapy, particularly in the tropics where hookworm infestation and poor diet are common and continuous medical care often impossible. Unfortunately the recent demonstration that much of the injected iron may remain in reticulo-endothelial cells and not be available for haemoglobin synthesis has raised doubts about the long-term results, particularly the possibility that subsequent iron deficiency anaemia may be all the more refractory (Henderson and Hillman, 1969). Until this problem is resolved one cannot really recommend 'Imferon' by 'TDI'.

In the interim it would appear that 'Jectofer' is the compound of choice when parenteral iron is necessary. It is particularly important in relation to pregnancy that 'Jectofer' should not be given to patients with urinary tract infection, as exacerbation of symptoms and presumably of pyelonephritis may occur; any parenteral injection of iron may occasionally cause severe anaphylactoid reaction particularly in allergic subjects and in asthmatics may stimulate bronchospasm. Adrenalin, an antihistamine and corticosteroids should be available when parenteral iron is being given. At Dundee Royal Infirmary one asthmatic pregnant woman with malabsorption of iron would accept that element parenterally only in the form of packed cells, as she developed severe bronchospasm with even a test dose of intramuscular iron.

5. REFRACTORY MEGALOBLASTIC ANAEMIA
In relation to pregnancy this may be defined as a failure of a megaloblastic anaemia to respond to therapeutic doses of oral folic acid or the development of a megaloblastic anaemia despite prophylactic oral folic acid. As far as the former is concerned several possibilities arise: malabsorption of folic acid; deficiency of cobalamin; the presence of infection or of an organic lesion; the rare megaloblastic change of neoplasms of the haemopoietic system on the basis of somatic mutation. Failure of prophylactic folic acid to prevent megaloblastic anaemia may be due to the patient's failure to take the supplement, to malabsorption, to cobalamin deficiency, to infection or organic lesions, to excessive demands for folic acid as in haemolytic anaemia or to anticonvulsant drugs. In relation to the last, large doses of folic acid carry a danger of precipitating fits and the situation requires careful supervision.

HAEMATOLOGICAL PROBLEMS IN GYNAECOLOGY

The main problem is of hypochromic anaemia from menorrhagia or metrorrhagia. Thrombocytopenia may be the cause of such bleeding and the lack of platelets may occur alone or as part of a disease involving all the blood cells. Leukaemic processes may cause such bleeding or occasionally may infiltrate the endometrium. It is important that patients with chronic uterine haemorrhage be given oral iron as soon as possible in an attempt to raise their haemoglobin level before diagnostic curettage and thus lessen the need for transfusion.

The leucocyte count and erythrocyte sedimentation rate (preferably by the Westergren method) may be useful in the diagnosis of inflammation and other organic lesions. A differential as well as a total leucocyte count may sometimes be of great value. Thus the finding of eosinophilia may give a lead to the presence of helminth infestation and this may occur in temperate as well as tropical communities, e.g. women infested with oxyuris vermicularis may suffer from widespread pelvic granulomata due to the presence of the threadworms and their ova. These are usually multiparous patients in a poor social environment with young children similarly infested.

The radiotherapeutic and chemotherapeutic management of advanced malignant disease of the uterus and ovary require monitoring of the haemoglobin level, leucocyte count and platelet count. The neoplasms themselves, particularly carcinoma of the cervix may cause anaemia through blood loss, secondary infection and renal failure from involvement of the ureters and bladder.

REFERENCES (SECTION 6)

Afifi, A. M., Banwell, G. S., Bennison, R. J., Boothby, K., Griffiths, P. D., Huntsman, R. G., Jenkins, G. C., Smith, R. G. L., McIntosh, J., Qayum, A., Russell, I. R. & Whittaker, J. N. (1966) Simple test for ingested iron in hospital and domiciliary practice. *Brit. med. J.*, **i**, 1021.

Barry, R. M., Diamond, H. D. & Craver, L. F. (1962) Influence of pregnancy on the course of Hodgkin's disease. *Amer. J. Obstet. Gynec.*, **84**, 445.

Blackledge, G. D. (1965) Unpublished. *The Serum folic acid levels of Dundee pregnant women.*

Bonnar, J. & Goldberg, A. (1969) The assessment of iron deficiency in pregnancy. *Scot. med. J.*, **14**, 209.

Brain, M. C., Dacie, J. V. & Hourihane, D. O'B. (1962) Microangiopathic haemolytic anaemia. *Brit. J. Haemat.*, **8**, 358.

Chanarin, I. (1969) *The Megaloblastic Anaemias*, Ch. 30, p. 815. Oxford: Blackwell.

Diggs, L. G. (1972) Rapid slide test for sickle haemoglobin. *Amer. J. clin. Path.*, **57**, 124.

French, E. A. (1972) Rapid test for sickle haemoglobin. *Amer. J. clin. Path.*, **57**, 123.

Giblett, Eloise, R. (1969) *Genetic Markers in Human Blood*, Ch. 10, p. 346 and Ch. 12, p. 443. Oxford: Blackwell.

Goodall, H. B. (1957) Microscopical examination of the 'buffy coat' from the haematocrit in the investigation of anaemia in pregnancy. *J. clin. Path.*, **10**, 248.

Goodall, H. B. (1961a) Haemoglobinuria in eclampsia and its relationship to hepatic damage. *7th Conf. Intern. Soc. Geograph. Pathol. Path. Microbiol.*, **24**, 602.

Goodall, H. B. (1961b) Megaloblastic anaemia of pregnancy and the puerperium. *7th Conf. Intern. Soc. Geograph. Pathol. Path. Microbiol.*, **24**, 682.

Goodall, H. B. (1970) Atypical bone-marrow changes in acute infections. Part 2. In *Myeloproliferative Disorders of Animals and Man*, p. 327. Edited by W. J. Clarke, E. B. Howard & P. L. Hackett. Oak Ridge, Tenn.: U.S.A.E.C., Div. of Tech. Info.

Henderson, P. A. & Hillman, R. S. (1969) Characteristics of iron dextran utilization in man. *Blood*, **34**, 357.

Hibbard, B. M. & Hibbard, E. D. (1963) Aetiological factors in abruptio placentae. *Brit. med. J.*, **ii**, 1430.

Hoffbrand, A. V. & Lewis, S. M. (1972) *Tutorials in Postgraduate Medicine*, Ch. 2, p. 39. London: Heinemann.

Hoover, B. A. & Schumacher, H. R. (1966) Acute leukemia in pregnancy. *Amer. J. Obstet. Gynec.*, **96**, 316.

Huehns, E. R. (1971) Biochemical compensation in anaemia. The scientific basis of medicine. *Annual Reviews*, Ch. 12, p. 216. Edited by I. Gilliland & Jill Francis. Brit. Postgrad. Med. Fed., Univ. of London, Athlone Press.

Huntsman, R. G., Barclay, G. P. T., Canning, D. M. & Yawson, G. I. (1970) A rapid whole blood solubility test to differentiate the sickle-cell trait from sickle cell anaemia. *J. clin. Path.*, **23**, 781.

Jackson, I. M. D., Doig, W. B. & McDonald, G. A. (1967) Pernicious anaemia as a cause of infertility. *Lancet*, **ii**, 1159.

Lehmann, H. & Huntsman, R. G. (1974) *Man's Haemoglobins*. Amsterdam: North Holland Publishing Company.

Lewis, R. A. (1970) *Sickle States: Clinical Features in West Africans*, Ch. 14, p. 77. Accra: Ghana Universities Press.

McKay, D. G. (1965) *Disseminated intravascular coagulation*. New York: Hoeber Med. Div., Harper and Row.

Scott, Jean M. (1963) Iron sorbitol citrate in pregnancy anaemia. *Brit. med. J.*, **ii**, 354.

Sheehan, H. L. & Lynch, J. B. (1973) *Pathology of Toxaemia of Pregnancy*, Ch. 38, p. 634. Edinburgh: Churchill Livingstone.

Sheehy, T. W. (1958) An evaluation of the effect of pregnancy on chronic granulocytic leukemia. *Amer. J. Obstet. Gynec.*, **75**, 788.

Valtis, D. J. & Kennedy, A. C. (1954) Defective gas-transport function of stored red blood cells. *Lancet*, **i**, 119.

Weatherall, D. J. & Clegg, J. B. (1972) *The Thalassaemia Syndromes*. Oxford: Blackwell.

Willoughby, M. L. N. & Jewell, F. G. (1968) Folate status throughout pregnancy and in postpartum period. *Brit. med. J.*, **ii**, 356.

Yawson, G. I., Huntsman, R. G. & Metters, J. S. (1970) An assessment of techniques suitable for the diagnosis of sickle cell disease and haemoglobin C disease in cord blood samples. *J. clin. Path.*, **23**, 533.

13. Blood Coagulation and Fibrinolysis

Following severance of vessels continued blood loss is prevented by temporary vasoconstriction and the formation of a haemostatic plug. Initially, the haemostatic plug consists of platelets and this is subsequently reinforced by fibrin. In the process of healing, when the fibrin has served its function, it is removed by the fibrinolytic system; and more permanent repair processes then occur. Changes in blood coagulation and fibrinolysis, which occur during pregnancy, may represent a physiological response to meet this challenge. In this account we are concerned not only with problems of bleeding at the placental site, but also with two derangements of the haemostatic mechanism: (a) disseminated intravascular coagulation—when fibrin may form widely throughout the vascular compartment depositing in small vessels; (b) thrombosis—this occurs as a consequence of inappropriate functioning of the haemostatic mechanism.

PHYSIOLOGY OF HAEMOSTASIS

Haemostasis has four main components: the vascular component, platelets, the formation of fibrin (blood coagulation), and the fibrinolytic mechanism for the removal of fibrin when it is no longer required.

Blood coagulation

On withdrawing blood by clean venepuncture and delivering to a glass tube, coagulation occurs in 10 minutes whereas in a tube containing some tissue, it clots in 10 seconds. The latter system is described as the extrinsic mechanism, because tissue is an essential component though plasma factors are also involved. It is quite possible that tissue from the placental site may cause intravascular coagulation by this mechanism. The system which operates to coagulate blood without tissue is called the intrinsic thromboplastin system. The following are the components which are involved in eventual fibrin formation:

Factor I—Fibrinogen; Factor II—Prothrombin; Factor III—Tissue factor; Factor IV—Calcium; Factor V, Factor VII, Factor VIII—Anti-haemophilic globulin (the factor missing in haemophilia), Anti-haemophilic factor; Factor IX (the factor missing in Christmas disease), Christmas factor; Factor X, Factor XI, Factor XII—Hageman factor; Factor XIII—Fibrin stabilizing factor.

The coagulation mechanism can be represented as follows:

Extrinsic system	Prothrombin	Intrinsic system
Factors V, VII X		Factors V, VIII, IX, X, XI and XII
Tissue		Platelet phospholipid
Ca + +		Ca + +
	Thrombin	

The action of thrombin in coagulating fibrinogen is described below.

Platelets in addition to provision of phospholipid make an important contribution in their own right by adhesion and aggregation to produce a mechanical seal.

The components of the coagulation mechanism almost certainly do not all react together at once but in some definite sequence. The evidence is that an activated factor X (X a) together with factor V and phospholipid (from platelets or tissue) are responsible for converting prothrombin to thrombin. Vascular endothelium must have unique properties in the maintenance of blood fluidity. As soon as blood comes in contact with a surface other than vascular endothelium activation occurs by the two routes mentioned. The extrinsic mechanism is triggered by tissue damage, the tissue reacting with factor VII to cause activation of factor X. By the intrinsic pathway factor XII or Hageman factor is activated by loss of contact with vascular endothelium. By a subsequent series of reactions involving factors XI and IX again factor X is activated leading to a prothrombin converting principle as happens along the extrinsic pathway.

These concepts can be represented as follows:

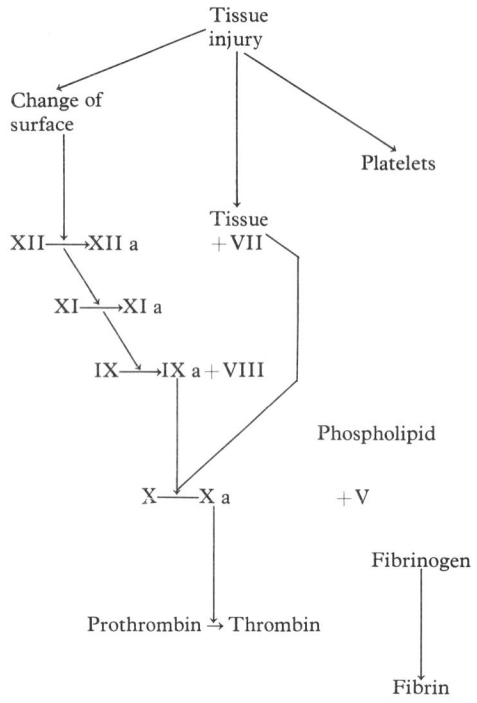

The letter 'a' added after a clotting factor means the activated form of that factor.

A deficiency of factors II, VII, IX or X is common as an acquired abnormality due to the administration of coumarin or indanedione drugs or as a result of vitamin-K deficiency such as may arise, for example, in obstructive jaundice, malabsorption or in haemorrhagic disease of the newborn. These vitamin-K dependent factors are synthesized in the liver, a process which is blocked by the administration of coumarin-like drugs.

Genetic deficiencies of any of these coagulation factors can occur but in the case of the female they are so rare that detailed consideration is not justified in this account. Patients with von Willebrand's syndrome are mentioned towards the end of this chapter.

A deficiency of fibrinogen may first be suspected when whole blood is found to be incoagulable in a glass tube. The formation of a small clot which fails to entrap the red cells and is therefore visible as separate from the main bulk of the red cells also suggests a severe deficiency of fibrinogen.

Fibrinolytic enzyme system

In recent years considerable research and clinical interest has been focused on the phenomenon of 'fibrinolysis'.

In 1933 it was found that the culture fluid of certain strains of haemolytic streptococci contained a substance now named streptokinase, capable of causing rapid lysis of human blood clots. The fibrinolytic enzyme system has four main components: plasminogen, plasmin, activators and inhibitors. Plasminogen, a plasma β-globulin is converted by activators to plasmin, a proteolytic

THE FIBRINOLYTIC ENZYME SYSTEM

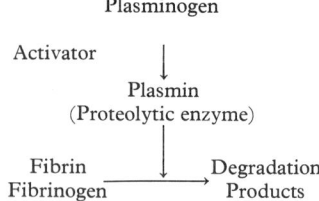

enzyme which under suitable circumstances digests fibrin to give soluble products. Activation of plasminogen, that is, its conversion to plasmin is an enzymatic reaction and is irreversible.

Plasminogen activators are widespread throughout the body; almost all body tissues with the exception of the liver and placenta contain activator, the activity being concentrated around blood vessels particularly veins and venules. Plasminogen activator activity is also present in the blood plasma and is responsible for physiological blood fibrinolytic activity.

Inhibitors of the plasminogen/plasmin system
A number of synthetic amino acids e.g. aminocaproic acid and tranexamic acid show anti-activator activity. These are available commercially.

FIBRINOLYSIS *IN VIVO*—THE SHERRY HYPOTHESIS
A possible mechanism by which the relatively non-specific proteolytic enzyme plasmin is restricted *in vivo* to digestion of fibrin has been proposed by Sherry and his colleagues (Sherry, Fletcher & Alkjaersig, 1959). According to their hypothesis when fibrin is laid down it carries with it sufficient plasminogen to ensure its subsequent lysis; plasmin is produced in close physical proximity to fibrin which is lysed.

CONVERSION OF FIBRINOGEN TO FIBRIN
The conversion of fibrinogen to the final coagulum is brought about by the proteolytic enzyme thrombin which splits off two small fragments (fibrinopeptides A & B) from a fibrinogen molecule to form fibrin monomer. Monomers of fibrin then polymerize to form a visible fibrin network. When fibrin is formed in purified systems, the polymers are held together loosely by weak electrostatic forces and are soluble in five molar urea. Under physiological circumstances in the plasma, stable fibrin is formed, insoluble in five molar urea, the molecules being linked by chemical bonds created by the enzyme plasma transglutaminase or fibrin stabilizing factor (factor XIII). This plasma enzyme is normally present in an inert form, and is converted to an active form by

thrombin in the presence of calcium ions. These reactions can be summarized as follows:

FIBRINOGEN

Thrombin

FIBRIN MONOMER + FIBRINOPEPTIDES

FIBRIN POLYMER (SOLUBLE)

Factor XIII

FIBRIN POLYMER (INSOLUBLE)

When disseminated intravascular coagulation occurs in addition to fibrin monomer, various split products of varying molecular size form from fibrinogen and/or fibrin. Complexes of fibrin monomer and a variety of degradation products of differing molecular size form. These can be detected as fibrin-fibrinogen degradation products (FDP) or fibrinogen/fibrin reacting protein (FRP).

The biological role of the plasminogen-plasmin system
It is possible that the plasminogen-plasmin system may be in dynamic equilibrium with blood coagulation, the two systems acting together to maintain an intact patent vascular tree.

Until more conclusive observations have been made, the concept of a dynamic equilibrium between clotting and lysis remains an attractive but unproved hypothesis. There can, however, be no doubt that the two systems react with one another at many levels, e.g. both systems can be activated by the activation of Hageman factor.

Platelet function

In normal human blood, platelets circulate as single disc-like fragments of cytoplasm at a concentration of approximately 200 000–250 000 per cu mm. In addition to providing a source of phospholipid for the blood coagulation mechanism the platelets play a vital role in haemostasis. When small blood vessels are severed or damaged the contraction of the vessels which follows is usually insufficient to arrest haemorrhage. At the site of vascular injury blood loss is prevented by the rapid accumulation of platelets to form a haemostatic plug which is subsequently reinforced by fibrin. Using electron microscopy it has been demonstrated that initially the platelets adhere to the collagen fibres in the connective tissue beneath the damaged endothelium.

Platelet-collagen contact provokes complex biochemical and morphological changes in the platelets. Adenosine diphosphate (ADP) is released from the platelets at the site of injury and causes further aggregation of platelets leading to the progressive occlusion of the vessel by the platelet mass. Simultaneously the vascular injury triggers the process of blood coagulation which leads to thrombin formation.

The main factor in the consolidation of the platelet plug is the formation at its periphery of increasing amounts of fibrin, and in a matter of hours to days almost all the platelets are replaced by fibrin.

In the puerperium and following operations increased platelet adhesiveness to glass has been reported by several authors and both the platelet count and adhesiveness are found to be maximal at the tenth post-operative day. Such patients have an increased number of young platelets in circulation in the post-operative period and these young platelets have been shown to be selectively adherent to collagen both *in vivo* and *in vitro*. The platelet changes in the puerperium and after surgery have therefore possible important implications in respect of thrombotic complications at these times.

BLOOD COAGULATION AND FIBRINOLYSIS IN PREGNANCY

The haemorrhagic complications of pregnancy and the increased incidence of thrombo-embolism during pregnancy and the puerperium have attracted many to investigate the effect of pregnancy on the haemostatic mechanism. In recent years with increasing improvement of assay methods a more definite pattern of change in the haemostatic system has been shown to occur in response to pregnancy. At the same time it must be appreciated that several of the conditions described have become very rare, particularly 'missed abortion' and 'abruptio placentae'. Changes in coagulation factors and in the fibrinolytic enzyme system appear to be minimal in the first trimester but thereafter an increase in the level of certain clotting factors develop and considerable deviation from the normal occurs in the components of the fibrinolytic enzyme system.

Blood coagulation changes in pregnancy

The plasma fibrinogen level increases in parallel with the period of gestation (Fig. 13.1) and levels of 400–600 mg/100ml are usually found in late pregnancy and during normal labour (Bonnar, McNicol and Douglas, 1969a). In addition to the rise of fibrinogen, the coagulation factors VII, VIII and X are also increased. Factor IX level is also said to rise in pregnancy.

Fibrinolytic enzyme system and pregnancy

In a recent study of the effect of pregnancy on the fibrinolytic enzyme system, the level of plasminogen was found to be elevated during pregnancy and the increase was shown to occur *pari passu* with that of fibrinogen (Bonnar *et al.*, 1969a); allowing for the expansion of plasma volume in pregnancy, the changes represent a doubling in the absolute amounts of circulating fibrinogen and plasminogen (Fig. 13.1). A diminished level of

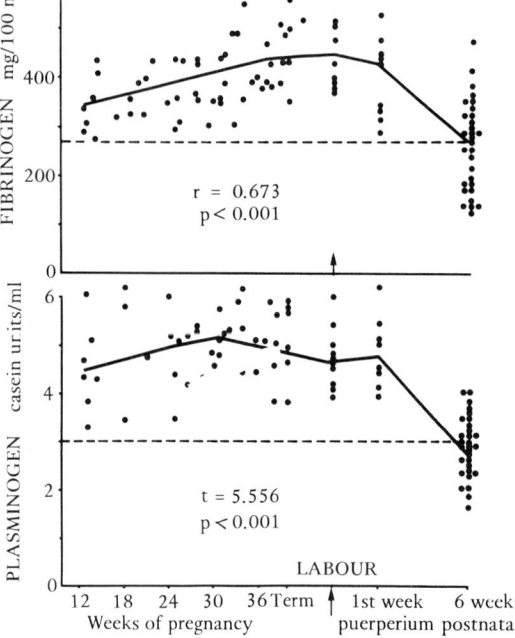

Fig. 13.1 The effect of pregnancy on the levels of fibrinogen and plasminogen. (From Bonnar, J., McNicol, G. P. & Douglas, A. S. (1969)—*Brit. med. J*, **iii**, 387.)

plasma fibrinolytic activity in pregnancy occurs in the presence of increased levels of both fibrinogen and plasminogen, suggesting that a decreased level of circulating plasminogen activator or an activator inhibiting mechanism is probably responsible for the decreased fibrinolysis.

Haemostasis during parturition

Although parturition presents a serious challenge to the haemostatic system it has generally been held that contraction of the myometrium —the 'living ligatures of the uterus'—is the mechanism which in the main controls blood loss at delivery. The effect of childbirth and placental separation on the haemostatic mechanism was recently investigated by serial observations in healthy women and striking changes were found to occur during the actual process of parturition (Bonnar, McNicol and Douglas, 1970). In the third stage of labour a significant shortening of clotting tests, a sharp increase of factor VIII activity, and a decrease of fibrinogen and plasminogen were found in the peripheral blood. Furthermore studies in the uterine circulation during placental separation at Caesarean section confirmed that sudden changes consistent with a local activation of the clotting mechanism take place in the uterus probably at the placental site during the third stage of labour (Bonnar, Prentice, McNicol and Douglas, 1970).

The decreased fibrinolytic activity of pregnancy is surprisingly not influenced by the physical exertion and mental stress of labour, although in other circumstances both stress and physical activity have been shown to provoke a sharp increase in fibrinolytic activity in the plasma (Sherry *et al.*, 1959). The change from reduced to normal fibrinolytic activity takes place between 15 minutes and 1 hour after placental delivery (Bonnar *et al.*, 1970a).

The mechanism by which fibrinolytic activity returns to normal after delivery is unknown. Placental extracts contain high levels of fibrinolytic inhibitors and the placenta itself has been suggested as one of the possible reasons for fibrinolytic inhibition in the mother. In simultaneous studies on maternal and cord blood taken at birth while the cord was pulsating we have found that the blood in the umbilical vein returning from the placenta has increased levels of inhibitors and also a very high level of fibrinolytic activity (Bonnar, McNicol and Douglas, 1971a). The high levels of fibrinolytic activity in the cord blood may be a consequence of the transient hypoxia which occurs in the baby during delivery or may be due to activator release from the endothelium of the umbilical veins.

The changes in the blood coagulation and fibrinolytic systems seem therefore to indicate that during parturition the haemostatic mechanism has an important complementary function to the unique process of myometrial contraction which by extravascular compression diminishes the blood flow to the placental site. The increase in the level of clotting factors which takes place during pregnancy may therefore represent a protective response to provide for rapid and effective haemostasis after delivery. The activation of the clotting mechanism during parturition would also seem to carry a risk of intravascular fibrin deposition and thrombosis. The abrupt return of fibrinolytic activity may provide a protective response to combat this hazard.

During the puerperium the incidence of thrombo-embolic complications is 3-4 times greater than during pregnancy. The changes in the haemostatic mechanism during this time may be one of the factors which predispose to thrombosis. In the first two weeks after normal delivery and after Caesarean section a secondary increase takes place in the level of fibrinogen, factor VIII remains elevated and the number of adhesive platelets shows a steep rise (Bonnar *et al.*, 1970a). Wright (1942) reported a striking increase in the adhesiveness of platelets after parturition. The high platelet count, and increased levels of fibrinogen and factor VIII together with the limited physical activity which may follow delivery, especially Caesarean section, are possible explanations of the predisposition to thrombosis during the puerperium. Early mobilization and active leg exercises would seem therefore to be of special importance following parturition and particularly operative delivery.

SEX HORMONES AND BLOOD COAGULATION

The mechanisms by which the changes in the levels of coagulation factors and in fibrinolytic activity are brought about in pregnancy are still obscure. From the third month of pregnancy the levels of oestrogen and progesterone gradually increase and during this same period the changes appear in the haemostatic mechanism.

The effects of the oral contraceptives, particularly the combined oestrogen and progestogen preparations on the coagulation mechanism may therefore be of relevance. Oral contraceptives can cause a rise of the fibrinogen level similar to that observed in pregnancy. It has also been reported that a significant rise of factors VII and X can occur and after two years on oral contraceptives the factor VII levels may be similar to those of

late pregnancy. Unlike pregnancy, oral contraception is not associated with any decrease of fibrinolytic activity, but an increase in the level of plasminogen similar to that found in pregnancy has been found.

Considerable evidence has now accumulated to confirm that the risk of venous thrombo-embolism is increased in women taking high oestrogen containing contraceptives; epidemiological investigations suggest that the risk of thrombo-embolism was multiplied by a factor of 6 or 7. Since the risk of thrombo-embolism is also increased after surgery and during long periods of immobilization, women taking these drugs may have an increased likelihood of post-operative venous thrombosis. The evidence is that the lower oestrogen content contraceptive pill now in common use carries a much smaller hazard of thrombo-embolism.

Coagulation defects in obstetrics

Defective haemostasis may arise in a wide range of obstetric complications but the most common conditions are abruptio placentae, intra-uterine death, septic abortion and amniotic fluid embolism. Massive transfusion of compatible routine bank blood may also precipitate a generalized haemorrhagic state. The pathogenesis of defective haemostasis in pregnant women has attracted considerable interest. The bulk of the evidence suggests that fibrinogen depletion results from enhanced utilization due to intravascular coagulation.

In recent years it has been demonstrated that the lack of circulating fibrinogen is only one part of a complex syndrome which involves both the coagulation and fibrinolytic systems and the function of the platelets. Abruptio placentae is the complication of pregnancy and labour most likely to give rise to serious coagulation failure and this condition has received most attention. Missed abortion is the next most frequent complication of pregnancy leading to fibrinogen depletion.

ABRUPTIO PLACENTAE

The incidence of fibrinogen depletion and defective haemostasis is related to the type and degree of placental separation and the severe concealed or mixed variety of abruptio placentae is nearly always accompanied by decreased levels of circulating fibrinogen if the levels are compared with those found in normal labour (Bonnar, McNicol and Douglas, 1969b). The visible bleeding in abruptio placentae may be negligible despite the presence of massive intra-uterine bleeding and a serious disturbance of the clotting mechanism. Indeed the latter may only reveal its presence when the blood sample taken for grouping does not clot or persisting oozing develops at the site of venepuncture.

The depletion of circulating fibrinogen in abruptio placentae has received great emphasis but in the context of defective clotting this is best regarded as only one aspect of the condition. In addition to low levels of fibrinogen, depressed levels of factors V and VIII and platelets have been found. We have confirmed these findings and also found that in severe cases factor II (Prothrombin) can be seriously depleted, the plasminogen level is decreased, platelet aggregation and adhesion are disturbed, and extremely high levels of fibrin degradation products can be detected in the serum (Bonnar et al., 1969b).

The main theories advanced in explanation of the haemorrhagic diathesis associated with abruptio placentae include:

1. Utilization of clotting factors at the site of intra-uterine coagulation.

2. Liberation of tissue thromboplastin from the placental site into the circulation producing disseminated intravascular coagulation.

3. Activation of the fibrinolytic enzyme system.

The local utilization of fibrinogen, other clotting factors and platelets in extensive intra-uterine clotting has been suggested as the main reason for the depletion of these factors in the circulation. This may be a contributory cause of the haemorrhagic state in some patients but is unlikely to be the total explanation.

The possibility of intravascular coagulation arising in abruptio placentae arose from the work of Schneider (1951) who suggested that thromboplastin could enter the systemic circulation from the damaged placental site and initiate widespread intravascular fibrin deposition. The placenta and decidua are particularly rich in thromboplastin and the injection of thromboplastin in the form of a tissue extract can produce intravascular deposition of fibrin with resulting depletion of plasma fibrinogen. In several fatal cases of abruptio placentae, fibrin-like material has

been reported in the pulmonary arterioles and in the veins of the uterus (Schneider, 1951). Many autopsies have not demonstrated intravascular fibrin deposition but this can be explained by fibrinolytic dissolution of thrombi in the vessels before and after death.

In studies on the pregnant hamster, Brown and Stalker (1968) have shown that during both spontaneous premature placental separation and the application of trauma to the placenta, white emboli are released from the placental bed not only into the maternal circulation but into the fetal circulation. During placental separation following Caesarean section we have found that the blood draining the placental site exhibits a striking shortening of clotting tests which could be explained by the entry of thromboplastin into the uterine circulation (Bonnar et al., 1970). The phenomenon found at Caesarean section is shortlived and normal clotting times are restored within 10–15 minutes of delivery of the placenta.

In abruptio placentae we have found high levels of FDP indicating that active fibrinolysis is taking place. As shown in figure 13.2, the

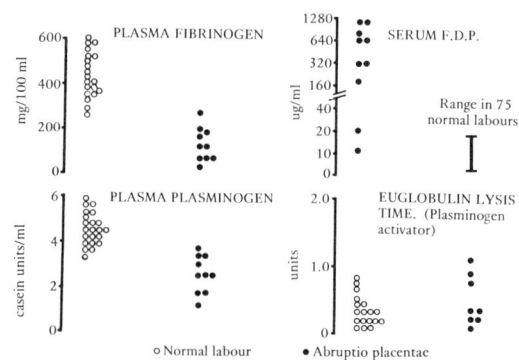

Fig. 13.2 The levels of fibrinogen, plasminogen, serum fibrin degradation products (FDP) and plasminogen activator in 10 patients with abruptio placentae prior to treatment as compared with the findings in 20 healthy patients in normal labour. (From Bonnar, J., McNicol, G. P. & Douglas, A. S. (1969) *J. Obstet. Brit. Cwlth.*, **76**, 799.)

high levels of FDP were accompanied by a low level of systemic fibrinolytic activity, as measured by the euglobulin lysis time. In the presence of diminished fibrinolytic activity in blood sampled from arm veins a high level of FDP suggests that these products are most likely the result of lysis of fibrin possibly in small blood vessels as opposed to lysis of circulating fibrinogen. The combination of low levels of fibrinogen and plasminogen and large amounts of FDP would seem to be consistent with the concept that intravascular coagulation, generalized or localized to specific target organs, is followed by activation of the fibrinolytic mechanism. Removal of fibrin deposits in such circumstances may be mediated, as already described, through adsorption of circulating plasminogen activator.

Haemostatic plugs formed at the placental site may be subject to the same lytic influences which are operating presumably at small vessel level causing the rise in FDP. Within 24–48 hours after delivery the elevation of FDP level has almost disappeared and the fibrinogen level has been restored to normal.

At present, it would appear that in the haemorrhagic state complicating abruptio placentae a complex interaction of the coagulation and fibrinolytic systems is responsible. The available evidence suggests that the haemostatic defect results from the entry of coagulant substances into the circulation from the placental site leading to intravascular clotting. The conversion of fibrinogen to fibrin in the vascular compartment would appear to be accompanied by a simultaneous activation of the fibrinolytic enzyme system which lyses the intravascular fibrin, this activity however is limited to small vessels.

Such a sequence of events would explain the depletion of fibrinogen, the associated decrease of plasminogen, platelets, and coagulation factors II, V and VIII, and the appearance of a large amount of fibrin-fibrinogen breakdown products in the circulation. The presence of high levels of the latter is likely to be a major factor in defective haemostasis and would readily account for prolongation of blood clotting tests and the impairment of platelet function.

INTRA-UTERINE DEATH AND MISSED ABORTION

Fetal death *in utero* is the second most common obstetric condition which can be associated with fibrinogen depletion. The coagulation defect following intra-uterine death is a gradual process and when delivery is delayed for over one month approxi-

mately one-third of patients can develop defective haemostasis with fall in fibrinogen level.

In most cases of fetal death spontaneous expulsion of the fetus takes place before any serious depletion of clotting factors has developed; the vast majority of patients with intra-uterine death go into labour spontaneously within 14 days of fetal death. The diagnosis of intra-uterine death may in some cases, however, be fraught with difficulty and in this situation delay may be the only certain way to establish that the fetus is not alive.

Correction of the coagulation defect by intravenous heparin infusion has given support to the concept of fibrinogen depletion by disseminated intravascular coagulation as the mechanism.

AMNIOTIC FLUID EMBOLISM
The clinical syndrome of amniotic fluid embolism was first described in 1941. As general maternal mortality is further reduced, the relative contribution of rare complications such as amniotic fluid embolism correspondingly increases. The catastrophe can occur during labour, at or shortly after delivery, and at Caesarean section. The typical case is characterized by the sudden development of profound shock, respiratory distress and cyanosis, usually following a period of vigorous uterine contractions. If the patient survives the primary phase of shock a haemorrhagic diathesis invariably supervenes with bleeding from mucous membranes and at venepuncture sites; severe haemorrhage from the uterus invariably follows when the placenta separates.

Abortion and intra-uterine infection

Infection of the uterus and products of conception in early pregnancy is usually the result of attempts to induce abortion. In late pregnancy intra-uterine infection may arise following surgical induction of labour or spontaneous rupture of membranes where delivery is delayed. Defective haemostasis with a fatal outcome has been described following criminal abortion. Coliform organisms may be obtained on blood culture and culture of the products of conception.

The clinical picture has been compared with the experimental Schwartzmann reaction, a condition in which disseminated intravascular coagulation and multiple micro-emboli are produced by two intravenous injections of bacterial endotoxin. McKay (1965) has produced considerable evidence that widespread intravascular clotting is the mechanism responsible for endotoxin shock and defective haemostasis.

In pregnant animals, only one exposure to bacterial endotoxin is necessary to produce the Schwartzmann reaction and this may be a result of the diminished fibrinolytic activity in pregnancy which facilitates intravascular fibrin deposition.

OTHER OBSTETRIC CONDITIONS
Occasionally a severe haemorrhagic state has followed uncomplicated Caesarean operations. The entry into the circulation of thromboplastic material from the placental site or amniotic fluid is the most likely explanation.

Pre-eclampsia and eclampsia
Electron microscopic study of tissue obtained by renal biopsy from patients with preeclampsia has revealed glomerular changes which appear to be specific for this disease. The lesion consists of swelling of the glomerular capillary endothelium, increase of intercapillary cells and deposition of an amorphous fibrinoid material within the cells and beneath the basement membrane. The amorphous substance in the glomeruli of pre-eclamptic patients using immunofluorescent techniques has been shown to be identical to fibrin. A prominent finding in some fatal cases of eclampsia is widespread fibrin deposition and in patients who survived eclampsia liver biopsies have shown fibrin thrombi.

In situations where the secretion or action of plasminogen activator is impaired, fibrin deposition would be more likely to occur and compensatory hypertension may develop to overcome increased peripheral resistance caused by intravascular fibrin.

Extensive fibrin deposition has been shown in the placental bed of patients with pre-eclampsia and this has previously been interpreted as the result rather than the cause of the hypertension. In 10 patients with severe pre-eclampsia we have found significantly higher levels of fibrin breakdown products than were present in normal pregnancy (Bonnar, McNicol and Douglas, 1971b) and following eclamptic seizures the level of breakdown products sharply increased.

DIAGNOSIS OF COAGULATION DEFECTS
The possibility of a coagulation defect should be considered in patients presenting with the predisposing obstetric complications discussed in the preceding part of this chapter. Screening procedures should be readily available at any time to give warning that the haemostatic mechanism is abnormal and alert the blood transfusion service to the need for obtaining adequate supplies of fresh compatible blood. An obstetrical service should have a staff panel willing to donate blood for these rare but catastrophic patient problems. Any patient who presents clinically with local or generalized signs of abnormal bleeding may have a haemostatic defect. In particular, profuse or intractable bleeding from the uterus before or after delivery and persistent oozing during operative procedures or afterwards from incised wounds are in many cases due to defective haemostasis. Prolonged bleeding at venepuncture sites, spontaneous haemorrhage into the skin and from the nose and mouth, and bruising or disproportionate haematomata developing around sutures and intramuscular injections are likely to be indicative of haemostatic failure.

Laboratory tests
The most convenient screening tests are concerned with the level and clottability of the plasma fibrinogen and with the platelet count. The appropriate laboratory service should be asked to provide information on the thrombin clotting time and the behaviour of the clot formed. Fibrinogen assay should be available both by a measurement of clottable fibrinogen and by precipitate produced chemically by heating. In practice these results are not as discordant as might be expected (Miller *et al.*, 1971). A measurement of fibrin/fibrinogen degradation products should be available. A blood film is needed. Measurements of plasminogen and plasminogen activator should be available (McNicol and Douglas, 1964). Patient management will often have to proceed without these results because of the urgency.

SCIENTIFIC BASIS OF THERAPY

This section deals briefly with the general principles and treatment of haemostatic failure in pregnancy. In many situations where this complication arises, with the exceptions of missed abortion and intra-uterine death, haemorrhage is the predominant clinical concern and the patient's condition often requires immediate treatment.

The following principles should be taken into account in the management of obstetric haemorrhage complicated by defective haemostasis.

1. The circulatory state of the patient is more important than the derangement of the blood clotting mechanism and restoration of the blood volume has first priority. In patients with serious haemorrhage and a severe coagulation defect the transfusion of a large volume of blood will be required. In bank blood the platelets can be seen in unreduced numbers during the shelf-life of the bank blood. However they rapidly become non-functional. Furthermore routine bank blood also becomes deficient in factors V and VIII. Therefore for transfusion of these particular patients this is one of the small number of situations when it is mandatory that the blood be fresh.

2. If vaginal delivery can be accomplished without damage to the genital tract, myometrial retraction will often control or greatly reduce bleeding from the placental site. Delivery by Caesarean section or by hysterotomy requires the same degree of haemostatic competence as any other abdominal operation. Therefore, unless the resolution of the underlying condition is being unduly delayed it is advisable to aim at spontaneous delivery rather than resort to surgical interference. If circumstances demand surgical intervention the clotting failure must be controlled prior to operation.

3. The acute coagulation disorder is the result of the obstetrical complication and expediting the process of delivery is of prime concern since this will allow the haemostatic mechanism to recover.

Abruptio placentae

This is now a rare disorder. In this condition, especially the severe mixed or concealed variety, the blood pressure and pulse rate do not always reflect the severity of the haemorrhage. Indeed, a normal blood pressure is often found in abruptio placentae when extensive placental separation and haemorrhage have taken place. A fulminating type of pre-eclampsia with hypertension and albuminuria may be found in patients with abruptio placentae; this condition which is provoked

by the placental separation may well be the result of disseminated intravascular fibrin deposition and vasospasm.

Central venous pressure studies in patients with abruptio placentae have confirmed that severe hypovolaemia often exists which is not reflected in the arterial blood pressure. During rapid and adequate correction of the depleted blood volume the central venous pressure should be monitored as this may be a factor in limiting the process of intravascular fibrin formation. Prompt replacement of blood loss is also of course of particular importance in the prevention of acute renal failure.

The delivery of the patient with abruptio placentae is usually followed by spontaneous and rapid correction of the coagulation defect. As soon as the perfusion of vital organs is restored by blood volume replacement, measures to expedite vaginal delivery should be employed. Many of these patients are of high parity and rupture of the membranes initiates good labour and accelerates the process. Early delivery may forestall an overt coagulation failure and it has been reported that the incidence of haemostatic failure bears a close relationship to delay in performing amniotomy.

Administration of fibrinogen is one of the traditional methods of treatment for the coagulation defect in abruptio placentae. The recent evidence is that when delivery is accomplished without trauma, fibrinogen therapy was rarely indicated. The most rational approach to treatment is the transfusion of fresh whole blood to provide a full complement of coagulation factors and viable platelets, rather than a large quantity of stored blood and plasma.

The use of plasma expanders, such as dextrans, is also to be avoided as these substances may aggravate the haemorrhage state by inhibiting platelet adhesiveness and aggregation. Triple or quadruple strength plasma infusions may produce cardiac arrest possibly as a result of their high potassium content and these preparations should not be used.

If surgery is contemplated careful screening of the patient's blood, including the platelet count, is vital. If marked thrombocytopenia or persisting coagulation failure is present the operation should be delayed until the blood clotting is restored and fresh blood containing viable platelets is available. In such circumstances a fibrinogen concentrate in addition to the fresh blood should restore the deficient haemostatic components to at least their minimum effective level. Fibrinogen 4–6g can be infused in 30 minutes; if fibrinogen concentrate is not available 1 litre of fresh or fresh-frozen plasma should be given as this contains 3g of fibrinogen and also factors V and VIII.

The evidence now available indicates that plasma fibrinolytic activity is reduced in late pregnancy and labour and a similar situation exists in abruptio placentae. This suggests that therapy with fibrinolytic inhibitors such as aminocaproic acid may be potentially hazardous in that such agents will inhibit plasminogen activation in intravascular fibrin deposits and therefore they may carry a risk of promoting vascular occlusion and hence such complications as renal failure.

Treatment with heparin has been suggested to inhibit intravascular deposition and so arrest the consumption of the coagulation factors. If the vascular compartment was intact this concept would be attractive but in women actively bleeding from damaged blood vessels at the placental site it is more than likely that heparin would seriously aggravate the haemorrhage and this would outweigh any beneficial effect on the overall situation.

Intra-uterine death and missed abortion

In contrast to abruptio placentae the coagulation defect with intra-uterine death becomes manifest gradually over an interval of several weeks and does not usually give rise to an emergency exsanguinating haemorrhagic state. The gradual onset of depletion of clotting factors allows a more detailed analysis, and coagulation studies should be performed at weekly intervals from the time that fetal death is suspected. Clinically significant coagulation changes do not usually arise unless the duration of intra-uterine death exceeds one month. In view of the efficiency of prostaglandins in evacuating the uterus in cases of missed abortion, steps to effect delivery can be taken as soon as the diagnosis is established. Intra-amniotic injection of hypertonic solutions of saline or glucose are best avoided in view of the serious hazard of introducing infection.

If a patient presents with evidence of abnormal haemostasis and she is not in labour,

steps should be taken to restore normal clotting before attempts are made to evacuate the uterus. As the primary process appears to be intravascular coagulation, the logical therapy in the undelivered patient with an intact vascular system is to give heparin to block the continuing fibrinogen-fibrin conversion. Heparin can be given as an infusion of 1000 units hourly. Serial fibrinogen estimations are necessary to determine the effect of the heparin and when the plasma fibrinogen level has been restored to over 200mg/100ml then heparin can be discontinued and steps taken to induce labour. The alternative treatment of repeated infusions of large doses of fibrinogen is possible but carries the risk of hepatitis.

In patients with intra-uterine death of long standing, fresh compatible whole blood should be readily available to meet the possibility of serious post-partum haemorrhage. Likewise if surgical intervention is contemplated a supply of fresh blood should be provided prior to operation.

The effects of aminocaproic acid have been studied in intra-uterine death and the therapy failed to correct or prevent deterioration of the haemostatic defect (Dubber, McNicol and Douglas, 1967). Aprotinin has been advocated in this condition but the summation of evidence now is that fibrinolytic inhibitors have no rational basis, unless potent and abnormal fibrinolytic activity can be demonstrated, and this is rare.

AMNIOTIC FLUID EMBOLISM
The mortality from this condition is over 80 per cent. A definite diagnosis however can usually only be made in fatal cases but in recent years a few reports have appeared in which the clinical syndrome has strongly suggested amniotic fluid embolism and with energetic treatment the patient has survived.

Cyanosis and severe hypotension are the two predominant features and oxygenation by the most efficient means available is immediately necessary. A major factor in the severe shock is intravascular clotting; in dogs, heparin administration prior to the intravenous injection of amniotic fluid prevents or greatly diminishes the fall in blood pressure. If the patient is undelivered and no bleeding is present to account for the severe state of shock then the immediate use of heparin is justifiable to prevent continued fibrinogen-fibrin conversion and progressive vascular occlusion of the pulmonary vessels.

SEPTIC ABORTION AND INTRA-UTERINE INFECTION

Infection with Gram negative organisms is the likely precipitating factor and effective bacteriocidal therapy will be required. With hypovolaemia and serious bleeding, fresh blood should be used to replace the depleted clotting factors.

Other haemostatic problems in pregnancy

THROMBOCYTOPENIA

This condition may occur as a feature of the acute coagulation disorders already discussed in which case the treatment is that of the primary disorder. Patients with megaloblastic anaemia of pregnancy may also exhibit a decreased platelet count which will be corrected within a few days of starting folic acid therapy.

Idiopathic thrombocytopenic purpura may present in pregnancy and treatment with steroids is indicated. If the platelet count returns to normal while the patient is on steroid therapy this should be reduced and discontinued if the platelet count remains adequate; it is unwise to maintain steroid therapy throughout pregnancy in idiopathic thrombocytopenic purpura. There is a risk of haemorrhage in the newborn child of a mother with idiopathic thrombocytopenic purpura, even in a mother previously 'cured' by splenectomy.

Normal vaginal delivery without excessive bleeding can take place in thrombocytopenic patients. When thrombocytopenia is known to be present at the time of onset of labour steroid therapy should be given. If operative delivery is contemplated, fresh blood, fresh platelet-rich plasma (or platelet concentrates) should be available.

VON WILLEBRAND'S SYNDROME

This genetic haemorrhagic disease affects both males and females and is characterized by a prolonged bleeding time and a deficiency of factor VIII. Menorrhagia, epistaxis and gastrointestinal bleeding are characteristic features. During pregnancy the level of factor VIII may markedly improve but in some patients no such increase occurs and this group appears to be especially liable to severe post-partum haemorrhage.

If the factor VIII level remains below 50 per cent in late pregnancy an infusion of cryoprecipitate should be given at the onset of labour to provide adequate haemostatic levels of factor VIII during and after placental separation. Cryoprecipitate therapy should be maintained for a few days after delivery.

Anticoagulant therapy in pregnancy

Drugs of the coumarin group cross the placenta and can be associated with fetal mortality as a result of haemorrhage in the infant before or during labour. Fetal abnormality has also been reported following the use of these drugs in early pregnancy. Heparin on the other hand with a molecular weight of 20 000 does not cross the placenta and is not associated with any known fetal hazard. The action of heparin can also be rapidly reversed by intravenous protamine sulphate, 1–1·5mg for 1mg (100 units) of heparin.

In a recent analysis of perinatal deaths associated with the use of coumarin derivatives in pregnancy, Hirsh, Cade and O'Sullivan (1970) found that the main hazard of these drugs arises from their administration in early and late pregnancy. The levels of factors II, VII, IX and X in the healthy newborn are lowered and fibrinolytic activity is markedly increased (Bonnar et al., 1971). Coumarin derivatives (molecular weight about 1000) will produce further depletion of these Vitamin K dependent factors in the fetus and so impair the haemostatic competence of the infant that serious haemorrhage may result from the trauma of delivery. Heparin is therefore the safest anticoagulant to use during pregnancy and is to be preferred particularly in early and late pregnancy.

Long-term parenteral therapy with heparin may not be practical and where anticoagulant therapy is believed to be mandatory from early pregnancy Hirsh et al. (1970) suggest that as a compromise, coumarin drugs can be used after the first trimester until 37 weeks' gestation. There would require to be a major indication for use. Such a regimen will allow the fetal clotting factors to return to their normal level before delivery.

The administration of sedatives and anticonvulsant drugs during pregnancy increases the incidence of haemorrhagic disease of the newborn and their concomitant administration with anticoagulant drugs would aggravate the bleeding tendency in the fetus. Hence, these drugs and indeed any drugs that cross the placenta should be avoided if possible during pregnancy. In the puerperium oral anticoagulant drugs can be employed but the baby should not be breast fed because the drug is excreted in the milk.

When the anticoagulant effect of the coumarin and indanedione drugs requires to be reversed vitamin K_1 should be administered under the standard dosage regime for these circumstances.

Eclampsia and Pre-eclampsia

Recent work in these topics has provided suggestive evidence that disseminated intravascular coagulation is an aspect of the pathogenesis. This does not mean of course that this is the primary cause of the disorder. *Oestrogens and thrombosis.* Much interest has been shown in recent years in the relationship between the occurrence of venous and arterial thrombosis with the administration of the contraceptive pill but this topic is outwith the consideration of this chapter.

REFERENCES

Biggs, R. & Macfarlane, R. G. (1962) *Human Blood Coagulation and its Disorders*. Third Edition. Oxford: Blackwell Scientific Publications.

Bonnar, J., Davidson, J. F., Pidgeon, C. F., McNicol, G. P. & Douglas, A. S. (1969) Fibrin degradation products in normal and abnormal pregnancy and parturition. *Brit. med. J.*, **iii**, 137.

Bonnar, J., McNicol, G. P. & Douglas, A. S. (1969a) Fibrinolytic enzyme system and pregnancy. *Brit. med. J.*, **iii**, 387.

Bonnar, J., McNicol, G. P. & Douglas, A. S. (1969b) The behaviour of the coagulation and fibrinolytic mechanism in abruptio placentae. *J. Obstet. Gynaec. Brit. Cwlth*, **76**, 799.

Bonnar, J., McNicol, G. P. & Douglas, A. S. (1970) Coagulation and fibrinolytic mechanisms during and after normal childbirth. *Brit. med. J.*, **ii**, 200.

Bonnar, J., Prentice, C. R. M., McNicol, G. P. & Douglas, A. S. (1970a) Haemostatic mechanism in the uterine circulation during placental separation. *Brit. med. J.*, **ii**, 564.

Bonnar, J., McNicol, G. P. & Douglas, A. S. (1971a) The blood coagulation and fibrinolytic systems in the newborn and the mother at birth. *J. Obstet. Gynaec. Brit. Cwlth*, **78**, 355.

Bonnar, J., McNicol, G. P. & Douglas, A. S. (1971b) Coagulation and fibrinolytic systems in pre-eclampsia and eclampsia. *Brit. med. J.*, **ii**, 12.

Brown, L. J. & Stalker, A. L. (1968) The maternal and foetal micro-circulation following placental separation or trauma. Proceedings of the international conference on Microcirculation, Gothenburg, Sweden. *Bibl. anat.*, p. 374.

Dubber, A. H. C., McNicol, G. P. & Douglas, A. S. (1967) Acquired hypofibrinogenaemia—the defibrination syndrome—a study of 7 patients. *Scott. med. J.*, **12**, 138.

Hirsh, J., Cade, J. F. & O'Sullivan, E. F. (1970) Clinical experience with anticoagulant therapy during pregnancy. *Brit. med. J.*, **i**, 270.

McKay, D. G. (1965) *Disseminated intravascular coagulation*. New York: Hoeber.

McNicol, G. P. & Douglas, A. S. (1964) The fibrinolytic enzyme system in '*Recent Advances in Clinical Pathology*', Series IV, p. 187. Ed. by S. C. Dyke, London: Churchill.

Millar, H. R., Simpson, J. G. & Stalker, A. L. (1971) An evaluation of the heat precipitation method for plasma fibrinogen estimation. *J. Clin. Path.*, **24**, 827.

Schneider, C. L. (1951) Fibrin embolism (disseminated intravascular coagulation) with defibrination as one of the end results during placenta abruptio. *Surgery, Gynaec. Obstet.*, **92**, 27.

Sherry, S., Fletcher, A. P. & Alkjaersig, N. (1959) Fibrinolysis and fibrinolytic activity in man. *Physiological Reviews*, **39**, 343.

Wright, H. P. (1942) Changes in the adhesiveness of blood platelets following parturition and surgical operations. *J. Path. Bact.*, **54**, 461.

FURTHER READING

An expanded version of this chapter with detailed references will be found in Scientific Basis of Obstetrics and Gynaecology. Ed. R. R. Macdonald. London: Churchill. Chapter 9. '*Blood Coagulation and Fibrinolysis*'. John Bonnar, G. P. McNicol and A. S. Douglas.

14. Surgical Conditions in Obstetrics

THE ACUTE ABDOMEN

All the likely causes of an 'acute abdomen' may occur in the pregnant woman but perforation of a peptic ulcer is rare.

Diagnosis is often confused by the enlarging uterus, the stretched abdominal wall is less likely to show resistance and organs may be displaced or hidden by the pregnant uterus. Moreover, the conditions specific to pregnancy—pyelonephritis; ectopic pregnancy; rupture of broad ligament vessels; retroplacental bleeding—may themselves produce an 'acute abdomen' and are important in differential diagnosis.

Acute appendicitis

Appendicitis is one of the commonest causes of acute abdominal pain from non-obstetric causes. The condition may be very serious in pregnancy if delay in diagnosis and treatment allows rupture or extensive peritonitis to occur. While, in general, the disease behaves as it does in the non-pregnant, the appendix may be displaced upwards and outwards in late pregnancy so altering the physical signs. The normal if somewhat high ESR and leucocytosis of pregnancy can confuse.

Abortion and premature labour may occur especially if peritonitis occurs.

DIAGNOSIS
In the first trimester of pregnancy the signs and symptoms are very similar to that in the non-pregnant, but if there is associated morning sickness preceding the condition this may lead to some difficulty in diagnosis. The pain is usually generalized abdominally to begin with and then localizes in the right iliac fossa and rebound tenderness is a marked feature in the area of McBurney's point. In retrocaecal and pelvic appendices the signs will be different as in the non-pregnant. In mid-pregnancy the appendix may be displaced upwards and to the right and tenderness will become more marked out towards the flank.

Examination of the urine may not always be helpful because in such cases pus cells are frequently found and a high bacterial count.

In the third trimester the pain and tenderness are maximal on the right side at about the level of the umbilicus or even higher under the costal margin. Acute pyelonephritis is usually the chief component in the differential diagnosis and also cholecystitis. Other conditions which might be confused with acute appendicitis later in pregnancy are abruption of the placenta, ruptured ovarian cyst and degeneration of a fibroid. If appendicitis occurs, as it can do during labour, the diagnosis may be missed because of the labour pains and vomiting. Persistent pain, a rising pulse, pyrexia and fetid breath should alert the clinician to the possibility.

Treatment of acute appendicitis
An emergency appendicectomy should be performed as soon as the diagnosis is suspected. In cases of doubt it is always wiser to do an exploratory laparotomy as the consequences of a ruptured appendix are so alarming. A right paramedian or pararectal incision is usually made and the uterus gently retracted with as little disturbance as possible to allow access to the caecum and appendix. After removal of the appendix in the routine fashion it is not usual to require drainage. Antibiotics are given and if dehydration is present intravenous fluids are administered. If labour commences soon after the operation the wound is quite safe, and there is usually no worry about dehiscence. If appendicitis occurs during labour it is preferable to await until after delivery before doing the appendicectomy as there is often delay in labour. It is preferable to avoid Caesarean section in cases of appendicitis because of the possibility of the infection spreading into the uterus.

Intestinal obstruction

This can occur because of volvulus (intussusception) colonic neoplasms or adhesive bands. Displacements of the uterus because of pregnancy can predispose to the development of intestinal obstruction, particularly if it is due to adhesions. Obstruction is suspected when there is persistent vomiting associated with colicky abdominal pains. In early pregnancy it is very important to distinguish the condition from hyperemesis gravidarum, but the pain is usually indicative of obstruction, and the abdominal distention also suggests the diagnosis. Volvulus is a rare cause of obstruction. It usually affects the left side of the colon and it may be necessary to do a Caesarean section in order to allow sufficient access to correct the volvulus. In acute intestinal obstruction in addition to the vomiting and colic there is distention, tenderness over a large area and also rebound tenderness. If the obstruction is low in the large bowel the vomiting may not occur until late. Auscultation reveals the high-pitched tinkling sounds and an X-ray of the abdomen may show fluid levels in the loops of intestine.

If the obstruction is incomplete the clinical picture is less definite and the pain may be intermittent as may also be the vomiting. In small bowel obstruction prompt surgical intervention is indicated. If adhesions are suggested by a previous scar or a history of pelvic infection it may occasionally be sufficient to pass a long intestinal tube to cause decompression and relief of symptoms. This is followed by conservative treatment with intravenous fluids, but if the symptoms persist surgical intervention must be proceeded with, and the obstruction relieved by dividing the adhesions or removing any other cause of the obstruction. If there is difficulty in gaining access then a Caesarean section must be performed to empty the uterus and reduce its size.

In large bowel obstruction a laparotomy is performed and any volvulus or intussusception is corrected. If a neoplasm of the left colon is found then a transverse colostomy is performed and resection is done a few weeks later. When the uterus is large it may be necessary to do a Caesarean section to gain sufficient access.

Diverticulitis

This can occur in pregnancy and is like a left-sided appendicitis. Mild attacks are treated conservatively with antibiotics and intravenous fluids, but if a perforation is suspected immediate operation and drainage is essential. After the pregnancy is completed definitive treatment of the diverticulitis can be carried out.

Rupture of the splenic artery

This is due to a rupture of splenic aneurysms and can occur in late pregnancy probably because of displacements of the spleen by the uterus. The rupture may cause a dramatic collapse because of severe internal haemorrhage and unless emergency laparotomy can be carried out quickly and the bleeding site located and ligated the patient will die. Sometimes the rupture is more gradual and a pulsating haematoma forms which will later rupture into the general peritoneal cavity. In early pregnancy rupture of an ectopic pregnancy is suspected. When laparotomy is performed there may be difficulty in locating the site of the bleeding because the abdomen is filled with blood. The bleeding may occur from many sources in the abdominal cavity. Immediate blood transfusion and urgent surgery is required. The pelvis is usually searched first being the most likely source of the bleeding, and it is then necessary to inspect the mesenteric vessels and the hepatic and splenic arteries. The bleeding vessel is ligated and splenectomy may be required. Traumatic rupture of the spleen may occur particularly in road accidents, but it can also occur in cases of splenomegaly. Again there is a rapid onset of shock and evidence of intraperitoneal bleeding. Laparotomy must again be carried out promptly and a splenectomy performed when the source of the bleeding has been determined.

Rupture of the liver

Although it is sometimes spontaneous especially after severe pre-eclampsia it is usually caused by trauma. There is severe epigastric pain with evidence of intraperitoneal bleeding with a marked fall in blood pressure. There is referred shoulder tip pain. Emergency laparotomy and control of the bleeding by packing or liver suture is performed.

Torsion of the Fallopian tube

This can occasionally occur and the symptoms are those of lower abdominal pain and a tender palpable mass lateral to the uterus. The treatment is surgical removal of the tube.

Torsion of the uterus

This is usually associated with fibroids, ovarian cysts or adhesions. There is severe abdominal pain and collapse. Laparotomy is performed and the uterus is untwisted and any pelvic pathology is dealt with. Usually torsion of the uterus would cause intra-uterine death of the baby. Hysterectomy may be necessary.

Rupture of uterine and ovarian vessels

This occurs rarely and appears to be spontaneous although it can sometimes be traumatic. There is acute abdominal pain and severe shock. A haematoma may form. Laparotomy is performed immediately and the bleeding vessel ligated. It may be necessary to do a hysterectomy in some cases.

Acute pancreatitis

In the majority of cases this develops in late pregnancy or early after delivery. The aetiology is as in non-pregnant, and gall bladder disease is a common association. The condition has been reported after chlorthiazide therapy. The condition is very rare but more extended investigation for raised serum amylase in the early stages and of serum lipase in the later stages might disclose more cases where mild digestive upset is all that is complained of. In mild cases the signs and symptoms resemble gall bladder disease with flatulent dyspepsia. Acute haemorrhagic pancreatitis classically produces sudden severe upper abdominal pain radiating to the back and shoulders: drowsiness, vomiting and lethargy may be presenting and later abdominal distension may supervene.

Conservative management as in the non-pregnant with nasogastric suction, fluid and electrolyte maintenance, addition of human salt-free albumin or blood transfusion along with the relevant antibiotic. Shock requiring adrenocorticosteroids is unusual.

Peptic ulcer perforation

Usually during pregnancy there is relief of ulcer symptoms and acute complications of peptic ulceration are rare during pregnancy. There is usually a history of peptic ulceration and the onset of perforation is associated with severe pain, tenderness and rebound tenderness with evidence of peritonitis. In late pregnancy the onset may be more gradual and the abdominal wall is not so rigid. The treatment is again immediate repair of the perforation. Haemorrhage from a peptic ulcer can occur but it is very rare during pregnancy. The patient is treated with blood transfusion and a partial gastrectomy may rarely be required.

Rupture of the rectus abdominis muscle

These usually occur in women who have had many pregnancies and occurs usually in late pregnancy or in labour, but may be associated with coughing. Pain occurs usually at the lower end of the rectus sheath and there is a swelling caused by the haematoma. The diagnosis may be made difficult if the haematoma is deep in the muscle. Minor tears are treated conservatively, but large haematomas are evacuated and the muscle is sutured.

Acute cholecystitis

This is less common than acute appendicitis and is almost always associated with gall stones. The onset of the symptoms is usually acute with pain in the right upper quadrant of the abdomen radiating through to the back and to the right scapular region. There is tenderness over the gall bladder and hyperaesthesia over the back. It is sometimes difficult to differentiate from acute appendicitis or pyelonephritis or pancreatitis. It is usual to treat cholecystitis conservatively during pregnancy with intravenous fluids containing electrolytes and glucose, and to relieve the pain with analgesics. Usually the acute condition will subside in 24 or 48 hours. Surgical treatment is postponed until after delivery, but in a few cases, because of persistence of pain, high fever and the development of empyema it may be necessary to operate during pregnancy and perform a cholecystectomy.

Hernias occurring during pregnancy

It is rare for external hernias to cause any trouble during pregnancy, but very occasionally a hernia may become incarcerated.

Inguinal hernias are observed carefully during pregnancy in case strangulation should occur. Usually during pregnancy the enlarging uterus pushes the contents of the sac away and the hernia gives no trouble.

Incisional hernias, particularly of the abdominal wall may become very large during pregnancy because of the intra-abdominal pressure, but conservative treatment is usually sufficient. Very occasionally strangulation of the bowel can occur.

Diaphragmatic hernias very commonly give trouble during pregnancy because of the oesophageal reflux of the gastric content. It is in the form usually of a sliding hiatal hernia. They respond well to postural treatment and alkalis.

Haemorrhoids

Because of the increased abdominal pressure and the tendency to constipation during pregnancy and also the effect of progesterone on the veins, haemorrhoids tend to be common during pregnancy. The haemorrhoids can give rise to pain, swelling and bleeding. Thrombosis of haemorrhoids can cause severe pain. Internal haemorrhoids may become prolapsed and are liable to trauma, ulceration and thrombosis. Haemorrhoids can usually be diagnosed on inspection alone, and a proctoscope should be used to inspect the anus and rectum. It is important not to miss some other rectal pathology if a bleeding pile is seen. Haemorrhoids can be treated by injection using phenol in almond oil if they are very troublesome and if they are very painful and troublesome they may require excision. During pregnancy most cases are treated by local applications such as anusol, and later ice or cold packs after delivery.

Anal fissure

This causes pain and irritation around the anus. These are usually treated conservatively with anaesthetic ointments, proctocaine injection of the sphincter or forceable dilatation, but if the fissure is very troublesome it may be excised.

Rectal prolapse

This is predisposed to by the increased intra-abdominal pressure but is treated conservatively during pregnancy and surgical correction is put off until after delivery.

CARCINOMA OF THE BREAST

Although it is often suggested that carcinoma of the breast is more common in pregnancy and that the condition is aggravated by pregnancy there is little evidence to support this. Carcinoma of the breast is hormone dependent in most cases but in spite of the high levels of oestrogens in pregnancy there seems to be little if any evidence that the condition advances more rapidly or becomes more invasive during pregnancy or lactation. Possibly the fact that many of the patients are young and the condition seems to be worse in the younger age groups is the reason for thinking that carcinoma of the breast is a more virulent disease in pregnancy.

The incidence from the survey of the world literature was found to be one in 3 200 pregnancies (Whyte and Whyte, 1956). There was about an equal distribution between those found during pregnancy and those found in the puerperium. If the cancer develops in early pregnancy it is usual to recommend termination of the pregnancy before carrying out treatment. This is carried out in the usual way with radical surgery and in some cases radiotherapy. If the condition is found in late pregnancy a few weeks delay may be allowed before inducing premature labour and delivering the baby. This is then followed by mastectomy with or without radiotherapy. In general the prognosis is poor, probably because of the young age group affected and the delay in diagnosis possibly because of the changes which occur in the breast during pregnancy masking the lesion. In the puerperium the condition may be mistaken for a breast abscess or for lactational engorgement. It is usual to advise that pregnancy should be avoided for at least five years after the carcinoma of the breast has been treated.

Carcinoma in other organs

Carcinoma of the alimentary tract is not affected by pregnancy and is dealt with as in the non-pregnant patient, but evacuation of the uterus may be desirable in order to obtain access, particularly if the tumour is in the colon or rectum. Pregnancy can mask the symptoms of both the upper and lower alimentary tract because of the common occurrence of vomiting and constipation in pregnancy. If symptoms and signs of obstruction develop the pregnancy must be disregarded and the obstruction relieved preferably by a transverse colostomy after emptying the uterus. It may be possible to do a resection and anastomosis as in the non-pregnant patient, but it will usually be necessary to do a colostomy and then the resection some two weeks later.

ORTHOPAEDIC CONDITIONS

Backache

This is a very common complaint during pregnancy and is probably due to what Shakespeare called the pride of pregnancy. To compensate for the weight of the distended abdomen the woman has to pull her head and shoulders backwards and stick out her abdomen. This compensatory lordosis causes a strain on the ligaments and intervertebral discs of the spine. In addition to this postural factor there is the softening and stretching of the pelvic ligaments due to the effect of progesterone and or relaxin. The ligaments affected are those of the symphysis pubis and the sacroiliac joints. The low back pain is across the buttocks and is most often due to this sacro-iliac joint strain and tenderness is elicited on pressure over the joints.

Backache due to postural alteration is usually a little higher in the spine and usually affects the dorsal or lumbar areas rather than the sacral areas. The backache is aggravated in future pregnancies and is worse in older women than in younger women who still retain good tone in their muscles.

Post-partum low back pain is very common and is due to the further changing in posture which occurs post-partum because of the spine returning to its normal curvature. There is also the aggravation at this time because of the stooping and bending which the woman has to do in lifting her baby. Occasionally the pain may be very low down in the sacrococcygeal region. This again is thought to be due to postural changes or possibly due to the woman sitting on the coccyx because of her changed posture. Pain in the coccyx occurs quite frequently after a difficult forceps delivery when the sacrococcygeal joint may be overstretched or the coccyx may be fractured.

Intervertebral disc herniation or prolapsed disc can occur at any time during pregnancy and causes acute back pain which is usually either cervical or lumbar. The pain is localized and severe and radiates either to the arms or down the legs. In severe cases there may be hyperaesthesia or muscle weakness. This is probably the cause of most sciatica which is seen during pregnancy.

TREATMENT OF BACKACHE

An important part of antenatal care is to ensure good posture and proper exercise. High heeled shoes are best avoided and a firm mattress should be advocated. Exercises carried out during the antenatal period should be supervised by a physiotherapist or someone competent to prescribe the exercises as injudicious exercise at this time can cause backache. If acute back pain occurs then all exercises should be stopped and complete bed rest should be prescribed for a few days to see how the backache responds. Occasionally backache may be so severe particularly from disc herniation that traction is required.

Separation of symphysis pubis

Because of the action of relaxin the ligaments joining the symphysis are relaxed and this allows the pubic bones to move freely. Severe pain over the symphysis can sometimes occur, but usually a firm corset is sufficient to control the movement and prevent the pain. If the pain is severe absolute bed rest may be necessary for a period. The condition is more often seen as the traumatic sequel to a difficult forceps operation.

Ankle sprain

Again because of the laxity of ligaments pregnant women are very liable to twist and sprain their ankles. This is treated in the usual way with firm binding and elevation.

OTHER ORTHOPAEDIC CONDITIONS

Fractures, dislocations and other injuries are treated as conservatively as possible during pregnancy. Fractures of the pelvis are particularly important because of the possible interference with delivery. Other orthopaedic conditions such as dislocations of the hip and spondylolisthesis can also cause distortion of the pelvis and give rise to cephalo-pelvic disproportion.

Varicose veins

Varicose veins often appear for the first time

during pregnancy and this is thought to be due to the effect of progesterone. There is also usually a strong family history of varicose veins. Pressure of the enlarging uterus on the inferior venacava probably also contributes to the development of varicose veins. They can vary in severity from a small area on one leg to extensive varicosities over both upper and lower limbs and on the vulva. When there are marked varicosities the woman complains of heaviness and discomfort in the legs. The legs and feet are often oedematous.

SUPERFICIAL PHLEBITIS

Superficial phlebitis quite commonly occurs. This is now thought not to be of serious importance and it is customary now to advocate full ambulation with supporting bandages to the legs. If, however, there is a spread to the deep veins then the treatment is as described in Chapter 21.

Varicose eczema and ulceration tends to occur in older women of high parity. Complete bed rest is essential in these cases until the ulceration clears up.

Treatment of varicose veins

As the varicose veins tend to regress after pregnancy many advocate conservative treatment only with supportive bandages. Elastic stockings are not so effective as broad elasticated bandages. Elastic tights have recently proved effective and minimize the risk of later complications and thrombosis.

Surgical treatment is seldom justified during pregnancy, but injections of sclerosing fluids are advocated by some. The disadvantage of the conventional type of injection technique of sclerosing fluids is that recanalization can occur. A technique introduced by Fagan depends on compression of the veins after the injection of the sclerosing fluid and he claims very good results with this. If post-partum sterilization is contemplated in such patients it is best to do this under anticoagulant cover or to postpone the operation for some months.

REFERENCES

Fagan, W. G. (1963) Continuous Compression Technique of injecting Varicose Veins. *Lancet*, **ii**, 109.
Walker, B. E. & Diddle, A. W. (1969) Acute Pancreatitis in Gynacologic and Obstetric Practice. *Amer. J. Obstet. Gynec.*, **105**, 2.
Whyte, T. T. & Whyte, W. C. (1956) Breast Cancer in pregnancy. *Ann. Surg.*, **144**, 384.

FURTHER READING

Medical Surgical and Gynaecological Complications of Pregnancy (1965) Ed. Ravensky, J. J. & Gottmacher, A. F. Edinburgh: Livingstone.

15. Immunology and Incompatibility

THE IMMUNOLOGICAL PARADOX OF PREGNANCY

To the contemporary student or doctor with a background in modern immunobiology, the most remarkable feature of placentate reproduction is that the feto-placental 'graft' is tolerated by the mother. It has a genetic—and therefore antigenic—constitution different from the mother's by virtue of the paternal contribution. By all laws of transplantation immunity the mother should react against these tissues causing rejection. The paradox that this does not happen has been the subject of much speculation and experimentation. If the mechanism can be discovered and artificially emulated, the problem of homograft rejection will be solved; failures of the mechanism may account for pregnancy and neonatal diseases and deaths.

Immunological responses to foreign tissues are of two varieties; (1) *humoral*, with the production of antibodies of various immunoglobulin types and (2) *cellular*, involving attack on the foreign tissues by certain members of the lymphocyte population. It is well known that humoral response to the conceptus can occur. The Rhesus antibody response in Rhesus-negative (d/d) women is the best example. It is extraordinary, of course, that despite the millions of differing genes—and consequent antigens—which mothers and their babies may possess the only one which causes trouble with any degree of regularity is the Rhesus system.

Any suggestion of cellular response is strikingly absent in pregnancy. Even with pregnancies of advanced maturity, lymphocytic infiltration around the placental attachment, such as occurs with homograft rejection, is not seen; and it is cellular activity which appears to be mainly responsible for homograft rejection. The main problem, therefore, is how does the conceptus avoid *cellular* attack? It is helpful to consider separately the situations (a) at implantation of the fetilized ovum and (b) after development of the placental trophoblast which acts as interface between conceptus and mother. There is much to suggest that quite different processes are involved.

a. IMMUNOLOGICAL FACTORS AT IMPLANTATION

The fusion of gametes apparently involves an abrogation of immunological laws but as it is at unicellular level with a haploid chromosome complement it may be regarded as a very special case. The implantation of the zygote in the decidua, however, raises inescapable immunological issues. Initially the zone pellucida might give protection to the paternal antigens but this appears not to be a vital role as eggs can survive even when it is dissolved prior to implantation. There is some evidence that decidua is capable of playing an immunological 'quarantining' role at about the time of implantation, probably interfering with the afferent pathway of the immunological reflex. Cytoplasmic interchanges between fetal and maternal tissue take place and may play a part in the ultimate acceptance of the trophoblast by the production of an immunological 'no man's land' or hybrid zone. Such a mechanism has been claimed relevant in relation to schistosomes surviving in the tissues. Fertilized mouse eggs are rejected by hyperimmune hosts if transplanted *before* trophoblast development suggesting that in the initial stage the conceptus expresses transplantation antigens but that the trophoblast is a special type of tissue lacking transplantation antigens or by some mechanism preventing their expression on the cell surface.

b. AFTER PLACENTAL FORMATION

The separation by the placenta of the fetal and maternal circulations is almost certainly the most important factor from an immunological viewpoint, even though fetal blood may escape into the maternal circulation from time-to-time. When this does happen, however, if there is immunologic incompatibility in respect of Rhesus antigens it is probable that an iso-immune reaction will be initiated.

An explanation is needed, however, for the

antigenically foreign trophoblast cells existing in direct apposition to the maternal blood and decidua. Four postulates have been advanced:

    a. Antigenic immaturity of the fetus;

    b. Depressed maternal reactivity;

    c. The uterus is a privileged site;

    d. A barrier between conceptus and mother.

a. The fetus does have antigenic competence as grafts of fetal tissue other than trophoblast are rejected though sometimes less rapidly than adult ones.

b. There is some evidence that maternal immunological responsiveness is reduced in a general way, possibly under the influence of steroid and chorionic gonadotrophic hormones.

Anderson and Benirschke (1964) working with pregnant armadillos concluded that a degree of maternal immunological inertia to the conceptus is important. Hormone levels must be particularly high at the trophoblast-decidua interface, the site of production, and their local effect may be greater than studies on peripheral blood reveal. There may be some specific unresponsiveness to paternal antigens, possibly a consequence of a humoral factor produced by primary exposure to small numbers of cells at implantation. Such an antibody might coat the trophoblast, hide its active antigens and allow its unmolested growth ('immunological enhancement' —a phenomenon known in experimental tumour research). Hulka *et al.* (1963) found anti-trophoblast antibody in post-partum serum against early and late placentae, both the patient's own and other women's. The idea therefore developed that such antibodies normally attach to the placenta while *in situ*, only becoming detectable in the circulation when this source of adsorption is extruded. Alternatively the maternal cells may be rendered unresponsive by the initial exposure ('immunological paralysis'). However, as mothers *do* reject grafts of tissue from their fetuses these hypotheses alone cannot explain failure to reject trophoblast.

c. The idea that the uterus is in some way an immunologically privileged site, like the anterior chamber of the eye, can be dismissed. Extra-uterine pregnancies occur and occasionally develop to full maturity while homografts to the uterine cavity share the fate of grafts elsewhere.

d. This leaves the 'barrier theory'. This theory in turn has literally 'holes in it'; fetal cells can be demonstrated in the maternal circulation in a high proportion of cases and though it was claimed a complete fibrinoid barrier existed round trophoblast cells, subsequent electron microscope studies have shown this to be incomplete.

However, even though incomplete it does seem to represent a major factor. The barrier may take several possible forms. The trophoblast may by some biological sleight of hand contrive to present a contact layer to the mother which lacks antigens, or at least the major histocompatibility ones. Alternatively it may be that the fibrinoid layer covering trophoblastic villi forms an effective functional barrier though anatomically incomplete. This fibrinoid is said to be rich in scialic acid and its digestion from the trophoblast has been claimed to remove the barrier effect. It may be that hydrational or electropotential influences make the anatomic gaps of little significance.

It may be pertinent to the problem that all the humoral immunologic responses of mother to her fetus which are commonly recognized (e.g. anti-red cell, anti-white cell, anti-platelet, anti-immunoglobulin antibodies) represent responses to antigen present in the *fetal blood* as distinct from the trophoblast. All these responses can be attributed, therefore, to placental 'leaks' rather than to the chorionic tissue itself.

In summary, it rather appears at present that a variety of factors contribute to the survival of the trophoblast in a hostile environment. Some form of 'blockage' at the trophoblast level of expression of transplantation antigens appears to be the main one but local hormone influences may also play a significant role as may 'enhancing' antibodies.

Much of contemporary thinking and work on immunology in pregnancy is based upon the negative approach of trying to explain 'How does the placentate fetus survive *despite* known immunological laws?'. This rather implies that whatever the function of tissue immunity it has none in relation to pregnancy. A more positive approach is to consider the converse—'How could placentate reproduction have developed without immunological defences existing to preserve the integrity of mother and fetus?' Grosser in 1933 defined the obligatory role of the placenta in preserving fetal and maternal individuality. It is not at all beyond the bounds of possibility that this represents the fundamental *raison d'être* of tissue immunity. The next section provides some evidence in support of this.

IMMUNOLOGIC MATURATION OF THE FETUS

1. HUMORAL IMMUNITY

It was previously assumed that the fetus existed in a state of immunologic immaturity. This was because in the newborn most of the immunoglobulin present was found to be of maternal origin. This degrades over the three months following delivery during which time the level falls only to rise subsequently as the baby manufactures significant quantities of

there has been a recent infection. IgA is not usually detectable at term but has been found in cord sera of infants born to mothers who have had viral or bacterial infections in pregnancy (*see* Jones, 1971).

The matter of placental transfer is apparently controlled by molecular form rather than size. All the immune globulins are made up from fork shaped units (Fig. 15.1) composed of two light (L) and two heavy (H) chains. IgM consists of five such units linked into a single molecular structure. Each L chain is united to one end of an H chain, forming the antibody's combining site (Fig. 15.1) while the two H chains are combined by a disulphide bond distant to this end. If treated with papain

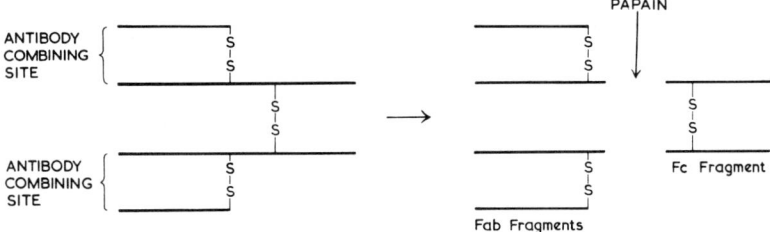

Fig. 15.1 Diagrammatic illustration of IgG molecule (*left*) consisting of two heavy chains (*centrally*) and two light chains (*above and below*) all united by di-sulphide bonds. After papain treatment (*right*) the molecule is split into 2 Fab and one Fc fragments, the Fc fragment only possessing the same capability as the whole molecule for placental transfer.

its own immunoglobulins. It was presumed that the mother supplied the fetus across the placenta to cover a period of inability to synthesize its own globulins. It was also presumed that this supply was boosted by immune globulins in colostrum on first suckling.

Recently, however, it has been discovered that contrary to earlier belief the fetus is at an early stage capable of responding immunologically to foreign antigens. It now seems that the reason for its failure to produce certain immunoglobulins while *in utero* is its isolation from extraneous antigenic stimuli combined with the presence of large quantities of maternally derived antibody.

Immune globulins, formerly known as gamma globulins, are now referred to as IgG (the original gamma globulin), IgA, IgM, IgD and IgE. IgG, IgM and IgA appear to be the most important. IgA is found particularly in secretions including colostrum. IgG which has a molecular weight of 150 000 and a sedimentation coefficient (S) of 7, crosses the placental barrier from mother to fetus whereas IgA which has a similar molecular weight does not, nor does IgM (molecular weight 900 000 19S).

Thus the finding of IgA or IgM in cord serum is presumptive evidence of their production by the fetus. IgM is frequently found towards term and may be present in greatly increased amounts if

the molecule splits as indicated into two Fab (antibody site fragment) and an Fc (crystallizable fragment). In most elegant animal studies Rogers Brambell and his colleagues (*see* Brambell, 1970) showed that if placental transfer of IgG was measured before and after papain digestion the Fc fraction crosses at the same rate as the whole molecule while Fab fragments, though a fraction of the whole molecular weight, cross much more slowly. This conclusively proved that some type of 'key to the lock' mechanism operates.

It follows from this that fetuses which carry antigens to which the mother possesses IgG antibodies may be damaged by these antibodies. These may be iso-antibodies—as in Rhesus disease—or auto-antibodies directed against antigens which the mother herself possesses as in auto-immune thyroid disease, myasthenia gravis and thrombocytopenic purpura.

The maternal transfer of IgG is probably not fortuitous for it will usually carry antibodies specifically protective against such illnesses as measles, rubella, diphtheria, etc., which if they do afflict a newborn baby tend to be extremely serious.

2. CELLULAR IMMUNITY

Human fetuses have lymphocytes evident from the 2·0cm stage, approximately seven weeks' gestation. There is a 'lymphoid surge' up to a peak level of about 7000 lymphocytes cu mm at about mid-pregnancy and it is about this time that the fetal thymus is largest in relation to total body size. Gut associated lymphocyte development ('B' lymphocytes) appears to be delayed until late gestation and it is presumed the early lymphocytes are thymus-derived ('T' lymphocytes).

Furthermore, from animal experiments and chance observation in humans it seems fairly certain that fetal lymphocytes are immunologically competent from about the second trimester. Studies on therapy with severe Rhesus disease (page 273) throw light on this matter; attempts at deliberately producing fetal chimeras by introducing Rhesus-negative marrow prior to mid-pregnancy have been uniformly unsuccessful (Browne, 1967). In addition, while blood containing lymphocytes has now been given at intra-uterine transfusion on very many occasions from mid-pregnancy onwards, colonization of the fetal system by donor lymphocytes with runt disease (retarded development, wasting and ultimate death due to 'graft-versus-host' immunological reaction) has only been recorded once (Naiman et al., 1966). This suggests that at this stage, the fetus is usually able to eliminate donor lymphocytes by the usual mechanism of allograft rejection. The occurrence of red cell and XX/XY chimerism, however, in dizygotic twins indicates that immunological tolerance* can be induced where there is interchange of tissue from a very early stage of development.

It is also possible that maternal immunologically competent lymphocytes may pass into the fetal circulation and, once past the placental barrier, these would attack the fetal system. Materno-fetal chimerism with runting has been recorded but in association with congenital absence of the baby's thymus. This points to a more positive role of the fetal immune system in intra-uterine life with the thymus producing cells capable of protecting the fetus from colonization by immunologically hostile maternal cells which may cross the placental barrier. Placental tissue may possess immunologic competence. In mice, placental cell suspensions produce runting in totally irradiated recipients. Douglas (1965) has suggested that an immunologically competent placenta protects the fetus from potentially injurious maternal cells.

3. THEORETICAL ASPECTS OF RESPONSE TO RUBELLA INFECTION

Much evidence on immunologic activity of the fetus can be obtained by study of pregnancies complicated by infective diseases—experiments of nature. The plasma cell proliferation found in mid-trimester fetuses afflicted with congenital syphilis provides an example.

One of the harshest but most informative of these experiments of nature is provided by the chance occurrence of rubella in pregnancy. The malformations which may occur if this happens in the first trimester and constituting the 'rubella syndrome' are dealt with in Chapter 23. Of more specific immunologic concern is the *expanded rubella syndrome* in which the babies are born with low birth weight, hepato-splenomegaly, thrombocytopenic purpura, etc., and secreting the rubella virus. This they continue to do chronically representing, of course, a hazard to other children in maternity units and especially to pregnant nursing staff and patients. Initially it was thought the persistent viraemia represented a manifestation of immunological tolerance but the regular finding of high levels of IgM in the cord blood, indicating fetal response to the infection, makes this unacceptable as the whole story.

Presumably the persistent viraemia is due to inactivation of some factor, probably cellular, which normally limits the spell of viral colonization. It may be that some form of partial immunological tolerance—cellular but not humoral—is involved. The latest stage of pregnancy at which rubella infection has been followed by the expanded congenital rubella syndrome is about the end of the fourth month.

4. INTER-RELATIONSHIP OF IMMUNOLOGIC AND COAGULATION SYSTEMS

For simplicity the body's various defence systems tend to be studied in isolation but nature does not recognize such compartmentalization and there is an overlap between the coagulation and immunologic systems which is particularly manifest in pregnancy. Perhaps the best known example of this interaction relates to the Schwartzmann phenomenon. In non-pregnant animals secondary injection of bacterial endotoxin, after a primary 'sensitizing' injection, will promote a state of collapse,

---

* Immunological tolerance refers to the induction of a state of non-reactivity to a foreign antigen by introduction of that antigen in appropriate dosage, usually *in utero* or the early neonatal period.

frequently fatal, associated with intravascular fibrinogen-fibrin conversion and fibrin deposition. The endotoxin appears to act as an antigen and antigen-antibody complexes trigger off the process. In pregnancy, however, the Schwartzmann phenomenon can be elicited by the *primary* injection, the pregnant state in some way altering reactivity. Thus an immunologic change may account for the great predisposition of pregnant individuals to develop intravascular coagulation.

A biologically active polypeptide, bradykinin, is released as a consequence of activation of both the clotting and the immunologic systems and there is a considerable amount of evidence to suggest that many profound influences are to a large measure mediated by bradykinin. Hageman factor (Factor XII) is activated by contact with glass and initiates clotting *in vitro*. *In vivo* it is probably activated by other substances. Its activation leads to a cascade of proteolytic enzyme activity ending in digestion of fibrinogen to fibrin. Hageman factor also causes production of a factor which influences vascular permeability. Another influence, mediated through the other pathways is the activation of kallikrein from kallikreininogen with consequent conversion of kininogen to kinins (including bradykinin) which exert a variety of effects—dilating peripheral vessels with consequent hypotension, producing pain, leucocyte migration, contraction of certain smooth muscles, etc.

The complement system in immunologic processes involves a cascade mechanism very similar to that operative in coagulation. Antigen-antibody complexes react with C′1 producing with one component of the C′1 structure (C′1s) an enzyme C′1 esterase. This catalyses subsequent reactions with other components of the complement system. In the *absence* of antibody complexes, however, Hageman factor (XII) can convert the C′1s fragment to C′1 esterase. Thus it may trigger off the whole complement cascade *without* the usual primary immunologic event.

ISO-IMMUNE DISORDERS

Rhesus haemolytic disease

INTRODUCTION AND HISTORY

Haemolytic disease of the newborn is the best known and most important immunological disorder of pregnancy. It is an example of isoimmunity. In the usual situation a Rhesus-negative (d/d) mother is sensitized by Rhesus-positive (D) blood of another individual—either by blood transfusion or from a fetus *in utero*. As a consequence anti-Rhesus antibodies develop and any subsequent children who are Rhesus positive (D) are liable to be affected by these antibodies crossing the placenta and haemolyzing the red cells. This is a unique situation in which an interaction between four individuals, counting the father, is required to produce disease in the fourth (*see* Fig. 15.2). An understanding of Rhesus haemolytic disease can probably best be obtained by a consideration of its history from the recognition of the

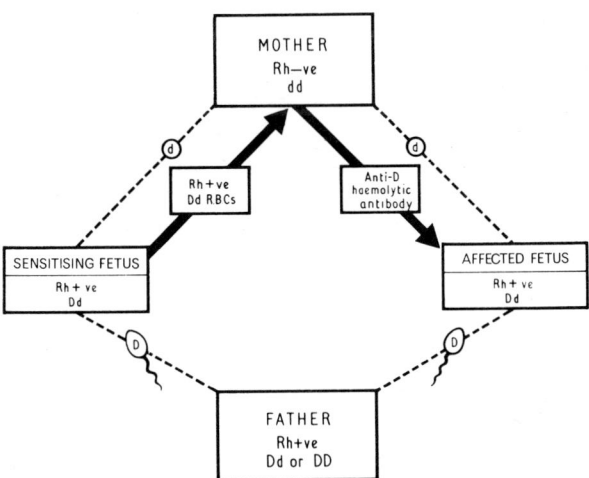

Fig. 15.2 Diagrammatic illustration of the mechanism whereby the involvement of four family members ultimately results in Rhesus haemolytic disease in the fourth. By courtesy of the Editor, *British Medical Journal*.

condition as an entity 30 years ago, the elucidation of its immunologic mechanism, the development of successful forms of neonatal treatment, of efficient means of antenatal prediction, of transfusing the baby while still in the uterus to the final development of means whereby the whole process may be prevented.

It was known that certain women bore babies who were anaemic at birth or became so soon after (haemolytic anaemia of the newborn); became seriously jaundiced soon after birth (icterus gravis neonatorum); were born in a state of congestive heart failure with gross oedema looking like a 'Michelin-man' (hydrops fetalis) (Fig 15.3) or died *in utero* before birth. It was shown that this process affected

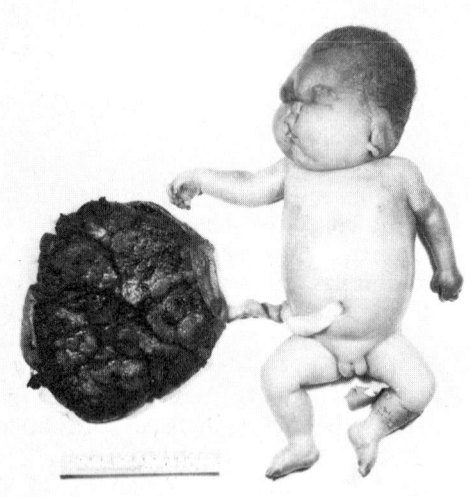

Fig. 15.3 Hydropic fetus and placenta showing gross subcutaneous oedema. There is also ascites and hydrothorax. The placenta is not only oedematous but enlarged by villous proliferation.

only the children of certain women and virtually never first babies. The usual pattern was of progression in successive pregnancies from haemolytic anaemia of the newborn to 'icterus gravis' to hydrops fetalis to intrauterine death. All these clinical types had in common the presence in the circulation of immature red blood cells and their marrow precursors and the term 'erythroblastosis fetalis' was coined. In 1939 Levine postulated that the disease was due to a blood group antigen and in 1940 Landsteiner and Weiner by immunizing rabbits with red cells from the

Macacus Rhesus monkey, produced an antibody which agglutinated the monkey red cells and also the red cells of approximately 85 per cent of European humans. It was deduced that these 85 per cent possessed an antigen universally present in monkeys and they were said to be 'Rhesus-positive'.

It soon became clear that the Rhesus factor was not a single antigen but a complex of linked antigens, one set maternally derived and the other paternal. The major Rhesus antigen is usually denoted by the capital letter 'D' for Rhesus-positive and small 'd' for Rhesus-negative. Along with these, each parentally derived antigen group has a 'C' or 'c' and an 'E' or 'e'—all inherited in a single CDE unit. Even this is some oversimplification as rare variants of the treble pair arrangements are found. The gene for the 'D' antigen is dominant over the 'd' allele. All Rhesus-negative individuals are d/d but Rhesus-positives may be D/D (homozygous) or D/d (heterozygous) and this difference may be of great importance.

This is known as the Fisher-Race terminology. An alternative designed by Weiner has been used in America. This takes such forms as Rho, rh^1 etc. Appropriate conversions will be found in Table 15.1.

Table 15.1 Nomenclatures for Rhesus antigens

Fisher-Race	Weiner
(CDE)	(Rh–Hr)
D	Rh_0
C	rh^1
E	rh^{11}
d	Hr_0
c	hr^1
e	hr^{11}

After discovery of the blood group systems involved, it was not long before it was realized that Rhesus-positive (D) babies with anaemia due to maternal antibodies could be treated by transfusing Rhesus-negative d/d blood which would not be lysed by the antibodies. The antibodies, which may persist for up to three months but have their maximal effect in the first few days, would still go on destroying the baby's own Rhesus-positive (D) cells and cause serious jaundice. This, if severe, is associated with deposition of the bile material in the basal ganglia of the brain—*kernicterus*—which has certain characteristic clinical features in the initial phase and ultimately results in a mentally retarded and often spastic child (*see* page 456).

The next development was a major therapeutic one—*'exchange transfusion'*. At birth or soon after, using a catheter into an umbilical or other vein, Rhesus-negative d/d blood is slowly injected and the baby's own Rhesus-positive (D) blood withdrawn. As a consequence most, but of course not all, of the positive cells are removed and replaced by negative cells which will persist in the baby's circulation until the antibodies have ceased to have significant haemolytic effect. In the process of exchange *pari passu* with the washing out of the Rhesus-positive (D) cells, most of the antibodies present in the plasma are also removed. Subsequently, the transfused cells are replaced by fresh Rhesus-positive (D) cells, manufactured by the baby's own marrow.

Bevis of Manchester then discovered that by studying specimens of liquor, collected by amniocentesis, one could tell how severely the baby was affected and this led to further great advances in management. In 1963 Liley of New Zealand introduced the technique of transfusing, while still *in utero*, babies so seriously affected at such an early stage of pregnancy that they stood no chance of survival otherwise. Finally from Liverpool and New York in the last few years has come a startlingly simple immunologic technique for the prevention of Rhesus sensitization in association with childbirth (*see* page 274).

Quite apart from the special interest of the disease and the practical problems involved in mastering it, the procedures which have helped achieve this have contributed indirectly to more general progress. Bevis's introduction of amniocentesis as a means of determining the state of the fetus was a 'breakthrough' in the literal and metaphoric sense. Previously the fetus was a surprise package, hidden in its wrappings from all assessment but the simple palpation of the obstetrician. Before Liley's introduction of intra-uterine transfusion the possibility was not entertained that the child in the womb could actually be treated specifically and effectively. The ultimate prophylactic mastery of Rhesus disease—one form of immunological rejection—has given encouragement, previously lacking, that immune problems can be dealt with in a fundamental way and that the homograft problem will ultimately be overcome.

AETIOLOGY

As explained above, Rhesus disease is caused by sensitization of the mother by another individual usually her own child, with resultant disease in subsequent D positive children due to antibody crossing the placenta and lysing the baby's red cells. This represents rather the *framework* of the disease and it still has to be explained how some Rhesus-negative (d/d) women are sensitized by D positive fetuses while others are not.

Information on this matter has accumulated as the result of the introduction of the Kleihauer technique. In this procedure films of maternal blood are treated with a citric-phosphate buffer which causes any fetal cells present to stand out as dark, refractile bodies in comparison with the maternal cells which appear as pale, transparent 'ghosts' (Fig. 15.4). The basis of the method is differential elution of fetal and maternal haemoglobin.

Application of this technique to the study of women during pregnancy and following delivery has shown that the majority of feto-maternal haemorrhages occur during delivery but they may also happen during the antenatal period particularly with mechanical complications or manipulation. Rhesus sensitization is commonest when the Kleihauer test on maternal blood collected after delivery shows a

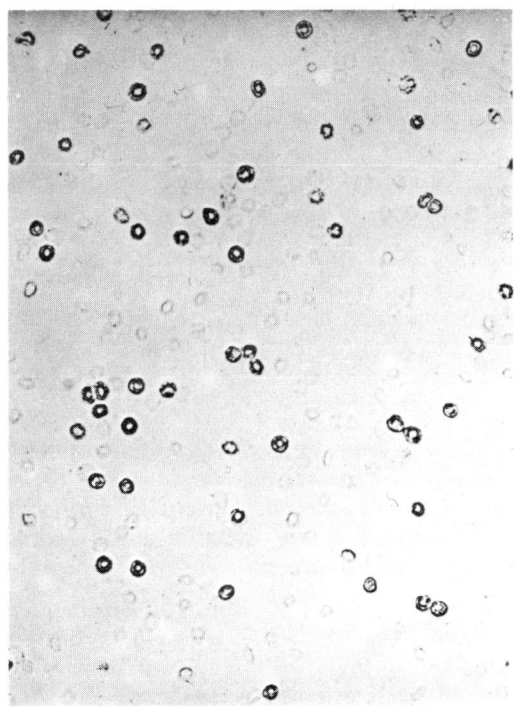

Fig. 15.4   Blood film treated by Kleihauer procedure. The fetal cells stand out as dark refractile bodies compared with the 'ghost' appearance of the maternal cells.

high fetal count. The risk is also related to whether or not the mother and child are ABO blood group compatible. Other unknown factors operate, some Rhesus-negative (d/d) individuals being persistently resistant to immunologic challenge by ABO compatible Rhesus-positive (D) cells.

MANAGEMENT OF PREGNANCY IN RELATION TO RHESUS DISEASE

Practically the problem involves consideration of (a) measures necessary for all pregnant women; (b) measures for those who are found to be Rhesus-negative (d/d); (c) measures for those who are found to be Rhesus-negative (d/d) with antibodies, and (d) prophylaxis.

a. *Measures for all pregnant women*

The first essential for dealing with Rhesus disease is to establish those patients at risk. This should be done at the first antenatal examination when a specimen of venous blood should be sent to the laboratory (usually in this country, that of the Regional Blood Transfusion Service) for ABO and Rhesus grouping. On the same specimen serological testing for syphilis, rubella and screening for irregular antibodies is normally performed. If this shows the patient to be Rhesus-positive (D) then there should be no further cause for concern unless she has a history of blood transfusions, unexplained stillbirths or jaundiced babies, or unless antibodies to Rhesus factors other than D or other abnormal antibodies are found in her blood at the first examination.

b. *Measures for the Rhesus-negative (d/d) pregnant women*

When a woman is known, or discovered on early antenatal testing to be Rhesus-negative (d/d) then two potential problems exist which must be catered for:

i. she may have antibodies and have a baby affected by Rhesus disease;
ii. she may become sensitized in the course of pregnancy or, more probably, at the time of delivery.

In relation to (i) blood must be tested for such antibodies and in regard to (ii) repeated antibody tests must be done and anti-D gamma globulin given as a prophylactic measure after delivery or any other episode with a high risk of sensitization.

If a woman is Rhesus-negative and antibodies have been demonstrated she must immediately come under the care of obstetricians particularly knowledgeable of the condition. She must be booked for confinement in a centre where intra-uterine exchange transfusion can be easily and efficiently undertaken.

Where antibodies are not demonstrated at routine checks (booking 22, 28 and 36 weeks), then there is no contra-indication to delivery under general practitioner care provided that samples of cord blood and maternal blood taken at delivery can be efficiently tested, as below, and anti-D immunoglobulin given where necessary (*see* (d) *later*).

If the initial tests are negative, antibody checks should be repeated on maternal blood specimens at 26–28 weeks and 34–36 weeks. If no antibodies are present at the second of these it is highly improbable that they will develop in sufficient concentration to significantly affect the fetus by term. At delivery in such a case two specimens should be obtained; (a) cord blood and (b) maternal venous blood. The cord blood should be sent for Coombs' testing.* It is also used for performing Rhesus and ABO grouping on the baby. If the baby is Coombs' negative and Rhesus-negative (d/d) no further action is required but if it is Coombs' negative and Rhesus-positive (D), then anti-D IgG should be administered to the mother with a view to preventing sensitization from occurring (*see later*). The maternal blood specimen is used for Kleihauer testing for the presence of fetal cells in her circulation.

Although the necessity for antenatal Rhesus screening has long been appreciated it was salutary to discover that at the time of the British Perinatal Mortality Survey of 1958 no fewer than 8·2 per cent of mothers had not had antenatal determinations done. A similar situation exists with regard to prophylaxis. Hibbard (1971, *personal communication*) showed that most failures of the prophylactic regime in Liverpool were due to failure of the system designed to administer it to all mothers at risk, rather than in failure in the efficacy of the preparation. *The moral of these facts applies to all aspects of the Rhesus situation—good*

---

* Coombs' test is an agglutination test with anti-human globulin which in its direct form detects any immunoglobulin which may be adherent to the fetal red cells. This would detect any cases in which the fetus was Rhesus-positive (D) and maternal antibodies had developed after the last antenatal test.

results are only obtained by the careful, systematic application of the established techniques to all patients.

c. *Measures for women found to have Rhesus antibodies*

Ideally, cases of Rhesus sensitization should be referred to a centre specializing in their care. In the Newcastle region excellent results were obtained by the centralization of all cases of Rhesus disease. If this could be achieved throughout the country the perinatal mortality from Rhesus disease could be expected to be reduced by an order of 75 per cent (Stabler, 1960). The need for such centralization is all the greater today when the number of cases of Rhesus disease is diminishing. This is due (a) to the reduction of the number of pregnancies in women of high parity, (b) to contraceptive and sterilizing procedures in women with high levels of Rhesus antibodies and (c) to the influence of prophylactic administration of anti-D IgG in preventing the disease. Also, the procedures which need to be performed occasionally in modern management are of such complexity that good results can be expected *only* where they are done with reasonable frequency. Centres should be established only in major obstetric units where the necessary expertise and experience can be obtained. Geography may dictate the number of centres.

At the outset of Rhesus sensitization as with most immune responses an IgM antibody is produced, detected in saline and inactive in producing fetal haemolysis as it does not cross the placenta. The laboratory report often refers to it as only being detected by enzyme techniques. Later IgG antibody, detected in albumen and able to cross the placenta, appears and the haemolytic process commences. Whenever Rhesus antibodies are detected for the first time it is essential to arrange for a titre determination. The laboratory may do this automatically or may require a further specimen.

Previously serial readings of titre were the only available and often misleading guide to the degree of fetal involvement. Now such serial readings are used more as a guide to the need for amniocentesis and as a monitor of the amniocentesis results especially in late pregnancy. If the titre remains low on serial estimation at fortnightly intervals throughout, especially in a first affected pregnancy, the baby is unlikely to be seriously affected and there is no necessity for amniocentesis. What is meant by 'low' must be established for the individual laboratory. In our Regional Transfusion Laboratory this is less than 1:40 (Tovey, 1969) or 15 international units/ml or 2·5mgm of anti-D IgG.

This very rough prognostic guide means that the number of cases requiring amniocentesis may be considerably reduced. Valuable as amniocentesis is, unlike simple venepuncture it carries *some* risk of increasing maternal sensitization and so if it can safely be avoided this is desirable.

If the titre stays low induction of labour at about 38 weeks is usually appropriate. If the titre is above the critical level or the mother has already produced a significantly affected baby it is wise to perform amniocentesis. When this should be done will depend (a) upon the history and (b) upon the time a *significant* antibody titre is detected. If there is a very bad history it may be wise to start amniocentesis at about 20-22 weeks' gestation. If on the other hand it is only at 37-38 weeks that a significant titre develops, there will be little point in doing other than induction amniotomy at 38 weeks. Generally, however, amniocentesis is started at about the 28-30th week.

Amniocentesis

Amniocentesis is performed with full antiseptic precautions with the patient reclining in the dorsal position with slight head elevation. It is essential that the bladder should be empty. A puncture site is selected usually in the flexure of the fetal trunk between upper and lower limbs. Placental localization by sonar as a preliminary is recommended by some, but this is not precise as to placental edge and does not give complete safety. Following injection of a small quantity of local anaesthetic a *very* sharp fine gauge lumbar puncture-type needle is inserted directly into the amniotic cavity at a depth of 3-4 inches. The stylette is then withdrawn and when fluid is seen to emerge an aspirating syringe is attached. The specimen (5ml approx.) is then transferred to a glass container and *protected from light* until analysis (ultra-violet light can degrade bilirubin and lead to falsely low readings).

Liquor obtained (approx. 5 ml) is sent to the laboratory for spectrophotometric analysis after appropriate filtration and dilution. Normal liquor amnii on spectrophotometric scanning with measure-

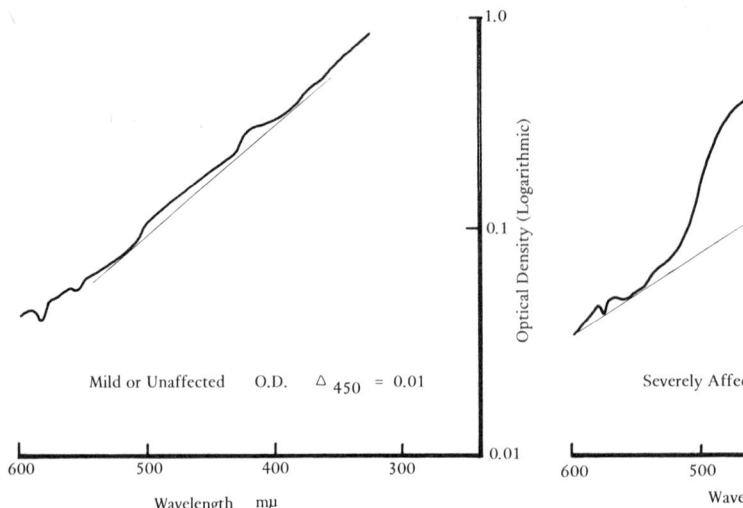

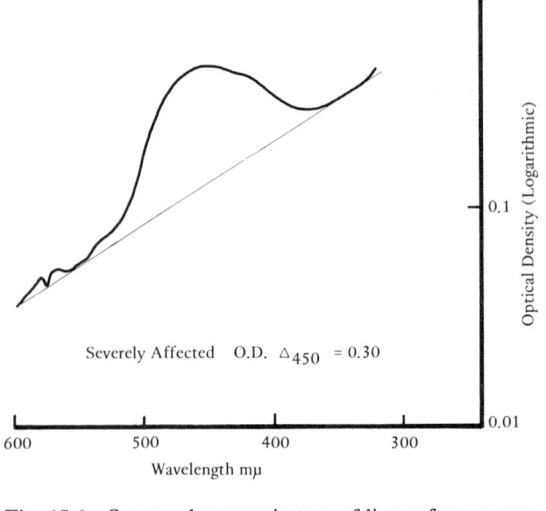

Fig. 15.5   Semi-log plot of spectrophotometric scan of liquor amnii specimen from fetus mildly affected or unaffected by Rhesus haemolytic disease. The slope is almost a straight line.

Fig. 15.6   Spectrophotometric scan of liquor from a case of Rhesus haemolytic disease in which the baby was severely affected. Note the optical density peak at 450mμ. The height of this above the double-tangent line drawn to where this curve leaves the normal slope measures in this case 0·30 on the log scale (O.D. 450).

ment of absorption in the range 350mμ to 700mμ gives an approximately straight, sloping line when plotted on semi-log paper (Fig. 15.5). If there is significant quantity of bilirubin-type products of haemolysis, this straight line becomes distorted by a peak, maximal at 450mμ. The height of this peak gives a good estimate of the degree to which the baby is affected. This may be measured from the base-line or from a double-tangent line drawn where the abnormal peak leaves the normal slope (*see*

Fig. 15.6). If this figure is plotted on a prediction chart derived from retrospective analysis of liquors from affected and unaffected babies, a very good estimation of the likely degree of severity of fetal involvement can be given. A chart widely used is that devised by Liley of Auckland (Fig 15.7). It will be seen that the slope of the various grades is downwards towards term. For reasons not understood, there is *normally* quite an amount of bilirubin-type material in mid-pregnancy liquor and this steadily

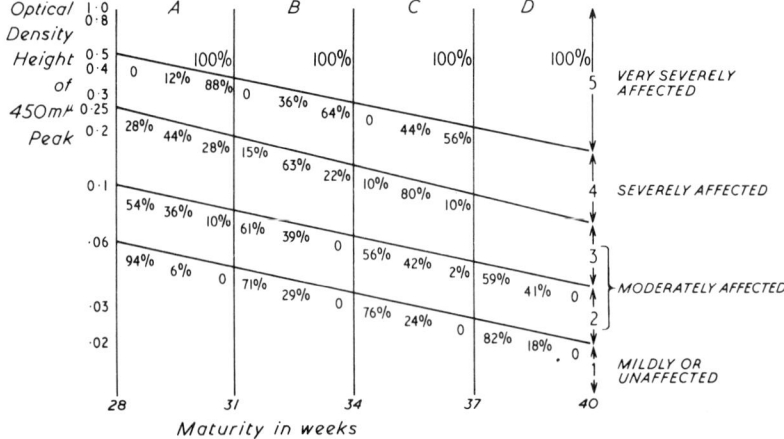

Fig. 15.7   Prediction chart devised by Liley. The optical density peak measurement is plotted on this chart in relation to maturity. The percentage figures recorded in each sector indicate the probability of the infant being 'mildly' or 'unaffected' (*left-hand number*); moderately affected (*central number*); severely or very severely affected (*right-hand number*). Mildly or unaffected implies a Coombs' test negative on cord blood or cord haemoglobin >14g/100ml; moderately affected—cord haemoglobin 8·0–13·9g/100ml; severely affected cord haemoglobin <8·0/100ml; very severely affected—intra-uterine death imminent.

decreases towards term. It is often extremely difficult to be certain at an early stage whether a baby is affected or the 450mμ peak is merely a physiological one. This, however, is usually easily resolved by doing a repeat amniocentesis in about two weeks; if the result is significantly lower, the baby is unlikely to be seriously affected but if it is even higher it is virtually certain that the baby is affected.

If yet another amniocentesis is done another two weeks later the spectrophotometric result will usually lie approximately on the projection of the line joining the points of the plotting of the first two predictions. Only rarely will more than three amniocenteses be necessary in the course of a single pregnancy. Separate but potentially confusing peaks from the base-line reading may be given by the presence in the liquor of other substances such as meconium or haemoglobin.

Liley's chart only indicates, *on the basis of probabilities*, how severely the baby is likely to be affected if delivered at the time indicated. The obstetrician has still to work out, rather intuitively, what course of action to follow, and when. A refinement introduced by Whitfield (1970) is an 'action line' which is superimposed upon the Liley chart (Fig. 15.8). By plotting two or more results and projecting the line through the points till it meets the 'action line' gives a guide as to when the obstetrician should be taking action. When the intersection occurs before delivery is feasible, intra-uterine transfusion is usually appropriate. From 33 weeks' maturity onwards it becomes progressively more reasonable to deliver the baby and pass it to the care of the paediatricians with prospect of a successful outcome. This is usually achieved by inducing labour unless some physical factor makes this particularly dangerous in which case Caesarean section will be indicated.

It is important to have close co-operation between obstetrician and paediatrician particularly at the time delivery is planned. Matters should be so arranged that the birth is likely to occur at a convenient time and a team of skilled, experienced paediatricians should be at hand to deal with the baby immediately it is born. Blood should be available so that exchange transfusion can be initiated at once if the baby's condition is critical.

Intra-uterine transfusion

If the severity of the fetal haemolytic process seems such that the baby will die *in utero* and immaturity precludes delivery then intra-uterine transfusion must be considered. For this procedure concentrated group O Rhesus-negative (d/d) red blood cells are used, cross-matched against the mother's blood. Blood should be freshly donated in order that red cells which reach the fetal circulation will possess maximal survival time. The value of prior localization of the placenta by placentography although performed in most centres is at least debatable; as with amniocentesis, if the placenta is demonstrated on the anterior uterine wall, the operator has very little choice but to go through it in order to effect the transfusion.

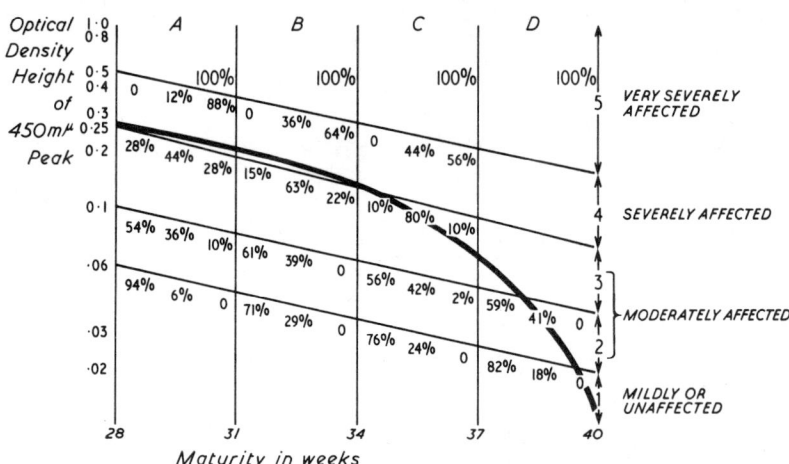

Fig. 15.8 'Action-line' of Whitfield superimposed on Liley prediction chart. Plotting the 'O.D. 450' of 2 or more successive amniocentesis scans and projecting the line joining these plots till it meets the 'action-line' gives a guide as to when the obstetrician should intervene. If this occurs before 33 weeks, or early plots are above the 'action-line', intra-uterine transfusion should be considered.

The procedure is made easier if the fetal tissues have been outlined by injecting a fat-soluble contrast medium such as iodophendylate (Myodil) into the amniotic cavity at least 25 hours prior to the procedure. This adsorbs on to the vernix caseosa on the fetal skin and so outlines the fetal contour. The transfusion is carried out on an X-ray table with television image intensifier facilities. The co-operation of an obstetrician and a radiologist with special experience of the technique is essential.

Premedication such as pethidine 150mgm is given 30 minutes previously as much to sedate the fetus as mother. With the bladder empty routine abdominal antiseptic skin preparation is performed. Appropriate leads may be attached to the abdominal wall to allow ECG, phonocardiographic or ultrasonic monitoring of the fetal heart. Disturbance of the fetus by palpation is avoided as far as possible. Sterile radio-opaque markers are attached to the abdomen to help with positioning during the procedure; a sterile plastic adhesive drape carrying a grid of radio-opaque threads may be used (Fig. 15.9). The fetus is then screened radiologically and an X-ray picture taken. If this shows a fetus which is obviously hydropic, the prospects of success are very low indeed. Poor as the prospects are, however, it is usually best to proceed.

The best line of approach to the fetal abdomen is then decided and the skin and abdominal wall are infiltrated with lignocaine 0.5 per cent along this line to secure analgesia. A Tuohy needle (which has the orifice on the lateral aspect of its tip) is then introduced, or a straight needle with 'Teflon' sheath. By feel the operator learns to recognize when the needle has passed through the maternal abdominal wall and uterus to reach the amniotic cavity. This can be confirmed by withdrawing the stylette temporarily to determine if the needle tip is in liquor. Then, exerting manual counter-pressure on the fetus as necessary, the needle is pressed onwards through the fetal abdominal wall into the peritoneum —aiming low to avoid liver and cord insertion. The stylette is again withdrawn and radio-opaque water-soluble dye injected under X-ray screening. If the position is correct the outline of the peritoneum is recognizable with indentation produced by loops of bowel (Fig. 15.10). Any fetal ascitic fluid present should be withdrawn before injection. It is often found that the needle is incorrectly placed and dye is injected elsewhere than the peritoneal cavity. This seems to cause little significant damage to the fetus. Even such extraordinary pictures as intra-uterine myelograms have been obtained and the baby survived apparently unharmed.

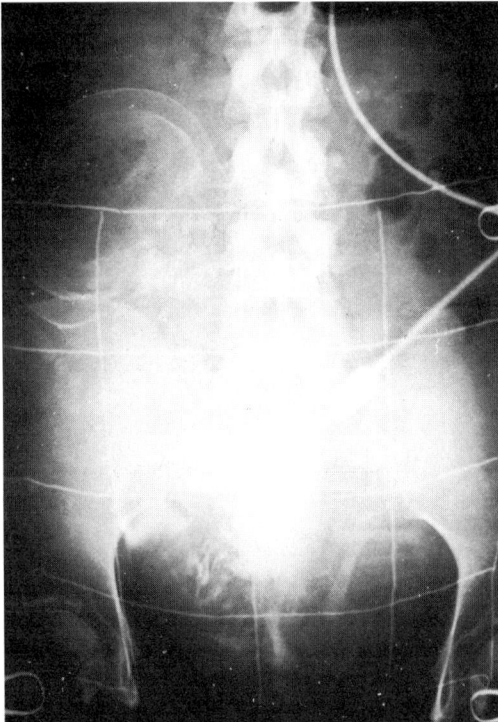

Fig. 15.9   Intra-uterine transfusion under X-ray control. The grid effect is produced by radio-opaque strands on sterile, adhesive abdominal drape. Fetal skin has been outlined by prior iodophendylate injection. Note the gap between scalp skin and skull, indicating that the fetus is hydropic.

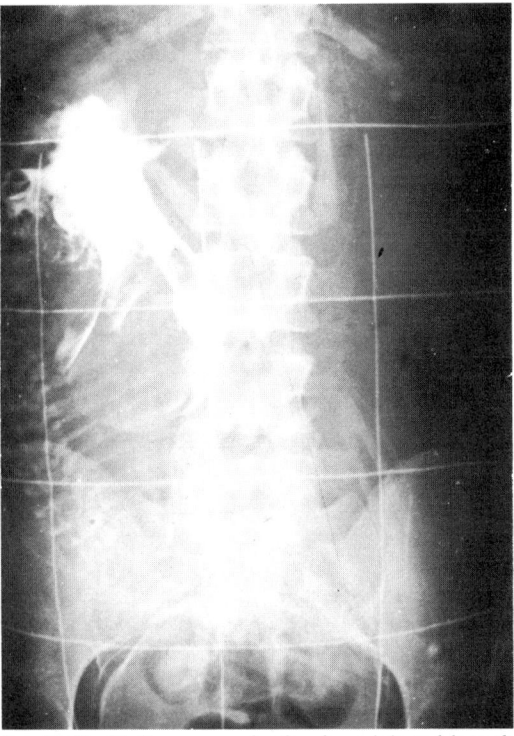

Fig. 15.10   Radio-opaque dye has been injected into the fetal abdomen. It is indented by bowel and has outlined the fetal liver. Note how close the fetal scalp outline is to the skull compared with Figure 9. This baby was not hydropic.

A fine polythene catheter may then be introduced through the Tuohy needle and the needle withdrawn or the core of the straight needle may be removed leaving the 'Teflon' sheath. Alternatively the blood injection may be performed directly through the needle. The quantity of blood given varies according to the fetal maturity, condition and response. It is usually of the order of 60–120ml. If fetal heart monitoring reveals signs of cardiac embarrassment, indicating overloading of the peritoneum, the transfusion should be stopped and possibly some blood withdrawn.

If the fetus is not hydropic, the blood from the peritoneal cavity will be absorbed, mostly over the subsequent 48 hours, and transferred via the thoracic duct to the fetal circulation. At the completion of the procedure ampicillin is usually injected. It cannot be over-emphasized that infection is a potentially disastrous complication of this procedure. The risk becomes perilous if the fetus should die—as it may well do if case selection has been stringent. Then any bacteria inoculated are left in a large mass of ideal culture medium (the dead fetus), incubated at body temperature. If a fetus dies after transfusion it is wise to expedite its delivery as rapidly as possible.

Further transfusion will be indicated approximately every two weeks until a stage of viability is reached when induction of labour is performed as with other cases of Rhesus disease, followed by appropriate paediatric management (see page 456).

The amount of X-ray screening time should be measured. With experienced operators using screening only at essential moments, the amount of radiation involved does not exceed acceptable limits.

At delivery after intra-uterine transfusion a Kleihauer test is performed on the cord blood in order to determine what proportion of the cells are of adult (i.e. donor) type. Frequently this is high—virtually 100 per cent. If Kleihauer assessment is not done routine cord testing may suggest the baby itself is Rhesus-negative (d/d), Coombs' negative and that it has been mistakenly transfused!

Several other types of intra-uterine transfusion of a more direct nature have been experimented with—canalizing a fetal vessel on the edge of the placenta or bringing out a fetal limb for cannulation of a vessel. While these approaches do involve direct entry into the fetal circulation and therefore the possibility of an intra-uterine *exchange* rather than 'top-up' transfusion, the increased technical hazards are such that they have not been widely used.

Experiments have been made in very severe cases, where even intra-uterine transfusion appeared to offer no real hope, of introducing Rhesus-negative (d/d) marrow into the Rhesus-positive (D) fetus at a stage of pregnancy when it is still immunologically immature. The fetus, it was hoped, might accept this marrow as 'self' and develop as a Rhesus-positive (D) Rhesus-negative (d/d) chimera, the latter cells being unaffected by the maternal antibodies. To do this the uterus had to be opened at an early stage, the fetus delivered for injection of the marrow, and the uterine incision closed. Technically the hazards are less than might be imagined and the pregnancy is usually undisturbed. It appears, however, that no ultimate successes have been obtained with this immunologically intriguing procedure which suggests that the fetus is immunologically capable of reacting to foreign cells even at that early stage (see page 264).

Therapeutic plasmapheresis
Plasmapheresis (see page 275) has been used during the pregnancies of women with very high levels of Rhesus antibodies in an attempt to reduce the antibody level. There is, however, no convincing evidence that it improves the fetal prognosis. Administration of corticosteroids and Rh-hapten has also been tried without convincing benefit.

Types of bilirubin and albumin binding
Jaundice does not occur before delivery because the bilirubin produced by haemolysis crosses the placenta. Bound to serum albumin, it is transported to the maternal liver where the enzyme glucuronyl transferase converts it from the indirect to the direct, excretable form, bilirubin glucuronide. The neonate's liver lacks adequate quantities of glucuronyl transferase and hence indirect bilirubin builds up rapidly after delivery, with obvious jaundice.

It is the free, unconjugated bilirubin not bound to albumin which tends to deposit in, and damage, the brain cells. It follows that anything which interferes with the albumin-binding capacity will have an untoward influence. Such substances include sulphonamides, especially sulphafurazole ('Gantrisin'), salicylates and caffeine. They should not be prescribed to mothers likely to give birth to babies with haemolytic disease nor, of course, to babies with the disease.

Paternal genotyping
A technique to discover whether the father is hetero- or homozygous for D (paternal genotyping) is of little assistance in managing pregnancies in which the mother has Rhesus antibodies but of considerable help in giving advice about future pregnancies. The anti-D antibodies will, of course, only be harmful if the baby has inherited the D antigen from its father. Anti-d serum is not available so direct

testing is not possible. However anti-sera are available against the five other antigens of the Rhesus system—c, e, C, D and E. By testing paternal cells with these antigens a phenotype is obtained, e.g. CCDee—red cells having reacted with anti-C, D and e sera but not with c and E. With this knowledge the possible genotypes can be calculated with their order of probability. In the example quoted the genotype could be CDe/CDe or CDe/Cde. The former has a frequency of 17·7 per cent and the latter only 0·8 per cent so it is *probable* that the genotype is CDe/CDe and the father therefore homozygous D/D. Be it noted that there is a calculable element of guess in this prediction. In the example quoted there is a 22·1 to 1 chance it is correct.

The doubt element in a genotype prediction may, of course, be removed if study of the father's children shows that some are D positive and others negative. He must then be heterozygous—unless, of course, his paternal role is in doubt!

Paternal genotyping is extremely helpful when there are antibodies other than anti-D particularly if there is a history of previous transfusion or pregnancy by another partner.

Family patterns
When Rhesus haemolytic disease develops two patterns of behaviour may be found. Each Rhesus-positive fetus may be progressively more seriously affected until early fetal death occurs or a 'plateau effect' is observed and after a certain degree of severity is reached subsequent babies are not significantly more affected. In general it is appropriate to work on the assumption that any Rhesus-positive fetus will be *at least* as seriously affected as its predecessor. From time-to-time, however, exceptions to this rule produce a pleasant surprise for the patient and her attendants.

Maternal syndrome with hydrops
One intriguing aspect of Rhesus sensitization is that when the fetus is so seriously affected as to have become hydropic the mother may show manifestations of an illness indistinguishable from pre-eclamptic toxaemia with hypertension, albuminuria and oedema. Such cases are rarely seen today on account of the efficient management which Rhesus cases receive. Their occurrence, however, does add one small piece of evidence to the problem of the aetiology of pregnancy toxaemia (*see* page 183).

d. *Prophylaxis*
Development. The ultimate chapter in the Rhesus story concerns prophylaxis which has recently become a practical procedure. Professor C. A. Clarke and his colleagues in Liverpool were interested in the fact that various diseases showed a variable incidence according to the ABO blood group of the individual. This was true of Rhesus haemolytic disease with a preponderance in AB as opposed to O mothers. They established that where the mother was incompatible with the fetus on an ABO basis in such a way that it would be expected that the mother would haemolyze any fetal cells that crossed into her circulation, sensitization virtually never occurred. They presumed that the cells were destroyed before they had been in the circulation long enough to evoke an antibody response. Accordingly, they postulated that if it could be arranged to introduce a haemolytic antibody effective against *all* Rhesus-positive (D) cells that entered the mother's circulation, the natural ABO effect might be reproduced artificially. They came up with the apparently paradoxical idea that anti-D antibody given soon after delivery (when most feto-maternal bleeds occur) might have this effect. Despite initial disappointments, they persevered and eventually showed that the method was highly effective. At first they proved its efficacy by treating only mothers who were ABO compatible with their babies and who were shown by the Kleihauer technique to have had significant fetal bleeds into the maternal circulation, i.e. those at very high risk of sensitization. Later this was extended to cover all at risk no matter how slight.

At the same time an American group worked on the same lines, though starting from a different hypothesis. They presumed an antigen would not evoke primary antibody response in the presence of adequate antibody of the same specificity. This led them to a similar regime and similarly encouraging results.

Current practice
In this country Rhesus-negative (d/d) women without antibodies who deliver Rhesus-positive (D) children are now given 100μg of anti-D immunoglobulin within 72 hours of delivery. Such women who have abortions before 20 weeks are given 50μg of immunoglobulin (100μg after 20 weeks). Maternal blood is screened by the Kleihauer test for fetal cells.

If a particularly large transfer of fetal positive (D) cells is noted a larger dose of immunoglobulin may be given. It is known that such a regime will prevent the great majority of cases of sensitization (about 98 per cent). At present the efficacy of smaller doses than those mentioned is not established. As the source of material is human, it follows that work urgently needs to be done on this in the hope that the dose can be lowered further. Enough is known now, however, to be able to say that Rhesus sensitization which has been one of the common and major obstetric problems over recent decades will soon become something of a rarity.

In Rhesus-negative women without antibodies who have incidents in pregnancy which it is known are likely to precipitate feto-maternal haemorrhage (e.g. external cephalic version or amniocentesis done for some purpose other than Rhesus diseases such as chromosome study or assessment of liquor for fetal maturity) it is wise to perform Kleihauer determinations before and after the procedure. If these show that a significant feto-maternal haemorrhage has occurred then anti-D IgG should be given as prophylaxis against the occurrence of sensitization. The quantity of antibody involved is so small that it will have no significant haemolytic effect on the fetus *in utero*.

It is still not entirely clear which of the two hypotheses for using the anti-D gammaglobulin explains its efficacy in practice. It may indeed be the case that both the red cell destructive effect and the blocking effect of presence of the specific antibody on the antibody-producing cells may each exert an influence.

Supply of anti-D
The supply of anti-D gammaglobulin depends entirely upon the availability of a pool of Rhesus-negative (d/d) human donors who possess anti-D antibodies in high titre. Such donors may be (a) women who have been sensitized during childbearing and (b) males, or post-menopausal women, who have allowed themselves to be sensitized artificially by injection of Rhesus-positive (D) cells. Injection carries some risk, though a very small one, of transfer of serum hepatitis. This source will, however, have to be relied upon increasingly in the future as the number of women naturally immunized by childbirth diminishes. Donors who have the necessary titre of anti-D can be bled much more frequently than routine blood donors by using the technique of plasmapheresis. In this procedure blood is withdrawn, red cells and plasma are rapidly separated by centrifugation and the red cells returned to the donor. Anaemia does not develop and the liver is capable of replacing very rapidly the protein removed. Donors may give two donations of blood yielding 600ml of plasma at a single session and repeat this up to four times per month. One such donor may provide enough anti-D to give protection to all 'at risk' Rhesus-negative (d/d) mothers in a population of one million.

OTHER CAUSES OF FETO-NEONATAL HAEMOLYTIC
    DISEASE
It must be understood that a woman can develop antibodies to any antigen she does not herself possess so that whilst Rhesus (D) negative mothers with anti-D antibodies compose 95 per cent of all serological incompatibilities other situations can arise. For example, a Rhesus (D) negative woman can develop antibodies to a fetal c antigen to such an extent that the fetus needs transfusion. Antibodies may develop to factors outside the Rhesus system e.g. Kell and Duffy, etc.

Of the many other blood groups which theoretically could be a source of iso-immune haemolytic disease, some only produce antibodies which are of IgM type and do not cross the placenta, while with others the antibodies are only weakly haemolytic.

Naturally occurring maternal anti-A and anti-B antibodies do not cause fetal haemolytic disease of A, B or AB fetuses as the antibodies are of IgM type. However in a small proportion of cases where mother and baby are ABO incompatible iso-immune anti-A or B antibodies, particularly anti-A, may develop and as these are of IgG type they can cross the placenta causing fetal haemolysis. These cases are detected by the paediatricians on careful investigation of so-called physiological jaundice of the newborn. Even when maternal anti-A or anti-B antibody of IgG type is present and crosses the placenta its effect on the fetus is usually relatively mild. This is because the A and B antigens occur on the tissues and in soluble form in plasma much of the antibody becomes bound to antigen present in these forms, causing no ill effects. While in European and white American populations most cases of fetal haemolytic disease are due to blood group incompatibility with iso-immunization this is not so in many parts of the world (e.g. Greece and the Far East) where an inherited deficiency of an enzyme, glucose-6 phosphate dehydrogenase, is the main cause of fetal and neonatal haemolysis. Hereditary spherocytosis or congenital haemolytic anaemia, galactosaemia and pyruvate-kinase deficiency are other causes of feto-neonatal haemolytic disease.

NON-RED CELL ISO-IMMUNITY
Iso-immunization to leucocytes may occur in preg-

nancy. In fact this phenomenon is utilized by collecting serum from patients of high parity in order to carry out grouping tests on white cells of potential organ donors. These antibodies may be detected in 15–20 per cent first pregnancies and 65 per cent subsequent pregnancies. Transplacental passage is common but there have only been isolated reports of neonatal neutropenia.

Platelet iso-immunization also occurs but again iso-immune neonatal thrombocytopenia is relatively rare and usually mild. However, it presumably carries some risk of intra-cranial haemorrhage in the newborn as is found with auto-immune neonatal thrombocytopenia (see p. 276).

In addition iso-immune antibody production occurs to immune globulins. These globulins possess a whole system of genetically inherited variables—akin to the well-defined grouping system of red blood cells. Babies in utero may develop anti-Gm antibodies (Gm is one of the grouping systems involved) to IgG which has reached it across the placenta from the mother. It does not appear, however, that such antibodies are in any way deleterious.

AUTO-IMMUNE DISEASES

In auto-immune diseases the outstanding feature is the presence of immune reaction by the individual's system to its own antigens. This may be a primary event or secondary to some primary pathological process. There is consequently dispute as to which diseases should be so graded. If, however, all diseases which have possibly an immune basis or at least a secondary immune mechanism are studied in pregnancy, inferences may be drawn which are relevant to the disease processes and their management in the pregnant and non-pregnant state. Hench's (1938) classic observation of the beneficial effect of pregnancy upon rheumatoid arthritis, a disease with an immunologic component, led ultimately to the discovery of cortisone.

Pregnancy can be thought of as an immunologic experimental system with the fetus (individual B) grafted on to the mother (individual A), existing in a state of constructive symbiosis. From an immunologic point of view B is isolated from A with the exception of the fact that IgG can cross the placental barrier. If a maternal disease process is produced by an abnormal IgG and the fetus bears antigens against which that IgG is active then it may be expected that some babies may show signs of their mothers' disease, thus pointing to the nature of the disease process.

This operates in the case of at least three well recognized medical conditions: (a) thyrotoxicosis; (b) 'idiopathic' thrombocytopenic purpura; (c) myasthenia gravis. In all of these the baby may show a transient form of the maternal disease which will rapidly regress after birth, never persisting longer than about three months. This is, of course, identical to the behaviour of haemolytic disease of the newborn and corresponds to the time taken for the IgG derived by transfer from the maternal circulation to undergo degradation.

In the case of thyrotoxicosis the IgG material which causes the neonatal disease is now identified as long-acting thyroid stimulator (LATS). This remarkable substance, chemically an immune globulin, stimulates the thyroid but with a different duration of action from thyrotropic hormone, which does not cross the placenta. It is only in recent years that the significance of LATS has been established but the clue to its existence and nature was provided by an obstetrician's observation of the transient neonatal syndrome over 50 years ago. The occurrence of the neonatal disease form is relatively infrequent; it may be the case that the abnormal IgG has to be present in very high concentration to affect the baby or is only present in some cases of thyrotoxicosis.

Transient neonatal involvement is commoner with 'idiopathic' thrombocytopenic purpura and myasthenia gravis. In the former there is a very high perinatal mortality from intracranial haemorrhage; small, normally self-limiting capillary bleeds extend into fatal haemorrhages because of the thrombocytopenia. In the latter, awareness of the possibility is essential as the presentation may be by neonatal apnoea, readily corrected by a fast acting anti-cholinesterase preparation such as edrophonium chloride.

In each of these three conditions the remarkable phenomenon has been recorded of a baby being born with a transient form of the disease to a mother who has been clinically cured of her own disease by surgery—thyroidectomy, splenectomy or thymectomy. The explanation for this is simple and illuminating. To produce the overt disease form there must be present not only the pathological IgG antibody but also a functioning end organ—thyroid, spleen or thymus.

Auto-immunity has also some relevance to the problem of infertility (see page 278).

Immunological considerations relating to

pre-eclampsia and the coagulation system are considered in the relevant chapters.

PRACTICAL ASPECTS OF RUBELLA IMMUNITY

Since the discovery of the influence of rubella infection in early pregnancy in relation to fetal malformation, the achievement of immunologic protection against the hazard has been a major objective. Until recently previous infection with the natural virus was the only effective protection which existed and this, of course, was entirely haphazard. The development of attenuated living virus vaccines ('Cendevax', Smith, Kline and French, 'Almevax', Burroughs Wellcome) has changed the situation. In the application of this resource different policies have been adopted in different parts of the world.

In the United States vaccination of the whole population of children aiming at 'herd immunity' has been the policy. It is, however, not known if the administration of the vaccine in early life will produce effective immunity persisting into adult life. Later checks are, therefore, necessary and 'follow-up' problems arise. In the United Kingdom a policy of protecting females between the ages of 11 and 14, regardless of whether or not they had previously acquired natural resistance by an earlier infection, has found favour. Inoculation given then is likely to continue to be effective at least through the early, and most fertile, years of reproduction.

The great current problem is the woman now in the reproductive age-group and potentially at risk from rubella. If rubella resistance is found to be absent prior to conception then vaccine may be offered. This should be checked on all women attending infertility clinics. The patient must be warned to avoid pregnancy for at least 2–3 months after vaccination and that, if pregnancy should occur in this period of time, the question of termination may arise. Information is lacking on the risk of fetal malformation if vaccination and early pregnancy inadvertently coincide; it is necessarily only acquired in a haphazard way and will vary with the timing of events and possibly the nature of the vaccine.

What is to be done when pregnant patients are encountered who are of unknown status with regard to rubella resistance? Positive or negative history of previous rubella infection is valueless in view of the high diagnostic error. Determination of haemagglutinin-inhibiting antibody titre is therefore necessary and should be done on the first antenatal blood specimen. If the titre is 1 in 20 or over (this figure will vary depending on the laboratory) previous infection and therefore resistance can be assumed. If less than 1 in 20 (as will be the case in approximately 15 per cent) the reverse must hold and in the absence of a safe vaccine for use in pregnancy, postpartum vaccination must be considered. This is a more suitable time than at first appears. The chance occurrence of another pregnancy is unlikely; most adult rubella infection occurs from intimate contact with childhood cases which is much more likely to occur when the woman has a toddler of her own. Thus puerperal vaccination of unprotected primigravidae can deal with most of the problem with minimal complications. In some centres it is suggested that all puerperal women should be vaccinated to save the need for early pregnancy screening.

Another problem is the mother who presents in early pregnancy as a rubella contact with the possibility of acquired infection. If possible serum should be obtained from the 'rubella' sufferer to check since many virus infections (e.g. echo) mimic clinical rubella. Serum must be obtained from the mother for antibody titre determination. If this is low at the outset and rises then infection may be presumed. *It cannot be overemphasized that the vital step in this situation is to get the initial specimen of blood at the earliest opportunity.* Any delay may make the dilemma impossible to resolve. If the serological evidence points to active infection then termination may be offered on the grounds of the fetal malformation risk.

There is no justification for the use of non-specific gamma globulin for the woman exposed to rubella risk but 'specific antibody' is possibly worthwhile immediately after exposure.

If the initial antibody titre is over the level taken as indicative of prior infection the problem remains as to whether re-infection may take place. There is no doubt that occasionally it may do. However, in relation to the main worry of fetal involvement, it seems to be the case that with secondary infection viraemia is unlikely to occur and if this does not happen the fetal risk is minimal. Differentiation of a secondary from a primary response may be done on the pattern of immune globulin changes. In a primary response there is an initial, transient development of IgM anti-rubella antibody preceding the rise in IgG, and persisting for about three weeks from the infection. In the secondary response the IgG alone rises. Complement-fixing antibody testing may also be helpful; this rises with infection but persists only for 6–24 months.

IMMUNOLOGY AND FERTILITY

A possible role of immunological factors has been sought to explain infertility when no other cause is evident and, quite differently, to provide means of curbing undesired fertility. Much experimental work has been done to demonstrate the immunogenicity of seminal fluid but this has produced little that has been of positive help to the infertile couple. While auto-immunization of the male occurs with production of antibodies which may agglutinate his own sperm, this appears in most cases to be a secondary reaction to testicular damage such as is produced by mumps orchitis or occlusion of the vas, and not a primary phenomenon.

Iso-antibodies to her male partner's sperms may be demonstrated in some infertile women but they are also present in a significant proportion of fertile women. Mononuclear cells in the cervix may phagocytose spermatozoa or their fragments and initiate the immune response. To what extent the findings of antibodies in maternal serum correspond with the situation in the cervical mucus is not at present entirely clear. It has been claimed that if by the male partner using a condom the serological findings revert to negative, pregnancy rates of 50–60 per cent can be achieved.

The problem arises as to the factors governing females' response to antigenically foreign spermatozoa. The evidence suggests that sperm deposited in the vagina rarely evoke a reaction. If directly injected into the uterine cavity, however, an immunologic response is much more probable. This suggests that the cervix may play a part, possibly limiting the number of sperms which ascend to a quantity insufficient to provoke an immune response.

Much excitement was aroused when Irvine et al. (1968) demonstrated antibodies active against ovarian granulosa and theca interna cells in women with amenorrhoea and auto-immune Addison's disease. This pointed to a new mechanism for anovulation but it does not seem from subsequent studies that this has a wide significance.

With regard to immunologic control of fertility, while much promising work has been and continues to be done in animals, it has not yet reached the stage of practical application to humans.

ABORTION

It now seems that ABO blood group incompatibility is in some way related to the chance of abortion occurring and that if an abortion occurs in an ABO incompatible mating there is a significantly increased chance that the abortus will be ABO incompatible with the mother (Clark, 1972). There is, however, no conclusive evidence that ABO incompatibility plays a major role in the problem of recurrent abortion. A small number of cases of very severe Rhesus iso-immunization, of course, may terminate as late abortions (20–28 weeks).

IMMUNOLOGIC ASPECTS OF CHORIONIC CARCINOMA

When trophoblastic tissue undergoes cancerous change to become chorionic carcinoma a unique biological situation exists (see p. 261). The trophoblast which has invaded decidua *physiologically* in order to provide the fetus with nutriments and oxygen, etc., has gone on to invade the mother's system in a *pathological*, destructive way. It is not known how the normal extent of trophoblastic invasion is controlled but it is possible that it has an immunologic basis. Immunologically, chorionic carcinoma may be regarded as the antithesis of Rhesus iso-immunization which has been described as 'the immunologic repudiation by the mother of her unborn child'; in chorionic carcinoma failure of maternal immunologic reaction may allow the trophoblast to destroy the mother.

If this were the case it might be expected that the greater the degree of immunologic incompatibility between mother and fetus (or mother and father as the foreign fetal antigens will be derived from him) the less would be the risk of uncontrolled trophoblastic invasion. A study of data on cases recorded in a central registry supported this (Scott, 1962). It was found that the blood group distribution of mothers with chorionic carcinoma showed a shift away from group O towards AB, i.e. towards the universal recipient situation in which the fetus would be more likely to be ABO compatible. Further studies have confirmed this tendency. Bagshawe et al. (1971) have shown an excess of A women and O men matings and suggest that O trophoblast is stimulated by the A antigens—a graft-versus-host type of reaction aimed at 'rejecting' the maternal host. Lawler et al. (1971) studied the HL-A (human leucocyte antigen) situation in chorionic carcinoma. They found no greater compatibility between patients and husbands but they did find a suggestion that compatibility reduced survival prospects.

REFERENCES

Bagshawe, K. D., Rawlins, G., Pike, M. C. & Lawler, S. D. (1971) ABO Blood-Groups in Trophoblastic Neoplasia, *The Lancet*, **i**, 553.

Bevis, D. C. A. (1956) Blood pigments in haemolytic disease of the newborn. *J. Obstet. Gynaec. Brit. Cwlth.*, **63**, 68

Brambell, F. W. R. (1970) *The Transmission of Passive Immunity from Mother to Young.* Amsterdam, London: North Holland Publishing Company.

Browne, J. C. M. (1967) Quoted in *Blood Transfusion in Clinical Medicine.*, p. 676 by Mollison, P. L. Oxford: Blackwell.

Clarke, C. A. (1972) Practical effects of blood group incompatibility between mother and fetus. *Brit. med. J.*, **ii**, 90.

Douglas, G. W. (1965) The Immunologic Role of the Placenta. *Obstet. Gynaec. Surv.*, **20**, 442.

Hench, P. S. (1938) Ameliorating effect of pregnancy on chronic atrophic (infectious rheumatoid) arthritis, fibrositis and intermittent hydrarthrosis. *Proceedings of the Mayo Clinic*, **13**, 161.

Hibbard, B. M. (1971) *Personal Communication.*

Hulka, J. F., Brinton, V., Schaaf, J. & Baney, C. (1963) Appearance of Antibodies to Trophoblast during the Postpartum Period in Normal Human Pregnancies. *Nature* (London), **198**, 501.

Irvine, W. J., Chan, M. M. W., Scarth, L., Kolb, F. O., Hartog, M., Bayliss, R. I. S. & Drury, M. I. (1968) Immunological Aspects of premature ovarian failure associated with idiopathic Addison's disease. *Lancet*, **ii**, 883.

Lawler, S. D., Klouda, P. T. & Bagshawe, K. D. (1971) The HL-A System in Trophoblastic Neoplasia. *Lancet*, **ii**, 834.

Liley, A. W. (1963) Intrauterine transfusion of foetus in haemolytic disease. *Brit. med. J.*, **ii**, 1107.

Naiman, J. L., Punnett, H. H., Destine, M. L. & Lischner, H. W. (1966) Yy chromosomal chimaerism. *Lancet*, **ii**, 590.

Perinatal Mortality. *First Report of the 1958 British Perinatal Mortality Survey* (1963) Eds. Butler, N. R. & Bonham, D. G., Edinburgh and London: E. & S. Livingstone Ltd.

Scott, J. S. (1962) Choriocarcinoma: observations on the etiology. *Amer. J. Obstet. Gynec.*, **83**, 185.

Stabler, F. (1960) Haemolytic disease of the newborn. *J. Obstet. Gynaec. Brit. Emp.*, **67**, p. 741.

Tovey, L. A. D. (1969) The Place of Antibody Titre Estimation in the Management of Women with Anti-D Antibodies. *J. Obstet. Gynaec. Brit. Cwlth*, **76**, 117.

Whitfield, C. R. (1970) A three year assessment of an action line method of timing intervention in rhesus isoimmunisation. *Amer. J. Obstet. Gynec.*, **108**, 1239.

FURTHER READING

Anderson, J. M. & Benirschke, K. (1964) Maternal tolerance of fetal tissue. *Brit. med. J.*, **i**, 1534.

Billingham, R. E. (1971) The Transplantation biology of mammalian gestation. *Amer. J. Obstet. Gynec.*, **111**, 469.

Brambell, F. W. R. (1970) *The Transmission of Passive Immunity from Mother to Young.* Amsterdam, London: North Holland Publishing Company.

Charles, A. G. & Friedman, E. A. (1969) *Rh Isoimmunisation and Erythroblastosis Fetalis*, London: Butterworths.

Douglas, G. W. (1965) The Immunologic Role of the Placenta. *Obstet. Gynec. Sur.*, **20**, 442.

Freda, V. J. (1962) Placental transfer of antibodies in man. *Amer. J. Obstet. Gynec.*, **84**, 1756.

Jones, W. R. (1971) Immunological factors in pregnancy. In *Scientific Basis of Obstetrics and Gynaecology*, ch. 8, p. 183, Ed. Macdonald, R. R. London: Churchill.

Queenan, J. T. (1971) The Rh problem. *Clin. Obstet. Gynec.*, **14**, No. 2, 489-646.

Ratnoff, O. D. (1971) The interrelationship of clotting and immunologic mechanisms. In *Immunobiology*, ch. 14, p. 135. Ed. Good, R. A. & Fisher, D. W. Stamford, Connecticut: Sinauer Associates Inc.

Scott, J. S. (1968) Pregnancy as an experimental system for the study of immunological diseases. *J. Reprod. Fert.*, Supplement 3, 41.

Solomon, J. B. (1971) *Foetal and Neonatal Immunology.* Amsterdam, London: North-Holland Publishing Company.

Wld. Hlth. Org. tech. Rep. Ser., No. 468 (1971) Prevention of Rh Sensitization.

16. Antenatal Care

Implantation, growth, development and delivery of a healthy mature baby is a highly complex process demanding, for the best results, a high degree of physical competence, adequate nutrition and a good environmental situation for the mother. The human race has, however, multiplied, despite poverty, malnutrition and poor environmental conditions, but babies produced in these conditions carry an appalling risk of perinatal, neonatal or infant death, or chronic disease. Inadequate development may produce grossly inadequate adults. We can do little in the pregnancy currently at risk to improve greatly the basic quality of the mother, but we can assess and correct obvious illness, recommend a high quality of diet, replace deficiencies and monitor progress, and thus probably exert some influence on the ultimate quality of the child.

HISTORICAL NOTE
(*ack*. Brown, F. J., 1946)

It is now universally recognized that there ought to be careful supervision of the expectant mother from the beginning of pregnancy by doctors and nurses specially experienced and trained in obstetrics. Healthy women sometimes fail to meet the demands of pregnancy, and anomalies may appear in pregnancy which can be diagnosed and corrected only by careful routine assessment. Very few of the earlier writers fail to make some reference to the 'hygiene' of pregnancy or to the treatment of its diseases and disorders. Much of the advice given by Reynold in his *Byrth of Mankynde* in 1540, by Mauriceau in *Des Maladies des Femmes Grosse et Accouches*, in 1668, and by Smellie in 1761, in *A set of anatomical tables and practice of midwifery—a collection of cases*, is in line with modern practice. There had been from time immemorial in Paris, special hospital refuges, even although of a primitive kind, available for pregnant women who were ill, in premature labour or who at term needed shelter—They were available to all—'a la femme légitime, à la femme dissolue et à cette infortuneé qu 'un instant de fragilité a rendeé mère' (Tenon, 1788).

Pinard in 1878 and in 1895 describing his work in the *Clinique Baudelocque* reported, as did the obstetricians with experience in the other refuges, that eclampsia could be prevented, malpresentation corrected and disease treated, and that the babies born to these girls who had shelter for sometime in those institutions were better and fitter and less frequently prematurely born than those of women often of better social groups who continued at work until delivery.

In 1899 the Lauriston Prenatal Home was opened in connection with the Maternity Hospital in Edinburgh, and to it were admitted unmarried pregnant women. They were under the supervision of Dr Haig Ferguson, one of the obstetricians to the Royal Maternity Hospital. He noted the benefits which followed medical care and supervision given to the girls and suggested that the ordinary patients who were admitted to the maternity hospital should have similar benefits. In 1901 Dr J. W. Ballantyne, of Edinburgh, who had been an assistant to Dr Haig Ferguson, published a paper entitled *A Plea for a Promaternity Hospital*. In this he deplored the lack of knowledge of the physiology and pathology of pregnancy and suggested that in a pro-maternity hospital problems of pregnancy might be studied. While he was concerned at first mainly with the causes of abortion, fetal deformity and stillbirth, he later showed interest in the preventive aspects of antenatal care, and many of his prophecies of the results to be obtained from antenatal care have been realized. Up until this time women with medical complications of pregnancy had been admitted to medical wards of general hospitals, where they were under the care of physicians who were not as a rule interested in the diseases of pregnancy. The admission of the patient was often secured with difficulty, and she was discharged as early as possible since births in the wards of a general hospital were inconvenient and upsetting to the routine.

In 1907 the Hamilton Bed in memory of Dr Hamilton, formerly Professor of Midwifery, was endowed and it was occupied for the first time by a patient suffering from hydramnios.

There was at that time, however, no suggestion

that routine examination of all pregnant women, normal as well as abnormal, should be carried out, as is the practice today.

In America, however, progress along these lines had occurred. In Boston, in 1901, the Instructive Nursing Association began to pay antenatal visits to some of the women in the outpatient department of the Boston Lying-in Hospital, and by 1912 this Association paid about three antenatal visits to each patient. In 1911 the pregnancy clinic of the Boston Lying-in Hospital was opened, and arrangements were made to visit patients in their own homes where advice was given as to preparation for confinements, the urine was tested and any danger signals reported to the medical staff. In 1912 an antenatal clinic was opened in Sydney, New South Wales. By 1915 an antenatal clinic was started at the Royal Maternity Hospital in Edinburgh, to be followed quickly by antenatal clinics at all maternity hospitals.

In Britain the Notification of Births (Extension) Act, 1915, allowed local authorities to make what provision they thought necessary for the care of expectant mothers, and the Maternity and Child Welfare (1918) Act allowed them to build maternity hospitals. By 1935 it was estimated that there were 1400 state-aided clinics in England and Wales alone. In many voluntary maternity hospitals part or all of the cost of treatment was borne by the government through the local authorities. The clinics not attached intimately to maternity hospitals were actually built by local authorities and staffed by salaried maternity and child welfare officers, assisted by health visitors or midwives paid by the local authorities. This was without doubt the quickest method of bringing medical and nursing advice to the large numbers of women and children who, not being insured under any scheme, were unable to afford fees to private practitioners. While this service did extremely valuable work, especially in the field of health education, it was handicapped by the fact that the medical officers were not on the staff of the maternity hospitals in which the women were confined and consequently did not have any experience of treating complications of pregnancy or labour. The National Health Service had not (before 1974) remedied this state of affairs, since the care of the expectant mothers could be undertaken by the Regional Hospital Board, the local authority or the general practitioner. If the patient books for confinement in a large maternity hospital antenatal care may be given by the specialist staff of the hospital, or by the general practitioner or the local authority medical officers working in co-operation with the hospital staff. If she books for confinement at home or in a small cottage hospital, antenatal care is given by the general practitioner or the midwife, or by both, but sometimes their work is not well co-ordinated. The family doctor may conduct the antenatal examination either in the patient's home or in his consulting rooms, and the midwife in the patient's home or she may arrange for her to attend a local authority clinic. The domiciliary and hospital organizations were not well co-ordinated as a rule and differences of opinion as to the merits and demerits of hospital or home confinement on the part of the officials of the organizations concerned often militated against the best interests and desires of the patient.

ORGANIZATION OF CARE OF THE MOTHER

For the last 60 years antenatal care has been organized throughout the world on the team concept of the midwife (or the public health nurse), the general practitioner and the specialist, and has been running at public health clinics, voluntary clinics, doctors' offices, hospitals and private consultant centres. Organization has depended on the area, the local practice and the determination of the profession or the public to secure improved results.

In Great Britain integration of the three arms of the Health Service as from 1974 may have in some areas, little or no effect on the organization of care, but in some others there will be real change.

The development of Area or District 'Divisions' or Program Committees for maternity (and gynaecological) care composed of trained specialists, specially trained and interested general practitioners, midwives, paediatricians specially knowledgeable in neonatal care, and advised by experts in community care, should, however, greatly improve the quality of the organization and therefore, quality of the care.

It will become obvious to the student that high quality antenatal care can be given to most patients by the trained practitioner who observes strictly certain simple rules. When, however, patients are involved who have a limited ability to reproduce safely or easily, or who have a serious physical handicap, quality care can be given only under the supervision of the expert.

The detailed organization of antenatal, labour, postnatal and neonatal care will obviously vary tremendously with the district and the country, with the attitudes of the people concerned and with those of the Government concerned, with the degree and extent of special care available and with the desire or ability of the women to avail themselves of it.

There is still much we do not know about the anomalies of pregnancy so that failures still take place despite supervision of high quality and sometimes without discernible cause. However, if current knowledge could be applied to the care of all pregnant women both fetal and maternal mortality and morbidity would fall to negligible levels. It is therefore the duty of every trained doctor or midwife to ensure that the individual patient, and every other pregnant woman whose care they can undertake or influence, receives such a degree of care as she requires or can be in the circumstances made available to her from as early in pregnancy as possible.

It is sometimes said that the antenatal care of a woman begins with her own birth or even with her own conception. This is intended to demonstrate that much of the ability of a woman to have a successful pregnancy and to bear a fit and healthy child is determined or influenced by the quality of her own upbringing and maybe influenced for better or worse, physically and psychologically by all that has happened to her herself as a fetus, as a child and in her adolescence. The animal breeder is concerned with pedigree and the record of his stock. In the human situation we must realize similar influences apply. It is, however, one of the duties of the doctor to seek, correct, influence, or compensate for, the inevitable deficiencies of his patient.

The father

In human reproductive physiology (in contradistinction to the high importance given the sire in animal reproduction), there is a tendency to ignore the father. It may be that we should look more clearly at the father (the heredity and the genetics) as well as at the mother who combines her own hereditary complement with the creation of an environment for the fetal development.

We must at least determine whether the father suffers from transmissible disease and is likely to be a carrier of any lethal or handicapping genetic trait. The quality of the father is, of course, particularly important where donor males are being selected for artificial insemination.

Routine care

Care of the pregnant woman should in all cases be undertaken by a person specially trained and specially skilled. In developed countries where limitation of family size is now seriously practiced, there is a real (some-

times unexpressed) desire that children born should be the best possible and mere survival is not necessarily success. In developing countries it may still be difficult to instil the belief that each pregnancy is precious and that special care of the mother is needed. Even in the Western world the mother and the husband often insist that the mother's prime duty is to her existing children or to the husband, and measures necessary to protect the wellbeing of the future or the developing fetus or even of the mother herself, are difficult or impossible to apply.

Under modern conditions the first antenatal visit is recognized as a visit of assessment, a visit at which plans are made for routine care throughout the pregnancy, arrangements put in hand for special investigations or ancillary help, the place of delivery discussed and facilities booked.

The patient should be seen as early as possible by those who are to be expected to care for her in labour. The details of the first visit will obviously vary with all local circumstances but we will here consider the routine to be expected in any developed country and to be attempted elsewhere when possible.

The patient

The woman must be first considered as an individual in terms of her past and present medical history, body build, state of nutrition and obstetric history, secondly as a member of a family with itself a history of hereditary traits such as tuberculosis, hypertension or hereditary anomalies, thirdly as a member of a community or group which might have religious beliefs or customs or taboos.

FAMILY HISTORY
Family history should include a record of hereditary or familial disease of any kind— genetic anomalies, diabetes, tuberculosis, hypertension and twinning, especially where the twins were non-identical. It would also be of some value to have records of special school attendance or any other proof of mental inadequacy of relatives or of siblings. The obstetric behaviour of the patient's sisters might be of interest.

HISTORY
A medical history should be sought down to the most intricate detail. Any condition may be significant, and distant disease may have

left sequalae, recent disease may still be active. The most obvious conditions are:

Heart disease—congenital or acquired with or without existing symptoms.

Tuberculosis—as an index of family risk and with a risk of recrudescence.

Renal disease—which might already have restricted her renal function or might so do in pregnancy.

Trauma—to spine or pelvis or legs with distortion or deformity.

Anaemia—especially if associated with abnormal haemoglobins. Even a simple iron or folate deficiency can be grossly exaggerated by pregnancy.

Hepatitis—which might recur in pregnancy if choleostatic or if viral be associated with fetal deformity.

Diabetes—which will produce a real and serious risk to mother and child.

Previous gynaecological operation—dilatation of the cervix, previous cone or amputation may lead to incompetence. Uterine scars or damage may lead to rupture in labour.

Pulmonary embolus—or phlebothrombosis would be very liable to recur in the existing pregnancy.

The problem is to be assessed, the degree of disability judged and if active the degree of activity fully evaluated. Expert help and advice may be needed to evaluate the risk of the pregnancy to the mother and of the disease to the pregnancy.

The situation may be such that the pregnancy may need to be terminated forthwith, if the maternity disease precludes successful pregnancy at this time with sterilization if the risk is permanent. The special remedial measures to correct the risk may be decided upon, or the precautions necessary to minimize the risk discussed.

In the presence of active disease, e.g. diabetes, asthma, chronic infections with helminth, malaria, special care or special therapy will be required and should be planned from the start and the special co-operation of a medical expert may be in the best interests of the patient.

OBSTETRIC HISTORY
A careful record should be made of previous pregnancies. This should include date, place of care and delivery, duration of gestation and of labour, method of delivery, sex, weight and condition of child. Any antenatal, labour or postnatal anomalies would be noted and information obtained of the progress of the child. Each pregnancy is to some extent its own isolated event, but women do establish patterns, good or bad, in reproduction. One abortion is more likely to be followed by another than if the first pregnancy had not aborted, one perinatal dead child is more likely to be followed by another, poor growth by poor growth, premature labour by premature labour, antepartum haemorrhage by antepartum haemorrhage, malpresentation by malpresentation, retained placenta by retained placenta, or deformity by deformity. A woman who is delivered easily vaginally of a 4000g baby must have a good pelvis but three babies of 2500–3000g do not indicate a normal pelvis and may be followed by disproportion with uterine rupture if the next child is large.

Where a woman has had previous children elsewhere than under the care of the present doctor, it is wise to write to the previous hospital or centre for the records of the previous pregnancy and labour, and certainly always if there is any reason to think that the previous pregnancies were in any way unusual or if the baby was in any way damaged.

MENSTRUAL HISTORY
This history is probably best taken with relevance to the existing pregnancy, rather than as an historical event.

Age at menarche, the normal cycle pattern and the history of cycles in the few months before pregnancy is specially noted.

The date of the first day of 'last menstrual period' is recorded and the details of that period discussed. Was it at the correct time and of normal duration and amount?

If the patient had been recently on contraceptive progestogens the facts and time of stopping are recorded.

Routine medical examination at first assessment

General.
1. Her *height* is measured and *weight* taken with minimal clothing.
2. Any physical anomaly is noted and assessed.
3. Physical examination is made with special reference to breasts, heart, lungs, central nervous and locomotive systems.
4. Varicosities of leg veins are searched for and any special examination made

if indicated. Ankle or more generalized oedema is searched for.

Urine. Specific gravity is noted and tests are made for albumin and sugar. A midstream or clean catch specimen should be taken for a check on urinary tract infection.

Blood. Venous blood preferably without stasis is taken for estimation of haematocrit, haemoglobin level, ABO and Rh grouping and checks for syphilis (Wasserman or VDRL), rubella immunity, Australia Antigen, other special routines may be required, e.g. checks for abnormal haemoglobins, alpha fetoprotein levels, malaria parasites, etc. depending on the local circumstances.

Blood pressure. This should be taken lying down and after a few minutes' rest.

Uterus. Fundal height above symphysis is recorded by some accepted measure, coded or measured in centimetres. While fundal height is notoriously unreliable as an absolute means of estimating gestation age, careful records of height and uterine mass generally give a good guide to uterine growth and therefore pregnancy wellbeing.

Estimation of uterine size by pelvic examination in early pregnancy is desirable as the best estimate of pregnancy duration can be made at this time. A note should always be made as to whether uterine size is compatible with clinical dates. Discrepancy should be recorded and reassessed at later visit. Hydramnios should be tested for if the uterus seems unduly large.

Fetus. If the fetus is large enough to be palpated, its size, lie, presentation and position should be noted. Multiple pregnancy may be suspected.

Vulva-vagina. Discharge if present should be noted, swabs taken if indicated, so that specific therapy can be given to any vaginitis.

Cervix. In many units, routine antenatal cervical cytological smear is taken on all multigravida and selected primigravida at first or later visits.

Where there is a history of recurrent abortion, vaginal pregnancy termination or of cone biopsy, or of amputation of the cervix, the risks of cervical incompetence must be remembered.

A Shirodkar type cervical suture may be necessary at 10–12 weeks as a prophylaxis, or later after 26 weeks if premature labour is imminent.

The damaged uterus. The uterus with previous classical Caesarean section or hystero-tomy, with perforation at termination or curettage, or with extensive myomectomy, or the uterus in which tubal or ovarian implantation has been done, or when Strassman or other utriculoplasty has been performed, have a risk of rupture during late pregnancy or early labour. Tenderness or pain or bulging suggests rupture or imminent rupture. Labour should rarely be allowed to occur.

The uterus with lower segment section, with extensive cervix repair, or after lower segment or cervix tears post delivery or post abortion may rupture in labour. Tenderness, pain and bleeding are significant. All such cases must have specialist supervision antenatally and in labour.

PLAN OF LATER CARE

Following the assessment and discussion at the first visit and once various reports of blood and urine examination are available, and there has been a review of old medical and obstetric records, various decisions fall to be taken. The actual decision will depend on the local circumstances and the various care systems available.

In general, whoever is to be responsible for delivery and therefore to a large extent for the outcome of the pregnancy, should select the main features of the antenatal care and perform such an amount of care sufficient to make him fully acquainted with all the features of the case. Selection of the proper place and quality of antenatal care is as important as selection of place for delivery. Care may be entirely general practitioner, entirely hospital or specialist, or a combination of the two. Patients in whom the problem is likely to be one of delivery need be seen only occasionally by the specialist. Where the problem is likely to be one of the antenatal period or prematurity, perhaps a tighter specialist control should be exercised. In general in the county areas of Scotland, some 25 per cent of patients have shared care and specialist delivery, some 25 per cent shared care and general practitioner unit delivery and some 50 per cent are looked after entirely by their general practitioners. Perinatal mortality under these circumstances is excellent.

Patients with a recent history of premature labour, poor fetal growth, antepartum haemorrhage, perinatal death, recurrent abortion or unduly difficult labour, Caesarean section, hysterotomy, therapeutic abortion or gynaecological operation, should clearly have antenatal care largely under specialist supervision.

Where the patient has some medical disease, specialist medical opinion should be combined with specialist obstetric opinion and care should always be shared. It is important, if possible, that care, say of the diabetic, should be shared between a physician specially knowledgeable in the care of diabetes in pregnancy and an obstetrician specially knowledgeable of the care of pregnancy in diabetes. Care should, if possible, in a major centre, be centred on a small group of experts. (This applies similarly to cardiac, hypertensive, thyroid patients and those with Rh or other serological incompatibility.)

Place of delivery

This decision is not usually made until the end of the first visit or even later. It is becoming throughout the world, the custom for institutional delivery, i.e. delivery in a centre specially equipped to make delivery safer for mother and child. The degree of sophistication varies from the village delivery centre in the African bush through the 24-hour centre in the 'big city', through the well equipped general practitioner maternity unit or nursing home to the University Hospital with every conceivable facility. (Delivery in the patient's own home is, as a general principle, not acceptable but is occasionally necessary for want of another facility or desired by the patient with the good home. In a modern society with all facilities available, domiciliary delivery should be allowed only to highly selected patients.) We should, in other words, if we must, 'select for home confinement'. It is significant that where adequate general practitioner maternity beds are available, home confinement is confined to the extremely wealthy or the unintelligent poor.

In general we should also select for general practitioner unit delivery cases which are almost certain to have minimal anomaly, tall healthy primigravidae, aged 18–25, or second or third gravida with a clear history.

In the reorganized British system the whole maternity service will be integrated such that all specialist, and general practitioner, obstetricians and midwives are part of a team planning and organizing care to the benefit of the patient. General practitioner units will be the responsibility of the integrated divisions and rules will be made by local agreement. Where the general practitioner unit is part of a major hospital obviously more freedom in booking is possible. However, in practice many mistakes in place of booking are still being unnecessarily made.

In countries where hospital facilities are limited by geography or by extent, selection out will have to be made for more expert care of those who must be in hospitals of various degrees of sophistication.

Visits after the first

In general visits should be monthly until 28 weeks, and fortnightly thereafter until term, after which weekly visits may be necessary. Where some abnormality is suspected or noted, even though minor, weekly visits may be necessary at any time and especially in primigravidae after the 30th week.

The purpose of care is to monitor the progress of pregnancy from the point of view of mother and child, to detect, diagnose and treat aberration from normal and later to judge the likely problems that might be met in labour (see Chapter 19).

The patient should have the whole pattern of her pregnancy care discussed with her and her wishes taken into account. She should be informed of the reasons for decisions, especially when they appear to conflict with her expressed wish. The facilities available to her in the way of special foods and allowances should be explained in full. She should be informed of special antenatal classes provided within the unit and whether or not her husband will be also invited. She should be encouraged to discuss her pregnancy and the problems created by it (medical or social) at any time and made to feel that her doctors, nurses, health visitors and physiotherapists and dieticians and social workers are actively interested in her welfare.

The pregnancy

At each visit the mother's general health should be discussed. Nausea, sickness, heartburn, constipation, sleeplessness assessed and advice or treatment given.

The uterine size and shape should be measured and recorded. While the fundal height may be inaccurate in relation to actual dates, it is an essential guide to growth of the uterus and the child, or may raise suspicion of multiple pregnancy, hydramnios, or associated intra-abdominal tumours. It is to be remembered that in primigravida the uterus enlarges after the 20th week as a long oval, and in multigravida rather as a round cyst. A multigravida may have a large capacious uterus without an unduly high fundus.

WEIGHT

Routine weighing (with minimal clothing) is an excellent guide to pregnancy wellbeing (*see* Chapter 6), and should be done at all visits. In general a steady rise of 1lb (say, 450g) per week from the 12th week to the 38th week, is the normal mean and is associated with the best results. Purposeful weight reduction by grossly retarding intake is *not* good antenatal care, but limitation of excess *gain* by dieting measures is acceptable. Encouragement of the poor undernourished to eat well may improve the quality of the child. The relation of weight gain to hypertensive disease are discussed in Chapter 10.

BLOOD PRESSURE

Routine blood pressure (lying down) at all clinic visits. The behaviour of abnormal blood pressure states is described in Chapter 10. The earlier the pressure is established in pregnancy the better we understand our patient. Certainly the level ought to be known before the 12th week, since by then most of the major haemodynamic changes have already occurred. As soon as the diastolic pressure rises by 15mmHg or reaches 90mmHg the clinical situation is one of hypertension and appropriate measures (*see* Chapter 10), should be taken.

OEDEMA

Oedema is common in the legs in pregnant women especially in hot weather, but may of course, be a sign of hypertensive, renal, cardiac or metabolic disease, or of anaemia. The aetiology must be sought. Unilateral oedema may be the first sign of antenatal deep vein thrombosis.

URINE

Routinely urine checks are done at most clinics for albumin and sugar. The importance and significance of various tests for sugar, is discussed in Chapter 12, as is the need for tests for ketones.

Culture of clean catch and midstream specimen of urine done routinely at first visit is necessary later only if symptoms of urinary infection appear. Special collection and transport methods are necessary. Other special tests, e.g. prophorins etc., as indicated.

Urine samples (12 and 24 hour) may be required for estimation of oestrogens, chorionic gonadotrophin, *see* Chapter 18.

BLOOD

Haemoglobin and other special tests sickling, fragility, buffy coat, etc., will be taken as indicated in investigation or therapy of abnormal states, but routinely haemoglobin levels should be taken at first visit, 24–26 weeks, 32–34 weeks and term. The level at which special study is indicated will vary from place to place, but certainly any level less than 75 per cent (11g per cent) requires investigation (*see* Chapter 12).

At first visit all bloods will be checked for Rh states, but also for the presence of non-specific red cell antibody so that any unusual antibody state will be picked up, e.g. Kell Duffy *et al.* If a patient is Rh (D) positive and no abnormal antibodies are found at first visit it is unnecessary, to repeat the test unless some unexplained problem appears, or of course, as a check in a subsequent pregnancy. If she is Rh (D) negative, and there are no antibodies at first visit a repeat should be done at 24 and again about 36 weeks. If abnormal antibodies are found then the titre level should be checked at *every visit*, i.e. monthly until 28th week and fortnightly thereafter, *see* Chapter 15.

Blood may be required for all sorts of reasons, but for fetal monitoring the special needs are detailed in Chapter 18.

BREASTS

The breasts and nipples should be examined to assess their suitability for lactation. If the mother has previously lactated easily, then she will be likely to need no special guidance. If she has had previous cracked nipples, mastitis or abscess she ought not to breast feed and will probably not wish to.

In general the ability to breast feed is usually associated with the degree to which the breasts increase in bulk during pregnancy, but this is difficult to assess. All that is required for care is gentle washing with soap and water and support gently by a brassiere. Shields and other special care suggested for the nipples and breasts to encourage lactation are probably of little value.

It must be remembered that in modern society a fairly large number of women are quite incapable of producing enough milk to feed a child successfully.

Minor ailments

The detection and care of most is discussed in the relevant Chapters 12, 16, etc.

CRAMPS

Common and annoying. Calcium deficiency is suggested but most cases respond to an increase in salt intake (up to plus one level teaspoonful per day), taken in a salty drink, e.g. Bovril or soup. Sometimes they are a sign of more serious vascular disease and this should be checked.

HAEMORRHOIDS

May be very painful in late pregnancy and certainly in labour and in the puerperium. Local application, cold compresses, lotion and ointments are useful and necessary.

CONSTIPATION

This is common during pregnancy, especially in the first half, and may be troublesome even in women not habitually troubled by it. It is due probably to bowel reaction to the endocrine changes of pregnancy, although in the later weeks mechanical pressure may play some part. In most cases the only treatment required is fluid, diet containing fruit and vegetables, some daily exercise and a regular attempt at evacuation. However, in the patients where this does not succeed, senna in some form is usually adequate, small doses being taken routinely, but if constipation had been present before pregnancy of course, the patient's usual drug therapy may be required. Drastic chemical purges should, of course, be avoided. There is some suggestion that liquid paraffin interferes with the absorption during pregnancy of vitamins, but in the minimal doses necessary, this is probably not terribly important.

FAINTING

In women with extensive varicose veins in legs and vulva, fainting when standing for any length of time is always possible. Later in pregnancy when a pregnant woman lies on her back she may of course, faint from interference with cardiac return due to uterine pressure on the inferior vena cava. She may find it best to sleep, in late pregnancy, on her left side.

REST AND SLEEP

In the early months the patient may complain of a tendency to faintness and fatigue, but this usually passes off by the fourth month and such extra rest as is necessary may have to be taken. Later on, when the uterus becomes large, and especially if there is any varicosities, she may feel tired and find her legs heavy. In general, in late pregnancy, afternoon rest and early to bed is advisable in so far as the woman's family commitments will allow.

Difficulty in sleeping in late pregnancy again is not uncommon, and there seems no harm in minimal doses of evening sedatives to allow sleep.

EXERCISE

Exercise in pregnancy is usually achieved by women in the normal course of work or housekeeping. Most multigravidae have no need of any routine extra exercise. However, to the primigravida who is not in employment, or the house of office bound multigravida regular short walks in the open air are advised. In general, more strenuous forms of exercise like swimming or golf would depend on the individual. If she is accustomed to such exercise, then there is no particular reason why in the first half of pregnancy at least, she should not continue. Most women, who are regular drivers, drive cars without difficulty until late in pregnancy, but the expressed dangers of some forms of lap-belt is relation to the fetus and uterus must be remembered. High-speed driving (with the risk of accident) or prolonged periods sitting in a car, are certainly contraindicated in late pregnancy.

The place of antenatal purposeful exercise in the form of physiotherapy classes is still open to debate. There is little doubt that in patients who desire this type of therapy, the exercises will assist circulation, breathing, gently mobilize joints, may keep the freedom of the muscle stretch available, and teach control and relaxation of the muscles of the pelvic floor. Where directly applied to labour such antenatal classes can do little but good. Especially where the patient has been properly schooled in those exercises continuation of the exercises in the first stage of labour is likely to be helpful.

There is no doubt at all, however, that the vast majority of pregnant women achieve adequate exercise in the ordinary course of a day's living and classes have value limited to a relatively small group, but this small group does benefit from them.

BATHING AND CLOTHING

The modern pregnant woman does not wear

special supports except for varicose veins and there is no doubt at all that elastic tights are a necessary part of the care of the pregnant woman with varicosities. These should be prescribed and worn. Otherwise clothing should be loose and free as is the accepted modern custom. Obviously hygiene and cleanliness is important. There seems little risk in daily showers and baths during pregnancy.

COITUS
Coitus during pregnancy is certainly not harmful, except perhaps in the presence of threatened abortion, or where there is a history of abortion or if premature labour threatens, when the orgasm associated with coitus may have adverse effects on the pregnancy. In the later months there is some risk of infection and it is usually suggested that in the last few weeks coitus should be avoided. Similar restrictions would apply if the membranes are ruptured or antepartum bleeding has occurred.

TEETH
Dental care of the pregnant woman is an essential part of antenatal care and dental examinations and advice should be part of all good antenatal clinic services. In the Dundee Teaching Hospitals of 2768 booked patients, 48 per cent were considered to have dental defects. Seventy per cent elected to be treated by their own practitioners and of the remaining 214, 496 fillings and 255 extractions were performed. General anaesthesia was necessary in 76 patients.

ALCOHOL
The risks of chronic alcoholism and smoking are outlined in the 'risk to the fetus' in Chapter 25. It is clear that cigarette smoking should be stopped during pregnancy. Alcohol in moderate amounts can do little if any harm.

VARICOSE VEINS
In the pregnant woman varicosities are common and often distressing by their appearance, by the feeling of weight or tiredness or even fainting if large amounts of blood pool. They are dangerous as a source of phlebitis or phlebothrombosis. Elasticated stockings or tights are essential and should be prescribed and worn. Varicosity of the vulvar area is helped by tights but probably not completely alleviated, and rest with the legs elevated or actually in bed is also required.

Active therapy by injection and compression is advised in several centres and if expertly done may give comfort. It is to be remembered, however, that the disability is greatly relieved after pregnancy is over and conservative therapy in pregnancy is usually sufficient.

THE FETUS
Antenatal fetal monitoring is described in Chapter 18. Throughout pregnancy and certainly from 28 weeks the fetus should be palpated and his size, lie, presentation and later position established and recorded. It is to be remembered that (in Britain) at the 28th week the mean weight of a baby is 1000g, by the 35th week 2500g and at term 3500g, and practice should be obtained in assessing the actual weight of the child in relation to those guidelines.

Undue size in relation to dates should raise suspicion of multiple pregnancy at least by 16 weeks and hydramnios may appear at any time after 24 weeks. The poor growth uterus or baby should certainly be suspected by 24 weeks if not earlier.

In late pregnancy it is extremely important to assess baby size (small, average or large, at least), as the risks of labour and delivery are high in the small and in the large child and intelligent anticipation may prevent tragedy. The small child should be born always in a centre with special nursery facilities and advance warning of the size would allow early transfer of the *mother* in labour. Similar provisions for maternal transfer apply also if labour begins before the end of the 37th week.

By late pregnancy the lie of the child should be longitudinal, the presentation cephalic and the position occipito-anterior. The head should be sitting close to the pelvic brim and may be engaged especially in the primigravida. Failure of engagement in the primigravida at term is not necessarily abnormal but should merit further check and discussion about place of delivery if this has not already been arranged for a major unit.

Multiple pregnancy would of course by now, be obvious.

BREECH
It is probably wise to apply external version to a child presenting as a breech at any time after the 32nd week, when it can be *easily* performed. The fetal heart should be checked afterwards. Version may be contra-indicated in severe hypertensive syndromes or in association with antepartum haemorrhage and

certainly when elective Caesarean section is already planned. Version under anaesthesia should be reserved for highly selected cases. The large breech baby in the primigravida at term should probably be delivered by Caesarean section.

TRANSVERSE OR OBLIQUE LIE

Oblique lie with the head or breech just failing to come into the midline may be significant of placenta praevia, or of a pelvic or uterine tumour, or of pelvic contraction or even of unsuspected twins.

A *transverse lie* may also be associated with these situations but is more likely, in the multigravida, to be associated with a lax round uterus in which the child may lie as it pleases (breech, vertex or transverse), varying from day to day. In the primigravida it almost always is associated with abnormality of uterine shape, abnormality of the child or a lower abdominal tumour.

The patient with transverse lie should be admitted to hospital about 38 weeks or so, especially when her home is distant, so that she will be in hospital when labour starts. Investigation for placental site, tumour, twins or pelvic contraction should be made and then labour awaited. When labour starts compaction occurs and the child almost always assumes the correct lie. If this does not happen, or if the membranes rupture with cord or arm prolapse, the necessary action can be taken.

Diet in pregnancy

The requirements of selected food materials during pregnancy have been very fully listed in Chapter 5.

It must, however, be realized that nutrient requirements have to be translated into available food, which can be properly absorbed and utilized. Correct foods must obviously be available when needed and the purchasing power of the mother must allow her to obtain the foods.

Relative starvation is very common throughout the world and the pregnant woman is extremely vulnerable. Absolute deficiency of protein is very uncommon in the Western world but certainly not so in countries where drought, famine and war are frequent. Calorie deficiency almost always runs parallel with protein deficiency. Serious malnutrition in a previously well nourished population, e.g. wartime Holland or Stalingrad, has a very different and much lesser effect than famine in an always malnourished population, such as Bangladesh; Southern Sahara; Central Africa or Central America. Populations are often malnourished because dysenteries: helminth infection and other chronic illness interferes with appetite or absorption and tribal taboos might exclude foods which are really essential. Even in Scotland malnourishment is not unusual in pregnant women and children, and poor dietary attitudes or financial stringency often makes vegetable or fruit intake and intake of fat soluble vitamins deficient in winter and early spring.

It would seem somewhat illogical in well nourished women to prescribe routine additions and there is no doubt that these are often overprescribed. Many healthy pregnant women are not iron deficient and do not benefit from extra iron. Iron therapy should always be given where deficiency is proven. However, it is strongly recommended that, in industrial cities of the Western world, a daily dose routinely of iron and folic acid (and possibly vitamin C), be given after the 12th week to avoid nausea and risk of teratogenesis, to meet the requirements of pregnancy. Almost certainly half the mothers will not need it, but the others will benefit and it is very difficult to select out these groups who have deficient intake or stores. If this is done, however, it is most important that the blood should still be tested routinely for iron and folate deficiency and reliance should not be placed on the women taking the supplements.

Minimal doses of 60mg elemental iron and 0·3mg folic acid are given. No serious attempt is made to restore haemoglobin levels. If these are low the reasons should be sought (*see* Chapter 12).

DIETARY ADVICE

The dietician, who should be part of all antenatal care can (*see* Chapter 5) by advice and discussion do much to guide the patient to good dietary habits, to correct food fads and to establish within the confines of the circumstances a diet adequate to the patient's needs. Pregnancy is possibly not a time when diet restriction in any drastic sense to reduce or hold weight is advisable. Maintenance of a minimal steady gain in the fat patient is debatable but a greater than average gain in the thin and undernourished is desirable if it can be achieved.

Education at antenatal clinics

The process of pregnancy should be a period during which the mother can be educated, not only with regard to her pregnancy and to its progress and its problems, but also in a general sense in relation to diet, clothing, habits, personal hygiene and newborn and later baby care. Much of this can be done by the individual doctor and midwife in his personal care of the individual patient. Certainly by so doing a great deal of personal trust is built up and the confidence of the patient and the comfort of her pregnancy and her labour will be that much increased. There is no reason, however, why in the modern busy antenatal clinic, such advice and guidance cannot be given. It is also of an advantage to establish special classes of instruction, seminars during the antenatal period available to the pregnant woman and to her husband. Talks on the principles and values of antenatal care, pregnancy diet, practical food advice, cooking demonstration, instruction on the purchase and preparation of easily available foods, on the clothing and personal hygiene during pregnancy, on baby care and of course discussion on the special problems of the area in which the patient may be living, or the special problems faced by her community.

Class instruction in relation to labour is probably best given to husband and wife together. The stages of labour are described and the general techniques and methods of caring for the woman in labour within the unit are described.

Questions should be freely asked and answered, so that the woman and, if she wishes, her husband have a reasonable knowledge of the organization of labour care and what normally is to be expected.

In the less advanced and more primitive situation it is intensification of care that is clearly necessary, and in the highly sophisticated situation a more balanced attitude to the outcome of such care is probably now indicated.

There is no doubt that modern labour is infinitely less distressing and certainly less prolonged than before. Where the unit undertakes special labour techniques such as routine syntocin following induction, or routine syntocin accelerated labour then these techniques should be explained to the patient and the reasons given. All methods of pain relief in relation to labour of all types should be discussed and apparatus for the patient's personal use, e.g. entonox demonstrated.

If the patient wishes her husband to be present during labour there is usually no contra-indication. The individual doctor or midwife conducting the labour can of course, make the rules about the circumstances in which the husband may be asked to leave. Distressing and difficult deliveries are probably not ideally witnessed, but this is for discussion, preferably before the labour begins. It is sometimes considered good practice that the antenatal mothers should visit the labour suite and meet the team that will be looking after them during labour. Certainly in the newer and more attractive hospitals this would be an excellent prophylactic measure. In the less attractive hospitals the quality and obvious efficiency of the labour suite team will go far to dispelling doubts or problems in the minds especially of the young primigravida.

Mothercraft teaching has become much more fully developed in more recent years and classes which instruct the actual or potential mother in care of the newborn and of young children have been of tremendous advantage in improving total child care in the community.

In most modern obstetric units, the paediatrician with special interest in the newborn undertakes routine care and long-term follow-up of babies delivered on the units. Such checks may be only of the abnormal or difficult, but perhaps from a research point of view more routine regular follow-up checks are arranged. This type of activity, with an emphasis on assessment of later child quality should enable the obstetrician to monitor the outcome of his own work. The principle should be explained to the patients, since with understanding of the aims and value, tremendous co-operation from and interest of the parents is usually achieved.

RESULTS OF ANTENATAL CARE

There is no doubt that in modern practice the quality of antenatal care is steadily increasing. If the simple rules outlined, of regular checks and of appropriate action in the presence of anomaly were followed, the overall quality would be better still. This improvement in results of care is reflected in the fall in perinatal deaths and in the general overall improvement in health and intelligence of young children. It is possible, however, that with the intensification of antenatal care, there might be an intensification of therapy to the point at which unnecessary therapy is given. For example, induction of labour is perhaps instituted where induction is not clearly indicated, and followed by the risks of induction failure. The undue anticipation of problems is dangerous where the risk of the problem is sometimes less than therapy advocated. Maternity units must exercise total vigilance in relation not only to the quality of care, but also to the extent of therapy apparently indicated by that care.

REFERENCES

Ballantyne, J. W. (1901) A plea for a promaternity hospital. *Brit. med. J.*, **1**, 813.
Pinard, M. (1895) Note pour servie a l'histoire de la puericulture intrauterine. *Bull. Acad. Méd.*, 593.
Tenon, M. (1788) *Memoires des hospitaux de Paris.*

FURTHER READING

Ballantyne, J. W. (1902) *Manual of Antenatal Pathology and Hygiene.* Vol. 1: The embryo.; Vol. 2: The foetus. Edinburgh: Green.
Brown, F. J. (1946) *Antenatal and Postnatal Care*, 6th edn. London: Churchill (from whom much of the material Historical Note has been borrowed).
Browne, F. J. & Browne, J. C. McC. (1970) *Antenatal and Postnatal Care*, 10th edn. Edinburgh: Churchill Livingstone.

17. Signs and Symptoms in Obstetrics

THE DIAGNOSIS OF PREGNANCY

Although the diagnosis of pregnancy is generally straightforward it is not always so and it is important to keep in mind that a mistake, either way, can have important consequences for the mother, the child and possibly for the doctor. For example, a patient long trying to become pregnant may be bitterly disappointed and even psychologically disturbed if wrongly told that she is not pregnant. Again, failure to diagnose pregnancy can seriously hazard the fetus if the mother is exposed to pelvic radiation or receives teratogenic drugs in the first trimester. On the other hand, when a woman is pronounced pregnant when she is not, a precipitate and ill-advised marriage may follow or there may be delay of weeks, even months, in establishing that the pelvic swelling is not, in fact, a pregnancy but an ovarian cyst —if it happens to be a malignant cyst the delay could be disasterous. In general, pregnancy is more easily diagnosed when the patient is young and slim and has hitherto had regular, monthly periods. Difficulties do tend to arise when the patient is older, more obese or has had irregular periods.

SYMPTOMS AND SIGNS IN EARLY PREGNANCY

Amenorrhoea

In a healthy woman who has been menstruating regularly the cessation of periods strongly suggests pregnancy. A second missed period makes the probability stronger. But it must be remembered that pregnancy can occur in a young girl who has never had periods and in nursing mothers who tend not to menstruate during lactation. And the reverse may happen: a patient who is undoubtedly pregnant can have cyclical bleeding which simulates menstruation. Apart from pregnancy there are other causes of amenorrhoea. Change of climate or environment; for example, in girls travelling abroad or taking up a new post may be the cause of amenorrhoea but this seldom persists for more than a month or two. In others the desire for pregnancy or fear of pregnancy may be so great that this by itself causes the periods to cease and is associated with other symptoms and signs of pregnancy —the abdomen may swell progressively and 'fetal movements' may be felt by the patient. Such a pseudo-pregnancy can continue for months and the patient be quite convinced that she is pregnant in spite of all advice to the contrary.

Amenorrhoea following discontinuance of the contraceptive pill has received increasing attention in recent years. Post-pill amenorrhoea was first reported in 1966. Many cases have since been recorded and the association with oestrogen-progestogen mixtures is strong enough for a causal connection to be presumed. It is now established that many of these patients respond to treatment with clomiphene or pituitary gonadotrophins and the presumption is that the fault lies in the hypothalamus and is due to some interference with the production of releasing hormones which control pituitary secretion. It has been suggested that women whose periods were previously irregular are more liable to this type of amenorrhoea but there is no doubt it can occur in women whose periods had been quite regular prior to their taking the contraceptive pill. Again the length of time on any particular oestrogen-progestogen mixture bears no relationship to the risk of amenorrhoea when the pill is stopped—its occurrence has been noted after only two to three months use. It is as likely to occur among younger as among older women and multiparous and parous women are equally affected.

In clinical practice it is important always to record whether a patient, thought to be pregnant, was on oral contraception prior to the last recorded menstruation. Where a patient has been taking oral contraceptives the accuracy of the last menstrual period should be questioned and indeed she may not be pregnant at all in spite of the amenorrhoea. In some of these cases the patient may have amenorrhoea lasting for several months or may never menstruate again without suitable treatment. Amenorrhoea, therefore, is no more than presumptive evidence of pregnancy but where the date of the last menstrual period is known precisely and pregnancy is confirmed by other means it does help to fix the date of conception and the expected date of delivery.

Nausea and vomiting

Many pregnant women are troubled to some extent by early morning nausea and even vomiting especially during the first two or three months of pregnancy. Several factors probably contribute to these troublesome symptoms. It is widely acknowledged that gastric tone and motility are reduced in pregnancy. It has been shown, for example, by Hansen (1937) that the emptying time for the stomach as shown by the disappearance of dye from aspirates after a test meal containing methylene blue, increased from an average of 50 minutes in non-pregnant women to between 80 and 130 minutes in pregnant patients. More recently Davison, Davison and Hay (1970) have confirmed that there is delay in the emptying time of the stomach in women who are pregnant. These findings are explained by the widespread relaxation of smooth muscle which takes place in pregnancy and commonly accepted to be related to increased production of progesterone. Wolf (1943) convincingly demonstrated that interruption of gastric contractions and decreased muscle tone of the stomach wall is associated with a feeling of nausea and even vomiting. These physiological considerations are important but it should be remembered that some individuals feel nauseated and vomit more easily than others. The sight, smell or even thought of certain foods are sufficient to make some pregnant women sick whilst others find themselves unduly sensitive to stress of any sort and their reaction is to feel nauseated or to be sick. Again nausea and vomiting are commoner in early pregnancy and, of course, are a feature of hydatidiform mole where levels of chorionic gonadotrophin are high. It is not surprising that high gonadotrophin levels have been suggested as a factor in the etiology of nausea and vomiting in pregnancy but the evidence is unconvincing.

Vomiting in later pregnancy is a different matter and likely to be associated with concomitant disease such as infection of the urinary tract. The possibility of appendicitis should always be kept in mind, for this is an important complication which must not be missed. Occasionally a diaphragmatic hernia, previously unsuspected, is found to be the cause of epigastric discomfort and vomiting.

The mouth

It is quite common for the gums to become swollen and 'spongy' in pregnancy and some patients complain that the gums bleed easily. Cohen et al. (1969) in a serial study of 16 pregnant women confirmed an increase in gingivitis and demonstrated increased 'tooth mobility'. The oedema of the gums in pregnancy is but part of the general change in connective tissue ground substance related to increased oestrogen production in pregnancy. There is undoubtedly a need for increased dental care in pregnancy.

An excessive secretion of saliva, ptyalism, is a rare complication but very troublesome when it does occur; mostly it is associated with nausea. In reviewing the etiology of ptyalism Hytten (1971) has noted that many textbooks in obstetrics suggest that 1 to 2 litres of saliva may be produced daily by these patients but this would be accepted as normal by most physiologists. Ptyalism is more likely to arise from a nauseated pregnant woman's inability to swallow her saliva as she normally would. Conclusive evidence of overproduction of saliva in pregnancy is lacking.

Heartburn

Heartburn, an uncomfortable retrosternal burning sensation, is a further complication of loss of tone in smooth muscle in the stomach wall. There is convincing evidence that the symptoms are due to a reflux oesophagitis arising from regurgitation of gastric acid. The cardiac sphincter, itself affected by the general relaxation, is less effective in controlling regurgitation, especially towards the end of pregnancy when intra-abdominal pressure is raised. Evidence for this view is strengthened by Castro's (1967) work in which he showed that acid, perfused into the lower oesophagus of pregnant women, gave rise to no symptoms in women who did not previously have heartburn but those with heartburn immediately developed the typical burning pain.

Varicose veins

Loss of tone in smooth muscle in leg veins, made worse in time by the pressure of the enlarging uterus, leads to distension and varicosity of veins in some women. The likelihood of varicose veins is greater in the later months of pregnancy, though as a rule the situation improves once the pregnancy is over.

Backache

The pelvic girdle becomes less stable during pregnancy due to softening of the lumbo-sacral and pubic ligaments. At the same time, there is a steady increase in weight and a gradual alteration in the patient's centre of gravity with compensatory lordosis. It is hardly surprising that many pregnant women experience some degree of lumbo-sacral backache which generally disappears once the pregnancy is over. Bad posture, ill-designed shoes and obesity tend to aggravate the situation and occasionally the separation of the sacro-iliac and pubic bones is so great that the patient has considerable difficulty in walking because of the excess movement at these joints. The pain, under these circumstances, can be very severe and cause great discomfort. This extreme degree of laxity of the pelvic joints with accompanying backache is known as sacro-iliac arthropathy.

Paraesthesia

Fluid retention and tissue oedema lead in some pregnant women to compression of the median nerve (carpal tunnel syndrome) or of the lateral cutaneous nerve of the thigh. These patients complain of 'pins and needles', and numbness of the hands or of the anterolateral aspects of the upper thighs.

Fainting

Some women in early pregnancy are troubled by vaso-vagal syncope, especially if they stand still for any length of time. Usually they have adequate warning in that they first feel light-headed, have nausea and sweat before they lose consciousness. Later in pregnancy the pressure of the large uterus on the inferior vena cava, when the patient is in the dorsal position, can interfere with the return of blood to the right side of the heart. This uncommon cause of fainting is relieved when the woman turns on to her side.

Bladder symptoms

As the uterus enlarges in early pregnancy it presses on the bladder and the patient complains of frequency and nocturia. In addition to this pressure effect, there is an increase in the output of urine. Hytten and Klopper (1963) have drawn attention to the extraordinary ability of the kidneys in early pregnancy to excrete water and diuresis of 30ml/minute after a water load are not uncommon. Excessive thirst and polyuria are commonplace in the first few months of pregnancy. In later pregnancy there is a decline in the ability to excrete water, so that towards term it is not unusual for slight oedema of the hands, legs and feet to appear and the face may appear fuller.

Occasionally an acutely retroverted uterus may become trapped in the pelvis around the 12th to 14th week of pregnancy and give rise first to difficulty in micturition and then to acute retention of urine. As pregnancy progresses the enlarging uterus becomes an abdominal rather than a pelvic organ and pressure on the bladder eases; but bladder symptoms may again become troublesome in the last few weeks of pregnancy as the fetal head settles in the pelvic inlet.

Constipation

A frequent complaint in the early months of pregnancy and due initially to loss of tone in the smooth muscle in the bowel wall aggravated later by the pressure of the enlarging uterus. Increased absorption of water in the colon may intensify constipation as pregnancy progresses.

Breast changes

About the time of the first missed period there is commonly a heavy sensation in the breasts accompanied by tingling and even soreness. In primigravidae the areola and nipple become more pigmented and Montgomery's tubercles (hypertrophic sebaceous glands) appear in the primary areola. By the end of the first trimester the breasts begin to enlarge and due to hypertrophy of the mammary alveoli the tissue becomes nodular and the breasts rather tender. Fine veins appear just under the skin surface, reflecting the increased vascularity of the breasts. The nipples become larger and more erectile and by the third or fourth month a thick, yellowish fluid, colostrum, can usually be expressed by gentle massage. Compared with milk, colostrum contains more protein (mostly globulin), more minerals but less fat and sugar. Colostrum also contains a number of antibodies which help to protect the new-born child against a variety of infections. Similar breast changes are occasionally seen in women with ovarian or intracranial tumours and it is not unknown for at least some of the changes to be found in women who imagine themselves to be, but in fact are not, pregnant.

Vulval and vaginal changes

Within a few weeks of conception the vestibule and vaginal walls take on a dusky, bluish tint and some varicosity of the veins around the vulva is sometimes seen. Further evidence of pelvic hyperaemia is the characteristic soften-ing of the vulval tissues, the vaginal walls and the cervix. The character of cervical mucus alters—it becomes thick, viscous and opaque and forms a plug that fills the cervical canal. This mucus, allowed to dry on a glass slide, does not show the 'fern' pattern associated with the first half of the menstrual cycle but gives a beaded or cellular picture. The ability to 'fern' is related to the concentration of electrolytes, chiefly sodium chloride, in the cervical mucus and this decreases under the influence of the increased production of pro-gesterone in pregnancy.

Uterine enlargement

By the sixth week in most patients it is possible to detect uterine enlargement on bimanual examination, though in obese women this may not be detected until later. From about the 8th to the 14th weeks the uterus has a very distinctive feel on bimanual examination. The soft isthumus of the cervix is easily compressed between the fingers in the anterior fornix and the fingers of the abdominal hand and the globular fundus of the uterus seems to bc quite apart from the vaginal portion of the cervix. This is Hégar's sign. After the 14th week the isthmus is incorporated in the gestational sac, the cervix is thereby shortened and Hégar's sign can no longer be elicited.

Skin changes

A characteristic feature of pregnancy is the increased deposit of pigment in the skin affecting chiefly the face, vulva, perineum, linea alba, the area around the umbilicus and the areola of the breasts. The brown pigmenta-tion becomes notably less after the pregnancy but generally persists in some measure. Stil-boestrol and some types of oral contraceptives can give rise to the same sort of skin pigmenta-tion. Striae gravidarum are more noticeable in some women than others and are seen chiefly over the anterior abdominal wall, in the flanks, in the breasts, thighs and buttocks. In the affected areas the elastic fibres in the connective tissue underneath the skin partially give way allowing localized stretching of the skin. In the initial stages the underlying vessels are more clearly seen and give the striae a purplish discoloration; at a later stage the striae become white and glistening and though they may, to some extent, regress after preg-nancy they never completely disappear. It is possible for these skin changes to be absent in pregnancy, and conversely they may arise in other conditions apart from pregnancy, for example, they may be associated with obesity or ascites.

SYMPTOMS AND SIGNS IN LATER PREGNANCY

Ballottement

During the fourth and fifth months of preg-nancy the fetus is relatively small in relation to the amount of liquor surrounding it. On gentle vaginal examination with the fingers in the posterior vaginal fornix a slight tap upwards with the fingers displaces the fetus, which soon settles back on to the examining finger. This internal ballottement is elicited some weeks before it is possible to demonstrate the same signs on abdominal examination.

Fetal movements

Movements of the fetus are first noticed by most patients around the 18th week (primi-gravidae a week or two later). Some describe a fluttering sensation, others sharp 'tappings' or even sinuous movements. As the pregnancy progresses the movements become more notice-able and can be felt and even seen abdominally.

Fetal heart sounds

The detection of fetal heart sounds on abdominal auscultation is indisputable evidence of the presence of a live fetus. The sounds cannot usually be detected by the fetal stethoscope until about the 20th to the 22nd week of pregnancy, and at this stage the heart rate ranges from 120 to 140 beats/minute. When first audible the fetal heart beat is best heard in the mid-line between the symphysis pubis and the umbilicus but as pregnancy progresses it is loudest over the area where the fetal chest lies under the uterine wall and this varies depending upon the presentation, position and attitude of the fetus. With the development of ultrasonics it is now possible to detect the movements of the fetal heart as early as the 10th to 12th week of pregnancy. Doppler, a 19th-century Viennese professor of physics, established that sound or radio waves return to a transmitting source at an altered frequency if reflected by a moving object. This principle is now used by various small ultrasonic machines to detect movement of the wall of the heart or larger arteries. The distinctive noise produced by the various Doppler recorders indicates the presence of fetal life long before the fetal heart can be heard by auscultation.

Braxton Hicks contractions

From an early stage the pregnant uterus produces regular, painless contractions and from mid-pregnancy onwards these can generally be quite easily felt on abdominal palpation. These contractions may also be felt where the uterine enlargement is due to such conditions as haematometra or a soft uterine fibroid.

Progressive uterine enlargement

As pregnancy progresses the uterus enlarges steadily and a rough guide to the height of the fundus at various periods of gestation is given in figure 17.1. Serial measurements of the height of the fundus (in centimetres) above the symphysis pubis can be of some help in monitoring the continuing growth of the fetus.

RADIOLOGICAL EVIDENCE OF PREGNANCY
Because of the well established risk that radiation in the early months of pregnancy may interfere with normal organogenicis, it is best to avoid any X-ray of the pelvis at this stage.

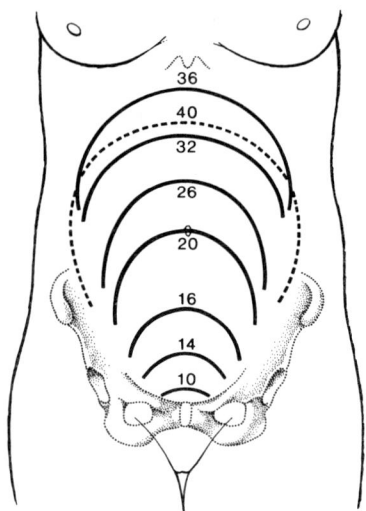

Fig. 17.1   Fundal height at various periods of gestation.

It is therefore unacceptable in modern obstetric practice for radiology to be used as the means of diagnosing pregnancy. But in later pregnancy radiology is of value in differentiating the pregnant uterus from other abdominal tumours. With an obese patient or where there is polyhydramnios it is occasionally difficult to be certain whether the fetus is alive or dead and an X-ray examination may be helpful. Overlapping of the fetal skull bones (Spalding's sign) or the presence of gas in the fetal heart or large vessels is firm evidence of death. Where radiology is used for some reason and fetal skeletal parts are identified then this is irrefutable evidence of pregnancy.

SONAR IN THE DIAGNOSIS OF PREGNANCY
So far as is known at present, this technique carries no risk for the early, developing embryo and Donald claims that most pregnancies can be diagnosed by sonar after the fifth or sixth week of gestation. Much depends upon the quality of the scan and the interpretation of what is seen. At this stage the gestational sac is seen as a white circle near the fundus of the uterus.

PREGNANCY TESTS
There have been many biological tests for pregnancy making use of such test animals as mice, rats, rabbits and female as well as male frogs. All of these tests took many hours and, because they involved laboratory animals, were quite costly. They are now largely of historical interest. Laboratory methods of diagnosing

pregnancy have advanced considerably over the past 10 years and *in vitro* immunological techniques are now widely used. The immunological tests in common use are based upon the detection of chorionic gonadotrophin in urine, preferably an early morning specimen where the concentration of gonadotrophin is relatively high. Human chorionic gonadotrophin is a species specific protein and can be used to produce antibodies in the sheep. The antibodies from the sheep are then used to coat tanned red cells or latex particles. When brought into contact with the specific antigen (human chorionic gonadotrophin in the urine of a pregnant woman) there is an antibody-antigen reaction clearly demonstrated by the behaviour of the particles to which the antibodies are adhering. Properly supervised and interpreted these tests are highly reliable. Hobson reports an accuracy rate of 99·2 per cent. An occasional source of error is the immunological similarity between chorionic gonadotrophin and luteinizing hormone secreted by the pituitary gland. In most tests involving immunoassay, luteinizing hormone cross reacts with antibody to chorionic gonadotrophin and if the test is so sensitive as to identify very small amounts of chorionic gonadotrophin it may give a positive result for luteinizing hormone excreted in the urine. Another cause of error is the tendency for the levels of pituitary gonadotrophin to rise as women approach the menopause; a false positive is more likely to be found in older women. As the level of chorionic gonadotrophin falls after the fourth month of pregnancy the accuracy of immunological pregnancy tests becomes progressively less reliable. Their reliability in abnormal pregnancies such as ectopic pregnancies is not very great because of the low level of chorionic gonadotrophin.

Progesterone induced withdrawal bleeding is occasionally used to differentiate pregnancy from other causes of amenorrhoea but it is an unreliable test. In a non-pregnant patient with the endometrium under the effect of oestrogen the administration of progesterone for three or four days should be followed by bleeding when the progesterone is withdrawn. But a false positive is obtained where the endometrium is not primed by oestrogen or where there is plentiful endogenous progesterone. An interesting, though not very reliable test is the examination of cervical mucus thinly spread on a glass slide. As the mucus dries it forms a distinct pattern. A fernlike pattern suggests that the patient is not pregnant whilst a cellular or beaded pattern is characteristic of the second half of the menstrual cycle or of pregnancy.

ABDOMINAL EXAMINATION IN LATER WEEKS OF PREGNANCY

The patient should be lying comfortably on a couch with a pillow supporting the shoulders and head and it is both courteous and helpful for the doctor to do everything he can to put the patient completely at ease. The examination room should be pleasantly warm and a light blanket or sheet arranged so that no more of the patient is uncovered than is necessary for abdominal inspection and examination. A nurse should always be present as a chaperon.

Inspection—it is most important to look carefully at the abdomen before making any examination. Old striae gravidaraum, white and silvery, suggest a previous pregnancy. There is a tendency for the skin to be lax in multigravidae and firm and more elastic in primigravidae. Previous surgery will be indicated by scars and the site of the scar will give some indication of the nature of the surgery. As a general rule the uterine size should relate to the gestational age of the pregnancy but with obese patients this may not be so. Discrepancy between the observed size of the uterus and the period of gestation may suggest the possibility of a multiple pregnancy or of a poorly grown baby that is 'small for dates'.

In later weeks of pregnancy the uterus should be ovoid with the long axis longitudinal

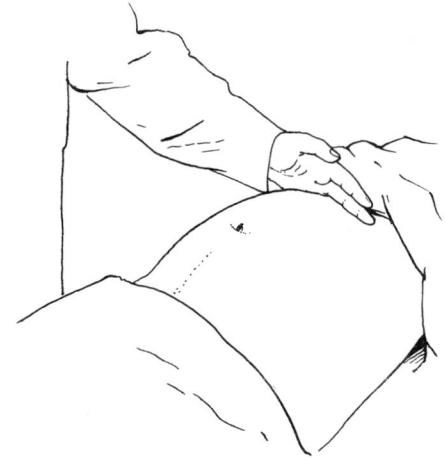

Fig. 17.2   Establishing the position of the fundus of the uterus.

though this may not be so obvious in multi-gravidae. Irregularity of the outline of the uterus may be due to a fibroid or an ovarian cyst, whilst broadening of the fundus raises the possibility of an arcuate uterus. Fetal movements can generally be seen quite easily during the last few weeks of pregnancy.

Palpation—this part of the examination should follow a set routine so that nothing of importance is missed. It is convenient to begin at the upper pole and to establish the position of the fundus (Fig. 17.2). Next, with two hands, the uterus is gently palpated from the fundus to the lower pole (Fig. 17.3). In this

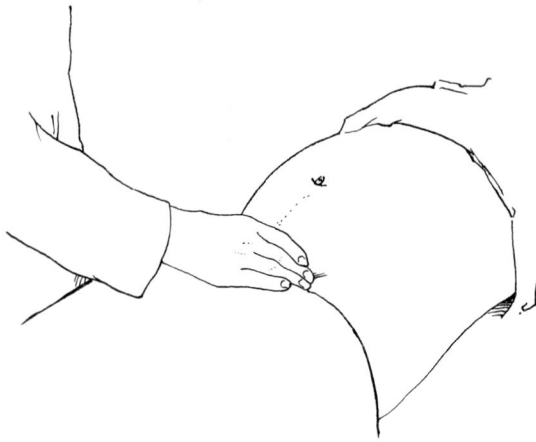

Fig. 17.4   Palpation of lower pole of uterus to establish presenting part.

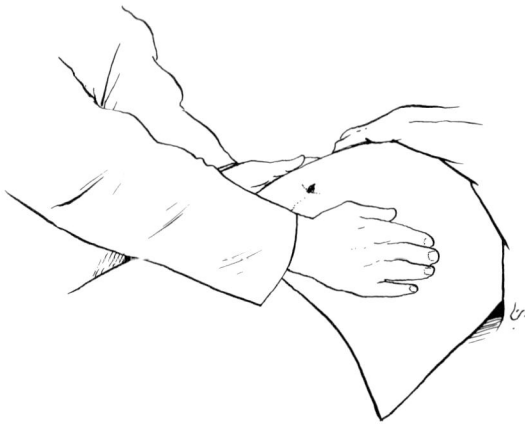

Fig. 17.3   Palpation of each side of the uterus from fundus downwards.

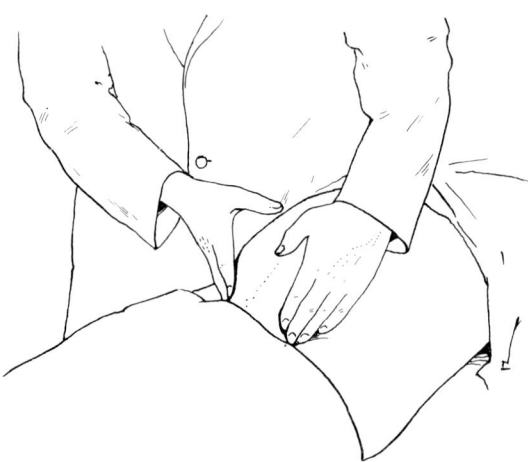

Fig. 17.5   Establishing the position of the presenting part in relation to the pelvic inlet.

way the firm, rounded breech can be felt in the fundus and as the hands pass downwards the fetal back is felt on one side and limbs on the other. At the same time, a good impression is gained of the size of the fetus but the ease with which this can be done will depend upon the amount of liquor present, the thickness of the abdominal wall and the degree of relaxation of the abdominal muscles. With a breech presentation the hard, round, fetal head is felt in the fundus and a distinguishing feature is that it ballottes more easily than the breech. Again, when the head is in the fundus the patient often complains of discomfort, even pain, in the subcostal region, and on palpation the fundus is tender. Examination of the lower pole (Figs. 17.4 and 17.5) confirms the presentation and the relationship of the presenting part to the pelvic inlet. The more gentle the examination the more will be felt. With a vertex presentation the hard fetal

head is usually quite easily felt. The head may be high and mobile or fixed in the pelvic brim (the greatest diameter of the head still above the inlet) or engaged in the pelvis (the greatest diameter being passed through the pelvic inlet). The height of the sinciput relative to the occiput is a good indication of the degree of flexion of the fetal head. When the head is well flexed the occiput is significantly lower than the sinciput. With a poorly flexed head the two are about the same level.

In primigravidae the fetal head generally engages in the last four weeks of pregnancy but in multigravidae it may well remain mobile until labour begins.

Auscultation—fetal heart sounds are better

heard with the special fetal stethoscope than with the ordinary physician's stethoscope. The sounds are generally best heard by placing the stethoscope over the child's back and the rate varies between 120 and 140 beats per minute. Where the placenta overlies the fetal back a distinctive soft blowing sound—the uterine souffle—may partially obscure the fetal heart sounds.

Differential diagnosis of pregnancy

Other pelvic tumours, notably a soft uterine fibroid or an ovarian cyst, may be mistaken for pregnancy or the error may be the other way. And it is important to remember that pregnancy may co-exist with either of these tumours. Pelvic inflammatory disease and occasionally haematometra may give rise to confusion. These conditions are not generally accompanied by amenorrhoea and, of course, an immunological pregnancy test is likely to help. Where there is doubt a very detailed history should be taken and careful pelvic examination made and if uncertainty remains then the passage of a few weeks, if it is possible to delay, should resolve the diagnosis.

The present, widespread, use of oral contraceptives does occasionally give rise to confusion, for these endocrine preparations may be associated with softening and blue discoloration of the vaginal walls and cervix, nausea and even amenorrhoea. But the uterus is not significantly enlarged.

Diagnosis of fetal death

The death of the embryo in the first trimester is generally followed by abortion but where the embryo is retained and forms a carneous mole the diagnosis can be difficult. The uterus, under these circumstances, ceases to grow and in time is distinctly smaller than it should be for the period of gestation. But if the patient is seen for the first time and there is no precise record of uterine size over the previous few weeks an accurate diagnosis is by no means easy. A negative pregnancy test strongly suggests that the embryo is dead but the placenta may continue to produce chorionic gonadotrophin for several weeks and a positive pregnancy test does not necessarily mean that the pregnancy is viable.

REFERENCES

Castro, L. de P. (1967) *Amer. J. Obstet. Gynec.*, **98**, 1.
Cohen, D. W., Friedman, L., Shapiro, J. & Kyle, G. C. (1969) *J. Periodont*, **40**, 563.
Davison, J. S., Davison, M. C. & Hay, D. M. (1970) *J. Obstet. Gynaec. Brit. Cwlth.*, 77, 37.
Hansen, R. (1937) Physiology of the stomach in pregnancy. *Zbl. Gynäk.*, **61**, 2306.
Hytten, F. & Klopper, A. (1963) *J. Obstet. Gynaec. Brit. Cwlth.*, **70**, 811.
Hytten, F. E. and Leitch, I. (1971) The Physiology of Human Pregnancy, Ed. Oxford: Blackwell Scientific Publications.
Wolf, S. (1943) *J. clin. Invest.*, **22**, 877.

18. Antenatal and Intrapartum Assessment of Fetal Growth, Maturity and Wellbeing

INTRODUCTION

Since the high peak of maternal mortality (nearly seven per 1000 in Scotland) some forty years ago, there has been firstly a dramatic, and later a steady, lessening of maternal risk. Maternal death is due now to the bizarre situation or to the occasional lapse from a quality of care that we know how to give.

Since the Second World War the outcome for the child as measured by perinatal death has continued to improve, so that perinatal mortality rates are falling steadily except in a few areas with relatively poorly organized care.

The improvement in perinatal death has been achieved largely by identification of *risk mothers*—e.g. small stature, high parity, very young or old, previous bad obstetric history, and of *risk situations* in the pregnancy under study—e.g. prolonged pregnancy, hypertensive syndromes, bleeding, diabetes, poor fetal growth, etc. Having identified risk groups, the obstetrician then pays particular attention to patients within these groups in an attempt to select out individual cases requiring special therapy. Selection of the patients in this way has obviously been efficient if measured by the drop in perinatal deaths but this often requires the obstetrician to make decisions based on an assessed statistical risk. He must, for example, know that if a patient is past dates with meconium staining of the liquor, there is a 10 per cent risk of the child dying in labour; but he would not be able to be sure of the risk to the individual child under study. He might not consider a 10 per cent risk a justification for interference, or he might perform a hundred Caesarean sections to save ten babies. He might not know how to assess the risk to the individual child.

Increasing emphasis on the extra risk carried by the child of *low birth weight* has greatly increased the study of factors likely to lead to this condition, of methods to differentiate between normal and poor intra-uterine growth and of methods designed to estimate or measure the intra-uterine gestational age of the baby.

Some twenty years ago the baby *born prematurely* was shown to be at obvious risk of blindness from therapy in high oxygen concentration, and since then there has been much concern of the special late hazard to the prematurely born especially since modern care of the neonate has ensured longer and more frequent survival. Hyaline membrane disease with respiratory distress has been intensively studied and methods of therapy and especially of prevention have a high priority in research.

Antenatal risk of external factors adverse to normal development have been postulated for centuries but such risks were highlighted by phocomelia and other defects which followed the extensive use of thalidomide in the years 1961–62. Since then there is continuous search to find external trauma of all types: drugs; chemicals; X-radiation etc.

For many years we have known that when the baby is affected by serological incompatibility, blood pigments are present in the *amniotic fluid*. This knowledge, although used as a monitor in a simple way some twenty years ago (Bevis, 1953) was not fully utilized nor the technique investigated until it became possible to treat the affected child *in utero*. (Lilley, 1963.) It is now considered important that the characteristics of the amniotic fluid be fully studied. (Chapter 9.)

Change in the abortion law in Great Britain has stimulated the search for techniques of very early *diagnosis of fetal anomaly* which have led to increasing awareness by the mother at risk that she could be reassured that she carries a normal child.

Modern obstetrics requires therefore, that we should be able to measure, throughout pregnancy, fetal growth, and where necessary fetal maturity, normality and wellbeing at any given time. We should be able to measure fetal age and perhaps maturity of certain tissues, e.g. skin or lung or kidney. We also require to measure accurately the stress which the individual fetus in labour may suffer, his likely ability to stand stress, and his actual reaction to it.

It is tempting in description to try to distinguish techniques designed to measure maturity from those designed to measure growth or wellbeing but in any consideration of such parameters it soon becomes obvious that it may be difficult to disentangle indices of growth from those of maturity, and of maturity and growth from those of wellbeing. As far as possible, however, the investigator should be clear what parameter his technique is measuring and what the measurements mean.

ANTENATAL

Monitoring by clinical method

While it is agreed that biochemistry, electronics and ultrasound may improve the quality of information available a great deal of monitoring can be done by meticulous clinical care.

At the first visit the information on last menstrual period should be assessed and evaluated (see Chapter 17) and the likely pregnancy duration recorded. The uterine size should then be compared with the assessed dates, any discrepancy noted and, if possible, investigated. At later visits the continuing growth of the uterus should be checked and constantly assessed against the dates so that the original estimations can be verified or growth variation discovered. By about twenty-eight weeks it should be possible to palpate the growing fetus and the steady growth of the baby should be checked and assessed at each visit. By care in these assessments a good idea of fetal maturity and adequacy of growth can be obtained in most cases. Difficulty arises with late first visits, uncertain dates (although 'clinical dates' should be assessed) but frequently because of inaccurate or insufficient observation or unwillingness of the observer to interpret his own findings adequately.

Maternal weight gain in early pregnancy is an invaluable guide to the wellbeing of the pregnancy and, in late pregnancy, to the continued growth of the fetus and placenta.

Failure of maternal weight to rise should be looked upon with real suspicion and failure to gain steadily at any time after thirty weeks is a very helpful guide that the fetus is not growing or that the pregnancy is not progressing well. The normal expected pattern of weight gain in pregnancy is described in Chapter 5 and the dietary advice in Chapters 5 and 16. A mother who for some reason is on a limited diet may in fact fail to gain weight and the dietary habit should be questioned where weight gain is poor. Temporary weight loss, of course, accompanies minor illness.

The response of the mother with 'positive health' certainly suggests a 'good pregnancy' and clear evidence of skin changes, slight oedema (without hypertension), and often worsening of varicose veins may be good signs of maternal response.

The pregnant woman who is carefully attended throughout pregnancy by one or a few intelligent doctors who carefully check and record routine antenatal clinical observation and whose labour is as carefully monitored by classical methods (see later) rarely needs special biochemical or electronic aid. The standard of care must be meticulous and findings must be intelligently assessed. Antenatal care is difficult to do well.

Monitoring in very early pregnancy

Hormones of the corpus luteum and feto-placental unit—

PROGESTERONE AND 17αOH PROGESTERONE

In very early pregnancy progesterone and oestrogen are produced by the corpus luteum and much of the success of implantation and of the pregnancy itself will depend on its function. There is a gradual fall in corpus luteum progesterone as the pregnancy approaches the tenth week by which time placental trophoblast progesterone production is established. *17αOH Progesterone* is produced in large amounts by the corpus luteum but *not* by trophoblast and the measurement of this substance in plasma (or of pregnantriol, its main metabolite in urine) may give a good indication of corpus luteum function. Levels reach a peak by the seventh week and fall steadily till the ninth or tenth week and then remain very low, but levels of oestrogen rise steadily from fertilization arising firstly from the corpus luteum and later from the feto-placental unit. Fully validated studies of the use of these substances as early pregnancy monitors is not available at this time (Holmdahl *et al.*, 1972).

HUMAN CHORIONIC GONADOTROPHIN

Production reaches a peak level in serum (and urine) about the tenth to the fourteenth week after which there is a fall followed by a rise again after the thirtieth week.

The estimation of this hormone to diagnose hydatidiform mole and to monitor the therapy of choriocarcinoma is well known (Chapter 9) but apart from that, studies of the value of measurement in pregnancy abnormality so far do not suggest great clinical value.

HUMAN PLACENTAL LACTOGEN

This material formed in the syncitio trophoblast is detectable in plasma from the sixth week and levels up to $1 \mu g/ml$ are present by the tenth week. Low levels in a case of threatened abortion are said to signify a poor outcome.

SONAR

The value of sonar in early pregnancy is fully described in Chapter 28 and by Donald *et al.*, 1972, and Hellman *et al.*, 1973.

By the eighth week the fetal head size also may be sufficient to allow the diagnosis of multiple pregnancy and quintuplets have been diagnosed at nine weeks. (Campbell and Dewhurst, 1970.)

The fetal heart may be detected early in pregnancy by use of the Doppler effect. Pulsed ultrasound, however, can detect the movement of the walls and valves of the fetal heart by the sixth week or so (Robinson, 1972) and this technique may prove of value along with other methods.

After the twelfth week placental growth has also been assessed (as a research study) by ultrasonic measurement of placental volume (Hellman *et al.*, 1970).

Monitoring after the first trimester

After the twelfth week we are concerned with measures of continuing fetal growth and wellbeing and at various stages with the maturity of the fetus itself or perhaps only with the maturity of one or other of its systems (e.g. pulmonary function). It is *essential* in some situations such as maternal diabetes and fetomaternal serological incompatibility and important in all pregnancies that the intra-uterine age of the fetus be known with some accuracy. As has been previously said, the knowledge may be relatively simply acquired when the patient has been seen from early in pregnancy, but often absolute or confirmatory measures of age would be very useful. Fetuses mature at different rates and individual fetal organs may lag behind the rest of the fetus. The fetus suffering intra-uterine growth retardation, i.e. poor growth syndrome, is behind in his bone development as well as his head size. One twin may show less advanced bone growth (ossification centres) than his brother. It is difficult to be absolute and certain but guides may be obtained by intelligent use of the methods available.

Good growth suggests wellbeing but slow growth may be compatible with a perfectly reasonable fetus provided the growth is progressive (Walker, 1967). The well grown baby, on the other hand, may become acutely anoxic in the post date period and studies of growth, maturity and wellbeing may be necessary each independent of the other.

Growth and maturity

Fetal growth may be implied from continued uterine growth in early pregnancy, and after twenty-eight weeks or so the continued growth of the fetus can be palpated. Where, however, early growth is difficult to assess or later growth seems slow or inadequate ultrasound or biochemical measures may help.

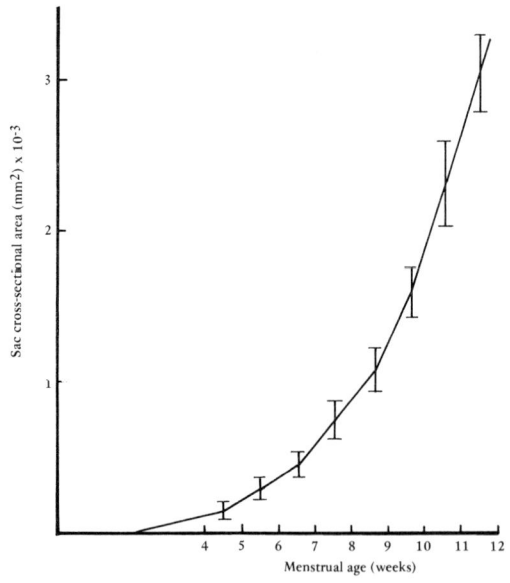

Fig. 18.1   Dimensions of gestation sac in early pregnancy (after Christie 1975).

In expert hands measurement of sac size may be a very early pregnancy guide (Robinson, 1975 and Fig. 18.1) and certainly after fourteen weeks the fetal bi-parietal diameter may be measured and its steady increase charted against the units 'standard curve' (*see* Fig. 18.2).

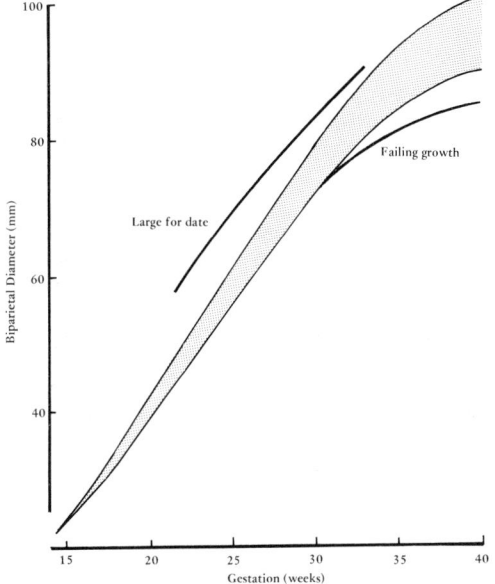

Fig. 18.2 Mean biparietal diameter of fetal head and the curve in a child large for dates or with incorrect dates and the curve showing slowing of biparietal growth in late pregnancy (after Christie 1975).

Serial readings close and parallel to the normal curve are to be expected. Readings parallel to the curve but some distance away suggest that the fetus is older or younger than expected. If the growth pattern of the individual fetus is oblique and falling away from the expected pattern a deteriorating growth situation is suggested. The growth rate may be helpful if only one or two readings are available. The biparietal increase at a rate of 2·5–3mm per week from the eighteenth to twenty-fifth week and slows to 1–2mm per week by the thirty-sixth week (Campbell and Newman, 1971). Such measurements require a high degree of skill and ability to interpret them can be found only by experience and constant check of the findings against head measurements at birth.

Fetal weight is somewhat more difficult to assess by ultrasound as the correlation between head size and weight is not too close. However, if the biparietal diameter is over 9cm there is a 90 per cent chance that the child weighs more than 2500g.

FETAL AGE AND FETAL MATURITY
There are many situations where an accurate measurement of the age of a fetus would be of immense value especially when it is necessary to interpret readings of urinary or plasma hormones or even biparietal diameters. Knowledge of fetal age is also an essential prerequisite to timing of induction of labour although in some cases this is considered unnecessary if fetal pulmonary maturity can be measured (*see later*).

In early pregnancy the proponents of *ultrasound* claim extreme accuracy in age determined by measurement of fetal sac size and later of biparietal diameter. It is claimed that up to twenty weeks or so biparietal diameter will correctly 'date' a fetus (Campbell, 1969), but this view should be regarded with some reservation unless several readings are available (Willocks and Dunsmore, 1971).

Radiological assessment of fetal age is discussed in Chapter 28. It must be realized that the information obtainable is strictly limited since it relies on ossification centres or bone density.

Amniocentesis
In the risk situation *amniocentesis* may be of more value to the fetus than the minimal risk of the operation. This procedure is not without some risk and in all cases must be preceded by identification of the placental site by ultrasound. Amniotic fluid contents may be used in several ways to estimate fetal age. Many substances have been measured and such measurements are still used with varying value.

Point screening systems based in a combination of biochemical and cytological features are said to give an estimation of fetal maturity accurate to within two weeks (Lind and Billewicz, 1971).

1. *Nile Blue Sulphate (0·1 per cent)* stains cells from fetal sebaceous glands a bright orange colour in late pregnancy and this is a measure of the maturity of these glands and, therefore, of skin maturity. There is a high rise to more than 50 per cent of such cells in the liquor after the thirty-eighth week. This is of some value as a check that the fetus is at term but of little further value. Staining with haematoxylin and eosin or the Papinocolaou technique is as effective.

2. *Urea, Uric Acid and Creatinine levels—*

Urea and uric acid levels are of doubtful value but creatinine levels are closely correlated with maturity. Levels greater than 2mgm per 100ml are normally found only after the thirty-eighth week. This test is, however, useless in some maternal hypertensive syndromes where the creatinine and urea may be much raised.

3. *Oestriol*—In late pregnancy it is likely that fetal urine is the main source of amniotic fluid oestriol, since the concentrations of free oestriol, oestriol sulphate and glucosidurinate are very variable. The absolute levels are probably of little use in gestational age assessment.

4. *Bilirubin*—The spectroscopic examination of amniotic fluid to detect the level of bilirubin is of value in cases of serological incompatibility and is discussed in Chapter 15. The level normally falls to zero by the thirty-sixth week and this fact is used occasionally as a guide to maturity.

5. *Phospholipids*—The maturity of the fetal lung in relation to surfactant and the child's likely ability to survive after birth can be assessed by measurement of the stable lecithin content or the lecithin: sphyngomyelin ratio. Both rise when such surfactant levels in the lung reach safe levels. The lecithin sphyngomyelin ratio is usually 1:1 before that time and rises rapidly to 5:1 (Gluck *et al.*, 1971) when safe levels of surfactant are reached. This is usually some time after the thirty-fifth week. In the risk baby who must be delivered or when knowledge of certain neonatal survival might be invaluable, ratio levels of 3:1 are taken as evidence that neonatal respiratory distress syndrome would be unlikely to occur (Bhagwanani *et al.*, 1972).

6. *Amniotic fluid* biochemistry and cytology in relation to fetal anomaly are discussed later.

CLINICAL METHODS
The clinician estimates maturity with some accuracy from uterine size in early pregnancy probably up to twenty to twenty-two weeks. After that the vagaries of growth make accuracy very low indeed.

In late pregnancy, however, he has better guides:
The maternal weight gain slows or stops after about thirty-eight weeks unless, of course, poor fetal growth or a poor pregnancy has distorted the pattern earlier, or sudden weight gain from fluid retention intervenes.

Amniotic fluid becomes relatively and actually less and 'more baby' seems to fill the uterus. After term the uterus may actually shrink and there appears to be no liquor.

In primigravida the head may engage about thirty-seven weeks or so but non-engagement is common and normal in multigravida.

As term approaches it is more and more likely that the cervix and lower segment will be soft, the cervix be taken up and partially dilated. This sign in the individual case is of little value as such findings precede premature labour and a tight closed cervix is common at term and more common after term since patients with a ripe cervix tend to go into labour sooner. Unripeness is part of the post-mature syndrome and does *not* indicate that the fetus need not be delivered.

FETAL PRODUCTS
It would be expected that the best source of information about the child would be from measurement of some material of purely fetal origin, present in the maternal blood or urine, or at least in the amniotic fluid. Various substances are available for study.

Oestriol. Ninety per cent of the oestriol in the maternal plasma or excreted in the maternal urine is an end product of a complex biochemical process which, beginning with maternal cholesterol, depends on the normal function of the placenta, of the fetal adrenal and of the fetal liver (Chapter 4). It, therefore, is an obvious monitor of fetal wellbeing and also to some extent a guide to fetal weight. It is best measured by the Brown and Coyle (1962) or similar technique. Unfortunately, the chemical techniques are tedious and require a high degree of skill. The need for methods more adapted to screen a large number of patients has led to the development of 'total urinary oestrogens by auto analyser techniques'. These measures are certainly less accurate and the results more difficult to interpret and they rely, as did the oestriols, on the accurate collection of a twenty-four or forty-eight-hour specimen or urine. Modern techniques of radioimmunoassay of plasma oestriol or oestradiol 17B promise to be more useful and certainly can be applied to a large number of patients (Masson, 1973).

Rising levels of maternal urinary oestriol indicate that the child is not at risk in hypertensive syndromes in maternal diabetes and in maternal fetal Rhesus incompatibility, and this latter fact is especially useful to assess fetal response after intra-uterine transfusion. In maternal hypertensive syndromes while ultrasound may measure the growth of the fetus, urinary or plasma oestriol can measure the fetal wellbeing. In general, low values, failure of late pregnancy rise or, at the worst, falling values suggest a deteriorating fetal condition. Low values, however, may rise after the patient is admitted for bed rest and this is a very helpful guide to the effects of treatment. The values which suggest imminent fetal death and at which delivery is imperative vary with the technique of estimation and should be established by the clinical unit in collaboration with the laboratory concerned.

In anencephaly and in fetal hepatitis oestriol levels are extremely low. In the first case the precursors are not formed in any amount and in the second, failure of fetal liver function stops the process before oestriol is formed.

Other oestrogens
The interest in the measurement of urinary oestriol relies on the fact that 90 per cent is fetal in origin. There are many more oestrogens of interest. Total oestrogens currently measured by many and varied techniques contain many oestrogen fractions and the significance of those is difficult to assess. In addition to the classical oestrogens, oestriol, oestrone and oestradiol, there are oestriols like Ring K ketolic oestrogens and labile oestrogens which are present in relatively large amounts. The significance of these is not known at this time but they all increase steadily during pregnancy. Towards term oestriol should occur for some 75 per cent of the total oestrogen in the normal situations but accounts for less than 50 per cent in diabetic pregnancies. Maternal plasma 17B oestradiol may be in future helpful if it is measured in pregnancy but 50 per cent is maternal in origin from maternal adrenal precursors.

Progesterone and pregnanediol
Progesterone in early pregnancy is produced by the corpus luteum and there is a gradual fall in corpus luteum progesterone production up to the tenth week by which time placental (trophoblast) production is fully established. 17α hydroxy progesterone is produced in large amounts in the corpus luteum but not in the trophoblast and is, therefore, not available as a late pregnancy estimate of fetal well-being. While plasma levels of progesterone will probably have real value in relation to

measurement and assessment of abnormal physiological states in late pregnancy and early labour, the techniques are not yet sufficiently established for other than research use but the main urinary excretion product of placental progesterone is pregnanediol which for a very long time has been measured to assess fetal and placental wellbeing.

Pregnanediol, though still useful, has fallen out of favour largely because techniques for testing are slow. Progesterone levels in the maternal plasma vary somewhat from day to day and during the day and presumably reflect changes in uterine blood flow and placental activity. The levels rise steadily in pregnancy. There is still doubt whether progesterone levels normally fall in late pregnancy (Turnbull *et al.*, 1974), or continue to rise as shown originally by Walker, 1963. The highest levels of progesterone are found in the fetal umbilical vein and also in the maternal veins draining the uterus.

Human placental lactogen
This is formed in the placental syncitio trophoblast and can be measured by radioimmuno-assay from the sixth week of pregnancy. Serial measurements may, therefore, be a useful measure of placental function which might replace pregnanediol which is measurable only by slow chemical means. It does not, however, appear to be a more reliable test except in threatened abortion where it has been found that low levels signify that the pregnancy may not be continuing. The levels rise from $1\mu g/ml$ at ten weeks to $4-10\mu g$ at thirty-eight weeks (mean $6\mu g$). There is some preliminary evidence that low levels below $4\mu g$ in late pregnancy are a sign suggesting fetal distress in labour and neonatal asphyxia. Serum HPL does not correlate with fetal weight. Levels, as seen in diabetes, pre-eclampsia, twins and Rh immunization, are not particularly helpful.

Human chorionic gonadotrophin
Reaches a peak level of some 60–70 international unit per ml in serum (and urine) about the tenth to fourteenth week. The level falls to 5–15 units to rise again after the thirtieth week and readings of 5–40 units may be seen at term (mean about 12). The estimation of this hormone to diagnose hydatidiform mole and choriocarcinoma is well known but as stated earlier the significance of abnormal levels is not studied (Yukorkala, 1973).

OTHER SUBSTANCES

Alpha Feto-Protein is produced by the fetal liver and yolk sac (it has, however, been shown to be present in small amounts in normal human serum) and levels are elevated in pregnancy rising from 18–119ng/ml early to 103–550ng/ml in late pregnancy levels *above* 550ng often up to 9000ng/ml are seen in fetal distress or after actual fetal death. In early pregnancy, especially in threatened abortion high levels signify fetal death but no advance information of outcome can be expected (before twelve weeks) in apparent normal cases. Since this test depends on the presence of a fetus, it has been used in differential diagnosis in a case of suspected hydatidiform mole.

Enzymes

It would appear that estimation of enzymes of placental origin should prove a useful guide to pregnancy wellbeing but these tests have in general proved disappointing.

Serum-heat Stable Alkaline Phosphatase

This has been the substance most frequently assessed and since it can now be measured by radioimmunoassay, the test can be done easily and quickly. Alkaline phosphatase arising in placental trophoblast is heat-stable and plasma levels rise steadily during pregnancy till term.

Measurement is in King Armstrong Units, and levels rise from less than 2 at twenty-six weeks to 4–14(8) at term—abnormally *high* levels are seen in hypertensive disease with placental damage with antepartum haemorrhage and with diabetes (Hunter, 1969).

Serum Cystine Aminopepsidase—Oxytocinase

This material is also produced by the placenta only, and only in pregnancy. The levels rise steadily. In diabetes the results are higher than normal but there is no evidence of value of the tests as a monitor of wellbeing.

Diamine Oxidase

Histaminase arises from the retro-placental maternal decidua and is an adaptive response to protect against fetal diamines. Measurement of this enzyme is relatively simple and levels rise rapidly to the twenty-fourth week and after this time fall gently. It was hoped that it would be a useful monitor for normality of early pregnancy but this hope has not been fulfilled.

It does not seem either to be of prognostic value in cases with poor growth, impending fetal death or pre-eclampsia.

5 Adenosine Triphosphate

ATP is an important source of energy in fetal carbohydrate metabolism and measurement of the levels in the fetal red cells should reflect anoxic conditions. High levels should be found in the cells of the umbilical artery blood where anoxic condition of the fetus exists.

OTHER INDICES OF MATURITY AND WELLBEING

The fetal ECG studied under standard conditions is said to have different characteristics at various stages of pregnancy and in expert hands can be used as a marker of maturity. Changes in the P Q wave have been described which are significant of postdates pregnancy with hypoxia. This is preliminary but promising work (Epszteyn, 1972). The growth rate of the fetus in late pregnancy can be assessed by measurement of the fetal uptake of ^{75}Se selenonethiomine an amino acid which emits gamma rays that can be measured with detectors of high sensitivity. This technique is said to pick out babies of recent or prolonged poor growth (Lee and Garrow, 1970).

ASSESSMENT OF FETAL STRESS

Under fetal risk situations, e.g. hypertensive syndromes, antepartum haemorrhage, threatened abortion earlier in present pregnancy, stillbirth or neonatal death in previous pregnancy, post dates pregnancy, high maternal age, maternal diabetes and in poor growth syndromes, the individual fetus may already, at the onset of labour, be suffering from anoxia or other transfer difficulty. The fetus may respond poorly to the stress of labour and in the extreme situation die *in utero* or very early in labour, with little warning. When such pregnancies show deteriorating clinical growth or there is an anomaly in the maternal oestriol excretion or there are other grounds for suspicion, further study may be helpful. Meconium in the liquor and variation of the fetal heart rate during uterine contractions are accepted clinically as evidence of 'fetal distress' and proof that the fetus is already under stress which he may not be able to combat if the stress should increase.

MECONIUM IN LIQUOR

It is sometimes worthwhile to search out before labour these fetuses already stressed, examining the colour of the liquor by amnioscopy through the cervix. This test is occasionally used in the risk situation to prove that the fetus is not yet stressed, i.e. the liquor is still clear. The presence of meconium may indicate the desirability of immediate delivery by Caesarean section or immediate induction depending on circumstances. A negative result, i.e. clear liquor, may mean absence of stress response at that time but not necessarily that stress may not occur in the future.

OXYTOCIN CHALLENGE TEST

The fetus already in anoxic difficulty may respond poorly to labour and it is possible to assess this risk by the use of the period of induction of labour with syntocin to observe the fetal response (an oxytocin challenge). Once adequate contractions are observed fetal heart slowing beginning at the height of the contraction and persisting for a short period is a positive result, and indicates that the fetus will respond poorly to continuing labour. This is a really valuable monitor.

ANOXIA CHALLENGE TEST

If the fetus is already somewhat oxygen deficient he is likely to show a definite response to maternal anoxia and this is the basis of the anoxia stress test (Bailie et al., 1973).

The mother is given a sedative, placed in a quiet room, and the fetal heart rate constantly monitored till a steady basal rate suggests 'fetal sleep'. Maternal ambient oxygen is then cut to 15 per cent and the fetal heart response recorded. A rising fetal heart rate indicates that the fetus has been already somewhat oxygen deficient and the added anoxic stress has produced a clearly measurable response. Such babies should be soon delivered.

This test although physiologically well chosen is still under research trial and may be somewhat risky to the child.

In the sheep it has been shown that if maternal anoxia is induced in this way, there is a decrease in uterine blood flow but some increase in haemoglobin concentration through the uterus. However, the pO_2 in the maternal uterine vessels falls sharply (Makowski et al., 1973).

Antenatal diagnosis of fetal anomaly

It is often important that any unusual or abnormal state of the child be diagnosed antenatally. This information is important in antenatal management as the possibility of intra-uterine therapy has been introduced by intra-uterine transfusion and it may not be long before other forms of intra-uterine surgery become possible. Moreover, changing attitudes to abortion have made more acceptable the concept of therapeutic termination following diagnosis of a deformed child.

There is rarely any external sign of fetal anomaly except hydramnios and oligohydramnios where anomaly should always be suspected and sought out. Very rarely the fetus

hydropic from *serological anomaly* will produce in the mother peculiar hypertensive 'toxemia' like symptoms and signs (Chapter 15), and with fetal *neuroblastoma* catacholamines crossing to the mother can produce minor symptoms of sweating, pallor, headaches and palpitations and tingling in the fingers and toes.

Skeletal anomaly can, of course, be diagnosed by radiography after about fourteen to sixteen weeks. In many of the babies at risk from thalidomide phocomelia was diagnosed in this way before twenty weeks. Radiography is mostly used to diagnose or exclude gross CNS deformity in late pregnancy. Care should be taken if minor degrees of hydrocephaly are suggested especially in breech where the projection of the head may suggest large diameters. Fetal position occasionally suggests, falsely, angulation of the fetal spine. Ultrasound is, of course, a good guide to hydrocephaly and microcephaly by careful combination of date accuracy and biparietal measurement and can with some accuracy diagnose anencephaly, but this diagnosis should be applied with some caution.

Biochemical anomaly of maternal urinary hormone excretion can be used in the diagnosis of anencephaly, neonatal hepatitis, congenital adrenal insufficiency. In neonatal hepatitis alpha, anti-trypsin levels in the amniotic fluid are low.

The value of amniocentesis in diagnosis and therapy of Rhesus incompatibility was pioneered by Bevis (1965) and is fully discussed in Chapter 15. Diagnosis of fetal genetic disease is now possible in a wide range of situations mainly by amniotomy in early pregnancy and by biochemical study of the liquor, by biochemical study or chromosomal study of cultured fetal or amniotic cells (Hareny, 1971). This is fully discussed in Chapter 7.

There is at this time an increasing demand for elective antenatal investigation of the risk of fetal mongolism where the mother is at risk (e.g. primigravida over 35). Provided the placenta is located (preferably by ultrasound in very early pregnancy), the risk of amniocentesis from the twelfth to sixteenth week should be small, but the study should be undertaken only when there is a clear risk of anomaly and with full knowledge that all facilities are available for the necessary tests. The technical procedures are in many cases very difficult

---

Alphafetoprotein is elevated in the amniotic fluid and maternal serum when the fetus has an open spina bifida or anencephaly (Walker, 1976).

and the service should be offered if it is efficient and accurate. Indiscriminate and emotional use should be resisted. There are, or ought to be, in all areas genetic counsellors and geneticists who can advise on the individual risk in a pregnancy and of the possibility of antenatal diagnosis and which laboratory centres are capable of the investigation.

Valente (1973) has suggested that fetal skin biopsy might be possible through an amnioscopy to enable more thorough analysis of fetal genetic material. Blood samples from fetal placental vessels may possibly allow diagnosis of haemoglobinopathy.

ASSESSMENT OF FETAL WELLBEING IN LABOUR

The traditional method of monitoring the fetus in labour was described in the last edition of this textbook as follows:

'The fetal heart rate should be counted at hourly intervals during the first stage. This should be done after the pain or at least in the intervals between the pains and not while the uterus is contracting as the heart is then difficult to hear and there is generally some slowing' and again 'In a normal labour where progress is satisfactory vaginal examination will often not be necessary . . .'.

In the years since, these statements have

four hours. Contraction strength and duration would be assessed by the attendant midwife or doctor palpating the abdomen.

Many new methods of obtaining information on intra-uterine fetal wellbeing and assessment of labour intensity have been developed and these are causing a revolution in intrapartum care. Indeed, such has been the impact in the understanding of fetal heart rate patterns that even in places where such instrumentation is not available attempts are being made to listen to the fetal heart in a different way particularly during and immediately after contractions often, contrary to the old beliefs, the very time when the most interesting information is available.

Fetal Heart Rate

One of the main advances in assessing intrapartum fetal wellbeing has been the change from intermittent listening to the fetal heart with a Pinard stethoscope to continuous recording by electronic means on a strip recorder.

There are three main methods of measuring electronically the fetal heart rate: the detection of sound with a microphone, the detection of movement by ultrasound using the Doppler effect and the detection of the electrical impulses from the QRS complex of the fetal ECG (Fig. 18.3). All the early work attempted

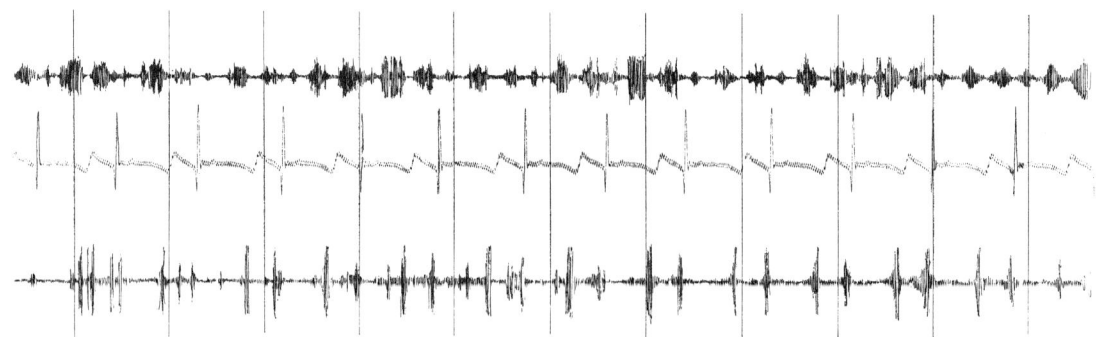

Fig. 18.3   Upper trace: Fetal Phonocardiogram
Middle trace: Fetal Electrocardiogram
Lower trace: Fetal Ultrasonocardiogram
Note the 'cleaner' signal from the ECG which is much easier to use as a trigger for a ratemeter.

become out-of-date even for traditional monitoring. It would be standard practice now in many units for a patient in established labour to have the fetal heart rate listened to at least for half a minute every fifteen minutes and for vaginal examination to be done at least every

to do this by phonocardiography i.e. by placing a microphone on the maternal abdominal wall and picking up the fetal heart sounds after suitable amplification. Even after highly sophisticated filtering has been carried out to reduce the extraneous noise inevitable in this method the signal is always of poor quality (although still an advance on the traditional method).

Ultrasonography also requires sophisticated filtering and although usually a better signal than that obtained by phonocardiography there are some 15 per cent of cases in which it is impossible to get a satisfactory ultrasonic tracing and the phonocardiograph may then still be useful.

Detection of the QRS complex of the fetal ECG may be detected by 'non-invasive' means but much the best quality signal requiring minimal filtering, is obtained by attaching an electrode directly to the fetal scalp (Fig. 18.4). In established labour especi-

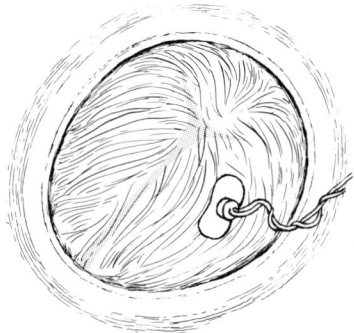

Fig. 18.4 View of a clip electrode attached to a fetal scalp as seen through a colposcope.

ally when there is concern for the fetus this method is to be recommended.

It is more convenient to calculate the rate of the fetal heart by generating a pulse synchronous with the appropriate signal and measure the interval between the pulses so generated and give the reciprocal of this as a rate. The commercial instruments now available work on this principle and generate such a synchronous pulse (Fig. 18.5) activated by the sound, the Doppler effect or the QRS complex and it is from the interval between each of the synchronous pulses that the rate is calculated.

It is important to remember that a rate at the bottom of a fetal heart dip of say sixty beats to the minute is not related to an auscultation record taken over half a minute showing a rate of sixty beats to the minute since during a dip the very slow rate may only be maintained for some two or three beats and the average over half a minute might well be one hundred and twenty or more (Fig. 18.6). To avoid such confusion it would be desirable to refer to fetal heart frequency in contra-distinction to an average fetal heart rate.

The instantaneous rate is traced on a pen-recording drum of paper activated by an instantaneous ratemeter voltage. By this method minute variations in instantaneous fetal heart rate undetectable to the human ear can be noted, more accurate estimate of the average fetal heart rate showing normal rate, bradycardia or tachycardia is possible (*see* Fig. 18.7) and, most important of all, fetal heart rate slowing over a short period, usually called dips, can be appreciated as can accelerations. Moreover the recording is equally as good during contractions as between contractions unlike the sounds heard with the Pinard stethoscope.

Uterine activity

There are two main clinical methods of measuring uterine activity (Fig. 18.8). An

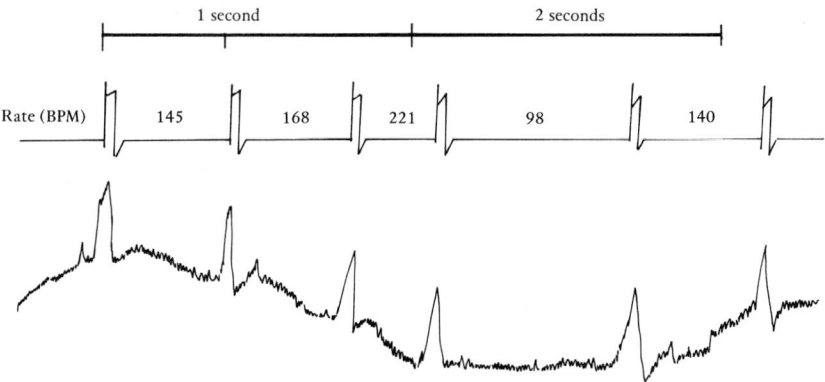

Fig. 18.5 Lower trace is an ECG. Upper trace is the derived synchronous pulse used to trigger a ratemeter.

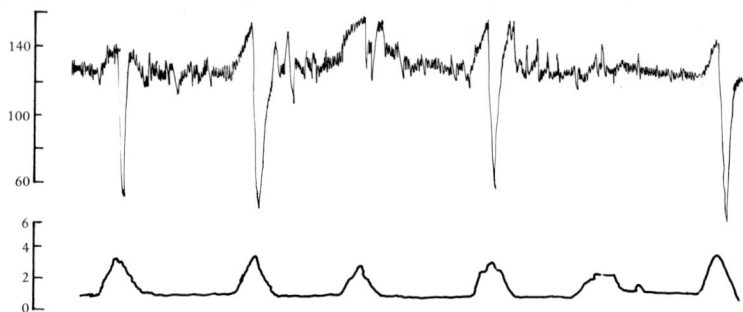

Fig. 18.6   During contractions (lower trace) the FHR slows to or below 60BPM but average FHR is above 120BPM.

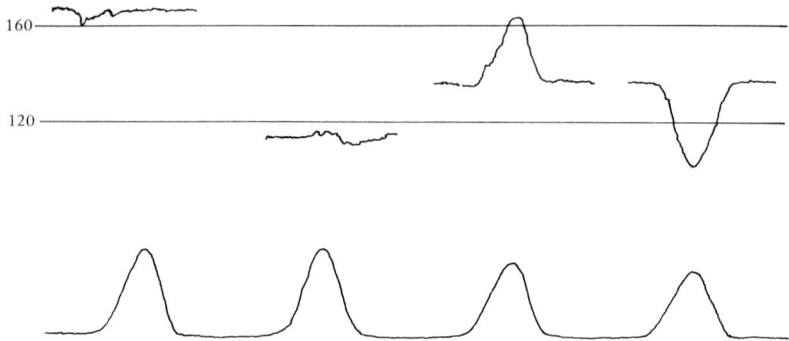

Fig. 18.7   Baseline tachycardia above 160BPM
Baseline tachycardia below 120BPM
Acceleration and dipping during contraction.

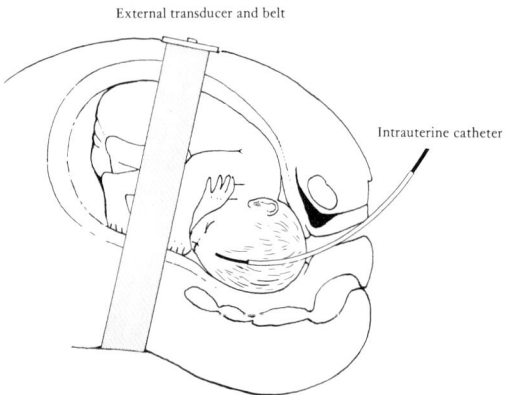

Fig. 18.8   External tocograph with strap recording uterine activity. Intra-uterine catheter attached to pressure transducer recording intra-uterine pressure.

external tocograph can measure the frequency of contractions and length of contractions. This method cannot, however, give a very definite measure of uterine contraction intensity. Such additional information can be obtained only by the use of invasive techniques

the usual one being an intra-amniotic catheter attached to an external pressure transducer. With careful technique it is then possible to measure the frequency, duration and the intensity of each contraction thus completely characterizing the energy the uterus is expending on the fetus. Information derived from either source is again put on to pen-recording paper and continuously recorded.

The exact time relationship between uterine activity and fetal heart rate response can be accurately noted and important information as to fetal wellbeing deduced (*see following*).

Clinical technique of monitoring fetus and uterus

To obtain the reliable information so necessary for clinical decisions to be made from continuous cardiotocography it is essential that the operator is familiar with the instruments he is using, is aware of the electronic basis on which they work and is able to recognize spurious signals and unsatisfactory signals.

To use the invasive techniques he must be skilled in applying the electrodes and inserting the catheters. It is obvious, therefore, that training and experience is essential before satisfactory results will be obtained.

When intra-uterine pressure catheters are used there are many possible pitfalls. The common assumption that they are either working or totally blocked is dangerous and could lead to tragedy. Partial blocking of catheters with attenuation and a reduction of the true signal does occur and could lead to over-stimulation of an already robust labour (Fig. 18.9).

ization of the scalp was necessary to apply it satisfactorily and as a consequence the cervix had to be at least some 3cms dilated (Fig. 18.10). Using the spiral electrode (Fig. 18.11), an experienced operator can attach it blindly by palpation, and the dilatation need be no more

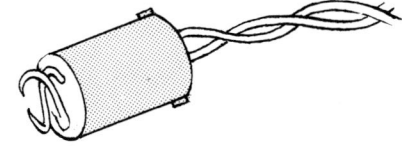

Fig. 18.11   Spiral electrode.

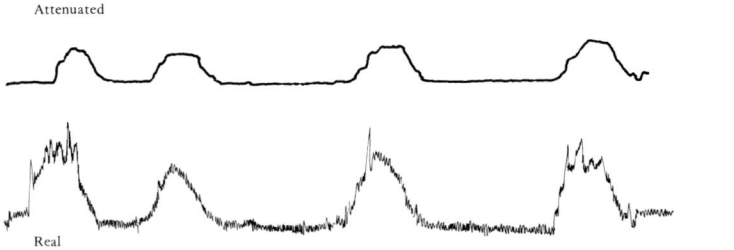

Attenuated

Real

Fig. 18.9   Simultaneous recordings from two intra-uterine catheters. Upper tracing is from a partially blocked catheter.

External cardiotocography requires the careful application of the abdominal belt, careful positioning of the tocograph and microphone or transducer and each time the patient moves a check is necessary to see that the signal is still satisfactory. With the invasive techniques well designed electrodes must be applied preferably without intervening membrane. With the original clip electrode visual-

than 1cm. Care should be taken to ensure that the attachment is made to a recognizable area i.e. over skull bones and obviously not over fontanelles or in abnormal presentations to unrecognized parts of the body lest damage to face or eyes should occur. Perfectly satisfactory signals can be obtained from breech presentations by attachment to buttock or leg.

The intra-amniotic catheters must be introduced with care particularly if there is a lack of liquor when the technique is more difficult. The traditional method is to pass the catheter introducer behind the baby's head in the manner of a 'Drew Smythe' catheter (Fig. 18.12a) and advance the catheter through the introducer. It is advantageous to flush the catheter continuously with sterile water during this procedure thus preventing the catheter becoming blocked and also creating a space in front of the catheter tip as it advances. This is usually straightforward in those patients whose labour is being induced and no liquor has escaped before the introduction of the catheter. In cases of long ruptured membranes or where there is very little liquor it is often easier to introduce the catheter anteriorly between the symphysis and the head thus getting into the uterine cavity much more easily and with less

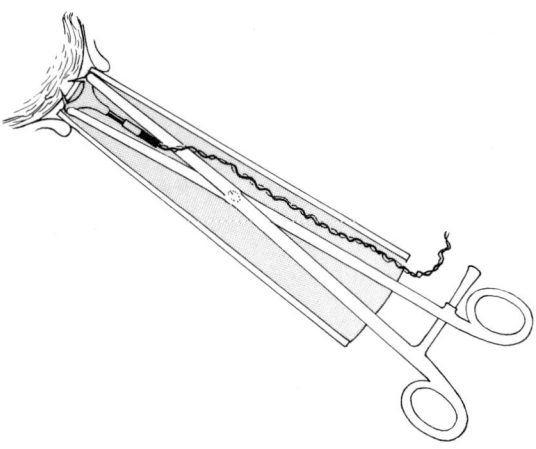

Fig. 18.10   Application of clip electrode to fetal scalp through a colposcope.

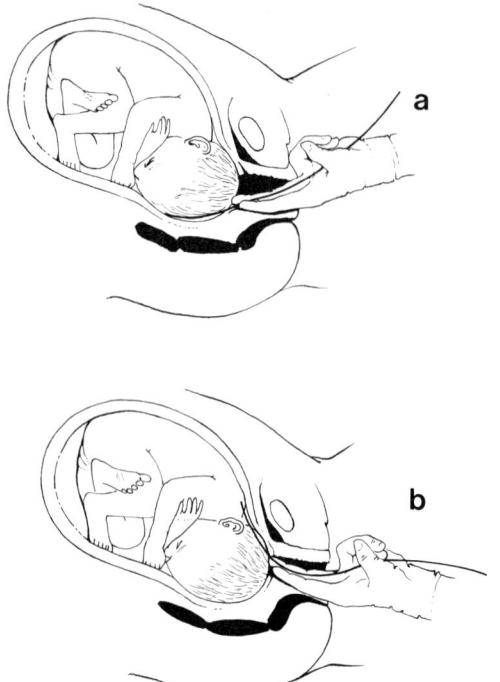

Fig. 18.12a. Catheter introduced traditionally behind the head.
b.   In some cases anterior insertion is easier.

bending of the catheter beyond the point of palpation (*see* Fig. 18.12b).

Clinical indications

Since the traditional methods of monitoring are imprecise and to some extent subjective it could be argued that continuous cardiotocography is indicated in all cases in which there is time to institute it. In practice, however, it is unusual for sufficient equipment to be available for all cases to be so managed and methods of selection becomes necessary.

It is easier to say which patients it is safest to leave not continuously recorded, e.g. multiparous patients in their second or third pregnancy who have had previous normal deliveries after going in to spontaneous labour at term are least at risk. At the opposite end of the spectrum is the patient with multiple indications for monitoring, e.g. a patient with a history of Caesarean section for fetal distress who is obese, suspected of poor growth syndrome and was being 'actively managed' in labour with epidural anaesthesia. To handle such a case in this way would make fetal

monitoring mandatory. The obesity makes palpation of the contractions unreliable, the epidural prevents patient discomfort indicating strong contractions. An intra-uterine pressure catheter is the only reliable guide to the efforts of the mother and the stress to the fetus. There is a high chance of fetal distress occurring both from the history and the suspected dysmaturity of the fetus and only continuous recording of the fetal heart rate would be sure of giving adequate warning of distress.

There is no doubt even an experienced midwife or obstetrician palpating contractions can be seriously misled in the obese patient as to the strength of contractions and if the patient is receiving epidural anaesthesia, disaster can occur without apparent warning. With continuous cardiotocography there is almost certainly a considerable time between the onset of danger signals and disaster.

To list the indications for continuous cardiotocography is almost to list obstetric complications:

Previous stillbirth neonatal death or morbidity.
Previous prolonged labour.
Post maturity.
Dysmaturity.
Pre-eclampsia and hypertension.
Elderly primigravidae.
Multiple pregnancy.
Borderline disproportion—'trial labour'.
Rh disease.
Induction—especially if syntocinon is to be used.
Syntocinon—to stimulate a lagging labour.
Epidural.
Obesity.
Diabetes.
Antepartum haemorrhage.
Meconium staining.
Clinical tachycardia or bradycardia.

Stimulation of labour with oxytocic drugs deserve special mention. Since there is no doubt over-stimulation can occur and since there is no set dose response relationship it is necessary to titrate the infusion against the labour. Since the active conduct of labour is now more common, short labours are coming to be expected and the risk of over-stimulation becomes greater. Satisfactory titration can only be carried out if a full objective measure of the quality of labour is available thus it is desirable that any labour being stimulated by syntocinon should be monitored with intra-uterine pressure measurements and this becomes more important if the fetus is for some other reason in a high risk category or the uterus has a scar upon it. In such cases the syntocinon can be increased until the strength of the contractions and/or the frequency of the contractions reach a satisfactory level and can be reduced or stopped if the strength or frequency exceed a limit. Such a 'stress' limit can be variable and will be set by clinical judgment. Thus a 'normal' fetus would have a higher limit than a 'high risk' fetus. At the same time whether that 'stress' limit were reached or not any sign of fetal distress would immediately indicate the need at least to reduce stimulation although additional measures might be indicated ranging from pH measurements to immediate Caesarean section.

Stress testing

Most continous cardiotocography is arranged during labour. However, continuous recording has been used in the pre-labour period in an attempt to forecast how the fetus is likely to behave when labour starts. This might be of use in a case of severe poor growth syndrome or a patient with a history of previous stillbirths after fetal distress. The objective here is to measure how the fetus behaves in the presence of stress and external cardiotocography is obviously the only method possible. Two methods of applying stress are commonly used, one method is to infuse syntocinon without rupturing the membranes inducing syntocinon contractions and observing the effect on the fetal heart. The implication being that if the fetal heart shows significant slowing particularly Type II dips (*see later*) then elective section would be indicated. A second method of causing stress is to try and create relative fetal anoxia by getting the mother to breathe a 15 per cent oxygen/nitrogen mixture again observing the effect on the fetal heart.

Monitoring

Many of the continuous cardiotocographs are referred to as 'monitors' incorrectly. Most of the ones in common use at present are *continuous recorders only* and monitoring is carried out, as before, by the attendant midwives and obstetricians interpreting the results obtained and correlating these results with other information such as observation of the

patient, measurements of the vaginal dilatation, measurements of scalp blood pH etc. There are, however, appearing on the market now some instruments which incorporate true monitoring devices with various degrees of sophistication most of which, at this stage in our knowledge, ought to be used with the greatest caution till more experience of how they behave in practice is built up. There is no doubt, that in the future many sophisticated monitors will become available which will greatly reduce the amount of information requiring to be processed by the obstetrician than is the case at present. Examples of such fetal monitors extend from the simple recognition of tachycardia and bradycardia by the Sonicaid FM2 to the more sophisticated 'Sentinel' of the Berkley Engineering Company and the Alert of the Corometrics Company. These instruments can, within limits, recognize not only bradycardia and tachycardia but extended contractions, prolonged contractions, too frequent contractions and fetal heart rate dips and even distinguish between Type I and Type II dips to some extent. Various warning devices are incorporated and switches can be included which shut off power to infusion apparatus. Thus the automatic control of labour by 'closing the loop' is theoretically possible.

Automatic control of labour

It is not uncommon in industry for instruments to control a machine and for the machine to give back information to the controlling instrument which thereby modifies its instructions. There are many examples of this 'closing the loop', one of the more sophisticated being an automatic pilot.

It is possible for the infusion of syntocinon to be controlled by an instrument in such a way as to increase the dose if the contractions are poor and thus alter the infusion rate according to the response of the uterus. The 'Cardiff Infusion Pump' in the automatic mode does this and with an intra-uterine pressure catheter in place the infusion pump propelling syntocinon along a special infusion set steadily increases the dose until contractions are satisfactory in intensity and in frequency. Various automatic alarm devices which stop the pump are incorporated to cope with such problems as catheter blockage, over-stimulation, etc. There is no doubt that this method, developed in the Cardiff Infusion Pump, though admirable in principle has some practical problems. Certainly the patient on such a pump should never be left without careful watch since one of the principal practical disadvantage is the possibility of a partially blocked catheter misleading the instrument and thereby over-stimulating a labour (*see* Fig. 18.9). A disadvantage is that this system is only able to increase, keep steady or stop the pump. It is unable to decrease the infusion rate.

Interpretation of cardiotocographic pen-recording tracings

This is a new skill obstetricians must acquire and the interpretation of these tracings is still a developing science. Various patterns are already described although unfortunately nomenclature is still not agreed and different descriptions for the same pattern are still used. Tachycardia and bradycardia are self-evident. The term base-line tachycardia or bradycardia means the average or unstimulated heart level (*see* Fig. 18.7). Beat-to-beat variation or fetal heart frequency variations is the change in the interval between one synchronous pulse and the next (Fig. 18.5), and loss of this is seen when there is very severe fetal depression or under the influence of

come on rather later and certainly wearing off after the contraction has worn off are considered to be much more serious, they are suggestive of fetal anoxia and definite distress. The former are called Type 1 or early decelerations and the latter, more clinically significant, Type 2 or late decelerations. However, even Type 1 dips are often of some significance and correlation has been suggested between the total area of dips (whether Type 1 or Type 2) and fetal outcome. Dips can occur not so definitely related to contractions, the so-called variable dips, and these are thought to be associated with various types of cord entanglement. At present the exact amount of emphasis to be put on the fetal heart rate tracing pattern in any given case is still by no means clear and more experience in many different centres is needed before definite rules can be laid down. At present the obstetrician must exercise his clinical judgment. There is no doubt that if Type 2 dips are present for any length of time then action of some kind is required even in an otherwise normal pregnancy and labour. This action might be no more than a fetal scalp pH though in the high risk situation it might well indicate Caesarean section or another method of immediate delivery which is appropriate.

Less attention has been paid to the tocographic tracing on its own although a well-

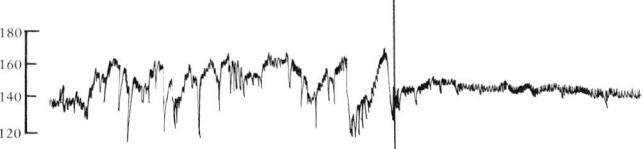

Fig. 18.13   Sudden loss of fetal heart rate fluctuation.

certain drugs (Fig. 18.13). Acceleration patterns are not uncommon particularly in relation to contractions. Their significance is not clear though it is certainly related to fetal stimulation e.g. flushing of a catheter with cold fluid is often accompanied by transient acceleration (Fig. 18.14). A great deal of significance is read into fetal heart rate dips. Those coincidental with contractions are considered to be caused very often by pressure on the fetal head with consequent stimulation of the vagus nerve. This effect can be abolished or at least reduced with atropine. Dips occurring with a close relationship to the contractions but tending to

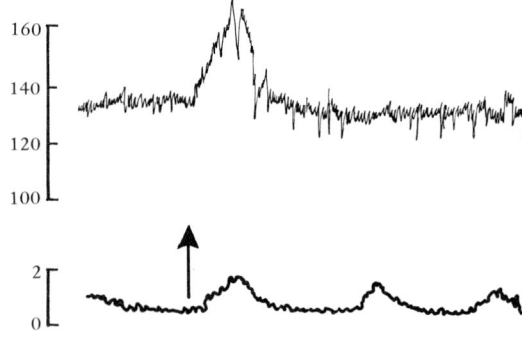

Fig. 18.14   At ↑ catheter was flushed with cold water.

placed catheter properly inserted and regularly flushed to ensure there is no blockage can give a tracing of uterine activity in the form of intra-uterine pressures which can give warning of problems even before the fetal heart rate tracings are giving rise for concern. The following dangerous situations can be recognized:

1. Too strong contractions, i.e. the acme of the contraction reaching levels in the first stage of labour above 100mm of mercury would always be serious and even levels below this could cause concern in the case of suspected fetal dysmaturity or a scar on the uterus.

2. Contractions which last longer than usual, certainly longer than a minute, would certainly be cause for concern and if syntocinon was being administered would be a reason for cutting back the speed and volume of infusion.

3. A rise in the base-line would also be a warning sign although a check should be made to see that the external transducer is in line with the mid-uterine area. This ensures the intra-uterine pressure is being measured correctly and no artefact is being introduced because of a column of fluid adding or subtracting to the base pressure because the transducer is at a different height.

4. Too frequent contractions with short intervals between should cause a close watch to be kept on the labour and particularly on oxytocic dosage.

The significance of abnormally shaped contractions is less clear but it has been noted that notched or even paired contractions can occur in the presence of a bicornuate uterus although often they occur in a uterus in which no abnormality is noted. Some abnormal shapes of contractions are associated with partial blockage of the catheter and this is where experience in the observer is valuable.

More subtle methods of analysis are becoming possible. Measurement of the area of the contractions enables the cumulative effect of the labour to be looked at closely and the rate at which energy is being expended on the fetus can be monitored. New forms of partograms can be constructed on this basis which can give a more detailed analysis of the labour but it is difficult to do this adequately without sophisticated equipment such as digital computers.

Fetal scalp pH

A further method of assessing fetal well-being in labour is to obtain a specimen of fetal blood for analysis. The technique for doing this is now well established, the steps are as follows: The membranes must be ruptured. The scalp is visualized by passing an endoscope through the cervix and pressing it firmly against the scalp. The scalp is cleaned and hyperaemia encouraged by spraying with ethyl chloride. An incision is made through the skin and free bleeding obtained. Silicon cream applied before incision is useful to keep the blood in a globule while a tube is filled by capillary attraction. The pH of the specimen is then read on special instruments designed to operate on small specimens of blood. Single results should not be relied upon and serial results are much more informative. Experience in collection and measurement is necessary. Although there is no doubt that a normal pH can be greatly reassuring in the presence of abnormal cardiotocographic findings it is not an absolute guarantee of good fetal outcome. The fetal scalp pO_2 and pCO_2 have been found less useful. One objection is their fluctuations are so much greater and faster, the pH having a much slower response and recovery and therefore a drop in value is much easier to pick up clinically with intermittent sampling.

FUTURE DEVELOPMENTS

This is a fast expanding area of technological development and various possibilities are being actively pursued at present. Most of the 'monitors' at present are analogue devices and digital monitors using computers are already being developed. Some more sophisticated intra-uterine methods of signal collection using intra-uterine transducers and electrodes are already available in an experimental form. Radio transmission from such devices will free the patient from the encumbrance of wires and catheters. The continuous measurement of pO_2, pCO_2 and pH in the fetus may yield worthwhile information in the management of labour. The possibilities are endless. The practical problem is to correlate the usefulness of results with the consequent expenditure though in dealing with unborn babies expenditure related to the reduction of morbidity both physical and mental during labour and delivery must surely have a high priority.

REFERENCES

Abdul Karim, R. W. (1974) (Ed.) Human fetal medicine. In *Clinical Obstetrics and Gynaecology*, **17**, No. 3. London: Harper and Row.

Baillie, P., Fisher, A. & Molteno, C. D. (1973) *Hypoxic Stress Tests*. Unpublished.

Bevis, D. C. A. (1953) The composition of liquor amni in haemolytic disease of the newborn. *J. Obstet. Gynaec. Brit. Emp.*, **60**, 244.

Bevis, D. C. A. (1956) Blood pigments in haemolytic disease of newborn. *J. Obstet. Gynaec. Brit. Cwlth.*, **63**, 68.

Bhagwanani, S. G., Fahny, D. & Turnbull, A. C. (1972) Prediction of neonatal respiratory distress by estimation of amniotic fluid lecithin. *Lancet*, **i**, 159.

Brown, J. B. & Coyle, M. G. (1963) Urinary excretion of oestriol during pregnancy—a shortened procedure. *J. Obstet. Gynaec. Brit. Cwlth.*, **70**, 219.

Campbell, S. (1969) The prediction of foetal maturity by ultrasonic measurement and the biparietal diameter. *J. Obstet. Gynaec. Brit. Cwlth.*, **76**, 603.

Campbell, S. & Newman, G. B. (1971) Growth of the fetal biparietal diameter during normal pregnancy. *J. Obstet. Gynaec. Brit. Cwlth.*, **78**, 513–519.

Donald, I., Morley, P. & Barnett, E. (1972) The diagnosis of blighted ovum by sonar. *J. Obstet. Gynaec. Brit. Cwlth.*, **79**, 304.

Epszteyn, L. (1972) The foetal E.C.G. *Ph.D. Thesis*. University of London.

Gluck, L. & Kulovich, M. V. (1973) *Fetal Lung Development Paed. Clinics of N. America*, **29**. Ed. Gluck, L. Philadelphia: Saunders.

Hareny, P. (1971) Prenatal cytological recognition of x-linked and chromosomal abnormalities. *J. Obstet. Gynaec. Brit. Cwlth.*, **78**, 1024.

Hellman, L. M., Kobayashi, M., Tolles, W. E. & Cromb, E. (1970) Ultrasonic studies on the volumetric growth of the human placenta. *Amer. J. Obstet. Gynec.*, **108**:5, 740–750.

Hellman, L. M., Kobayashi, M., Cromb, Ellen (1973) Ultrasonic diagnosis of foetal malformation. *Amer. J. Obstet. Gynec.*, **115**, 615.

Holmdahl, T. H. & Johansson, E. D. B. (1972) Peripheral Plasma Levels of 17α-Hydroxyprogesterone during human pregnancy. *Acta endocr.*, **71**, 4, 765–772.

Hunter, R. J. (1969) Serum heat stable alkaline phosphatase: an index of placental function. *J. Obstet. Gynaec. Brit. Cwlth.*, **76**, 1057–1069.

Klopper, A. (1968) The assessment of feto-placental function by estriol assay. *Obstet. Gynec. Sur.*, **23**, 813–838.

Lee, P. & Garrow, J. S. (1970) A clinical evaluation of the selenomethionine uptake test. *J. Obstet. Gynaec. Brit. Cwlth.*, **77**, 982.

Lilley, A. U. (1963) Intrauterine transfusion on haemolytic disease. *Brit. med. J.*, **ii**, 1107.

Lind, T. & Billewicz, W. Z. (1971) A point-scoring system for estimating gestational age from examination of amniotic fluid. *Brit. J. Hosp. Med.*, **5**, 681.

Makowski, E. L., Hertz, R. H. & Meschia, G. (1973) Effects of acute maternal hypoxia and hypoxia on the blood flow to the pregnant uterus. *Amer. J. Obstet. Gynec.*, **115**, 5.

Masson, G. M. (1973) Plasma oestriol during normal pregnancy. *J. Obstet. Gynaec. Brit. Cwlth.*, **80**, 201–205.

Robinson, H. P. (1972) Detection of fetal heart movement in the first trimester of pregnancy using pulsed ultrasound. *Brit. med. J.*, **2**, 466.

Turnbull, A. C., Flint, A. P. F., Jeremy, J. Y., Patten, P. T., Keirse, M. J. N. C. & Anderson, B. M. (1974) Significant fall in progesterone and rise in oestradiol levels in human peripheral plasma before onset of labour, *Lancet*, **i**, 101.

Valenti, C. (1972) Endoaminioscopy and fetal biopsy: a new technique. *Amer. J. Obstet. Gynec.*, **114**, 561–564.

Walker, J. (1963) The clinical circumstances at the time of labour in *Initiation of Labour*. U.S.P.H. Service 1390.

Walker, J. (1967) The 'Small for Dates' Baby. *Proc. Roy. Soc. Med.*, **60**, 877.

Walker, J. (1976) Prognostic value of antenatal screening. *Amer. J. Obstet. Gynec.*, **124**, 30.

Willocks, J. & Dunsmore, I. R. (1971) Assessment of gestational age and prediction of dysmaturity by ultrasonic fetal cephalometry. *J. Obstet. Gynaec. Brit. Cwlth.*, **78**, 814.

Yukorkala, O. (1973) Maternal serum HPL levels in normal and complicated pregnancy as an index of placental function. *Acta Obstet. Gynaec. Scand.*, Supp. 26.

FURTHER READING

Abnormal Uterine Action in Labour—A symposium (1952) *J. Obstet. Gynaec. Brit. Emp.*, **59**, 617.

Beard, R. W., Filshie, G. M., Knight, C. A. & Roberts, G. M. (1971) The significance of the changes in the continuous fetal heart rate in the first stage of labour. *J. Obstet. Gynaec. Brit. Cwlth.*, **78**, No. 10, 865.

Caldeyro-Barcia, R. & Poseiro, J. J. (1959) Oxytocin and contractibility of the pregnant human uterus. *Amer. New York Acad. Sc.*, **75**, 813.

Caldeyro-Barcia, R., Poseiro, J. J., de Paiva, C. N., Rogers, C. G., Lathan, A. F., Zambrana, M. A., Hernandez, G. A., Beaquis, A., Leigones, F. A. & Filler, N. (1961) Effects of abnormal uterine contractions on a human foetus. *Mod. Probl. Paed.*, **8**, 267. Basle: Karger.

Effects of labour in the fetus and newborn (1965) *Wld. Hlth. Org. tech. Rep. Ser.*, No. 300.

Fetal Medicine (1974) Clinics in Obstetrics and Gynaecology. Ed. Beard, R. W. London: Saunders.

Hammacher, K., Huter, K. A., Bokelmann, J. & Werners, P. H. (1968) Foetal heart frequency and perinatal condition of the foetus and newborn. *Gynaecologia*, **166**, 349.

Hon, E. H. (1968) *An atlas of fetal heart rate patterns.* Connecticut: Newhaven Harty Press.

Hon, E. H. (1969) *An introduction to fetal heart rate monitoring.* Connecticut: Newhaven, Harty Press Incorporated.

Methods for monitoring fetus in pregnancy and labour (*Proceedings of the second study group of R.C.O.G.*) (1971) Ed. Clayton, S. & Beard, R.

Perinatal Medicine (1969) *Proceedings of the 1st European Congress.* London: Verlag Acad. Press.

Perinatal Medicine (1971) *Proceedings of the 2nd European Congress.* London: Karger.

Perinatal Medicine (1972) *Proceedings of the 3rd European Congress.* Vienna: Hans Huber.

Perinatal Medicine (1973) *Proceedings of the 4th European Congress* (in print).

19. Labour

The uterus normally delivers the fetus when the child is fully mature and capable of the degree of independent existence normal to the species. This varies from the total dependence in the marsupial to the relative independence of the young of most four-footed mammals.

Early delivery may be 'abortion' in up to 25 per cent in the human, delivery before term (i.e. before the end of the 37th week), in another 5 per cent (7 per cent of those reaching viability) and postponed after 42 weeks in probably another 5 per cent. Abortion or premature delivery is often due to changes not identical with those operating at normal term and prolongation may be due to failure of normal functions for reasons currently ill-understood.

In the lower mammal, labour seems to be associated with changes in the relative levels in the maternal serum of oestrogen and pro-gesterone triggered off by a surge of *fetal* cortisol (Liggins, 1972). The fall in proges-terone is associated with a rise in the levels of prostaglandin F2α (Flint *et al.*, 1974).

The oestrogen rise cause, after thirty min-utes, a rapid increase in uterine blood flow (Killam *et al.*, 1973).

Although confirmatory results are not yet accepted in the human, it is possible that the pattern established in the sheep may, in a modi-fied way, apply to the human. The timing and levels occurring are, however, very different.

In the sheep, ACTH from the pituitary promotes increased corticosteroid produc-tion from the fetal adrenal and is associated with increased oestrogen precursor (DHAS) with a secondary rise in circulating maternal oestrogen. There is associated a rise in mater-nal prostaglandin F2α. This may stimulate the uterus directly into action or activate the fetal or maternal pituitary. There is also at this time a surge of fetal pulmonary surfactant production. Oxytocin is present only in spurts associated with contractions.

In the sheep this new activity develops in a very few days. There is evidence in the human, however, that all these functions; (i.e. rise in oestrogen and in prostaglandin F2α and fetal pulmonary surfactant and a possible fall, on progesterone levels) begin apparently some *weeks* before labour actually starts.

The absence of a normal pituitary/adrenal axis in a fetus still alive is associated with failure of labour to begin. In the human this is seen in the anencephalic (without hydram-nios) (Malpas, 1933) and in the sheep or cow in genetically determined syndromes of pro-longed gestation. Pituitary/adrenal deficiency in lambs whose mothers have been poisoned by veratrium californicum (in the Idaho Hills) or by salsola tuberculata (Kirrakul lambs in S.W. Africa), is also associated with failure of maternal labour and the loss of the lambs. In the Idaho situation, there is always a degree of cyclops deformity and the condition was first investigated because of the extent of commercial loss of the lambs.

LABOUR

Labour is the process by which the uterus expels the fetus through the birth passages. Labour to be normal must continuously pro-gress. Progress is measured by dilatation of the uterine cervix and (variably) by descent of the presenting part.

In normal circumstances the onset of labour is dictated by the feto-placental unit and labour is maintained probably also by fetus and plac-enta with some help from the mother, but final delivery of the child is completed usually by the expulsive effort of the mother herself.

The duration of labour, even in completely physiological situations, varies with the age of the mother and whether it is a first or later baby. In primigravidae the mean duration is some 12–14 hours (of which the first five to ten hours are a slow latent phase, the next four to five hours a stage of active dilatation, the next hour an adjustment phase before the last hour of final expulsion). In multigravidae the mean duration is seven to eight hours (with the phases lasting five hours, two hours, twenty minutes, and thirty minutes on average).

Labour to the mother begins with an increasing intensity in frequency, duration and force of the contractions which have been a characteristic of the pregnancy since the early weeks. The patient herself in late pregnancy notices these contractions as an intermittent hardening of the uterus, which tends to stand firmly forwards. Such contractions are even in early labour at first not painful except to individuals with a history of primary dysmenorrhea who may interpret these early labour contractions as causing discomfort. Gradually, however, as the strength of the uterine action increases the degree of discomfort experienced by the patient becomes such that pain may be considered to occur. The word 'pain' as given to a uterine contraction is perhaps significant of the normally expected result.

Contractions or 'pains' are felt first in the abdomen and perhaps later also in the small of the back, but low back discomfort is more likely to be associated with pelvic stretching associated with descent of the fetal head.

Contractions slowly increase in frequency and strength over the period of the initial latent phase until the preliminary dilatation of the cervix is achieved. This latent stage is usually considered to be completed when the cervix is some 2–3cm dilated and fully taken up.

At this time the head is usually loosely applied to the cervix and the membranes are still intact with a small bag of forewaters intervening between head and cervix.

By the end of the latent phase, when the cervix is 2–3cm dilated the labour, if normal and smooth, is, *in time*, half way through the first stage (i.e. half way to full dilatation of the cervix). Even if the latent phase is slow and long, the active phase after 3cm lasts usually only two to six hours.

The active period of dilatation to 10cm progresses at a rate of 0·5–2cm per hour. At some point during the active phase (usually towards the time of full dilatation) the membranes which have preceded the head with a thin 'bag' of forewaters rupture and the head sits firmly on the cervix.

At the end of the first stage (i.e. just after full dilatation) the greatest diameter of the fetal head is usually through the cervix and the head is lying deeply within the cavity of the pelvis. (There are exceptions in some multigravida where descent of the head does not occur until full dilatation has been achieved).

Once the head reaches the pelvic floor (and this is usually 15 to 20 minutes after full dilatation of the cervix) the mother has an instinctive reflex need to assist in expulsion of the child and this she does by active (bearing down) contraction of her abdominal muscles coincident with the uterine contractions. Mothers who have lost this reflex due to disease may expel the fetus by voluntary action or if this is also lost by uterine action alone, but in the patient completely paralysed help by forceps extraction is usually required. Similar help may be needed when epidural anaesthesia is used.

The tissues of the vagina and perineum have usually become softened and distensible, and the lower vagina and vulva gradually distend by the intermittent pressure of the head and the head is ultimately delivered. There is often a short rest after delivery of the head and the shoulders and body follow with the next contraction. The uterus contracts down after the expulsion of the child and usually there is rapid placental separation. The placenta is gradually released firstly into the upper segment of the uterus and then expelled into the vagina after five to fifteen minutes.

PHYSIOLOGY OF LABOUR MECHANISMS

'Normal labour' in the human is best defined as labour *which ends in the spontaneous cephalic delivery, at or about term, of a live mature child requiring minimal resuscitation after a labour lasting less than eighteen hours and with minimal damage to the mother*; all other labours and deliveries being considered abnormal.

Labour, characterized by the uterine contraction and upper segment retraction with cervical dilatation and descent of the fetus with the reflex production of maternal expulsive effort once the head reaches the pelvic floor, depends for its normal onset and progress on several factors.

FACTORS INFLUENCING LABOUR

1. *The fetus*, who probably by his biochemical reaction induces labour when best suited to himself and to the stage of his development (*see* page 318). He is also concerned as a passenger through the pelvis, and his size, lie, presentation, and position, will determine the ease or difficulty of his passage.

2. *The uterus.* Studies in the sheep suggest that the uterine muscle responds biochemically to the stimulus of cortico steroids from the fetus and placenta with the production of prostaglandin. The efficiency of muscle action function depends on its anatomy, its biochemistry and the resistance to its forces.

3. *The bony and soft tissues* of the passages through which the fetus must pass determine by their capacity, and ability to stretch, the likely success of the labour. Moreover, the hormone status and responsiveness of the soft tissues is also important.

4. *The mother.* The physiological acceptance by the mother of the feminine role, her expectation and acceptance of discomfort, her response to her attendants and her reaction to environment will often influence the pattern of her labour or the safety of the delivery. Her age, parity and past obstetric experience may greatly influence her efficiency.

5. *The attendant.* The response of the mother and the pattern of her labour can be influenced by the attitudes of the attendant and the quality of care given. Quality of care may be determined by sympathy, understanding, explanation and obvious care for the fetus as well as the provision of adequate surroundings, pain relief, and operative delivery where necessary.

THE FETUS

The full time fetus measures some 48–52cm in length, but in the uterus lies curved with its legs, arms and head flexed. *Attitude* is the term applied to the relative position of the fetal parts to one another and the normal attitude of the fetus is therefore, one of flexion. The body of the child is compressible and the limbs readily undergo the displacement required to render the delivery of the body

easier. The body itself can bend freely in almost any direction demanded for its easier descent during labour.

The fetal skull

In the great majority of cases the child is born head first and when the head is free of the maternal passages the birth is easy as a rule. When the child is very large difficulty with the shoulders may occur.

From an obstetrical point of view the head may be divided into the base, the face and the vault. The base and face are composed of bones which by the time of birth are firmly joined together. The solidity of those areas protect the medulla against the shearing strength to which the vertex is subjected during labour. The vault of the skull is composed of one occipital, two parietal and two frontal bones (Fig. 19.1). The bones

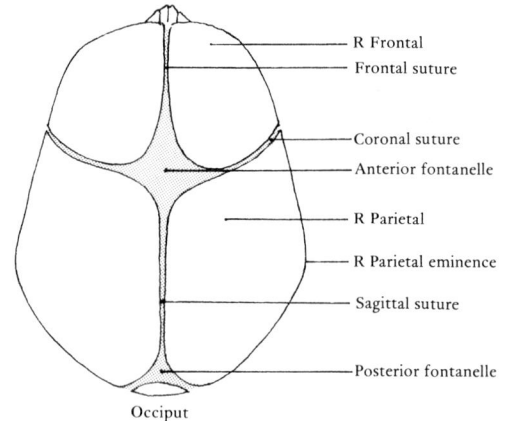

Fig. 19.1 The bones, sutures and fontanelles of the vault of the fetal skull.

comprising the vault are at birth incompletely ossified, the edges being membraneous and joined to one another by fibrous tissue. The space between each bone is called the 'suture'. These areas of fibrous tissue are of great importance since in labour when the head is under pressure they allow considerable overlapping of the bones to alter the shape of the head. This change is called 'moulding' and the capacity of the head to mould enables it to become longer and narrower and may permit it to pass more easily through the birth canal. The combination of particularly strong contractions in association with disproportion between skull and bony pelvis may cause excessive moulding and so distort the skull that damage to the supporting tentorium with tears of major veins may occur. In normal moulding the occipital and frontal bones are driven under the parietals and the leading parietal is driven under the other (*see* Fig. 19.2). The sutures between the bones are

fontanelle to just behind the occipital protuberance. This is the engaging diameter when the head is fully flexed in a vertex presentation and the area enclosed by this and the biparietal diameter is the functional vertex. The length of both the biparietal and the suboccipito bregmatic is 9·5–10·0cm in the normal term fetal skull. When the head is fully flexed the

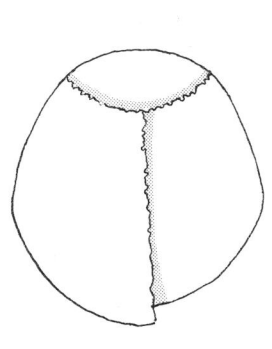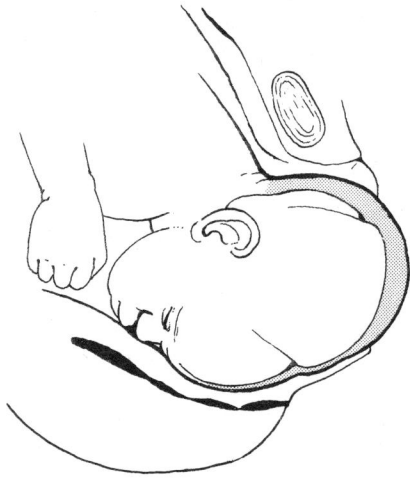

Fig. 19.2   Moulding of the fetal skull associated with the difficulty of the head negotiating the bony pelvis.—Note that the occipital and frontal bones slide under the parietal and the posterior parietal under the other.

frontal between the halves of the frontal bones, *sagittal* between the parietal bones, *coronal* between the frontal and parietal bones, *lambdoidal* between the occipital and parietal bones.

The fontanelles are the spaces formed where the sutures meet. The anterior fontanelle or bregma is a lozenge-shaped area of varying size between frontal and parietal bones and always clearly palpable. It is, of course, maintained for several post-natal months. The posterior fontanelle, triangular, lies between the parietal and the occipital bones. This fontanelle is often occluded in labour by moulding or obscured by caput.

A certain knowledge of the diameters of the fetal skull is necessary to a proper understanding of labour and of the mechanisms of labour. The main diameters with which we are concerned are those associated with various degrees of flexion or extension of the head associated with various presentations and positions of the head in relation to labour itself. (Fig. 19.3.)

1. The *suboccipitó bregmatic diameter* is from the posterior aspect of the anterior

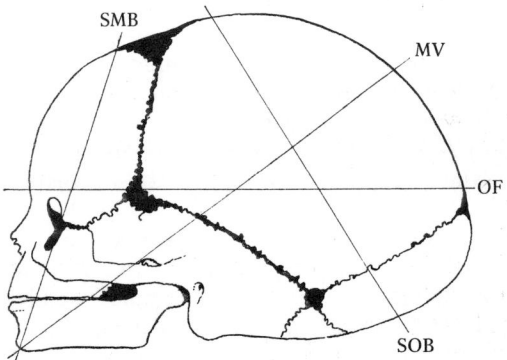

Fig. 19.3   The diameters of the fetal skull used in obstetrics.

area and shape of presenting part, the vertex, is therefore, a circle.

2. The *occipito frontal diameter* runs from the anterior aspect of the posterior fontanelle to the root of the nose. This diameter of 11·5–12cm is the engaging diameter in a badly flexed head presentation often where the position is occipito posterior. The corresponding transverse diameter remaining the biparietal.

3. The *mento vertical diameter* runs from midway between the fontanelles to the tip of the chin and measures 13·5–14cm. This very large diameter is the engaging diameter in a brow presentation.

4. The *sub mento-bregmatic diameter* runs from the chin to the anterior end of the anterior fontanelle. This is the engaging diameter when the face presents and like the suboccipital bregmatic measures 9·5–10cm so that the fully extended face presents a somewhat similar engaging circle to the fully flexed vertex.

The presentation and position of the fetus

The 'presentation' is that part of the child which occupies the lower pole of the uterus, i.e. the part which 'presents' during labour. The 'lie' of the child is its direction in relation to the long axis of the uterus. If the lie is longitudinal the presentation will be cephalic or breech, if the child is lying transversely or obliquely then the presenting part may be a shoulder or an arm. If the cord should precede the child and lie in advance of it this would then be a cord presentation.

The 'position' of the child is defined as the relation of a particular area of the child, the 'denominator' to a particular part of the pelvic brim of the mother. In vertex presentations the occiput is chosen as the denominator, in face and brow presentations the chin and in breech the sacrum. During pregnancy and until the onset of labour the presentation and position of the child may vary but in the majority of circumstances the child takes up his final lie and presentation about the thirty-fourth to thirty-fifth week of pregnancy. In the primigravida after that time for example, the child can rarely turn because of the development of the primigravid uterus in a long oval. In the multigravida the uterus may be a round and the instability of the child may persist into the very late weeks since the child has enough room to lie in any way it chooses. In some instances the final lie or presentation is not determined until early in labour.

VERTEX PRESENTATION
Normally in late pregnancy the child lies with the head leading or presenting and in a degree of semi-flexion so that probably the occipito frontal diameter will present. However, preceding labour or at the very beginning of labour the first movement of the fetal head

is one of flexion and the vertex with the sub-occipito bregmatic diameter would then present. In many cases the child tends to face its own placenta so that the actual position of the body of the child *in utero* is to some extent determined by the position of the placenta. However, in late pregnancy as the child's head enters the pelvis it tends to do so in the transverse diameter of the brim and the head is then said to be in the right or the left occipital lateral position. As the head descends into the pelvis before or during early labour it is most usual that the sagittal suture of the head should be slightly in front of the lateral position. The commonest of all final positions is the *left occipito anterior* (Fig. 19.4). Left or

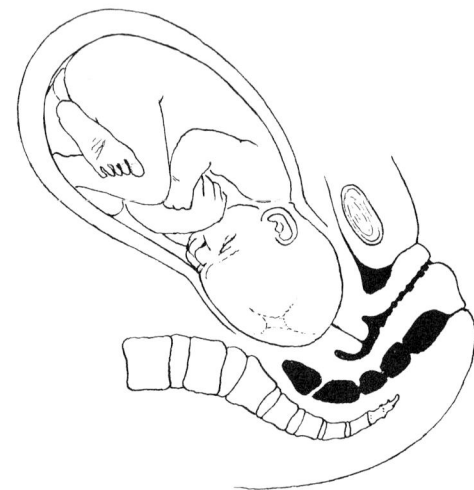

Fig. 19.4   The head in left occipito anterior position.

right occipital anterior positions are more common and relatively more normal. Occasionally the head takes up the position before or after labour with occiput rotated towards one or other sacro iliac joint. These occipito posterior positions are associated more commonly with abnormal labour partly because of the malflexion of the head associated with them and, therefore, a larger (occipito frontal) engaging diameter.

Occasionally the head may fail to rotate at all and will descend into the pelvis still in the occipito lateral position and often also associated with malflexion. The head may fail to rotate forwards.

THE POWERS
The uterine contractions and the maternal expulsive effort constitute the driving force.

In recent years the physical biochemical and endocrine peculiarities of uterine function in late pregnancy have been extensively studied. Turnbull (1957) and Turnbull and Anderson (1968) and Friedman (1967) are amongst the recent authors who have described in great detail the clinical pattern of uterine behaviour in labour and have measured and recorded uterine function.

The tocograph of Lorand (1933) was applied to the abdomen and recorded uterine contractions by a small piston which moved with the hardness of the uterus. The actual record was taken on paper on a small drum driven by clockwork. More recent external devices have been the strain gauge toko dynamometer of Reynolds (1948) and others.

In more recent years, however, most of the studies, especially in labour, have been by intra-amniotic catheter. The technique originally described by Williams and Stallworthy (1952) measures the intra-uterine pressure by a catheter passed into the amniotic sac behind the head (using the Drew Smythe catheter as a guide). Caldeyro-Barcia and Alvarez (1957) studied intra-amniotic pressure by a catheter inserted by transabdominal amniocentesis but studied also pressures in the uterine muscle by the placing of small balloons on catheters within the muscle itself. There is some recent suggestion that the high figures of intra-myometrial pressure recorded by this method during contractions are not correct.

Some co-ordinated uterine activity, usually known as 'Braxton Hicks' contractions, commences at about the twentieth week of human pregnancy. At thirty-two to thirty-four weeks' gestation further increase in activity occurs, but the magnitude of the increase and the subsequent pattern of change depends on the stage of gestation at which the spontaneous onset of labour will ultimately occur. If labour is to start before full term, uterine activity, on average, rises steeply between the thirty-second and the thirty-sixth week with little increase thereafter, whereas if the onset of labour is likely to be after term the increase in activity after the thirty-second week is slight and by thirty-eight weeks is only one quarter of that seen in the group due to begin labour before term. The clinical state of the cervix also relates to the time of onset of labour. In those primigravidae in whom labour starts by the thirty-eighth week of pregnancy, the internal os in most cases admits at least one finger by the thirty-second week, but in only 10 per cent of those in whom pregnancy will be prolonged to the forty-second week or more.

It appears that generally speaking the time of gestation at which labour starts may be determined many weeks before. Most writers consider that a certain amniotic pressure and a certain frequency of contraction is necessary to successful progress of labour. It is, however, also clear that cervical or lower segment 'resistance' play a role in determining the strength needed and perhaps in preventing dilatation even with adequate contractions. Lindgren (1973) for example found that there was no cervical dilatation unless the intra-uterine pressure with the contraction reached 25mm of mercury and that the contractions were at least 12 per hour. There is no absolute agreement of the actual pressure and frequency required but the principle is accepted.

A single contraction wave in early labour (measured by its effect on uterine pressure) begins with a resting pressure of some 10mm Hg. The contraction rises fairly fast to its peak. It can be felt by the attendant once the pressure reaches 20mm Hg and by the patient by 30mm Hg. Similarly as the contraction passes off, sensation is first lost by the patient and then by the attendant. The maximum pressure reached varies with the stage of labour and the activity of the uterus but ranges in labour from 30mm Hg to 60mm Hg. Superimposed maternal voluntary effort may increase the pressure on the fetus up to 150mm Hg in the second stage.

As the uterus in labour contracts the muscle mass exhibits an unique characteristic (which has been insufficiently studied) that of retraction. As labour contractions continue the uterus gradually becomes divided into two distinct areas—an upper segment which becomes shorter and more bulky and a lower segment (including the cervix) which becomes longer and thinner. The lower uterine segment; arising initially from that area of the uterus called the isthmus; probably is formed sometime after thirty weeks and allows the head to become accommodated in the lower part of the uterus, ultimately to engage in the pelvis. At this stage this accommodation is probably from some stretching of the area of the isthmus but also some uptake of the upper definitive cervix and internal os. The whole pattern becomes grossly exaggerated where there is mechanical resistance to descent of the baby. Contraction and retraction of the upper segment has the effect of pulling the cervix open and upwards over the presenting part. This effect is aided somewhat by the thrust downwards of the presenting part through the opening cervix. Turnbull (1957) has shown that a reduction in the concentration of hydroxyproline in the cervix and a dissociation of the collagen fibres into fibrils increases the softness and distensibility of the cervical tissues. In late pregnancy this change is associated with a greater softness of the tissues of the lower segment and vagina and para-vaginal tissues which can be palpated as a guide to ease of labour. As a result of the retraction the upper segment becomes progressively shorter and thicker and the lower segment progressively longer and thinner. Provided the cervix dilates and is pulled up over the head and especially if the head descends there is no undue lengthening of the lower segment. The varying behaviour of the various segments of the uterus is essential to normal progress of labour.

As the uterus contracts the fundus pushes the abdominal wall forwards and this is helped by active contractions of the round ligaments which act as stays. This has the effect of lining the baby up to the pelvic inlet which is angled to the vertical, *see* Figure 19.12.

At the onset of labour the cervix may still be firm, long and closed or more usually soft, partially taken up and dilated (Fig. 19.5). As labour progresses the cervix becomes fully taken up and then dilated, the membranes bulge and ultimately rupture. Cervical dilatation does not usually become complete and total until the presenting part descends and the cervix is pulled up past it. The cervix recedes further and further during labour and the vaginal fornices also rise. As the head descends after or close to full dilatation the cervix is pulled up past and may in fact rise as high as the pelvic brim and the vagina accommodates the whole of the fetal head. Most cases of disproportion especially with occipito-posterior or transverse position never quite reach full dilatation.

THE MEMBRANES

In late pregnancy the membranes, amnion and chorion, are lightly attached to the lower uterine segment and as it forms accommodates to the presenting part. Normally there is no

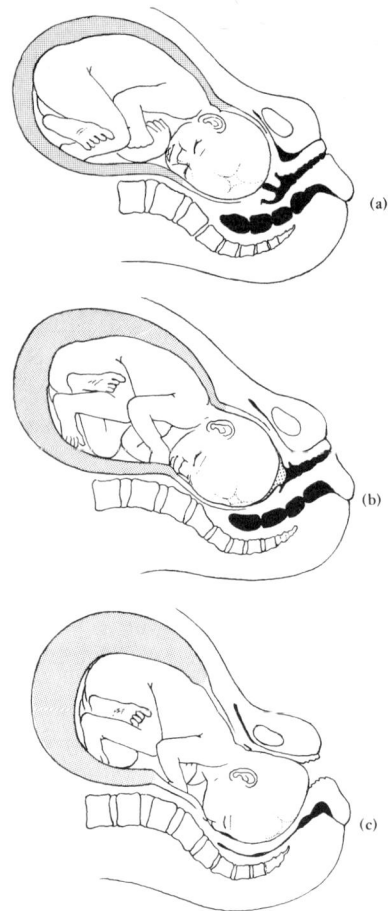

Fig. 19.5   The stages in dilatation of the cervix.

tendency for the membranes to bulge through the cervix even with the contractions which occur during pregnancy. If, however, the cervix dilates unduly or if 'incompetent' then the membranes may bulge and rupture with this onset of premature labour.

Normally as labour progresses the membranes bulge in front of the presenting part producing a bag of waters of greater or lesser extent. Where the presenting part fits well the bag is thin and distended only during a contraction, where there is a poor fit the bag may present through the partially dilated cervix and rupture early.

The bag of membranes probably assists in the movement of the cervix over the head, but the modern techniques of induction where the membranes are ruptured early do not seem to delay labour. Just occasionally especially in the multigravida an unruptured bag of membranes at full dilatation prevents descent of the head. The child may actually be born with the membranes intact over the head—'a caul' said, in fishing communities, to prevent later death from drowning.

THE PASSAGES
The soft tissues and the bony pelvis.

The softness and distensibility of the vagina and paravaginal tissues have already been briefly discussed. There is hyperaemia loosening of connective tissue, increase in mucosal thickness and hypertrophy of smooth muscle cells. This softening which makes the tissues feel like soft rubber is already obvious by the last few weeks and to some extent extends to the muscles of the perineal body. It is quite essential that the vagina should distend and dilate and lengthen to accommodate the presenting part after full dilatation of the cervix and that the perineum and the vulvar orifice should gradually stretch to allow the birth of the child.

As the head descends into the pelvis after full dilatation it reaches the pelvic floor. The muscles of the pelvic floor are mainly the group forming the levator ani (the coccygeous and ileo coccygeous) but the pyriformis and the obturator fascia contribute to the shape of the walls and floor of the cavity.

Viewed from above the pelvic floor is a funnel with a somewhat short anterior side but converging towards the vagina. As the presenting part reaches the pelvic floor the uterine contractions plus the elastic resistance of the muscles force the leading area of the presenting part to rotate to the front. So that a head presenting as an occipito lateral or occipito anterior will rotate so that the occiput is anterior. An occipito posterior may rotate in the opposite direction. A badly flexed head may meet the pelvic floor equally and, therefore fail to rotate.

After the occiput rotates to the front the presenting part lies at the level of the ischial tuberosites. The head is still well flexed. The cervical and thoracic spines start to extend once the head (still well flexed) moves downwards and forwards. It is at this time well back from the subpubic arch. Extension of the head does not occur until it is ready to come through the vulva and if an episiotomy is done it virtually does not extend at all. As the head comes down well posterior the perineum is distended and the anus when distended becomes D shaped and the anterior rectal wall is exposed. As the head distends the vulva, the vulvar opening is diverted upwards and forwards. The perineum can become very thin indeed.

THE BONY PELVIS
The bony pelvis has been described in Chapter 2 and some of the commonly seen bony abnormalities are described.

The obstetrical ideal pelvis, as described in Chapter 2, is essential to normal labour and delivery but minor aberrations are common. The real importance of the really round pelvis is that the whole of the area of the brim is available to the fetal head for engagement since the greatest transverse diameter being in the mid-pelvis is also the greatest available diameter.

Where there is posterior segment flattering with a shortened AP diameter (the commonest abnormality), there may be a reasonably good transverse diameter but it is not all available to the head in view of the flattening posteriorly.

If the pelvis is of the shape described as normal or ideal difficulty in labour can come only from an unduly large child, a malpresentation (e.g. brow), or occasionally with a malposition of the head with malflexion where there is failure of a large head to descend and rotate to the front. There may, however, be in some tall women with adequate dimensions in round or long oval pelvic brims and a copious cavity some contraction of the pelvic outlet with the pubic spine and alae of the pubis being pushed medially and some forward displacement of the lower sacrum. Where the pelvic brim is adequate it is unusual for outlet contraction to be severe. If the brim is long and oval there may be relative narrowing of the pelvis throughout. If, in such a pelvis, the head engages as an occipito anterior in the antero-posterior diameter it remains thus and is delivered naturally. If it engages in the occipito posterior it may deliver spontaneously, require forceps assistance or obstruct especially if the lower sacrum comes forward at all.

Pelves which have characteristically triangular or flattened brims are usually smaller, flattened certainly in the anterior posterior diameter and often have a contracted cavity and outlet. Classically the rachitic pelvis is contracted (flattened) only at the brim and is exceptionally roomy in the cavity (which is short) and the outlet. (This is seen often in pelves with posterior segment flattening which is a minor degree of the true rachitic pelvis.) In such cases disproportion at the brim, once overcome, is followed by easy delivery.

THE EFFECT OF LABOUR ON THE MOTHER

A labour which is smooth and relatively easy has often a most uplifting and joyous effect on the mother who is able to participate in and take pleasure from the final birth of her child. A labour which is long, painful and associated with disproportion or malpresentation may kill the mother or, at the best, leave her mentally and physically scarred for life. The risks and dangers of labour arise throughout labour but vary with the stage of labour.

Premonitory stage

This may last for several days or a week or two before labour. The woman, especially the primigravida, may experience the sensation of 'lightening', when the head engages in the pelvis and the uterus sinks to a lower level. Discomfort which she may have had in breathing due to the pressure of the uterus on the diaphragm may disappear. On the other hand, pressure on the bladder with frequency of micturition may be aggravated, and there may be greater difficulty in walking as a result of relaxation in the joints of the pelvis.

In late pregnancy in the primigravida with the softening and formation of the lower segment and some loss of liquor the head sits deep in the uterus and may, therefore, 'engage' in the pelvis. The greatest diameter is then already through the pelvic brim. Failure of the head to engage in a primigravida may be due to failure of the lower segment to soften and distend, failure of the head to flex, to a posterior position, to some degree of disproportion or occasionally in a very tall primigravida where there is already adequate space in the abdomen.

In many primigravidae and multigravidae the upper part of the cervix becomes 'taken up' in the latter weeks, i.e. the cervical canal is obliterated from the internal os downwards.

In addition to these changes, progressive softening of the vaginal walls and the vulva occurs and there is usually an increase in exudation from the vaginal walls.

Whilst the uterine contractions that precede the onset of labour are generally painless it sometimes happens, especially in multigravidae, that for several days, or even some weeks, they may be so powerful as to cause discomfort, to disturb sleep and even to suggest that labour has actually started. Such contractions (the so-called false pains) differ from those of true labour in that they do not dilate the cervix. Moreover, they are felt mostly in the abdomen and vary greatly in their site, intensity and periodicity. The painful contractions seem to be most troublesome at night and by interfering with sleep cause exhaustion unless sedatives are given.

There is some danger that the obstetrician may consider the mother to be in labour, and take unnecessary action to stimulate apparently inadequate contractions. On the other hand, if the false labour is sufficiently annoying and distressing to the multigravidae, he should induce labour by rupture of the membranes close to term. Certainly false labour after term in the multigravida is a clear indication for induction.

The first stage up to full dilatation of the cervix

This is characterized, as we have discussed, of a relatively slow latent phase and then a phase of acceleration when the cervical dilatation proceeds rapidly often without any apparent increase in the strength of the contractions or even of frequency.

The most obvious effect on the mother is that produced by the pain of the contraction. The degree of pain is determined by the person feeling it and labours vary greatly in the amount of discomfort they produce and women vary tremendously in their response to labour pain.

It is true that in some labours the actual labour contractions are relatively painless, and cervical dilatation occurs without undue tension and expulsion gives satisfaction rather than great and painful effort. Some women achieve this but this is certainly not common and even normal to the modern woman. The greatest single help to the mother that can be given in labour is relief of pain.

Pain is due probably to uterine muscle ischaemia, cervical stretching, stretching of the pelvis especially rotation about the ileosacral joints and later to soft tissue resistance.

Contraction pain is felt, as previously described, after a certain intra-uterine pressure is reached, and then disappears, ileosacral pain is constant when the head is tightly engaging, pain between contractions over the uterus suggests retroplacental bleeding, or undue lower segment or scar stretching.

CARDIAC FUNCTION IN LABOUR

Experimental studies have been mainly under epidural anaesthesia (Lees et al., 1970), but show that there are marked increases in left ventricular work. With the contraction the cardiac output rises by some 25 per cent due to a rise in stroke/volume and without any rise in heart rate. The CVP rises by 3–5mm/Hg just before the uterine pressure rise is detectable. The arterial blood pressure rose by some 10mm/Hg, possibly because of the removal of the low resistance of the chorio decidual space (see later), the cardiac pulmonary blood flow increases, and there is a rise in pulmonary arterio-venous oxygen difference.

In the normal situation there is no cumulative effect of labour and the cardiac output changes seem less if the patient is nursed on her side. Animal experimental work which extended the human studies (Lees, 1970), showed that with the contraction the uterine component of the cardiac output seems to increase markedly. Immediately after delivery there is a sustained rise in cardiac output and in arterial pressure, the heart rate remaining unchanged.

If there is a cumulative change in cardiac pattern during labour this is due to pain and apprehension, and that this can be greatly relieved by proper relief of pain (see Buchan et al., 1973). Much of the serious rise in cardiac output following delivery from the lithotomy position depends on the sudden release of caval pressure and a greatly increased cardiac return. There is of course, a blood loss of between 3 and 500ml during delivery, which successfully relieves any undue autotransfusion back from the uterus to the maternal circulation.

UTERINE AND PLACENTAL BLOOD SUPPLY

If the mother lies on her back in late pregnancy or in labour the uterus may compress the pelvic veins and the inferior vena cava and prevent adequate venous return to the right heart with consequent maternal hypotension. This effect is more definite during a contraction. Similarly the common iliac artery may be occluded at the height of a labour contraction in the full term uterus with the mother on her back or right side but this is probably not itself an added hazard as the placental circulation will have already ceased by this time due to interference with venous outflow.

Uterine contractions cause a fall in total uterine blood flow roughly proportional to the strength and duration of contractions. The venous channels in the uterine wall are first closed off and the intervillous space tends to fill with blood and the blood is dispersed through the cotyledons. The arteries of the uterine wall, and therefore, the muscles are well supplied normally (at a pressure of 60–80mm Hg) but the placental flow falls markedly. There is still argument of the effect of the uterine contractions on pressure within the myometrium and on freedom of muscle flow. Certainly frequent powerful contractions will interfere with uterine myometrial filling.

With the contraction blood squeezed out amounts to some 250ml and this causes a slight rise in CVP and in right auricular pressure. There is a rise in arterio venous oxygen differential a slight rise in cardiac output and a rise in systolic blood pressure. Femoral vein pressure rises with the contraction—especially with the mother on her back. The maternal blood pressure rises during a contraction but not usually to great degree until the expulsive efforts of the second stage, when the pressure rise may be quite high. It is, however, essential that the maternal blood pressure should be monitored as occasionally a rapidly rising pressure is the first and only warning of impending eclampsia.

The normal maternal adrenocorticoid response to the pain and apprehension of labour is seen by a rise in the hydroxycorticosteroid levels in the blood. These levels rise high with the stress of the second stage. This response is abolished where epidural anaesthesia deletes maternal pain. Buchan et al. (1973).

Adverse circulatory effects of anaesthetic or other agents may increase the effects by themselves causing hypotension. Maternal hypovolaemia associated for example, with the dehydration of a long labour has a similar and often added effect.

RESPIRATORY FUNCTION

Andersen and Walker (1970) have shown that apart from the distress of the contraction there is no change from pregnancy in the stimuli to ventilation in labour. With each contraction with some over breathing the maternal pO_2

and pH rise and though in the second stage severe degrees of maternal hypocapnia can be demonstrated there is certainly no progressive maternal acidosis in normal labour.

During the second stage of labour especially with overbreathing—panting—or excess effort, the maternal pCO_2 may fall to very low levels (16mm Hg).

Although theoretically the fetal arterial pO_2 may suffer because of very low maternal pCO_2, the short duration of such levels (confined to the later second stage normally) does not seem to have a serious effect on the normal child.

GENERAL

If the mother is, however, asked to undertake a long and painful labour there will be interference with electrolyte balance and carbohydrate intake and dehydration and starvation and all the sequelae of excess effort without adequate supporting intake will appear.

The effects of labour on the fetus

Since normal mammals are born by a process of labour, it must be assumed that, apart from the fact of achieving birth, the forces applied to the fetus in labour should confer some benefit on the baby. If we consider labour, there are firstly those factors directly concerned with the mechanical problems of parturition, and others coincidental with labour which are preparatory to birth and for extra-uterine life. Since labour may obviously vary in its difficulty, it is to be expected that the baby should be able to compensate to some degree for adverse effects temporary to labour—but it is difficult to define the limits within which no damage will occur.

PARTURITION

The first effect is one of *compaction*. The child before labour lying relatively freely in the uterus has, in late pregnancy, suffered some degree of compaction by the relative loss of liquor and is usually forced to lie longitudinally. With the onset of labour, however, compaction is tighter and the child is lined up towards the brim and his limbs are *flexed* and compressed close to his body. Minor degrees of oblique or transverse lie are corrected, and the fetal spine straightens with the contraction to take the downward drive of the uterine contraction. His head is flexed when descent occurs and the whole child then becomes a 10cm elongated cylinder with the folds and creases greased by vernix.

Intra-uterine pressure due to contraction is first effected on the whole child but as the cervix dilates and the head fits firmly into the dilatating cervix and lower segment, there is increasing downward pressure on the body, and on the head laterally within the cervix. There is less pressure on the leading scalp which may then distend with oedema (the caput succedaneum).

Moulding of the head (*see* Fig. 19.2, page 321) is a normal process designed to allow smaller diameters to be presented by the descending head. Moulding is due mostly to soft tissue resistance and, therefore, little or none may be present in the child of the multigravidae. In the primigravida, however, and especially where there is also bony resistance and a long and difficult progress through the pelvis moulding may be extreme. While extra dural haemorrhage and fracture are uncommon unless difficult or failed forceps delivery is added to an already moulded head, tears of the tentorium with or without rupture of the straight sinus or of the unsupported great vein of Galen may occur (Fig. 19.6). It is pressure on the head and moulding at the brim

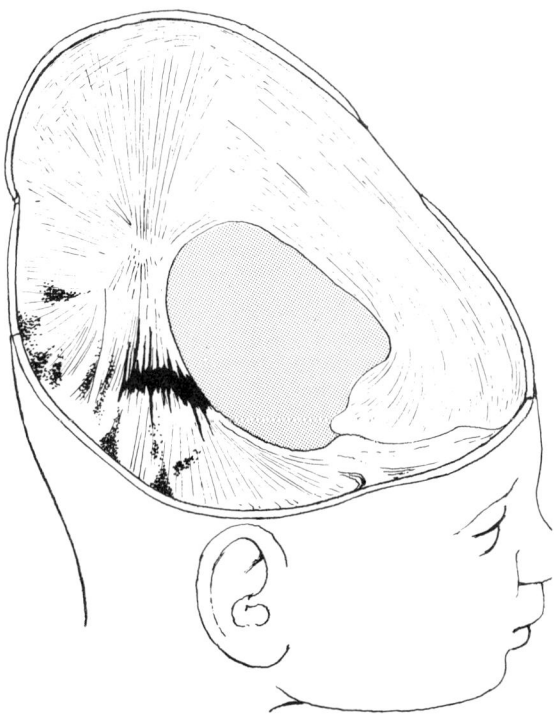

Fig. 19.6   Tear of the tentorium with minor haemorrhages in the falx following undue moulding.

and the pelvis or resistance at the outlet that is often responsible for the fetal bradycardia that may accompany contractions (Type 1 dips).

Especially in the presence of disproportion between head and pelvis, excessive or sudden 'moulding' is a risk to the after-coming head of a child born as a breech when the sudden pressures applied to a head delivered quickly through the pelvis may kill or damage. In the child born prematurely with a soft mouldable head it is probably the sudden release from pressure at the moment of birth which is most harmful, for this reason wide episiotomy with or without guided forceps delivery is advised.

THE EFFECT OF THE UTERINE CONTRACTIONS

During uterine contractions the intervillous space normally is filled with blood which is widely dispersed through the space by the contractions so increasing the area of uptake for oxygen and transfer of CO_2 lactate.

The principal determinant of immediate fetal tolerance to excessive and frequent uterine contractions is the quality of oxygen stored in the intervillous space blood and the rate of oxygen utilization of the fetus. Complications such as partial placental separation or interference with fetal cord circulation are, of course, overriding factors.

EFFECT OF LABOUR ON CARDIAC FUNCTION

In discussing the effects of labour, Dawes (1967) has pointed out that the fetus is clearly not a passive partner. His studies reported mainly the various changes in the fetal cardiac output, and in feto-placental uterine respiratory change. Any deterioration in fetal oxygen levels often with occurrence of metabolic acidosis causes redistribution of the output of the fetal heart, so that umbilical flow is maintained while pulmonary and femoral flows may be reduced. Active dilatation improves the flow in the coronary and cerebral vessels. Ability to undertake these reflex mechanisms appears during the latter half of gestation in the sheep, long before the fetus is 'viable'. By virtue of those responses to adverse conditions the supply of glucose to the heart and brain and the distribution of the products of anaeroboic glycolysis is made easier. Provided that the blood arterial fetal pH can be maintained at a reasonable level fetal survival will still occur even in the adverse circumstances.

THE EFFECT OF LABOUR ON FETAL BLOOD GASES

It is likely that normal labour has little effect on the oxygen supply to the fetus except perhaps momentarily during second stage contractions. The principle determinant of the effect of such contractions depends on their duration and frequency and on the quantity of oxygen available in the intervillous space blood, on the preceding oxygen status of the fetus and on the rate of oxygen utilization of the fetus itself. Saling (1967) has shown that if one considers only mean changes in scalp blood there is a fall in pO_2 and a rise in pCO_2 by the end of labour. It has, of course, been shown by many previous writers that up to 50 per cent of babies have low blood levels of oxygen in cord vessels at birth and that in 25 per cent the Apgar score is low. Clinical fetal distress will be seen in 6 per cent of women in labour before term and some 12–15 per cent after term.

Studies between animal and human have shown that during or just after a contraction the fetal oxygen levels are lowered. Most babies who are subjected to some lowering of levels can compensate for temporary lowering of available oxygen and do not suffer.

FETAL RISK

There are many factors which may influence the fetal risk in labour:

Maternal hypoxia or hypovolaemia are preventable or correctable states. The mother should never be given a gas mixture to breathe with less than 21 per cent available oxygen or encouraged to hold her breath for long and tense periods in the second stage (nor for that matter should excessive or prolonged panting be encouraged).

Maternal hypotension which is associated with the supine position, with anaesthesia or with haemorrhage, is dangerous but correctable, but may be an unsuspected source of 'fetal distress'.

Fetal cord compression or entanglement with interference with umbilical venous flow will cause an irregularity in fetal heart rate along with bradycardia or tachycardia and, of course, a fall in oxygen levels if the pressure is frequent or prolonged.

The oxygen state of the fetus. There is very little animal experimental evidence of the effect of labour on the already anoxic fetus. Clinically, fetuses from pregnancies where the risk of anoxic death is likely often stand labour badly. It is possible that these fetuses are already close to the limits of their ability to compensate for a deteriorating oxygen supply or in a situation where any further deterioration will be unsupportable. Pregnancies complicated by maternal hypertensive syndromes, antepartum haemorrhage, diabetes or prolonged pregnancy are particularly at risk.

Oxytocin infusion. Oxytocin used in excessive dosage may produce uterine contractions that are too strong or too frequent and produce asphyxial effects on the fetus just as do the excess contractions of natural labour. Moreover such contractions can also produce fetal cerebral damage by an undue drive effect on the head and undue compression as does sudden moulding.

Serious fetal effects do not usually occur until the fetal arterial pO_2 drops from its normal 20-32mmHg to some 10-15mmHg at which time the fetal arterial blood is some 15 per cent saturated. Partial or minor effects may be produced by lesser degrees; such are difficult to measure but most studies suggest a less good oxygen and pH environment in babies delivered after augmented labour.

The fetal heart. Most of the observations made by the expert clinical observer have been quantified and experimentally studied by physiologists. Caldeyro Barcia (1963).

Characteristically the fetal heart shows a 5-7 per cent beat to beat variability in rate and this variability is evidence of normal physiologic control mechanisms. Beat to beat variability is abolished by the application of atropine to the mother which drug also increases the fetal heart rate.

Bradycardia. Continuous monitoring of the fetal heart has shown that sometimes the rate may dip from the normal 140 per minute to below 110 per minute synchronous with the uterine contraction with recovery of rate as the contraction passes off (Type 1 dips). This type of transient bradycardia is due almost always to pressure on the fetal head or to intermittent cord pressure. Mostly it does not result in fetal anoxia and fetal scalp pH is unchanged, but as shown by Walker (1959) and later writers, *prolonged* pressure on head or cord with bradycardia may result in low fetal arterial pO_2.

In other circumstances the fetal heart rate begins to slow as the contraction passes off and the slowing persists for one or more minutes after the contractions has disappeared (Type II dips). This type of bradycardia is due probably to a degree of fetal myocardial anoxia. It is likely a sign of interference with transfer at the placental site and suggestive that the contractions either themselves (or because of a secondary effect on the cord) are interfering with fetal oxygenation. Some 20 type II dips, or situations where 35 per cent of contractions cause type II dips, will cause definite depression in the fetus.

Normally the arterial pO_2 falls during a contraction to reach its lowest some thirty seconds after the peak of the contraction. Only if the pO_2 falls far enough and long enough can the heart rate follow with bradycardia.

Fetal tachycardia with a rate over 155 beats per minute and especially if sustained, is the first sign of lowered fetal oxygenation when inadequate oxygen is available to the mother. When the mother is asked to breath a low oxygen mixture there is a steady rise in fetal heart rate. In babies who are already compromised and already suffering some degree of oxygen defect, the fetal heart rate will fall under such circumstances. This is sometimes used as a test of antenatal fetal compromise. (*See* Chapter 18.)

OTHER EFFECTS

Meconium. Passage of meconium by the fetus is generally accepted as a sign that the fetus is compromised. However, clinically meconium remains in the liquor once passed and may be evidence of old compromise now past. However, if present at all, it must be looked upon as a sign of importance, and must be viewed seriously and further action and investigation initiated.

It is difficult to be certain of the actual immediate physiological or biochemical cause but in general as has been realized for over 100 years it is probably evidence of interference with respiratory interchange. It tends to appear when fetal arterial pO_2 falls. Alone it is a worry, with fetal tachycardia or irregularity or bradycardia it carries serious prognostic significance.

Effects of difficult labour

Persianinov (1967) noted that certainly during the first stage in normal labour fetal cardiac activity undergoes no measurable change, and especially no change during contraction. The heart beat may fall during expulsive pains due to head pressure, and especially in the presence of any degree of disproportion, but also in the more severe situation of maternal straining with undue pressure effects on the placental circulation. Prolonged expulsive pains following each other at short intervals promote undue head pressure and a more marked and prolonged fetal bradycardia which may be in time accompanied by very low pO_2 in the fetal artery since the slowing of the circulation allows a much greater oxygen clearance (Walker, 1959).

Surgical interventions; internal version and breech extraction, the application of forceps, the use of vacuum extractors, all cause reflex changes of the fetal cardiac activity of varying degrees with changes in loudness and duration of sound, appearance of murmurs and disappearance of rhythm. With forceps application there is very strong reaction in fetal cardiac activity in response to the introduction of the blades, and also during the period of traction. There is also some changes in the configuration of the ECG.

Obstetric version, fetal breech extraction, bringing down the fetal leg in an incompletely dilated os, are always accompanied by marked disturbances of cardiac activity at times leading to complete block of the fetal heart.

If therefore, the labour is long, the contractions strong with little rest between, or where there is disproportion due either to pelvic contraction or to fetal malposition, or where fetal malpresentation requires manipulation, then labour may exert many and different effects on the baby.

Perhaps one of the most interesting effects described is that of undue pressure on the fetal head on the perineum. Where the fetal head is allowed to be held up by a rigid and resistant perineum without episiotomy, or where, after delivery, the head is allowed to lie at the vulva waiting for the next pain, there may be a very severe bradycardia associated with marked deoxygenation (Walker, 1959) and sometimes obvious congestion of the fetal head, this is accompanied by difficulty in resuscitation and very real long term effects on child intelligence and behaviour.

The actual damage to the child associated with the techniques and method of delivery has already been described in Chapter 23. The effects of various forms of anaesthesia and drugs on the fetus have been described in Chapter 25.

CORD CLAMPING

If the child is delivered of its mother when squatting the child is persistently below its own placenta and blood cannot run back out of its body by the patent umbilical vein. In clinical practice varying degrees of transfusion of placental blood to the child may occur. The effects of such transfusions have been studied by Yao and Lind (1974) who have reviewed the physiology. They found that (provided the infant is not held above the level of its placenta and provided that the placenta is sited in the upper contractile portion of the uterus) the first placental transfusion of blood occurs with the final contraction which normally expels the child and that little change in the placental transfusion takes place over the next 15–45 seconds. After about 45 seconds, a second contraction occurs expelling the placenta and this greatly increases the transfer of fetal blood and this second transfer occurs earlier and in greater amount where an oxytocic has been given immediately after, or at the time of, birth.

The umbilical arteries normally constrict at about 40–45 seconds and no more blood is pushed out from the baby. However, the umbilical vein remains open and blood can run back to the placenta if the child is held up especially if clamping is unduly delayed. They studied 'early clamping' which is clamping in *less than 30 seconds* after the child is born and 'later clamping' which is at about two minutes or so when the second contraction and the second transfusion has occurred. No relation was found between the amount of placental transfusion and the onset of first breath and first cry or with later baby blood volume or haematocrit.

The 'later clamped' babies suffered from a certain amount of over-transfusion and systolic blood pressures were higher for some 1–3 hours after the baby was born and after that time, fairly marked transudation of plasma out of the circulation occurred. Neither factors were found in the babies clamped round about 25–30 seconds after delivery. Late clamping appeared to produce increased stress to the child. The babies tend to be more sleepy. 'Early clamped' babies, that is where the cord is clamped at about 25–30 seconds after birth are more awake in the first few hours allowing better maternal nursing relationships. They breathe sooner and have less respiratory grunting possibly in view of less transudation of the excess fluid from the pulmonary vessels. They have a higher PO_2 and a lower PCO_2 in the first three hours. Although they have somewhat lower Apgar scores at birth they have a much better nursery course partly because of less distended circulation.

It is, therefore, recommended in general that:

1. The child must not be held above its own placenta.

2. With normal healthy babies (and premature babies who show no difference in their behaviour pattern), the cord should be clamped at about *20–25 seconds* after birth, the child being held at or below the level of its own placenta.

3. If the child is asphyxiated or plethoric with anoxic distress it usually has already a greater blood volume. There is no point in delaying clamping, and the cord should be clamped fairly soon.

4. Where the infant is pale or shocked, it is well worth delaying clamping for 2–3 minutes to allow the second transfer of placental blood if resuscitation can be continued while the child is still attached. If not, the child should be clamped and resuscitated and there may be a point in collecting its own placental blood aseptically for later transfusion.

At birth

Pulmonary maturity

For sometime before or coincident with the onset of labour the fetal lung is stimulated to increase in surfactant production and the fetal adrenal is alerted to meet any demand on it. There seems little doubt that surfactant is more actively present when the onset of labour is spontaneous or labour has in fact taken place. There is still some evidence that while surfactant is largely an age phenomenon a child after elective Caesarean section is more likely to develop respiratory distress.

The fetus is preparing for extra-uterine existence and much of his capability to survive depends on his respiratory function. The developing *lung* is full of *fluid* and during the later part of labour and after the head is born the compression of the thorax allows expression of some of that fluid and helps lung expansion at birth. The remainder of the fluid is removed via pulmonary lymphatics after respiration begins.

OTHER FACTORS

During labour there are many and varied alterations in transfer of nutrients which have been ill explored. It has been shown for example, that the levels of various serum proteins in the newborn depends on whether the child has been delivered before labour, i.e. by elective Caesarean section or when the normal labour has preceded sampling. The finding is particularly true of the broad group of gamma globulins most of which are transferred from the mother and which are much higher in the child born after labour. Other blood constituents of the child may be different after labour.

Endocrine status

The fetus is at the end of labour in a state of potential excitability ready to meet the challenge or accept the stimulus of external factors during and after birth. Certainly after birth the withdrawal of progesterone releases the fetus from the calming effect of that hormone.

Survival in adverse circumstance

The ability of the fetal or newborn mammal to survive long periods of partial asphyxia without brain damage depends in large part on the very large reserves of glycogen in its heart and liver and of course, on the low energy utilization of its brain. The successive relatively short periods of asphyxia which may occur during abnormal labour will however steadily deplete fetal glycogen stores, in both liver and heart, and while this depletion may not have an obviously severe effect on the baby *in utero*, it will tend to lead to fetal hypotonia and neonatal hypoglycaemia, especially in premature infants.

CONDUCT OF LABOUR

Care of the woman in labour may have to be undertaken in bizarre or grossly unsuitable surroundings which might be the normal or usual surroundings in an undeveloped or primitive society. Labour is the subject of many taboos and the customs and beliefs of the patient and her relatives must always be observed. It is obviously, however, the responsibility of the trained attendant to try to alter the circumstances if they are obviously disadvantageous to the patient.

In the advanced countries of Western

Europe and the United States, medical participation in, and responsibility for, labour care is increasing and the midwife is becoming more and more an expert partner. For nearly two-thirds of the world's people the quality of labour care available is frontier in the extreme, and serious damage and death are common.

Labour, which is essentially a period of psychological and physical strain to the mother, and of immense importance to the child, cannot be physiological to the mother who is undergrown, under-nourished, anaemic or diseased, and might be the final insult to a child itself poorly grown and perhaps already infected. It is fortunate for the mother that in the primitive situation the small under-nourished mother often produces prematurely a small undernourished child since an adequately grown child could not be vaginally delivered.

Preparation for childbirth begins when the mother herself is born and requires provision of adequate nutrition, prevention from infection and proper medical care during her growth. If those features can be coupled with public health measures to permit a pure water supply and freedom from epidemic and insect borne disease, the girl should grow well nourished to her full stature. Her pelvis will, with growth, be large and well formed, her uterus and its blood vessels well grown and capable of an adequate response to pregnancy.

Care of the pregnant or labouring mother depends on the quality of organization of care within the community and the provision of the necessary trained personnel—midwives or doctors—to administer such care.

In the clinical situation preparation for labour will begin with the mothers first antenatal visit (which might be already late in the period of gestation).

Attitudes

The attitude of the patient to labour depends on the attitude of her society, her community or group, and especially in some communities on her own experience in serving women in labour. To most women, labour is a natural and necessary part of childbearing, is accepted as likely to be painful but not unbearable and, in the modern world, no longer dangerous. Maternal mortality in England one hundred years ago was six per thousand and it was still at that level in Scotland in 1927. Since then the rate has fallen steadily till its present level of less than three per ten thousand.

However, most women nowadays expect help for their labour and certainly all should have such help. The type of help she wishes is firstly the presence of an intelligent sympathetic attendant, who will be with her, talk to her, and relieve her from undue discomfort. She wishes also the assurance that skilled help will be at hand for her and for her child, if needed. Most of the fear of childbirth is fear that she will be left alone, that the pain will be unbearable, that she will not have help immediately or that she and her child will suffer.

It is becoming more and more expected that the wife will request the presence of her husband with her in labour and sometimes even at delivery. The motivation here, especially of the husband, is sometimes difficult to unravel but many women obtain security and comfort from their husbands presence and many husbands experience a new dimension which may bind the marriage. The fashion is probably to be accepted and should be welcomed if both earnestly request it.

In general, the woman in labour should not be left alone except perhaps when she needs the peace of early sedation; certainly not at all when she is in late labour, having real discomfort, or of course, under oxytocin stimulation. In general the continuous presence of an intelligent attendant minimizes the need for early sedation and reinforces the efficacy of planned sedation later. Some form of additional pain relief should always be available and commonly used.

The woman should always have her labour and delivery in a place where her total forseeable labour care is possible. In other words, if she is in premature labour she should, if possible, be delivered where facilities are available to care for her baby (in other words, move the mother in labour rather than the baby afterwards).

If antenatal care has suggested that labour might be difficult or in some other way hazardous to mother or child, labour should always be arranged in the requisite place.

PREPARATION FOR LABOUR

In the last 20 years an increasing number of women in all countries have been provided with, and have elected to utilize, expert antenatal care and hospital or delivery centre for delivery. There are however, many situations where delivery in the patient's own home is essential, indicated or desired. It is customary however, in most advanced societies now to select out those cases suitable for home confinement rather than, as previously, select out abnormal patients for hospital.

The patient's home

Inadequate housing is a clear deterrent to home confinement. The minimum requirements for home confinement are that the patient should have a bed and preferably also a room to herself. The house should have preferably inside sanitation and a safe water supply. Care should be taken to see that no obvious source of infection is overlooked, such as acute or severe chronic pyogenic infection in any member of the household.

The room

If any choice is available the room chosen should be reasonably spacious, well lit and ventilated.

If possible, the room should be prepared in advance, by cleaning and the removal of unnecessary furnishing and hangings which harbour dust. One large table for basins and two smaller tables are required. If labour comes on unexpectedly before the room has been cleaned it is better to leave it undisturbed to avoid stirring up dust, and to cover with clean dust-sheets. The carpet should be protected by sheets of plastic sheeting or glazed brown paper under, and a yard beyond, the near side of the bed.

The bed

A single bed, not too low and not too narrow, is best. Most mattresses tend to sag when the patient lies on them. This can be overcome by slipping a board 4 feet by 2 feet over the sides of the bed-frame and under the mattress at the level of the patient's pelvis. It should of course, be removed as soon as the delivery is completed.

It is important that the bed be placed so as to be in a good light both by day and by night, and to give easy access to both sides.

Fresh laundered sheets and clean blankets should be used. A large impervious sheet should be placed next to the mattress. Over

this a sheet is placed, and over it polythene sheeting projecting beyond the near edge of the bed and covered by a draw-sheet. Sheets of clean brown paper or newspaper may have to be substituted.

Bath

Ideally the patient should have a shower at the onset of labour but if shower equipment is not available she should be washed in the kneeling position to prevent water entering the vagina. This is essential if the membranes have ruptured.

Evacuation of bowels

It is very important that the lower bowel should be well emptied early in labour. Suppositories are used but probably the most effective method is to use a disposable enema package with nozzle. This contains sodium diphosphate 10g, sodium phosphate 8g, distilled water 9g. Unless there is likely to be time for the enema to act completely it is better omitted.

Clothing

The clothing of the patient should consist of a short easily laundered nightdress. The gown is tucked up to the waist when the patient goes to bed during the second and third stages of labour. Clean clothing put on after the labour is completed.

ACTION EARLY IN LABOUR

If the patient has been adequately instructed in the antenatal period she will call the midwife or doctor or come into hospital whenever she feels that labour has begun or if there is bleeding, show, or loss of liquor. When called the midwife or practitioner should proceed to assess the situation as soon as reasonably possible. When the patient arrives in hospital assessment is made immediately.

The antenatal record is checked to ensure that there are no features for special care, and antenatally recorded instructions are carefully noted, e.g. 'consider elective Caesarean section': 'husband wishes to be present': 'for PPS', etc. It is quite essential that at first examination in labour special care is taken and positive decisions are made to define the range of care likely to be needed in the individual labour. Special decisions are made in the abnormal or unusual situation—e.g. *primigravidae* are likely to require operative delivery in up to 25 per cent of cases, cases of breech or other malpresentation, multiple pregnancy, associated medical disease, etc., are likely to need the presence of an anaesthetist and/or a paediatrician at delivery, blood may need to be available or other special drugs needed.

The patient is then questioned on the time and onset of painful contractions, their frequency. She is asked about show, or bleeding, or leaking of liquor. Her general condition is noted, her pulse, blood pressure and temperature taken, her urine checked for albumin, sugar and acetone. The size, lie, presentation of the baby and position of the presenting part are noted and the fetal heart located and the rate counted.

MANAGEMENT OF NORMAL LABOUR

Normal labour as defined earlier (p. 319) is smooth and there is steady progress. The difference between the primigravidae and the multigravidae is essentially one of time in all all stages though some primigravidae have shorter and easier labours than some multigravidae.

ANTISEPSIS AND ASEPSIS
As a rule, in cases of severe infection the pathogenic organism is derived from the doctor, midwife or someone else in contact with the patient, and may be introduced by the fingers during swabbing or a vaginal examination. The hands must therefore be thoroughly washed before the patient is touched. Since clothing may also be a source of infection, sterile or at least freshly laundered gowns and sheets must also be used. At the same time, since the vulva and vagina cannot be rendered sterile, reliance must also be placed on the use of antiseptic creams and lotions.

Infection is therefore prevented or minimized by the exclusion of possible carriers and the wearing of masks and of the use of sterile gowns, gloves and dressings, masks and antiseptic lotions and creams.

CLEANSING OF THE VULVA
The vulva, perineum, pubis and inside of the thighs are much more difficult to keep clean than almost any other area of the body. Most of the organisms present on the skin and anal region are of low virulence and unlikely to cause serious infection unless laceration of tissues allows entry, so that normal confinements carried out in poor home conditions are not likely to result in severe infection unless virulent organisms are introduced from outside. The use of sterilized instruments and gloves and plenty of antiseptic of adequate strength are the most important means of preventing puerperal infection. It is still customary to shave the vulva and wash down with soap and water. The patient should be told to avoid touching the vulva with her hands. This might be very dangerous if she had an upper respiratory tract infection when haemolytic streptococci might be transferred direct to the vagina.

During labour, pledgets of wool soaked in antiseptic lotions may be used to wipe away discharge. These pledgets should be drawn only from before backwards to avoid bringing infection forwards from the anus. Before vaginal examination or other manipulation, the vulva and inside of the thighs should be again cleansed.

MASKS
Masks should be worn by doctors and midwives, but they must be used with intelligence if they are not to become an additional source of infection. *They are worn only when the vulva is exposed*, that is for catheterization and during the delivery of the child and when sterile equipment (dressing or instruments) is being set out. Once it has been applied the mask should not be touched. When being removed it should be handled by the tapes and dropped into an antiseptic solution in a container. It should never hang round the neck or be carried in the pocket. A large supply should be kept outside the door of the labour room and before each episode of use examined a fresh one should be donned. Masks are now made of paper, and therefore supplied in large numbers and should be changed frequently and not worn for periods of more than one hour.

DIET
The problem of food intake during labour is a difficult one. On the one hand it is important that intake of calories and of fluid should be adequate. On the other hand digestion in the stomach is often delayed, and if an anaesthetic

is required there may be difficulty and danger from vomiting with the grave risk of aspiration pneumonia. In normal cases, that is to say, if the patient is unlikely to require a general anaesthetic, the following regime may be found suitable.

Give fruit juice and/or water on locker.
Provide a plastic drinking straw to allow patient to drink with minimum effort.

Breakfast
Tea, toast (thinly cut and lightly buttered; 'jelly' marmalade), lightly boiled egg if patient wishes it.

Lunch
1. Strained chicken broth or tomato juice.
2. Sieved meat or fish which contains no fat, no stringy vegetables.
3. Sieved fruits—apple, banana, pear, peach. N.B. no citrus fruits.

Supper
Tea, toast, as for breakfast. Lightly boiled egg if patient wishes it. Milk and ice-cream are apt to form a tough curd and are best avoided.

In those likely to require a general anaesthetic the intake should be restricted to the following:
1. When early in labour:
   Strained chicken soup, sieved fruit.
   Tea, toast and lightly boiled egg, fruit juice.
2. When labour is well established:
   Stop all fluids by mouth and give:
   a. Mouth washes
   b. Ice and/or barley sugar to suck
   c. Magnesium trisilicate, 1 teaspoonful every two hours. (This is given with a view to neutralizing the acid gastric secretion).

An intravenous drip containing dextrose 4·3 per cent and sodium chloride 0·18 per cent or dextrose 5 per cent is necessary when inadequate fluid can be given by mouth and certainly in late labour.

BLADDER
During labour the bladder is drawn up into the abdomen, and even when it contains as little as 3 or 4 ounces of urine it can be seen as a swelling above the pubes. When full it might possibly prevent engagement of the head and may cause the uterine contractions to be poor. Before the head descends deeply into the pelvis the patient is usually able to empty her bladder and should be encouraged to do so. A bed-pan is most uncomfortable for the pregnant woman, especially in labour, and a commode placed beside her bed is much more suitable, or easy access to a toilet. She should empty the bladder at not more than three-hourly intervals and the urine should be measured and tested for sugar, albumin and acetone on each occasion. Catheterization may be necessary. Later, especially when she is unable to get out of bed because of the effect of sedatives, also when the head is deeply engaged, catheterization will be necessary. If the head is deeply engaged it may be necessary to push it back and up slightly by means of a finger in the vagina before the catheter can be passed. A metal catheter is often best but force should not be used because of the risk of damage to the urethra.

REST AND SLEEP
Every effort should be made to see that the patient gets sleep at night especially in very early or doubtful labour and much can be done by simple measures to facilitate this. A light meal should be given and the bladder emptied. If the bed is comfortable, the room darkened and quiet and the patient reassured and given a mild sedative then sleep will often follow. Mogadon (Nitrazepam) or Valium (Diazepam) are suggested.

COMFORT AND CLEANLINESS
The patient's morale will be greatly helped if attention is paid to personal toilet. She should have her face and hands washed at intervals and her hair combed and brushed. Washing of the buttocks and thighs with changing of soiled sheets and clothing will add greatly to comfort. Showers can be taken in the first stage.

OBSTETRIC CARE
In the early part of the first stage, the mother should be encouraged to move about, to busy herself with minor tasks, knit or watch television. She usually best adjusts herself to the discomfort of the contractions and may close her eyes, breathe deeply or relax totally depending on her attitude or training. As soon as the discomfort becomes real, sedation is needed, the membranes rupture, or she has a pressure deep in her pelvis she should be in bed with a constant attendant.

Modern labour care involves routine *assessment* of the progress of labour and constant monitor of the wellbeing of the child. Such monitoring may, as we will later discuss, be done routinely (or only in special cases) by electronic instrumentation, but nevertheless in simple routine practice especially in the normal case there is no reason to expect that expert monitoring cannot be achieved by clinical means, but the checks must be carefully and regularly performed.

CONTRACTIONS

The strength and frequency of the contractions should be checked by abdominal palpation and the frequency and duration of each recorded. Contractions are felt by the patient for only a part of the duration of the contraction, but as labour progresses become steadily longer, more frequent and stronger the uterus standing out hard against the examining hand. The quality and success of the contractions can be judged by the constant change in their character. As the labour progresses and the head sinks deeper in the pelvis there may be constant backache associated with pelvic stretching and sacral joint tilting. As the second stage approaches the contractions are most painful and often most frequent. Just after full dilatation the head reaches the pelvic floor and the patient has an intense desire to 'push' as the head presses on the pelvic floor muscles. Strong voluntary abdominal muscle effort often with breath holding the flexion of the legs accompanies the latter part of the second stage.

ANALGESIA

Chapter 24 is an essential part of good labour care. Relief from pain is now a right but total relief from all discomfort is not necessarily desirable or possible. The need for excessive sedation to the detriment of the fetus is limited to a very few unusual situations. Epidural anaesthesia has offered new possibilities of total relief from pain.

ASSESSMENT OF THE MOTHER

Regular checks of the maternal condition should be made. At the onset of labour basal maternal pulse rate, temperature and blood pressure should be recorded and urine checked for albumin, sugar and acetone bodies. Throughout labour temperature should be recorded at least four hourly and always if fetal tachycardia occurs. All urine specimens should be checked. Maternal blood may require to be taken for crossmatching, for check-ing Rhesus antibodies, for elective tests for research purposes. Pulse and blood pressure should be taken very frequently.

Pelvic examination

Examination by the vagina is an essential part of the conduct of any labour and certainly should be done in the normal case whenever labour is clearly established and when the first sedation is required. In many cases several examinations will be necessary to define the pattern of labour and are an essential part of modern techniques of monitoring (Chapter 18). Properly performed vaginal examination is not dangerous and is probably less hazardous than rectal examination. The examination should be preceded by cleansing of the perineum and buttocks, washout of vagina with antiseptic lotion and draping with a sterile towel and an antiseptic cream should be freely used. (Rectal examination with a clean glove may occasionally help in assessment of descent of the head.)

Pelvic examination in labour is used to assess the progress of the labour but full information is obtained only if certain clear routines are followed.

The experienced examiner usually makes a composite examination of pelvis; cervix, and fetus in a routine developed by himself but he should record his findings under headings.

Pelvis

Shape, size of pubic arch, prominence of spines, length of sacro sciatic ligament, space in mid cavity, diagonal conjugate if head high, prominence of upper sacrum, and degree of forward protrusion of sacral tip and coccyx. In general in labour the cavity and outlet are easily assessed and the head may be the best pelvimeter for brim and upper pelvis.

The cervix

The position, the effacement (sometimes recorded as whether or not the cervix is 'taken up' into the lower uterine segment) and the degree of dilatation, in centimetres, is noted. A fully effaced cervix i.e. flush with the lower uterine cervix may not yet be dilated but in a multigravida a partially effaced cervix may be distinctly dilated.

In general in early labour the cervix is at least beginning to dilate and is partly taken up further and dilatation is steady, slow, till about 2–3cm, and fast thereafter.

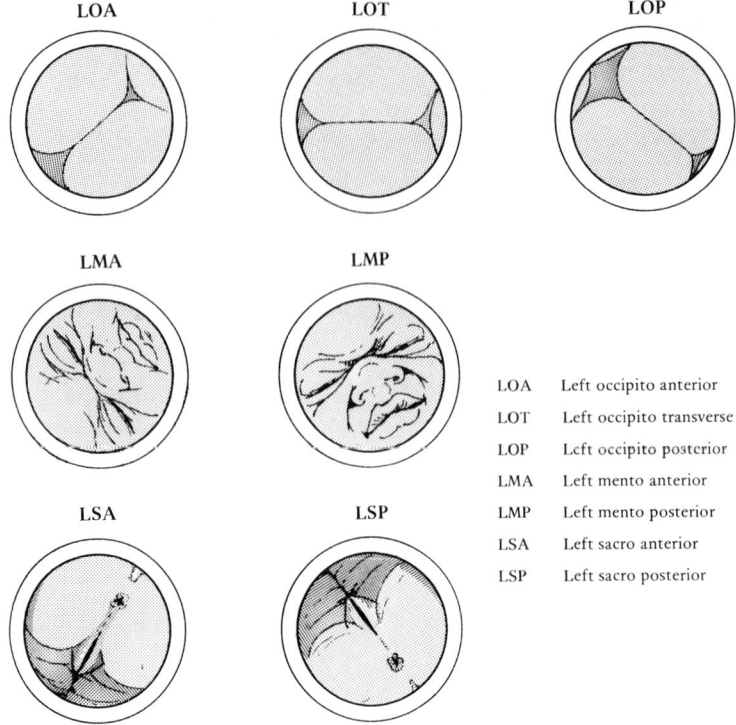

LOA	Left occipito anterior
LOT	Left occipito transverse
LOP	Left occipito posterior
LMA	Left mento anterior
LMP	Left mento posterior
LSA	Left sacro anterior
LSP	Left sacro posterior

Fig. 19.7   The areas palpated by the examining fingers in various positions and presentations.

The membranes
Intact or ruptured, as a thin film over the presenting part or as a large fluid filled bag (*see* Chapter 9).

The presenting part
Should be identified by the touch picture (*see* Fig. 19.7). Presentation has of course, been also determined on abdominal examination but is confirmed on pelvic examination and the actual position determined. Unusual situations like a presenting or prolapsed cord or a compound presentation of vertex with a hand or foot may be discovered.

The station
Degree of descent is determined in relation to the ischial spines (Fig. 19.8). When the leading part of the head is at the spines this is station O and distance above or below the spines may be recorded in centimetres or preferably as −1,2,3 or +1,2,3, or sometimes in other arbitrary divisions. Unless there is undue moulding or a particularly shallow pelvis (e.g. in the rachitic pelvis) the head at O or +1 station is usually engaged, i.e. the greatest diameter is through the pelvic brim. This is not necessarily so in face or brow presentation.

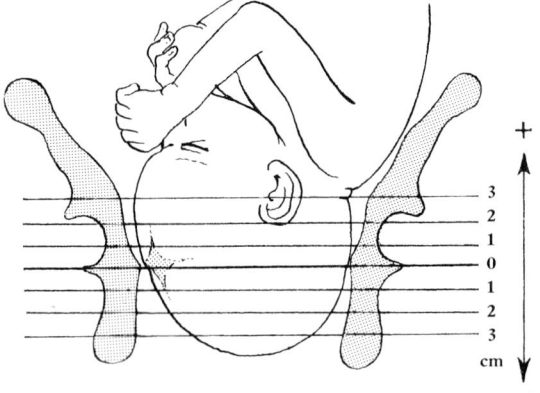

Fig. 19.8   Method of recording the degree of descent of the head in the pelvis.

Caput and degree of moulding
Caput is a measure of soft tissue resistance largely from the cervix and may seriously obscure land marks or confuse the assessment of the degree of descent.

Moulding
Moulding is due to a mixture of soft tissue and bony pressures and is in part a measure of the

points to the symphysis. At this stage the head may be easily felt under the symphysis but the leading part is well back and the cavity of the sacrum is empty. *At this level the head is not to be delivered from below.* As the head descends it fills the cavity of the sacrum and in the mid pelvis when the leading part has reached the spines, or a little below, the head points straight at the operator. This is the situation of most OP and transverse arrests and the head may be delivered by forceps after rotation but often with difficulty. As the head descends further it starts to point more and more upwards (Fig. 19.10). By the time the head is

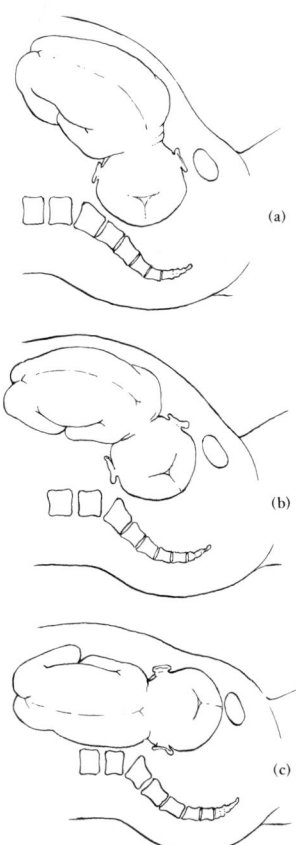

Fig. 19.9 The various inclinations of the head in asynclitism. (a) anterior parietal, (b) normal, (c) posterior parietal presentation.

degree of disproportion though obviously also of the force of the contractions and the ability of the head to mould. A seriously moulded head with palpable overlap of bones and obscured fontanelles will, depending, on its station and direction be an indication of undue disproportion and prove very difficult to deliver vaginally.

The direction of the head

The actual direction in which the head is apparently pointing is an excellent guide to its level within the canal and also the ease or otherwise of forceps delivery. Assessment of direction may be confused by asynclitism but this must be remembered when the head is high (*see* Fig. 19.9).

When the head is engaging and the greatest diameter is not yet through the brim the head clearly points backwards, an anterior parietal presentation exaggerates this and posterior obscures this, since then the head apparently

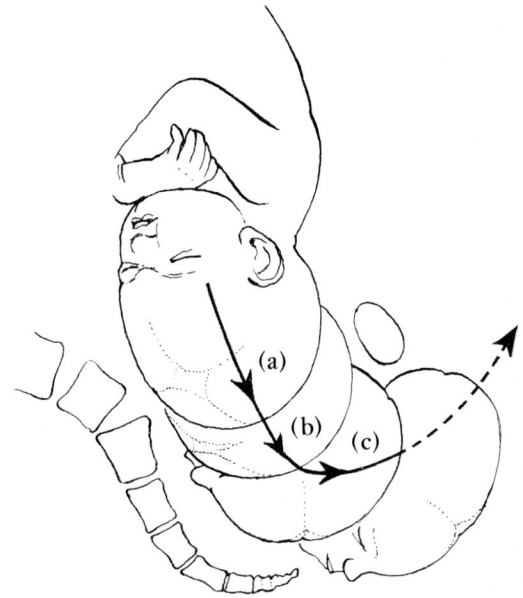

Fig. 19.10 The different 'directions' of the head as it descends through the pelvis. (a) High, (b) Mid, (c) Outlet.

on the outlet in the low forceps position it is clearly pointing up and forwards.

ASSESSMENT OF THE FETUS

During the antenatal period the wellbeing of the fetus will have been assessed and at the time of onset of labour the likely degree of risk should be known (Chapter 18). Where labour is likely to be mechanically difficult for the child or distressing to the mother an added degree of risk can be considered present.

Where the risk is seriously present then all modern techniques of monitoring should be available and used as discussed in Chapter 18.

The fetal heart rate is the most reliable guide to the state of the fetus and certainly before rupture of the membranes normally the only guide. The fetal heart should be listened to regularly during labour and certainly after each pain in the late first and second stage.

The modern practice of conducting labour with the patient lying on her left side makes auscultation of the heart difficult and the patient may well have to be in many cases turned on her back. This is where the use of some of the modern devices e.g. sonicaid and other instruments working on the Doppler principle have proved useful, but there is no reason why the patient cannot be regularly turned on to her back so that the fetal heart can be properly listened to.

During the early part of labour the fetal heart will normally run between 120 and 140 beats per minute, the regular beat to beat variation is not normally easily noticeable on auscultation but the regularity of mean rate is basal and uniform. During the ordinary contraction of the first stage and even of the early second stage there is no change in the fetal heart rate although the heart may be difficult to hear at the height of a contraction. If there is pressure on the fetal head or if there is interference with cord circulation, slowing of the fetal heart may occur at the time of the contraction and coincident with it. The rate may drop as low as 80 beats per minute. Normally where the bradycardia is due to head pressure the heart rate returns rapidly to normal, almost before the contraction has completely passed off—the so-called Type I dip. This is fully discussed in Chapter 18. When the pressure on the head is rather more severe or there is serious interference with cord function, and having a further effect on oxygenation the fetal heart fails to pick up at the end of the contraction and only very slowly returns to normal. There is also a slowing which begins with the height of the contraction and continues for sometime afterwards—the so-called Type II dip.

In addition to the more typical slowing of the fetal heart, irregularity of rate and rhythm is seen fairly frequently when there is interference with cord circulation (cord round the neck, cord tanglement). A pattern of trills of rapid beats followed by slow beats is fairly typical of this problem.

Tachycardia
Increase in heart rate is the first response to interference with fetal oxygenation. The rise is usually steady to about 160 beats per minute and is maintained as a basal tachycardia between contractions. Fetal tachycardia often precedes the serious bradycardia of anoxia, but also is seen in the cord entanglement. It is false evidence of fetal distress in the presence of maternal pyrexia, and in the presence of a rapid fetal heart the maternal temperature should always be taken. Fetal tachycardia may also be the only evidence of intra-uterine fetal infection.

In the older texts it is advised that the fetal heart should be listened to only between contractions since slowing which may occur with the contraction is not of itself significant. This is to a large extent true if one is assessing the degree of fetal anoxia, since the pressure associated with slowing limited to the contractions (is Type I dips) does not interfere with fetal oxygenation unless the pressure is unduly prolonged and in that case the heart rate fails to recover quickly.

In the risk baby, it has been recommended that in late pregnancy and certainly in early labour, examination of the *state of the liquor* should be made by amnioscope through the cervix. This is to exclude the presence of meconium staining or to detect the presence of meconium as an index of interference with fetal respiratory interchange.

Once the membranes rupture of course, the presence of meconium is usually obvious, but it is to be remembered in the late first stage especially that the head is often firmly jammed against the cervix and deep in the pelvis and any meconium passed is locked into the hindwaters only. The absence of meconium in this situation cannot be taken as evidence that no meconium is being passed. The significance of meconium is always difficult to interpret. It is clearly accepted by most workers as a sign of some loss of fetal status, probably associated with interference with respiratory interchange. Meconium alone without any alteration in fetal heart rate or regularity is significant but probably does not justify serious action, except in the high risk baby or in the premature baby or in the baby of the elderly primigravida who is not yet in labour. Meconium before the onset of labour or early in labour is clearly worrying, especially where labour is likely to be long or difficult. Meconium associated with alteration in fetal heart rate is clearly a sign requiring action. This is more fully discussed in Chapter 18, page 306.

In general the first stage should be conducted in an atmosphere of happy anticipation. The patient should be allowed to move about early on, once the membranes have ruptured or if there is discomfort and sedation is required she should be allowed to rest in bed and most of the time being on her left side. This is usually more comfortable, it tends to improve the quality of the contractions and also lessens the risk of a supine hypotension. The quality and nature of the pains is recorded and the fetal heart auscultated, the maternal state is constantly monitored, the fluid and certainly glucose intake are regularly maintained. Sedation is given as and when indicated and the progress of the labour are regularly assessed. As has been outlined early in this chapter, it is to be expected that in the primigravida, the first stage of labour would take something from 10-12 hours and in the multipara perhaps from 4-8 hours. If labour is progressing normally over these relatively short spaces of time, the serious discomfort of the late first stage is approached fairly rapidly, but the patient by this time will still be in very good condition and not exhausted. Normal labour is a tiring but not an exhausting experience. By the late first stage the discomfort is becoming more real, the head is beginning to descend usually deeply into the pelvis (although in some multipara it is still high until almost or nearly full dilatation), and it is at this stage that support from an adequate and intelligent attendant, adequate sedation and encouragement are probably most important. At this stage it is often likely that the earlier sedation of pethidine or other drugs of this type is wearing off, and that we can bring in the use of the nitrous oxide oxygen analgesics, which also provide adequate oxygenation to the baby.

Deterioration in the maternal condition is usually heralded by a rising maternal pulse (the maternal pulse rate does not normally rise in labour except occasionally at the height of a contraction). Vomiting and the restlessness with some oliguria and acetonuria are evidence that the mother is having a stressful labour.

Management of the second stage

To the experienced practitioner or midwife the onset of the second stage is clearly obvious in the general pattern of behaviour of the patient. There is an increase in intensity of the contractions and increasing backache, and a general attitude of frustration on the part of the patient until the cervix is fully dilated and the head begins to descend. Second stage contractions (in other words those associated with bearing down), increase in 'show', perhaps a little bleeding from the fully dilated cervix, and the patient with a feeling of fullness and tenseness in the area of the rectum, are evidence that the second stage is well established and appears perhaps 15-20 minutes after full cervical dilatation. In most labours the membranes rupture just before the onset of the second stage, but in many instances of course, rupture has taken place long before, and in others the membranes bulge as a large bag in front of the baby's head and sometimes the child is actually born with the forewaters intact.

Coincident with the onset of the second stage, careful records of fetal heart should be taken as at this stage sudden distress due to either undue pressure or to cord prolapse may occur. It is probably wise to undertake a pelvic examination if the membranes rupture at this time as occasionally hidden prolapse of the cord may occur. If the head is deeply engaged in the pelvis at the time of the apparent appearance of second stage contractions and the patient has a strong desire to 'bear down', this usually means that the cervix is fully dilated and the head is pressing on the pelvic floor. Occasionally however, especially in primigravida, with an elongated head, and sometimes in multigravida who have been taught to bear down in previous labours, apparent second stage bearing down contractions occur before the cervix is fully dilated. If there is any doubt that there is full dilatation or if the head fails to appear fairly quickly following the onset of 'second stage' contractions then pelvic examination ought to be made. Occasionally in the primigravida the lower segment is thinned out over the head and the cervix is a small 1cm dilated dimple somewhere at the apex. This then would indicate an inert labour state and would be treated by heavy sedation and the patient allowed to progress somewhat later.

Bearing down efforts are usually reflex and spontaneous in the second stage of labour. It is questionable whether they should be over encouraged especially where the patient herself does not have a strong desire to bear down. Traditionally the patient is expected to hyperflex her legs which has the effect of improving the dimensions of the outlet and to take a deep breath, usually of an analgesic mixture with the first feeling of the contraction or even to be encouraged so to do by the midwife palpating the abdomen. Two or three quick breaths of analgesic are taken and then the patient encouraged to hold her breath and bear down strongly with the height of the contraction. This type of encouragement and coaching is often helpful but such extra effort should be of relatively short duration, should certainly be intermittent. A careful record should be kept of the fetal heart between expulsive efforts. It is often more advisable to consider a lift-out forceps delivery rather than have unduly prolonged expulsive efforts in the second stage.

As the head descends through the pelvis small particles of faeces are frequently expelled and these should be sponged off with fresh pledglets of wool soaked in antiseptic solutions and at this point when the vulva is exposed all attendants should be properly gowned, masked and those directly handling the mother should of course, be fully equipped with sterile gowns and gloves.

By the time the head has reached just below the spines preparatory to moving upwards and forwards it should be visible in the mid cavity at the height of the contraction—a small area about 2·5cm across. At this time the head is still in the mid cavity and may still fail to progress. With each contraction more and more of the head should be seen, the perineum should begin to stretch, the anterior aspect of the anal canal to bulge and be exposed, the anus forming a D shape, and as the head comes forward there is increasing stretching of the perineum especially in the primigravida. In the multigravida especially where previous adequate episiotomy and repair have not been done, the head usually delivers fairly easily through the gaping vulva, but in the primigravida and in the multigravida with a previous adequate episiotomy a serious degree of perineal stretching can occur. The need for episiotomy depends firstly on the age of the patient. In relatively young primigravida the perineum usually stretches fairly smoothly and evenly without damage but certainly in primigravida over twenty-five and in multigravida with previous episiotomies a repeat episiotomy is advisable to maintain the integrity of the pelvic floor and prevent undue stretching or undue tearing. The technique of episiotomy is fully described in Chapter 27.

In British obstetrics in general the patient is not usually put into lithotomy position with stirrups for routine normal delivery. She is delivered either in the dorsal position or fairly often in the left lateral position. This second position has much to command it in view of its lesser risk of supine hypotension. In the dorsal position however, it is simpler and easier to control the head and to assess the general progress of the delivery and the position tends to be more frequently used. The risks of supine hypotension have however to be remembered.

PREPARATION FOR DELIVERY

In the primigravida delivery is imminent once the head can be seen to be coming on to the pelvic floor, with a slight advance movement with each contraction. In the primigravida as soon as the second stage appears or even late in the first, full preparation should be made for delivery since in many instances progress from 4–5cm dilatation can be very rapid indeed. Advance preparations will have been made to receive the child and for the presence of an anaesthetist or a paediatrician as likely to be necessary. The child's cot would be at the ready, blanket warmed, resuscitation equipment available. In almost all multigravida and the majority of primigravida spontaneous delivery is to be expected. Older primigravida and multigravida with previous episiotomy are likely to require episiotomy or low forcep delivery. Undue insistence on spontaneous delivery is a mistake but it is difficult to insist on expedition forceps delivery where the practitioner or midwife are not experienced. Since episiotomy is now a routine in most primigravida and in multigravida where there has been a previous episiotomy or where there is an unduly large child, perineal laceration to any extent is uncommon.

PERINEAL LACERATION

The causes of such lacerations are usually (1) disproportion between the size of the head and the soft tissue outlet, and (2) too rapid expulsion of the head due, either to very strong pains or to undue exhortation on the part of the attendant, and (3) a somewhat tight and rigid perineum which fails to stretch easily.

In general it is to be hoped that the perineum will stretch easily and allow delivery of the head.

The delivery of a smaller diameter of the head can be assisted by avoiding undue extension of the head until the occiput is clear of the undersurface of the arch and the biparietal diameter has passed through the vulva. This can be attained by some degree of pressure with the left hand of the operator on the head as it begins to extend.

It is important to realize that the mechanism of labour includes intermittent pains and the intermittent pressure on the perineum allows normally some degree of stretching without undue risk of tearing.

Once the head is nearly born (the biparietal diameter just about through the vulva), it is quite important to stop any secondary efforts on the part of the patient and to encourage her to pant with the contractions. The obstetrician should gently deliver the head with a mild expulsive effort on the part of the patient between contractions. This allows the possibility of the head being guided through the vulva. The head should be allowed to come up to crowning gradually. If unduly slowly an episiotomy would be wise and the head delivered between contractions by a moderate push from the patient.

As soon as the head is born a finger should be passed up round the child's neck to search for a loop of the umbilical cord. If present, the loop should be gently drawn down and passed over the head from the occiput towards the face, or sufficiently loosened to allow the child's head to pass through. If the cord is too tight to permit movement then the cord should be cut between two pairs of artery forceps. If this is necessary however, care should be taken to deliver the child moderately quickly.

At this time the child's eyes should be cleansed (if possible before they open), by wiping with a sterile swab to remove discharge.

The delivery of the shoulders requires as much care as that of the head. The anterior shoulder delivered with the first contractions after the head, should be assisted by downward and backward traction on the head which is held between the flat of the hands or with one hand on the occiput and the other under the chin (see Fig. 19.11). If there is any delay at all, then the child should be delivered by traction and perhaps by some assistance with fundal pressure. In the occasional case with the large child, where there is some shoulder dystocia, then it is advisable to put the patient into lithotomy position over the side of the bed or alternatively into the left lateral position,

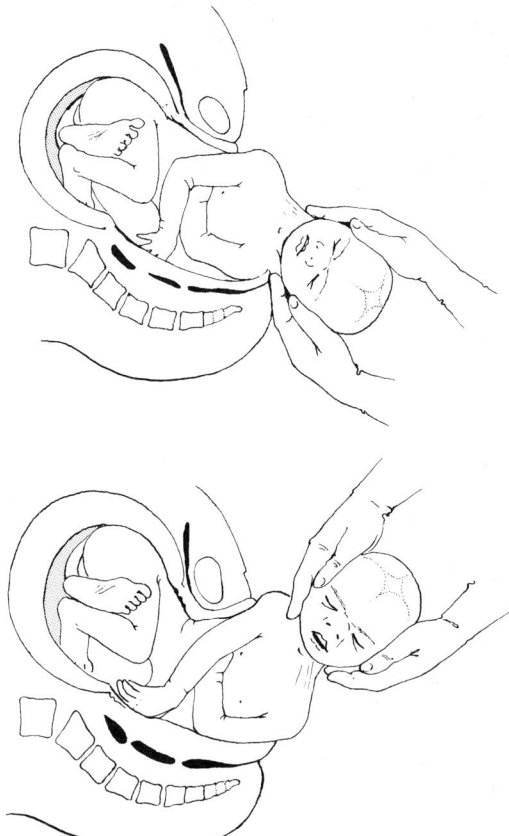

Fig. 19.11   Techniques of delivery of the shoulders.

this is followed quickly by an episiotomy and then the anterior shoulder delivered by strong downward and backward traction and once the anterior shoulder is delivered, the posterior shoulder by sweeping the head up over the perineum. Fundal pressure will help in the difficult situation.

With the delivery of the anterior shoulder, syntometrine is given intramuscularly. If the patient has been delivered in the left lateral position she should be rolled on to her back for the *third stage*.

THE BABY

If the child's face and eyes have been wiped just after the head is delivered there is no need for any special care of the face at this time as there will be no loose mucus or meconium to impede adequate respiration. It is usual to suck out the mouth and naso pharynx. The child should be left on the bed fractionally lower than the uterus and the placenta so that it can receive some transfusion of placental blood as the placenta separates and the uterus contracts. It is probably embarrassing to the child's physiology to milk the blood from the placenta or to lower the child much below maternal level to allow excess of placental blood to drain. The physiology of early and late clamping and the effects on the child are discussed earlier on page 331. In the normal circumstance the child should begin to breathe and perhaps to cry within 10–15 seconds of actual delivery. It often starts by stretching and extending its legs and arms, and provided the airway is clear respiration should start.

It is good practice to leave the separation of the cord until such times as crying has occurred or breathing is established.

If, after 30 seconds or so, it is not clear that the child is going to cry or breathe spontaneously, or if it is obviously unduly blue or unduly pale, then cord separation should be undertaken and full resuscitation as discussed in Chapter 23, instituted.

CLAMPING OF THE CORD

The cord should be occluded by two clamps placed together about 6 inches from the child's umbilicus and perhaps in modern practice by a third plastic clamp within about quarter to half an inch from the umbilicus itself (the cord being finally trimmed). The initial separation can take place between the first two metal clamps. In the absence of clamps there is no reason why the cord should not be tied off, but it must be tied in at least two places.

If the child's condition is satisfactory it is wrapped in a warm flannel or a towel and put into its cot.

In hospital some technique of identification of the baby is essential and the modern system of plastic bands round an arm and a leg is probably the best method. This must be done while the child is still in the delivery room with the mother and of course, labels should be previously prepared.

Cord blood samples for Coombs and other testing are best taken from the placenta.

Management of the third stage

There are two accepted simple techniques of third stage management and both will be described.

At this time the perineum and vagina should be inspected for laceration. In the majority of primigravidae there will be some minor tearing and certainly if there is an episiotomy there may be some extension, especially after difficult delivery. The suture of the laceration and/or episiotomy is as described in Chapter 27. Where local infiltration anaesthesia has been used for episiotomy then a little extra to the skin edges may be necessary for the repair. It is probably wise to omit repair of the perineum especially in the primigravidae until after the placenta is delivered, but any bleeding from the tear or episiotomy could be dealt with during the waiting period.

In some primigravidae the cervix is lacerated even when labour has been normal and certainly after forceps or other operative delivery inspection of the cervix should be routine.

The third stage was in the past (and still can occasionally be) the most dangerous stage because of the risk of sudden and uncontrolled bleeding. The disappearance of long, difficult and exhausting labour and of deep anaesthesia with ether or chloroform and with the automatic use of syntometrine in the latter part of the delivery process, has greatly minimized the chance of severe haemorrhage.

Separation of the uterus from the placenta depends on regular contractions and after separation firm contraction of the interlaced muscle prevents bleeding from the open sinuses at the placental site. The placenta usually separates with the first contraction after the child is expelled, and sometimes is already beginning to separate as the body is passing through the birth canal. Syntometrine should encourage this process and quite often the placenta will be separated within a minute or two of the actual birth of the child. At the first part of its separation, either under the influence of the syntometrine or normally, the placenta remains in the body of the uterus, and only after a variable time is expelled from the fundus into the vagina and the signs of so-called separation appear. Those are fresh bleeding, rising of the fundus into the abdomen above the placenta, the fundus becoming narrower and harder and some of the cord slips out of the vaginia.

In the first technique the separation and expulsion is allowed to occur spontaneously under observation, either visually or with a hand on the abdomen to guard the fundus and prevent it filling. The danger is that there may be interference with the fundus in an attempt to rush the separation process. If during the waiting period there should be trickle of blood from the uterus, this means that some placental separation is taking place, it may mean that the placenta is already separated. In the absence of clear signs of separation, very gentle finger tip massage of the uterus should encourage it to firm up and stop the bleeding, but only if the bleeding is unduly excessive should action be taken to remove the placenta expeditiously. Once the placenta is obviously separated and expelled into the lower segment and with the appearance of the signs of 'separation', the patient may be asked to bear down. The fundus of the uterus can be used as a piston to expel the placenta from the upper vagina and lower segment and this expulsion can be assisted by gentle cord traction. The danger of using the uterus as a piston to expel the placenta is real only where the uterus is soft and flabby and undue force is used. There is some slight risk of inversion at this time.

In the second 'Brandt Andrews' Technique soon after delivery and even before the signs of final separation appears the cord is firmly twisted round the operator's fingers and firm traction applied to the cord. Meanwhile the opposite hand is holding the fundus up in the abdomen and providing some degree of counter traction. If the placenta is separated already it will gradually ease out of the uterus and vagina. Care should be taken not to exert undue force, to pull unduly on the cord if the placenta is obviously not beginning to give, but with steady traction there is usually little problem. The function of the opposite hand is to prevent the fundus following the placenta down into the vagina or to invert. Moreover in both methods pushing the fundus up into the abdomen improves venous drainage and to some extent lessens uterine bleeding by minimizing uterine congestion.

The placenta once received, should be collected in to the cupped hands, the membranes twisted into a rope (care be taken that they too are complete) and gently extracted from the vagina. The placenta should be quickly inspected for gross abnormality or gross areas of deficiency.

There should now be no bleeding and the operator can proceed with perineal repair. It is important that there should be thorough inspection of the vulva and the vagina to decide on the extent of damage or tearing and that the repair should be properly done under good conditions.

THE VULVA
The vulva and any soiled areas of the thighs should then be wiped clean with a warm antiseptic lotion and dried. A sterile pad is placed over the vulva, soiled bed clothes removed and clean ones placed in position. The patient is covered with warm blankets and given a warm drink.

The temperature and pulse should now be taken. The pulse rate should be clearly under 100 and the temperature should be normal. A rapid pulse may be a sign of an exhausted patient or in fact, of bleeding, and care should be taken that the fundus of the uterus is inspected for firmness and hardness and that there is no external bleeding from episiotomy or tears.

After delivery the doctor should not leave the patient for half to one hour until he is satisfied that the uterus is well contracted, there is no bleeding from the perineal wound, the pulse and temperature are normal.

ACCELERATED AND AUGMENTED LABOUR

Since the early part of this century an increasing number of obstetricians have begun to explore the possibility of using oxytocic drugs in labour to improve uterine action and especially to shorten the total duration of labour. The interested reader is referred to an excellent review article by MacVicar (1973). In the last five or six years there has evolved a belief that labour should be short and efficient and that shortness and efficiency of labour should if necessary be achieved by the active stimulation of the uterus with oxytocic drugs. The claims of different workers are somewhat variable and it is probably best to review the pattern as first described by O'Driscoll and his colleagues (1970), by Turnbull (1957) and by Barber (1972). It is probably to Turnbull and Anderson that much of the credit for the more recent developments of acceleration should go, although the work out of which their method grew and the application of their techniques is different from those of other workers. They were more concerned with the direct stimulation of the uterus following amniotomy to minimize the waiting period following rupture of the membranes. Initially it was thought that it was best to use oxytocin to start labour contractions off but it was then clear that continuation of labour function was much more efficient if the oxytocin were continued.

In general the idea that the inert uterus or the uterus in whom the contractions were inadequate should be stimulated is of old standing and many workers including Friedman (1967) have advocated such action for a fairly long time. It is generally true that poor quality contractions and infrequent contractions will not permit labour to progress since it has been suggested that an adequate amount of power is essential to achieve full dilatation and ultimate delivery. Turnbull (1957) showed however, that even in normal labour the pattern and apparent strength and frequency of contractions seem to bear no relation to the ultimate pattern of the labour and even within the same labour the cervix could dilate at varying rates with apparently the same pattern of contractions. Moreover in the multigravida the mean intra-uterine pressures were less than the primigravida although labours were of course, faster. Occasionally however, as shown, when the uterus met fixed resistance to the passage of the head and the continued dilatation of the cervix the contractions ultimately become weak and irregular. This has of course, been shown previously by Friedman as part of the pattern of late labour disproportion.

Initially in the stimulation of labour rather small doses of oxytocin were recommended, e.g. some 2–6mμ per minute of syntocinon the synthetic preparation. By the end of the 1950s several authorities were firmly convinced of the safety and usefulness of this degree of stimulation. Gradually however, an increase in the amount of oxytocin was recommended. Turnbull and Anderson for example, in discussing the use of oxytocin intravenously for induction of labour recommended that the dose should be gradually increased over short intervals until strong regular uterine contractions were established—the technique being that of 'Oxytocin titration'. Once adequate uterine contractions are achieved the infusion is continued until delivery and for some hour or so afterwards. As pointed out by many authors, there is no method of inducing labour which is completely certain of its effects and completely safe for mother and fetus. On the other hand the process of labour itself, cannot be said to be without risk. Once induction of labour is decided upon in maternal or fetal interest, delivery should be expedited by the safest possible means. It must be, however, clear that the acceleration or augmentation of natural labour by the use of oxytocics also carries with it certain dangers. Two of the major possible hazards are those of excessive pressure on the fetal head and the risk of uterine rupture in the presence of some degree of disproportion and especially if the uterus is previously scarred.

Stimulation and augmentation of labour is suggested in approximately three different clinical situations.

1. Induction

It is generally believed that the risks of induction are largely those connected with infection after prolonged rupture of the membranes, and it is suggested that, if labour has failed to begin within twelve hours of artificial rupture of the membranes the uterine contractions should be stimulated by oxytocics. This situation is somewhat different in spontaneous rupture of the membranes and especially where this should occur rather early in pregnancy. Certainly where spontaneous rupture of membranes occurs late in pregnancy when the child is mature enough to survive independently, the case should be treated similarly to artificial rupture.

In recent years it has become customary in some units to induce labour by artificial rupture of membranes and followed immediately by the use of oxytocin to stimulate the onset of labour and to increase the quality of the contractions. There is certain virtue of waiting for an hour or so after artificial rupture of membranes, as artificial rupture is followed by slowing of uterine blood flow and it seems a little rash to add on the risks of oxytocin immediately. However, by whatever method is used it is now customary to escalate the dose of oxytocin fairly rapidly until adequate and regular contractions are obtained. As will be seen in Chapter 18, it is wise in conditions of escalation or stimulation of labour that the quality, strength and frequency of the uterine contractions should be monitored either by the immediate and close attendance of a nurse, of doctor, or by the use of intra-uterine pressure monitoring devices. There should, in addition, be either careful auscultation of the fetal heart or regular monitoring of the fetal heart by scalp electrode. In other words *whenever the escalation of labour, augmentation of labour, acceleration of labour is considered, careful monitoring of the quality and the strength of the contractions and of the fetal response is essential either by clinical or by electronic means.*

2. It is advocated by O'Driscoll, who considered that since prolonged labour presented a picture of mental anguish, risk of infection and of damage to the child, that it is essential that labour should not be allowed to remain prolonged. As we have seen previously, labour should follow a rapid curve. After 2–3cm cervical dilatation has been reached further dilatation should take place at the rate of approximately 1cm per hour. Where a labour is considered to be slow and dilatory oxytocin (10 units per litre of 5 per cent dextrose) is erected to stimulate and drive the labour, the rate of infusion regulated to ensure steady dilatation of the cervix preferably along the normal mean rate of dilatation (i.e. 1cm per hour) and limited only by signs of fetal distress. Barber similarly considers that oxytocin should be administered in pharmacological amounts to augment labour that is not progressing satisfactorily. Both authors consider that occipito posterior position, abnormal descent pattern, secondary inactive phase of labour, prolonged latent phase with a favourable cervix are *not* contra-indications to the use of oxytocin to stimulate a failing labour.

3. There is a third group where attempts are made to stimulate labour which is already prolonged and inert and often at a stage of failure of continuing dilatation with the cervix some 3–4 fingers dilated. This is a much more dangerous group of cases and the secondary inertia at this stage usually means that there is some degree of disproportion between head and pelvis.

The risks of accelerated augmented labour are essentially those of undue damage to the fetus because of undue pressure associated with a rapidly driving uterus and similar to the risks of precipitate labour in the multigravida. There is secondly a risk of uterine rupture if the uterus is unduly stimulated against disproportion or where there is a previous uterine scar.

CONTRA-INDICATIONS

There are few if any contra-indications to the use of oxytocin to initiate the onset of labour, except perhaps with a fetus highly sensitive to the stimulation of syntocinon. This sensitivity of course, can be checked as part of the study of the early effects of syntocinon stimulation. When we consider the question of 'augmenting labour' then there is a certain problem of contra-indications.

It is fairly clear that the Irish School (O'Driscoll and his colleagues) believe that there are virtually no contra-indications unless one is faced with absolute disproportion, gross malpresentation or transverse lie. There is perhaps a certain risk in the grand multigravida, or where there is a history of previous extensive cervical or pelvic floor repairs, or cone biopsy, or previous extensive operation in the uterus. No one would however use stimulated labour in such cases in any case. Moderate degrees of apparent disproportion and some malposition are not contra-indications provided careful and constant monitoring of the child is available. Where it is considered advisable to undertake augmented labour it is probably important to follow certain very carefully observed guides:

1. The degree of cervical dilatation, the position and firmness of the cervix, the presenting part, the degree of flexion or extension, the station of the head and the pelvic capacity are determined as a first and primary assessment. If there is any suspicion of cephalo pelvic disproportion, pelvimetry may be undertaken, but clinical examination is usually adequate and careful observation of the progress of the labour should certainly help to elicit clinical disproportion as it develops. The two bottle technique is best used, one bottle containing 5 per cent glucose connected to the infusion needle close to the arm, the other bottle containing 10 units of syntocinon in 5 per cent glucose. It is perfectly straightforward to use a simple drop technique although an infusion pump or a contraction controlled pump system is perfectly acceptable. Infusion should be started at relatively low dosage at something of the order of 5–7mμ per minute (something like 8–10 drops of a 10 per cent solution), the rate of infusion being gradually increased every 20–30 minutes until the uterine response is optimal. The optimal response should be not more than 2 to 3 contractions every 10 minutes, and of moderate intensity accompanied by a low uterine tonus. Care is taken to monitor the intensity, frequency, quality and duration of the contractions either by clinical or electronic means and maternal heart rate, blood pressure and general response to the contractions are noted. The child should be carefully monitored by regular auscultation of the fetal heart both during and with contractions or preferably by continuous electronic monitoring. It must be made

absolutely clear that *no unit should undertake augmentation of labour without the most careful routine techniques of monitoring being available for both mother and child.*

One other major point to consider in the presence of augmented labour is that everything happens *faster.* There can be no question of allowing labour to become unduly prolonged when oxytocin is being used, and certainly progress of dilatation and descent must be continuous, smooth and straightforward, otherwise there may be present some serious degree of disproportion and the risk of uterine rupture is very real. Dilatation should take place at least 0·7 to 1cm per minute in primigravida and somewhat faster in multigravida.

The use of augmented labour in the presence of a malflexed head or occipito posterior can often improve the quality of the contractions in such a way that adequate flexion occurs, the head comes down through the pelvis, rotates, and either a low forceps or spontaneous delivery can be achieved. Oxytocin should not be used to overcome what is clinically considered to be disproportion or it must be used with great care.

The major risks to the mother are those of uterine tetanus, uterine rupture, separation of the placenta, precipitate labour, cervical laceration, amniotic fluid embolism. Risks to the fetus are hypoxia due to the strength and frequency of contractions, or actual physical damage due to the unduly rapid labour.

Oxytocin drip should be continued after delivery to ensure reasonably adequate contraction in the third stage but bleeding may still occur, and it is probably wise to add ergometrine in the third stage rather than to increase the dose of oxytocin. If the bleeding does not quickly stop, some other source of the bleeding must be considered, for example, cervical tear or serious vaginal tearing.

The combined use of oxytocin stimulation and epidural anaesthesia can produce very smooth labour in the carefully controlled cases, *but monitoring must be that much more complete and accurate.* It is certainly very dangerous to use oxytocin with epidural anaesthesia in the presence of a uterine scar in view of the risk of silent rupture.

'DYSTOCIA' OR DIFFICULT LABOUR AND DELIVERY

Normal labour, page 319, is defined as 'labour which ends in a spontaneous cephalic delivery, at or about term, of a live mature child requiring minimal resuscitation, after a labour lasting less than eighteen hours and with minimal damage to the mother'. It will be seen from this that labour and delivery are different or abnormal if the delivery is not spontaneous and instrumentation or manipulation is required; if the delivery is premature or post term; if the child is not fully grown and developed or if the labour is prolonged and where there is undue damage to mother or child. While in general the course of labour is affected by the efficiency of the uterine contractions, the size, presentation and position of the baby and the shape and size of the pelvis, and to some extent by the custom and attitudes of the mother and her attendant, some anomalies may predominate and so dictate the ultimate outcome. For example, a grossly contracted pelvis will not permit the vaginal delivery of the child, a serious degree of malpresentation such as a transverse lie, or the presence of some obstructing feature in the pelvis in the nature of a cervical fibroid, will automatically dictate the pattern of the labour and the method of delivery. Similarly there may be factors in the mother such as severe heart disease, chronic respiratory disease, diabetes, previous pelvic floor operation which again would dictate the whole pattern of labour, care and of delivery, and each of these factors is discussed in the relevant areas of the text.

However, there are broad features which influence the pattern of labour in various maternal groups which merit some consideration.

PARITY

Difficult labour and the need for operative delivery is much more likely in the mother having a first baby as against the mother who has already had one or two vaginal deliveries. For example, the indicated forceps rate in first pregnancies is now about 20 per cent, but in second and subsequent pregnancies less than 5 per cent. The Caesarean section rate is not particularly different throughout the parities, and varies between 5 and 7 per cent the more parous women requiring Caesarean section for, of course, different reasons.

High parity tends to be associated with difficulty due to malpresentation, prolapsed cord, placenta praevia and very occasionally uterine rupture. It will be realized that the frequency of such complications of labour is decreasing as the large family becomes increasingly rare. However, the difficulties of the primigravida are relatively more frequent than they were in the past. This is somewhat offset by the fact that there are much larger numbers of young women having a first baby and youth, as we will see, is very much on their side.

AGE AND PRIMIPARA

In the human species in the more developed countries, menarche has been reached by the age of thirteen, and there is now a relatively much longer period before general maturity is also reached, both in the physical development of uterus and bony pelvis and to some extent in psychological attitudes and abilities to marry and raise a family. The young primigravida tends to reproduce badly, having a higher incidence of abortion and pre-eclampsia, and premature labour but her labour tends to be much more smooth and easy as her tissues are softer and stretch more easily, uterine function is better; her pelvis tends to stretch more easily and often because of malnutrition her child is not unduly large.

In general the incidence of Caesarean section or prolonged labour is low in young women, and becomes progressively greater with advancing maternal age. In the mother over thirty-five in first pregnancies the incidence of Caesarean section may be as high as 35–40 per cent, but this high rate is dictated somewhat by the often associated infertility, sometimes poor fetal growth or hypertension and other complicating factors associated with rising age.

It is interesting that in the upper social groups especially in those women who have had the opportunity of higher education, childbearing comes in the late twenties and their labours suffer somewhat because of advancing age, however, the difference is less than might appear at first sight. In Scottish communities now, the primigravida over thirty accounts for less than 5 per cent of all primigravida. With increasing age greater rigidity of the pelvic joints and ligaments, can explain some increase in mechanical difficulties and some ageing of the uterine muscle and loss of elasticity of the tissues of the pelvic floor might account for the greater incidence of dysfunction and so arises the problem of prolonged labour.

In the older multipara the uterus tends to have some greater difficulty in initiating and establishing labour and a somewhat greater risk of rupture in the presence of disproportion or any other form of obstruction. The classically dangerous cases is the multigravida with several previous normal sized children who might have an unusually large child or a hydrocephalic child and after a relatively silent obstructed labour, uterine rupture occurs. It is also important to remember that while a young primigravida may drive a moderately sized child through a contracted pelvis aided by good uterine function and some degree of pelvic stretching, she will fail as an older multigravida to deliver a similar sized or even smaller child since her pelvis is more rigid and there is relatively poor uterine function.

HEIGHT AND PHYSIQUE

The relationship between height and difficult labour is primarily that associated with pelvic contraction. Serious difficulty due to mechanical causes in labour was in the past very much more common in small women under 5ft 1 inch (155cm) in height, than in tall women 5ft 5 inches (165cm) or upwards. The incidence of dysfunction is of course, unaffected by height.

As we have seen previously, contraction and malformation of the pelvis is much more common in short than in tall women. Height, of course, is closely related to social class and is largely a function of adequate nutrition in childhood although there are women who are genetically small who are of course, well nourished. In the average industrial city of Scotland there are still some 22 per cent of women less than 155cm in height and this to a large extent dictates the degree of pelvic contraction seen.

Maximum stature is attained and pelvic deformities avoided if conditions for growth and adequate nutrition are present in early childhood. Primigravidae in the upper social groups therefore have advantages in the terms of height and physique and disadvantages to some extent in terms of age. Those from less favoured classes who may be undersized are more often young and tend to have smaller babies. There is no doubt that difficult labour in primigravidae is least often seen in those primigravida under twenty-five and more than 165cm in height.

LENGTH OF GESTATION

The percentage of difficulty in labour increases progressively the longer pregnancy is prolonged beyond 40 weeks. This increase effects difficult labour due both to mechanical causes and to uterine dysfunction. There is an obvious increase in fetal head size even after term and many more babies weigh more than 8 pounds (3·25kg). Those factors lead to disproportion with secondary dysfunction. There is however, an increase in uterine dysfunction associated with prolonged pregnancy. This situation is to some extent established even by 32–33 weeks when (as previously seen) uterine activity normally begins to develop in those patients who will go into labour at or about the correct time, but not in those where pregnancy is going to be prolonged. Post date pregnancy is, therefore associated with a failure of uterine activity of the normal pattern in late pregnancy and therefore with a failure of cervical softening and dilatation, so that at or after term the cervix is still long and closed. A cervix of this type cannot be taken as an indication that the patient has not yet reached term, but only that there is an element of dysfunction present. This problem creates difficulty when the question of induction arises and sometimes raises doubts in the mind of the obstetrician of the degree of prolonged pregnancy. *The state of the cervix is not a guide of any reliability to the duration of the pregnancy.*

ATTITUDE

The attitude to reproduction has already been discussed to some extent. The attitude is developed within the group or class concerned, but within each group especially in the more sophisticated western world attitudes to reproduction are developed personally from all sorts of sources. Women in the upper social groups who are taller and healthier as a rule are more likely to postpone marriage and limit childbearing to smaller families and to have much more positive attitudes. They are much more likely to expect special care in labour and they are much more likely to expect a minimum of discomfort. This inevitably influences not not only the attitude of the obstetrician but the type of care given.

High quality care now includes a large element of monitoring and a need for adequate analgesia (epidural or the use of inhalation analgesic with high oxygen content (entonox)), and episiotomy or low forceps with pudendal block. The ability of the obstetrician to relieve discomfort, to shorten labour and to minimize maternal damage has made a tremendous difference to the problem of the mother and to some extent to her attitude. The knowledge that these measures are available makes the mother much more likely to insist that she has them offered to her.

Prevention of difficult labour

The type of difficult labour occurring in any community varies somewhat with the standard of living, the customs of the community, but of course, adequate nutrition during pregnancy in a woman with a contracted pelvis may produce disproportion which would not have existed if her malnutrition had continued poor. It is obvious therefore, that adequate nourishment of the child from birth will prevent subsequent mechanical and functional difficulties in labour, but more perhaps can be done to anticipate the possibility of difficult labour by high quality antenatal care, by recognizing that certain groups of the community, certain heights and certain situations will make labour much more likely to be difficult and require much more meticulous care. O'Driscoll, K. (1972) claims that the use of oxytocics to stimulate poor labour progressively reduces the incidence not only of prolonged labour but also of cephalopelvic disproportion, posterior position, operative interference and trauma to the fetus.

PLACE OF DELIVERY

At some stage during antenatal care the decision has to be made as to place of delivery. In those areas where delivery always takes place in the confines of a specialist hospital, either in a general practitioner unit or in a specialist unit itself, the problem of selection is less. Where however, booking is being made for peripheral general practitioner units, or for some place where full delivery care in the nature of operative delivery cannot be easily obtained, then selection for booking must be specific. Safe outcome in relation to labour itself and the outcome of labour is seen in mothers having 2nd or 3rd babies who have had a previously perfectly normal history, in tall primigravida under the age of 25, and where delivery occurs between the end of the 37th and the end of the 41st week. The outcome for labour is likely to be less favourable in primigravida over the age of 25, in fourth or later births especially if there is any abnormality in the history, in all patients under 5ft 1in, and obviously where labour occurs before the end of the 37th or after the end of the 41st week. Of course, even although delivery is planned in the major centre action can be taken in the correction of malpresentation, in the recognition and correction of malpresentation and in obtaining knowledge of the co-existence of abnormal uterine pelvic tumours or pelvic bony deformity.

Difficult labour due to faults in the pelvis

The shape and size of the pelvis has been very fully discussed in Chapter 3. With the decline and virtual disappearance of rickets and grossly contracted pelvis becoming more uncommon, increasing attention has been focused on minor variations in pelvic size and shape. However, much of this minor difficulty has been offset in recent years by the increasing use of augmented labour (page 345).

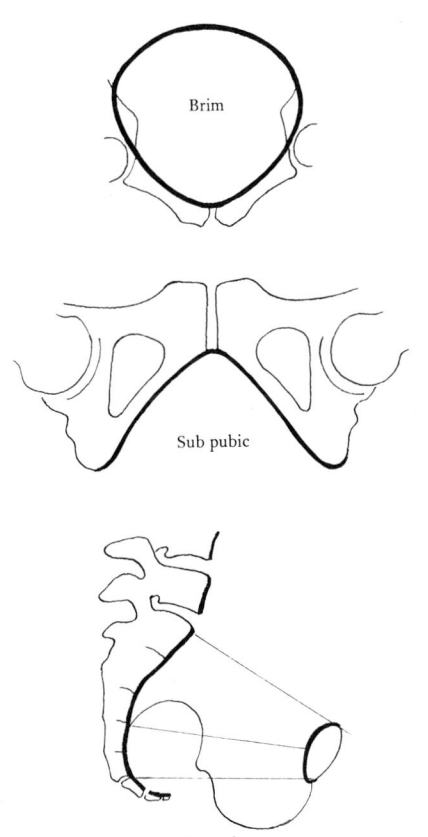

Fig. 19.12 Outline diagrams of the radiological appearances in lateral, brim and sub pubic arch views.

The normal gynaecoid pelvis described in Chapter 3 has round or slightly long oval brim and its appearance is shown in outline in Fig. 19.12. It will be noted that the diameters throughout the pelvis are wide and adequate.

Occasionally in tall primigravida, the pelvic brim is long oval—the anthropoid pelvis—and while the pelvic brim is almost certain to have adequate measurements the lower cavity and outlet may be contracted. This should be checked on digital examination of the pelvis in early labour.

The classical flat pelvis typical of childhood malnutrition is still common, with mainly posterior segment flattening. In any pelvis distorted by congenital anomaly, disease, fracture or new growth difficulty in labour is certain and elective Caesarean section is usually indicated.

MECHANISM OF LABOUR IN DISPROPORTION AT THE BRIM

At the pelvic brim in normal labour the head descends through an axis which bisects the pelvis or lies a little behind its mid-point. If the brim is round, the head usually engages in the occipito lateral position with its longer diameter in the transverse diameter of the brim. Occasionally some asynclitism (Fig. 19.9) exists with lateral tilting of the fetal head. The posterior parietal mostly presents but this is corrected as the head descends into the pelvis. In the long oval brim with a relatively narrow transverse diameter the head often engages directly mento-posterior. Measurement in this shape of pelvis are usually ample. However, if the head happens to engage with the occiput posterior there may be difficulty in ultimate delivery. If the brim is *flat* the head again engages in a transverse position but there is relatively less room between head and symphysis and disproportion may well occur. Occasionally in the slightly flattened pelvis especially of the multigravida acute extension may occur when the pains begin with the head rotating into full extension with the fulcrum at the area of the biparietal eminences, so that a face or brow presentation may develop.

Below the brim, the head previously entering the brim in the occipito lateral position descends if the cavity is round into the roomy posterior segment until it reaches the level of the ischial spines and then reaches the pelvic floor when the occiput rotates forwards.

Prominent ischial spines may arrest the head at this stage, but this arrest in the relatively normal pelvis is not unduly serious and flexion and rotation of the head may be obtained either manually and followed by forceps delivery or by use of forceps rotation. Undue contraction of the outlet or forward prolongation of sacrum may make funnelling situation through which the head can pass only with difficulty or not at all.

Arrest of the head in the cavity may take place at any level and in the occipito anterior, lateral or posterior position—and these are described on page 363.

PELVIMETRY

X-ray pelvimetry has been described briefly in Chapter 28 but for more recent discussion of the value and techniques the reader is referred to Russel (1973). X-ray pelvimetry is currently much less often performed or even required but it is still of sufficient interest to afford some discussion. It is clear that this method provides factual information about the dimensions and shape of the pelvic cavity. However, recent considerable criticism has been levelled against antenatal radiography particularly pelvimetry because of the radiation received by the fetus and the ultimate risk of fetal leukaemia or malignant neoplasm. However, there are situations where pelvimetry is of great value. This is for example, seen in the patient already in labour where some degree of disproportion and malpresentation or malposition is suspected which cannot be fully assessed clinically, and secondly, post-natally in patients who have had difficult labour leading to Caesarean section and/or difficult forceps where the pelvimetry result may be a guide to management in subsequent pregnancies. It is also of course, now possible to take anteroposterior measurements of the pelvic brim by ultrasound and this technique is likely to prove a great advantage once adequate experience is obtained by the operators.

Radiology will identify that tiny majority of women with very small pelves, e.g. the bispinous of less than 9cm or a sagittal outlet of 10cm or less, who are likely to have difficulty in labour. However, pelvimetry following difficult labour will suggest that the majority of pelves are apparently adequate. The simplest measurements which give the information required are—

1. Conjugate of the Inlet (the obstetrical diameter).
2. The transverse diameter of the Inlet (and the available transverse).
3. The Bi-spinous diameter.
4. Sagittal diameter of the Outlet (and the available diameter).

These measurements can be obtained by taking a standing lateral, a brim picture, and a view of the pubic arch.

STANDING LATERAL VIEW OF THE PELVIS

This is the best view when taken to assess the progress of the difficult labour antenatally or post-natally to determine the quality of the pelvic shape and size. In the lateral view (see Fig. 19.12) the features to be observed are:

1. The angle of inclination of the pelvic brim. This depends to some extent on the degree of maternal lordosis. The degree determines the difficulty or otherwise of the head engaging. With an inclination near the vertical the head on engagement may extend into the brim in the posterior position.
2. The shape and size of the sacro sciatic notch. A wide or rounded notch suggests a good cavity and bony outlet, narrow notch suggests some degree of funnelling.
3. The shape and curvature of the sacrum. The sacrum should be slim and nicely curved presenting a concave surface to the cavity making for room within the cavity itself. The lower part should not come unduly forwards and therefore producing some degree of funnelling. Occasionally the coccyx itself comes forwards and this may produce some minor difficulty at the outlet, but the coccyx is usually ignored in the first instance in assessing outlet measurement.
4. *Measurements* are then taken (a) of the obstetrical conjugate at the brim. This reads from the upper posterior aspect of the symphysis to the promontory of the sacrum, (b) from the lower end of the third piece of sacrum to the mid-point of the symphysis which is the mid-cavity measurement, and (c) from the tip of the sacrum to the lower aspect of the symphysis a guide to the anteroposterior of the outlet (see page 353).

THE ANTEROPOSTERIOR SUPINE VIEW

The technique described by Borell and Fernström allows measurements of the widest transverse diameter of the inlet and interischial spinous diameter with a minimum of radiation to the fetal gonads. The patient lying in the supine position, the X-ray beam suitably coned, is centred at a point 5cm above the

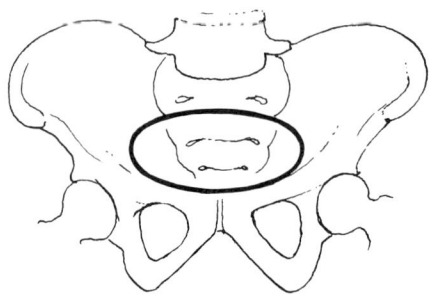

Fig. 19.13 The foreshortened view of the pelvis by this technique does not give a picture of the antero-posterior diameter.

symphysis in the midline and a magnified brim film obtained. A true lateral view is taken without altering the patient's position and various correction factors are applied to give the proper measurements of the magnified brim view taken in the supine position (Fig. 19.13).

If it is essential to know the exact shape of the brim, anteroposterior films are taken with the patient lying at an angle of 35° to the horizontal, bringing the plane of the brim parallel to the film. This view should of course, be restricted to post-partum cases, but on it alone can the true available transverse be obtained.

Data established from radiographs

PELVIC INLET

1. Conjugate diameter from lateral film.
2. Transverse diameter from AP brim film.
3. Brim Index =
$$\frac{\text{Conjugate diameter of brim}}{\text{Widest transverse diameter}} \times 100$$
4. Brim Area $= \pi \times \dfrac{d_1}{2} \times \dfrac{d_2}{2}$

where $d_1 = \frac{1}{2}$AP diameter, $d_2 = \frac{1}{2}$ widest transverse diameter.

5. Brim Shape. Unless films are available with the brim parallel to the film no true assessment can be made.

MID-PELVIS

1. The curvature of the sacrum, the inclination of the brim; the depth of the sciatic notches and sacralization of the fifth lumbar vertebra or coccyx may all be seen on the lateral film.

2. The diameter between the ischial spines may be read from the AP film.

PELVIC OUTLET

1. *Subpubic angle*. This is obtained from the radiograph of the pubic arch, and lies between tangents drawn from the symphysis pubis to the ischial tuberosities.

2. *Anteroposterior diameter of the outlet*

The total distance from the tip of the sacrum to the under aspect of the symphysis is obviously not all available to the fetal head and there are various methods (Morris, 1947) and (Gillanders, 1959) to measure the available space. Morris' technique seems best.

In a radiograph of the pubic arch a transparency representing the 9·5–10cm fetal head diameter is placed between the pubic rami allowing the transparency to touch the rami Fig. 19.14. The distance from the under surface of the symphysis to the top of the circle is then the 'waste space'. This is measured off on the lateral film along the pubic rami and the available AP drawn.

TRANSVERSE DIAMETER OF MID-PELVIS

Measure distance between tips of ischial spines on AP or brim view and correct for magnification.

SUBPUBIC ANGLE

Obtained from the radiograph of the pubic arch. The apex of the angle is the inferior margin of the symphysis and the sides are tangents to the ischial tuberosities.

SHAPE OF SACRUM AND COCCYX

Note on the lateral radiograph whether the sacral curve is reduced. If the coccyx is tilted forward observe whether its base is fused with the last piece of the sacrum.

Assessment of results of pelvimetry and obstetric forecast

PELVIC INLET

The use of a single measurement to assess inlet

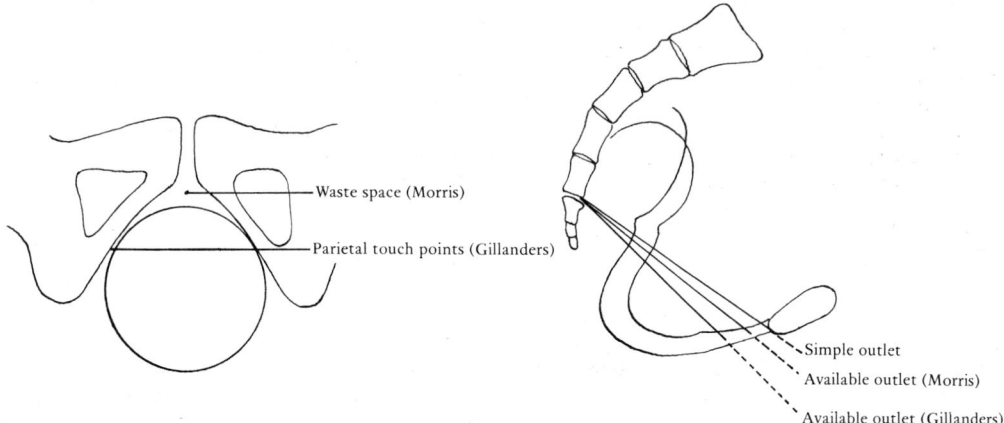

Fig. 19.14   Calculation of the waste space and the available anteroposterior diameter. After Morris (1947) and Gillanders (1959).

contraction is misleading but if a lateral film only is available some indication of the obstetrical outcome can be obtained by measurement of the true conjugate. It is unlikely that any difficulty will arise if this measurement is greater than 11cm (Borell and Fernström, 1960).

Allen's Guide is based on measurement of the brim conjugate and the brim area with a fetal skull diameter of 10cm. Allowance must be made of course, for fetal skulls above and below this measurement.

the fetal skull, in particular the sub-occipito-bregmatic diameter, the average length of which is 9·5cm. Gillanders therefore suggests that this figure, 9·5, should be subtracted from the available antero-posterior diameter giving a figure which he calls the 'free space at the outlet'. If this final figure is less than zero then outlet disproportion is present and its degree is indicated by the numeral. Pelves with figures greater than 2cm allow spontaneous delivery; those with figures less than −1·5cm will require forceps if vaginal delivery is contemplated. The

Table 19.1 Allen (1947)

Probable Mode of Delivery	Brim Conjugate cm	Brim Area sq cm
Vaginal delivery certain without any evidence of disproportion	over 13·0	over 130
Vaginal delivery reasonably certain, but there may be evidence of minor disproportion requiring forceps	10·5–13·0	105–130
Vaginal delivery uncertain and, if possible will show clear evidence of disproportion	9·0–10·5	85–105
Vaginal delivery extremely unlikely. Elective Caesarean section justified	under 9·0	under 85

Nicholson has also used the brim area as a prognostic index. With a brim area of 110sqcm 99·9 per cent of heads will pass, with an area of 100sqcm 97 per cent of heads will pass but if 90sqcm only 70 per cent will pass.

Occasionally separation of the symphysis pubis is seen which will alter the transverse but not the AP diameters.

DISTAL PART OF THE PELVIS

The ideal pelvic cavity is one in which the sacrum is well curved without forward shelving, with wide sciatic notches and ischial spines which are not prominent. This allows adequate room for rotation of the head during descent. In the flat pelvis the sacral curve is diminished or may even be reversed. There may be convergence of the side walls, narrowing of the sacro-sciatic notches and backward tilting of the symphysis. All these changes interfere with the descent and rotation of the fetal head.

An indication of the size of the mid-pelvis can be obtained from a study of the mid-pelvic area which is the multiple of the anteroposterior diameter of the mid-pelvis and the inter-spinous diameter. Allen considers that vaginal delivery is unlikely when the area falls below 70 to 75sqcm. The normal inter-spinous diameter is 10·5cm. If it is less than 9cm vaginal delivery may be difficult but if below 8cm extremely unlikely.

The position of the outlet plane is determined by the available subpubic space and by the diameter of

normal subpubic angle is approximately 80° but measurement of this becomes unnecessary if Gillander's method is used.

The presence of a forward projecting lower sacrum and/or coccyx may reduce the available AP diameter but the degree of reduction cannot be accurately assessed as movement at the sacro-coccygeal joint may occur to a variable degree during parturition, unless it is arthrodesed. The available AP diameter may be increased by tilting of the sacrum at the sacro-iliac joint during labour.

Deep transverse arrest is likely to occur due to failure of rotation of the head as a result of transverse contraction, prominent ischial spines with reduced inter-spinous diameter and convergent side walls, without compensatory increase in the available outlet diameter. The hooked sacral tip and rigid coccyx will interfere with the normal descent of the head rather than rotation. In a considerable number of cases with a normal pelvic brim forceps delivery will suffice but where the brim is abnormal and in addition the sacrum is flat with converging side walls resulting in serious obstruction to rotation of the head, Caesarean section will be required. If marked funnelling is present this mode of delivery is obligatory.

In the rickety flat pelvis the outlet is usually adequate, and if the head can pass the abnormal flattened and kidney-shaped pelvic brim spontaneous delivery is likely.

VALUE OF RADIOGRAPHY

Augmented and accelerated labour has rendered disproportion much less common but of course, where it does exist it appears clinically much sooner. X-ray pelvimetry tells much more accurately the shape and size of the pelvis than any other method, and such additional accurate knowledge should increase the confidence of the obstetrician in managing cases of prolonged labour. It provides a good guide to the best technique to be employed in forceps delivery. The experienced obstetrician will argue that careful palpation under an anaesthetic before applying the forceps will give all this information. He can also point out that it is in the border-line cases of disproportion, especially when this occurs in the cavity and outlet that X-rays give the *least reliable* forecast. In these cases the mode of delivery is often decided by such factors as uterine inertia, the age and temperament of the patient, and the occurrence of fetal distress. X-ray pelvimetry before the onset of labour might still be used in the following types of cases:

1. Women who have had disease of the lower spine and pelvic girdle or any abnormality affecting the lower limbs during growth such as tuberculosis, poliomyelitis, unilateral hip joint disease. These conditions may result in transverse contraction of the pelvic brim which may be impossible to diagnose without examination under anaesthesia.

2. Persistent or recurrent breech presentation where version has failed even under anaesthesia. The decision as to whether or not to allow vaginal delivery or perform Caesarean section may be greatly facilitated if X-ray pelvimetry has been done. A sagittal of 11cm with a transverse of 12cm is usually adequate.

3. Multiparae with a history of difficult labour resulting in a stillbirth, neonatal death or severe maternal injury and all cases of former Caesarean section for actual or alleged disproportion. Ideally, of course, X-ray pelvimetry would have been done immediately after the previous difficult labour.

The obstetrician should never act only on the forecast of the radiograph or radiologist. There is much to be said for the obstetrician doing his own interpretation. In this way he can correlate the X-ray findings with the clinical course of labour and improve his ability to make an accurate prognosis and to manage labour efficiently.

CEPHALOMETRY

Accurate cephalometry is now available by ultrasound, *see* Chapter 28. Where the biparietal diameter of the fetal head is actually 0·5cm less than the sagittal of the pelvic inlet, inlet disproportion should not occur. In view of the varying accuracy of the technique in practice 1cm should be allowed.

Dystocia due to faults in the uterine forces

Clinical results obtained by the techniques of acceleration and augmentation of labour have demonstrated clearly the role of efficient uterine action to ensure vaginal delivery. It has always been understood that in certain cases dysfunction in labour was often associated with minor degrees of disproportion although it was not always clear which was the primary fault. Previous information suggested that dysfunction of the uterus in labour increase with age in primigravida and (apart from the possibility of a less good uterine muscle function with age (Caldeyro Barcia and Poseiro, 1954)) it was suggested that there was, in the older primigravida a greater resistance of the cervix to dilatation. Resistance of the cervix was of course, according to the work of Turnbull, modified by the effects of hormones on the basic collagen tissues, but this facility to loosen and reorientate the collagen fibrils seemed to be less efficient with increasing age in primigravida.

The condition of a rigid cervix where the cervix fails to dilate despite strong natural or induced pains is however a very real entity and has never been satisfactorily explained. It does of course occur, following previous cone biopsy or cervical repair and is due then of course, to scar tissue, but occurring in an apparently undamaged cervix in a primigravida it is an unusual phenomenon. There is a vague possibility that in the induced cases this may be a secondary effect of a syntocinon causing cervical and lower segment spasm.

Apart from age, various other factors are associated with increasing difficulty in labour. Labour is more likely to be prolonged and difficult where the pregnancy is prolonged. Turnbull and Anderson have shown that uterine activity preparatory to labour begins normally about the 32nd week where labour will occur at the normal time. Where, however, the labour is likely to be postponed post dates, the activity is less and may be very poor indeed until a little before labour actually starts. It then continues poor in labour.

The problem of dysfunction labour in the post dates patient especially in primigravida is of course, complicated by the fact that the child is clearly larger, so there is a combination of dysfunction and disproportion.

The emotional stresses which accompany labour have also got a clear role. Crammond (1954) clarified the psychological aspects of uterine dysfunction, where he found that those having an abnormal and prolonged labour were of a different temperament from those having a relatively short normal labour. The abnormal patients were characterized by a tendency to rigid conventional behaviour and although with a pleasant and co-operative manner this concealed an extremely reserved attitude. There was very little overt anxiety but a high incidence of peptic ulceration. He considered the psychological makeup might predispose the patient towards dysfunction, but it was only one factor in a condition of multiple aetiology. He did not think that any type of antenatal preparation could change the patient's personality and influence the incidence of uterine dysfunction.

MEASUREMENT AND CLASSIFICATION OF
    DYSFUNCTION

The older classifications of dysfunction followed clinical observation and experimental evidence obtained by tracings of uterine function taken from various parts of the uterus by various investigators. It is however, clear that clinically there are two forms of dysfunction which effect the first stage.

Inertia

Uterine contractions are infrequent and weak and the cervix dilates slowly if at all. It is very often difficult in the primigravida, to decide whether or not labour has begun and certainly until the cervix is 2–3cm dilated there is no clear evidence that labour will in fact progress. The pain caused by those contractions is normally distributed but does not distress the patient, and the fetus shows no signs of distress provided the membranes remain intact. This type of inertia is not infrequent in primigravida, or for that matter, in multigravida especially with twins or hydramnios. Usually after a period of time the labour satisfactorily progresses and it is perfectly feasible to wait for this within reason. It is, however, also now accepted practice to rupture the membranes

and if this fails to improve the quality and frequency of the contractions to initiate syntocinon stimulation. Stimulation should be used only where, however, it is clear the patient is in labour and the cervix is soft and dilated. The clinical picture is indistinguishable from the so-called false labour where the pains will pass off and of course, the cervix has not dilated.

Inco-ordination

It is suggested that occasionally, especially in the presence of some degree of disproportion, the uterus may become inco-ordinate, and some areas show hypertonicity. Tetanic spasm of the uterus is seen of course, in the multipara especially in the presence of obstruction when very frequent and strong contractions precede imminent rupture.

Constriction ring

An annular area of the uterus may become persistently contracted and tense and it may grip the fetus so tightly as to prevent its birth, even when the cervix is fully dilated. This condition is seen mostly in a presentation where there is prolonged labour in a breech presentation and is especially difficult in this circumstance since the head is often above the ring and only Caesarean section can allow delivery. Such constriction ring is not infrequently seen where oxytocin has been exhibited in the presence of disproportion or where there has been some intra-uterine manipulation.

The retraction ring of Bandl

Appears as an oblique line across in the uterus. It is that area between the upper and lower segments which in the presence of an obstruction with elongation of the lower segment rises higher and higher into the abdomen. It is usually slightly oblique and with the upper higher side on the same side as the occiput. If the ring rises almost to the umbilicus it is significant of an extremely stretched and tense lower segment which might soon rupture.

Oedematous anterior lip of cervix

There is a condition where the cervix is nipped between the head and the symphysis, often with strong uterine contractions. It is possible that pressure necrosis may occur and an annular ring of cervix be detached and born with the head. This occurs only after a very prolonged and difficult labour situation. It is more likely that the cervix will in fact tear as the head descends. Those situations occur in the presence of minor degrees of disproportion where there is prolonged and strong uterine contraction. If early recognized the lip can be pushed up past the head if pressure is exerted during a contraction.

Excessive sedation
Excessive sedation specially with narcotic type drugs clearly slows labour and occasionally will cause arrest of progress even in the late first stage. In the second stage pudendal block anaesthesia may remove the response to pressure on the pelvic floor and lessen the expulsing effort of both uterus and mother.

Faults in forces of the second stage of labour

Inadequate contractions of the first stage may continue into the second. Quite often however, there is an associated constriction ring which is evidence of a tired and exhausted uterus and this complication is not at first obvious and it may be considered that the uterus is inert. Great care must be taken in such circumstances as syntocinon stimulation will tend to exaggerate the condition.

Inefficient second stage 'bearing down' effort by the mother may relate to poor uterine contractions or again the effect of a series of drugs on the mother so that she cannot be persuaded to bear down. Again the mother may be exhausted, frightened or in some other way unable to take active part in the expulsion of the child.

Bearing down effort on the part of the mother is not essential to the ultimate delivery of the child but if this is obviously inadequate, forceps delivery should be undertaken. Care should be taken however, to ensure that the apparent inadequacy of the bearing down effort is not due to the fact that the head has not yet fully reached the pelvic floor, or alternatively that it is held up on a prominent coccyx.

Resistant perineum
Quite often the perineum is resistant to stretch. This is a quality of the perineum of the older primigravida or in the multigravida with a previous episiotomy. In both instances adequate episiotomy under local anaesthesia is an essential part of the delivery.

RECOGNITION OF UTERINE DYSFUNCTION
In early labour the recognition of dysfunction of the uterus is difficult, and it is sometimes impossible to tell whether the patient is actually in labour or not. Uterine contractions are apparently present and those contractions are associated with patient discomfort. They are often regular but the cervix fails to dilate. If, after a reasonable period, cervical dilatation is obviously failing to occur it is best to offer adequate sedation to the patient, and after a period of sleep the discomfort and the active uterine contractions will apparently cease and the 'labour' will settle. Occasionally however, after a period of adequate maternal rest labour clearly progresses and cervical dilatation begins to occur. This condition of a 'slow starter' in labour or of the maternal awareness of a short early prodromal period of labour is very real in primigravida and often precedes active labour by 6–48 hours.

Once however, labour is clearly established dysfunction is best recognized if the observer remembers that labour must continue to progress.

The demonstration of uterine and other labour patterns by the recording of cervical dilatation against time was clearly described by Friedman (1967), where the slow dilatation characterizing a protractive active phase of primarily dysfunctional labour is seen in contrast to the mean rate of dilatation to be expected. The use of a graph to chart cervical dilatation and descent of the presenting part against time; a 'Partograph' allows visual monitor of the progress of labour. This use has become much more common since the advent of augmented and accelerated labour, Phillpott and Castle (1972) advise the use of an 'alert and action line' to dictate action in abnormal labour states in more primitive communities where labour progress can be monitored by relatively unskilled personnel and help called when labour is clearly abnormal. Phillpott's charts are based on the Friedman studies but it is interesting that he should record that in apparently normal African primigravida the rate of progress at the period of maximum acceleration is roughly half that of American patients, suggesting a higher prevalence of mild cephalopelvic disproportion amongst the African women. A similar situation is seen in Scotland, where Patel (1973) has shown that the speed of active dilatation in unselected Dundee women primigravida in unstimulated labour varies between 0·6 and 1cm per hour, as against the suggested speed of 1–1·5cm an hour of the Friedman charts (Fig. 19.15).

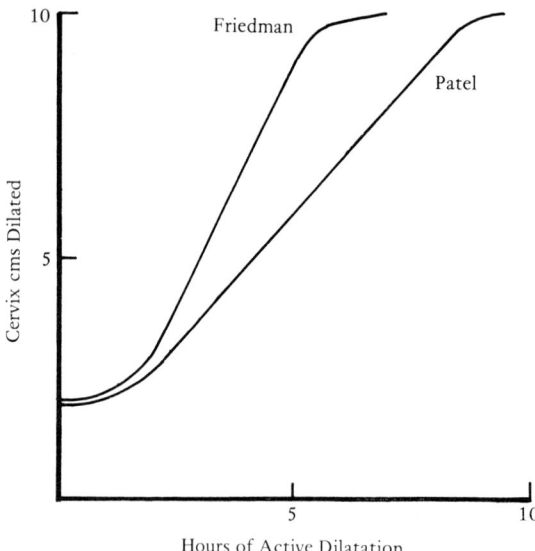

Fig. 19.15 Normal cervical dilatation in the primigravida against time (Friedman). The slower dilatations in communities with a similar greater incidence of pelvic contraction is seen in the main pattern if added to a thousand primigravida in Scotland (Patel).

FAILURE OF PROGRESS

From clinical and partograph evidence of labours compared with the normal mean rate of progress to be expected, it is clear that lack of progress can be defined (Fig. 19.16):

1. Primary inert labour with a prolonged latent phase—when there may be some doubt that labour is truly established.

2. A primary dysfunction when there is a slow but progressive slope in the acceleration phase once labour is established.

3. A secondary failure of dilatation where there is a clear halt in progress of dilatation after say 6–7cm.

MANAGEMENT OF DIFFICULT LABOUR

It is generally accepted that until the cervix is clearly 2cm dilated and continuing to dilate with contraction that labour cannot be considered to be established. This is a good general rule and if followed will prevent unwise attempts at stimulation. There is one group in which this general rule is difficult to apply and that is where attempts are being made to induce labour or stimulate labour with oxytocics and cervical dilatation fails to occur

despite very strong contractions with high monitored intra-uterine pressure. The problem is especially difficult where the apparent 'pains' are associated with fetal tachycardia, or meconium on amnioscopy, and certainly even more acute where the membranes have been ruptured artificially or spontaneously.

Once the accelerated phase has begun the degree of slope is a clear guide and failure to continue increasing dilatation will indicate secondary arrest.

The gradual descent of the presenting part is of course, part of the partograph evidence, (Fig. 19.16). The partograph also charts frequency and strength of contractions and the fetal heart rate at least during and between contractions.

Chapter 18 discusses the whole question of monitoring in labour and such action is especially needed where some labour anomaly has appeared.

Cases of primary or secondary inert labour are cared for under certain very general principles:

1. The fetus already at risk, i.e. associated with antepartum haemorrhage; hypertensive syndrome; prolonged pregnancy etc., should should not be hazarded unless with extremely efficient monitoring systems.

2. Prolonged rupture of membranes before or during labour create the further hazard of intra-uterine infection, which can of itself be fatal for the fetus.

3. A mechanical reason for the inert labour should always be sought.

4. Secondary inert labours with cessation of dilatation and often descent after 6–7cm particularly require careful assessment.

5. Difficult vaginal delivery is not acceptable.

Careful examination of the patient and careful assessment of the pattern of labour with particular regard paid to the condition of the child usually allows the experienced clinician to decide when the amniotomy should be performed, oxytocin stimulus should be instituted, or more sedation should be offered, epidural anaesthesia should be exhibited or immediate delivery should be undertaken.

Probably the biggest difference in the conduct of labour in the last few years has been the increased frequency of assessment by pelvic examination. Knowledge of the progress of dilatation, of descent, of moulding, of caput

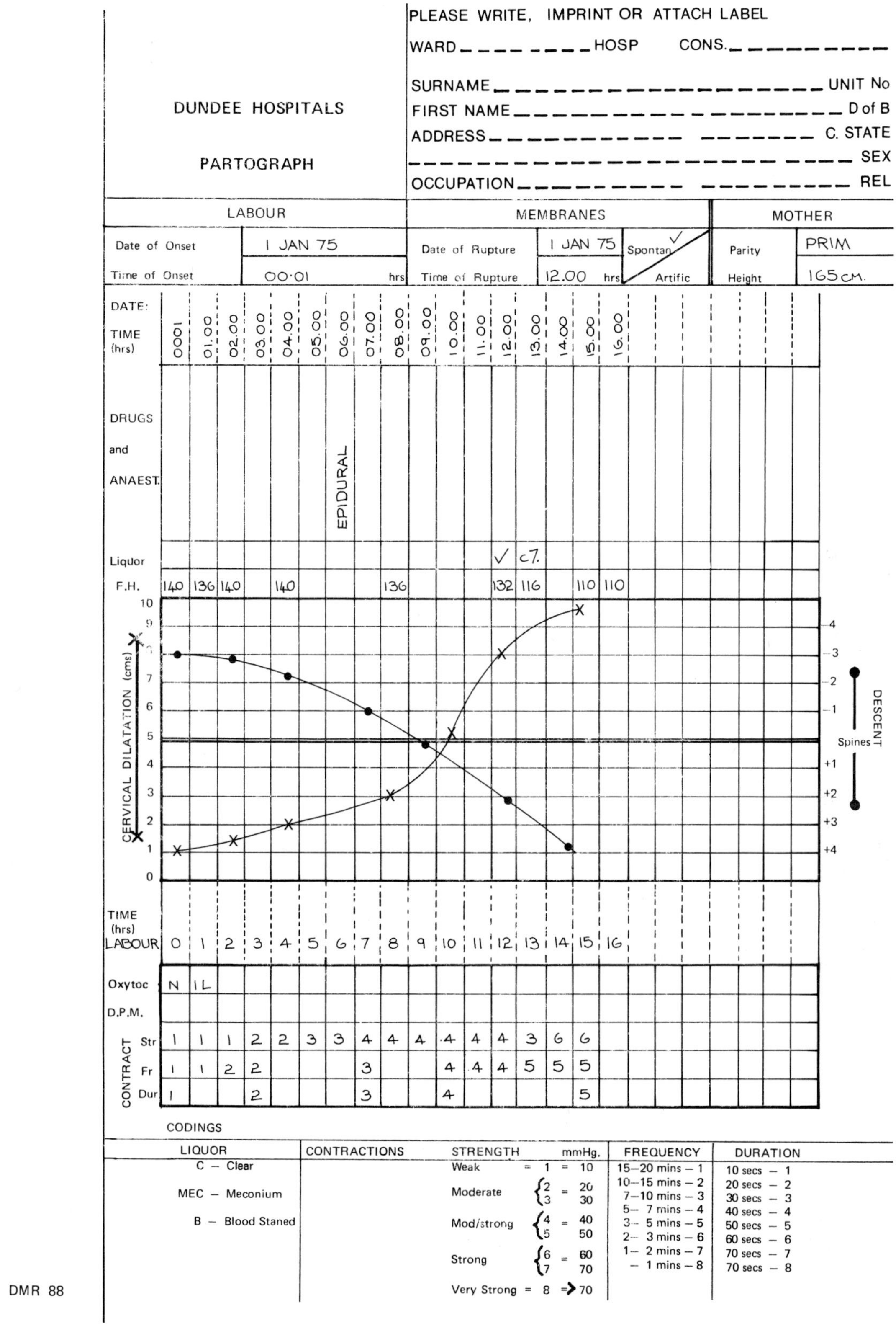

PLEASE WRITE, IMPRINT OR ATTACH LABEL

WARD _ _ _ _ _ _ _ _ HOSP   CONS._ _ _ _ _ _ _ _

SURNAME _ _ _ _ _ _ _ _ _ _ _ _ _ _ _ _ UNIT No

FIRST NAME _ _ _ _ _ _ _ _ _ _ _ _ _ _ _ _ D of B

ADDRESS _ _ _ _ _ _ _ _ _ _ _ _ _ _ _ _ C. STATE

_ SEX

OCCUPATION _ _ _ _ _ _ _ _ _ _ _ _ _ _ REL

DUNDEE HOSPITALS

PARTOGRAPH

LABOUR		MEMBRANES			MOTHER	
Date of Onset	I JAN 75	Date of Rupture	I JAN 75	Spontan ✓	Parity	PRIM
Time of Onset	00·01 hrs	Time of Rupture	12.00 hrs	Artific	Height	165 cm.

DATE:

TIME (hrs): 0001 01.00 02.00 03.00 04.00 05.00 06.00 07.00 08.00 09.00 10.00 11.00 12.00 13.00 14.00 15.00 16.00

DRUGS and ANAEST.   EPIDURAL

Liquor   ✓ c7.

F.H. 140 136 140 140 136 132 116 110 110

CERVICAL DILATATION (cms) 0–10

DESCENT / Spines +1 +2 +3 +4 / 1 2 3 4

TIME (hrs) LABOUR: 0 1 2 3 4 5 6 7 8 9 10 11 12 13 14 15 16

Oxytoc: N IL

D.P.M.

CONTRACT																	
Str	1	1	1	2	2	3	3	4	4	4	4	4	4	3	6	6	
Fr	1	1	2	2			3		4	4	4	5	5	5			
Dur	1			2			3		4				5				

CODINGS

LIQUOR	CONTRACTIONS	STRENGTH	mmHg.	FREQUENCY	DURATION
C — Clear		Weak = 1 = 10		15—20 mins — 1	10 secs — 1
MEC — Meconium		Moderate {2 = 20, 3 = 30}		10—15 mins — 2 / 7—10 mins — 3	20 secs — 2 / 30 secs — 3
B — Blood Staned		Mod/strong {4 = 40, 5 = 50}		5—7 mins — 4 / 3—5 mins — 5	40 secs — 4 / 50 secs — 5
		Strong {6 = 60, 7 = 70}		2—3 mins — 6 / 1—2 mins — 7	60 secs — 6 / 70 secs — 7
		Very Strong = 8 ➤ 70		— 1 mins — 8	70 secs — 8

DMR 88

Fig. 19.16   Partograph showing the information recorded in the course of a relatively normal labour.

and of presentation as well as knowledge of pelvic capacity can be obtained only in this way. Simple estimation of progress can be made by junior staff or by inexperienced midwives, *but at some stage of labour probably about 6–7cm dilatation or after 12 hours a very full and careful evaluation should be made by an experienced clinician to allow decision of the continued conduct of the case.*

The risks of difficult labour

Prolonged and difficult labour due to any cause will in the poorly attended cr unattended patient cause death or severe damage to mother and child.

TO THE MOTHER
Death in labour from exhaustion, infection, uterine rupture.

Damage due to extensive laceration of cervix, vagina, rectum, bladder or later slough, fistulae involving bladder or rectum where the head is arrested in the vagina for long periods. Serious morbidity may follow the therapy given especially where the mother is already exhausted, dehydrated or infected. In England and Wales in 1967–69 where the death rate for Caesarean section is 1·2 per 1000 (Report on Confidential Enquiries into Maternal Death. HMSO) there were 57 deaths following Caesarean section done for 'difficult labour' of which 19 were considered due to the anaesthesia and 12 to pulmonary embolism. There were in addition 18 deaths due to rupture of the uterus which in England and Wales is estimated to have a death rate of 7·7 per million deliveries but six times that in the age-group 35–39.

Whilst many deaths were avoidable the serious risk of difficult labour and of delivery of the already compromised patient should be obvious. Interestingly there were no deaths due to nerve blocks, epidural caudal or pudendal emphasizing once more the greater safety of these procedures over general anaesthesia in obstetrics.

TO THE CHILD
Death or serious damage from excessive or prolonged uterine contractions, due either to anoxic or undue pressure, to mechanical difficulty in delivery, or to intra-uterine infection.

The particularly serious risk suffered by the child already compromised has been previously noted.

The long term effects on the child are discussed in Chapter 25.

Effects in subsequent pregnancy
In a follow up study of 1105 women who, as primigravidae had suffered prolonged labour with or without operative delivery, Walker (1970) found that when the mother was under 25 at the time of delivery some 80–90 per cent were pregnant again within five years no matter the type of labour or delivery. There was clear evidence of voluntary infertility in the mother over 25 especially after Caesarean section which had followed long or difficult labour. Involuntary sterility was higher in the older women but many did not want to have another child. In some the reason for this was not clear, but fear of another difficult labour and over-anxiety were much more common in the older age-groups. Financial worries were also more frequently given as reasons for not having more children by the older women despite the fact that, on the whole, their social circumstances were superior to those of the younger women. They were also much more concerned about maintaining living standards and giving their one child 'every advantage'.

The number of children born subsequently may be affected by the form of delivery in the primigravida, but in modern obstetric practice very few women are having more than two children so it is only in the older women who voluntary decide to have one child that the limitations are seen.

It will be noted too that even where a mid-cavity forceps or rotation is required in a first delivery subsequent delivery is spontaneous in a high proportion of cases. This is not an absolute rule however and it is wise policy to book for specialist care any one who has had a difficult mid-forceps or rotation forceps in a first delivery. There is also the patient who has a second child after a long gap often where pregnancy has been postponed because of difficulty with first labour or delivery. These women are a particular problem and must have specialist care.

Dystocia due to faults in the child

Fetal dystocia in vertex presentations

EXCESSIVE SIZE OF THE FETUS
It is impossible to define in absolute terms what constitutes excessive size, since almost any baby may be too big if the maternal pas-

sages are small enough. In the absence of other complications it is unusual to find dystocia due to the size of the baby unless it weighs more than 8lb (3628g), and it is unusual to have an entirely uncomplicated delivery with a baby weighing more than 10lb (4535g).

Aetiology

We know little of the factors which determine that a child should be very large. Small women with a small uterus and therefore a limited blood supply grow small babies. Certain women habitually deliver large babies, and in others there is a tendency to produce a larger baby with each successive gestation, a fact which must be kept in mind when assessing the prognosis of labour in a parous patient. Diabetic mothers are prone to have quite unusually large children, indeed weights as high as 24lb have been recorded; and it is also interesting that many women who deliver large babies show blood sugar curves of a 'prediabetic' pattern and many of them develop true diabetes in later life. Maternal nutrition exercises some influence on the fetal weight; the child of a grossly undernourished mother tends to be small.

The importance of prolonged pregnancy is constantly under debate. The rate of growth of the fetus slows after 42 weeks. There is a wide range in the weight of babies in prolonged pregnancy but they have larger heads and are heavier.

Diagnosis

Excessive development of the fetus should not escape detection until difficulty or delay arise in labour, for it is an elementary point in antenatal care to maintain a watch on fetal growth and for misfit between the fetus and the maternal passages. The detection of disproportion between the head and the maternal passages can be made as already described under contracted pelvis. It should be recognized, however, that excessive development of the baby may not be associated with any strict bony disproportion between the head and the pelvic brim, and may yet cause serious dystocia. In such circumstances the condition may at least be suspected from the following findings:

1. Excessive enlargement of the abdomen may be present. Obvious fallacies are the possible existence of a twin pregnancy or hydramnios, which may simulate the growth of a single fetus, but a less obvious trap lies in the fact that women of differing stature show a different degree of abdominal enlargement. Thus a tall woman can carry a large child with very little protrusion, whereas a short woman may show considerable bulging with quite a small baby.

2. The fetus itself may seem larger than usual on clinical examination. In addition, a large baby, filling the uterus, is more rigid than a less developed child. Furthermore, an excessively large child, even in a tall woman, will often displace the xiphoid process of the sternum more or less directly forwards.

The ultrasound estimate of the degree of maturity of the fetus, based on measurements of the biparietal diameter, may be helpful.

Course of labour

In the delivery of a head which is overdeveloped but not otherwise abnormal, arrest occurs most often in the pelvic cavity with the leading part at the plane of least pelvic dimensions. Dystocia in the perineal stage of labour is unusual.

Difficulty during the birth of the trunk of the child is maximal at the delivery of the shoulders. When these are very broad there is a tendency for the anterior shoulder to become arrested at the upper border of the pubis, while the posterior shoulder slips into the pelvis but is unable to descend until its fellow is freed from the impaction at the pelvic brim. This type of dystocia is usually preceded by some difficulty in the delivery of the head, but, especially in multiparous patients with widely dilated soft parts, a large head may emerge without difficulty, the impaction of the shoulders following as an altogether unexpected complication which often kills a baby is skilled delivery is not immediately accessible.

Prognosis

The maternal prognosis is influenced unfavourably, not only by the difficulty in the completion of labour by the natural forces but also by the increased need for operative intervention. The maternal passages are more prone to laceration and, even when this does not occur, the stretching may be severe enough to cause later prolapse and stress incontinence. The stillbirth and neonatal death rates due to trauma are increased. There is a special liability to brachial plexus damage when the shoulders give rise to difficulty. The baby's weight loss during the first few days is usually excessive and neonatal infections are more common.

PROPHYLACTIC MANAGEMENT

If the existence of an overdeveloped fetus is certain, and especially if the patient has habitually delivered very large children with difficulty, it is justifiable to induce labour at some time after the thirty-seventh week of pregnancy.

MANAGEMENT IN LABOUR

If disproportion exists at the pelvic brim then the management is essentially the same as for contracted pelvis. It may even be necessary to carry out a Caesarean section in a patient who has already had successful vaginal deliveries. In the absence of brim disproportion, Caesarean section is rarely called for unless there be other complications, but delivery by forceps will very frequently be necessary, usually when the head is still in the cavity, a procedure which should rarely be attempted in domiciliary practice. In the primigravid patient an episiotomy should usually be performed prophylactically to prevent serious perineal lacerations.

If the shoulders become impacted, usually the anterior shoulder, one must act quickly if the baby's life is to be saved. The patient must be placed immediately in the lithotomy or left lateral position. The subsequent steps are as follows:

1. A wide and deep episiotomy is made under local infiltration. (There is rarely time for pudendal block.)

2. The head is grasped from side to side with both hands. The fingers are disposed so that the tips of two fingers from each hand are placed over the suboccipital region and the remaining two fingers of each hand over the submental region but not to the mid line.

3. Without in any way rotating the child's head, traction is made in a direction downwards and backwards in the axis of the pelvic brim. This involves carrying the head far back towards the anus. The traction force required is often considerable, but should of course be the minimum consistent with progress. The traction is made intermittently for some four to five seconds at a time, the degree of force being increased gradually with each pull. The brachial plexus is fully stretched and will be very liable to tear *if the neck is twisted*. The danger to the plexus may be reduced by getting the conscious patient to bear down strongly with each traction effort, or by manual pressure from the abdomen by an assistant if the patient is anaesthetized.

4. In favourable cases dislodgment of the anterior shoulder from its position of impaction at the pelvic brim allows of its rapid descent into the pelvis (Fig.

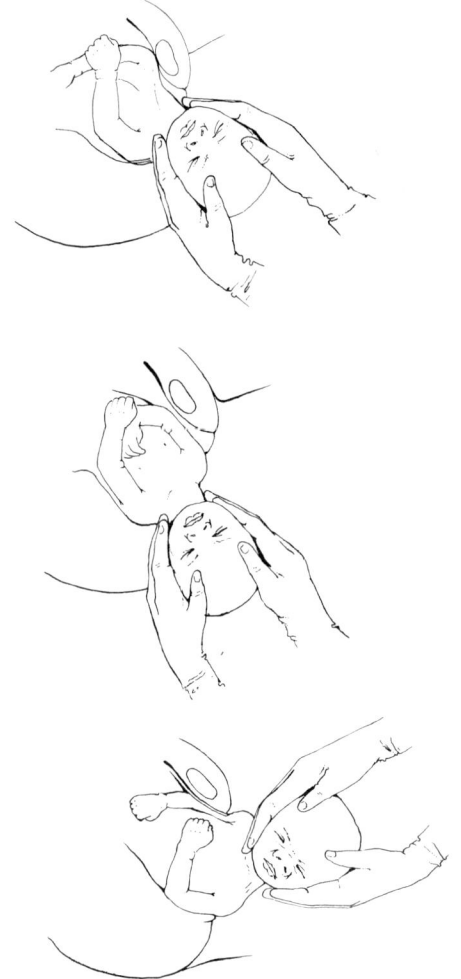

Fig. 19.17   Delivery of impacted shoulders.

19.17). The direction of traction is then altered, the head and neck being swung forwards until the posterior shoulder sweeps over the perineum, when the trunk of the child follows readily.

5. In less favourable circumstances strong traction fails to dislodge the anterior shoulder. The most effective plan is then to bring down the posterior arm. Pudendal block or general anaesthesia are needed. Introducing the whole hand into the vagina, under general anaesthesia which may require to be hurriedly induced, the attendant defines the posterior shoulder, and the hand is passed along the humerus of the child until the elbow is reached. If the elbow joint of the child is not already flexed, flexion is now secured by manipulation of the baby's forearm (Fig. 19.18) after which the child's hand is drawn down across the thorax and anterior aspect of the neck until it is delivered from the vulva, when gentle traction upon the hand delivers the posterior shoulder, the axilla of which now lies in contact with

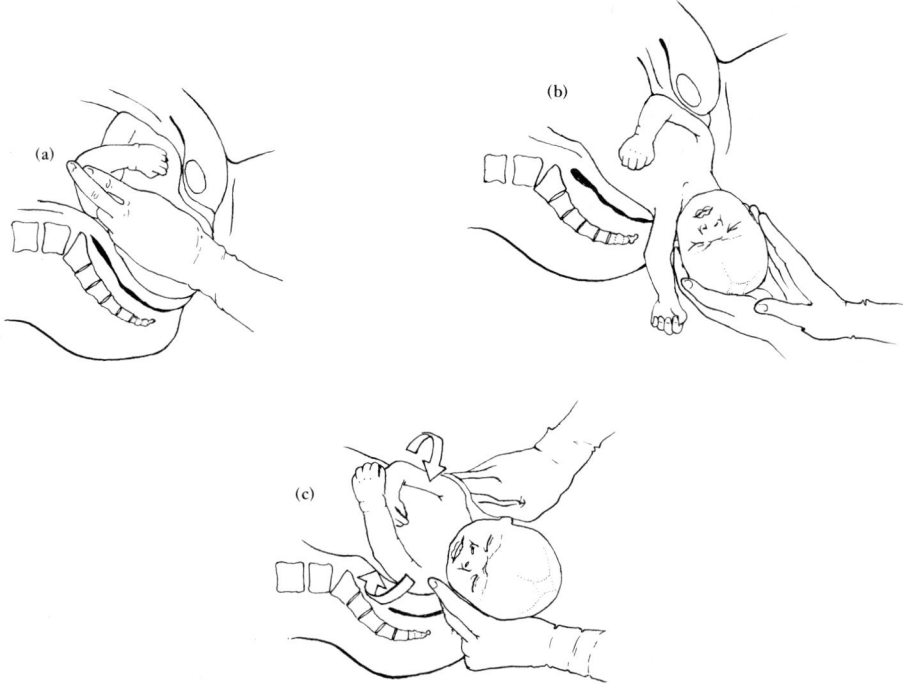

Fig. 19.18   (a) (b) Techniques of the delivery of the arm where the shoulders are impacted. (c) The end result of rotation of the shoulders.

the posterior commissure of the vulva. The traction on the baby's head in the axis of the pelvis is now resumed and rarely fails to deliver the anterior shoulder quite easily, when the remainder of the trunk causes no difficulty. Rotation of the body can be done here, using the delivered arm as a point of traction.

The manipulation of the posterior arm across the thorax of the child is not always easy, and in such circumstances other expedients may be adopted.

6. An attempt may be made to rotate the posterior shoulder to an anterior position, Fig. 19.18, taking care not to dislodge it from the pelvis. The shoulder which was originally anterior can then enter the pelvis quite readily.

7. Without such rotation, traction may be made on the posterior shoulder of a dead child by means of a finger, or even with a blunt metal hook. (This is a procedure of some desperation and is liable to produce damage to the axillary vessels or the lower trunk of the brachial plexus, the shoulder joint, humerus or clavicle in the living child.)

8. If the child is dead, the posterior clavicle or both may be divided by scissors in the operation of cleidotomy (Chapt. 27).

OCCIPITO-POSTERIOR POSITIONS OF THE
VERTEX

The term occipito-posterior is used to de-scribe the position of the head in relation to the maternal pelvis in those cases where labour commences with the vertex presenting and the occiput lying in either posterior quadrant of the pelvis.

About 20 per cent of labours commence with the occiput placed obliquely posterior, and it is more frequent to find the occiput in the right posterior quadrant (right occipito-posterior) than in the left posterior quadrant (left occipito-posterior). Such oblique posterior positions of the head may be found in any type of pelvis, but are less frequent when the shape of the pelvic brim is flat.

A direct occipito-sacral position is uncommon but is sometimes found in the long oval or anthropoid pelvis.

Aetiology of occipito-posterior positions
The majority of heads present initially with the occiput directly lateral, the long axis of the head being in or parallel to the transverse diameter of the pelvis. So long as the head has not entered the birth canal, deviations from this position are always liable to occur but seldom develop once the head has engaged in the pelvis.

Anything which serves to delay the easy engagement of the head—e.g. pelvic contraction, lax abdominal wall, uterine obliquity, constipation, excess liquor or twin pregnancy—increases the opportunities of chance deviation of the occiput from the occipito-lateral position. It has been suggested that a very bulky placenta may so alter the shape of the uterus as to force the fetus to assume a position in which the convexity of its back is directed away from the bulging placenta. The presence of the colon in the left posterior quadrant of the pelvis tends to prevent deviation of the occiput to that side and to favour the occurrence of the right occipito-posterior position. The fact that the occipito-posterior position occurs frequently where the pelvic brim is round in shape and that it does not tend to recur in successive pregnancies suggests that chance plays an important part in its causation.

The mechanism of labour in occipito-posterior positions

In oblique occipito-posterior positions the head lies initially at the brim with the occiput in the neighbourhood of the sacro-iliac joint, and the sinciput directed towards the opposite pectineal eminence. The long axis of the head lies in the oblique diameter. The attitude of the head should ideally be one of full flexion but in many cases the convexity of the maternal lumbar spine, being opposed to the convexity of the child's vertebral column, produces some deflexion of the head, so that the anterior fontanelle becomes the leading part of the head during labour and it is this factor of malflexion that is most important in the behaviour of the labour.

As labour progresses the head descends through the pelvic brim. If this is roomy or the head well flexed there is usually no difficulty. If the head is partially deflexed the occipito-frontal rather than the suboccipito-bregmatic circumference must pass through the brim. Delay is therefore probable until the head moulds or until full flexion occurs.

Once past the plane of the pelvic brim the head usually descends through the pelvic cavity in the occipito-posterior position without particular difficulty, until the leading part impinges upon the pelvic floor at the level of the plane of the least pelvic dimensions, where the pelvic axis swings sharply forwards. At this level rotation usually occurs.

In most cases the occiput rotates from the posterior position to the mid-line in front, thus moving through an angle of from 90–135°. This is usually called long rotation. The use of the term long rotation does not imply that the rotation will necessarily take a long time. Indeed, although occasionally the process may be tedious, rotation of an occipito-posterior position during the descent of the presenting part may be produced quickly.

When long rotation occurs, the further mechanism of labour is exactly as in normal cases.

PERSISTENT OCCIPITO-POSTERIOR POSITION

This is the name applied to those occipito-posterior cases (some 10 per cent) which do not show long rotation. There are three possible errors or failures in rotation:

1. The occiput may rotate backwards into the hollow of the sacrum. This is sometimes referred to as 'short rotation' of the occiput.

2. Forward rotation of the occiput may commence, but may cease especially if flexion is poor when the sagittal suture of the head comes to lie in the transverse diameter of the pelvis, with the occiput directly lateral. This is sometimes referred to as 'deep transverse arrest', a term which includes all cases of arrest in this position, irrespective of the original position.

3. The occiput may fail to rotate at all, remaining obliquely posterior.

In any of these three abnormalities the head may become completely impacted. If the head rotates into the hollow of the sacrum spontaneous delivery is possible, but may be accompanied by much soft tissue damage which can be avoided by wide episiotomy. The head descends to the outlet in the direct occipito-posterior position. The frontal region of the skull becomes a pivot at the lower border of the symphysis pubis, after which the head is delivered by a movement of flexion which sweeps the occiput over the perineum, the long occipito-frontal diameter distending the vulva in the process. Thereafter the face slips down from behind the pubes, giving the name of 'face to pubes' to this type of delivery. After the head is born the trunk of the child is expelled in the usual manner.

Aetiology of persistent occipito-posterior position

More than one factor is probably responsible for persistence of an occipito-posterior position. It has been customary to suggest that the determining factor in long rotation of the head is the spontaneous correction of the extension in the pelvic cavity or at the pelvic floor, and, conversely, the persistence of deflexion is responsible for the malrotation into the sacral hollow. This is undoubtedly an oversimplification, for X-ray examinations during labour have now confirmed impressions gained previously by clinical examination that persistence of the occipito-posterior may occur in the presence of good flexion.

While deflexion of the head may contribute to some cases of persistent occipito-posterior position, it is likely that at least equal importance should be allotted to certain other factors as follows:

1. When a head presents abinitio with the occiput opposite the hollow of the sacrum, the occiput very commonly remains in the same location.

2. When a head presents with the occiput obliquely posterior but between the sacro-iliac joint and the sacral promontory, short rotation to bring the occiput into the sacral hollow is the usual result.

3. When the head presents with the occiput obliquely posterior, but with the occiput placed

opposite the sacro-iliac joint, or between it and the pectineal eminence, the tendency is to long rotation. This may be interfered with, however, by factors which diminish the natural tendency to internal rotation. These are:

Feeble uterine contractions or a deficient pelvic floor. A diminished curvature to the birth canal, resulting from narrowing of the anterior portion of the pelvic outlet, which is then denied to the head.

A uterus tightly contracted around the child's body owing to the liquor amnii having entirely drained away.

Diagnosis of occipito-posterior position

The early diagnosis depends chiefly upon the findings on abdominal examination, for until some cervical dilatation has been achieved in labour, vaginal diagnosis lacks precision.

Inspection. With posterior positions of the occiput the anterior uterine wall (especially below the umbilicus), is frequently observed to be flattened or even concave.

Palpation. Occipito-posterior position may be suspected justifiably if the fetal head remains mobile from side to side in a primigravida during the last few weeks of pregnancy. A further finding pointing to this possibility is the simultaneous recognition of (a) difficulty in locating the back of the child together with (b) the presence of limbs on both sides of the mother's abdomen. When the back is eventually located, a sign of more direct diagnostic importance is the observation that the prominence of the head opposite to the side on which the back is found (i.e. the brow) lies much nearer to the anterior abdominal wall than the other cephalic prominence (i.e. the occiput). It may also be noted that the occiput and brow are very nearly on the same level, indicating some degree of deflexion, which in itself may arouse justifiable suspicions of occipito-posterior position.

Auscultation. There is sometimes difficulty in hearing the fetal heart-sounds. Generally they are best heard well round to the side towards which the back is directed, but if there is very marked deflexion of head and trunk, the fetal heart-sounds may be heard best over the ventral aspect of the child.

Vaginal examination. As the head does not fit the pelvis so exactly as in occipito-anterior positions, it may be difficult to reach the presenting part early in labour. Therefore the markings by which the position of the head is determined are difficult to define until the head has descended some little way into the cavity. If the anterior fontanelle is easily felt an occipito-posterior position should be suspected. In a right occipito-posterior position the anterior fontanelle in the right posterior quadrant, with the sagittal suture crossing the pelvis obliquely between them (Fig. 19.7).

Uterine inertia in first stage. The association of occipito-posterior position with uterine inertia has already been stressed and the observation of poor uterine action or of secondary failure of cervical dilatation after say 6–7cm with a head which remains above spines should raise the suspicion of an occipito-posterior position with positional disproportion.

Later in labour. In a patient who is not obese the diagnosis should be made by abdominal palpation without difficulty, but in plump patients it may never be made at all if long rotation occurs. In fact diagnosis late in labour is largely a matter of the recognition of the persistent occipito-posterior.

One of the most important indications is unexpected delay in the second stage of labour. If the head remains invisible after 20 minutes of second stage contractions in a primigravida, or in a parous patient, an abnormal position or presentation should be suspected and vaginal examination made to determine the exact presentation, position and attitude. This is not always easy since although the sutures and fontanelles are much more accessible than in earlier labour, they may be largely obscured by a caput succedaneum. In such circumstances the head may obviously be high and there may be such moulding that disproportion is diagnosed and Caesarean section indicated. However if vaginal delivery appears likely it will be necessary to palpate the fetal head with the assistance of a general, spinal, epidural or caudal anaesthesia to make a precise diagnosis. The free border of the pinna of the fetal ear is then the most generally useful landmark. With the ear flattened against the baby's head it points towards the occiput.

Sometimes even an experienced obstetrician may fail to diagnose the position correctly. Unexpected difficulty developing during forceps traction may be an important clue to the missed diagnosis, especially if the perineum begins to tear before the crowning of the head, if the head appears to be emerging very much farther backwards than usual, or if the forceps commence to slip.

Prognosis of occipito-posterior position

In occipito-posterior positions the prognosis is less favourable than in anterior positions both for mother and for child. Nevertheless the gravity of the condition should not be overestimated, so long as the medical attendant resists the temptation to resort to premature vaginal delivery and elects to use Caesarean section more often.

Opinions differ about the frequency with which occipito-posterior positions correct themselves spontaneously during labour. Probably about 90 per cent of occipito-posterior positions recognized at the onset of labour, given time, will correct themselves during labour, often in the second stage.

Some degree of uterine inefficiency in the first stage is common in occipito-posterior positions, but it generally yields to sedatives or stimulation. The difficulties and dangers of the malposition are largely part of the problem of disordered uterine action which is very much less common with augmented or accelerated labour (*see* page 345).

It is rarely possible to predict which case will undergo long internal rotation and which case will become a persistent occipito-posterior. The only clear exceptions are those cases where from the beginning of labour the occiput has lain opposite the sacrum or between the sacrum and the sacro-iliac joint. In such circumstances the head rotates into or remains in the hollow of the sacrum in a very high proportion of cases, especially when the pelvis is of the anthropoid type.

In persistent occipito-posterior position the prognosis is worst in those cases which become impacted with the occiput obliquely posterior. When the occiput rotates into the hollow of the sacrum the outlook is slightly better, in that spontaneous delivery is possible. The maternal soft tissues, however, are exposed to considerably increased risks of damage, since, as has been noted, it is common for the occipito-frontal diameter of the baby's head to have to pass the vulvar introitus.

In deep transverse arrest the prognosis resembles that of impacted oblique-posterior position, in that spontaneous delivery with the head remaining in the transverse position is unlikely to occur. Diagnosis of the position of the occiput is somewhat difficult and if the position of the head is mistakenly diagnosed as occipito-anterior, and forceps delivery attempted without rotation of the occiput, avoidable damage will be caused.

To sum up: it may be said that when the pelvis is ample and the forces of labour are reasonably efficient, either naturally or by stimulation, the prognosis for mother and for child is good. Pelvic contraction and uterine inertia influence the prognosis unfavourably. Given a second stage of labour of adequate duration, spontaneous rotation occurs in 90 per cent of cases. In the remaining 10 per cent the prognosis is not necessarily unfavourable unless operative delivery is unskilled.

Management of occipito-posterior positions

Modern techniques of augmented labour suggest that little attention need be paid to position of the head. However, where in early labour an occipito-posterior position is clearly present, the attendant is forewarned, especially where the occiput lies between the sacro iliac joint and the lateral aspect of the pelvis. Failure of progress of dilatation would early indicate stimulation especially where monitor suggested inadequate uterine action.

Second stage of labour. It is of great importance to allow an adequate time, since rotation will occur spontaneously in a high proportion of cases managed conservatively. Further, even when the head becomes impacted, if a conservative management has been adopted it is usual to find that the occiput has at least rotated to the more favourable location of a deep transverse arrest. On the other hand, it is unwise to delay too long. In surroundings favourable for operative intervention a patient should seldom be allowed more than forty minutes of second stage contractions; and, in a parous patient, anything over a half hour may become dangerous. These figures are only a rough guide, however, and cases require to be judged individually by the maternal and fetal reactions. Constant fetal heart and uterine pressure monitor is very helpful.

If intervention becomes necessary, correction of the malposition under epidural general anaesthesia, followed by the immediate extraction of the fetus by forceps, should be performed *provided Caesarean section is not indicated*.

Manual rotation of a persistent occipito-posterior position

Deep general anaesthesia is required. The operation is really a combined abdominal vaginal manipulation and for this reason the lithotomy position is generally preferred to the left lateral.

After gently stretching the perineum or after episiotomy for access the whole hand is introduced into the vagina to determine exactly how the head is lying. This should never be omitted even when the diagnosis seems certain. It also allows palpation of the pelvic shape and size. It is not of much importance which hand is employed in the vagina, but some operators feel more confident when the right hand is used for a left occipito-posterior position and the left hand for a right position. Once it has been decided to rotate, episiotomy allows manipulation. It is usual to hold the head with the thumb on one parietal eminence and the fingers on the other. The head having been slightly flexed by pressure on the sinciput, rotation then begun by using the whole hand to twist the head into the occiput into the mid-line

(Chapter 27). The first step is to press on the sinciput so as to increase the flexion and to diminish the diameters of the head which can now be rotated. This usually causes the head to disimpact and recede a little and it thus becomes easier to rotate. (It is tempting to push the head back to the level of the brim where it is often very easy to rotate, but this should be resisted since the head, in its corrected position, may not re-engage easily, or prolapse of the cord may occur, especially if the anaesthetic is rather light and the patient strains.) The head is grasped with the thumb over the anterior parietal bone and the fingers posteriorly and rotated in the appropriate direction. By placing the other hand on the mother's abdomen the baby's anterior shoulder is pulled round in the same direction at the same time. The rotation is continued until the occiput either lies directly anteriorly, or even lies in the contralateral anterior quadrant of the pelvis. It is of vital importance to attempt rotation of the trunk, for otherwise rotation of the head through 135° may cause the baby's neck to be twisted, and even if this does not often cause damage to the child it makes it certain that the head will take up its old position when the hand is removed. In the obese patient, or if the uterus is tightly applied to the fetal body, the abdominal manipulation may be difficult. In all cases after the rotation is completed, it is desirable to withdraw the vaginal hand for a few seconds and then re-insert it to check that the head is still in its corrected position. It may be necessary to hold the head in its new position until the first forcep blade is applied.

Even with the patient deeply anaesthetized the method outlined above sometimes fails and the fetal skull bones may be felt to 'dimple' under the fingers. In such cases the hand should be passed right into the uterus till it grasps the posterior shoulder. With the aid of the external hand on the anterior shoulder the trunk is now turned and the head turns with it or can be rotated easily with the vaginal hand as it is withdrawn. This is a major procedure and should not be attempted unless Caesarean section cannot be done. It nearly always results in a recession of the head up to or beyond the pelvic brim, with risks already noted. In such circumstances the head should be pushed back into the pelvis by suprapubic pressure before applying the forceps.

Face to pubes delivery

In persistent occipito-posterior position, with the occiput directly or obliquely posterior, it may not be possible to carry out a manual rotation, and forceps delivery in the face to pubes position may be considered. If the pelvis is ample, especially if it is of the anthropoid type, the fetus suffers little harm, but the risk of damage to the perineum and lower vagina is considerable and a deep episiotomy should usually precede forceps delivery. In the case of a *small pelvis* great force would be required to complete the delivery and Caesarean section would almost always be preferred.

Rotation and delivery by forceps

Where there is arrest in the deep transverse or occipito-posterior positions rotation by forceps is now standard procedure.

Successful use of Keilland's forceps depends, as with all technical procedure, on intelligent appreciation of the problem plus experience. This is indeed an instrument for the specialist. Keilland's forceps are ideal for delivery of the head in the occipito position or transverse position when the head is in the cavity of the pelvis and there is no outlet funnelling to prevent lower rotation and delivery; and especially where it is judged that the difficulty is a positional one mainly.

The forceps are applied ultimately to the sides of the head and once the exact position of the occiput is determined, the forceps should be held in the hand in the exact position in which they will lie once applied. Adequately lubricated with cream the anterior blade is then applied directly between head and symphysis starting almost in the vertical position. Once that blade is applied the posterior may be applied directly or be rarely 'wandered' into position having been first inserted over the face. Once the blades are in position the sliding lock is used to correct any asynclitism and some effort might be made to flex the head.

Rotation is gently attempted at the first level but often the head must be brought down to the pelvic floor before rotation is possible. It is dangerous to push the head up to rotate as it may not come down again but this may be the last resort before removal of the forceps and Caesarean section.

Keilland's forceps are dangerous to the mother in that severe tearing and occasionally bladder damage may occur after delivery. Cervical tears and bladder damage should be looked for. Such a delivery can be very traumatic to the baby and follow up studies of babies show some disturbing cases. Over-enthusiasm to deliver from the high pelvis should *not* be allowed.

Arrest in the lateral position

Arrest of the head in the lateral position deep in the cavity follows a similar pattern to arrest in the posterior position and may be a sequel to partial rotation, from the posterior position. However, the head may arrest in the lateral position in the high cavity having failed to descend usually because of a poor sacral curve and still be in a position of asynclitism. An anterior parietal presentation may suggest that the head is engaged since the head is difficult to feel above the brim and easy to feel in the anterior position vaginally. The clue is found in the empty posterior pelvis. Such cases can be delivered only by Caesarean section. Delivery from the lateral position deep in the pelvis is as described for posterior position by manual rotation or Keilland's forceps.

Fetal dystocia in malpresentation

Normally the head presents in varying degrees of flexion but once labour starts flexion occurs and the vertex leads. All other presentations are abnormal e.g. face, brow, breech, transverse or shoulder. When the cord leads in front of any presenting part 'cord presentation' is stated to be present. (Cord prolapse if the membranes are ruptured.) Compound presentation, head and arm or leg; breech and hand etc. do occur.

Malpresentation is due—

Mother: Uterine malformation
Pelvic contraction
Pelvic tumours
Lax uterus and abdominal wall altering the axis of the fetal body.
Fetal: Prematurity
Plural pregnancy
Hydramnios
Intra-uterine Death
Fetal Deformity
Placenta Praevia may be a predisposing cause.

Course of labour

Disproportion with obstructed labour is likely where there is malpresentation and is inevitable in transverse or shoulder presentation with a large child. However, until this obstruction occurs labour is no different than in vertex presentation although premature membrane rupture is a little more likely. Once obstruction appears labour may be strong and tetanic or secondary inertia may supervene.

For the mother the risk of anaesthesia and operative intervention is high and for the child damage and death are likely unless adequate obstetric action is taken. In modern units the risk to the mother or child should be slight.

Dystocia in association with abnormal cephalic presentations

The cases are those in which the attitude of the fetus has become so much extended that the leading part is either (1) the brow or (2) the face (Fig. 19.19). It is generally said that face presentations occur in about 1 in 400–500 births and brow presentations 1 per 1000.

VARIETIES OF FACE AND BROW PRESENTATION
In classifying face presentations the chin (or mentum) is used as the denominator. As in vertex presentation, the denominator may be found at the beginning of labour in any of the four quadrants of the pelvis, or it may be directly lateral, with the long axis of the head occupying the transverse diameter of the pelvis. The lateral position is not so common as in vertex presentations, and it is therefore usual to restrict the descriptive terminology of face presentations to four classical positions each of which may be taken to correspond to a vertex position in which, for some reason, the head has become completely extended until the face presents and the occiput lies

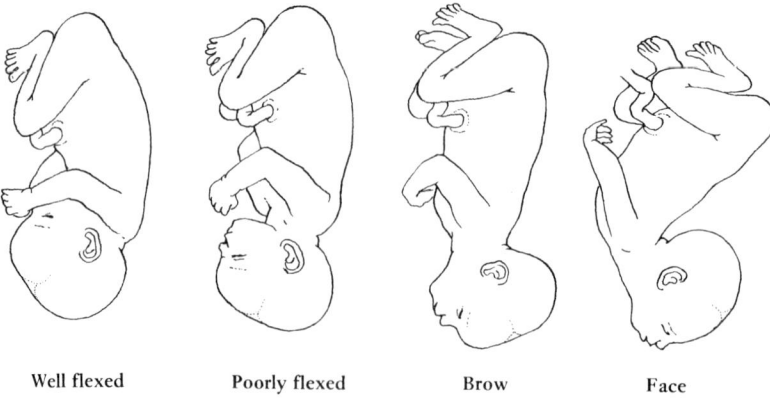

Well flexed   Poorly flexed   Brow   Face

Fig. 19.19   Varying degrees of extension of the head from vertex to face presentation.

more or less in contact with the back of the baby's neck. Thus for example the right mento-posterior (RMP) variety of face presentation may be regarded as resulting from the complete extension of a vertex presentation, LOA. Again a left mento-anterior (LMA) may result from the complete extension of the vertex presentation, ROP (Fig. 19.19).

Occipito-posterior position predisposes to extension of the head, and it is therefore not surprising that mento-anterior positions are much commoner (about six times) than mento-posterior positions.

It is usual in describing the position of a brow presentation in relation to the maternal pelvis to use the same notation as for face presentations, e.g. brow presentation, RMP.

Aetiology of face and brow presentation

In addition to the general causes of malpresentation listed above (p. 368) certain conditions are prone particularly to favour the presentation of the face or brow. Of these, exaggeration of the deflexion of an occipito-posterior position is rather common, such exaggeration being particularly predisposed to by the uterine obliquity of multiparity. Spasm of the fetal muscles of the erector spinae group undoes the spinal flexion in some cases. In others, face presentation is favoured by fetal lordosis, the result of spina bifida at almost any level. Other fetal deformities such as anencephaly, encephaloceles and bronchoceles are said to be present in 10 per cent of face and brow presentations. An occasional case is clearly attributable to multiple coils of umbilical cord looped round the fetal neck.

FACE PRESENTATION

Diagnosis—Palpation

The most striking feature on abdominal palpation is a depression between the occiput and back of the child. This, however, is not always easy to determine, and is especially difficult if the back of the child is directed posteriorly. The lower pole of the uterus may be sensitive and the fetal parts are consequently difficult to define. In this presentation the hand directed towards the chin can be sunk deeper down than the hand which palpates the occiput (Fig. 19.20). But here again difficulty may be experienced and a radiograph may be necessary. The limbs are particularly easily felt in mento-anterior positions in which the thorax is pushed forwards.

Auscultation. The fetal heart is heard below the umbilicus to one or other side. In mento-anterior positions the point of maximum intensity is much nearer to the middle line than in mento-posterior positions. In addition, in mento-anterior positions the clarity of the sounds is most striking, since the stethoscope is often placed directly over the precordium of the arched fetal chest at the point where it is thrust into closest contact with the abdominal wall. Indeed in many cases the observation that the fetal heart-sounds are usually loud

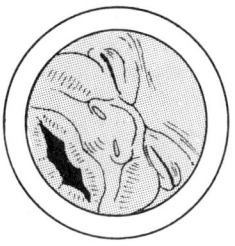

Fig. 19.20   The touch picture in RMP.

rouses the first suspicion that a face presentation may be present.

Vaginal examination. The landmarks of the face are the orbital ridges, the eyes, the bridge of the nose, the nostrils, the lips, the chin and the gums (Fig. 19.20). Although in theory these should enable a face presentation to be recognized quite readily the situation is far different in practice, since caput succedaneum may obscure all landmarks and since in many cases the presenting part remains high and inaccessible until late in labour. The 'touch picture' of oedematous cheeks is extraordinarily like that of buttocks and the swollen lips are often mistaken for external genitals, so that an incorrect diagnosis of breech presentation may be made. The most important adjunct to the differential diagnosis of face presentation is the recognition of the firm alveolar processes of the jaws when the finger is pressed into the mouth. Meconium on the examining finger diagnoses 'breech'. Despite this, mistakes are still possible, and may have to be excluded by examination carried out under anaesthesia with the whole hand in the vagina. X-ray examination is a valuable alternative.

Mento-anterior positions

These positions are the more favourable and fortunately occur six times as often as mento-posterior positions.

The head starts its descent in an attitude of extension often as a brow, and this is increased owing to the resistance of the pelvic canal. As the head descends in this attitude and meets with the resistance of the pelvic floor the chin rotates forwards, so that the long axis of the face rotates into the conjugate diameter of the pelvis, with the chin to the front. This movement is exactly similar to and produced by the same causes which bring about this rotation in vertex presentations. Finally the chin is driven under the arch of the pubis, and then the face, vertex and occiput pass over the perineum. Thus in a face presentation the actual birth takes place by a movement of flexion of the head instead of by extension as in vertex presentations. The last movement, as in vertex presentations, is an external rotation of the head brought about by the rotation of the shoulders when they reach the pelvic floor. One of the problems is that the face may reach the pelvic floor before the biparietal diameter has passed the brim and rotation is apparently very late. There is

7cm between face and parietal eminences and in a shallow pelvis the face may be on the floor with the parietal diameter not engaged.

Mento-posterior positions

These are comparable to the occipito-posterior positions of the vertex. As the face descends it may take the long rotation, in which extension becomes more marked and the chin rotates forwards until it comes behind the symphysis pubis. Thus it will be observed that the movement is exactly comparable to the long rotation observed in occipito-posterior positions. This is the most favourable termination.

Unfortunately, sometimes the chin rotates into the hollow of the sacrum, a condition known as persistent mento-posterior position. This is a most unfavourable occurrence, because the head, already extremely extended, with the chin behind, cannot be delivered. Caesarean section is necessary.

The caput succedaneum and moulding in face presentations

The caput succedaneum in face presentations forms over the malar bones and round the angles of the eyes and mouth. The result is that the child born in this position presents a bruised appearance, somewhat alarming to the mother. The bruising, however, provided no injury has been done to the child, soon disappears, and in a day or two is entirely gone. The moulding which occurs is typical. There is great elongation of the head which may persist for a few days. Very frequently, also if the child is placed in bed it will be observed that the head assumes the attitude of extension which it occupied during its passage through the canal. This is only temporary, however, for in a day or two the overstretching of the anterior muscles and the spasmodic contractions of the posterior muscles of the neck disappear.

Prognosis in face presentation

In general, the prognosis for mother and for child is worse than in vertex presentations. It is influenced not only by the malpresentation itself, which adds to the difficulty of labour even when all other factors are favourable, but also by the various aetiological factors which may in themselves be dangerous.

The chief danger to the mother is damage to the soft tissues due to the fact that as the head extends and moulds backwards a large diameter made up of the combined thickness of the head and neck has to pass through the introitus. The stillbirth rate may be as high as 30 per cent, since not only is the risk of severe injury to the fetus great but serious deformity, such as anencephaly, is frequently present. The risks are highest in mento-posterior positions, which so often call for operative delivery. The severe moulding of the fetal head, which occurs when it is passing through the pelvic brim, probably explains the fact that death of the fetus may occur suddenly early in labour. The face and neck are naturally more exposed to damage than usual and the eyes, sternomastoid muscles and trachea are most liable to be injured.

Management of face presentations

Prophylactic management. Face presentation is rarely diagnosed before the onset of labour, and even if it were little could be done to correct it. If it is recognized an X-ray examination should be considered to exclude fetal deformity and a standing lateral pelvimetry to estimate pelvic capacity. Should contraction be found and the baby appear normal, there is much to be said for an elective Caesarean section, especially in a primigravida.

Management in labour. Even in the absence of pelvic contraction Caesarean section may be performed in elderly primigravidae to secure a live baby, but in young women vaginal delivery should be aimed at in accordance with the principles detailed below.

1. *Mento-anterior positions.* No attempt should be made to alter the position, for in most cases spontaneous delivery occurs. Should this not take place the child can be extracted with forceps provided the pelvis is adequate.

2. *Mento-posterior positions.* In many cases a Caesarean section is by far the best treatment for mother and child alike, although 'long rotation' may occur.

Where Caesarean section is impossible some cases may sometimes be treated successfully in the second stage of labour by converting the face presentation into a vertex by manipulation, the operation is far from easy and there is a serious risk that the uterus may be ruptured, or the presentation converted to a brow. The essential step is to make quite sure that the attitude of the child's trunk is successfully converted from one of extension to one of flexion. This is done by pressing over the front of the fetal chest with a hand passed into the uterus while the child's buttocks are swung in the opposite direction by manipulation through the abdominal wall. If this procedure succeeds, the occiput may be hooked down with the fingers as the intra-uterine hand is withdrawn. Forceps delivery should follow immediately.

Manual rotation to anterior face may be tried.

If manipulations are to succeed, deep anaesthesia is necessary to relax the uterus fully. Should they fail, there is still a place for Caesarean section if the child's condition is good. Persistent strong traction should not be used. If the child is dead, craniotomy will be necessary.

BROW PRESENTATION

This is the most unfavourable of cephalic presentations. The attitude is midway between the complete extension of a face presentation and the flexion of a normal vertex (Fig. 19.21), and may arise as the head enters the pelvis in early labour. The large occipito-mental circumference engages in the brim, and, if

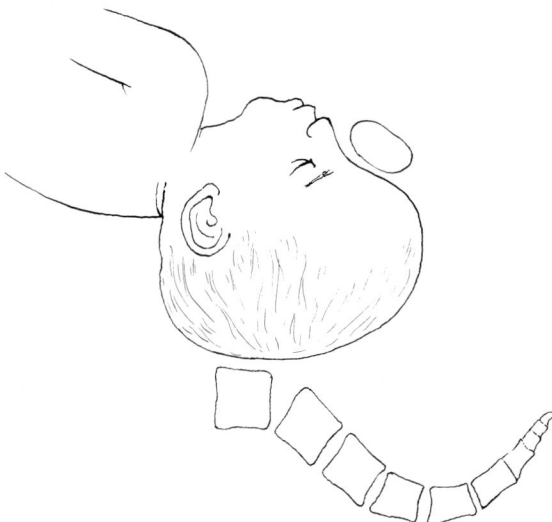

Fig. 19.21 A baby in brow presentation attempting to enter the pelvis—mento vertical diameter attempting to engage.

the child is normally developed, an impasse results unless the pelvis is exceptionally roomy. It should be noted, however, that a brow presentation discovered in early labour is not necessarily of such serious significance, because in a number of cases spontaneous correction to an attitude of full flexion occurs. In others, spontaneous conversion to full extension takes place, when the presentation becomes a face, with a much more favourable outlook— at least in those cases where the position is mento-anterior.

In cases seen later in labour such a favourable conclusion cannot be expected. The forehead of the child becomes impacted in the pelvic cavity, and the whole shape of the head is distorted by extreme moulding of the type shown.

Diagnosis
By abdominal palpation the presentation more closely resembles a face than a vertex, the resistance of chin and occiput being encountered at approximately the same level. Since the forepart of the head becomes engaged in the pelvic brim comparatively early one is apt to be deceived into thinking that the condition is quite satisfactory.

On vaginal examination the 'landmarks' felt are the frontal eminence, the orbital ridges and very generally the bridge of the nose and the nostrils. But the mouth, gums and chin can only be distinguished if the examining fingers are passed well up beyond the nose. If the labour has been in progress for some time the 'landmarks' referred to are very much masked by the oedematous condition of the forehead and face.

Treatment
Should the diagnosis be made while the membranes are intact or soon after they rupture, no active

treatment may be necessary, since within an hour or two spontaneous adjustment of the attitude may result. If strong pains are present here is a risk of rupture of the uterus, especially in multiparae, and intervention is necessary.

In the case seen for the first time late in labour, or when conservative management has failed, Caesarean section is best for both mother and child. Before Caesarean section is undertaken the child's condition must be satisfactory.

If it is decided to attempt vaginal delivery the choice is between conversion to a vertex or to a face presentation, followed by forceps; or conversion to a breech by podalic version. All these manipulations require deep anaesthesia if performed late in labour and carry a risk of uterine rupture. The procedures are essentially similar to those described under face presentation and podalic version.

When it is decided that the risks of these intra-uterine applications are too great a 'tentative' application of forceps may be employed (as in the mento-posterior face presentations). If this is unsuccessful, craniotomy is usually the only alternative.

PROLAPSE OF ARM WITH CRANIAL PRESENTATIONS
This complication is not common. However, its significance should be appreciated, for the accoucheur is apt, should he feel a hand or arm at the brim of the pelvis, to conclude that he has to deal with a shoulder presentation and to proceed immediately to perform the operation of version. With a prolapsed arm in front of the head this is not necessary. The correct treatment is to push up the arm beyond the head and allow the head to engage.

A very rare and particularly complicated condition is nuchal displacement of the arm, where it lies in the nape of the neck. Here the head sinks well down in the pelvis but is arrested at the outlet. It is specially difficult to recognize, but it should be suspected if there is difficulty in delivering the head with forceps where position of head and the pelvic outlet are normal.

The correct treatment is to anaesthetize the patient, dislodge the head and push the arm over the face to its normal position and apply forceps.

BREECH PRESENTATIONS
Breech presentation occurs in some 3-4 per cent of all deliveries. If premature deliveries are excluded, the incidence is 2·5 per cent. Breech presentation can often be corrected during pregnancy by manipulation through the mother's abdominal wall. This operation is known as external cephalic version. Its indications and contra-indications are discussed below (p. 377).

Varieties of breech presentation
Breech presentations are classified (1) in terms of the precise *attitudes* of the lower

limbs of the child and (2) in respect of the *position* adopted by the breech in relation to the maternal pelvis. The first of these classifications is much the more important.

Attitudes
The most significant attitude and in the primigravida at term the most frequent (70 per cent) one is the *breech with extended legs*. In this the thighs are flexed on the abdomen and the legs are extended at the knee joints (Fig. 19.22(a)).

Another attitude somewhat commoner in parous patients than primigravidae is the *breech with flexed legs*. In this the knees are flexed and the feet of the child present along-

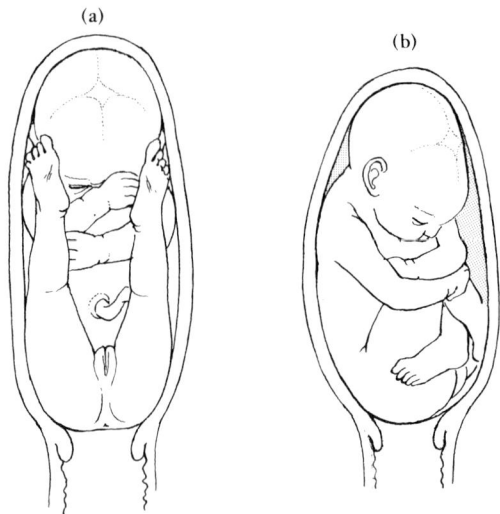

Fig. 19.22   (a) Breech with extended legs.
(b) Breech with flexed legs. (RSP).

side the buttocks. A breech with flexed legs is rather bulky in contradistinction from the breech with extended legs which is compact. Generally speaking, the breech with flexed legs is less capable of descent into the pelvis prior to the onset of labour (Fig. 19.22(b)).

Knee presentations occur as rather infrequent variants, and the *footling* presentation is also rather unusual. Their names are sufficiently descriptive.

Positions
It is customary to describe four classical positions of the breech in terms of the fetal sacrum (as denominator) in relation to the quadrants of the maternal pelvis. These four positions are left sacro-anterior (LSA), right sacro-anterior (RSA), right sacro-posterior

(RSP) and left sacro-posterior (LSP). Cases are also found where the breech presents with the sacrum directly lateral.

The precise diagnosis of position of the breech is comparatively unimportant. The mechanisms of labour differ only very slightly, and prognosis is not influenced by the position.

Aetiology of breech presentations
The general factors already enumerated as causes of malpresentations also operate in breech presentations.

Up to the thirtieth week of pregnancy a baby is almost as likely to present by the breech as by the vertex. This is the reason why at premature delivery the breech often presents. Between the thirtieth and thirty-fourth week, however, some factor operates which enables the fetus spontaneously to adopt the vertex presentation in all but a very few cases. It is noticeable that the babies who fail to do so nearly all show some undoing of the attitude of universal flexion so characteristic of the unborn child. Most commonly, this is found to affect the lower limbs, one or both knees being partially or completely extended. The effect is to convert the fetus from a rounded oval to a wedge-like body, the mobility of which within the uterus is probably restricted. This theory receives practical support from the well-known fact that it is often rather difficult to convert a breech with extended legs into a vertex by manipulation during pregnancy.

Some women have breech presentations in successive pregnancies. Here the breech presentation is evidently normal and serious difficulty is rarely experienced.

Diagnosis of breech presentation
It is of very great importance that a breech presentation should be recognized by 32 weeks or so, so that the presentation can be corrected by external version.

Near term the pregnant woman in whom the fetus presents by the breech complains not infrequently of discomfort in the upper part of the abdomen—for example, she states that she feels something hard pressing on her stomach, or that she has pain, under the ribs when stooping or that she has great discomfort about the region of the stomach when the fetus moves. Such symptoms should arouse suspicion that a breech presentation exists.

Palpation. The diagnosis of this presentation in the later weeks of pregnancy is generally possible by careful palpation. The presenting fetal part is felt to be softer, less regular and globular, than the hard head. The fetal part at the fundus, on the other hand, is felt to be hard, round and smooth. Sometimes the patient complains of pain on palpation over the head. At the fundus there is another important sign—namely 'ballottement' of the head between the palpating hands (Fig. 19.23). We emphasize this sign because it is

pronounced extension of the legs, they often displace the upper limbs from this situation, so that it is possible to feel small parts on a level with the head at the fundus of the uterus.

Auscultation. The fetal heart is usually heard with greater distinctness above the umbilicus than below, but in a breech engaged in the pelvis, the point of maximum intensity of the fetal heart-sounds may be at or even below the umbilicus.

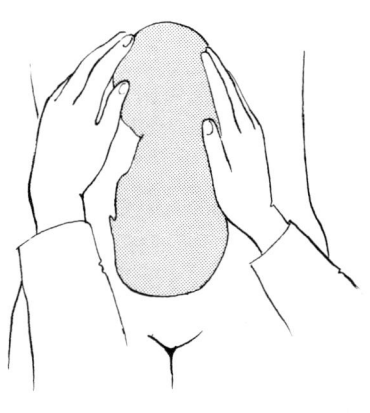
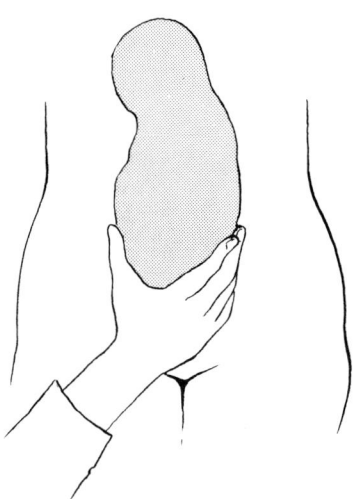

Fig. 19.23 Ballotment of the fetal head and palpation of the presenting breech.

frequently the first to arrest attention during the examination. In most cases it can be made out comparatively easily; but where the liquor amnii is scanty, the head well flexed and the trunk dorso-anterior, or the extended legs splint the head movements it is more difficult.

The back and limbs of the child are felt to either side of the uterus. The back can be traced down into the breech as a continuous unbroken curved line; but upwards towards the head there may be a slight break and the occiput may be felt if the head is not flexed. Where the dorsum of the child is posterior the limbs are felt in front.

It is important in a breech presentation at term to form an opinion as to whether or not the legs are extended. Assistance in this respect may be obtained from the facts that (1) in most cases a breech with flexed legs remains mobile above the pelvic brim until the onset of labour, whereas when the legs are extended, in primigravidae at any rate, the breech tends to sink into the pelvis; and (2) when the feet come to lie below the chin of the foetus in

Radiography or ultrasound. In cases in which after careful examination there is still uncertainty regarding the presentation, by the thirty-sixth week of pregnancy a radiography or ultrasound examination should be taken. Even the most experienced obstetrician may find this necessary, especially if the patient is fat or is a primigravida and the abdominal walls are very rigid. A radiograph will also show whether the legs are flexed or extended.

Vaginal examination. By vaginal examination it may be possible to distinguish the hard round head in the brim but the outline of a breech is difficult to define through the vaginal vault. When labour is well established, and a finger can be passed through the cervix, the softness and irregularity of the presenting surface should arrest attention.

Whenever the breech can be reached with ease its characteristic 'landmarks' are easily felt. These are the tuberosities of the ischia, between which is the anus and in front of this the genitalia and behind the all-important 'landmark' of this presentation—*viz.* the rough surface of the sacrum and tip of the coccyx (Fig. 19.7). After the membranes have ruptured and the breech has sunk into the pelvis, these 'landmarks' become more distinct, and the examining finger may enter the anus, recognizing the muscular tonus of its sphincter, and possibly showing meconium on withdrawal.

Still later, as the breech descends into the pelvis and the uterine wall during a contraction compresses the trunk, thick meconium may be forced out of the anus.

A number of factors combine to make labour in breech presentations a great deal more difficult than in vertex presentations. These factors operate to some extent irrespective of parity, but they are all at their most dangerous in the primigravida. The breech, a soft and to some extent a malleable structure, may slip out through soft parts which have been but partially dilated, after which the wider body of the child must pass. So far as the belly and thorax of the child are concerned, these structures are compressible and rarely cause much difficulty. But with the shoulder girdle and the head, the situation is different.

Shoulder girdle dystocia arises only if the arms are displaced from their normal position of flexion over the baby's thorax. Various degrees of 'extension of the arms' occur, and a 'nuchal displacement' is also described. Such displacements, except with the tiny child, may be a bar to spontaneous delivery.

The delivery of the head is generally the most critical phase of the labour. Though no larger than the parts of the child already delivered, its resistance is greater since it adapts itself less readily to the contours of the birth canal.

An entirely spontaneous delivery is uncommon, even in parous patients. However, we propose to describe the mechanisms, and will later take note of factors which may interfere with the mechanism of spontaneous birth. One of these is extension of the legs. It will therefore be assumed that labour commences with a breech with flexed legs presenting at the pelvic brim.

Mechanism of labour in breech presentations
Descent of the breech into the pelvic cavity occurs until the resistance of the pelvic floor is encountered, at which point the axis of the birth canal turns sharply forwards. At this level two events take place—*viz*: (1) internal rotation of the fetus to bring the sacrum into a directly lateral position with the bitrochanteric diameter of the fetus in the middle line, and (2) lateral flexion of the trunk to allow of the fetus accommodating itself to the curvature of the birth canal.

Further descent expels the anterior buttock, which emerges from the vulva and becomes fixed posterior to the apex of the pubic arch, with the lateral aspect of the buttock in the neighbourhood of the baby's iliac crest in contact with the symphysis pubis. Further descent and lateral flexion now occurs, as a result of which the anal region of the child followed by the posterior buttock appears at the posterior commissure of the vulva, and the breech is born (Fig. 19.24).

Sometimes a movement of the delivered breech now occurs similar to that of restitution in vertex presentations, the sacrum rotating slightly towards the quadrant of the pelvis which it originally occupied. This movement is seldom very marked, however, and as further descent occurs the back of the child usually lies very definitely to one side. After the feet, the abdomen and the thorax have emerged, the head usually enters the cavity with its long axis in the transverse diameter of the pelvis. It descends into the pelvic cavity, and there rotates in such a way as to carry the occiput forwards, the chin and face passing into the sacral hollow. The suboccipital region of the head then emerges through the vulva at the apex of the pubic arch, and the head thereafter pivots around the suboccipital region, the chin emerging at the posterior vulvar commissure, followed by the mouth, nose and forehead, after which the vertex and occiput slip out easily. The widest antero-posterior diameter passing in a favourable case is the suboccipito-frontal. This is the same as the widest diameter in vertex presentations, but whereas in the vertex the length of this diameter has been diminished by gradual moulding, the measurement of the unmoulded after-coming head is very often greater than the 4 inches (10cm) usually recorded for the suboccipito-frontal distance in the vertex-first baby.

FACTORS WHICH MAY INTERFERE WITH MECHANISM

Maternal factors
1. Faults in the forces.
Arrest of the process may occur at any point should the forces fail. Defective abdominal

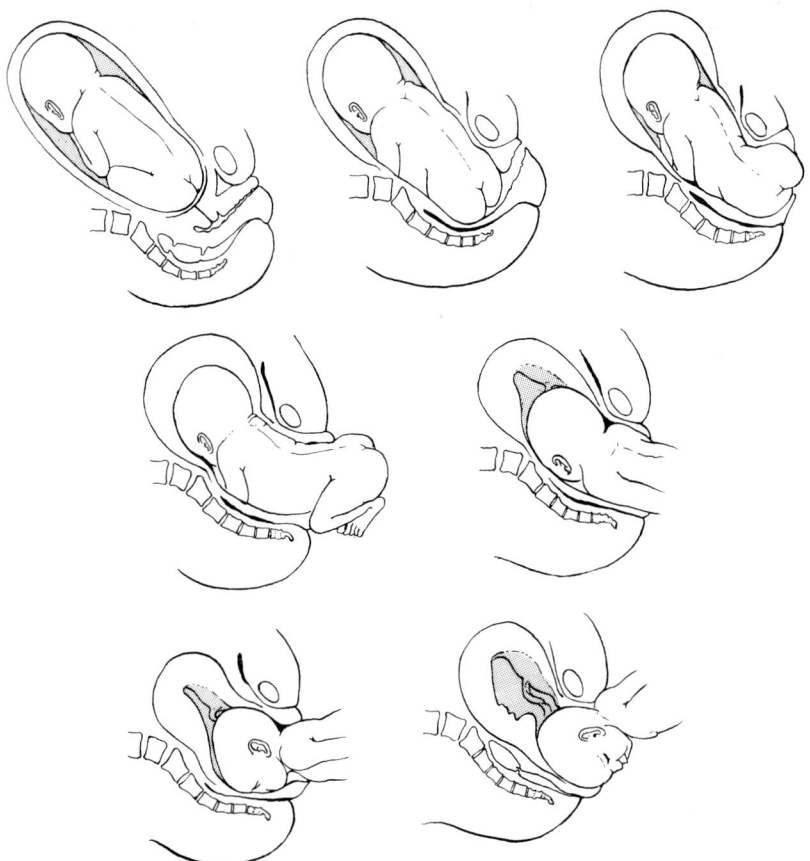

Fig. 19.24   Mechanisms of labour in breech.

powers are particularly unfortunate in the delivery of the head. This is usually the moment of greatest mechanical difficulty, which occurs at a time when the head has left the contractile portion of the uterus.

2. Faults in the passages.

Either bony contraction or tight soft parts may cause arrest. So long as the obstruction is moderate, the breech may emerge with comparatively little difficulty, although the shoulders or head may become impacted. Sometimes the partially dilated cervix may allow the escape of the breech, especially in footling presentations and if the baby is small.

Fetal factors

1. Extended legs.

The main effect of extension of the legs is to produce a splinting of the child's vertebral column, which prevents or interferes with that lateral flexion which is an important feature of the mechanism by which the child adapts itself to the curve of the axis of the birth canal at the level of the pelvic floor (Fig. 19.24). Two results are to be noted. Firstly, impaction of the breech at the level of the plane 'of least pelvic dimensions' is rather common. Secondly, when sufficient lateral flexion is present to allow the breech to pass from pelvic cavity to outlet, it is nevertheless insufficient in many cases to allow the anterior buttock to come as far forward as usual, and the posterior buttock may then be held up on the perineal tissues, and will certainly have to emerge much farther back in the pelvis than would be the case if full lateral flexion were possible. Severe perineal damage may result but deep episiotomy solves this situation.

2. Displaced arms.

If the arms are displaced, either in extension or in the uncommon nuchal displacement, arrest of the shoulder girdle takes place, usually at the pelvic floor or at the pelvic brim, if it is contracted.

3. Large fetal head.

This may be due to a large head as in hydrocephalus, or to imperfect flexion of the head, which throws the occipito-frontal circumference across the birth canal. A large fetal head may become impacted either at the brim or at the pelvic floor.

4. Malrotation of fetal head.

In this event the chin rotates anteriorly, while the occiput becomes impacted in the hollow of the sacrum, so producing an impasse. It is fortunate that although sacro-posterior positions of the breech are not uncommon the head of the child very seldom undergoes this form of malrotation.

THE COURSE OF LABOUR IN BREECH PRESENTATION

As in malpresentations generally, there is some tendency to prolongation of the first stage with early rupture of the membranes. Much of the liquor amnii drains away at once, since the breech plugs the cervix and lower segment inefficiently, and for the same reason prolapse of the cord may occur.

In the second stage the pains tend to be variable, and the uterus is apt to become 'exhausted' if the breech meets any considerable obstruction. Indeed the process of 'impaction' of the breech is nearly always associated with a more or less complete uterine inertia. Defective uterine action is also prone to develop after the birth of the breech but before the delivery of the trunk, and frequently calls for manual assistance.

The child is inevitably subject to a period of anoxia in breech deliveries. This commences just after the birth of the breech, at a time when the umbilical cord begins to be pressed upon by the close girdle of contact with the maternal passages. Possibly as a result of this anoxia the fetus is often seen to make respiratory efforts whilst the head is still in the birth canal and in some cases this results in the inhalation of mucus deep into the pharynx, or sometimes even lower into the respiratory tree. As a result, even in the most favourable of breech deliveries, the baby may be born in a condition of asphyxia.

Prognosis in breech presentation

Mother. In primigravidae this is not quite so good as in vertex presentations, due to the more tedious labour, the increased need for operative intervention and, above all, to the extensive soft tissue damage which could occur. Complete tearing of the perineum is more common than in vertex deliveries. In parous women the soft tissues are rarely damaged unless the baby is very large.

Fetus. The outlook for the fetus is much worse than in vertex presentations. Even when malformation is excluded, along with such intercurrent conditions as antepartum haemorrhage, contracted pelvis, cord prolapse and prematurity of the fetus, there remains a final mortality figure of some 3–4 per cent in many large maternity hospitals. This mortality is due principally to intracranial damage occurring as the head is made to transverse the pelvic canal rapidly without sufficient time for moulding, or to cord prolapse.

The fetus is also liable to a variety of non-fatal injuries, many of which give rise to serious and permanent damage. Amongst these may be mentioned non-fatal intracranial injuries; brachial plexus injuries; fractures of femur, humerus or clavicle; dislocations of limbs or jaw; and injury to sternomastoid muscles.

Vaginal delivery of a breech in a primigravida can be very difficult and great skill and experience are necessary if the best results are to be obtained. Although the actual delivery in the parous patient is much easier, the mortality figures do not differ as much as is to be expected from these in primigravidae, for the baby is subjected to certain additional accidents peculiar to the parous patient. For example, many parous patients have labour so easy and rapid that the child may be born to the neck in the absence of any attendants; prolapse of the cord is commoner; the trunk of the child may slip through a partially dilated cervix which then imprisons the arms or the aftercoming head; and breech presentation may develop in the lax multiparous uterus during the last days of pregnancy so that the breech delivery may come as a complete surprise.

The antenatal management of breech presentation

EXTERNAL CEPHALIC VERSION

The outlook for any individual baby is so much better when it presents by the vertex that attempts should be made to correct breech presentation in all primigravidae who have reached at the latest the 34th week of pregnancy, and even in the majority of multiparae.

After the 34th week of pregnancy version becomes increasingly difficult, since the baby is larger and the quantity of liquor amnii relatively less. Nevertheless we believe that even at this late stage or even later it should be attempted.

Technique of external cephalic version
The steps of the operation are shown in the accompanying illustrations with their legends. There are, however, some points which require special emphasis.

1. *Relaxation of the abdominal wall.* It is essential that the abdominal wall be completely relaxed. Much can be done by reassurance and explanation combined with extreme gentleness in all manipulations. Warm hands are essential. In very nervous patients the administration of a mild sedative, e.g. Valium about half an hour before operation is helpful. The use of general anaesthesia is generally *not* justified.

2. *Mobilization of the breech.* This, as shown in the illustrations, is the first important step in the operation. It may be made easier by putting the patient in the Trendelenburg position for half an hour beforehand.

3. *Direction of turning.* The baby should usually be rolled round in the direction to which its face is directed. This is designed to increase the flexion, and thus to reduce the baby's bulk. To turn the baby in the opposite direction would tend to cause some extension of the attitude and might result in a brow presentation. Nevertheless it is justifiable to attempt a 'backward' version when the orthodox 'forward' version fails, since it sometimes succeeds, especially when the long axis of the child lies obliquely towards the side of the abdomen occupied by the baby's back. Brow presentations produced in this way generally correct themselves within a few hours.

4. *Auscultation of fetal heart.* The fetal heart-rate and rhythm is carefully noted before and during the version, and if the operation is proving difficult the attempt should be discontinued if any irregularity of the rhythm be detected. If such irregularity disappears in a few moments, a fresh start should be made; but if it persists for some minutes it is safer to abandon the attempt altogether. Again, the fetal heart should be listened to after the successful completion of aversion. It may be slowed by as much as forty beats per minute, but the rate is usually back to normal within five minutes. If not, and especially if there is any abnormality of rhythm, cord obstruction

may have developed. To treat this it may be justifiable to push the baby back to a breech presentation, or in some cases immediate Caesarean section may be indicated.

5. *After-treatment.* The mother should report for examination in *one week's time so that the presentation may be checked*, and if it is again a breech, version should be performed again.

6. *Difficulties of version.* The most common cause of difficulty is a tight abdominal wall. Another cause is failure to mobilize the breech adequately. Of the fetal causes, extension of the legs often prevents version by splinting the child's body and preventing the increase of general flexion which is so helpful. Nevertheless, version should be attempted, and will often succeed. In some cases (in which, incidentally, the very diagnosis of breech presentation may be extremely difficult) the head is found to be tucked under the costal margin, inaccessible to the fingers. In such circumstances success may attend a modification of the usual technique whereby the operation is commenced by securing control of the head by dipping the fingers deeply under the costal margin, after which an assistant pushes up the breech from the vagina (*see* Fig. 19.36). Version is generally impossible, in the presence of twin pregnancy, uterine developmental abnormalities such as a single horn uteri, and in the rather rare condition of oligohydramnios.

Dangers of external version
1. *Placental separation.* If the placenta is on the anterior uterine wall the abdominal manipulation may produce a partial separation and haemorrhage. This is rarely dangerous to the mother but may lead to the intra-uterine death of the fetus from asphyxia. It may be prudent to locate the placenta first by ultrasound.

2. *Premature rupture of the membranes.* If the cervix is already partially dilated the membranes may give way during the manipulation, the onset of labour being an early sequel. Actually this accident is rare unless the patient is already on the verge of labour, and it is not a serious one unless the baby is lying transversely (when a shoulder presentation may result unless the attendant can push the baby back to a breech presentation), or unless prolapse of the umbilical cord occurs.

3. *If the umbilical cord* happens to be

wrapped round any portion of the fetus it may, during a version, be drawn so tight that its circulation becomes obstructed, or it may obstruct the fetal circulation to some vital part—e.g. cord around neck. Very rarely it may be ruptured.

4. *Compound presentation of head* with small parts sometimes results, but usually rights itself before labour.

5. *Cord presentation*, i.e. prolapse of the cord within the intact waters, sometimes develops.

6. *In the presence of a point of weakness in the uterine wall*, usually due to previous Caesarean section, version may precipitate a rupture of the uterus.

Contra-indications to external version

These include antepartum haemorrhage, where serious haemorrhage may result, twin pregnancy, fetal monstrosity, and cases where a previous Caesarean section has been performed. It should not be attempted, of course, in any case where delivery is to be by Caesarean section for other reasons, such as age, relative infertility, hypertension or previous stillbirth.

Management of uncorrected breech presentation in the primigravida

If version fails or is not attempted the pelvis should be examined carefully. Otherwise it may be better to have the pelvis measured radiologically. Standing lateral pelvimetry may be required or ultrasound pelvimetry. The fetus should also be examined radiologically if anomaly is suspected.

CHOICE OF MANAGEMENT
There are three possible alternatives—*viz*: (1) to allow labour to commence naturally, (2) to induce labour at or before the expected date of delivery, (3) to carry out an elective Caesarean section.

For all normal young primigravidae, with a good pelvis and a moderate sized child, only the first alternative is considered. Induction of labour is justifiable for other obstetric reasons.

In older primigravidae (past the age of 30) *there is much to be said for elective Caesarean section* because of the increased risk of stillbirth and damage to the mother and also because of the brevity of opportunity of later children. Contracted pelvis even of minor degree may justify Caesarean section at any age provided the baby is normal and of good size. (When Caesarean section is performed for such conditions as placenta praevia and hypertensive pregnancy toxaemia the child may lie as a breech, but in these cases the position of the fetus has not usually influenced the decision as to the mode of delivery.)

MANAGEMENT OF LABOUR
First stage—As in other malpresentations the membranes frequently rupture before or early in labour. If they do rupture vaginal examination should be performed at once to exclude prolapse of the cord. Unless the first stage is smooth, easy and progressive with steady descent Caesarean section should be considered.

Second stage—Undue prolongation of the second stage is less common than might be expected. If the maternal condition is good, the fetal heart satisfactory and progress occurring nothing need be done. Nitrous oxide and air should be offered as an analgesic, but stronger anaesthetics likely to result in diminished mental alertness should be withheld. Epidural is, of course, ideal.

The delivery—When the anterior buttock appears at the vulva the patient should be placed in the lithotomy position. No other position offers the advantages of the full litho-

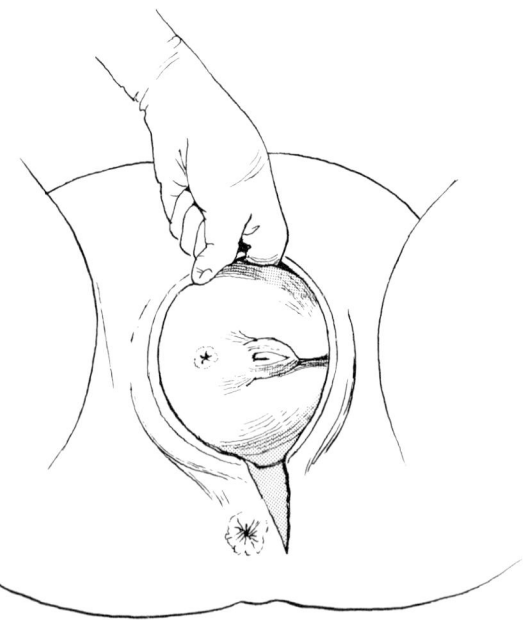

Fig. 19.25   The timing of episiotomy.

tomy position. The skin is sterilized and sterile drapes applied.

Pudendal nerve block is then made (Chapter 24) and in addition the area of deep episiotomy infiltrated. The episiotomy is best on the side the limbs are to allow easier access to the examiners hands and should be performed as soon as the anterior buttock shows (Fig. 19.25).

Following the block the contractions may ease off for a little.

When they recommence, the advance of the presenting part is watched until the anterior buttock is showing, with the perineum beginning to be distended by the posterior buttock. The perineum is boldly divided with scissors through the anaesthetized area so as to perform a very deep episiotomy, extending from the posterior commissure in the middle line backwards, and to one or other side almost to the level of the anus. This is perhaps the most important step in the conduct of the delivery. It removes much of the resistance of the primigravid soft tissues, and allows the breech to escape in an axis corresponding much more with that of the pelvic cavity than with that of the outlet, thus minimizing the need for lateral flexion.

The next contraction brings the anterior buttock down and may drive the posterior buttock out. At this stage the baby may pass much meconium and may avoid urine. The accoucheur should now urge the patient to bear down with her next contraction. A skilful midwife watching with her hand on the abdomen can yield invaluable service by noticing the onset of the contraction and by encouraging the patient to bear down.

The succeeding contraction will usually expel the belly and thorax of the child until the angle of the scapula is visible. Should this not be achieved, it will become necessary to assist the birth of the body of the child, preferably by means of pressure applied from the abdomen at the sides of the uterus, or by traction best applied by pulling from the feet or by traction holding the child's pelvis. It is to be preferred that the patient manage this expulsion with her own efforts.

When the angle of the scapulae is visible the body of the child is swung gently backwards—i.e. towards the floor. As a result, it is common to see the remainder of the anterior scapula with the acromion appear at the apex of the pubic arch, from which the anterior

arm can be readily disengaged by passing two fingers along the humerus as far as the elbow and making gentle downward pressure. Access to the arm can be helped by pressing the angle of the scapula backwards. The body of the child is then swung forwards, the posterior scapula passes over the perineum, and the arm is disengaged as in the case of its fellow.

Alternatively the Lövset manoeuvre (page 383) may be used as a routine for delivery of the shoulders.

The most crucial stage of the delivery is now reached namely the delivery of the after-coming head, which is at this point entering the pelvic cavity. Its passage of the brim and cavity is facilitated by allowing the child's body to hang down towards the floor, so that the weight of the child makes gentle traction on the head (Fig. 19.26). Quite often in a favourable

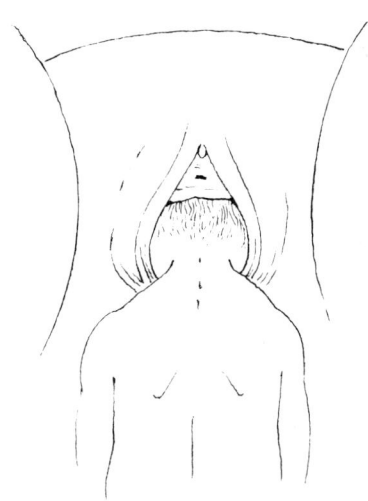

Fig. 19.26 The child allowed to hang.

case, as the head gently passes into the cavity and rotates into the antero-posterior diameter of the pelvis, one sees a smooth, steady, apparent elongation of the child's neck, and the hair of the suboccipital region of the child's head becomes visible at the apex of the pubic arch. This stage should not be hurried unduly. There is a temptation to accelerate the passage of the head by applying suprapubic pressure, and this may have to be done if the suboccipital hair does not appear spontaneously within, say, half a minute.

By far the most successful method of bringing the head through the outlet is the

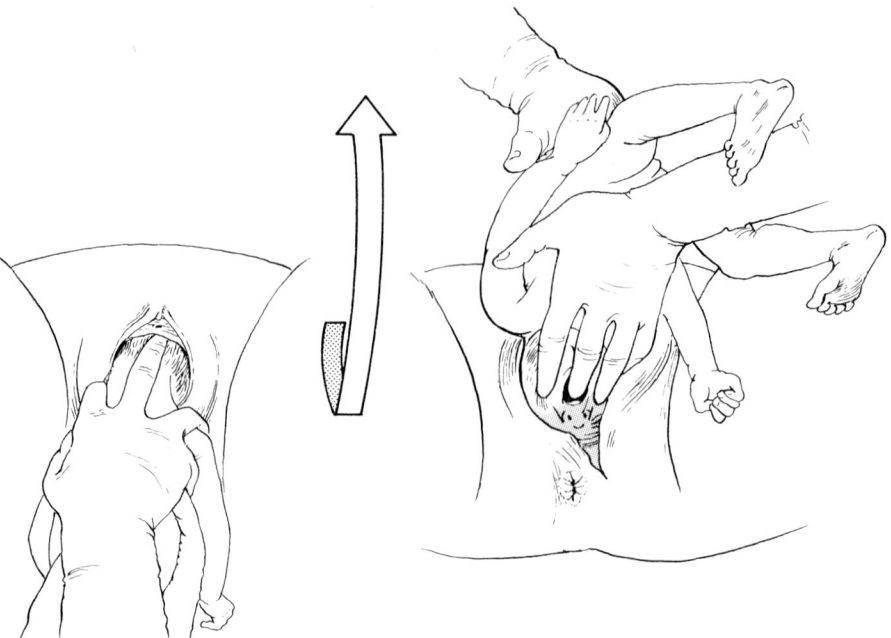

Fig. 19.27   The Mauriceau–Smellie–Veit manoeuvre.

application of obstetrical forceps (Chapter 27). There is however, a place for the use of un-assisted hands (the Mauriceau-Smellie-Veit grip). The middle finger of the fully pronated hand should be placed in contact with the baby's sub-occipital region while the thumb is introduced into one axilla and the little finger into the other, the index and ring fingers being passed over the posterior aspects of the appropriate shoulders (Fig. 19.27). The other hand, in full supination, is now applied over the face of the child, with one finger in the mouth and two others pressing over the malar bones at either side of the nose. This second hand is used to assist flexion of the baby's head while traction is made on the baby's shoulders by the index and ring fingers of the first hand, whose middle finger on the occiput splints the neck and encourages flexion. Traction is applied smoothly and steadily in the axis of the pelvis—i.e. initially downwards and backwards towards the floor, and then slowly changing to a traction (i.e. directly towards the accoucheur) followed by downwards and finally upwards, until the child's body is vertical or even slightly inclined towards the mother's abdomen. It is important to make traction all the time and not simply to lever the child forwards, as this might lead to injury to the neck.

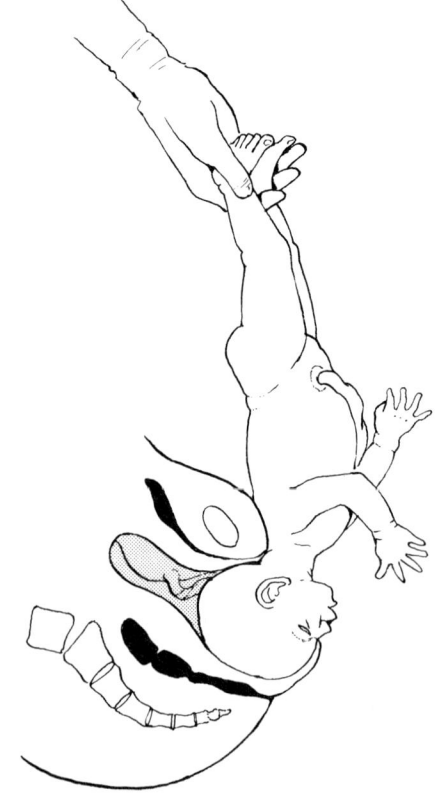

Fig. 19.28   The technique of manipulation of the child in the Burns-Marshall Manoeuvre.

In most cases the chin, face and forehead emerge slowly so that damage to the mother's soft tissues is avoided.

An alternative method for delivery in the multigravida is that described by the Burns and Marshall (Fig. 19.28). This technique can be used only when the head is well into the pelvis and there is a wide episiotomy or no perineal resistance. It should not be used for a premature child. It is the method by which mothers may deliver themselves. The child is grasped by the feet and swung upwards in an arc over the mother's abdomen. The body is kept taut and slight traction is also exerted. As the mouth is freed it is wiped clear. Care must be taken that the head does not 'pop' out of the vulvar introitus.

The foregoing manipulations are planned to take place with the patient fully conscious, pain being relieved by epidural or by pudendal block analgesic combined with nitrous oxide oxygen inhalation. However, as serious complications develop suddenly in many cases, it is essential to have a skilled anaesthetist standing by in case rapid induction of general anaesthesia should become necessary.

It is usual to refer to a delivery completed as described above as an 'assisted' breech delivery.

The third stage of labour is conducted along usual lines. It is quite possible to repair the episiotomy during the third stage without further anaesthesia.

THE MANAGEMENT OF UNEXPECTED COMPLICATIONS ARISING DURING ASSISTED BREECH DELIVERY

1. *Extended legs.* It is best to disengage extended legs as soon as the popliteal fossae are visible at the vulva. Although most women will succeed in expelling the child with the legs fully extended, the completion of the delivery of the trunk during a single uterine contraction is more likely to be attained if extended legs are flexed artificially. Attempts to achieve this rarely succeed prior to the appearance of the popliteal fossae at the vulva. The accoucheur places two fingers in the popliteal fossa and pushes the thigh against the belly of the child, at the same time slightly abducting it (Fig. 19.29). This simple manipulation has the effect not only of flexing and abducting the hip joint but also results in the knee joint becoming slightly flexed, the proximal portion of the tibia appearing outside the vulva. A finger is then placed along the tibia, by direct pressure on which the flexion of the knee joint is completed, the foot being disengaged from the vulva in the process. On no account should a finger be passed between the thigh and the baby's abdomen, as this may cause damage to the knee joint, or even fracture of the femur.

2. *Extended arms.* Extension of the arms is not usually a result of mismanagement, since X-ray studies have proved that extension of the arms can occur prior to the commencement of labour. It is important to recognize the existence of this complication promptly. The first sign is that the trunk of the child is expelled as far as the costal margin but may not descend farther. This is an indication to insert a single finger along the ventral surface of the child's thorax, and if the elbow cannot be palpated the arms are probably extended and should be brought down as soon as possible.

The child's trunk should be pulled down gently until the scapular angles are visible. By pushing the angle of the scapula backwards the arm may come down and the elbow can be located—the arm may then be delivered in the usual way. The traction should be applied to the child's pelvis, to avoid crushing the abdominal viscera. Alternatively the child may be held by the feet. It is generally easier to deal first with the arm which lies posterior. The body of the child is swung forwards (Fig. 19.30), and two fingers of one hand are inserted into the vagina along the aspect of the posterior humerus corresponding to the back of the child until the elbow is reached. The finger-tips are then manoeuvred round the humerus until they lie curved round the elbow, and the palmar surfaces of the fingers are made to lie along the shaft of the humerus. Firm, steady, uninterrupted pressure is now made upon the humerus, the fingers acting as a splint to prevent its fracture, the pressure being directed in such a way as to swing the elbow towards the mid-line of the child's body and to sweep it downwards over the front of the chest of the child. This procedure is not easy even in practised hands. It is important to avoid efforts to bring down the elbow by force with a single finger hooked round the humerus, and to remember the need to carry the humerus towards the mid-line of the child's body. If this last manipulation is used it will be found that the elbow flexes automatically to some extent. The posterior arm delivered, the body of the child is swung backwards

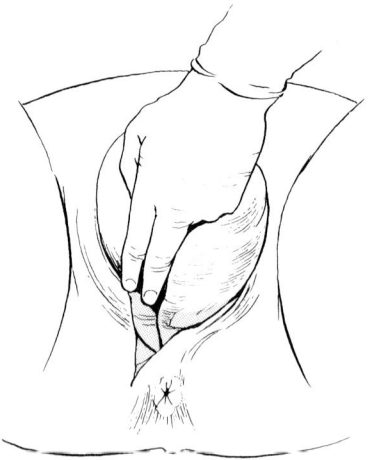
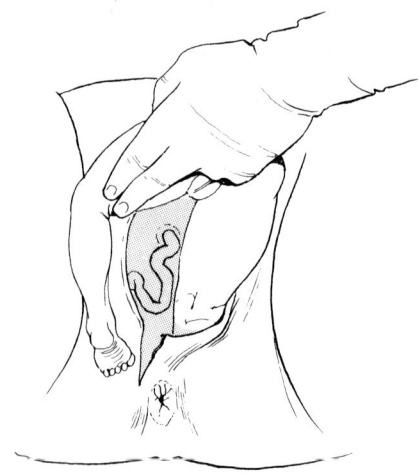

Fig. 19.29   Delivery of extended legs at the vulva.

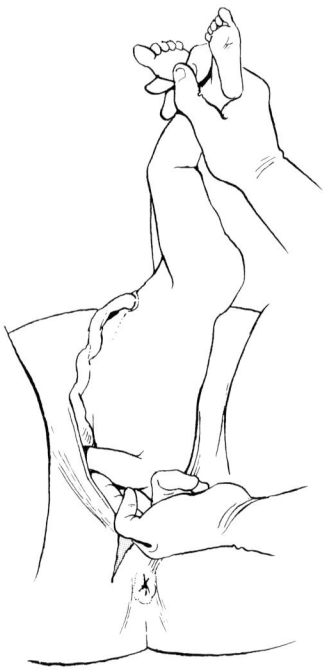
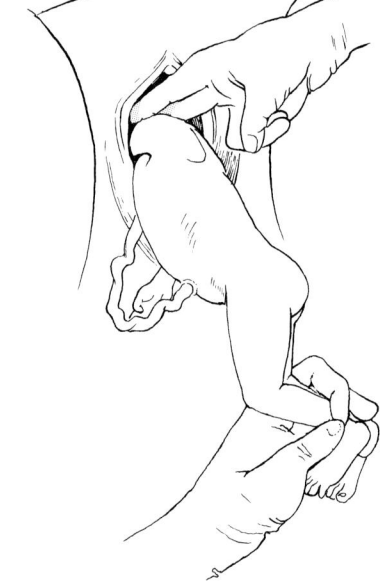

Fig. 19.30   The techniques of delivery of the extended arms.

towards the floor and the anterior arm is brought down in a manner precisely similar to its fellow.

Very occasionally the scapular angles may not come into view even with very strong traction. This is a very serious matter, for it indicates that the arms are arrested at a fery high level, usually by some degree of narrowing of the pelvic brim. The child will die unless the extension of the arms is relieved, but the treatment is in itself dangerous, for it in-

volves the introduction of the whole hand into the birth canal at a time when the thorax of the baby occupies the vagina. This is not only technically difficult but prone to cause much damage to the maternal soft tissue and to the child. However, the risk must be accepted if strong traction has been unsuccessful. The patient is anaesthetized and the four fingers of one hand, well lubricated, are introduced into the vagina between the body of the child and the posterior commissure of the vulva. The hand is passed gently along the child's body until the posterior arm is encountered, the thumb being introduced into the vagina if the limb is found to be beyond the reach of the fingers. When the arm is definitely located it is swept towards the middle line of the child and brought down over the front of the child's thorax and withdrawn from the vagina. The effort to draw down the trunk of the child to deliver the anterior scapula is now resumed and usually succeeds, and the anterior arm may be delivered by swinging the child back towards the floor and carrying out the manoeuvres already described. Occasionally, however, it is still impossible to produce any advance of the trunk. The thorax of the child should then be grasped firmly with both hands, the thumbs being placed parallel to the baby's spine, with the fingers encircling the thorax, the finger-tips reaching up the anterior wall of the chest as far as possible, aiming to reach the clavicles.

It is precisely this situation or when the arms are extended or nuchally displaced that the Lövset manoeuvre is designed to deal with and it is especially useful if one shoulder is already below the brim (usually the posterior) (Fig. 19.31).

The child is held by the pelvis with the thumbs over the sacrum and the fingers over symphysis and upper thighs. Care must be taken not to compress the abdomen. Traction is exerted during the process of rotation. The child is usually lying with its back to the right or left of the mother. It is then rotated with downwards and backwards traction so that the posterior arm trails across the chest, i.e. if the child's back is to the mother's left the rotation would be anticlockwise (and vice versa). The posterior shoulder is now under the symphysis and the arms can be delivered as usual. If necessary after one arm is delivered a second rotation will make the other arm more accessible.

3. *Nuchal displacement of the arm.* This rare complication is recognized when an attempt is being made to bring down an extended arm. The elbow is discovered to be flexed, with the forearm and hand lying behind the head. The body of the child is rotated in the direction in which the hand and forearm of the child are pointing. Friction of the maternal soft tissues tends to prevent the child's forearm from taking part in the movement, and as a result the forearm becomes extended at the elbow joint, and the condition can then be dealt with as an ordinary extended arm.

4. *The impacted after-coming head.* From the practical standpoint, difficulty with the after-coming head may occur at the brim and at lower levels.

Arrest at the brim rarely occurs except where there is a degree of pelvic contraction or when the baby is hydrocephalic (*see* page 392).

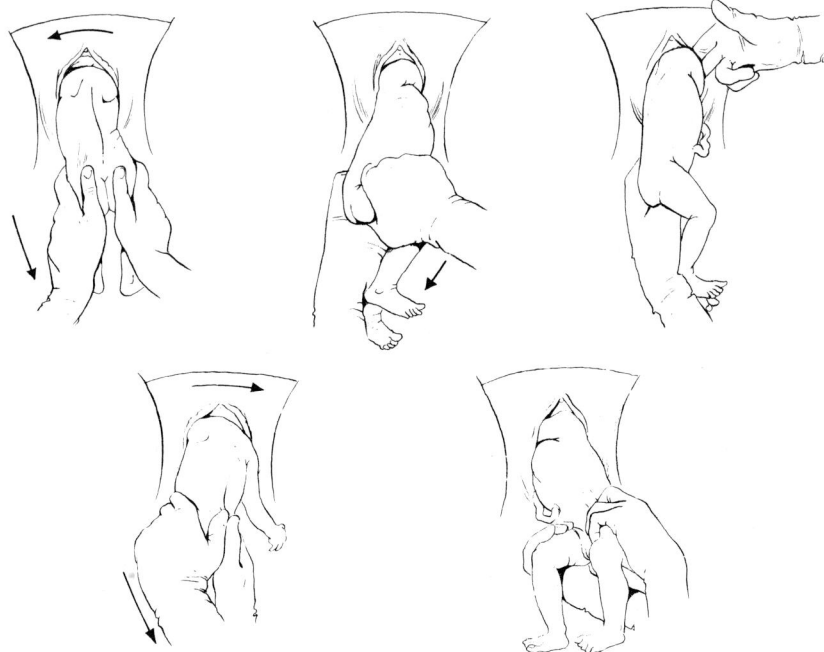

Fig. 19.31   Steps in the Lövset manoeuvre.

If the child's head is normal, suprapubic pressure should be applied to push the head slowly through the brim. The movement is controlled by placing one hand above the pubes and the other in the vagina. Two fingers of the vaginal hand should be passed into the mouth of the child, being used to maintain the flexion of the head, which serves to reduce the diameters which have to pass, care being taken to avoid dislocation of the mandible. This manoeuvre is often referred to as the Martin procedure. It is important to make the suprapubic pressure in the axis of the pelvic brim—i.e. backwards and slightly downwards. It is hardly possible to make traction in the correct direction by pulling on the body of the child, since the curve of the lower sacrum interferes. Similarly, it is inadvisable to use forceps at this stage. In favourable cases the firm pressure advised above squeezes the head slowly past the pelvic brim into the cavity, from which it may be delivered by other methods. In some cases, however, the head cannot be pushed through the pelvic brim and craniotomy is necessary.

Impaction at a lower level (i.e. in the cavity or outlet) is recognized when, after the head descends satisfactorily into the pelvic cavity (where almost invariably it undergoes internal rotation which carries the occiput to the front), it proves difficult with moderate traction by the Mauriceau-Smellie-Veit method to lift the head from the cavity. The treatment should be instantly to swing the child's body forwards, have it held by an assistant, and apply forceps (Fig. 19.32). The delivery is usually quite

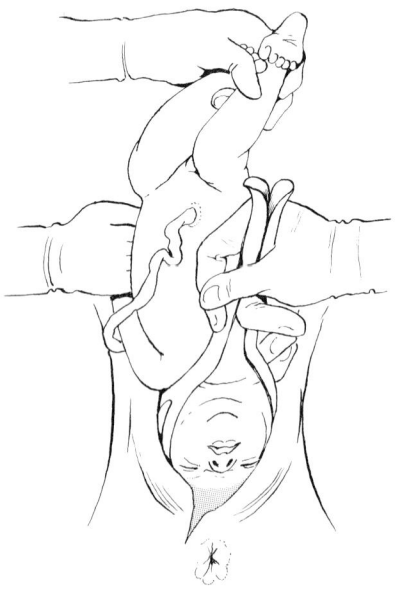

Fig. 19.32   Forceps to after coming head.

straightforward, using only moderate force, intermittently if necessary (*see* 'Forceps').

Where the occiput rotates into the sacral hollow it is nearly always possible by rotating the trunk of the child to correct this malposition, but, if not using the Mauriceau-Smellie-Veit grip, very strong traction is made backwards until the chin and face are born, when the body of the child is swung forwards to complete the delivery. The chin of the after-coming head should emerge first, but very occasionally, if the head is much extended, it is impossible to deliver the chin in this way and forceps should be applied to the head as it lies with the occiput in the hollow of the sacrum. If this fails, craniotomy should be performed.

MANAGEMENT OF IMPACTED BREECH PRESENTATION

The term *impacted* conveys the impression that the breech is arrested deep in the birth canal because of mechanical disproportion, whereas in most cases the arrest is due to failure of the uterine powers. The term may be used to describe arrest at the brim, but most often the breech is arrested with the legs extended at the plane of least pelvic dimensions, as a result of failing uterine contractions. The cervix may be fully or partially dilated.

Some cases are much better dealt with by Caesarean section. Some can be delivered by simple traction upon the baby's groin; while yet others are treated by bringing down one or both legs, after which the delivery is usually completed at once by traction on the child's feet (Fig. 19.33).

The method used depends upon the physical condition of the mother and the fetus, the stage of labour, and the size of the pelvis. In assessing the last two factors, great assistance can be obtained by a careful vaginal examination under full anaesthesia. Caesarean section will probably be called for if the pelvis is found to be contracted, otherwise vaginal manipulations aimed at producing quicker progress may well suffice provided no damage occurs to the child.

OTHER MANIPULATION

Bringing down a leg

After the examination under anaesthesia which precedes the planning of treatment, the anaesthetic is continued, and, if necessary, deepened to secure full relaxation of abdominal wall and uterus. The hand is inserted so that the palm lies along the ventral surface of the child—the right hand when the belly of the child is directed to the maternal left, and the left hand when the belly of the child is directed towards the maternal right.

The breech is gently displaced upwards sufficiently to allow entry of the fingers being introduced into the uterus, and as many fingers as the cervix will admit are passed along the flexor surface of the child's thigh until the popliteal fossa is recognized, when pressure is made upon the popliteal fossa with the finger-tips in such a way as to cause a movement of further flexion and slight abduction at the hip joint. This is the same manoeuvre as has been described already for dealing with extended legs at the vulva, and its effect within the uterus is the same, namely to cause flexion at the knee joint (Fig. 33). As this occurs a finger may be slipped over the tibia, by pressing on which the flexion of the knee joint is completed, the foot can be grasped (Fig. 19.33) and

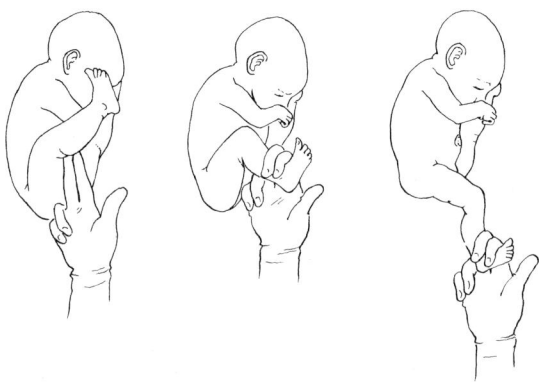

Fig. 19.33   The technique of bringing down the leg.

drawn down to the cervix, into the vagina, down to and through the vulva.

Measures to secure immediate delivery—during first stage

If immediate delivery is essential, Caesarean section should be performed since the risk of damage to the cervix and lower segment when an after-coming head is pulled forcibly through the cervical canal is too great.

During the second stage. Caesarean section may again be considered. It is probably the safest course in the presence of a pelvic contraction, or of a large child in an elderly primigravida. In such circumstances Caesarean section is the treatment of choice and should not be undertaken as a last resort when other methods fail.

If the decision is in favour of vaginal delivery the possible lines of treatment are as follows:
1. One leg, or both legs, should be brought down. It is usually better to bring down both when immediate delivery is contemplated. Thereafter, traction is made upon the feet in the axis of the pelvic cavity, an episiotomy being carried out as the buttocks begin to

distend the perineum. (Some operators prefer to make the episiotomy even before the legs are brought down.) When the pelvis of the child is delivered, the traction may be applied to the iliac crests of the baby and continued until the scapulae become visible, when the arms are dealt with as already described in connection with assisted breech delivery. The arms are usually extended when the child is pulled out in this manner, but the degree of extension of the arms may be slightly lessened by pressing on the sides of the uterus during the delivery of the trunk of the child. The foregoing procedure constitutes the classical *breech extraction*.

2. Groin traction may be applied when the impaction of the breech has occurred virtually on the perineum, and may be quite successful, with the traction applied by a single finger passed between the fetal thigh and the abdomen. The anterior groin is chosen, so as to reproduce the normal mechanism of expulsion, but sometimes it is possible to obtain access to both groins, which makes things easier. A wide and early episiotomy is desirable, except in those cases where impaction occurs on the perineum; finger traction will rarely be sufficient to overcome the resistance of the maternal passages, and a metal hook would be necessary. The risks of bony and soft tissue damage are so considerable that the breech hook is used only when the baby is dead or where it is impossible to bring down a leg owing to the uterus being very tightly contracted around the body and the limbs of the child, as sometimes happens in neglected cases.

3. If it is impossible either to bring down a leg or to secure delivery with groin traction, the obstetrical forceps may be applied to the breech with a bitrochanteric grip. The instrument very frequently slips off, in which case the complicated operation of breaking up the child may have to be undertaken.

MANAGEMENT OF BREECH PRESENTATION IN PAROUS PATIENTS

The general principles of management are the same in both parous and primigravid patients. The following are the more important differences:

1. *Antenatal management*

Since the fetal mortality is high in multiparae as well as primiparae, correction of the presentation by version before labour should be attempted routinely except in the few cases where there is some other contra-indication. Even in hospital it is possible for the baby to be partly born before the arrival of a doctor and thus to be asphyxiated.

2. *Management in labour*

Delivery may need little assistance but an experienced doctor should always be present if possible, since assistance may be needed at short notice especially if cord prolapse should occur.

The greatest danger to the child, apart from cord prolapse, is that before the doctor or even the midwife arrives, the partially dilated cervix may allow the breech to slip through but may cause arrest of the shoulder girdle or of the head. The arms can usually be disengaged, but the birth of the head is much more difficult. Gentle continuous traction on the shoulders of the child should be tried. In emergency the cervix can be incised at three and nine o'clock with guarded scissors and great care should be taken to resuture the cervix properly afterwards. Violent traction will certainly kill the child, and may cause grave maternal laceration. Many babies are unavoidably lost in such circumstances.

Caesarean section is rarely necessary except where there is some other factor such as placenta praevia or a previous stillbirth, or again with prolapse of the cord early in labour.

FOOT AND KNEE PRESENTATIONS

These are simply pelvic presentations in which the foot or knee has prolapsed. The foot may be distinguished from the hand by the presence of the heel.

Presentations of the *foot* should be left alone. It is a mistake to drag upon the limb and bring the trunk through the partially dilated cervix, for, as we have seen, this results in the arms and after-coming head being caught by the partially dilated cervix.

Knee presentations are very rare. The knee resembles the elbow but is to be distinguished from it by the presence of two prominences, with a slight depression between. If any difficulty arises, the foot is brought down and labour allowed to progress.

TRANSVERSE OR OBLIQUE LIE SHOULDER
    PRESENTATION

Abnormality of the lie is seen in some 0·5 per cent of women in late pregnancy.

Oblique lie is, if persistent, due usually to some anomaly failing to allow the head to occupy the lower pole of the uterus, for example cervical tumour, placenta praevia, pelvic brim contraction, and should be carefully investigated.

Transverse or unstable lie especially where the lie is constantly changing may be due to similar causes but usually is due to extreme uterine laxity and adequate liquor. Persist-

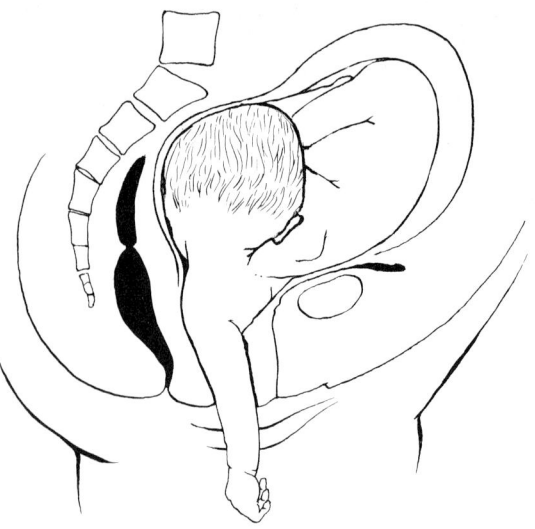

Fig. 19.34   Shoulder presented with prolapse arm.

ently transverse lie which will not correct is often due to a uterine abnormality bicornuate or cardiacus.

Shoulder presentation or arm presentation with or without cord prolapse follow failure of the malpresentation to correct in early labour (Fig. 19.34).

Diagnosis

The diagnosis is comparatively easy in most instances. The uterus is seen to be unduly wide transversely and to present an irregular outline, higher to one side than the other. This becomes more marked after rupture of the membranes. On *palpation* the bulky breech is felt to one side and the round, hard, globular head to the other.

On *auscultation* the fetal heart-sounds are best heard slightly above the brim of the pelvis, and consequently at a lower level than in vertex presentations.

Vaginal examination. In labour an arm may present or prolapse and, if not actually seen, may be felt in the vagina. It is not easy by touch to differentiate a hand from a foot. The absence of a heel is the most useful diagnostic point; others are the greater length of the fingers and the mobility of the thumb which contrasts with the relative fixity of the great toe. The presence of a hand in the vagina is not positive proof of a shoulder presentation but if the hand and forearm protrude from the vagina or can be drawn out as far as the elbow, then the diagnosis of shoulder presentation is almost certain. The axilla is recognized by the 'grid-iron' touch picture produced by parallel ridges felt as the finger crosses the ribs on the medial wall of the space. In practice it is often extremely difficult to reach the axilla, at least in early labour, and examination under anaesthesia may be necessary. Radiological examination is an alternative procedure in hospital.

Prognosis

The risk to the *mother* in *neglected* cases is very serious indeed. With very few exceptions, an uncorrected shoulder presentation produces a complete obstruction to delivery and rupture of the uterus. If the condition is recognized *early* and promptly treated, the prognosis, although serious, is much better.

The prognosis for the *child* is equally grave in the neglected case. When the condition is recognized and treated early, the outlook is very much better. Unfortunately prolapse of the cord occurs very frequently in transverse lie, and the baby may succumb to this before the diagnosis is made. Apart from this accident, the prognosis is only slightly worse than that for the baby which presents by the breech.

Mechanism of labour

Rarely the spontaneous expulsion of a child persistently presenting by the shoulder may be achieved by either of two bizarre mechanisms referred to as *spontaneous evolution* and *partus corpore conduplicato*. Both these processes necessitate a very large pelvis and a tiny child with a flexibility of the spine which is rarely seen before the child has been dead and macerated for some time. In spontaneous evolution the body, breech and legs slide past the presenting shoulder, after which the other shoulder and head are born. In the alternative mechanism the child is expressed in a doubled-up attitude. It must be again emphasized that both these mechanisms are excessively rare.

Management of transverse lie—Antenatal management

Up to the 32nd week of pregnancy a transverse lie usually requires no treatment. Between the 32nd and 36th week the discovery of a transverse lie is important, and calls for investigation to exclude placenta praevia, preferably by ultrasound. In the last four weeks of pregnancy, cephalo-pelvic disproportion will also have to be considered as a cause. In some cases no pathological condition is found, but it is essential to refer to a specialist hospital any patient who is discovered in the last eight weeks of pregnancy to have a transverse lie, especially if it persists or recurs.

Even if the position of the fetus is corrected by external cephalic version, the transverse lie is prone to recur. The most useful measure, therefore, is to admit the patient to hospital for the last two weeks of pregnancy. At the onset of labour the lie very often becomes longitudinal—either vertex or breech—except in those cases attributable to such abnormalities as bicornuate uterus.

Management during labour. In early labour uterine function usually straightens out the fetus to a longitudinal lie or gentle version can achieve this.

However, pelvic examination once labour is established should be done to confirm that the presentation is now breech or vertex.

If the transverse lie persists after membrane rupture or cannot be corrected then there is in the normal child no alternative to Caesarean section. Where the child is abnormal or where Caesarean section cannot be performed, internal version must be done under deep general anaesthesia. If the cervix is not quite fully dilated it is not essential to deliver the child immediately and only one leg need be brought down. It must be emphasized that internal version carries a very high mortality and is not acceptable as a routine procedure for delivery except perhaps in a second twin.

Unfortunately, *neglected transverse lie* is still seen occasionally as an emergency. When the shoulder is deeply impacted in the pelvis with the uterus tightly contracted around the child's body, there is a grave risk of uterine rupture unless Caesarean section is undertaken. The cervix is usually sufficiently dilated for any necessary manipulations, but the wall of the lower uterine segment is so thin that it is very easily damaged by hands or instruments. The child is usually dead, and it may be better to cut through its neck and deliver the trunk and decapitated head separately (*see* Chapter 26) than perform internal podalic version and breech delivery. Whatever method of vaginal delivery is adopted, the hand should be passed into the uterus immediately after the birth of the child to determine whether or not the organ is ruptured. Indeed some obstetricians feel that the chances of uterine rupture occurring are so grave in such cases that they are prepared to carry out a Caesarean section even in late and infected cases, and even though the baby is dead. This attitude may be rather extreme, but if the child is still alive and version impossible, Caesarean section is no more dangerous than vaginal delivery—but the classical is usually the operation of choice.

COMPOUND PRESENTATION

This term is applied to a condition in which an extremity prolapses alongside the presenting part. We have already referred to prolapse of the arm in vertex presentation. More complicated is the case in which a foot and arm present along with the head. This is a very rare occurrence, and is generally associated with a premature or macerated fetus.

The treatment is to push up the prolapsed limb or limbs and allow the head to enter the pelvic cavity. If the os uteri is fully dilated, forceps should be applied to the head and the delivery completed slowly. If replacement fails, podalic version or Caesarean section should be done. When an arm and leg prolapse in a shoulder presentation, version is easy as the leg can be readily grasped and the breech brought down—in such a case the arm should be ignored as it will move upwards as the child is delivered.

PROLAPSE (OR PRESENTATION) AND OTHER ANOMALIES OF THE UMBILICAL CORD

Prolapse of the cord is said to have occurred when any portion of it lies in advance of or alongside the presenting part.

The term *presentation* of the cord may be when the descent of the cord is recognized prior to rupture of the membranes. The word *prolapse* is now however generally used to cover all cases of descent of the cord, whether before or after rupture of the membranes.

Varieties. Cases are classified 'prolapse' (where the cord lies clearly in front of the presenting part) or *'occult' prolapse* (where the cord lies *alongside* the presenting part, and is more difficult to recognize by vaginal examination).

Frequency. Prolapse of the cord is said to occur once in about 1600 uncomplicated vertex deliveries—0·6 per cent. In contracted pelvis, in malpresentations (especially breech and shoulder presentation 6–7 per cent) with abnormal fetus, and other cases of marked fetal or uterine obliquity, the incidence is greatly increased.

Aetiology

Some cases arise from chance, but there is usually some misfit between the presenting part and the lower uterine segment which allows a loop of cord to prolapse, for example, malpresentation, malposition, hydrocephalus and anencephaly. Contracted pelvis, placenta praevia, plural pregnancy and hydramnios also contribute. In many multiparae the lower uterine segment has become softer as a result of repeated pregnancies. This may be an aetiological factor, but a lax abdominal wall permitting malpresentation may be of even greater importance. Cord prolapse also occurs as a complication of certain obstetrical operations in which the presenting part is intentionally or accidentally displaced from the pelvis—e.g. internal version or manual rotation of an occipito-posterior position. Spontaneous or artificial rupture of the membranes at a time when the presenting part is not yet engaged is a predisposing factor.

Diagnosis

As the child's life is immediately endangered by prolapse of the cord, early diagnosis is of very great importance. Unless the cord is visible at the vulva, the diagnosis can be made only by feeling the umbilical cord during vaginal examination. A routine vaginal examination should therefore be made at the time of rupture of the membranes where a clinical condition likely to predispose to prolapse of the cord is present. Nevertheless, using the usual method of vaginal examination, occult descent of the cord will often be undetected, and the prolapse may occur some time after the rupture of the membranes. The possibility of prolapse of the cord should therefore be considered in all cases where signs of fetal distress develop.

Tumultuous fetal movements in association with slowing and irregularity of the heart beats are highly suggestive of pressure on the cord. The tumultuous movements are often followed by a short series of extremely fast beats, not sustained sufficiently long to increase the rate recorded over a full minute. (Irregular irregularity.)

On vaginal examination a pulsating umbilical cord is readily recognized. A pulseless cord is less easily felt and may be overlooked altogether. Less frequently prolapse of the cord may be diagnosed erroneously. The digits of the fetus may resemble the convolutions of the funic vessels and, if the membranes are intact, they may sometimes recede from the palpating finger in a way which may simulate pulsation. (A prolapsed loop of fetal bowel (in exomphalos) and, rarely, maternal small intestine in cases of rupture of the uterus may be mistaken for umbilical cord.)

The absence of pulsation in a prolapsed

cord does not necessarily indicate that the fetus is dead. It may survive for a few minutes after the arrest of funic circulation. While pulsation in the cord indicates that the child is still alive, the examiner must however be careful not to be deceived by the pulsation in his own fingers. Ultrasound 'Doppler' techniques are helpful.

Prognosis

With modern treatment the perinatal mortality should be less than 20 per cent. The fetus, being already suboxygenated, is ill fitted to withstand rapid delivery. So long as the membranes are intact—i.e. in funic presentation—the prognosis is better. The fetal prognosis is slightly better in malpresentations, since a soft irregular presenting part such as the breech is less effective as a compressor than is the hard spherical head. When the malpresentation is a shoulder and, to a lesser extent, when it is a face or brow, the complete absence of engagement of the presenting part at the time of rupture of the membranes may result in survival of the fetus for a surprisingly long time as the cord is often uncompressed. Similarly, in contracted pelvis with disproportion compression is slow to develop. The portion of the pelvis through which the cord prolapses may also influence the prognosis, a cord placed in the pelvic bay beside the sacro-iliac joint being less liable to compression than one which lies directly between the presenting part and the pubes.

The maternal prognosis is not affected by prolapse of the cord *per se*, but the necessary operative treatment increases the risk of shock and sepsis resulting from the laceration of tissue and haemorrhage which are liable to occur if the delivery is hurried in an attempt to save the baby.

Management

When on pelvic examination the umbilical cord is felt through the intact membranes to present, there is little point with the mature fetus or if delivery is to be expected immediately in a premature baby of temporizing—elective Caesarean section is the treatment of choice. If the cord has clearly prolapsed and the child is alive, its best interests are served by immediate delivery. The method employed depends on the stage of dilatation of the cervix, the factors responsible for the prolapse of the cord and whether the patient is at home or in hospital. If the child is dead, in other-wise uncomplicated cases, the labour may be left to complete itself.

An immediate vaginal examination is necessary in all cases. During this examination complications such as hydrocephalus and contracted pelvis should be excluded, and the stage of dilatation of the cervix and level of the presenting part should be noted.

If the cervix is fully dilated and the presenting part is low in the pelvis, the child should be extracted at once by forceps or by breech extraction, according to the presentation. Episiotomy should be done to allow easy delivery.

If the cervix is fully dilated and the presenting part is high there is no alternative in the primigravidae to Caesarean section. In the multigravida the operator should consider why the presenting part is high and he may have to perform Caesarean section because of disproportion or a serious malpresentation. If he feels that vaginal delivery is possible, version and breech extraction is a possible alternative in the transverse lie, but if attempted in the cephalic presentation probably carries a very high mortality and section is still better. The overall Caesarean section rate should certainly be well over 60 per cent. If the cervix is incompletely dilated there is little alternative to Caesarean section if the child is to be saved. Replacement of the cord has a place where operation is not possible.

If the patient is at home or in a ward distant from the operating theatre it is good practice, especially if she is in labour, to position her in the exaggerated *Sims position* to allow the head to fall back from the presenting part. An assistant can hold the presenting part away from the cord with the hand in the vagina and two fingers pressing on the presenting part. General anaesthesia with a high oxygen content should be given soon on arrival in the labour suite.

Cord entanglement round body, limbs or neck, or short cord

Occasionally the cord is so short that it will not allow the child to be born and relative shortness due to looping round the child has a similar effect. Apart from the failure of the child to descend there is with the contractions acute fetal heart slowing and irregularity which tends to persist. Cord complication of some type is responsible for nearly half of all cases of fetal heart anomaly at and after term.

The cord is tangled round the neck or body in very many instances, but very often is slack without signs of fetal distress. Walker (1959) confirming earlier workers has shown that if there is fetal heart irregularity in association with cord anomalies or if the cord is tightly round the neck, there were low oxygen levels in the umbilical artery, clear evidence of poor fetal oxygenation. Undue tightness of the cord especially if several coils are tangled round the child will certainly kill it as the tightness increases with descent. Extensive tangling probably can kill antenatally.

Occasionally several loops round the neck can cause face or brow presentation. Fetal distress in such a situation would indicate operative delivery.

Undue length of the cord predisposes to tangling and prolapse and knotting. *True knots* do occur but rarely pull tight and the thick Wharton's jelly prevents the circulation becoming impeded.

OTHER ABNORMALITIES OF THE CORD

Abnormal attachment

Normally the cord is attached about the centre of the placenta. Very frequently, however, it is placed more to the side. In the *battledore placenta* the cord is attached to the edge of the placenta. Another fairly common abnormality is the so-called *velamentous insertion* of the cord, where the vessels are embedded in the membranes and spread out on their surface before they reach the placenta. If the placenta is situated relatively low in the uterus, the vessels may spread out on the membranes in the region of the lower uterine segment or cervix. This condition, termed *vasa praevia*, may be of serious consequences to the child, since a vessel may be torn when the membranes rupture and the child bleeds to death. Fortunately it is a very rare occurrence.

PREMATURE LABOUR

The degree of fetal maturity in relation to normal time of delivery varies greatly among mammals. The human fetus delivered at term is somewhat prematurely born in terms of enzyme maturity and the ability to survive unaided. Human pregnancy is however maintained by a series of hormone interactions between corpus luteum, placenta and the fetus itself, which is a relationship peculiar to the higher mammals.

Labour is premature if it occurs before the end of the 37th week of pregnancy, i.e. before 259 days from first day of last menstrual period.

Early onset of labour occurs in some 6–7 per cent of cases in single pregnancies but very much more often in multiple pregnancy, *see* Chapter 22.

The causes in the United Kingdom are in single pregnancy:

Antepartum haemorrhage	25 per cent
Intra-uterine death	
Pre-eclampsia	
Fetal deformity	each about
Rhesus incompatability	8 per cent
Premature rupture of membranes	
Other	

In over 30 per cent of cases there is no apparent clinical anomaly associated with premature onset, but some may be due to over stretching, failure of the uterus to accommodate the developing fetus, incompetent os, uterine abnormality etc.

The problems of premature labour to the mother are minimal. She may of course, be acutely ill with abruptio placenta or pre-eclampsia or pyelonephritis but the labour itself rarely causes problems unless the membranes have been ruptured for a long time, when there is a serious risk of infection.

To the child the main risk is that of being born too soon before organ maturity is such that independent survival is possible. With proper care survival is certainly possible with delivery after 26 weeks and is increasingly more likely as maturity increases. As we have seen (page 304) the ability of the newborn to maintain respiration depends to some extent on the surfactant production in the fetal lung. If premature labour threatens it is often possible to check the liquor for the lecithin levels and where levels are low attempts can be made to stimulate surfactant production by the giving of betamethasone to the mother (Liggins and Howie, 1973). The full effect of the drugs requires 48 hours.

Betamethasone acetate 6mg and betamethasone phosphate 6mgm by injection on two occasions 24 hours apart, are most effective in labour before 32 weeks. These drugs should probably not be given if the fetus is already distressed.

The child is often already compromised by the conditions causing the premature labour and may be anoxic and poorly grown with little ability to withstand further insult. For the delivery episiotomy is mandatory and especially in the primigravidae low forceps or forceps to the after-coming head may be necessary to protect the head from undue compression by the vaginal introitus.

The risk to the child of delivery as a breech is serious. Firstly, the small body may deliver through the partially dilated cervix, and the head be held up, or the cord be compressed, and secondly, the soft head may be too strongly squeezed within the birth canal or damaged by sudden release of pressure on delivery. An experienced obstetrician, a paediatrician and an anaesthetist should always be available.

The outcome for the child can be much improved by firstly arranging to book for specialist antenatal care (shared at least) and specialist unit delivery all mothers who have by virtue of past history or present complications any risk of premature labour. Secondly, all mothers in or possibly in labour before the end of the 37th week should always, if time at all permits, be transported to a unit where specialist paediatric facilities exist to care for the baby at and after birth.

Paediatric flying squad ambulances for the transport of premature babies to special units should be rarely required where the standard of antenatal care is high and there is intelligent use of resources.

Suppression of premature labour
Premature labour which would be prejudicial to the child in question may frequently be suppressed by bed rest and sedation to the mother. Unfortunately the sedative employed may of itself be grossly detrimental to the fetus if the labour should progress. Other methods should be used. These methods are valid before membrane rupture and wherever further time is required *in utero*, but are mostly useless if the cervix is 3–4cm dilated. Maternal cardiac disease and evidence of intra-uterine infection are contra-indications to suppression.

Alcohol
Fuchs (1963) showed that oxytocin release from the rabbit pituitary could be suppressed by alcohol, and clinical use of this technique has developed.

Currently alcohol is given by the intra-venous route. Initially a loading dose of 1·5g per K body weight of ethanol dilution in 500mls of 10 per cent dextrose is given every two hours. Following this a maintenance dose of 0·15g of ethanol per K body weight is infused over four hours until labour stops or it is obvious that it is going to continue in spite of alcohol.

Isoxsuprine (Duvaladin) acts on smooth muscle and causes relaxation of peripheral and cerebral blood vessels. It is alpha sympatholytic and beta sympathomimetic. To suppress labour it is given in dosage of 20mgm (250–750μg per min) by slow intravenous infusion and then 10mgm three hourly intramuscularly.

It is an excellent suppressor of uterine activity. There is a risk of hypotension if dosage is too high. It is suggested that it also has an indirect effect on fetal lung maturity, perhaps by stimulating surfactant activity.

Salbutamol is a B adrenergic stimulant used for smooth muscle inhibition in asthma. In control of premature labour it is given by intravenous infusion in dosage of 2–20μg per minute titrated against uterine response. It is a safe, well tolerated and effective uterine relaxant and can be used similarly to alcohol.

Ritodrine Hydrochloride (Utopar) is a B mimetic uterine relaxant given as an intravenous infusion. Initially 200μg per minute of the drug is given over a period of 24–48 hours reducing the dosage depending on uterine response. Oral dosage is 5–10mg four times a day. Side effects are palpitations, nausea and increased tightness of the chest. Animal experiments have shown an increase in uterine blood flow following the administration of the drug. This is probably the drug of choice in the management of premature labour at the present time.

Orciprenaline (Alupent) is a B mimetic. When properly used it reduces and inhibits uterine contractions even those stimulated by oxytocin and prostaglandin E. This is achieved by a direct adrenergic action. Maternal cardiovascular disease is a contra-indication. Side effects are palpitation and nausea. Intravenously, 10μg/minute is infused, diluted in Dextrose or Saline initially; and the dosage increased up to 60μg/minute depending on uterine response. Orally 0·02g can be given four hourly for seven days.

Cervical suture. Just as incompetence of the cervix may predispose to mid trimester abortion so it will occasionally be responsible for premature labour. If the cervical dilatation can be discovered before contractions have started or the membranes have ruptured a Shirodkar type stitch may be applied at the level of the internal os. This can be done even at 27–30 weeks when the membranes are bulging. If the patient is placed in the lithotomy position the cervix can be drawn down the suture inserted.

Abnormal uterus. Premature labour is like abortion (page 141) occasionally due to uterine abnormality, certainly where more than one premature labour has occurred, hysterosalpingogram is advised.

Premature rupture of the membranes

This term is used when membrane rupture occurs before the onset of labour. The main risk of the condition to mother and to child is of intra-amniotic infection leading to fetal intra-uterine infection and perhaps to serious maternal illness.

As we have already said if rupture is proven to have occurred, say after the 37th week, with a child of good size, then there is little point in attempting to continue the pregnancy and contractions should be induced with syntocin or Caesarean section performed. Where the membranes rupture before this time a quick check of lecithin content may be useful, surfactant production may be stimulated by corticosterones to the mother.

In the United Kingdom infection is relatively rare and it is often possible to maintain a pregnancy by bed rest in hospital for many weeks to allow the child to reach maturity. Elsewhere infection is often already present and immediate delivery may be indicated. This is required in most urban communities of the United States.

Precipitate labour

Very occasionally in the multigravidae labour may be extremely rapid, due to excessive strength of uterine contractions. In some the rapidity may be only apparent since the first stage has been completely painless and unnoticed by the patient; only a very short and dramatic second stage of a few minutes occurs. In general, precipitate labour rarely does serious damage to the mother as the tissues can easily be stretched, but occasionally serious tears may occur and sometimes there may be third stage bleeding due to inadequate placental separation. The main problem is to the child where rapid transit

through the bony pelvis may produce cerebral trauma. In many instances such babies are born unattended and delivered in strange places. In these circumstances, damage may occur to them immediately after birth or, alternatively no help is available for resuscitation. If strong uterine contractions occur when a woman is already under attention, the wisest thing is to assist delivery. It is dangerous indeed to try to hold back the delivery but it may be possible to guide the child.

Fetal dystocia due to errors in development or disease of the fetus

The antenatal diagnosis of fetal abnormality by amniocentesis and by X-ray and by ultrasound is discussed in Chapter 28.

LOCAL ENLARGEMENT OF FETUS
1. Head: hydrocephalus, encephalocele, meningocele.
2. Neck: congenital bronchocele; other tumours.
3. Shoulder: tumours.
4. Thorax: hydrothorax; tumours.
5. Abdomen: ascites; distended bladder; tumours of kidney, spleen, liver.
6. Pelvis: tumours.

Occasionally in the multigravidae labour can be obstructed by such lesions and uterine rupture can occur. Similar damage can be caused by forcibly extracting the child by forceps or traction on the limbs without first determining the cause of the delay and difficulty in the labour. Such errors in judgment are unfortunate since in practically every condition to be described the child's condition is incompatible with survival and operative procedures to facilitate delivery are very simple.

Hydrocephalus

In this condition the cerebral ventricles are distended with cerebrospinal fluid. The quantity may reach as much as 6–9 litres (10–15 pints), and the circumference of the head may be very much increased. The trunk of the child is generally puny, and face small although well formed: but the vault of the cranium is enormously distended, the individual bones being separated by wide sutures and fontanelles. Other abnormalities in the fetus, such as spina bifida, talipes, etc., often occur (Fig. 19.35).

Although by careful abdominal palpation

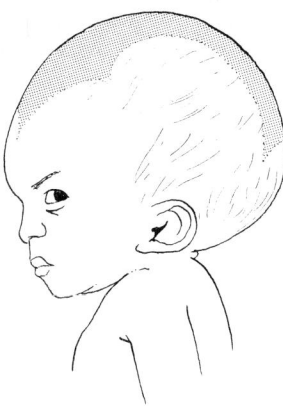

Fig. 19.35   The hydrocephalic head.

the enlarged head may be felt, especially when it is the presenting part, the condition may not be recognized until labour is well advanced. If hydrocephalus is suspected, an exact diagnosis can be made by radiography; this may in addition show a spina bifida deformity.

The fetus may die shortly before or during labour, the fetal heart may be heard throughout labour and occasionally the baby is born alive if the hydrocephalus is so slight as to offer no difficulty in delivery. Breech presentation occurs in about 25 per cent of cases. Other malpresentations also occur.

Fetus presents by the head. Recognition of hydrocephalus when the head presents is not difficult, since the presenting part remains above the pelvic brim. It is felt by abdominal palpation to be larger, more globular and softer than the normal head. There is no descent of the head even after labour has been in progress for some hours and the membranes have ruptured.

As soon as the fingers can be passed through the cervix the elasticity of the presenting head and the fact that the sutures and fontanelles are widely separated should lead to a correct diagnosis. If the fetus is dead or the head not tensely distended with fluid the hydrocephalus may be mistaken for the bag of unruptured membranes, for in such cases a portion of the fetal head projects through the cervix.

Once the diagnosis is made, the head should be perforated when the cervix is 4–6cm dilated, scissors, or a perforator can be used. It is often however, a good idea to insert a thick long needle and tube and allow the fluid to drain slowly. Alternatively the head may be punctured through the suprapubic portion of the mother's abdominal wall with a needle

after first emptying the bladder. Spontaneous delivery usually follows quickly.

Fetus presents by the breech

Here difficulty occurs only with the after-coming head, which is arrested at the pelvic brim. On vaginal examination the condition may not be suspected, for the base of the skull is more or less normal, but palpation of the abdomen should reveal an undue distension of the lower part of the uterus. If the trunk of the child is puny, and other malformations such as spina bifida or talipes are present, hydrocephalus should always be suspected if there is difficulty in delivery of the head.

Attempts to deliver by traction on the trunk and suprapubic pressure are dangerous, since if persisted it will cause rupture of the thinned-out lower uterine segment of the uterus.

The head may be perforated through the abdominal wall (bladder empty) with a long needle and sufficient fluid drained off to allow delivery. The head may be perforated behind the ear again with needle or scissors. This is not difficult and the escape of fluid is followed by collapse of the skull and rapid delivery. An alternative treatment is the withdrawal of the fluid by inserting a firm plastic or metal catheter into the spinal canal when a spina bifida or meningocele allows access in this way.

Meningocele and encephalocele

These cystic growths consisting of the meninges with or without brain tissue are usually found in the vicinity of the posterior fontanelle. They are often difficult to recognize, because being 'tucked away' behind the occiput they are inaccessible to the examining fingers in both cranial and breech presentations. When the head presents they tend to produce a brow presentation, while if the breech presents they prevent descent of the after-coming head.

The treatment is to perforate the sac with scissors or other pointed instrument. This allows the meningocele to collapse and delivery is easy. Some children with this condition may be delivered alive, but only if the meningocele is small and the stalk narrow.

Tumour of the neck of the child

The commonest tumour of the neck is congenital bronchocele. The diagnosis of the condition can be made by feeling the tumour just below the chin. It should be suspected in face or brow presentation or when difficulty with the aftercoming head is experienced in breech presentation.

The difficulties associated with congenital bronchocele are due not so much to the size of the tumour, for it is seldom extremely large, but to the fact that it produces an extension of the head and brings about a face or brow presentation. In breech presentation the extraction of the after-coming head may be rendered difficult because the tumour interferes with flexion of the head. Occasionally the tumour must be broken up and the head perforated.

Tumour of the shoulder

This complication is a great rarity. It favours a shoulder presentation. As the tumour is almost invariably a sarcoma the child need not be considered, and consequently the delivery should be terminated in the manner safest to the mother. It may be necessary to break up the tumour by a perforator or long scissors and decapitate the child.

Distension and tumours of the thorax

Complications of this nature are very great rarities. Occasionally, however, distension of the pleura with fluid, tumours of the pleura, lungs or thymus gland have led to extreme distension of the thorax.

The correct procedure is to perforate the chest. If the distension is caused by fluid, this is all that is necessary. A tumour may have to be broken up before the child can be extracted.

Distension and tumours of the abdomen

This complication is more common than the condition referred to in the two previous paragraphs. The fetal conditions which give rise to it are ascites, distension of bladder with atresia of urethra, hydronephrosis, and tumours of the abdominal viscera. The first three mentioned are the commonest causes and are incompatible with the child's survival.

Head presenting. Delay occurs after the head escapes. The complication should always be suspected where there is difficulty in extracting the trunk, and especially if the child's head and thorax appear puny. The obstruction is easily recognized by passing the hand up over the child's thorax, when the distended abdomen can be felt.

Breech presenting. Here the difficulty occurs at an earlier stage of the delivery than usual, for if the abdomen of the child is extremely distended the breech may not descend into the pelvis. The accoucheur may have difficulty in feeling the abdominal distension until he brings down a foot or both feet and introduces his hand into the uterus.

The treatment consists in opening the abdomen with a perforator or scissors. If the condition is ascites the abdomen immediately collapses and completion of the delivery is simple. The same applies to distension of the fetal bladder. If, however, there is a tumour such as hydronephrosis or retroperitoneal sarcoma, it may be necessary to make a larger opening into the abdomen and remove the tumour and some of the abdominal viscera.

Tumour of sacrum

This is a relatively rare complication. Generally the tumour is a sarcoma or teratoma. Where the head presents there is seldom much difficulty in extracting the breech. Where, however, the child presents by the breech there may be difficulty in determining what is presenting. Indeed, until the hand has been passed into the uterus a correct diagnosis is often impossible.

GENERAL FETAL DROPSY (HYDROPS FETALIS)

This condition, due usually to the most severe type of serological incompatibility (or occasionally to other factors) occasionally produces some degree of dystocia.

Diagnosis

Radiography may show the fetus occupying an unusual attitude the so-called Buddha position. Due to the gross distension of the abdomen, the arms are displaced upwards and outwards and the thighs pushed downwards and outwards with marked flexion of the knees. There may be a halo shadow round the skull, and the fetal scapula may be displaced laterally increasing the width between the scapula and the ribs due to the subcutaneous oedema.

It is rare in the modern unit that a child should be allowed to reach the stage of hydrops due to serological incompatibility since active investigation and intra-uterine transfusion would have occurred. However, other causes of fetal dropsy exist and the emergency case due to undiagnosed serological incompatibility can occur, and the diagnosis is made only following the birth of a dropsical baby and its enormous placenta or when delivery of the trunk of the fetus proves difficult. This is due to the presence of the subcutaneous oedema or to free fluid in the baby's peritoneal cavity.

Management

Since the child never survives in any case, it is quite permissible to facilitate the delivery by perforating the child's abdomen with scissors to allow the escape of the free fluid.

Since the placenta is usually extremely large and very friable, portions may easily be retained and cause post-partum haemorrhage. If bleeding does occur manual exploration of the uterus should be performed. If a blood transfusion is necessary particular care must, of course be taken in obtaining compatible blood.

DOUBLE MONSTERS

Double monsters are examples of uniovular twins in which the common blastoderm has not completely divided into two. They may be joined by only a thin band of tissue or there may be very intimate fusion.

These disomata may be asymmetrical where the fetuses are united by dissimilar parts, or symmetrical where the two are united by corresponding parts (head to head, etc.).

ASYMMETRICAL DISOMATA
These are often of very unequal sizes, the smaller appearing sometimes as a parasite of the other.

SYMMETRICAL DISOMATA
These are generally of equal size and there are three main varieties: (1) Thoracopagus, where the two fetuses have their trunks united, but have distinct head and limbs; (2) Dicephalus, where the fetuses have two heads, four upper limbs, but usually only two lower limbs; and (3) Syncephalus, where the two heads are fused; there is often only one set of upper limbs, but always four lower limbs.

Diagnosis
It is obvious that especially with symmetrical disomata, great difficulty may be experienced both in the diagnosis and the delivery, especially in cases in which the head presents. Some can be diagnosed by radiography, but in the thoracopagus variety, if the union between the two is slight, the radiograph may present the picture of a simple plural pregnancy.

Treatment
The syncephalus variety gives least trouble in labour and if the head presents it should be perforated and the rest of the child extracted. If the breech presents and the limbs are brought down, the abnormality, as in hydrocephalus, should be suspected if the head is found to be unusually large. Craniotomy should be performed.

The thoracopagus and the dicephalus varieties give most difficulty in labour, especially if the heads present. The time-honoured treatment is to perform internal version and bring down the lower limbs. Steadying the trunk and heads by traction, the mass of the fetus can then be broken up with strong scissors and a perforator. This may be very difficult and take a long time, and if the diagnosis is made radiologically before labour or in labour before prolonged attempts at vaginal delivery have been made Caesarean section is safer for the mother.

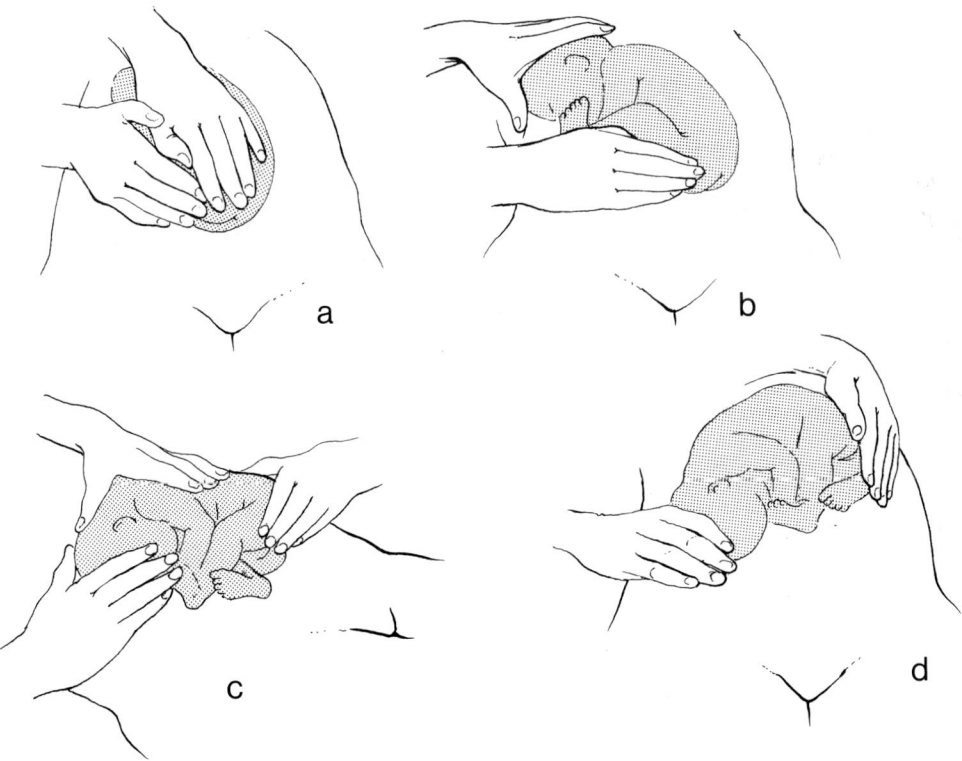

Fig. 19.36 Technique of external version from breech. (a) Breech mobilized at pelvic brim (b) Child flexed—breech pushed to one side (c) Rotation begun (d) Nearly completed.

REFERENCES

Anderson, G. J. & Walker, J. (1970) The effect of labour on the maternal blood gas and maternal base states. *J. Obstet. Gynaec. Brit. Cwlth.*, 77, 289.

Barber, H. R. Graber, E. A. & Orlando, A. (1972) Augmented Labour. *Obstet. Gynaec.*, **39**, 933.

Borell, U. & Fernstrom, I. (1960) Radiologic Pelvimetry. *Acta. Radiol. (Stockh) Suppl.*, **191**.

Buchan, P. C., Milne, M. K. & Browning, M. C. K. (1973) The effect of continuous epidural blockage on plasma 11-Hydroxycorticosteroid concentrations in labour. *J. Obstet. Gynaec. Brit. Cwlth.*, **80**, 11.

Caldeyro Barcia, R. (1963) in *Neonatal Respiratory Adaption*. US Dept. Health Educ. Welfare.

Caldeyro Barcia, R. & Alvarez, H. (1957) Abnormal uterine action in labour. *J. Obstet. Gynaec. Brit. Emp.*, **59**, 646.

Caldeyro Barcia, R. & Poseiro, J. J. (1954) Oxytocin and contraction of the pregnant human uterus. *Ann. N.Y. Acad. Sci.*, 75, 813.

Crammond, W. (1954) Pathological aspects of uterine dysfunction. *Lancet*, **ii**, 1241.

Dawes, G. S. (1965) in The effects of labour on the fetus and new born. *Wld. Hlth. Org. Tech. Rep. Ser.*, **300**.

Dawes, G. S. (1967) Physiology of the Fetus in normal labour in *Proc. 5th Wld. Cong. Gynaec. Obstet.*, Butterworth. Ed: Wood, C. & Walters, W. A. W.

Flint, A. P., Andersen, A. B., Patten, P. T. (1974) Control of utero ovarian venous prostaglandin F during labor in sheep: acute effects of vaginal and cervical stimulation. *J. Endocrinol.* **63**, 253.

Friedman, E. A. (1967) *Labour*, New York: Appleton.

Fuchs, A. R. (1963) in *Initiation of Labour*. p. 43. Ed: Marshall, J. M. and Burnett, W. M. US Dept. Health Educ. Welfare.

Gillanders, L. A. (1959) Radiological evaluation of the pelvic outlet. *Brit. J. Radiol.* **12**, 193.

HMSO Report on Confidential Enquiries into Maternal Deaths (1973).

Killam, A. P., Rosenfeld, C. R., Battaglia, F. C., Makowski, E. L. & Meschia, G. (1973) Affect of Oestrogens on the Uterine Blood Flow of Oophorectomized Ewes. *Amer. J. Obstet. Gynec.*, **115**, 1045.

Lees, N. H., Scott, D. B. & Kerr, M. G. (1970) Haemodynamic changes associated with labour. *J. Obstet. Gynaec. Brit. Cwlth.*, 77, 29.

Liggins, G. C. (1972) Foetal participation in the physiological controlling mechanisms of parturition in Foetal and Neonatal Physiology. *Proc. of Sir Joseph Barcroft Centenary Symposium.*, p. 562.

Liggins, G. C. & Howie, R. W. (1973) *Prevention of respiratory distress syndrome by antepartum corticosteroid therapy in fetal and neonatal physiology.* p. 613. Cambridge University Press.

Lindgren, L. (1973) Influence of uterine motility on cervical dilatation in labour. *Amer. J. Obstet. Gynec.*, 7, 117, 530.

Lorand, S. (1933) Uber ein neuen Uehenzeichnenden Apparat (Tokograph) *Zbl. Gyneak.*, 57, 554.

MacVicar, J. (1973) Acceleration and augmentation of labour. *Scot. med. J.*, **18**, 201.

Malpas, P. (1933) Post-maturity and Malformation of the Foetus. *J. Obstet. Gynaec. Brit. Cwlth.*, **40**, 1046.

O'Driscoll, K., Jackson, R. J. A. & Gallagher, J. T. (1970) Active management of labour and cephalopelvic disproportion. *J. Obstet. Gynaec. Brit. Cwlth.*, 77, 385.

O'Driscoll, K. (1972) Abolition of prolonged labour. *Proc. R. Soc. Med.*, **65**, 697.

Patel, N. (1973) Personal communication.

Persianinov, L. S. (1967) Effects of abnormal labour in the fetus, in *Proc. 5th Wld. Cong. Gynaec. Obstet.*, Butterworth. Ed. Wood, C. and Walters, W. A. W.

Philpott, R. H. & Castle, W. M. (1972) Cervical graphs in the management of labour in primigravidae. *J. Obstet. Gynaec. Brit. Cwlth.*, 79, 592–599.

Reynolds, S. R. M., Heard, O. O., Brans, P., Hellman, L. M. (1948) *Bulletin Johns Hopkins Hospital.*, **82**, 466.

Russel, J. G. B. (1973) *Radiology in obstetrics and antenatal paediatrics*, London: Butterworth.

Saling, E. (1966) Fetal and neonatal hypoxia in relation to clinical obstetric practice, London: Arnold.

Savage, E. W., Kohl, S. G. and Wynn, R. M. (1970) Prolapse of the Umbilical Cord. *Obstet. and Gynec.*, **36**, 502.

Turnbull, A. C. (1957) Uterine contractions in normal and abnormal labour. *J. Obstet. Gynaec. Brit. Emp.*, **64**, 321.

Turnbull, A. C. & Henderson, A. B. M. (1968) Uterine contractions and oxytocin sensitivity during human pregnancy in relation to onset of labour. *J. Obstet. Gynaec. Brit. Cwlth.*, 75, 278.

Walker, J. (1959a) *The Influence of Clinical Conditions on Oxygen Available to the Baby*, in *Oxygen Supply to the Human Fetus*, Ed. Walker, J. and Turnbull, A. C. T. Oxford: Blackwell.

Walker, J. (1959b) Fetal Distress. *Amer. J. Obstet. Gynec.*, 77, 1.

Walker, J. (1970) Obstetric Sequelae of Difficult Labour in Primigravidae. *Proc. 6th Wld. Cong. Gynaec. Obstet.*, Abstract 147.

Williams, E. A. & Stallworthy, J. A. (1952) Abnormal uterine action in labour. Proc. 13th British Congress (1952) *Lancet* i, 330. *J. Obstet. Gynaec. Brit. Emp.*, **59**, 217.

Yao, A. C. & Lind, J. (1974) Placental Transfusion. *Amer. J. Dis. Child.*, **127**, 128.

20. The Puerperium

It has taken forty weeks for the maternal organism to respond to the structural and functional demands of pregnancy. In the newly delivered woman all the pregnancy adaptations except those related to lactation have suddenly become redundant. The period during which these changes are reversed to the non-pregnant state is called the puerperium. This process of re-adaptation to the non-pregnant state has been traditionally taken to last six weeks, and in fact, most of it is completed within this period. The magnitude of the process and the speed with which it is completed makes the puerperium a period of physiological tumult.

I. STRUCTURAL CHANGES IN THE PUERPERIUM

a. Involution of the uterus

Immediately after the delivery of the placenta, the uterus weighs approximately 900g. The fundus is palpable 2·5cm below the umbilicus. The rough area of the placental site, uncovered by epithelium, is clearly distinguishable. The cavity of the uterus is in direct continuity with the vagina, and the cervix hangs as a curtain from the body of the uterus into the vagina. The vessels formerly supplying and draining the placenta are compressed by continuing uterine retraction, and also contribute to haemostasis by contraction of the vessel wall. The uterine contractions of labour continue, but, for some reason as yet not understood, are usually felt as 'after-pains' only in women who have previously borne children.

Involution or shrinkage of the uterus proceeds with remarkable speed. By the tenth day of the puerperium the uterus is no longer palpable in the abdominal cavity; it now weighs less than 500g. At the end of five to six weeks it has shrunk to almost its pre-pregnancy size, and now weighs less than 100g.

During this process of involution the number of myometrial cells does not diminish greatly, but there is a great reduction in the size and volume of each muscle cell. The connective tissue framework also diminishes in amount, but, at the end of the puerperium, the uterus contains more connective tissue than it did before the onset of the pregnancy.

We are indebted to Sharman (1966) for a meticulous study of the changes in the endometrium and in the former placental site. Apart from studying in detail ten uteri obtained at post-mortem, he carried out 626 endometrial biopsies from 285 women at varying times from the fifth day to nine months after parturition.

Within three days after parturition, the superficial layer of the decidua becomes necrotic, and is shed in the lochia. The deeper layer of the decidua, containing the base of the glands, is retained. Proliferation of epithelial cells from these glandular remnants together with the adjacent stroma is rapid and results in the reformation of an intact endometrial surface within seven to ten days of parturition, except over the former placental site. The restoration of an endometrial covering over the latter takes approximately three weeks.

Serial endometrial biopsies in Sharman's studies showed no evidence of secretory changes in the endometrium until the forty-fourth day. He therefore maintains that ovulation is not resumed before the fortieth day, and this has useful implications so far as contraceptive advice to the recently delivered patient is concerned. He also noted small degenerate decidual remnants and stromal inflammatory cell infiltration for two months after delivery. These are not to be taken as evidence of infection, but are part of the physiological process of tissue degeneration and repair.

The full repair of the former placental site takes up to six weeks. The contracted blood vessels become thrombosed and later organized by fibrous tissue. Some recanalization eventually occurs in some of the blood vessels.

In the myometrium, the larger blood vessels are obliterated by hyaline change, and are replaced by new, smaller vessels.

The cervix is torn to some extent in normal parturition, hence the difference in the shape of the external os in the non-pregnant parous and nulliparous cervix. The cervix is open and readily admits two fingers for a few days following parturition, but, in the absence of infection, it has narrowed by the end of the first week, making it difficult to introduce even one finger.

b. The lochia

This is the normal discharge from the genital tract in the puerperium. For up to three days it is red in colour (lochia rubra) and contains a variable amount of fresh blood as well as decidual debris. It then becomes pink in colour (lochia serosa) containing still some red cells, but predominantly leucocytes and necrotic decidua. By the end of the first week it is yellowish-white in colour (lochia alba) consisting now principally of serous fluid and leucocytes. It has a characteristic sweetish odour, and the discharge gradually diminishes in amount. It may last for three to six weeks.

c. Other structural changes

The abdominal wall may remain soft and flabby for some weeks. The striae gravidarum gradually become white in colour, but this process takes six to nine months. Permanent laxity of the abdominal wall, possibly with separation or divarication of the rectus abdominis muscles, may result in a woman who has had above average abdominal stretching, e.g. in twin pregnancy.

Baird (1935) carried out cystoscopic examinations of the bladder following parturition. He found oedema and hyperaemia of the mucosa with frequent submucous extravasation of blood. The puerperal bladder is readily distensible and relatively insensitive to volumes of urine which would ordinarily cause strong detrusor contractions. It is therefore vulnerable to over-distension and incomplete emptying. Residual urine, i.e. urine left in the bladder following micturition, predisposes to cystitis and ascending urinary tract infection, both

common complications in the puerperium. The ureters and renal pelves remain dilated and easily distensible, and these changes can take as long as eight weeks to revert to normal.

II. THE BREASTS AND LACTATION

Changes in the breasts are among the earliest symptoms of pregnancy. Increased vascularity in the substance and over the surface of the breasts gives a feeling of tingling, swelling and enlargement. Further progressive enlargement of the breasts occurs in the last two trimesters of pregnancy. This is presumed to occur under the control of oestrogens, progesterone and placental lactogen. Hytten (1971) has shown how extremely variable the degree of breast enlargement can be between different individuals. The increase in breast volume of a single breast ranged from zero to as much as 880ml with a mean value of about 200ml. Moreover, he showed that the increase in breast size in primigravidae was related to maternal age, older women having, on average, only one quarter of the increase seen in young women. He also showed that milk yield on the seventh day of the puerperium was related to the growth in size of the breasts, so that the younger primigravida is more likely to produce an adequate volume of milk than a woman having her first baby in her late twenties or later. Further evidence of decreased efficiency of the mammary gland with increasing maternal age is the steady decline in fat content of seventh day milk from a mean of 3·25g per cent in primiparae under 20 to 2·83g per cent in primiparae of 30 and over.

In the same study measurements of the size of the areola, and of the size and mobility of the nipple were made. It was shown that, at the beginning of pregnancy, inadequate protrusion of the nipple was present in about 60 per cent of primigravidae, but that, at the end of pregnancy, and in the absence of any specific antenatal treatment, this was present in only 16 per cent; and in only about one-third of the latter was there difficulty with the nipples when breast feeding was subsequently initiated.

The colostrum secreted in the breasts during pregnancy and available for the baby during the first two or three days of life, contains more protein and minerals, but less sugar and fat, than milk. Antibodies are readily demonstrable in colostrum. IgA may offer protection against neonatal enteric infection.

The exact mechanism by which milk secretion is initiated in the human remains unproved. In part, at least, the sudden fall in level of circulating oestrogens, progesterone and placental lactogen which occurs following the delivery of the placenta is associated with a release of prolactin from the hypothalamo-pituitary axis. The adequacy and duration of lactation are controlled in large part by the stimulus of suckling and by the completeness of emptying of the breast. Hytten, however, suggests that genetic influences may also be very important in determining the quantity, quality and duration of milk production.

Prolactin is an important stimulus to milk secretion. Oxytocin release from the neuro-hypophysis is stimulated by suckling or even the preparations for suckling, and is inhibited by fright or stress.

A raised circulatory oxytocin level causes contraction of the myoepithelial cells in the alveoli and small milk ducts. At the beginning of a feed at least 60 per cent of the milk is stored there, and failure of this let down mechanism can obviously cause the baby to receive only that fraction of milk stored in lactiferous ducts and sinuses.

On the second to fourth days after delivery, the breasts become larger and firmer. This enlargement, due to vascular engorgement, signifies the commencement of milk secretion. When very marked it makes the breasts heavy, tense and painful and temporarily flattens the nipples, making it difficult for the baby's jaw to 'bite' on the areola. Indeed in such a situation it is advisable to take the baby off the breast for 24 hours and relieve symptoms with analgesics, breast support and by means of emptying the breasts with a gentle breast pump.

Human milk is bluish-white in colour, slightly alkaline, and has a specific gravity varying between 1·026 and 1·036. The milk contains approximately 87 per cent water and 13 per cent solids (proteins 1–2 per cent, fats 3–4 per cent, sugar 8 per cent, minerals 0·1 per cent). Most drugs given to the mother appear in the milk. This certainly applies to antibiotics, sulphonamides, alcohol, alkaloids and those laxative drugs which are absorbed into the maternal circulation.

III. CLINICAL PHYSIOLOGY OF THE PUERPERIUM

a. Body weight

The average primigravida, eating to appetite, gains about 12·5kg body weight during pregnancy. A number of measurements made during early labour and just after delivery indicate that she loses, on average, 6kg in weight at parturition, leaving a surplus of around 6·5kg still remaining at the start of the puerperium.

When patients are weighed daily under standard conditions (Dennis and Bytheway, 1965) it is found that body weight usually rises or is held steady for three to four days before beginning to fall. In cases where oedema is present in late pregnancy (about 40 per cent of the total cases in the study) progressive weight loss from delivery is more common, though even in such patients the daily loss in weight is less in the first three than in the subsequent seven days of the puerperium (Fig. 20.1). The administration of oestrogens

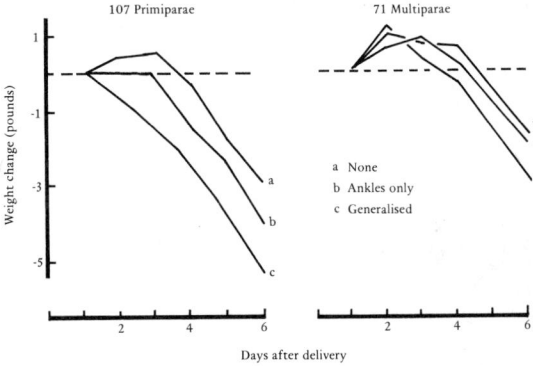

Fig. 20.1   Body weight changes in the first six days of the puerperium, related to the presence and type of clinical oedema in late pregnancy. None of the subjects was given any hormone for lactation suppression.

to suppress lactation increases the tendency to gain weight in the early puerperium. Weight gain in the early puerperium is more marked in multiparous patients (Fig. 20.2).

Body weight tends to stabilize about ten weeks after delivery (Figs. 20.3 and 4). At this time there is still a positive balance of about 2·25kg compared with the assumed pre-pregnancy weight. This positive balance is, on average, 0·7kg less in women who have continued to breast feed their babies than in those who have not lactated.

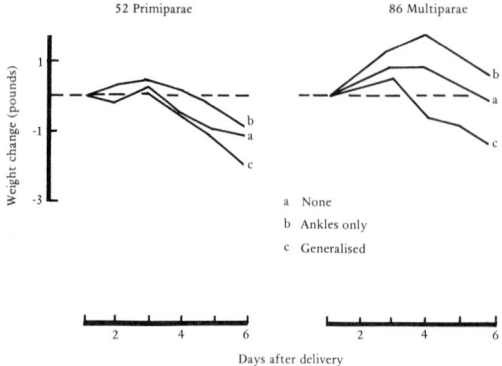

Fig. 20.2 Body weight changes in the first six days of the puerperium, related to the presence and type of clinical oedema in late pregnancy. All subjects were taking Stilboestrol tablets to suppress lactation.

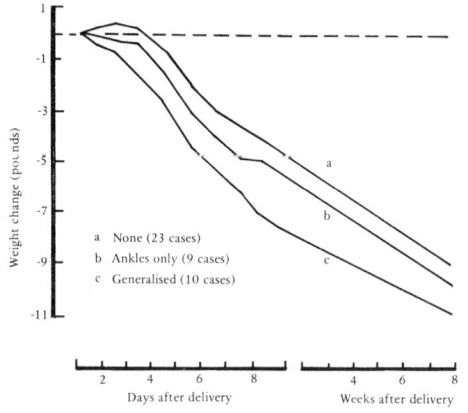

Fig. 20.3 Body weight changes from delivery until eight weeks later, in a group of 42 normal primiparae by the presence and type of clinical oedema in late pregnancy. None of the subjects was given any hormone for lactation suppression.

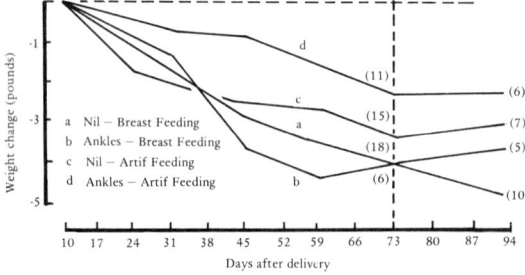

Fig. 20.4 Body weight changes between the 10th and the 94th days after delivery in a group of 50 normal primiparae, related to the presence and type of clinical oedema in late pregnancy, and to whether the subjects were or were not breast feeding throughout the period. (Number of subjects in each group in brackets.)

b. Water balance

It has for long been assumed that a diuresis commences immediately after parturition, and that this continues for one to two weeks until all the additional water stored during pregnancy has been eliminated. This pattern of water metabolism is indeed what happens in women who have accumulated demonstrable oedema in late pregnancy. In the 60 per cent who have not, the diuresis is usually delayed until the third or fourth day. In

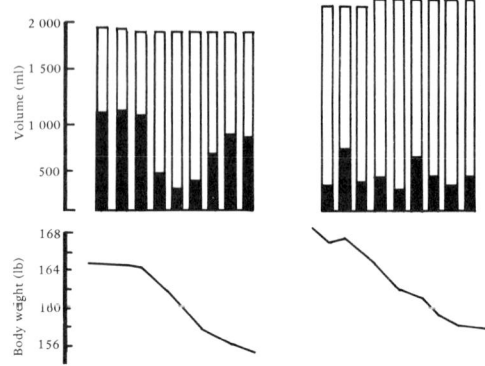

Fig. 20.5 Partial water balance and body weight change in two subjects during the first nine days of the puerperium. Both subjects were healthy normal primiparae, the subject on the left having no oedema in late pregnancy, whereas the other had generalized oedema. Each day's water intake is shown in the histogram measured upwards from the base-line. The measured output of water in urine, milk and lochia is represented by the clear part of the histogram. (No measurement was made of water loss through skin, lungs or faeces.) The subject who had had no oedema retained fluid until the fourth day, and only then began to show a fall in body weight, whereas the woman with generalized oedema had a much greater water loss from the first day.

figure 20.5 two water balance experiments are shown to illustrate this feature.

c. Haematological changes

Daily estimation of the haemoglobin concentration of peripheral venous blood shows an initial rise on the first day of the puerperium as compared with a late pregnancy measurement. This is followed by a sharp fall to a minimum level on the fourth and fifth days. Thereafter the haemoglobin level rises again, without any haematinic being administered. The haematocrit of peripheral venous blood behaves in a similar manner. The fall in haemoglobin concentration in the early puerperium is probably due to haemodilution, as the mean corpuscular haemoglobin concentration remains constant (Fig. 20.6). Indeed, when serial measurements of plasma volume

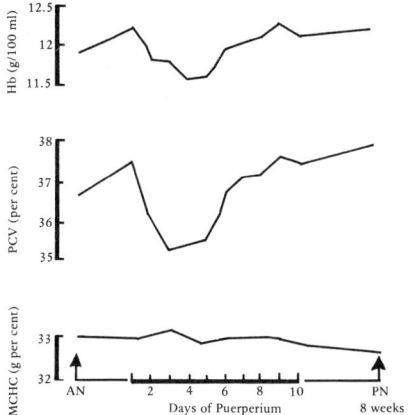

Fig. 20.6 Mean levels of haemoglobin, haematocrit and mean corpuscular haemoglobin concentration in peripheral venous blood in late pregnancy and in the puerperium in 42 normal primiparae. None of these subjects showed clinical oedema in late pregnancy nor were they given any hormone for lactation suppression.

and total circulating red cell volume are performed, a rise in plasma volume in the early puerperium can be shown. This has implications in the treatment of patients with heart disease. It also suggests that haemoglobin levels should be measured on the first rather than on the third day of the puerperium if anaemia is not to be over-diagnosed.

During and immediately after labour, a leucocytosis occurs, with counts ranging from 10 000 to 30 000/ml^3. The increase is made up predominantly of granulocytes. The erythrocyte sedimentation is very variable for 10–20 days post-partum, largely due to the high levels of circulating fibrinogen, and cannot be usefully employed as a diagnostic tool. Other pregnancy induced changes in blood coagulation factors persist for variable periods of time after delivery.

IV. CLINICAL MANAGEMENT

a. Attention in first few hours

Even in normal cases, the obstetrician or trained midwife should remain with the patient for at least an hour. During this time repeated checking of the continued contraction of the uterus is carried out by gentle abdominal palpation, and a check is made of the vulva to ensure that only slight bleeding is occurring. At the end of the hour the pulse rate, temperature and blood pressure are measured.

If the uterus becomes soft during this time a contraction can be stimulated by abdominal 'rubbing', and, if necessary, an oxytocic drug, e.g. ergometrine 0·5mg or syntocinon 5 units, or both can be administered parenterally. In such a situation the patient will have to be observed carefully for several hours until the obstetrician is certain that no further uterine relaxation and/or bleeding will occur.

b. Bladder function

When the danger of genital bleeding has passed care must be taken to avoid bladder distension. The urinary output should be noted and the patient should pass at least 100ml urine at a time within eight hours of delivery. If this does not occur, abdominal palpation may reveal the bladder as a vague swelling between the uterine fundus and the pubic symphysis. An injection of carbachol may be tried at this time, but, if this fails to restore adequate micturition, the bladder should be catheterized. If overdistension of the bladder has been permitted, a repeat catheterization may be required. In that case an indwelling catheter may have to be left in the bladder for 48–72 hours, though this will increase the chance of developing a urinary infection.

c. Care of the vulva

Shortly after the placenta has been delivered and any tear or episiotomy repaired, the external genitalia are bathed with a mild antiseptic solution and a sterile pad is applied. The sterile pad is replaced whenever possible, and the vulva is cleansed, preferably using a bidet, after bowel motions. If there is undue pain, the vulva should be inspected in a good light for infection or haematoma formation. If non-absorbable perineal sutures have been inserted, they are removed on the fifth or sixth day.

d. General care

The temperature, pulse and blood pressure are measured at least once per day. A rise in temperature during the first 24 hours only and not above 38 °C may be taken as physiological, but subsequent or more serious pyrexia requires investigation. 'After pains' due to uterine contractions, may require the administration of simple analgesics, such as aspirin. Early ambulation is now everywhere accepted, and even women who have been delivered by Caesarean section are encouraged to get up and walk a little on the first day. No special dietary measures are required, and there is no good evidence that the fluid intake affects the quantity or quality of breast milk.

e. The establishment of lactation

If a woman has decided to feed her baby, it should be put to the breast within 8 hours of birth, and preferably much sooner. The anxious primipara will require some help to ensure that the baby 'fixes' on to the areola, and only two or three minutes of suckling is required at this stage. Thereafter the baby should be placed in a cot, preferably beside its mother and put to the breast on demand; but the mother's sleep should be ensured by removing noisy babies to a small nursery at night.

During the first three or four days some complementary bottle feeding, using a milk formula, may be advisable, but thereafter artificial milk complements should be avoided until the sixth or seventh days, when the adequacy of lactation can be assessed. This is done preferably by seeing that the baby is contented and starting to gain weight. However, if the mother or the midwife are uncertain about this, 'test weighing' can then be done. By weighing a baby immediately before and after feeding at every feed for 24 hours, an idea of the volume of milk the baby has consumed can be obtained. If this is over 300ml, lactation will probably be adequate. In a woman who wishes to breast feed, this should only rarely be abandoned before the end of the first week unless the nipples become blistered or cracked. Breast engorgement and its management have been described in the previous section.

If the mother cannot or does not wish to breast feed, lactation is quickly inhibited if the breasts are not emptied. They should be supported by a brassière or binder. Fullness and discomfort occur in only a proportion of women and rarely last more than 48 hours. Simple analgesics are given. The use of oestrogens to suppress lactation has fallen from favour since it has been shown that their therapeutic efficiency is not high, and that their use may be associated with an increased hazard of deep vein thrombosis.

f. Emotional support

After the feeling of elation when the process of parturition is complete, there often follows a spell of mild depression—'the fourth day blues'. It is important that this is explained during pregnancy. It is normally short-lived, but in some women it may last for several weeks. Similarly, resumption of libido may take several months, and much marital misery could be avoided if the couple knew that a temporary loss of sexual drive is a common feature, often lasting for several weeks and sometimes even longer.

g. Discharge from hospital

In Western society the trend towards 100 per cent hospital confinement continues. Once the period of maximal risk has passed, and if home circumstances are favourable, there is an increasing trend towards early discharge from hospital. However, this is not appropriate if domestic help is inadequate, and many women with three or four children welcome the opportunity of staying in hospital for five to seven days before resuming their domestic responsibilities.

h. Resumption of menstruation

If the woman does not breast feed her child, menstruation usually recommences within six to twelve weeks of delivery. In Sharman's study this occurred in 91 per cent of cases. However, resumption of menstruation is much more variable in lactating mothers, where it may occur as early as six weeks, or as late as two years after confinement.

i. The post-natal period

After delivery and discharge from hospital regular post-natal visits by midwife, health visitor and general practitioner are essential to supervise the continued wellbeing of mother and child. Breast feeding often falters with return to home and reassurance and patient guidance may be necessary.

Return of the mother to full recovery may be slow psychologically or physically and perineal or abdominal wounds may give trouble.

Sleepless nights with a restless new baby are commonplace, and sympathetic help may be needed.

Lochia changing to a blood stained or brown discharge may persist for four to six weeks, but usually disappears before that time.

Occasionally sharp or serious bleeding with a still open cervix declares the presence of retained placental products or occasionally of an exuberant healing placental site. Urgent transfusion and curettage may be necessary.

Mastitis or breast abscess may occur especially if bottle feeding is begun and there is inadequate suppression of maternal breast function.

j. Post-natal examination

Routinely at six to eight weeks post delivery a formal post-natal examination is undertaken. By that time involution should be well established, menstruation may have returned, all wounds should be healed and medical complications exacerbated by pregnancy should have regressed.

The physical condition is checked, weight noted, breast, abdomen and perineal involution recorded; urine is checked for albumin and sugar, haemoglobin blood levels and blood pressures recorded.

Pelvic examination is done to ensure adequate healing and normality of the cervix and that the uterus is involuted, mobile and preferably anteverted. A routine cervical smear is taken unless it has been done in the antenatal period.

Where there has been difficult pregnancy, labour or delivery, or there has been any complication whatsoever, a full and explanatory discussion is held with the mother, questions answered, and the likely behaviour in the next pregnancy assessed.

Desire for, and technique of, contraception is discussed and the necessary action taken to establish a method satisfactory to wife and husband.

If there has been a perinatal death, or birth of a premature or deformed child, full explanation is given where possible, genetic counselling (if necessary) is arranged, and the outcome of the next pregnancy is discussed. Where desired, arrangements are made for later sterilization of husband or wife.

It is immensely important at that time that previously abnormal or difficult pregnancy is fully discussed, explanations given, and the likely 'next time' outcome explained.

REFERENCES

Baird, D. (1935) The upper urinary tract in pregnancy and in the puerperium. *J. Obstet. Gynaec. Brit. Emp.*, **42**, 733.
Baird, D., Hytten, F. E. & Thomson, A. M. (1958) Age and human reproduction. *J. Obstet. Gynaec. Brit. Emp.*, **65**, 865.
Dennis, K. J. & Bytheway, W. R. (1965) Changes in body weight after delivery. *J. Obstet. Gynaec. Brit. Cwlth.*, **72**, 94.
Hytten, F. E. (1971) Preparations for breast feeding, from *Physiology of Human Pregnancy*. Oxford: Blackwell.
Sharman, A. (1966) *Reproductive Physiology of the Post-Partum Period*. Edinburgh: E. & S. Livingstone.

21. Puerperal Infection

One of the most fascinating although tragic stories in the history of medicine is that of puerperal sepsis. Because of prejudice and ignorance the doctors who suggested that it was carried from one patient to another were subjected to ridicule and were unpopular amongst other doctors and midwives. There was considerable rivalry over the claims to the original observation that puerperal fever was contagious. The names usually associated with the original observation on the aetiology and prevention of puerperal sepsis are Semmelweis of Vienna and Oliver Wendall Holmes of Boston, but about half a century before Alexander Gordon of Aberdeen had published his Treatise on the Epidemic Puerperal Fever of Aberdeen in 1795. He pointed out the similarities between erysipeles and puerperal fever. The former occurring in an open surgical wound and the latter in the raw area in the uterus after separation of the placenta. The popular theory of the time was that the infection was caused by noxious substances in the atmosphere, but Gordon pointed out that the disease infected only women who were visited or delivered by a practitioner or taken care of by a nurse who had previously attended a patient with puerperal fever. His views were far from popular particularly amongst the local midwives who were so incensed that Gordon had eventually to leave the city. His fate, however, was mild compared to that of Semmelweis who was driven from Vienna in 1849 because of the jealousy of his superiors and he became so affected by this that he was driven insane and died in an insane asylum from a septic wound he sustained while doing a dissection. In Vienna the puerperal sepsis rate was very much higher in the hospital where medical students worked compared with the hospital where midwives trained. This Semmelweis reckoned to be due to the fact that the students came straight from the post-mortem rooms to deliver the women. He instituted a system of washing of the hands with chlorinated water before undertaking deliveries and in a short time the mortality from puerperal sepsis fell from 16 per cent to 1 per cent, which was much lower than in the midwives' hospital. It was not until the end of the 18th century, however, before general recognition was given to the infectious nature of puerperal fever. This was due to the work of Pasteur who showed that the infection was due to streptococci and later Lister demonstrated the value of antiseptic methods.

Puerperal sepsis was such a serious condition that it was made a notifiable disease and indeed it is still notifiable, although since the advent of chemotherapy it is now rarely a serious disease. In Scotland puerperal sepsis is notifiable if the temperature rises to 38°C (100·4°F) within 21 days (14 days in England and Wales). After an abortion or childbirth the temperature must be sustained at that level during a period of 24 hours or recur during that period.

Puerperal infection is defined as a post-partum infection of the genital tract which is usually localized to the endometrium but can often extend to other surrounding tissues. Although puerperal sepsis is rarely a serious disease nowadays there is no room for complacency as some cases still end fatally. This

Table 21.1 Maternal deaths from sepsis

	1952–54	1955–57	1958–60	1961–63	1964–66	1967–69
Abortion with sepsis	91	82	77	74	66	62
Puerperal sepsis	42	46	24	18	28	12
Sepsis after surgical treatment	26	30	23	19	29	14
Total	159	158	124	111	123	88

is seen from the table (21.1) which shows the numbers of cases dying from sepsis associated with pregnancy from 1952 to 1969. Although the number of deaths has fallen compared to pre-chemotherapy days there has not been a dramatic fall since 1952. Of the 12 deaths due to puerperal sepsis the majority followed spontaneous delivery, manual delivery of the placenta being performed in only 1 patient. The clinical diagnosis of sepsis was frequently not made before death and in many cases the bacterial cause was only looked for and determined at the post-mortem. In 12 of the cases dying of puerperal sepsis in 1967–69 the causative organisms were staphylococcus aureus (2), Esch. coli (4) and Cl. welchii (3). In the other three cases the organism was not stated. Fourteen deaths followed surgical treatment, of these 11 followed Caesarean section. The majority of the Caesarean sections were performed following prolonged labour.

BACTERIOLOGY

The common infecting organisms are:

a. *Escherichia coli*
Infections with E. coli have become increasingly common both post-partum and post-abortum.

b. *Staphylococci*
These are also becoming increasingly common as causes of puerperal infection. Because of their resistance to the action of sulphonamides and penicillin they have become relatively more dangerous pathogens than formerly.

c. *Streptococci*
Haemolytic streptococci were the commonest cause of puerperal sepsis but now they are a rare cause. The anaerobic form is one of the commonest causes of puerperal infection. The organisms are frequently found in the vagina of normal pregnant women and they quickly invade devitalized tissues. Streptococcus faecalis usually occurs with other organisms in puerperal sepsis.

d. *Miscellaneous organisms*
Pneumococci, clostridium welchii, anaerobic bacilli belonging to the bacteroides group, gonococci, salmonella typhosa and diptheroids can all occasionally cause puerperal sepsis. Quite often multiple organisms are found on the swabs from the vagina particularly in post-abortum infections.

Source of infection

Infection can come from the patient herself but is more likely to come from exogenous sources. When there has been trauma and the tissues are devitalized the organisms which are usually present in the vagina such as the anaerobic streptococci can cause the infection. The infection is more likely to come from an endogenous source either the doctor, nurse or other persons coming in contact with the patient. The infection may be from the respiratory tracts of those contacts or a direct contamination of hands, instruments or dressings.

SEPTIC FOCI OF THE SKIN OR THE THROAT
In some cases particularly infection with E. coli the organisms are carried up from the skin of the perineum which is heavily infected from the bowel. Occasionally the infection can come from the urinary tract.

PREDISPOSING FACTORS
The general resistance to infection may be reduced by poor diet, fatigue, debility or severe anaemia. The local resistance in the vagina may be reduced, particularly during labour if it is prolonged. The vagina is ordinarily protected by the lactic acid which is produced from the glycogen in the epithelial cells of the vagina by the Döderlein bacillus. The acidity of the vagina prevents the proliferation of pathogenic organisms. In pregnancy the pH of the vaginal secretion may fall well below 4. During labour, however, Döderlein's bacilli disappear and the acid is neutralized by the blood and liquor amnii, so that the natural protective mechanism is temporarily overcome.

During labour the dilatation of the cervix causes the loss of the plug of mucous (operculum) which prevents the passage of organisms through the cervix. The longer the labour the greater the likelihood of organisms multiplying in the vagina and passing up through the cervix. If there has been haemorrhage and trauma this also predisposes to infection. The chance of infection is greatly increased if there has been bruising of the tissues which might be caused either by instruments or by manipulation. Caesarean section particularly after the patient has been in labour for a long time can predispose to infection. If the placenta or even a small part of it is retained infection is liable to occur, either because of attempts at manual removal or because the placental tissue is retained and undergoes necrosis.

Pathology

The lesion of puerperal sepsis is basically that of wound infection with local inflammatory reaction in the pelvic organs and then extension through the lymph vessels or blood vessels. The widespread and early use of chemotherapy nowadays, however, in cases of puerperal sepsis usually prevents the development of the classical pathological features with endometritis and spread of the infection from the placental site through the blood vessels and lymphatics to involve the pelvic cellular tissue, the tube and ovaries and the peritoneum. The infection is usually treated nowadays before it can spread beyond the local site.

Infection is still likely to occur in the perineum, vulva, vaginal walls but again these local lesions are usually treated before the infection can spread up into the uterus and beyond. If the perineum, vulva or vagina became infected either because of lacerations or from an episiotomy the tissues become red and swollen and a discharge which occurs may be either sero-sanguineous or purulent. Lacerations of the cervix or of the vaginal vault may be associated with the formation of haematomata which predispose to infection.

When intra-uterine infection occurs there is a rise in temperature and in pulse rate. The lochia is usually heavy and offensive. There may be some tenderness of the lower abdomen and the uterus may be larger than would be expected.

When pyrexia occurs in the puerperium a high vaginal swab is taken so that the infecting organism can be identified and the sensitivity to antibiotics determined. Infection of the urinary tract is excluded by sending a mid-stream specimen of urine for bacteriological examination. If it is suspected that pieces of membrane or placenta might have been retained then an exploration of the uterus should be performed as soon as the infection is brought under control by chemotherapy.

Septicaemia is now very rare and is recognized by high fever, restlessness, sleeplessness and exhaustion. Peritonitis is rare except in cases of Caesarean section performed after a prolonged labour. Pelvic cellulitis can arise from infection spreading outwards from the uterus into the parametrium, but it is more likely to occur if there has been tearing of the cervix either in a spontaneous delivery or a forceps delivery. The pelvic veins may also be involved in the infection and phlebitis of the uterine veins can spread to the femoral veins and even to the inferior vena cava. Pelvic cellulitis can give rise to severe pain in one or both iliac fossae. In cases of septic pelvic thrombo-phlebitis infected thrombi may embolize to the heart, lungs or abdominal viscera. Acute salpingo-oophoritis occurs when the infection spreads from the uterus. As well as the signs and symptoms of endometritis there is marked lower abdominal pain and tenderness.

Endotoxic or bacterial shock can occur in some cases of puerperal or post-abortal sepsis. This condition of shock is produced when large numbers of Gram negative organisms (e.g. E. coli, proteus, vulgaris, Cl. welchii or enterococci) enter the circulation. Endotoxins are released from lysed bacteria which can be alive or dead. The clinical features are those of shock with hypotension and collapse but in addition there may be peripheral vasodilatation and flushing present. The mottled cyanosis and sub-normal temperature can occur in severe cases and death may result from hepatorenal failure. As adrenal insufficiency is likely to occur in these cases corticosteroid therapy is given as well as the other measures to combat shock.

Diagnosis

As soon as a rise in temperature is noted in the puerperium steps should be taken to establish the cause. It should be assumed that the infection is genital until proved otherwise, although it is equally important that the other common sites of infection in the puerperium are also carefully examined. The common extragenital infections in the puerperium are respiratory, renal, breast and venous. If possible the source of genital infection should be determined in case it is exogenous and therefore a risk to other patients. As well as taking high vaginal swabs for bacteriological investigation a mid-stream specimen of urine should be sent.

A general physical examination should be carried out with particular attention to the lungs, the kidneys, breasts and the lower limbs. The perineum is examined and the cervix inspected at the time of taking the vaginal swabs, and the uterus should be palpated abdominally to determine whether involution is proceeding normally. The erythrocyte sedimentation rate and leucocyte count are not very helpful in the puerperium because they are both raised during pregnancy. In some cases anaerobic and aerobic blood cultures may have to be carried out. Blood cultures should be collected while the temperature is rising or during a rigor and it is usually necessary to repeat blood cultures because it can be difficult to obtain a sample at a time when the organisms are circulating in the blood.

The prognosis for cases of puerperal sepsis has been completely revolutionized since the advent of chemotherapy. Even in cases which formerly had a poor prognosis such as those with septicaemia respond remarkably quickly to antibiotics, but in cases of generalized infection with the anaerobic steptococcus, staphylococcus pyogenes, or clostridium welchii the response may not be so good to the usual antibiotics, but there is now a sufficient number of wide spectrum antibiotics to ensure a good prognosis in the great majority of cases. It is important that supportive therapy such as adequate nutrition and rest and freedom from pain should be ensured and also that efficient drainage of any infected areas is carried out.

Prevention and treatment
Even though wide spectrum antibiotics will almost certainly cure infection it is nevertheless essential that every effort should be made to prevent the infection occurring. Infections around the vulva or in the vagina should be treated before the patient goes into labour. Probably not enough attention is paid to the treatment of vaginitis during pregnancy or preceding labour. It is essential that nursing and medical personnel attending on puerperal patients should not have any focus of infection particularly of the skin. Routine nasal and throat swabbing of staff is no longer carried out as pathogenic organisms are so commonly found. Masks should be worn by the attendants during labour but anyone with an upper respiratory infection should not enter the delivery rooms. Strict aseptic precautions as are observed in an operating theatre should be employed during labour and delivery. As lacerated tissues are so liable to

infection they should be avoided or repaired as soon after delivery as possible. Anaemia should be treated before labour commences, but if there is blood loss during labour this should be treated by blood transfusion as severe anaemia predisposes to puerperal infection. Drainage of the uterus can be encouraged by early ambulation and by putting the baby to the breast to stimulate contractions. If the lochia is heavy and the uterus remains large a retained portion of placenta should be suspected and an exploration of the uterus may be necessary. This should be done after antibiotic therapy has been commenced, and it should be done with as little disturbance of the uterus as possible. Most uterine infections respond to penicillin and this should be given at once while awaiting a report on the sensitivity to the infecting organism. Pain must be relieved and adequate fluids given.

The usual procedure is to start treatment with penicillin, streptomycin or tetracycline until the laboratory reports are available. Most infections will respond to this therapy but there are several other broad spectrum antibiotics which are available. If the infection seems serious and it is considered advisable to start treatment with something which is likely to be more effective than the usual antibiotics a mixture of ampicillin and cloxacillin can be tried before the sensitivity is available from the laboratory. Some of the other broad spectrum antibiotics available are:

Cephaloridine. This resembles ampicillin in its effect on Gram negative bacilli. It is well tolerated and is suitable for patients who are sensitive to penicillin, but it must be given intramuscularly or intravenously.

Lincomycin. This antibiotic is active against Gram positive bacteria and has a range resembling erythromycin. It is usually given orally, has a low toxicity and is active against most strains of staphylococcus aureus.

Nalidixic acid. This synthetic antibacterial is active against many coliform and proteus organisms. It is also given orally and is most extensively used in urinary tract infections.

Fusidic acid. This is another antibiotic which is effective against penicillin resistant staphylococci. It has a low toxicity and is well absorbed from the alimentary tract.

Kanamycin. This is also used for resistant forms of staphylococci.

Gentamicin. This is effective against Gram positive or Gram negative organisms which are resistant to other antibiotics. It is given intramuscularly.

EXTRAGENITAL CAUSES OF PUERPERAL PYREXIA

MASTITIS

Inflammation of the breasts is most likely to occur in women who are breast feeding and particularly in primigravidae. The usual infecting organism is the coagulase positive staphylococcus aureus, but the infection can also be caused by streptococcus pyogenes or E. coli. The organisms enter through fissures in the nipples and travel along the lymphatics or in the blood stream. Usually only one breast is affected. Engorgement of the breasts due possibly to blocking of the ducts with colostrum or to venous and lymphatic distention predisposes to the infection. Inflammation tends to occur in the areola around the nipple, but it often becomes diffuse throughout the breast. If the infection is not treated promptly an abscess may form. The infection tends to occur some weeks after delivery. The breast becomes engorged and painful and one area or quadrant of the breast becomes hard, reddened and very tender. Antibiotic therapy should be started at the first indication of infection in the breasts. If treatment is not instituted early there is extensive destruction of breast tissue. The inflamed area becomes softened and fluctuation and oedema of the skin indicates that there is underlying pus formation. In such cases the temperature may be very high and accompanied by rigors. The patient becomes very ill and the infected breast is very painful.

Treatment

Fissuring of the nipples is prevented by careful routine care of the breasts which is particularly concerned with keeping them clean. If fissuring occurs then this would be promptly treated with tincture of benzoin or a commercial preparation. A nipple shield may be required if the nipples become too tender to allow the infant to nurse directly. When the breasts become engorged or inflamed they should be well supported by a firm binder. Feeding should be discontinued from the infected breast and antibiotic therapy started. Analgesics must be given to relieve pain and if an abscess forms surgical drainage should be carried out. The incisions should be made radially and should be wide enough to give adequate drainage.

URINARY TRACT INFECTION

The subject of pyelonephritis and cystitis of pregnancy is considered elsewhere (page 221). Infection of the urinary tract is a common cause of pyrexia in the puerperium. The infection may have arisen during pregnancy and persisted or occurred intermittently during pregnancy. In such cases where there have been recurrent attacks a thorough investigation of the urinary tract should be carried out a few weeks after delivery. Infection of the urine may occur for the first time in the puerperium, particularly if catheterization has had to be carried out. The infecting organism is usually coliform, but other organisms particularly staphylococci may be found. Dysuria may be present but in some cases there are no symptoms and it is therefore important that a mid-stream specimen of urine should be sent for examination in any case of pyrexia in the puerperium. Renal angle pain may or may not be present if infection has spread to the kidneys. Rigors may occur and pain occurs over the renal angle usually on the right side. Chemotherapy and a high intake of fluids will usually clear up the infection quickly.

Other extragenital causes of infection

It is important to remember that a pyrexia arising in the puerperium may be due to an infection quite unconnected with the pregnancy or childbirth. Respiratory infections due to influenza or pneumonia can develop at this time. Bowel infections are also quite liable to occur. Appendicitis occurs not infrequently in the puerperium. It may arise without any previous history or it can be an exacerbation of a chronically inflamed appendix. The condition is very liable to be confused with a puerperal uterine or tubal infection, but if there is any doubt laparotomy is usually advisable.

Isolation of patients with puerperal pyrexia is not considered necessary nowadays because chemotherapy is so effective. If however pyrexia persists despite treatment and particularly if there is any discharge of pus patients should be isolated and 'barrier' nursed.

THROMBO-EMBOLIC DISEASE

Although not all cases of venous thrombosis

are due to infection and it is the usual practice to divide the cases into non-septic venous thrombosis or phlebo-thrombosis as opposed to thrombo-phlebitis, nevertheless there is bound to be some inflammation of the veins in both types. Most of the cases of venous thrombosis seen now are not due to pelvic sepsis but are more likely to be due to spontaneous intravascular clotting. In these cases of phlebo-thrombosis there is probably minimal inflammation of the veins. The mechanisms involved in intravascular thrombosis are not completely understood and clinical signs and symptoms of deep vein thrombosis are very variable, so that prevention and treatment are not easy.

Although deaths from pulmonary embolism are not very frequent they nevertheless constitute one of the main causes of maternal death. In the Report on Confidential Enquiries into Maternal Deaths in England and Wales in 1967–69 (Ministry of Health, 1972) there were 75 deaths from pulmonary embolism, twenty-two of which occurred antenatally and 53 occurred post-natally. The comparable figures for the three year periods from 1952 onwards are shown for comparison in the table (21.2). Deaths from pulmonary embolism

(phlebo-thrombosis) affecting usually the ileo-femoral vessels. It is not always possible to differentiate the inflammatory from the aseptic types.

SUPERFICIAL THROMBO-PHLEBITIS

The saphenous vein is the most commonly affected and the condition is predisposed to by varicose veins. The affected vein is tender and hard, and there is a red line along the skin overlying the veins. There is little or no systemic disturbance and usually there is no fever. There is little danger of any of the thrombus becoming separated and the risk of embolism is therefore slight. The thrombosis may occasionally spread from the superficial veins to the deep femoral vein giving rise to deep thrombo-phlebitis. The treatment for superficial thrombo-phlebitis is rest, supporting bandages with pressure exerted over the line of the vein and elevation of the foot of the bed. Local heat may be helpful in relieving the pain. As soon as the pain is relieved the patient is encouraged to move the limb and become ambulant. Anticoagulants may occasionally be indicated and sometimes antibiotics are used, but it is worth noting that aureomycin and terramycin accelerate clotting while pen-

Table 21.2 Maternal deaths from pulmonary embolism and rates per million maternities for each of the Triennial Reports 1952–69

Report period (in years)	Deaths from pulmonary embolism	Total Maternities	Rates per million maternities
1952–54	138	2 052 953	67·2
1955–57	157	2 113 471	74·3
1958–60	132	2 294 414	57·5
1961–63	129	2 520 420	51·2
1964–66	91	2 600 367	35·0
1967–69	75	2 457 444	30·5

are second only to abortion as the cause of death associated with pregnancy. Most of the cases are not associated with infection but are due to a coagulation defect. There is a steady increase in the incidence with increasing age. Obesity also seems to be a predisposing factor and anything which causes a decrease in the rate of venous flow for example, bed rest can predispose to the condition.

Venous thrombosis may be superficial or deep. If superficial it may be an inflammatory process and is sometimes called thrombo-phlebitis, but it probably results just as often from a coagulation defect. The deep variety is most often nowadays of an aseptic nature

icillin prolongs it slightly so that it is the latter drug which should be used.

DEEP THROMBO-PHLEBITIS

This is always an inflammatory lesion and is associated with pelvic sepsis. The sepsis spreads from the tissues to involve the pelvic veins and then can spread to the veins in the legs. The condition is best prevented by avoiding pelvic sepsis or treating it early. Besides antibiotic therapy anticoagulants are given in the active treatment. Anticoagulant therapy is usually started with heparin and continued with one of the dicoumarin drugs. Heparin is administered as a continuous infusion intravenously and control is maintained by estimating the clotting time of the blood aiming at a time of 15 to 20 minutes. It is particularly useful in cases of pulmonary embolism where a quick action is required. Pain is relieved by analgesic drugs. Anti-coagulant therapy is continued with one of the dicoumarin drugs (e.g. Tromexan, Dindevan or Warfarin) orally. The effect reaches its maximum about 18 to 24 hours after admin-istration of the drug and control is effected by estimating the prothrombin time. The dos-age should be adjusted so that the concentra-tion of prothrombin is kept at about 40 per cent of normal. These drugs have less danger-ous side effects than heparin and are much cheaper with apparently comparable clinical benefits. The antidotes to these drugs are vitamin K_1 and whole blood transfusion. It these drugs are used for antenatal phlebo-thrombosis they should be discontinued and replaced by heparin in the few weeks before delivery as they cause considerable damage to the utero-placental site, with in some cases death of the fetus. Heparin is quickly neutral-ized by the intravenous injection of pro-tamine sulphate. If the limb is cold, cyanosed, swollen and painful parasympathetic nerve block has been advocated to relieve the spasm of the artery and vein at the site of the thrombus. In some cases there has been dram-atic improvement after this form of treatment.

PHLEBO-THROMBOSIS

This is an aseptic condition and is due to a coagulation defect which affects the deep veins of the lower extremeties and sometimes the pelvic veins. The posterior tibial, femoral and external iliac veins are the ones usually affec-ted, and the thrombus can extend down into the veins of the calf muscles and of the foot. The immediate danger of phlebo-thrombosis is fragmentation of the clot with pulmonary embolism. The emboli if large may be instantly fatal due to occlusion of the pulmonary trunk at its bifurcation. If they are smaller they can cause infarction of the lung substance to a greater or lesser degree. Repeated emboliza-tion has a serious prognosis and in such cases surgical intervention is usually indicated. The remote effect of venous occlusion depends on the sufficiency or otherwise of the collateral circulation. Occlusion of the opening of the profundifemoris into the main femoral channel causes oedema of the legs if the collateral veins are not adequate. The veins of the glutei and the skin of the lower abdom-inal wall become distended. Poor venous circulation leads to disturbance of the oxygena-tion and nutrition of the tissues of the leg so that the leg becomes chronically thickened, easily tired and if it is severe the skin may eventually become ulcerated. Deep venous thrombosis after spontaneous delivery is un-common and death from pulmonary embolism is rare. Phlebo-thrombosis is more common after operative delivery, particularly Caesarean section and in older women, and prophylaxis with anticoagulants such as macrodex or heparin is advocated in such cases by some obstetricians. Antenatal phlebo-thrombosis can occur but it is less common than the puer-peral variety. Phlebo-thrombosis usually ap-pears at the end of the first week after delivery. The calf of the affected leg becomes painful or tight when the patient walks and there may be a slight pyrexia. Tenderness can be elicited on deep palpation in the posterior mid-line of the calf and pain can be produced in the calf by dorsiflexing the leg (Homan's sign). Oedema occurs in the lower leg and the circumference of the affected leg will be found to be greater than the other leg. The circumference of the legs should be measured daily so that the progress of the condition can be assessed. In a few cases the phlebo-thrombosis may be clinically silent and only detected after a pulmonary embolism has occurred. Prophy-laxis is most important in the prevention of phlebo-thrombosis and pulmonary embolism. Oestrogens, particularly in large doses, for the suppression of lactation should be avoided in older women, particularly if they have had operative deliveries and if they are obese. Early ambulation and leg exercises while in bed should be advocated. Dehydration should be avoided and pillows should not be placed under the patient's knees. The active treat-ment with anticoagulant therapy is the same as that described for deep thrombo-phlebitis, but in some cases surgical treatment will also be indicated. When the thrombus is spreading or where there has been a second embolism the femoral vein or the ileo-femoral vein is explored and the thrombus evacuated by suction. The vein can either be repaired or ligated.

REFERENCES

The Department of Health and Social Security, London (1972). *Report on Confidential Enquiries into Maternal Deaths in England and Wales 1967-69*. London: HMSO.

FURTHER READING

Cruickshank, R. (1963) In *Mod. Trends Obstet.*, 3rd edition. Kellar, R. J. London: Butterworth.
Porter, I. A. (1958) *Alexander Gordon, M.D. of Aberdeen 1752-99*. Edinburgh and London: Oliver & Boyd.
Thoms, H. J. (1935) *Classical Contributions to Obstetrics and Gynaecology*. Springfield, Illinois: Thomas.

22. Multiple or Plural Pregnancy

In some primitive societies twin births were regarded as proof of infidelity and the mothers were ostracized and regarded as impure. In other societies it was the twins who were considered impure and it was not uncommon for one or both to be left to die. The Scottish missionary, Mary Slessor, gained renown because of her work in saving such twins in Calabar in West Africa. There are many references in history and mythology to twinning. Rome is said to have been founded by Remus and Romulus, the twins who were suckled by a shewolf. Shakespeare, himself the father of twins, develops the theme of twins in *Twelfth Night* and *Comedy of Errors*.

In the smaller mammals large litters are common, but in large mammalia, including man, multiple births are relatively uncommon. It is very rare for a woman to have more than four babies (quadruplets) although the highest number reported has been seven (septuplets). Administration of gonadotrophins and other ovulation stimulators can cause multiple births and nine babies were produced in this way in Australia in 1971. In species with long gestation periods there is less likelihood of multiple births and animals with a long life span usually have only single births. The number of breasts is also related to the number of offspring and species with two breasts usually produce only one offspring at a time. The incidence of multiple births varies in different parts of the world, being more common in Africa than Europe and less common in Japan. From American life insurance figures the incidence per million births is 10 539 twins (1 in 95 births), 93 triplets (1 in 10 750 births) and 1·1 quadruplets (1 in 909 090 births) (Metropolitan Life Insurance Co., *Statistical Bulletin*, 1960). These figures give quite good support to Hellin's Law (1895) which states that twins occur once in every 89 births, triplets in 89^2, and quadruplets in 89^3. The most remarkable number of offspring was that credited to the Countess of Hagenau who was supposed to have produced 365 children at the one birth, but this was almost certainly the number of vesicles in a hydatidiform mole. Several authenticated reports of sextuplets have been recorded and there are many quintuplets on record. The first to survive to adult life were the Dionne quintuplets who were born in 1934 in Canada. Others have been born and since survived in Buenos Aires, South America in 1943, South Dakota in 1964, South Africa in 1966, and Scotland in 1972.

The chances of survival of the babies are less and the risks to the mother greater in multiple pregnancies than in single pregnancies. For these reasons multiple pregnancy in man is usually considered to be pathological.

TYPES OF MULTIPLE PREGNANCIES

One fertilized ovum may split to form, eventually, two or more babies which will be 'identical'. This is known as a monozygotic or uniovular multiple pregnancy. When two or more ova are fertilized at the same time the babies will be non-identical. This is known as a dizygotic (trizygotic, etc.) or binovular (triovular, etc.) multiple pregnancy. When several babies are formed as in quintuplets or sextuplets these usually result from a mixture of multiple zygotes, some of which develop singly and others splitting to form two or more fetuses. For example, sextuplets could arise from 4 fertilized ova, 3 of which continued to grow singly and one which split to form 3 identical fetuses. For simplicity only the features of the two types of *twin* pregnancies will be discussed.

Monozygous twins

Corner, the famous American embryologist, has shown that monozygotic twins can be produced either by a *separation* of early blastomeres, by duplication of the inner cell mass, or by duplication of the embryonic rudiment of the germ disc.

Coming as they do from one ovum, monozygous twins are bound to show certain physical and mental similarities but the degree of similarity depends on the stage of development at which division takes place. The later the division occurs in development, the more identical will the twins be. Monozygous twins are of the same sex and have the same blood groups and blood enzymes, but the finger and palm prints, although often of the same pattern, are not identical. The colour of the hair

shown all over the world in a circus. The union in conjoined twins may be at virtually any site and the amount of union may vary from slight skin fusion to the creation of a double monster in which limbs, trunks and organs are shared (Fig. 22.1).

Examination of the placenta and membranes is helpful in determining whether the twins are monozygotic or not. This will show that usually the vessels from the two cords anastomose so that the whole 'placenta' can be injected from either cord. There is usually only one chorionic membrane and usually two amniotic membranes (Fig. 22.2). If fusion occurs very

Thoracopagus Dicephalus Syncephalus

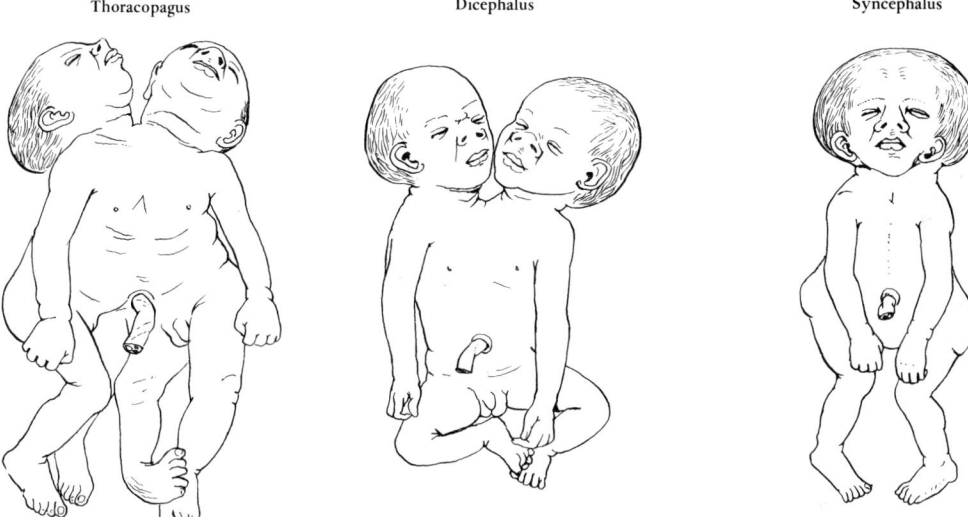

Fig. 22.1 Various forms of conjoined twins.

and eyes can also be different. The diagnosis of zygosity can be made by determining the blood groups, ABO, Rhesus, Duffy, Kell, MN, and Ss, and by a study of the red cell enzymes by electrophoresis. The enzymes which can be distinguished are 6 phosphogluconate dehydrogenase, adenylate kinase, acid phosphatase and phosphoglucomutase. It is also possible to distinguish the placentas by identifying the six different phenotypes according to the electrophoretic behaviour of their alkaline phosphatases. When a skin graft or indeed an organ transplant is grafted from one monozygotic twin to his co-twin then the graft behaves like an auto-graft.

Occasionally complete division does not take place and this results in conjoined twins. These are usually called Siamese twins after the conjoined twins Cheng and Eng who were

early two independent placentas with different membranes may form from the single zygote so that placental examination alone is not a completely reliable method of establishing the zygosity of twins. An exception to this is the rare monoamniotic twin pregnancy in which the two fetuses develop in a single amniotic sac and must be monozygotic. The intercommunication between the two circulations of monozygotic twins may allow an unequal pressure of blood to the fetuses so that occasionally the heart or the head of one fails to develop properly resulting in a fetus acardiacus or a fetus acephalus.

In Europe the frequency of monozygous twinning is remarkably constant at about 3 to 4 per 1000 births. The rate is about the same in Japan, but it is higher in Gambia (6·7 per 1000), Nigeria (5·0 per 1000) and S.

India (8·3 per 1000). The incidence is not affected by parity or age of the mother. Although the overall incidence of twinning is influenced by heredity there is no good evidence to show that either maternal or paternal influences play a part in producing monozygotic twins.

Dizygous twins

Twins arising from two ova are no more alike than siblings from separate pregnancies and may or may not be of the same sex. Dizygotic twins are much more common than monozygotic twins. The formula (Weinberg) for the distribution of dizygotic and monozygotic twins in a total population is:

Number of dizygotic twins = 2 × number of different sex

or Number of monozygotic twins = Total number − 2 × number of different sex.

Each ovary may produce an ovum or two ova may come from one ovary. Two distinct placentas usually form with two chorions and two amnions (Fig. 22.2) or the placenta may be fused to form one placenta with four layers of membranes between the two fetuses.

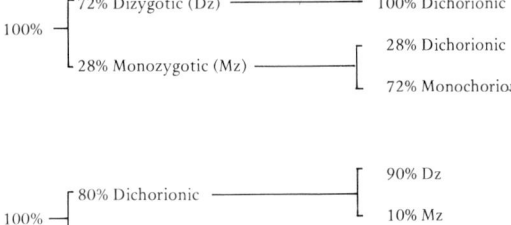

Fig. 22.3 Distribution of zygosity and placentation in the Birmingham Twin Study.

The Birmingham study (Cameron, 1968) of 668 pairs of twins showed that 80 per cent were dichorionic and 90 per cent of these were dizygotic, but 20 per cent were monochorionic and all of these were monozygotic. Twenty-eight per cent of the total twin pairs were monozygotic and 28 per cent of these were dichorionic (Fig. 22.3).

In a study of 326 twin births made by Corney, Robson and Strong (1968) the zygos-

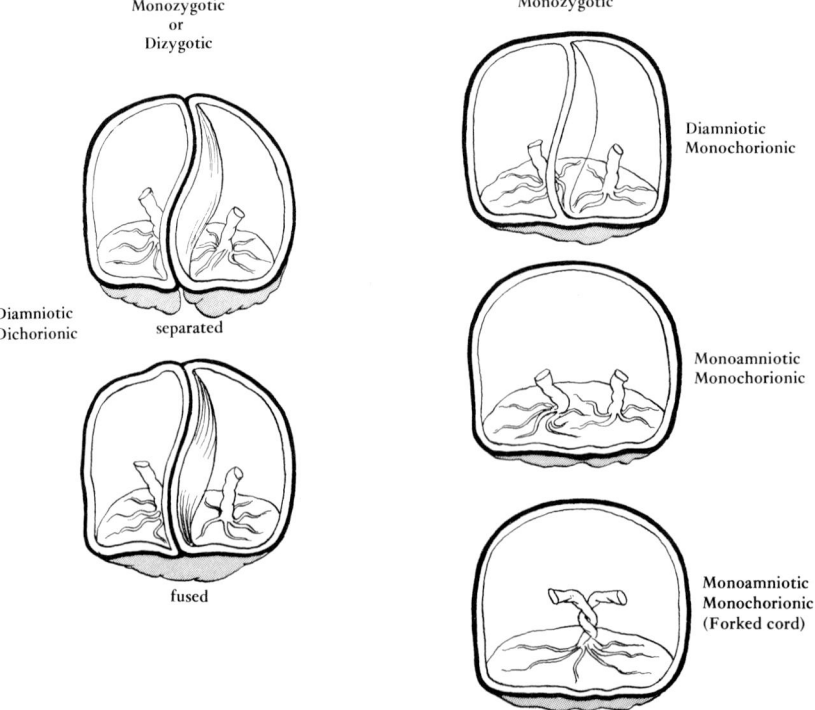

Fig. 22.2   Diagrammatic representation of zygosity and placentation.

ity determinations were based on sex, red cell antigens, ABO, MNSs, Rh, LUa, K and FYa, the red cell enzymes ACP, 6PG, PGM1 and AK and placental alkaline phosphatase. The results indicated that whereas dizygotic twins are always dichorionic between 15 per cent and 20 per cent of monozygotic twins may also be dichorionic. Of course, unlike sex twins must be dizygous and they are no more alike than brothers and sisters. If the two placentas are fused together the circulations do not mix to any great extent, however, so that a fetus acardiacus cannot occur. A condition, on the other hand, which does occur in dizygous twinning as well as monozygous is fetus compressus or papyraceus. In this, one fetus dies early in pregnancy and if it is not expelled it becomes compressed between the uterine wall and the membranes of the surviving fetus.

Blood chimerism in dizygous twins can occur when there is circulation of blood cells from one twin to the other through a small area of vascular anastomosis in a fused placenta, thus there is a mixture of blood groups in the twins with one group predominating in one twin and the other group in the second twin. Similarly chromatin bodies can be found in the nuclei of some leukocytes of males with female co-twins. There are, however, no reports of freemartins in humans. Freemartins are the female co-twins of bull calves, and in them the uterus and ovaries are usually absent.

There is a remarkable ethnic difference in the incidence of dizygotic twins. In European countries the incidence per 1000 births varies from 5·9 in Spain to 10·9 in Greece, while in Nigerians the rate is 39·9 (Bulmer, 1960) and in Japan 1·3 (Morton, 1955). Increasing parity causes an increase in dizygous twins (Fig. 22.4).

Matthews Duncan, the famous Scottish obstetrician, noted in 1866 that there was an increasing incidence in the age of twinning until forty years when the incidence fell off because of the diminished fecundity. The dramatic rise in the incidence with increasing age of the mother, until between 35 and 39 years, with a subsequent fall occurs in dizygous twins (Fig. 22.5). Multiple pregnancies are also thought to be more common in highly fertile women.

Anderson (1956) found that the incidence of twinning in Aberdeen primigravidae was almost twice as high in those who were tall (64 inches or more) as in those who were small (less than 61 inches). Tall, older primigravidae

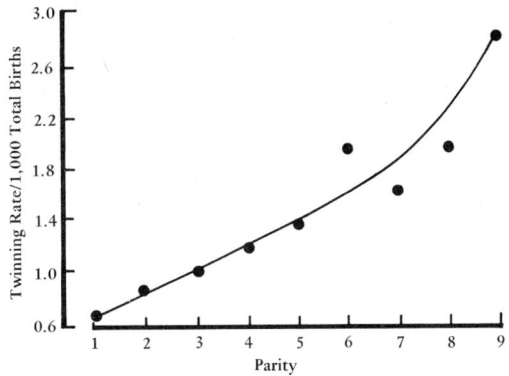

Fig. 22.4 Graph showing the increasing twinning rate with increasing parity.

come typically from the upper social classes. Millis (1958) found that in poor Chinese women in Singapore the twinning rate was low. Bulmer (1959) reports that the twinning rate fell in France, Holland and Norway during the Second World War, but not in Denmark and Sweden. There were severe food restrictions in the former countries but not in the latter. Data furnished by the Central Bureau for Statistics in the Hague shows that the decline in the incidence of twinning was in dizygotic twins and was most marked in the year 1945 which could be related to the occurrence of the six-months' period of hunger associated with the withdrawal of the German military forces from Holland. The incidence of twinning in Scotland (Fig. 22.6) has been

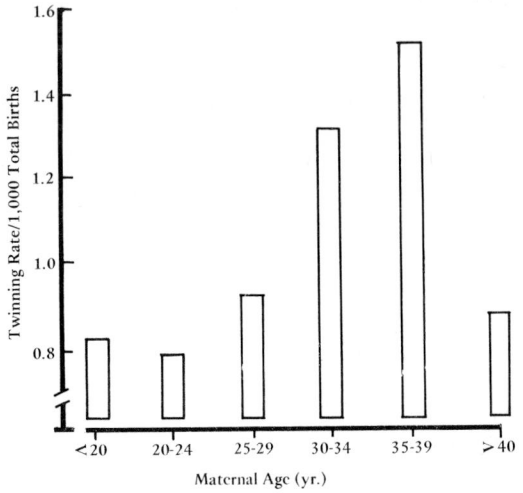

Fig. 22.5 Graph showing the increasing twinning rate with age up to age 35–39 and the decline thereafter.

falling since 1957. This is due to women having their babies when they are younger and to the fall in the number of high parity women.

A familial predisposition to dizygous twinning was found by Greulich (1934) and Bulmer (1960) found that 4 per cent of mothers of twins were themselves twins, but only 1·7 per cent of fathers. Probably the most informative study on inheritance in human dizygotic twinning was that of Whyte and Wyshak (1964). They used the data from more than four million genealogic records on file at the Genealogical Society of the Church of Jesus Christ of Latter Day Saints at Salt Lake City, Utah. A single record contains information about the children borne by a specified woman to a specified husband. They found that when women who are dizygous twins become parents they produce twins at the rate of 17·1 sets per 1000 maternities. On the other hand the wives of men who are dizygous twins have a twinning rate of only 7·9 per 1000 maternities. The female sibs of dizygous twins behave like female twins and the male sibs like male twins so far as the frequency of twins among the offspring is concerned. This is consistent with the hypothesis that the genotype of the mother affects the frequency of dizygous twinning, but that of the father does not.

Aetiology
Apart from such predisposing factors as age, parity, ethnic group and heredity, little is known about the causation of multiple pregnancy except that there is a low incidence in some countries with a low standard of living, in conditions of severe food restrictions and in short lower social class women compared to upper social class women. These factors suggest that standards of physical development and nutrition may affect the likelihood of twinning. A small South American animal, the armadillo, produces several monozygotic fetuses and this is thought to be due to delayed implantation causing slowing of growth. Development of the armadillo begins in the Fallopian tubes and continues until the egg passes down into the uterus as an early blastocyst. Development then stops in the armadillo for a period of several weeks with the blastocyst lying free in the uterus. Stockard (1921) considers that the arrest of the progress of the armadillo at this stage is probably on account of an exhaustion of the original oxygen supply derived from the ovarian blood and is not due to any temperature change. The uterus fails to react immediately to the presence of the blastocyst, implantation is delayed and no means of obtaining the oxygen necessary for continuing development is possible until the egg becomes implanted. After the delayed implantation has taken place development is slowly resumed in a way which gives rise to multiple embryo formations or budding. The quiescent period in the armadillo egg is probably the result of lack of oxygen.

Artificial stimulation of the ovaries has, however, recently become recognized as a cause. In the treatment of the infertile woman with amenorrhoea human pituitary follicle stimulating hormones, followed by chorionic gonadotrophin, is used to induce ovulation. If the dosage is not carefully controlled several ova may be liberated and fertilized. Twins, triplets and even nontuplets have been reported following the use of this therapy. The synthetic non-steroid agent, clomiphene citrate, is also used to induce ovulation in anovulatory patients and the incidence of multiple pregnancies is increased tenfold when conception occurs during a cycle in which clomiphene therapy is given. Such multiple pregnancies are due to the fertilization of two or more ova. Liberation of more than one ovum at the time of ovulation is predisposed to by heredity.

Two ova from two different cycles could, in theory, be fertilized giving rise to twins of different ages. This is superfetation. Two ova shed during the same cycle may be fertilized by spermatozoa from two males giving rise to superfecundation. It is known that superfecundation definitely occurs in animals, for example, a mare mated with a horse and then a few minutes later with a jackass produced twins one of which was a horse and the other a mule. Superfecundation probably also occurs in humans. Superfetation is also known to occur in the mare, but has never been demonstrated in women. It would be necessary for ovulation to occur during the course of pregnancy and as yet this is unproved in humans. Cases which have been claimed to be human superfetation have been shown to be due to the early death of one fetus and the continuing growth of the twin.

Diagnosis
The diagnosis is sometimes not made until after the first baby has been delivered and the

large size of the uterus makes it obvious that there is another baby. However, multiple pregnancy can be suspected from about 10 weeks of gestation if the *uterus is recognized to be larger* than is expected for the duration of amenorrhoea. A multiple pregnancy should be suspected if there is excess weight gain. It is important to make the diagnosis as early as possible during pregnancy so that preventive measures can be taken which may reduce the chances of complications in pregnancy and labour.

On abdominal palpation in late pregnancy there is frequently an impression of *multiple small parts* but this is an unreliable guide as a baby lying occipito-posterior can also give this impression. Three large parts may be felt, such as two heads and one breech or two breeches and one head. This is more likely when the babies are lying side by side *in utero* but is not usually possible when one baby lies behind the other (Fig. 22.7). When a head is felt which seems small in relation to the amount

to listen over the two areas. In practice a difference of more than ten beats in a minute is generally accepted as diagnostic of twins. It is very rare to obtain such a clear finding. A Doptone (Sonicaid) can give a better indication because it detects the flow of blood in the babies' hearts rather than the sound.

A false suspicion of multiple pregnancy is most commonly caused by the woman mistaking the date of her last menstrual period so that the uterus seems unduly large. Less commonly, fibroids, ovarian cysts or a hydatidiform mole may cause confusion over diagnosis. Hydramnios is also a factor which causes difficulty in differential diagnosis.

Clinical course
Almost invariably the course of a twin pregnancy is not smooth. Even though the complications may not be serious they can, nevertheless, be very trying for the patient. Many of the discomforts are mechanical from

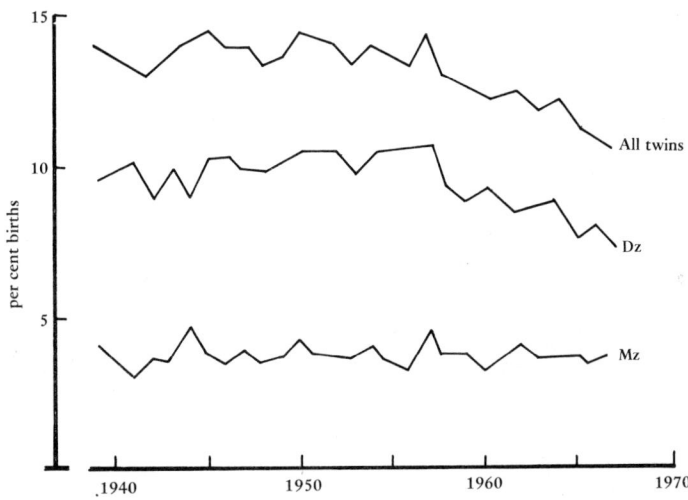

Fig. 22.6   Figure showing the declining rate of twinning in Scotland from 1957. The decline is in the dizygotic twins and the monozygotic rate is unchanged.

of baby present multiple pregnancy should be suspected. Palpation is made difficult by the presence of hydramnios which frequently complicates twin pregnancy. Vaginal examination can be of help in the diagnosis if one head is engaged in the pelvis and another head can be felt clearly in the abdomen.

Auscultation of two fetal hearts over two widely separate areas is suggestive but not diagnostic. For a definite diagnosis based on auscultation it is necessary for two observers

the over-distension of the uterus and the pressure of it on the pelvic vessels and organs. Lower abdominal pain and backache are very common as are frequency, constipation and varicose veins. Oedema of the abdominal wall, vulva and lower limbs is also probably due to pressure although lowered plasma protein concentrations may play a part. Near term the woman may have great difficulty in walking, partly because of locomotor difficulties and partly because of breathlessness.

The maternal physiological response is

greater than in a singleton pregnancy. This is evidenced by the greater increases in serum volume, in total body water, in oestriol excretion, and in cardiac output in twin pregnancies compared to singletons (Rovinsky and Jaffin, 1966; MacGillivray, Campbell and Duffus, 1971).

The greater demands for iron often cause anaemia and the haemoglobin concentration is further lowered by the greater increase in serum volume than in single pregnancies. Megaloblastic anaemia is more common in twin pregnancies. The incidence of detachment of the normally situated placenta is not increased but there is more chance of a placenta praevia.

The incidence of pre-eclampsia is much greater than in single pregnancies but is not significantly greater in monozygotic than dizygotic twins. Hydramnios is common and the acute form almost always occurs in the monozygotic rather than the dizygotic type.

Multiple pregnancies usually end prematurely whether they are complicated or not and this is one of the main causes of the high perinatal mortality rate in twins.

MANAGEMENT DURING PREGNANCY

Once the diagnosis is made efforts must be made to ensure that the woman has adequate rest and diet. The onset of premature labour may be avoided or delayed by rest. This is most readily achieved in hospital, but the patient may be unwilling to stay in hospital or there may be too few hospital beds available to make this possible. The woman should rest almost completely from about the 32nd week onwards, if possible. The value of hospital admission and bed rest in the prevention of premature onset of labour in twin pregnancies is very difficult to assess and no really satisfactory prospective study has been carried out. Most workers have recommended that patients found to have a multiple pregnancy should be admitted to hospital before the 34th week for rest, but the great majority of perinatal deaths in published series occur before the end of the 32nd week. If premature labour and perinatal deaths are to be avoided by rest then the woman must be admitted to hospital probably at the 28th–30th week. A major difficulty in determining whether rest prevents premature labour is to have a proper control group and in most series the control group has been composed of either undiagnosed cases or of women who refuse to come in for rest. If beds are available and the woman is willing to come in it is probably useful to take the patient in for observation and to ensure that she has an adequate diet. Otherwise it is probably desirable to advise the woman to take as much rest as possible at home. She should report to the hospital as soon as she thinks labour is starting.

Weekly vaginal examinations from the 30th week onwards might reveal that taking up and/

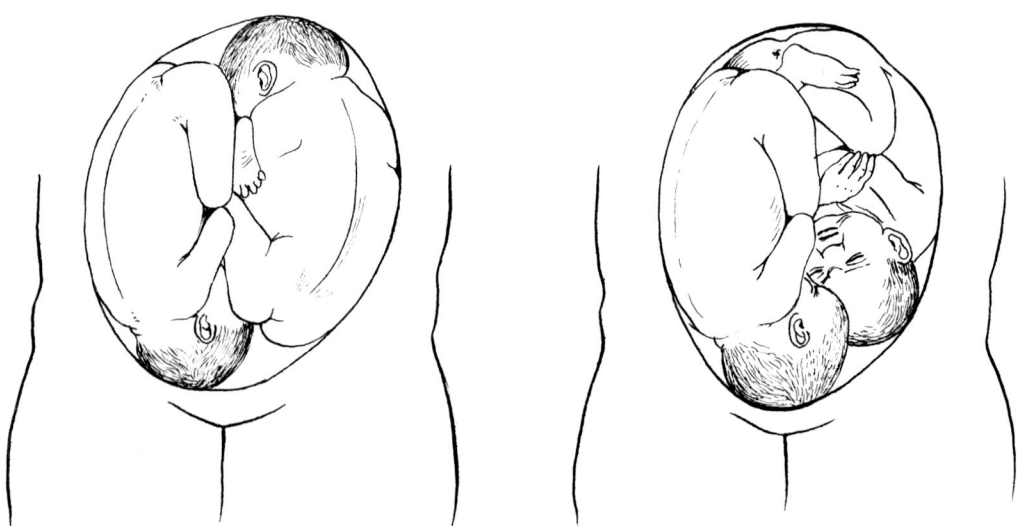

Fig. 22.7   Multiple small fetal parts are more readily felt when the twins lie alongside each other but may not be felt if one twin lies behind the other.

or dilation of the cervix is occurring and in some cases a Shirodkar or MacDonald suture can prevent premature delivery. If there is uterine activity and the membranes are intact an isoxsuprine or alcohol infusion might be valuable.

An added advantage of having the woman in hospital is that frequent observations of the blood pressure and urine can be made more easily. The onset of pre-eclampsia will be detected earlier and it is possible that the onset might be delayed by rest.

A good balanced diet with adequate proteins, minerals and vitamins should be ensured.

Some believe that labour should be induced before term on the theoretical grounds that placental insufficiency may occur earlier than in a single pregnancy. There is, as yet, no clear evidence that this occurs in all twin pregnancies but in any case no twin pregnancy should be allowed to go beyond term.

MANAGEMENT OF LABOUR

The presentations are usually as follows:

Vertex/vertex	40 per cent
Vertex/breech	26 per cent
Breech/vertex	10 per cent
Breech/breech	10 per cent
Longitudinal/transverse	8 per cent
Both transverse	6 per cent

Because of the small size of the babies compound, brow and face presentations and prolapse of the umbilical cord sometimes occur. Malpresentations of the first baby may necessitate delivery by Caesarean section but if it is considered that the presentation is suitable for vaginal delivery and there is no other indication for Caesarean section labour is allowed to proceed as usual.

It is desirable that at least one paediatrician and an anaesthetist should be available at the delivery. A pudendal nerve block should be induced when the second stage is reached, particularly if labour is premature and the babies are likely to be small. An episiotomy is performed as for the birth of any small baby. Forceps can be applied if required or if the baby is presenting as a breech the delivery can be assisted. When the first baby is born the cord is tied as usual, making quite certain that the placental end is tied as the second twin can bleed through the placenta of the first when the placentas are fused.

The lie of the second baby is then determined and if it is transverse it is corrected by external version to a cephalic presentation. It is not necessary to correct a breech presentation as the dilated birth canal allows an easy delivery. The fetal heart rate of the second baby is then checked and if there is fetal distress the second baby must be delivered at once. If the fetal heart is satisfactory the labour is allowed to progress. Should the uterus not begin to contract again soon after the birth of the first baby the membranes of the second sac are ruptured artificially. It has been clearly shown that after some 15 minutes the risk to the second child rises and there is no virtue in awaiting the onset of labour. If uterine contractions are not stimulated there is a risk that the cervix will close and the second twin will be retained *in utero*. This is very unlikely to happen nowadays but an interval of 56 days has been reported between the birth of the first and second babies. Very occasionally the uterus may fail to contract when the membranes are ruptured and a Syntocinon infusion should be used to initiate contractions.

If it has been necessary to deliver the first twin under general anaesthetic it is, of course, correct to proceed immediately to extract the second baby rather than allow the woman to come round from the anaesthetic. When the head is presenting it can either be pushed into the pelvis and delivered with forceps or, if the head does not come down easily it can be drawn down with the ventouse or internal podalic version can be performed, followed by breech extraction. Undue haste must be avoided as the babies are usually small and easily traumatized.

Where the first baby presents as a breech, difficulty may be experienced in delivering the after-coming head because suprapubic pressure cannot usually be effectively applied. This is seldom serious as the baby is usually small. Forceps should be used to deliver the head when it is brought into the pelvic cavity if there is still difficulty. Very rarely difficulty in delivering the head of the first baby may be due to interlocking with the head of the second baby. In such a case the head of the second baby is pushed upwards out of the pelvis and the first baby delivered. If this is not possible the first baby is extracted as far as possible and held out of the way while forceps are applied to the second head and traction exerted. If this fails decapitation has to be performed.

The babies are usually born before the placenta or placentae are delivered. If the first placenta is delivered before the second baby is born no harm results unless there is union of the circulations. The heart of the second child should, therefore, be auscultated carefully and if there is fetal distress or evidence of haemorrhage the second baby should be delivered forthwith.

A dangerous situation is created when ergometrine or syntometrine is given with the delivery of the first baby in an undiagnosed twin labour. The uterus contracts down causing impairment of the placental circulation and possibly placental separation. The cervix also begins to close. The second twin must be delivered promptly if it is to survive. The delivery may be difficult if the cervix is closing, particularly if it is a breech delivery and the cervix closes around the neck of the baby.

Triplets are dealt with in a similar manner to twins and vaginal delivery is usually achieved unless Caesarean section has been necessitated by some complication such as antepartum haemorrhage, pre-eclampsia or prolapsed cord. Delivery of quadruplets and quintuplets in recent years have mainly been by elective Caesarean section in the absence of other complications presumably because it was thought by the obstetrician that there was likely to be too much risk of asphyxia to the last baby to be delivered. Vaginal deliveries of quintuplets (e.g. the Dionnes) seemed to illustrate how remarkably safe this is for all the babies but in view of the theoretical risks most multiple births over three will continue to be delivered by Caesarean section.

Prognosis for babies

Morbidity and mortality are commoner in the babies of multiple than of single pregnancies. This is, in part, due to the obstetric complications such as haemorrhage and toxaemia which occur during pregnancy, and partly to the premature onset of labour. One twin is often larger and stronger than the other and the second to be born is at greater risk than the first. The male of co-twins is usually larger than the female.

Multiple births usually result in abnormal fetal growth. The combined fetal weights, however, exceed the weight of singletons. McKeown and Record in 1952 demonstrated that women can on average support fetal growth up to nearly 3000gm of combined

weight without evidence of growth retardation. The placenta is probably not causally involved in the subnormal growth since its weight is normal or even relatively high in multiple births (Pankamaa and Aschen, 1958). Daw and Walker (1973) found that the total fetal weight added from 32 to 40 weeks was 1800gm in single and some 2000gm (1000×2) in twin pregnancies suggesting a uterine supply and stretch limitation (Fig. 22.8). Naeye, Benirschke, Hagstrom and Marcus (1966) confirmed

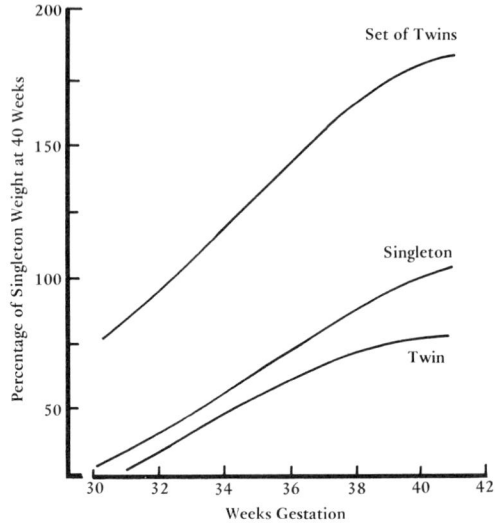

Fig. 22.8 Figure showing that although the combined weights of twins are greater than singletons, individual twins are lighter. The levelling off of the growth curve occurs earlier in twins than in singletons.

McKeown and Record's observation that fetal growth is independent of litter size until 30 weeks. The growth pattern supports McKeown's view that environmental rather than genetic factors are primarily responsible for the abnormal growth of twins in later fetal life.

Among human twins discordance for birth weight as well as for other factors is greater in monochorionic than in dichorionic pairs (Fogel, Mitowsky and Gruenwald, 1965). This does not appear to be due to zygosity. Naeye and his co-workers (1966) found monochorionic twins are both smaller and have a greater intrapair variation in birth weight than dichorionic twins. Intra-uterine environmental influences and the action of a variety of exogenous agents are all possible mechanisms in the production of intrapair differences between presumed isogenic individuals. There is no difference between like sexed and unlike sexed dichorionic twins, even although some of the former must be assumed to be monozygotic.

Almost all monochorionic twin placentas have vascular anastomosis between the twin circulations, but their effectiveness in equalizing supplies is variable. Some anastomosis may cause inequality of blood flow leading to the so-called transfusion syndrome in which one twin is anaemic and the other hypervolaemic with a high haematocrit value. The former twin is usually but not always considerably smaller than the latter. In the transfusion syndrome there is hydramnios in the sac of the plethoric baby and probably about one-third of monochorionic twins are affected. Some authors consider the risk to the second child is no greater than to the first (Potter and Fuller, 1949; Aaron et al., 1961) but others found a much greater death rate in the second twin (Guttmacher and Kohn, 1958; Farrell, 1964; Law, 1967).

The high perinatal mortality in monoamniotic twins is usually due to knotting of the intertwining cords.

In the 1958 British Perinatal Mortality Survey there was an excess of deaths of second born twins before, during and after delivery. Delay in delivering second twins is often thought to be a contributory factor to their overall higher fetal and neonatal mortality. In the 53 pairs in this series in which the first twin had survived and the second succumbed, 61 per cent had been delivered more than 30 minutes after the first, which was significantly more than the 21 per cent in the 38 pairs in whom the second twin had been the sole survivor.

The risks are particularly great in babies of women from the lower socio-economic classes who tend to have light-weight single babies. Anderson (1956) found that babies whose aggregate weight was less than 8lb occurred in 32 per cent of short women and 13 per cent of tall women. Over 10 per cent of the tall women had babies which together weighed 14lb but none of the short women achieved this.

The weight of the baby is of far greater importance than the method of delivery in determining the chance of survival. Death of both twins before the onset of labour is most likely to occur if they are both male. The smaller twin is at greater risk of antepartum asphyxial death and of mental handicap, possibly from chronic growth retardation in utero. Intrapartum death is more likely with the first child especially due to breech delivery.

Congenital malformations are twice as common in twins as in singletons. Monozygotic twins have more malformations than dizygotic twins. Monozygotic twins are isogenic while dizygotic twins are genetically different. Abnormalities are more often concordant in monozygotic than dizygotic twins, but the incidence of discordant abnormalities in monozygotic twins is surprisingly high. Genetic alterations resulting from gene mutations or chromosomal rearrangements in the embryos following cleavage, developmental accidents occurring during the formation of the twin embryos, intra-uterine environmental influences and the action of a variety of exogenous agents are all possible mechanisms in the production of intrapair differences between presumed isogenic individuals. There are between five and ten times as many twins among patients with cerebral palsy as in the general population. There is a very high perinatal mortality among the co-twins of children with cerebral palsy, suggesting an unfavourable uterine environment before birth. The combination of twin pregnancy and severe pre-eclampsia is the most common obstetrical complication associated with neurological damage in mentally handicapped children.

REFERENCES

Aaron, J. B., Silverman, S. H. & Halperin, J. (1961) Fetal survival in twin pregnancy. *Amer. J. Obstet. Gynec.*, **81**, 331.
Anderson, W. J. R. (1956) Stillbirth and neonatal mortality in twin pregnancy. *J. Obstet. Gynaec. Brit. Emp.*, **63**, 205.
Bulmer, M. G. (1959) Twinning rate in Europe during the war. *Brit. med. J.*, **i**, 29.
Bulmer, M. G. (1960) The twinning rate in Europe and Africa. *Ann. hum. Genet.*, **24**, 121.
Cameron, A. H. (1968) The Birmingham twin survey. *Proc. R. Soc. Med.*, **61**, 229.
Corney, G., Robson, E. B. & Strong, S. J. (1968) Twin zygosity and placentation. *Ann. hum. Genet.*, **32**, 89.
Daw, E. & Walker, J. (1975) Growth Differences in Twin Pregnancy. *Brit. J. clin. Pract.* In Press.
Daw, E. & Walker J. (1975) Biological Aspects of Twin Pregnancy in Dundee. *J. Obstet. Gynaec. Brit. Cwlth.* In Press.

Farrell, A. G. W. (1964) Twin pregnancy: a study of 1000 cases. *South African Journal of Obstetrics and Gynaecology*, **2**, 35.

Fogiel, B. J., Mitowsky, H. M. & Gruenwald, P. (1965) Discordant abnormalities in monozygotic twins. *J. Pediat.*, **66**, 64.

Greulich, W. W. (1934) Heredity in human twinning. *Amer. J. phys. Anthrop.*, **19**, 391.

Guttmacher, A. F. & Kohl, S. G. (1958) The fetus of multiple gestations. *Obstet. Gynaec.*, **12**, 528.

Hellin, D. (1895) *Die Ursache der Multiparitat der Uniparen Tiere uberhaupt und der Swillings-schwangerschaft beim Menchan insbesonderer.* Munchen: Seitz and Schaner.

Law, R. G. (1967) Standards of obstetric care: *the report of the North West Metropolitan Regional Obstetrical Survey*, **94**, 131, 164, 200 and 228. Edinburgh: Livingstone.

MacGillivray, I., Campbell, D. & Duffus, G. M. (1971) Maternal metabolic response to twin pregnancy in primigravidae. *J. Obstet. Gynaec. Brit. Cwlth.*, **78**, 6, 530.

McKeown, T. & Record, R. G. (1952) Observations on fetal growth in multiple pregnancy in man. *J. Endocr.*, **8**, 386.

Millis, J. (1958) The frequency of twinning in poor Chinese in the Maternity Hospital, Singapore. *Ann. hum. Genet.*, **23**, 171.

Morton, N. E. (1955) The inheritance of human birth weight. *Ann. hum. Genet.*, **20**, 125.

Naeye, R. L., Benirscke, K., Hagstrom, J. W. C. & Marcus, C. C. (1966) Intrauterine growth of twins as estimated from live born birth weight data. *Paediatrics*, **37**, 409.

Pankamaa, P. & Aschen, E. (1958) Ueber das Verhaetnis zwischen Frucht und Plazenta bei Zwillingsschwangerschaften. *Annls. Chir. Gynaec. Fenn.*, **47**, 81.

Potter, E. L. & Fuller, H. (1949) Multiple pregnancies at the Chicago Lying-in Hospital 1941–47. *Amer. J. Obstet. Gynec.*, **58**, 139.

Renkonen, K. O. (1967) The birth order of twins. *Annls. Med. exp. Biol. Fenn.*, **45**, 174.

Rovinsky, J. J. & Jaffin, H. (1965) Cardiovascular haemodynamics in pregnancy. 1. Blood and plasma volumes in multiple pregnancy. *Amer. J. Obstet. Gynec.*, **93**, 1. (1966) 2. Cardiac output and left ventricular work in multiple pregnancy. *Amer. J. Obstet. Gynec.*, **95**, 781. (1966) 3. Cardiac rate, stroke volume, total peripheral resistance and Central blood volume in multiple pregnancy. Synthesis of results. *Amer. J. Obstet. Gynec.*, **95**, 787.

Stockard, C. R. (1921) Developmental rate and structural expression: an experimental study of twins, 'double monsters' and single deformities, and the interaction among embryonic organs during their origin and development. *The Amer. J. Anat.*, **28**, 115.

Whyte, C. & Wyshak, G. (1964) Inheritance in human dizygotic twinning. *New Engl. J. Med.*, **271**, 1003.

FURTHER READING

Bulmer, M. G. (1970) *The biology of twinning in man.* Oxford: Clarendon Press.

Mittler, P. (1971) *The study of twins.* Harmondsworth: Penguin Books.

MacGillivray, I., Nylander, P. P. S. & Corney, G. (1975) *Human Multiple Reproduction*, London and New York: Saunders.

23. The Newborn Infant

At the moment of conception a new being is created whose genetic characteristics differentiate him from all others of his kind. During his early growth and development in the uterus, he is acted upon by many environmental influences which further shape him so that by the time of birth every infant has a combination of genetic and acquired attributes which renders him unique. Hitherto, although a distinct individual, he has been protected from the full impact of the external world and dependent on his mother for nutrition, excretion and much of the metabolic processing associated with these. The sudden and violent shock of birth thrusts him into a hostile environment, while the severing of the umbilical cord throws the full burden of metabolic activity on to his own organs. While he will still rely to a considerable extent on his mother for food, warmth and protection, his survival depends increasingly on his own efforts. It is little wonder therefore that the newborn period is critically important, for if the infant does not regulate his functions in response to new demands or is unable to resist the attacks of micro-organisms, he will succumb or at best will survive with lasting disability. Perhaps the surprising thing is that so many human infants do make the necessary adjustments and that only a small minority, mainly those born too early, fail to adapt unaided.

Good neonatal care thus consists to a great extent of the provision of nourishment and suitable surroundings for large numbers of normal infants, and active help for those few who are finding adaptation difficult. It also implies the difficult decision to withhold such help when an infant is so abnormal as to have no chance of ultimate survival.

CARE IMMEDIATELY AFTER BIRTH

When the head is born the eyes should be wiped, each with a separate dry sterile wool swab, from the inner to the outer canthus: any external mucus or blood should be removed from the mouth and nose. The practice of instilling antiseptic drops into the infant's eyes at birth has been discontinued as a routine since gonococcal ophthalmia is much less common; but the disease is reappearing. As soon as the infant is born, he should be held with his head down to let fluid drain from the respiratory tract. Often he will cry at once but if not the mouth and nasopharynx should be sucked clear of secretions. Usually the umbilical cord is still pulsating strongly and it should not be divided for 30–60 seconds. During this time the infant is held below the level of the placenta and the pulsations of the cord gradually cease as gravity and uterine contractions aid the transfer of 50–100ml of blood from the placenta to the baby. Increasing the blood volume in this way increases the infant's iron stores and avoids the hypovolaemic state which may be associated with a higher incidence of respiratory difficulties in the newborn period. However, if the infant is pale and limp, if the cord is tightly round the neck or if serological incompatibility is present, the cord should be cut immediately. To divide the cord it is ligated in two places— 5 and 10cm from the umbilicus—with sterile nylon tape or twisted linen thread and then cut with sterile scissors between the ligatures. Just before the cord is cut, a wrist name tape or other means of identification should be securely fastened to the infant.

If the baby is breathing satisfactorily, he should be inspected quickly from head to foot for signs of abnormality and the number of vessels in the cord should be carefully noted. The wet newborn infant loses heat very quickly so no time must be lost in placing him in a cot wrapped in warm towels and blankets, with the head down at an angle of 15 degrees. If the baby is not breathing when the cord is cut, measures of resuscitation should be immediately instituted as described below. If there was hydramnios during pregnancy, an oesophageal tube should be passed to confirm that the oesophagus is patent, and to empty the stomach of swallowed liquor.

As soon as possible after birth, the infant must be carefully weighed. Biparietal diameter ought to be measured. The head circumference and crown-rump length are measured at the 24-hour examination, since these are used primarily as basic growth measurements forwards. If crown-heel length can be recorded, this is also useful.

ESTABLISHMENT OF RESPIRATION

Respiration is initiated and maintained by centres in the brain stem. The two main types of respiration, rhythmic breathing and intermittent gasps, originate in different parts of the respiratory centre. The centre responsible for rhythmic breathing responds to neurally transmitted stimuli from peripheral thermal and tactile receptors, especially those in the skin area served by the trigeminal nerve. If this centre is depressed by hypoxia, single gasps are initiated chemically when central and peripheral chemo-receptors are stimulated by falling oxygen tension and rising carbon dioxide tension following division of the umbilical cord. Single gasps allow sufficient oxygenation to revive the depressed centres, so that rhythmic breathing soon follows, provided that the respiratory centre has not been damaged. Animal experiments suggest that a baby who does not breathe at birth may be in primary apnoea, i.e. before gasping starts, or in secondary apnoea, i.e. beyond the last gasp so that no further gasping will occur spontaneously. The difference between the two is not recognizable clinically though the difference in their prognostic significance is obvious.

The lung of the fetus at term is full of fluid. Some of this may be expelled by compression of the chest during delivery and may be replaced by a little air when the chest wall recoils passively after the compression is released. Despite this, the alveoli remain unexpanded and considerable opening pressure (as much as 40cm of water) may be required to overcome the effects of surface tension. Some of the remaining fluid drains away by gravity and the rest is absorbed mainly through the lymphatic system. The pulmonary alveolar cells secrete a surface-active phospholipid (surfactant), which has the property of reducing surface tension and so preventing the alveoli from collapsing completely, as would otherwise occur after each breath. The infant born before term (38–42 weeks) may lack adequate surfactant and this partly accounts for his predisposition to respiratory disorders (see page 440).

When breathing starts, the pulmonary alveoli expand and this mechanical effect, added to the effects of rising oxygen and falling carbon dioxide levels in the plasma, results in a rapid fall in pulmonary arterial pressure, due to active dilatation of arterioles. This permits blood to flow through the lungs rather than through the ductus arteriosus, which closes functionally in response to the changes in blood gas tensions. The blood returning from the lungs to the left atrium increases pressure in that chamber and the foramen ovale in the interatrial septum closes, so that all right to left shunting of blood ceases.

Once breathing is established it is mainly abdominal and diaphragmatic: the rate is usually 40–45 per minute, but is often irregular. The lungs should be fully expanded within two days.

RESUSCITATION OF THE NEWBORN INFANT

Most infants start to breathe as soon as they are born and the great majority within a minute or two of birth. They may cry almost immediately, or, after a brief period of apnoea, may gasp a few times before starting to breathe rhythmically. All that is required is clearance of the air passages, if possible before the first breath is taken: this is achieved by aspirating fluid from the mouth and pharynx and by holding the baby upside down, when fluid drains out by gravity. The infant's condition may be assessed by means of the Apgar score, usually recorded at one minute and again at five minutes after birth. The attendant counts the heart rate using a stethoscope and while doing so observes the infant's colour and respiratory effort. The resistance to passive movement of the limbs indicates muscle tone while the response to the stimulus of pharyngeal aspiration may be a grimace or a cry. A score is allocated for each characteristic as

Table 23.1 The Apgar score

Score	Heart rate	Respiratory effort	Muscle tone	Response to stimulation	Colour
0	Absent	Absent	Flaccid	None	Blue or pale
1	Less than 100 per min	Slow and irregular	Some flexor tone	Grimace	Body pink; Extremities blue
2	100 per min or more	Strong cry	Active movement	Cry	Pink all over

shown in Table 23.1 and the five scores are added together to give a total score. A baby who is in good condition and cries at once usually has a score of 8, 9 or 10, whereas a severely asphyxiated infant may have a score of 3 or less. The time of the first breath and the time to sustained respiration (TSR) should also be recorded.

In a small proportion of infants, breathing does not start spontaneously and for these active measures of resuscitation are required. In large obstetric units, an experienced member of the paediatric staff should be present at delivery whenever difficulties are anticipated, so that his whole attention can be directed to resuscitation of the infant. Since difficulties cannot always be anticipated, and since every second after delivery of an asphyxiated infant counts, the paediatrician should be in the hospital and instantly available at all times of the day and night. In smaller units this will not always be possible, and then the baby must be resuscitated by the most experienced person available. Whether this is midwife, paediatrician, anaesthetist or obstetrician is less important than that those undertaking resuscitation should be trained and experienced in the techniques. It is useful to have a small committee of paediatrician, obstetrician, anaesthetist and midwife to keep techniques under review and to supervise the training of staff in the necessary skills.

Principles of resuscitation

Failure to initiate breathing at birth is due to depression of the respiratory centres by asphyxia, drugs or trauma, or by a combination of these. Even if respiratory efforts are made, the lungs may not expand because the airways are blocked or congenitally abnormal. The lungs of the infant born long before term may be too immature to expand effectively.

If apnoea persists the newborn infant will eventually die but he can live for a remarkably long period and spontaneous breathing may start after 20 minutes or more, even without any attempts at resuscitation. Should the infant survive such prolonged apnoea, however, he may not emerge unscathed. At first he is protected by anaerobic glycolysis of carbohydrate reserves in the heart and liver but these are rapidly used up and severe lactic acidaemia develops. Although individual resistance to the effects of asphyxia varies greatly, all infants probably sustain some injury to brain cells after a few minutes of apnoea and brain damage is likely to increase with the passage of time. The aim of resuscitation is therefore not only to prevent death by establishing respiration but also to avoid brain damage by establishing it at the earliest possible moment. Time after birth must be measured in seconds and active measures of resuscitation instituted as soon as it is apparent that the infant is not going to cry or gasp spontaneously.

Obstruction to the airway must be cleared initially and efforts may then be made to stimulate the respiratory centres. If these are not quickly successful, the lungs must be ventilated by artificial means. The immediate objective is to oxygenate the infant's arterial blood as rapidly and efficiently as possible: thereafter the aim is to maintain oxygenation until adequate natural respiration is established. During these procedures, action may be required to prevent or correct extremes of biochemical and thermal deviations from the normal.

Practice of resuscitation

As soon as the infant's head is delivered, the mouth and nasopharynx must be sucked clear of mucus, amniotic fluid and other secretions. A mechanical aspirator may be used or the attendant may suck through a disposable mucus extractor or a sterilized soft rubber mucus catheter with a glass trap. When birth is complete, the infant is held upside down to allow fluid to drain from the respiratory tract. Flicking of the feet or further pharyngeal aspiration provides reflex stimulation to gasping. If the infant is not breathing by this time, oxygen may be administered using a small face mask or funnel. This serves the dual purpose of stimulating the face in the area of the trigeminal nerve and of providing an atmosphere rich in oxygen in readiness for the first breath. If this does not follow within two minutes, or if there is reason to suspect obstruction in the larynx or lower respiratory passages, an endotracheal tube should be passed under direct laryngoscopy without further delay. After careful aspiration of the tracheal contents, oxygen or air is administered intermittently by repeated, brief occlusion of one limb of the Y-piece adaptor attached to the endotracheal tube. The pressure should not exceed 30cm of water and each puff should last for less than a second, with 2 seconds in between. Since chilling occurs very readily, the infant should be kept warm throughout the period of resuscitation. This may be achieved by maintaining the temperature of the delivery room at not less than 20 °C, avoiding draughts, keeping the infant's body covered whenever possible, and providing additional heat by means of a warmer either under the mattress or above the resuscitation area. If the infant is obviously limp and pale at birth, with an Apgar score of 3 or less, it should be assumed that he is in secondary (terminal) apnoea and no time should be lost in intubating the trachea and insufflating oxygen. Since the accumulation of lactic acid is a feature of neonatal asphyxia, correction of the resulting acidaemia by injecting 10ml of 8·4 per cent sodium bicarbonate solution followed by 10ml of 10 per cent glucose into the umbilical vein may aid recovery when the Apgar score remains low. If the heart beat is absent, cardiac massage should be started by applying brief pressure once every 1–2 seconds to the left of the sternum using two fingers.

Narcotic drugs administered to the mother shortly before delivery may cause anoxia in the baby, due to depression of his respiratory centres. When this occurs, levallorphan, 0·02mg per Kg, or nalorphine, 0·2mg per Kg should be injected into the umbilical vein. Analeptic drugs such as vanillic acid diethyl-amide are of doubtful value in resuscitation, though their administration to an infant in primary apnoea may be followed by a gasp. Since primary and secondary apnoea cannot be distinguished clinically, however, there is no justification for postponing intubation and positive pressure ventilation in the hope that the drug will be effective. Prophylactic antibiotic treatment may be given if there has been much instrumental interference with the airways.

With the treatment outlined above, which should be undertaken only by those trained in the techniques, most asphyxiated babies soon start to gasp. The respiratory centres then reach the level of oxygenation at which they will respond and rhythmic respiration begins. Occasionally, however, intermittent positive pressure ventilation must be continued for 30 minutes or more before breathing starts. If there is no sign of spontaneous respiration after this period, it is likely that the infant's central nervous system is seriously damaged or abnormal and the decision to continue ventilation by mechanical means should be taken only after careful consideration of the possible outcome (Fig. 23.1).

The baby delivered in domiciliary practice should normally need little resuscitation as most complicated labours are now conducted in hospital. In the home, provided an asphyxiated baby is placed in the head-down position and his airway gently cleared, respiration will usually begin even if a supply of oxygen is not available. A bulb resuscitator, such as the Blease-Samson, may be used if breathing does not start after a few minutes. All doctors undertaking domiciliary or general practitioner unit obstetrics should be proficient in the technique of endotracheal intubation and intermittent positive pressure respiration so that they can deal efficiently with the occasional case of prolonged apnoea.

LATER CARE OF THE NEWBORN INFANT

During the few hours following birth, the infant should be kept under very close observation, either in the delivery room or in a special observation nursery. As soon as convenient the umbilical cord is clamped with a sterile plastic clip about 1cm from the umbilicus and the excess removed: it should be inspected

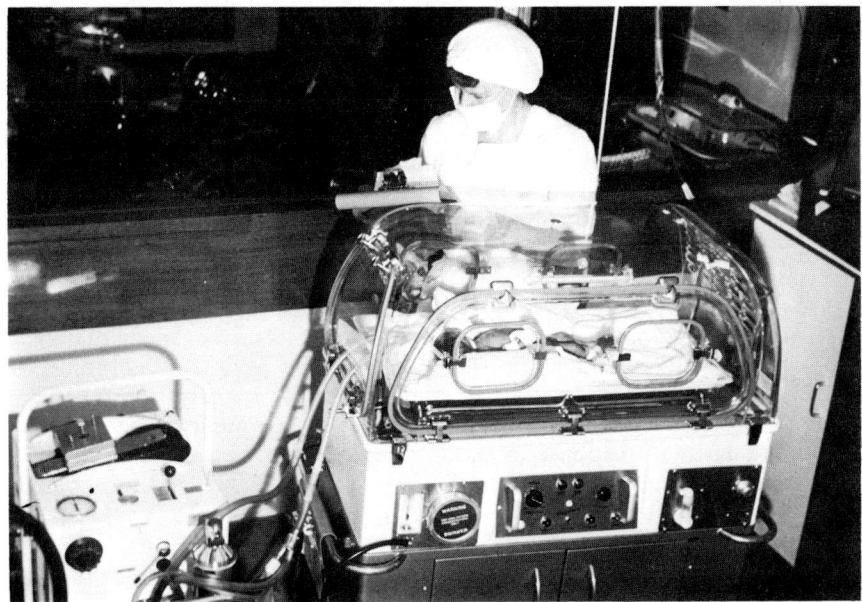

Fig. 23.1 Intermittent Positive Pressure Ventilation of a pre-term infant with respiratory distress, using an East Radcliffe ventilator.

frequently in the hours after birth to detect any leak of blood, though this is rare with the modern type of clip which exerts continuous pressure on the stump. After 24 hours the clip can be removed and thereafter the cord is treated with an occlusive paint or spray, or alternatively powdered and covered with a sterile dressing, until it dries and falls off.

Some hours after birth, when the mother has recovered from the immediate effects, the infant is transferred to a cot at her bedside and thereafter should only be removed to a nursery if he is crying enough to disturb his mother's rest. Communal nurseries can be dangerous places, especially if they are overcrowded, and they should be used as little as possible. In modern hospitals, contact between infants and the risk of cross-infection are reduced by use of single rooms or individual nurseries, by nursing patients in cohorts delivered at the same time, or by similar devices.

The infant should be nursed in a well-ventilated room, kept at 21 °C (70 °F). Though many types of cot are available, a suitable one in common use consists of a perspex bassinet on a mobile stand with built-in locker, which contains bath, dusting powder, thermometer, clothing and so on, for the infant's personal use. He should wear a simple vest, gown and soft napkin and should be protected from draughts. In the home, additional blankets and hot-water bottles may be required to prevent chilling, especially in the early hours of the morning when the temperature of the room is likely to fall. After the first few days, the clothing and heating will vary according to the place and the season.

Napkins should be changed frequently, certainly before and after feeds, and the buttocks should be washed with soap and water, mopped (not rubbed) with soft towelling, and then lightly dusted with powder or smeared with a suitable cream. Frequent washing and bathing of the newborn baby is unnecessary and may be harmful since accidental abrasion of the skin may open the way to infection. The infant can be gently cleansed following birth and thereafter no bathing is required until shortly before the baby goes home. At that time, when the mother is being instructed in the care of her baby, the opportunity can be taken to show her how the baby should be bathed.

THE NORMAL NEWBORN INFANT

Adjustment to extra-uterine life

At birth the fetus suddenly assumes a separate

existence as an infant and usually has little difficulty in making the many necessary adjustments to neonatal life. The lungs and kidneys take over many of the functions of the placenta, and the heart and circulation quickly adapt to the new system of gaseous exchange (*see* Chapt. 6). Within an hour or two of birth the adult type of circulation is established and the relatively large heart soon pumps 500ml of blood per minute in 120–140 beats, the blood pressure being about 85/45mm/Hg. During fetal life the haemoglobin is of a special type (Haemoglobin F) which, in comparison with adult haemoglobin (Haemoglobin A), takes up oxygen more readily at low tensions and releases it more easily in response to falling pH levels. This facilitates oxygenation of the tissues under the conditions of fetal life. The infant born at term has about two-thirds of his haemoglobin in the fetal form, but this proportion rapidly diminishes in the ensuing weeks. The mean haemoglobin concentration in umbilical venous blood is 17g per 100ml: after a first-day rise, it falls to about 14·5g per 100ml within a month and still further later. The red cells, which are larger in size than the adult type, fall gradually from about 5 million per cmm at birth to just over 4·3 million at one month. These values refer to venous blood and the examination of capillary blood gives higher and more variable results, which may explain contradictory results in the literature. There are, however, considerable normal variations from baby to baby. During the first week there is a reticulocytosis of 3–5 per cent and a few nucleated red cells are seen, but the reticulocytes fall to less than 1 per cent, and the nucleated red cells disappear within a week. Striking changes in the leucocytes occur. The total count rises from a mean value of 11 thousand per cmm at birth to 19 thousand per cmm at 24 hours and thereafter falls to 10 thousand per cmm at one week. Neutrophil polymorphs predominate for a few days, but thereafter there is a relative lymphocytosis, which persists throughout infancy.

The bilirubin level in plasma (normally less than 1mg per 100ml) is raised to 1–2mg in all newborns and rises by the third to the fifth day to 3–10mg. At levels above about 4mg the baby appears jaundiced and the urine may occasionally contain bile. Jaundice may be seen in nearly half of all babies on the fourth day, though the proportion varies with different observers. It fades gradually and has usually disappeared within a week, although it may persist for a fortnight or longer and raise suspicions of more serious disorders.

The occurrence of physiological jaundice in normal newborn infants, and especially in those born before term, is due mainly to inefficient hepatic function. The glucuronyl transferase system which is necessary for the conjugation of bilirubin has low activity at birth and excretory mechanisms by the hepatic cells may also be inadequately developed. During the period of jaundice, the infant's behaviour is usually normal but he may be drowsy and disinclined to feed for a day or two. *Visible jaundice on the first day of life is never physiological.* While all these changes are going on, the newborn baby is beginning to feed and to excrete meconium and later faeces. He is also regulating his body temperature and metabolism.

The newly born infant is a partial homeotherm, in that he can to some extent maintain his body temperature despite changes in environmental temperature. He is very susceptible to heat loss, however, because of his low thermal insulation and relatively large surface area. In response to cold, body heat is conserved by cutaneous vasoconstriction. As the ambient temperature falls to a critical level, the metabolic rate starts to rise and continues to do so until a maximum rate of heat production is reached. Should the environment become yet colder, the body temperature will start to fall. It is believed that a major site of heat production in the newborn infant is the brown adipose tissue widely distributed throughout the body. Immature infants respond more variably to cold, but in general their critical temperature is higher, they increase heat production earlier and reach the maximum rate sooner, so that they are less efficient homeotherms than infants born at term. The kidneys secrete urine from about the fourth month of intra-uterine life, and by 40 weeks are able to adjust water, electrolyte and acid/base balance efficiently enough for ordinary requirements. Any unusual demand may overtax their capacity, however, and so the newborn infant is predisposed to oedema and acidaemia. The blood glucose falls rapidly from levels of 80–100mg per 100ml at birth to about 50mg a few hours later and this low level may persist for several days, but is seldom accompanied by clinical signs of hypoglycaemia. The glycogen reserves of the newborn infant's liver are readily mobilized to meet energy needs and this is especially important at a time when the infant's ability to utilize fat and protein is still limited.

The gastrointestinal tract is almost fully functional soon after birth, though it may be deficient in some of the digestive enzymes, notably amylase. The healthy infant born at term can therefore suck, swallow, digest and absorb milk and can excrete meconium and subsequently faeces.

The endocrine glands undergo considerable changes at birth. The adrenal cortex, which produces distinctive neonatal steroids, rapidly involutes and the pattern of steroid excretion soon approaches the normal for adults. The adrenal medulla secretes mainly noradrenaline at birth, while the thyroid produces quantities of hormone which in the adult would be considered as representing hyperthyroidism. It is not known whether the baby's own hormones play any part in the so-called genital crisis of the newborn, which is probably mainly due to withdrawal of maternal oestrogens. It is characterized by enlargement of the breasts in both sexes, possibly with secretion of a little milk on the third day, and sometimes by vaginal bleeding in female infants (Fig 23.2).

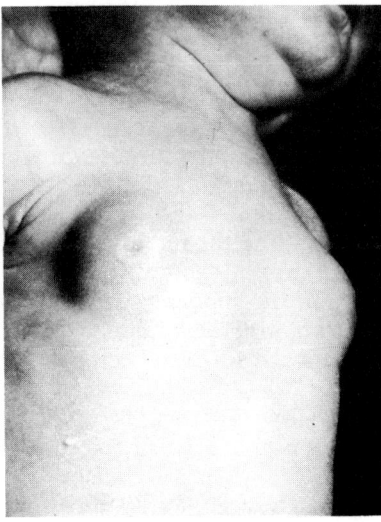

Fig. 23.2   Neonatal enlargement of breasts.

While many of the infant's functions rapidly become efficient after birth, his ability to defend himself against micro-organisms is slow to develop. He will be protected to some extent by antibodies, mainly IgG, transferred through the placenta from his mother, but it will be some months before he begins to synthesize his own immunoglobulins in any quantity. During this time there is gradual disappearance of maternal antibody, so that his protection is at its lowest when he is about three months old.

Examination of the newborn infant

The infant will be inspected generally as soon as he is born, but he should also be carefully and systematically examined by an experienced doctor about 24 hours after birth. The family and maternal history should be available and must be scrutinized for any indication of possible genetic or prenatally acquired abnormality. A history of hydramnios during pregnancy or a single umbilical artery observed at birth will alert the examiner to the possibility of congenital malformation. The examination should be conducted in a warm, well-lit nursery and the infant should be lying unclothed on a firm flat surface. It is helpful to have the mother present, as she will be reassured by seeing the careful examination of her infant and can have any anxieties resolved by explanation at the time. Observations should be recorded on a standard examination form as they are made and any abnormality should lead either to further investigation and treatment if necessary or to later re-appraisal before the infant goes home. The following account describes some of the many normal variations which may be encountered but only experience will enable the examiner to judge when further action is required. When minor variations are considered to be within the limits of normal, this should be carefully explained to the mother, who will often worry over supposed abnormalities which are in fact quite harmless.

Infants vary in size according to sex, birth order and gestational age, and to the parents' race, type and socio-economic status, as well as to intrinsic differences. The average British baby weighs just over 3400g ($7\frac{1}{2}$lb) and has a crown-heel length of 51cm (20 inches), a crown-rump length of 34cm (13·4 inches) and a head circumference of 34cm (13·4 inches). Centiles for birth weight according to sex, birth order and gestational age, and allowing for maternal height and weight, are given by Tanner and Thomson (1970). The face and body become ruddy as soon as respiration is established and there should then be no cyanosis, pallor or jaundice. Slight blueness of the hands and feet due to sluggishness of the peripheral circulation may persist normally for a few days. Slight degrees of oedema are not uncommon, especially about the dorsal aspects of the feet and hands, the pubes and the eyelids. The hands should be examined for palmar creases as a single palmar crease (Fig 23.3) suggests Down's syndrome.

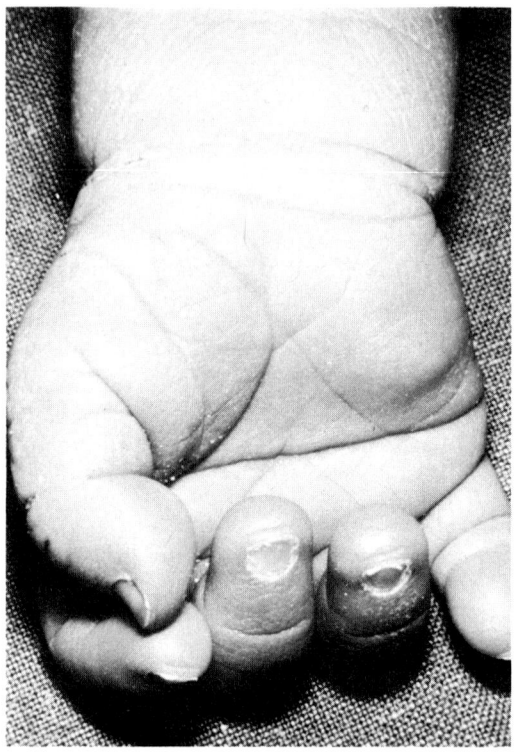

Fig. 23.3   Horizontal palmar crease.

Varying amounts of whitish, greasy *vernix caseosa* cover the soft velvety skin. Greenish-yellow vernix is indicative of fetal stress and anoxia, or of haemolytic disease. The fine hair (lanugo) that may cover areas of the body usually disappears in a week, as does the powdery desquamation that is commonly seen soon after birth. In the flexures, erythema and scaling is sometimes excessive and these areas should be watched for infection. The epidermis is loose and excessive heat and clothing can cause the innumerable tiny vesicles called miliaria. Some infants develop a blotchy erythematous rash, with tiny white vesicles containing many eosinophil cells, within a day or two of birth. This is probably a sensitivity reaction ('erythema toxicum') and should not be mistaken for an infection. Nevertheless, the ease with which the skin of the newborn can be infected must not be forgotten.

Small white spots or milia, due to enlargement of sebaceous glands, may be visible on the nose and cheeks: they disappear spontaneously. Petechiae about the face and back are not uncommon and are occasionally so numerous as to be almost confluent, producing a resemblance to cyanosis. Faint telangiectatic naevi ('stork bites') are often seen about the nape of the neck, in the glabellar region and on the upper eyelids. They worry mothers, who can be assured that they will disappear in a year or less. A large pigmented spot may be seen over the buttocks of an infant of African or Asian race and is known as a 'Mongolian blue spot'. It gradually becomes less noticeable as the skin colour darkens.

A healthy newborn infant exhibits *flexor tone*, lying with all limbs flexed. He sleeps for long periods of day and night, but is active when awake and hungry. His cry is loud and vigorous, and should not be whining, feeble or shrill. He can see and hear and may respond to light or sudden sounds by turning his head and eyes in their direction. Various other responses can be elicited by appropriate stimuli. Stroking away from the mouth will produce searching, sucking movements towards the stroking finger (the rooting response). The *Moro reflex* consists of sudden extension of the upper limbs with opening of the hands, sometimes followed by partial flexion of the limbs and crying. It can be elicited by holding the infant up and allowing the head to drop a short distance relative to the trunk or by suddenly striking the cot. This reaction may be diminished or absent in the infant with abnormal cerebral function.

The *anterior fontanelle*, which varies in size from baby to baby, is open and not bulging. The eyes are usually closed for much of the time: the irides are bluish. Occasional squinting may be seen, for good co-ordination of the eye movements does not come for weeks. The optic discs are normally clear-cut and greyish-white and the retinae paler than in the adult.

The *chest* is round and respiration is mainly abdominal. Lung expansion may be incomplete on the first day but breath sounds should be heard on both sides. The heart rate varies with the infant's activity from 100–160 beats/minute. It is usually possible to say if the heart is on the normal side, for the apex beat can be felt. Cardiac murmurs heard in newborn babies do not necessarily mean that the heart is abnormal: conversely, the absence of murmurs in the first few days does not rule out the possibility of a congenital cardiac malformation. The femoral arterial pulses should be carefully palpated, for their absence may indicate coarctation of the aorta.

The *abdomen* of the newborn is usually protuberant: the edge of the liver can often be felt below the costal margin; the spleen and the kidneys may also be palpable. Normally the prepuce is partly adherent to the glans penis and may not be retractable for many months. Routine circumcision or stretching of the prepuce is quite unjustifiable. The testicles are palpable or can be drawn down into the scrotum in nearly all infants born at term: a small hydrocele is frequently present but usually disappears within a few weeks. The labia minora and clitoris of the female infant are prominent, as the labia majora are under-developed and do not cover them. A mucoid discharge from the vagina is very frequently seen and there is often a small tag at the vaginal orifice, which will disappear without treatment in a month or so. The anus should be examined for patency. Lastly, the range of movements of the muscles and joints of the limbs should be tested. Full extension of arm and leg joints is not always possible in the newborn. If the hip joints are normal, the flexed lower limbs can be abducted almost to 90 degrees. In many newborn infants, the hip joints feel slightly unstable during the first few days, but when the femoral head can be moved in and out of the acetabulum with a distinct 'clunking' sensation, dislocation is present. Apparent bowing of the legs is normal in the newborn. A slight calcaneo-valgus deformity of the feet is often present in the first few weeks but only requires orthopaedic treatment if it is severe.

The body temperature of infants born at term falls about two degrees in the first hours of life but rises to normal within 8–12 hours. The size of the heart is relatively greater than in later life and this should be remembered when X-ray films are being examined: and the cardiac output, 500ml per minute, is twice as great per unit of body weight as in the adult. Blood volume varies somewhat according to the amount of placental blood the infant receives, but a good working rule is that the volume is usually about 85ml/kg of body weight.

The assessment of maturity

An infant born many weeks before term is extremely immature and likely to suffer from certain consequential disorders, so that he has clinical problems quite different from those of the baby born at or near term. For this reason it is important to try to assess the maturity of the newborn infant. The organs and tissues of the fetus mature at different rates but, in general, maturity is related to gestational age, as calculated from the first day of the last menstrual period. This is not always known, however, and even when it is stated mistakes readily occur, e.g. due to irregularity of the menstrual cycle or the use of contraceptive drugs. It is sometimes valuable therefore to determine maturity by means other than the estimation of gestational age.

The *fetal nervous system* is much less affected by adverse influences on intra-uterine development than are body weight and abdominal viscera, which may be considerably reduced in size. Neurological function is therefore closely correlated with post-menstrual age and can be used as an indirect indication of maturity. The presence or absence of certain neurological reflexes, which first appear at characteristic periods of fetal life, affords a comparatively simple method of clinical assessment. For example, the pupillary reaction to light develops about the 30th week, the glabellar tap reflex appears about 33 weeks and the neck-righting reflex about 35 weeks. By eliciting several of these reflexes, an approximate assessment of neurological age can be made (Robinson, 1966) but the result is influenced by the nervous state of the baby and may be quite erroneous if he has sustained damage to the central nervous system during birth.

External physical characteristics of the infant, such as the appearance of the skin, cartilage formation in the external ear, the development of the nipples, breast tissue, and external genital organs, and the skin creases on the soles of the feet, also give a good indication of maturity. Precise definitions of the different degrees of these characteristics and a method of deriving a total maturity score are given by Farr and her colleagues (1966a & b). The method has the advantage of being virtually independent of the infant's general condition at the time of assessment, usually about 24 hours after birth. Radiological determination of osseous development is of some value in judging maturity, but is less precise than evaluation of physical characteristics. Other methods which have been used are the appearance of the fundus oculi, the velocity of conduction in motor nerves and analysis of the EEG record, but all these require skill and special apparatus and they are not in general use.

With care, neurological reflexes and external characteristics, separately or in combination (Dubowitz and Goldberg, 1970), can be used as indirect measures of gestational age to an accuracy of $\pm$ 2 weeks: marked discrepancy between gestational age as measured in this way and that calculated from the stated date of the last menstrual period should alert the clinician to the probability that the latter is erroneous.

Screening procedures

Neonatal screening consists of routinely examining every newborn infant in the population for evidence of existing or future abnormality. It is costly in time, money and skill, so that it is only justified if the rewards are commensurate with the effort required. If the abnormality sought occurs very rarely, the enthusiasm of staff and therefore the accuracy of screening is likely to wane rapidly: if mistakes occur because the method is not simple, reliable and specific, screening becomes discredited: there is a danger that subsequent signs of abnormality will be disregarded because the baby is known to have been screened. For these reasons, screening of the newborn must be employed with discretion and limited to what is reasonable and feasible.

Physical examination, including testing for dislocation of the hip (*see* above), is the most important form of screening. Newborn infants are also screened for the presence of one or more metabolic errors. The Guthrie blood test for hyperphenylalaninaemia, which may

be an indication of the disorder phenylketonuria, is widely used in this country and the method, which depends on inhibition of specific bacteria, can be extended to screen for other metabolic errors: in this test a few drops of capillary blood obtained by heel prick are absorbed on specially prepared paper, which can then be transmitted by post to a central laboratory. Positive tests should be checked by biochemical estimation of the plasma concentration. In some hospitals, the urine is routinely tested for reducing substances to detect inborn errors of carbohydrate metabolism, especially galactosaemia. Galactose in urine gives a positive reaction to Benedict's solution but its identity must be verified by chromatography, since traces of lactose, fructose or other reducing substances may appear in the urine of newborn infants.

Whenever screening methods are used, care must be taken to ensure that parents understand the purpose of the test and the implication of a positive result. Much unnecessary anxiety can be generated if doubtful positive cases are reported without adequate explanation.

Progress in the first week

The newborn infant, having survived the stresses of birth and made the sudden change from almost complete physiological dependence to a separate existence, now undergoes more rapid and extensive growth and development than at any period during later life. He sleeps much of the time, unless he is prompted to waken by hunger, thirst or the discomfort, for example, of a soiled napkin. There are considerable variations in behaviour between different babies, however, some being more wakeful than others.

Urine is often passed during or soon after birth but none may be seen for 24 hours or longer. Palpation of the abdomen often stimulates micturition. Very little urine may be passed during the first two or three days but the daily amount soon increases and by the end of a week may total 200ml or more, passed in small quantities at a time. Dark greenish viscid meconium is passed several times daily during the first two or three days. If none is passed in the first 12 hours, the baby should be examined carefully to exclude the possibility of obstruction. About the fourth day the stools change and become yellowish-green in colour and less homogeneous, often containing slime and undigested milk ('changing stools'). If the milk intake is adequate the stools quickly become pasty and yellow, with a sour non-offensive odour: the colour in a breast-fed baby will be golden-yellow and the reaction usually acid, while on cow's milk the stools are paler yellow, alkaline and greater in bulk. Great variations in the number of stools occur and one to six a day may be passed by normal infants. Later, some breast-fed babies may have a stool only every two or three days but this need not cause concern if the baby is thriving and the stools appear normal when passed.

During the first three or four days of life, the weight of the healthy infant falls, probably due to diminution in the body fluids, since the fluid intake is less than that lost in the urine and stools and through the skin and lungs. This physiological loss of weight varies from 5 to 10 per cent of the birth weight; the lost weight is regained by the seventh to fourteenth day. The vernix disappears naturally in a few days. The stump of the umbilical cord dries and shrivels up and the mummified remains are usually shed within a week, leaving a small moist granulating area. This soon heals but till then is a potential portal of entry of infection.

INFANT FEEDING

Most doctors agree that breast feeding is the method of choice for the nutrition of the human infant and indeed in many parts of the world it is vitally important for the infant's survival and well-being. Breast feeding, especially when prolonged after the first year as is common in unsophisticated communities, may prevent the grosser manifestations of protein malnutrition when food is short. Feeding an infant on the breast protects him to some extent from infection, especially infantile gastro-enteritis, provided that no additional food or other material is conveyed to his mouth. Lack of cleanliness, the inability to store milk under satisfactory conditions, and local or tribal practices all militate against successful artificial feeding and in countries where these conditions pertain, mortality among bottle-fed babies is appallingly high. In this country, however, babies thrive perfectly well on many different kinds of milk and methods of feeding,

if due attention is paid to hygiene and technique, and the wishes of the mother should therefore guide the doctor. Some mothers will want to breast feed their infants, while others will prefer to feed them on cow's milk. Whichever method is chosen, the mother should be carefully instructed in the proper techniques. There is an advantage in breast feeding initially even for as little as two weeks, since thereby the risk of neonatal tetany caused by excess phosphate consumption is reduced.

Certain principles must be borne in mind in all systems of infant feeding.

The infant must receive enough food—This obvious fact is frequently forgotten and more babies suffer from underfeeding than is generally realized. After the first few days, the newborn baby will need about 120 calories per kg of body weight. Milk provides about 70 calories per 100ml and sugar about 4 calories per gram. Reconstituted half cream dried milk provides about 60 calories per 100ml. With these few facts the sufficiency of an artificial feed can often be checked in a few moments.

Sufficient fluid must be given—Infa⊥s readily suffer from fluid lack, for they lo⊥e relatively more from the bowel, lungs and skin than the adult, and poor concentration by the newborn kidney makes necessary a larger urinary output. An infant needs at least 150ml of fluid per kg body weight per day.

The diet should contain the proper amounts and kinds of protein, fat and carbohydrate—Presumably the proportions and characters of these in human milk are right for the human infant. Even with dilution and the addition of sugar, cow's milk only approximates to this ideal.

The infant's food should be readily digestible—Human milk is easily digested by the infant. Its curd is not tough and its fats are well tolerated. The same is not true of cow's milk, which requires modification of the tough curd and for some babies slight reduction of the fat content. These objectives are both achieved in the dried milks used widely for infant feeding in this country.

The food must be free from pathogenic organisms—Human milk from healthy breasts satisfies this criterion although of course the nipple will harbour whatever organisms are present on the surface of the breast. Poor social circumstances, in which there is difficulty in keeping cow's milk under hygienic conditions, argue in favour of breast feeding. Gastro-enteritis is rare in breast-fed babies.

Vitamins and minerals must be sufficient—To protect against rickets, an infant needs 400 i.u. of vitamin D daily. Most dried milks contain vitamin D as added calciferol in sufficient quantity to supply the infant's requirements. Especial care must be taken to see that infants fed on fresh cow's milk or on the breast receive additional vitamin supplements as cod liver oil or vitamin concentrate, which will also supply adequate vitamin A. Most milks contain sufficient vitamins of the B group. Unless fed on a dried milk fortified with vitamin C, both breast and bottle-fed infants should be given ascorbic acid daily in the form of fresh orange juice or orange juice concentrate; a few infants vomit orange juice and they may be given rose hip syrup or ascorbic acid. The daily requirement of vitamin C is about 15mg. Mothers should be warned not to boil orange juice since vitamin C may be partly destroyed in this way.

With the exception of iron, the minerals in both human and cow's milk will be sufficient. No additional iron is needed if the infant starts a mixed diet by four to five months, but if there is delay or if the infant is born before term, supplemental iron should be given unless he is fed on a proprietary dried milk with added iron. Syrups containing iron in a chelated form are available commercially; these do not have the unpleasant astringent taste of the iron mixtures formerly in use.

Breast feeding

Breast feeding is an individual physical and emotional experience for each mother, which can give intense personal satisfaction. Encouragement and help by a knowledgeable doctor will often be the deciding factor in successful breast feeding. It has been estimated that about two-thirds of mothers are capable of producing enough milk with a sufficient content of fat. Outputs are very variable, but, in general, young mothers have higher outputs than older mothers.

Colostrum, secreted by the breasts in the first two days or so after parturition, is a yellow fluid containing up to 8 per cent of protein. By the third day usually the change to milk begins ('the milk comes in') and the amount secreted rises rapidly to a mean output of about 450ml (15oz) at the end of the first week. Thereafter the milk yield increases more slowly. Mothers worry sometimes because breast milk looks bluer and more 'watery' than cow's milk but appearance is not a reliable guide to composition, and should not induce the mother to wean her baby if he is contented and gaining weight satisfactorily. Sometimes the full secretion of milk is delayed for a week or so and complementary feeds of diluted milk should then be given to make up the quantity required until adequate lactation is established. These should not be sweetened with sugar in case the infant starts refusing the breast. In hot weather, plain boiled water should be given after or between feeds to prevent dehydration.

There are certain conditions in which breast feeding is contra-indicated.

1. If the mother has active or recently healed tuberculosis she must not feed her baby, for her own condition might be made worse and she will probably infect her infant. The baby should be removed from the mother and vaccinated with B.C.G., separation being continued for at least six weeks or longer if still infective.

2. In mental disease, such as puerperal insanity, since the mother may injure her baby.

3. When the mother has chronic disease, such as cardiac or renal disease; these are not complete contra-indications, the decision depending on the individual circumstances.

4. When another pregnancy supervenes during lactation.

5. In post-partum disorders, such as post-haemorrhagic states or infection, it may not be possible for the mother to feed her baby in the early days; similarly immaturity or illness of the infant may prevent breast feeding. In such cases, the breasts may be expressed until the mother's health improves or until the infant is strong enough to suck from the breast. Few mothers can maintain their milk supply in this way for more than two or three weeks, unless they are very determined.

Suppression of lactation. In recent years there has been a decrease in the percentage of mothers who breast feed, so that in Scotland today only 30 per cent of babies are ever breast fed. While in the past many women were unable to produce enough milk to satisfy the baby, there is no reason to believe that the percentage of these women has increased. There are probably many reasons for the unpopularity of breast feeding. The increasing safety of bottle feeding, the discomfort experienced in the initiation of breast feeding, the uncertainty as to whether the baby is getting enough, physical distaste for the procedure, the known risk of breast abscess and in some cases the need or the desire to go back to work. The incidence of breast feeding is highest in women who have held professional jobs.

Techniques of suppression of lactation and post-natal care of the breasts in general are discussed in Chapter 20. The antenatal care of the breasts is fully described in Chapter 16, on antenatal care.

Techniques and times of breast feeding. The baby should be put to the breast for the first time 6 to 8 hours after birth for one to two minutes at each breast. The time allowed is increased gradually until he is having not more than ten minutes at each breast. During this period, any difficulties in fixing and sucking should be overcome and soon the secretion of breast milk becomes established. The draught or let-down reflex is conditioned and the mother becomes aware of the milk being 'let down' by the tingling sensation in the breast when she begins to feed her baby. The infant plays an active part in the establishment and maintenance of lactation. He draws the nipple into his mouth, his gums champ on the areola, and his tongue and palate play on the nipple. A good nurse and a calm atmosphere are of great help in establishing lactation. The nursing mother should take adequate fluids and a liberal diet but so-called lactagogues are not effective.

When feeding is established, a healthy baby of average size may be fed every four hours, say at 6 and 10 a.m., 2, 6 and 10 or 11 p.m. A feed between 10 p.m. and 6 a.m. may be necessary if the baby wakens during the first few weeks. For smaller infants six or seven three-hourly feeds may be required at first. In self-demand feeding the baby is allowed to determine when and for how long he is fed. This may mean ten or twelve demands daily in the first week or so, but soon the demands decrease until the baby has chosen for himself a three- or four-hourly schedule. Both breasts should be used at each feed, the breast used second at one feed being given first at the next to ensure emptying. The mother must be comfortable and relaxed at feeding times. It is important that the breast should not obstruct the baby's nose and breathing, for successful breast-feeding implies co-ordinated breathing and swallowing. All babies swallow air with their feeds and must be sat up to break wind once or twice during and again at the end of the feed.

Difficulties in breast feeding. Various conditions in the *infant* may cause difficulty. He may be small and feeble; he may suffer from cerebral irritation; he may have a malformation such as cleft palate, cleft lip or micrognathia. Nasal obstruction or oral thrush may prevent adequate sucking.

In the *mother* there may be difficulties from the size and shape of the nipples but these can sometimes be prevented by good antenatal care. Engorgement of the breasts may occur during the first week of the puerperium probably from the rapid withdrawal of inhibiting oestrogen from the mother's blood. It can usually be prevented from becoming extreme if, at the onset, milk is removed by the baby feeding or manual expression.

If this is not done, the breasts become hard, painful and oedematous, and the infant can no longer fix on the nipple. Stilboestrol will often relieve the tension and swelling and meanwhile the infant should not be put to the breast. Cracked nipples are most frequent during the first week, especially in primiparae. There may be an almost invisible fissure or small abrasion and either is very painful. The baby must not be put to the affected breast, which should be emptied by manual expression. Cetrimide cream or other application will usually cause rapid healing and the infant can often resume feeding after 24 hours.

Mastitis and breast abscess, usually staphylococcal, may follow cracked nipples or engorgement, but sometimes arise from no obvious cause. The mother develops fever and her breast becomes tender, red and swollen. The baby should not be put to the affected breast during treatment, but may continue to feed from the other side, though in most cases the mother decides to stop breast feeding.

Underfeeding on the breast—The healthy baby who is underfed fails to gain weight, often sleeps badly and cries a lot. Constipation is common at first but if the underfeeding is prolonged or severe, the stools become frequent, loose and green. Test weighing the baby before and after each feed for 24 hours will confirm the diagnosis. The cause is usually inadequate lactation, which may only be temporary. The mother should be assured that the baby is healthy and care should be taken to see that she is getting sufficient rest and a suitable diet. Giving an unsweetened complementary feed of half-cream milk (say, as much as he wants up to 50ml) will allow the baby to start gaining weight. This in turn, by encouraging the mother, will aid the secretion and flow of milk, and gradually the complementary feeds can be omitted. Underfeeding may of course be due to infection or other disorder in the infant and a careful examination should always be made to exclude infection if the baby shows a disinclination to take the breast.

Overfeeding at the breast—This is seldom a problem, but may occasionally cause vomiting and loose stools. Adjustment of the feeding-time, with a little chloral to the baby if necessary, will usually be all that is required.

Artificial feeding

If the mother cannot or does not wish to feed her infant, suitably modified cow's milk is usually substituted. In some countries goat's milk is used; and for babies with allergic sensitization to cow's milk, a milk freed of lactalbumin or a soya-bean 'milk' is sometimes tried. Various other specially modified milks are available for the treatment of specific disorders in the infant.

COMPARISON OF COW'S MILK AND HUMAN MILK
There are quantitative and qualitative differences between the constituents of the two milks. The *protein* content of human milk is just over 1 per cent, two-thirds being lactalbumin and one-third caseinogen. Cow's milk contains 3·5 per cent protein, of which about four-fifths are caseinogen. Hence cow's milk contains seven times as much caseinogen as human milk, producing a larger, tougher curd in the infant's stomach.

In both milks the average percentage of *fat* is around 3·5, but there are considerable variations. The fat particles of human milk are formed largely from neutral fats and are smaller and more easily digestible than those of cow's milk. Lactose is the *carbohydrate* in both milks and is the most constant constituent—7 per cent in human and 4 per cent in cow's milk. The *mineral* content of human milk is approximately 0·2 per cent, one-quarter that of cow's milk, which contains much more calcium and phosphorus, as well as more sodium, potassium and chlorine. Neither milk contains much iron, but human milk has slightly more. The vitamin content of both is very variable.

Cow's milk requires modification to render it more suitable for infant feeding, and care must be taken that it is completely sterile. The protein can be made more digestible by heat or dilution, and is also suitably modified by modern processes of drying or evaporating milk. At present, dried milk is most frequently used for feeding babies in this country, but evaporated milk and boiled whole fresh milk are also used. Babies will usually thrive equally well on any of these but the keeping qualities and convenience of dried milk make it particularly suitable when domestic facilities are limited. Modern dried milks are fortified with vitamins and iron, so that supplements are not needed, and some are modified by replacing butter fat by vegetable fat (filled milks). If the mother changes to fresh cow's milk without seeking advice about additional sources of vitamins, there is a risk of nutritional deficiency in her baby. For these reasons, the use of fresh cow's milk for infant feeding is discouraged as a national policy.

In 1974 the Department of Health and Social Security recommended that the sodium content of dried milks should be reduced to avoid the risk of hypernatraemia and such dialysed milks are now available.

PRACTICAL DETAILS OF FEEDING
The metric system is widely used in hospitals in this country for calculating feeds, but directions for reconstituting milks for infant feeding are usually given in ounces on the container and British mothers understand this system more readily, so it will be used here.

The fluid requirement of an infant is $2\frac{1}{2}$ fl oz per pound body weight per day (approximately 150ml per kg) but this will vary with changes in metabolic and environmental conditions. Dried milk is reconstituted by adding one level measure of milk powder to 1 fl oz of water—e.g.—a 10-lb baby requires $10 \times 2\frac{1}{2} = 25$ fl oz per day, to which would be added 25 measures of milk powder if feeds are made up in bulk for the day. If each feed is prepared separately, five measures of powder should be added to 5 fl oz of water.

Some proprietary brands of dried milk contain added sugar already, but *not* National

Dried Milk. Both modified (half-cream) and full-cream National Dried Milk and all feeds made from liquid milk require added sugar (cane sugar is satisfactory for this purpose). Add one and a half level teaspoons per feed up to the age of 3 months, and reduce to one level teaspoonful thereafter. Half-cream milk may be used up to the age of 2 weeks, but between 2 and 4 weeks a gradual change should be made to full-cream which should always be used after 4 weeks. Both varieties should be used at full strength for the normal baby. Feeds should be brought to body heat before being given. Feeding is started at about 6 hours after birth, giving boiled water only for one or two feeds. Half-strength milk may be offered thereafter and the strength and quantity rapidly increased until the infant is receiving his full requirements. Most term infants can be fed four-hourly from the start, though small infants may require three-hourly feeds at first. Feeding times should not be rigidly adhered to, even if demand feeding is not practised—e.g. if baby wakes up an hour earlier and is obviously hungry, he should be fed. A few babies may require an extra feed during the night for the first few weeks. In hot weather, the infant should be offered extra boiled water once or twice a day.

The most satisfactory guide to successful feeding is regular weight gain. If the baby is not gaining weight and appears unsatisfied, increase the amount of feed, and go on doing this until he appears satisfied and is gaining weight. If an infant is to be artificially fed, the mother should possess at least three feeding bottles, a bottle-cleaning brush, several teats, containers for sterilizing the bottles and teats, and a glass funnel. All bottles and teats must be cleaned immediately after feeds by frequent rinsing with cold water and by the use, if necessary, of a cleaning brush. Sterilization is effected by boiling or by immersing in a solution of sodium hypochlorite or sodium dichloroisocyanurate. If the boiling method is used, the bottles and teats should be left covered in the water in which they were boiled.

In feeding the infant the bottle should be held so that the teat is always full of milk. When dried milk is used, the fat may separate out during the act of feeding and so the bottle should be shaken once or twice during the feed. Particular attention should be given to the following points of technique:

1. See that the baby is held in a comfortable position while feeding and that the mother is also comfortable and relaxed.

2. See that the hole in the teat is large enough for the milk to drip out slowly when the bottle is inverted.

3. Make sure that the infant breaks wind in the middle of the feed and again at the end. The whole procedure of feeding should not take longer than twenty minutes.

4. All utensils used in the preparation or giving of feeds should be regularly cleaned and sterilized between feeds.

The average weight gain during the first three months of life is 30g (1oz) per day after the first 10 days. After the age of three months the average weight gain is 120g (4oz) per week. Introduction of solid food (weaning) is usually started between one and three months in this country; there is no need to do so before four months but many mothers like to wean earlier, and with normal healthy infants considerable latitude can be allowed.

INFANTS OF LOW BIRTH WEIGHT

An infant born before term may be so immature as to require more than ordinary care and may have disabilities which prejudice his chances of survival or his future development. Gestational age is the best indication of the degree of immaturity but it cannot always be determined and so the body weight at birth has been used as a guide to the quality of care needed. By international agreement a 'premature' infant has been defined as one weighing 2500g ($5\frac{1}{2}$lb) or less at birth, and this definition has proved useful for medical and social comparisons between different communities. Body weight is not a good indication of maturity at birth, however, since about one-third of infants weighing less than 2500g are born after 37 weeks of pregnancy, being small for reasons other than short gestation. An expert committee of the World Health Organisation (1961) recommended that 'low birth weight' should be used in preference to 'premature' to describe these small infants. This term includes infants of body weight appropriate to gestational age who are born early, and so are immature ('pre-term') and also infants born at or near term whose weights are low for gestational age ('light for dates'), usually defined as below the 10th centile.

Table 23.2   Incidence of low birth weight (per cent) by social class*
(All Aberdeen primiparae 1967–70, legitimate single births)

Husband's social class	Wife's father's social class			All classes
	I or II	III	IV or V	
I or II	5·5	6·4	3·3	5·9
III	8·0	8·0	6·6	7·4
IV or V	10·0	10·2	11·7	11·1
All classes	7·3	8·2	8·0	8·1

* Excluding 5·6 per cent of low birth weight infants in whom the wife's father's social class could not be determined.

Table 23.3   Birth weight, gestation period and husband's social class
(All Aberdeen primiparae 1967–70, legitimate single births)

Husband's social class	I or II		IV or V	
Gestation period (weeks)	37 or less	38 or more	37 or less	38 or more
BIRTH WEIGHT (g)	%	%	%	%
Less than 2000	0·8	0·5	2·3	0·5
2000–2499	1·7	2·4	3·4	4·8
2500–3499	3·3	53·2	4·3	52·6
3500 and over	0·5	37·6	0·6	31·6
All weights	6·3	93·7	10·6	89·5

Incidence

The incidence of low birth weight in Scotland is between 7 and 8 per cent but the rate is influenced by many factors, such as the age, health and physique of the mother. For example in Aberdeen primiparae in the years 1967–70, the rate of low birth weight in each 5-year age-group between 15 to 19 and 35 plus was 9·4, 7·8, 6·2, 8·4 and 15·3 per cent respectively. It is difficult to assess accurately the levels of maternal health and physique by direct clinical examination but an indirect measure of these can be obtained by using the Registrar-General's social classification. The justification for the use of this information is based on the observation that those women whose fathers or husbands belong to Social Classes I and II (business and professional men) are healthier and better nourished than those whose fathers and husbands belong to Social Classes IV and V (men with semi- or unskilled jobs). For example, while 8·1 per cent of all Aberdeen primiparae have babies of low birth weight, the rate varies from 5·9 per cent where the husband is in Social Class I or II to 11·1 per cent where he is in Social Class IV or V (Table 23.2).

Table 23.3 shows the relationship of these rates to the duration of pregnancy. It will be seen that in Social Classes I and II, and IV and V the percentages of pregnancies lasting 37 weeks or less were 6·3 and 10·6 respectively. About one quarter of all the babies weighing less than 2000g were born in the 38th week or later and more than half of those weighing between 2000 and 2500g. The table shows that the percentage of babies weighing 3500g or more is greater in Social Classes I and II. Thus the superior health and physique of the women in Classes I and II has two effects: (1) a lower incidence of early onset of labour and (2) heavier babies at all stages of gestation. Of the two, the tendency to heavier babies at each stage of pregnancy does much more to produce the low overall rate of low birth weight in Social Classes I and II than the diminished risk of early onset of labour.

Aetiology

Table 23.4 shows that in about one-third of all firstborn low-weight babies, there is no recognizable obstetric abnormality. There is little doubt that severe toxaemia of pregnancy, antepartum haemorrhage, malformation of the fetus and maternal disease such as diabetes, cardiac or pulmonary disorders, predispose to low birth weight, but it is unlikely that mild toxaemia—i.e. a rise of blood pressure to

Table 23.4   Liveborn infants of low birth weight, 1967–70
Associated maternal conditions
(All Aberdeen primiparae, legitimate births)

Maternal condition	Single births %	Twin births %
Normal	36·2	28·6
Severe toxaemia	5·6	14·3
Moderate toxaemia	7·2	28·6
Mild toxaemia	14·8	14·3
Antepartum haemorrhage	12·8	9·5
Threatened abortion	18·4	0·0
Maternal disease	4·9	4·8

140/90mm occurring for the first time after the 20th week of pregnancy with not more than a trace of albumin in the urine—has any effect on the weight of the baby. In fact in the years in question, there were 35 infants of low birth weight in 749 cases where mild toxaemia was the only detectable obstetric abnormality, giving the low rate of 4·7 per cent. The factors responsible for low birth weight in the 36·2 per cent of cases where the pregnancy seemed normal are difficult to determine but attention has already been drawn to the influence of age and social class, which also have an effect in the cases where there are important obstetric factors. It is clear therefore that where the standard of obstetric care is uniformly high the incidence of low birth weight is determined more by general factors such as the type of patient and her state of health than by the medical complications of pregnancy.

Characteristics of pre-term infants

Infants born at less than 37 completed weeks often weigh very much less than 2500g (5½lb), are likely to be less than 46cm (18·2 inches) in length, and are small and frail with relatively big hands and head. The ears are soft and poorly formed. The skin is fine, often lanugo-covered, delicate and easily infected. The labia minora are relatively large. The abdomen is protuberant and thin-walled. The cry is feeble. Sucking and swallowing are weak, and may be absent in very immature infants. Mucus gathers in the mouth and the cough reflex is poor; regurgitation, which easily occurs even before food is given, involves the danger of aspiration pneumonia. Expansion of the lungs is difficult, breathing may be irregular with apnoeic periods, and cyanosis readily occurs with handling and feeding. Bones and muscles are softer than in the term infant. The temperature is unstable and is not a good guide in prognosis. Antenatal storage of minerals, vitamins, and general body constituents is deficient, and this causes, among other things, tendencies to rickets and anaemia. The immune response is poorly developed: infections are readily acquired and may give rise to few signs. Staphylococci, colon bacilli, monilia and respiratory viruses constitute a greater threat to pre-term than to term babies. Jaundice is more common and more intense as enzyme systems in general, and that for bilirubin conjugation and excretion in particular, are poorly developed. The stomach capacity is small, fat is poorly absorbed (but not sugar and protein) and the stools are variable in frequency and consistency. Diarrhoea rapidly produces dangerous depletion of water and electrolytes. There is some functional immaturity of the kidneys and hence care must be exercised in the giving and in the withholding of fluid and electrolytes. In the first week the pre-term infant has a greater percentage of loss of his birth weight and regains it more slowly than the term baby.

Though the skull is thin and excessive moulding may occur, haemorrhage resulting from birth trauma is uncommon. The danger of cerebral haemorrhage is increased, especially in the presence of anoxia, by the fragility of the capillaries. Malformations are more common than in term babies and may affect any organ but chiefly the central nervous system, gastro-intestinal tract and heart—in that order. The pre-term infant, then, has many disadvantages, the greatest being immaturity of the respiratory mechanisms; survival largely depends on the degree of development of the lungs at birth.

Characteristics of light-for-dates infants

Infants whose birth weights are disproportionately low for gestational age vary greatly in their characteristics, since there are many causes of their low weight. Some are apparently normal, being light in weight for genetic reasons, and have no distinguishing characteristics apart from their small size. The growth of others has been retarded by placental or maternal disorders, especially those affecting blood supply to the fetus. Congenital malformations of genetic or intra-uterine environmental origin may also be associated with poor growth. Such different aetiologies account for the differences between light-for-dates infants: these have not yet been clearly related to causes, however, and light-for-dates infants are still considered as one group, though it must be realized that it is not a homogeneous one.

Many light-for-dates infants appear alert and active and seem neurologically mature. Some show loss of subcutaneous fat, appearing thin and wizened, and there may be meconium staining of the skin, which is dry and peels readily. Though these changes may occur in babies of any gestational age, they are most often seen in those born after term and have therefore been attributed to failing placental function. However, their relationship to the efficiency of the placenta and to low birth weight is far from clear. In some cases, meconium passed before birth has been inhaled, giving rise to difficulties in establishing breathing. Respiratory difficulties are also liable to arise from massive intrapulmonary haemorrhage, to which light-for-dates infants are especially prone.

Prolonged intra-uterine hypoxia is likely to cause serious post-natal acidaemia, while an adverse prenatal environment causes depletion of carbohydrate stores, leading to neonatal hypoglycaemia. Depression of the blood glucose level may be rapid and prolonged, often to 10mg per 100ml or less. Frequent estimation of the blood glucose following birth, with intravenous administration of glucose if necessary, is therefore essential if cerebral damage from hypoglycaemia is to be avoided.

Although the light-for-dates baby is particularly liable to acidaemia and hypoglycaemia, in other respects he is metabolically at an advantage compared with the pre-term infant. It must be remembered, however, that a light-for-dates infant can be born at any stage of gestation and can therefore also be pre-term, in which case he will suffer from all the disadvantages of immaturity as well as those of fetal growth retardation.

COMPLICATIONS OF IMMATURITY

The respiratory distress syndrome—The pulmonary alveoli of the newborn infant at term are lined with a surface-active phospholipid (surfactant) which prevents complete alveolar collapse on expiration, so that the residual air necessary for satisfactory ventilation is retained in the lungs. Pre-term infants may lack adequate amounts of surfactant and so are prone to atelectasis and consequent respiratory difficulties. Transudation of fibrin-containing material from the pulmonary capillaries into the alveoli adds to the respiratory distress and the infant may die within a few hours or days of birth. At necropsy the lungs show patchy atelectasis and the alveoli are lined with the fibrinous transudate (hyaline membrane). It is not yet clear whether the transudation is due to increased permeability of pulmonary capillaries or is a secondary effect of deficiency of surfactant. Infants who die in respiratory distress commonly have associated haemorrhage into the cerebral ventricles (intraventricular haemorrhage).

The respiratory distress syndrome is characteristically seen in immature infants who may have been difficult to resuscitate and who show increasing difficulty in respiration within a few hours of birth. There is progressive indrawing of the ribs and sternum with each inspiration, the respiratory rate rises to over 60 per minute and there is an audible respiratory grunt. As hypoxia and hypercapnia develop the pulmonary vascular resistance increases and there is reduced pulmonary blood flow, with right to left shunting of blood through the ductus and the foramen ovale. Deficient oxygenation is accentuated by blood flow through unaerated areas of the lungs, which increases the total right to left shunt. The infant becomes cyanosed, respiratory and metabolic acidosis develop and death may ensue usually within 36 hours.

Respiratory distress may also result from pneumonia, intra-pulmonary haemorrhage, pneumothorax or diaphragmatic hernia: radiological examination of the chest will often help in diagnosis, since infants with respiratory distress associated with hyaline membrane show a characteristic diffuse granular appearance of the lung fields, the bronchi being clearly outlined with air (air bronchogram).

About one-third of all infants who develop respiratory distress syndrome are likely to die, the mortality rate depending on the number of very immature infants, the frequency of associated intraventricular haemorrhage and the quality of care given. In addition to all the ordinary measures in the management of low birth weight, attempts should be made to increase oxygenation by raising the ambient oxygen concentration or by continuous positive airway pressure (CPAP): to diminish the metabolic component of the acidosis by infusing alkali: and possibly to remove carbon dioxide by artificial ventilation (Fig. 23.1), though the clinical indications for this have not yet been established.

Despite improvements in management, respiratory distress syndrome remains the most important cause of neonatal death in this country.

Inhalation of feeds, mucus, or regurgitated stomach contents readily occurs, sometimes even with the most careful handling and feeding. Aspiration pneumonia is found at necropsy more often than it is diagnosed clinically. Any baby who suddenly has breathing difficulty should be suspected of having inhaled food or vomitus and the nasopharynx should be aspirated carefully. Oxygen is given if required and antibiotic prophylaxis should be started.

Cyanotic attacks occur with cerebral haemorrhage, with pathological lung states, and with congenital heart disease, but are often simply signs of immaturity. In very small babies, apnoea readily follows handling and feeding, or may occur spontaneously. Breathing may start again after some seconds, but if the episode lasts longer than half a minute there is a risk of brain damage. Close and continuous observation is essential if apnoeic attacks are to be detected and cut short by peripheral stimulation, or by intubation and ventilation if necessary. A baby subject to apnoeic spells may be nursed on an apnoea alarm mattress, which gives an audible indication when the baby's respiratory movements stop.

Pre-term infants are deficient in the enzyme which conjugates bilirubin (glucuronyl transferase), have low levels of plasma albumin, which binds bilirubin, and have other physiological disabilities, all of which render them liable to *hyperbilirubinaemia*, and to kernicterus if the unconjugated bilirubin in the blood rises to about 20 to 25mg per 100ml. Untreated babies who develop kernicterus show, towards the end of the first week, rolling of the eyes, head retraction and lethargy, and many die in a few days with increasing jaundice and fever. In others recovery may seem to take place but most of these show residual athetoid cerebral palsy with high-tone deafness. With modern methods of treatment, kernicterus should seldom if ever occur. Overdosage with vitamin K and sulphonamides leads to increased jaundice and must be avoided. A rise in plasma bilirubin to dangerous heights may

often be prevented by exposing the infant to light (phototherapy), taking care to protect the eyes from the light source. In some cases, however, an exchange transfusion will be required to prevent the bilirubin rising above 20mg per 100ml; some paediatricians prefer to transfuse at lower levels.

Intracranial haemorrhage may occur during delivery, or early in the first week, especially after breech or other difficult deliveries. It is often intraventricular, subarachnoid, or subependymal in site, and may give rise to respiratory difficulty or to twitching and convulsions.

Anaemia is common and has many causes, as in any newborn infant. The pre-term infant is particularly liable to anaemia, however, because the red cell mass at birth is small and the rate of post-natal growth relatively rapid. Additional factors are the accentuated post-natal fall in the number of red cells, inadequate erythropoiesis due to immaturity of the bone marrow, and insufficient stores of iron. The anaemia is commonly normochromic and the haemoglobin may fall to 7g per 100ml or less a month after birth. Infants born many weeks before term are especially likely to develop megaloblastic anaemia as a result of folate deficiency.

Rickets may occur in the rapidly-growing pre-term infant and may not be entirely prevented by giving vitamin D, since the intake of calcium and phosphorus may be the limiting factor.

Hypothermia or cold injury occurs in small newborn infants subjected to environmental cooling, as may happen in the home during the night. The baby is apathetic and refuses to feed. The red face contrasts with the pale, oedematous body, which feels very cold. Recovery may follow gradual re-warming and treatment with glucose, oxygen and antibiotics as necessary, but mortality is high.

Retrolental fibroplasia is due to the use of oxygen in greater than 30 to 40 per cent concentration over too long a period. The vessels of the retina become dilated and tortuous and haemorrhages appear. The retina becomes detached, especially at the periphery, a fibrous mass is formed in the vitreous, and blindness results. Both eyes are usually involved. In the early stages the condition is reversible but nothing can be done when the retrolental mass has formed.

Care of low birth weight infants

Whenever the birth of a low weight infant is anticipated, arrangements should be made for it to take place in a fully-equipped hospital and a member of the paediatric staff should be in attendance at the delivery. Drugs and anaesthetics that depress the infant's respiratory centre should be used as sparingly as possible. When the baby is born, the umbilical cord should not be cut until it has stopped pulsating. If he is in poor condition, however, or if he does not breathe readily, it may be preferable to divide the cord at once and accept possible disadvantages of a smaller red cell mass. The baby is then received into a warmed sterile towel and laid on his side with the head slightly lowered. The airways should be cleared gently and an intramuscular injection of vitamin K_1 given. Resuscitation if required must be exceptionally gentle and skilful. Since loss of body heat occurs very rapidly, no time must be lost in transferring the baby to a warm cot or incubator.

Infants of low birth weight should be under the care of nurses and doctors with special experience and training. They must be handled with great care and observed constantly, by day and night. The smaller infants, whether pre-term or light-for-dates, are best cared for in a special care nursery provided with incubators, a piped supply of oxygen, air and suction, facilities for intensive care and an adequate number of nursing and medical staff. Such nurseries are costly to equip and run and must be of a reasonable size to function efficiently. They should therefore be limited in numbers and serve relatively large populations, catering both for infants of low birth weight and for other newborn infants requiring special care. Those infants whose low weight at birth has not been anticipated and who are born in smaller hospitals or at home, should be transferred to the special care nursery as quickly as possible after birth. Larger infants who seem normal may be nursed with their mothers in ordinary post-natal wards or at home, but the danger of unsuspected hypoglycaemia in a light-for-dates infant must not be forgotten, nor must the large immature baby of the woman with latent or chemical diabetes be overlooked. While the baby is in the special care nursery, his mother should be encouraged to visit and handle him frequently, so that she gains confidence and establishes the desirable close relationship with her baby.

Control of environment. For larger infants nursed in cots the temperature of the room should be 21-24 °C (70-75 °F). A relative humidity of 60-65 per cent is best but in practice infants tolerate drier air and in this country humidity is not carefully controlled unless the baby is in an incubator or receiving oxygen therapy. Smaller infants should always be cared for in incubators in a nursery at 27 °C (81 °F), the temperature in the incubator being adjusted to between 32 and 35 °C (90-95 °F) according to the condition of the infant, aiming to maintain the body temperature as near to 36·5 °C (97·7 °F) as possible. A perspex shield within the incubator helps to diminish loss of heat by radiation. In general, the pre-term infant requires a higher ambient temperature than the light-for-dates infant of the same body weight. The infant should be naked except for a soft napkin so that he can easily be observed. The hands are only covered if there is a risk of his pulling out a nasogastric tube; tubular gauze without threads should be used, since a thread from a glove can cause gangrene if it becomes twisted tightly round a finger.

Oxygen in a concentration not exceeding 40 per cent is used for babies who are cyanosed, the concentration being lowered as soon as cyanosis is dispelled. Exceptionally a higher concentration may be required but should be used for as brief a period as possible. The passage of all gases through or over water ensures that humidity is kept at 65 to 70 per cent, or higher if there is respiratory difficulty.

When the baby reaches a weight of about 2000g and is thriving, he may be transferred to a cot in a warm room, and finally to a cooler room. From there he will go home when he has reached a weight of 2300 to 2700g, depending on his general condition, the capability of his mother and the circumstances of his home environment. A few days beforehand, it is desirable to admit the mother to hospital to learn how to look after her baby, especially as regards feeding, bathing and care of the skin. The family doctor and the health visitor or district nurse should be informed of the impending discharge.

Prevention of infection. The most important single factor is a high standard of nursing. The nursing staff should be supervised by a specially trained sister or midwife, and there should be a total nursing staff ratio of one nurse to each infant in the nursery. No one with a cold, sore throat or other infection should ever enter a special care nursery. It is not necessary to put each baby in a separate cubicle to obtain good results, although single cubicles have certain advantages. A convenient arrangement is to have 4–8 incubators or cots in a room with a floor space of 30 sq ft for each. Glass walls should line the corridors for easy visibility. Each room or cubicle should contain a wash-hand basin, piped oxygen, air and suction, and a weighing machine capable of weighing to the nearest 5g. The walls must be kept clean and floors should be oiled and dry-sweeping prohibited to minimize the risk of contamination of the air with dust. Each infant should have his own bath, linen and nursing equipment in the locker of his cot. All nurses and doctors must wash their hands on entering the nursery and also before and after every handling of an infant. The nurse should put on a special gown or other form of protection when attending to an infant to prevent his coming in contact with her clothing. Soiled napkins and clothes must be dropped straight into special containers and taken to the laundry by porters. Nurses must on no account sort out, count or wash soiled linen, and 'sluicing' should always be done by non-nursery personnel. The work of the milk-kitchen (formula-room) should be done by a special staff, the nurses in training taking duty in rotation.

Babies suspected or known to be infected should be isolated in single cubicles in a self-contained part of the nursery, and looked after by nurses who do not come in contact with other babies. All examinations and treatment should be carried out in the baby's cubicle.

The skin of pre-term infants is easily abraded and infected and is probably washed, rubbed, anointed and powdered too frequently in most nurseries. All that is needed at birth is to remove blood from the face, and thereafter to keep the napkin area clean. Bathing can be omitted during the first few weeks, and started only when the baby is over 2000g in weight. Hexachlorophane powder may be applied to the body, especially to the perineum, groins, axillae and umbilicus, but should be used sparingly since accumulation of hexachlorophane on the skin may be absorbed and is potentially neurotoxic.

Feeding—This requires infinite care; there are dangers in delaying feeding and also in feeding too early and in giving too much in the first days of life. Late feeding carries the risks of hypoglycaemia, hyperbilirubinaemia and unnecessarily prolonged acidaemia. Vomiting, cyanotic attacks and inhalation pneumonia may be caused by feeding too early, or by poor feeding techniques. More mature infants will be able to suck and to swallow from the beginning: less mature ones may be able to swallow but not suck, and some can do neither. Babies with poor sucking and swallowing reflexes will have to be fed by gavage; this is done by passing a soft catheter (size 8 to 10 French Gauge) through the mouth into the oesophagus for a distance equal to that between the bridge of the nose and the xiphisternum and allowing the feed to run in by gravity from a funnel attached to the tube. The baby should not cough or choke if the tube is inserted properly. The feed is given slowly; and the tube is then pulled out slowly and pinched while being withdrawn to avoid fluid dripping from the end of the catheter and entering the larynx. The head of the cot should be raised while the feed is being given and for 10–15 minutes thereafter. Alternatively, an indwelling nasogastric catheter (5 FG) can be used, especially where disturbance of the baby is particularly undesirable. It is passed down the nose into the stomach and can be left in place for a few days at a time, the feeds being put in by a syringe. In very tiny or seriously ill infants, the initial feeds may have to be given intravenously.

Whatever the method of feeding used, it should be started within 12 hours of birth; in general, light-for-dates infants can be fed earlier and given larger quantities than pre-term ones. Starting with small amounts, the feeds are gradually increased according to the infant's tolerance. The first feed is usually given a few hours after birth and consists of 5 or 10 per cent glucose in water. Thereafter feeds of breast milk or modified dried milk are given, the latter at half strength for a day or two and then at full strength. A suitable quantity is 60ml per kg in the first 24 hours of feeding, starting with 5 to 10ml per feed and giving a feed every 2 hours. The quantity is gradually increased and later the intervals between feeds may be lengthened. By the end of the first week, the baby should be receiving 150ml per kg daily in 8 feeds. Very small vigorous infants may require as much as 200ml per kg daily. If tube feeding is necessary initially, the change to bottle feeding should be made when the baby begins to suck the tube and when a trial bottle feed has been successful.

Even if the dried milk is fortified, additional vitamins will be required, for the baby will have started life with low reserves and needs an increased supply in view of the rapid growth that occurs. After the first week 50mg of ascorbic acid and 400iu of vitamin D are needed daily, usually combined with other vitamins in an aqueous concentrate. In this way rickets and scurvy can be prevented but it may be more difficult to prevent anaemia, especially in the first three months. Iron should be given from the age of one month and continued until the infant is on a full mixed diet. A preparation of iron in chelated form is often tolerated better than ferrous sulphate. Infants weighing less than 1500g at birth should also receive folic acid for a few weeks.

Prognosis in low birth weight
The outlook, immediate and remote, depends on the birth weight and degree of maturity, and also, to a less extent, on the presence of malformations, the occurrence of complications, the medical and nursing care in the neonatal period, and the home conditions thereafter. Death occurs usually in the first 48 hours of life and the prognosis improves with each day of survival thereafter. Half of the deaths occur on the first day and a fifth of them on the second day. The mortality rate rises steeply as birth weight declines. The importance of low birth weight as a lethal factor is shown by the fact that, although only 7 per cent of babies are 2500g or less at birth, this group contributes about two-thirds of the deaths in the first week.

The improvement in mortality rates in recent years has many causes and the influence of each factor cannot be isolated and assessed accurately. In general, it is the result of rising standards of obstetric and paediatric care and always in the background the long-term educational and preventive work of community health departments. Rising standards of living, better nutrition in consequence, younger age at marriage and a decreasing incidence of the very large family are imponderable factors which have nevertheless been of great importance.

Death rates and morbidity in infants of low birth weight throughout the whole of the first year and even up to four years of age are relatively high—mostly due to congenital defects and infections (respiratory and gastro-intestinal). It should be noted that, in general, death rates for infants born at term whose birth weights are well below the 10th percentile for gestational age are higher than for infants of the same birth weight born early. Asphyxia, pneumonia and pulmonary haemorrhage are the principal causes of this increased mortality.

Infants of low birth weight are later than usual in reaching the physical and mental milestones, even when age calculated from the date of conception is used, and as a group they are still smaller and lighter than children of good birth weight (over 2500g) on reaching the age of school entry. The smallest babies have an increased risk of mental subnormality and neurological defect.

Although better methods of management are reducing death rates in infants of low birth weight and morbidity among those who survive, the aims must still be to prevent pre-term birth and to promote healthy fetal growth. These constitute major problems of obstetrics and human ecology.

PERINATAL ASPHYXIA AND TRAUMA

Pathogenesis of asphyxia

Anoxia, or more accurately *hypoxia*, denotes inadequate oxygenation of the fetus or newborn infant. The term *asphyxia* was formerly used to describe the clinical condition of the infant who did not breathe at birth but now encompasses the changes which follow failure of respiratory gas exchange, *viz.* falling oxygen levels, rising carbon dioxide levels and falling pH of the blood, as a result of respiratory and metabolic acidosis. *Apnoea* is failure to breathe spontaneously and may be a cause of neonatal asphyxia.

Anoxia may be present before birth, during labour or after delivery and may or may not be accompanied by the other changes of asphyxia, depending on the cause. Until recently it was believed that the fetus existed in an oxygen environment well below the levels of extra-uterine life but new experimental evidence indicates that the level is only a little below that of normal adult life and that the fetus does not normally suffer from oxygen lack.

Anoxia of the fetus in utero may occur for a variety of reasons. Such conditions as toxaemia of pregnancy, accidental haemorrhage, maternal anaemia or heart disease, and abnormal placental function may lower the oxygen saturation in the fetal blood. When the fetus is anaemic, as in erythroblastosis, the anoxia is of a different type (anaemic anoxia) and the lesions are different. Compression of the umbilical cord, which occurs if it prolapses or is wrapped round a part of the fetus, may cause cessation of its circulation so that the oxygen supply to the fetus is cut off abruptly. Unless the compression is released quickly the fetus will die.

Normal labour diminishes gas exchange across the placenta but this hardly affects the healthy newborn infant. However, a fetus suffering from anoxia from one or other of the causes enumerated above may not be sufficiently oxygenated to survive even a normal labour. Prolonged labour, particularly if it is associated with irregular hypertonic uterine contractions, may lead to more severe asphyxia. Undue compression of the fetal head as in cephalopelvic disproportion causes kinking of the main cerebral veins with local congestion and intracranial anoxia.

It is impossible to estimate the degree of anoxia which will prove fatal or cause permanent damage to the fetus. It is known, however, that a baby can be born alive and vigorous and survive apparently undamaged with the oxygen saturation of the haemoglobin in the cord blood well below 20 per cent, and even below 5 per cent. The duration of asphyxia, as judged by pH and PCO_2, is probably more important than the oxygen saturation at birth.

Pre-existing asphyxia may be of such severity that *after delivery* the heart progressively slows and stops and respiration is not established. If less severe, the respiratory centre is not so depressed and breathing becomes regular after a few preliminary gasps. Asphyxia may develop *after delivery* even if the oxygen saturation has been good both before and during labour. This may be due to depression of the respiratory centre by a rise in subtentorial pressure following traumatic haemorrhage or by anaesthetic or analgesic drugs given to the mother during labour or at delivery.

Even if the respiratory centre has not been depressed before birth, blockage of the larger air passages by material inhaled during labour may cause asphyxia to develop after birth. The obstruction may be in the finer bronchioles so that circulation of air in the alveoli cannot take place, but in such cases respiration is usually established. It must be emphasized that mechanical obstruction to respiration constitutes a much more serious risk to the already asphyxiated baby than to the one without depression of the respiratory centre.

When there is inadequate oxygenation either *in utero* or after birth, the infant is able to utilize his faculty for anaerobic metabolism and can live for 20 to 30 minutes without oxygen and for longer periods with a very deficient supply. The duration of survival may depend on reserves of glycogen in the body and these may have been depleted by asphyxia operating for some time before birth; if so, the infant will die quickly unless adequate oxygenation can be achieved soon after birth.

The mildly asphyxiated infant is usually cyanosed, the pulse strong and regular and the muscle tone good. The mouth is often firmly closed and a finger inserted to the soft palate or beyond causes the baby to tighten the muscles of the pharynx in an attempt to expel it.

In severe asphyxia the baby is paler and may be slightly blue or grey-white. The heart usually beats very slowly and the force is very poor; in fact, the impulse on the chest wall may be difficult to feel. The muscle tone is poor so that the baby is very limp and stimulation of the soft palate produces no response.

In the absence of treatment, recovery may be delayed for many minutes. It starts with the onset of respiratory efforts. To begin with irregular gulps or gasps occur, sometimes at quite long intervals, and gradually give way to more regular respirations at shorter intervals and later to crying. As soon as breathing begins the baby's colour improves and gradually becomes pink, but the extremities and the area round the mouth may remain pale or slightly blue for some time, especially in the more severely shocked babies, indicating that the peripheral capillary circulation has not yet returned to normal. The severely asphyxiated infant is especially liable to intracranial haemorrhage, since haemostasis may be deranged due to disseminated intravascular coagulation.

Treatment of asphyxia

Asphyxial changes arising *in utero* may be anticipated and prevented by induction of labour, for instance, in severe toxaemia, in diabetes or in the elderly primigravida, especially if pregnancy is prolonged unduly. Where asphyxia has developed, immediate Caesarean section may be necessary. If it is believed that hypoxia is developing as the result of fetal anaemia, intra-uterine transfusion may be valuable, while if there is maternal hypoxia, the administration of oxygen to the mother may help.

Preparations should always be made for the resuscitation of a newborn infant, but when the risk of asphyxia is increased, special facilities should be available. If at all possible the birth should take place in a large maternity hospital with adequate paediatric facilities. Meconium staining of the liquor amnii in cephalic presentations or in the first stage of labour in breech presentation is evidence that the fetus is receiving insufficient oxygen and if, in addition, the fetal heart-rate becomes slow and irregular the oxygen lack is probably critical. There is some evidence that the passage of meconium is characteristic of slowly developing asphyxia, e.g. due to placental failure. On the other hand, sudden slowing and irregularity of the fetal heart without the passage of meconium is more likely to result from obstruction of the umbilical vessels because the cord has become tangled round the neck or limbs or has prolapsed. Unfortunately the degree of hypoxia cannot be measured accurately by either of these signs and sometimes the fetal heart stops beating with little or no warning. Sampling of fetal blood for analysis during labour and assessment of meconium staining by amnioscopy are currently being evaluated and hold out some hope of improving diagnosis. Until better methods of assessing the state of the fetus are available, however, clinical management of the labour will continue to be difficult.

On delivery oxygen must reach the vital centres in the baby's brain as quickly as possible and it is important that the general principles of resuscitation be clearly understood and promptly applied. If the respiratory centre is depressed by anoxia it will not respond to any stimulus until oxygenated blood reaches it. If it is depressed by traumatic haemorrhage or drugs the baby must be kept alive until the centre can respond. It is self-evident that respiratory interchange can only take place if the air passages are clear of mucus, amniotic debris, or inhaled material. Chilling should be avoided, but the baby should not be warmed too vigorously as this increases the need for oxygen. The techniques of resuscitation are described on page 425.

Perinatal trauma

Injury to the baby is most likely to occur with abnormal presentations or positions and in cases of disproportion between the head or shoulders of the baby and the birth canal. At one time cerebral birth trauma was probably the most frequent cause of stillbirth. For example, Holland in 1922 estimated that about 50 per cent of stillbirths were due to this cause.

The incidence of serious birth injury is now low in countries or communities where living standards are high, since contracted pelvis is rare and the obstetric services are usually well developed. Good antenatal care and the wider use of Caesarean section and low forceps delivery have greatly reduced the risk to the baby. On the other hand, in some underdeveloped countries or in the poorer districts of many large cities malnutrition with associated contracted pelvis is common. Birth injury in such areas is still frequent, particularly where the standard of obstetrics is poor.

Bruises and laceration of skin—These are usually slight. The scalp may become oedematous and easily bruised if the fetal head is allowed to remain too long on the pelvic floor

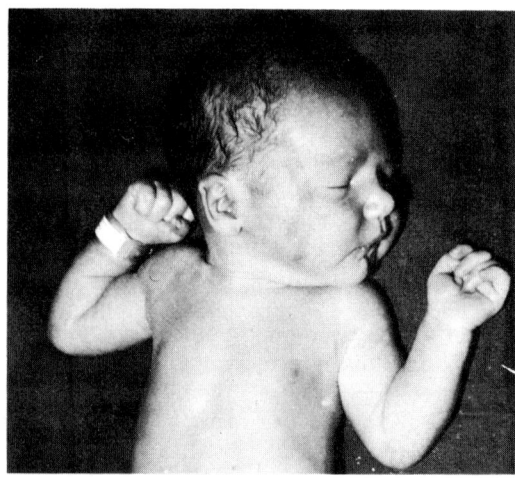

Fig. 23.4   Mark of forceps on face.

or distending the perineum in the second stage of labour. The baby's genitalia or buttocks in a breech presentation, or the eyelids, nose and lips in a face presentation, may become very oedematous and congested. Forceps blades are liable to abrade the skin (Fig. 23.4) and the use of the ventouse may cause local swelling and ecchymoses. As a rule such injuries heal very quickly: gentian violet, 1 per cent aqueous solution, should be applied and the area kept as dry as possible. If redness or other signs of infection develop the appropriate antibiotic should be used. Deeper cuts or lacerations should be stitched.

The caput—The presenting part of the fetus is usually surmounted at birth by a localized area of oedema formed from pressure of the soft tissues of the birth canal. The caput may be sited over any of the skull bones, on the anterior buttock, on the face, the brow, or the shoulder of the infant at birth. There is exudation of blood into the subcutaneous tissues and, where the resistance of the mother's birth canal is high or labour prolonged, the caput may be extensive. Usually the tissues return to normal in a few days, but superficial breaks in the skin may need treatment.

Cephalhaematoma—This is due to a localized extravasation of blood between the periosteum and the skull bones and is therefore usually limited to the area of one bone, although several bones may be separately affected. There may also be a linear fracture. The swelling may not be obvious until one or two days after birth but may then become quite large so that the head appears deformed, especially if the swelling is bilateral (Fig. 23.5). The blood is fluid at first but the serum soon collects in the centre and the clot round the edges of the haematoma may then be invaded by osteoblasts derived from the displaced periosteum. The hard ridge so formed may simulate a depressed fracture. The blood usually takes some weeks to absorb but recovery is complete and there is no residual thickening. No treatment is necessary as a rule but if there are any abrasions of the scalp over the area special care should be taken to prevent infection, since bacterial invasion of the extravasated blood might be serious. The cause of cephalhaematoma is obscure and while it may occur in normal labour it is more liable to happen after difficult vertex or breech delivery.

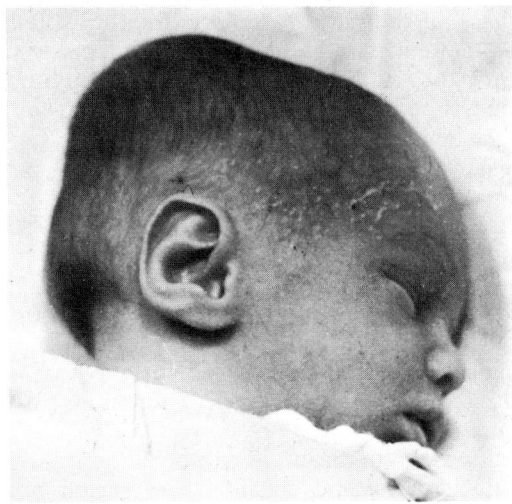

Fig. 23.5   Cephalhaematoma.

Sternomastoid 'tumour'—About a week to ten days after birth a firm swelling may appear in one or other sternomastoid muscle, usually about the middle. It is believed to be due to exuberant formation of fibrous tissue following necrosis of muscle fibres at birth. There is little likelihood of later torticollis but the mother can avoid this possibility by stretching the muscle several times daily. The swelling disappears after about two months.

Injury to bones
Fracture of the clavicle, usually unilateral, is not uncommon even in relatively easy labours, although it occurs most often where there has been difficulty in delivery of the shoulders.. It may not be recognized, for pain appears to be slight. The arm may not be used as freely as it should be or a swelling from the callus which forms in large amounts may be noted after a week, usually near the centre of the bone. Crepitus is seldom felt and should not be sought. The bone soon heals and treatment is not usually necessary, though the arm may be bandaged lightly over the chest for a few days if desired.

The *humerus* or the *femur* may rarely be broken in difficult breech delivery—the humerus just below the deltoid insertion and the femur about the centre of the shaft. There may be radial nerve injury associated with fracture of the humerus. The striking deformity makes diagnosis easy. Adhesive strapping, 5cm wide, can be put round the arm at the site of fracture and the arm lightly bandaged to the chest for ten days. A femoral fracture should be treated more energetically and to prevent permanent anteroposterior bending the limbs should be put up in traction-suspension for a fortnight.

Multiple fractures are seen in the rare condition *osteogenesis imperfecta congenita,* a disease inherited recessively. There may be widespread fractures of the limbs, which are grossly deformed, and of the skull, which is soft, has wide membranous spaces, and often bulges in the parietal regions. Many of these babies are stillborn, others survive two or three weeks, a few for years. There is no treatment.

The *spine* of the infant is rarely injured as it is able to withstand considerable tension provided traction is in the long axis. Strong traction, however, on the hyperextended spine or strong lateral traction, as may occur when there is difficulty with delivery of the shoulders or with the after-coming head, may cause fracture and separation of the vertebrae, usually the seventh cervical and first thoracic. The degree of spinal cord injury depends on the degree of displacement of the vertebrae and complete transection of the cord with subsequent paralysis can occur. Most infants so damaged die soon after birth from this or other associated injuries but in those who survive the degree of permanent paralysis is much less than that present in the first few days.

The *skull* of the infant is rarely fractured but furrows or spoon-shaped depressions may arise, even during spontaneous delivery, from pressure on the promontory of the sacrum or on irregular bony areas in the pelvis. There is no true fracture and no pressure symptoms. The depressed area may need elevation by operation if it does not rapidly right itself. True fractures can occur when there is undue compression of the skull in forceps delivery in cases of cephalopelvic disproportion. Although serious the condition is not necessarily fatal.

Injury to viscera
The *liver* and *adrenal* glands may very occasionally be damaged by compression, especially during breech deliveries. It used to occur when some of the older methods of resuscitation involving vigorous flexion and extension of the infant's trunk were used. Haemorrhage into the adrenal gland or intraperitoneal

haemorrhage from rupture of the liver may cause death from shock.

Injuries to nerves
The facial nerve is unprotected after its exit from the stylomastoid foramen and may be compressed by the tip of a forceps blade at that point or where it crosses the ramus of the mandible. Injury may also occur in spontaneous deliveries. The external muscles of the mouth and eye are rendered immobile but sucking is not interfered with (Fig. 23.6).

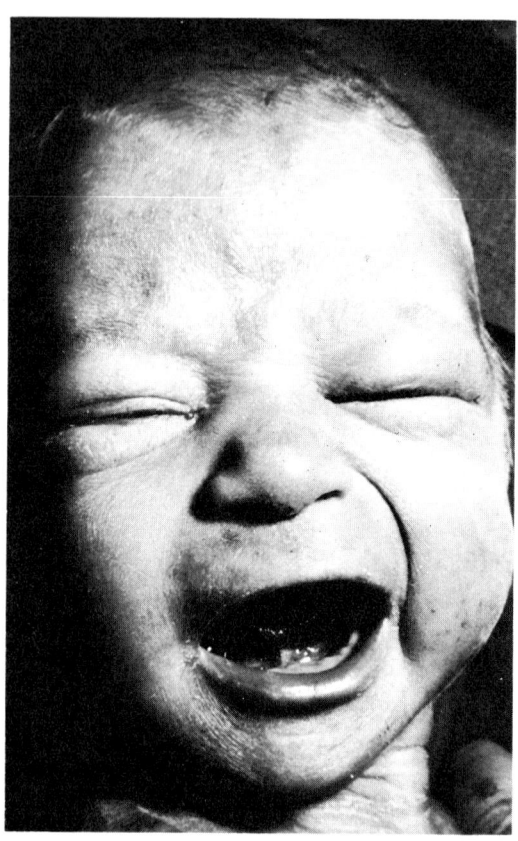

Fig. 23.6　Right-sided facial paralysis.

Recovery usually takes place in two weeks since the lesion is most commonly due to haemorrhage and oedema round the nerve trunk, and the only treatment necessary is to protect the eye until the muscles regain their power.

The nerve roots or trunks of the brachial plexus may be damaged by extreme lateral traction of the head on the shoulders. Excessive digital pressure against the axilla or forceful extension and abduction of the shoulder during delivery of an arm may have the same result. The fifth and sixth cervical roots are those most commonly injured with subsequent paralysis of the upper arm, a lesion known as *Erb's palsy*. The affected arm is rotated inwardly at the shoulder and is held in extension and adduction. The forearm is pronated and the palm directed posterolaterally. If the seventh and eighth cervical and first thoracic are also damaged the whole arm and hand are affected. If, rarely, the damage is limited to the lower roots and the hand alone is affected, the lesion is known as *Klumpke's paralysis*. The phrenic nerve is derived in part from those same roots of the brachial plexus and unilateral paralysis of the diaphragm, with recurrent attacks of cyanosis, may co-exist with the arm lesion.

Treatment is directed at resting the affected muscles. The arm should be externally rotated, abducted, flexed and fixed above the infant's head by passing a band of adhesive strapping round the wrist and pinning it to the sheet at head level for a few days, after which gentle massage and passive movement may be started. Generally, the damage is limited to laceration of the nerve sheath, with oedema and haemorrhage, and recovery is complete in a few weeks or months.

Intracranial haemorrhage

Bleeding within the cranial cavity may be the result of direct trauma or of asphyxia and vascular congestion: commonly both factors operate since cerebral birth trauma may cause apnoea and lead to asphyxia, while the difficulties in delivery which may lead to perinatal hypoxia also increase the risk of direct injury to the brain. Moreover, the venous congestion accompanying asphyxia increases the severity of haemorrhage following minor degrees of injury.

Intracranial birth trauma may result in tears of the tentorium cerebelli or the dural venous sinuses, contusion of cerebral tissue, or bleeding into the substance of the brain. The bones of the cranial vault at birth are softer and less well calcified than in the older infant and they are joined together by membranous tissue which allows the bones to override and also allows the head to alter its general shape to fit more easily into the birth canal. In this process of moulding and descent through the cavity of the pelvis the head may be compressed but

increase in intracranial pressure is lessened by outward bulging of the membranous layers joining the skull bones, especially over the fontanelles. The septa of the dura mater, *the falx and the tentorium*, may be regarded as a protective system of stays or ligaments restraining excessive moulding.

Excessive or too rapid moulding may put the tentorium, or occasionally the falx, beyond its limit of stretch and one or other or both leaves may rupture (Fig. 23.7). Haemorrhage

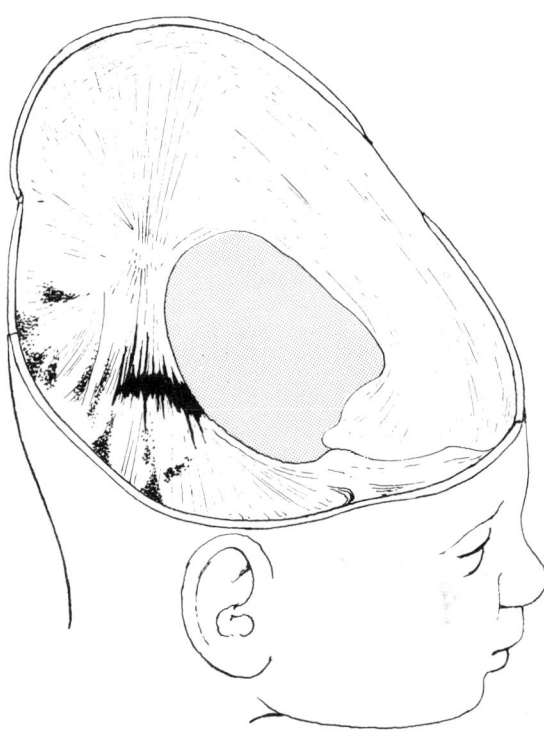

Fig. 23.7 Rupture of tentorium cerebelli on right side with haemorrhage into the tentorium and falx cerebri. A large collection of blood was removed from the region of the tentorial tear before the specimen was mounted.

from the site of rupture is usually slight, but when the tentorium tears the whole of the moulding force is thrown on to the great cerebral vein (of Galen) or its tributaries, which run unsupported to the point of entry into the straight sinus. These veins or the straight sinus itself may then be torn with resulting subdural and subtentorial haemorrhage which is often fatal from compression of vital centres. Occasionally the original tentorial tear, following the use of excessive force, may extend direct into the straight or lateral sinuses with resultant massive bleeding.

Tentorial tearing with subdural or subtentorial haemorrhage is the classical lesion of cerebral birth trauma. Such injury is most likely to occur in difficult breech delivery, especially where the fetal head is forced rapidly through the bony pelvis. It is also liable to occur in a vertex presentation where there is disproportion, especially if a strong pull with the forceps is necessary to deliver the head. Malposition of the head, leading to oblique application of forceps and a strong pull to complete the delivery, will also increase the risk of cerebral birth trauma. Occasionally the lesion occurs in an easy spontaneous delivery and there seems little doubt that some babies are more easily damaged than others. There is some evidence to suggest that the baby of the healthy well-nourished woman is better able to withstand the hazards of a difficult labour than that of a poorly nourished woman.

Perinatal asphyxia may cause intracranial haemorrhage, usually intraventricular or subarachnoid, especially in pre-term infants. In intraventricular haemorrhage, bleeding arises from the choroid plexus or vena terminalis and may be contained at first by the ependyma lining the ventricles. A small subependymal haematoma may be reabsorbed but usually, after a few hours or days, the ependyma gives way under pressure and blood floods the ventricular system, causing distension of the lateral ventricles.

Subarachnoid haemorrhage may spread over the whole surface of the cerebral hemispheres but is usually limited to the area of the major vessels. Petechial haemorrhages may also be found in the brain substance of both pre-term and term babies dying from asphyxia.

CLINICAL FEATURES

In severe intracranial haemorrhage, the newborn baby will be shocked and in a state of asphyxia pallida—pale and grey in colour, difficult to resuscitate and then unnaturally quiet. Death may occur in a few hours. Most babies survive but some of these, usually within the first 24 hours, show signs of cerebral irritation such as restlessness and irritability, a whimpering incessant cry or an occasional high-pitched one, open eyes, local or general convulsions, abnormal movements of the eyes, poor sucking and swallowing, irregular respiration and cyanosis. Sometimes general rigidity is present. The anterior fontanelle may be tense and bulging. Lumbar puncture gives equivocal results and is nowadays less commonly done than formerly: it may be dangerous if the intracranial pressure is great. Bulging fontanelle is seen in some cases of subdural haematoma and subdural tapping should usually be carried out to exclude this possibility in cases of cerebral birth trauma.

With careful nursing, quiet and warmth, maintenance of a clear airway, the use of humid oxygen in some cases, and sedation with chloral hydrate or phenobarbitone, the infant's condition improves within a few days, abnormal signs disappear and normal feeding behaviour is established. In most cases recovery is complete but long-term follow-up is necessary, since some infants will develop late sequelae. If signs of cerebral irritation have not subsided by the end of a week, the prognosis must be very guarded.

Clinically, it is difficult to distinguish the signs of asphyxial intracranial bleeding from those of severe uncomplicated asphyxia, especially in the pre-term infant. Extensive intraventricular haemorrhage is usually present when a small pre-term infant fails to establish respiration or dies rapidly within a few hours of birth. When a subependymal haematoma has formed, there may be no abnormal features until rupture suddenly occurs, when the baby may die or develop cyanotic attacks with or without twitching or convulsions. Very small infants may simply show diminished activity and grey pallor. Rupture of a subependymal haematoma often accounts for sudden deterioration and death in a pre-term baby who has been making satisfactory progress for a few days after birth. There is no effective treatment for intraventricular haemorrhage, but the incidence may be reduced by transfusion of fresh frozen plasma when the thrombotest level is under 10 per cent.

INFECTION IN THE FETUS AND NEWBORN INFANT

On rare occasions the fetus may be infected from his mother before birth but in general he is protected by maternal defence mechanisms and by the placental barrier. The uterus is no longer as safe as it was, however, for modern methods of prenatal diagnosis are increasingly invading its sanctity and inevitably carrying with them the risk of introducing infection.

As soon as he is born the infant begins what will be a lifelong battle against micro-organisms. Despite newer techniques of prevention and treatment, infections remain a menace to the newborn, especially those due to Staphylococcus pyogenes and Escherichia coli. The child will always have to live with these organisms as commensals on his skin and mucous membranes respectively, but in the newborn period they are especially liable to cause local inflammation, sometimes leading to septicaemia and death. While both fetus and infant have some defences against infective agents, they are poorly developed and feeble so that infections are a greater danger than at any other time of life.

Protective mechanisms

The newborn infant is protected against many infections by antibodies derived from his mother. These are nearly all IgG antibodies actively transferred across the placenta and the specificity of the immunity thus conferred depends on the maternal immunity. The newborn baby is usually protected against diphtheria, tetanus, pertussis, measles, poliomyelitis and herpes in varying degree: this passive immunity rapidly wanes and has virtually disappeared before the infant begins to produce his own immunoglobulins in sufficient quantity, so that at about three months after birth the infant is at his most vulnerable.

The fetus does form some immunoglobulins, mainly IgM, but only in minute amounts, and fetal immunoglobulin is therefore almost entirely maternal IgG. The virtual absence of IgM in the newborn infant except in rare cases of intra-uterine infection, may account for his special susceptibility to E. coli. A few weeks after birth, synthesis of IgM increases and shortly afterwards formation of IgG and IgA starts, although adult levels are not reached for several years. Cellular immunity mediated through the lymphocyte-thymus system develops between the third and fifth months of intra-uterine life and may be a more important protective mechanism in the fetus and newborn than circulating antibodies. Local tissue inflammatory reactions also play a part but are poorly developed in the newborn infant.

Prenatal infection

Infection may reach the fetus transplacentally from the maternal blood stream, the most common route, or occasionally by ascending vaginal infection or through infected endometrium.

The time of infection of the embryo or fetus is very important, since infection in the period of embryogenesis, roughly the first 12 weeks, may result in major malformation, while later infection cannot, although it may damage the formed fetus and so produce congenital or other abnormalities.

Rubella in early pregnancy has been proved to cause serious fetal malformations, especially of the heart and central nervous system, though it more frequently causes abortion. Infected infants may excrete rubella virus for many weeks after birth and are therefore a risk to attendants. Infection later in pregnancy can still result in fetal rubella and virus excretion; the infant often appears normal, though he may have hepatosplenomegaly.

Other virus diseases, such as measles, chicken-pox, smallpox and hepatitis, are sometimes transmitted to the fetus. Cowpox virus can cross the placenta, and the danger of vaccinating pregnant women is now realized. Neonatal fibro-elastosis of the heart may be due to prenatal infection with Coxsackie virus. Cytomegalovirus may pass to the fetus from a mother who herself shows no clinical signs of the disease.

Tuberculosis, syphilis and listeriosis of congenital origin are rare and with good antenatal care should seldom occur. Protozoa can cross the placenta and toxoplasmosis is an important prenatal disease, causing hydrocephalus or microcephaly, while malaria is not uncommon in endemic regions, especially when the mother is not immune.

When the membranes have been ruptured for some time before delivery, either because of prolonged labour or delay in the onset of labour, bacterial invasion is likely to occur and the infant may develop pneumonia from inhaling infected amniotic fluid. During the passage through the birth canal, the infant may also be infected from the mother, e.g. with gonococci. When such risks are apparent, antibiotics may be given antenatally to the mother and to the baby after birth.

Post-natal infection

The newly born infant is rapidly colonized with bacteria from his environment, such as staphylococci and diphtheroid bacilli. About 50 per cent of adults carry staphylococci on their skin and in their noses and by the end of the first week, 60 to 90 per cent of infants have been colonized. In infants born in hospital, a high proportion of the staphylococci are resistant to penicillin and sometimes to other antibiotics as well. These organisms can be readily grown from the umbilical stump, the conjunctival sacs and the nares; when colonization is heavy, bacterial infection is more likely to ensue. Where anti-staphylococcal measures are practised, colonization may be by Gram negative organisms such as Pseudomonas aeruginosa and Proteus strains, and in some hospital units, the growth of Ps aeruginosa in moist apparatus such as incubators and ventilators constitutes a real threat to the newborn infant.

CONTROL OF INFECTION

Local infections are apt to become generalized and no infection, however slight, should be ignored although it should not be over-treated. Doctors and nurses must be constantly on their guard against infections of the newborn. As few persons as possible should come in contact with a newborn baby, and those with any respiratory or skin infection should stay away. In hospital, there should be an adequate nursing staff, day and night. Hands should be washed before and after treating any infant, and protective clothing should be worn when nurses have to handle babies, e.g. when carrying babies to their mothers at feeding-times. Care should be taken to avoid the slightest trauma to the skin, nose or eyes of newborn infants. If an infant shows any sign of infection, he should be isolated and nursed by a special team. Since the floor and walls of a room in which an infected patient has been nursed will usually be impregnated with staphylococci, they should be thoroughly scrubbed with soap and water and the room well ventilated before another patient is admitted. Bowel infections are more common in bottle than in breast-fed babies, and prevention of bowel infections is a good argument for breast feeding. It will not, however, prevent the spread of epidemic diarrhoea in a nursery. Such epidemics are rare, and may be due to viruses or to special types of *Esch. coli* (such as 0111B4 and 055B5). Scrupulous cleanliness in the preparation of feeds and the cleansing of bottles and teats will help to avoid certain infections, notably thrush. Lastly, to prevent infection, antibiotics may be used in certain conditions, *viz.* (1) in cases of early rupture of the membranes, (2) where liquor amnii is meconium-stained or is offensive, (3) where there have been instrumental forms of resuscitation, (4) where a newborn baby is ill and yet no focus of infection can be found. Ampicillin and cloxacillin may be given intramuscularly; 50mg of each every six hours. Alternatively penicillin and kanamycin may be used; 20 000 units per kg and 5mg per kg respectively, twice daily for five days.

Some local infections may easily be recognized clinically, for example, the sticky eyes of conjunctivitis, staphylococcal skin foci and the white spots of thrush in the mouth; but generalized infection may ensue without a focal infection being noticed. The newborn infant reacts to generalized infection in his own way, and this should be suspected if after a few days the baby begins to feed badly, to become drowsy, to show a little fever or a fall in temperature, to vomit, to show signs of dehydration or to have loose stools. Indeed, any abnormal sign whatsoever in a newborn infant should first of all make one think of infection. Routine investigation in such cases should include culture of the urine and blood, and examination of the cerebro-spinal fluid.

Septicaemia in the newborn

Infection of the bloodstream may follow the introduction of organisms via the nose, throat or lungs; the skin; the eyes; the bowel; and the umbilicus. The most usual infecting organisms are staphylococci, *Esch. coli*, pneumococci and streptococci, while in some hospitals *Ps aeruginosa* is not infrequently the cause. The signs and symptoms of septicaemia vary in type and intensity. An overwhelming infection may kill a previously healthy baby within a day. On the other hand a baby with osteomyelitis and staphylococcaemia may nevertheless be sleeping and feeding well. There is usually some fever with septicaemia, but the temperature may be normal or even subnormal. There may be apathy, refusal to feed, vomiting, diarrhoea, greyness and lack of the normal skin turgor. Examination may reveal a focus of infection such as an abscess: the spleen is often enlarged, and in some cases the liver. Jaundice, haemorrhage, cyanosis and convulsions may occur in severe cases. Culture of blood from a peripheral vein is essential for diagnosis and should be repeated as often as necessary, at least three times if the first culture is negative. The appropriate antibiotic is given if an organism is grown and its sensitivities can be determined: if not, ampicillin and cloxacillin or kanamycin are probably best. Dehydration will have to be overcome and oxygen given if necessary. Corticosteroids may occasionally be life-saving. A resulting anaemia may justify blood transfusion, which may also be used in the acute phases.

With the newer antibiotics the outlook is not so serious as it was, but deaths still occur, and necropsies often reveal unexpected evidence of infection where none was recognized clinically.

Skin and subcutaneous infections

Minor infections are very common. The incidence of pustules in babies varies in different hospitals from 2 per cent up to 10 per cent if every case, however slight, is recorded. Staphylococci are usually cultured from the pus. Deeper infections, such as paronychia, are usually due to the same organism. Septicaemia occurs occasionally, probably more commonly than is recognized: it may be quickly overcome or give rise later to more serious staphylococcal lesions, such as pneumonia or meningitis. Staphylococcal pemphigus sometimes occurs in institutions as a small epidemic: occasionally a case of exfoliative dermatitis is seen during an epidemic of pemphigus neonatorum.

Cellulitis sometimes occurs as a hard, red, inflammatory lesion, which clears up without surgery, and sometimes as a localized abscess which needs drainage. True mastitis, usually staphylococcal, may occur in either sex; this is not unexpected in view of the activity of the breasts in the newborn.

All babies with skin infections in hospital must be isolated. If only a few pustules are present, they may be painted with 0·5 per cent hibitane in spirit. Deeper and more widespread lesions call for systemic treatment after bacteriological examination of the pus and of blood. Cloxacillin may be given until the appropriate antibiotic is determined.

Conjunctivitis

Gonococcal ophthalmia is rarely met with nowadays, and routine prophylaxis with silver nitrate at birth is no longer advised. When it does occur, there is a serous discharge which becomes purulent, and the lids become red and swell so that the eyes cannot be opened voluntarily. Treatment is with intramuscular penicillin, and by irrigations with saline and instillation of penicillin drops.

Simple conjunctivitis, usually due to staphylococcal infection, is very common and occurs in babies at home or in hospital in 3–10 per cent of cases. Generally there is only a slight discharge and a little conjunctival redness ('sticky eye'), but more severe inflammations can occur. Many cases clear up with simple cleansing by saline. If not, an ophthalmic ointment containing antibiotic should be applied. In severe cases systemic therapy should be used. All babies with infected eyes should be isolated, though it should be noted that slight stickiness of the eyes in the first 24 hours is not necessarily due to infection.

Umbilical infections

Staphylococci or gram-negative bacilli can often be grown from the umbilical stump, but spread to the liver with abscess formation is rare; the danger should not, however, be forgotten. Treatment of a mild inflammation is as for other skin infections. Any excess of granulation tissue that follows a mild omphalitis should be treated with a silver nitrate stick.

Rarely in this country, but commonly in some tropical countries, *tetanus of the newborn* follows the application of umbilical dressings contaminated with tetanus bacilli. The signs of irritability, muscle rigidity and convulsions may be confused with those of cerebral damage or of septicaemia, but the picture is often typical and the condition easily recognized if it is borne in mind. Recovery may follow treatment with penicillin, antitoxic serum, sedation and artificial respiration, but mortality is very high.

Respiratory infections

Pneumonia in the first two days of life may originate antenatally or as the result of inhalation of infected material during birth. It is not easy to distinguish such an infection from pneumonia due to aspiration of polymorph-laden amniotic fluid by the asphyxiated fetus or of gastric contents by the newborn infant. The various atelectatic lung conditions also give rise to diagnostic difficulty. Pneumonia is a not uncommon finding at necropsy: often the symptoms have been those of a general infection, and clinical pulmonary signs have been absent. The treatment is as for septicaemia.

After the first three days the commonest neonatal respiratory infection is the 'common cold', either a simple coryza or an obstructed nose causing difficulty in feeding. Symptoms usually clear up in four or five days, but occasionally bronchitis or pneumonia supervenes. The diagnosis is easier if it is known that other members of the family at home have just had a 'cold', or if there should be a small epidemic in a nursery. The infant may be given 1 per cent ephedrine in saline nose drops for two or three days if there is feeding difficulty.

Aspiration of feeds may lead to a severe haemorrhagic and suppurative pneumonia. This occurs more commonly when nursing staff are inexperienced but is not completely avoidable even with the most skilled nursing. The airway should be cleared in any baby who suddenly develops breathing difficulty, and antibiotics and humid oxygen should be given.

Staphylococcal pneumonia occurs apparently as an airborne infection and also as part of a more general staphylococcal infection. Lung abscesses, empyema and pneumothorax may ensue.

The different types of pneumonia in the newborn are all difficult to diagnose; and radiology, while confirming the presence of localized or diffuse opacity, cannot always differentiate the various lung lesions found at this age.

Meningitis

Meningitis in the newborn is most frequently due to Esch. coli and occurs as part of a septicaemia. As with other neonatal infections, however, a wide variety of organisms can be responsible. Signs of meningitis may be present and the fontanelle may be tense, but the clinical picture may be only that of the septicaemia. Convulsions may occur. As in any ill newborn infant, lumbar puncture and blood culture are essential. If the cerebrospinal fluid is abnormal, treatment is started at once with, e.g. ampicillin and gentamycin or kanamycin, the appropriate combination of antibiotics being substituted as soon as the organism is identified. Since death or neurological damage are common sequelae of neo-

natal meningitis, treatment must be prompt, vigorous and prolonged.

Alimentary infections

Thrush due to infection with candida albicans is the commonest type and comes from the vagina of the mother. It is spread by the hands of attendants and by the utensils used in artificial feeding. It is said to be more common in babies previously treated with antibiotics. Small white plaques appear on the buccal mucosa, the tongue and the palate; in some cases this fungus infection may spread to the oesophagus, a simple infection thereby becoming severe. The condition is more serious in pre-term babies. Removal of a spot reveals a raw area on the mucous membrane. Mycelium and spores can be seen microscopically if a patch is examined. Treatment with nystatin (200 000 units per ml) or with 1 per cent gentian violet in water for a few days usually cures the condition. The occurrence of an epidemic of thrush in a nursery calls for a review of the nursing techniques. It should not be forgotten that a rash in the napkin area may be due to thrush.

Diarrhoea due to dysentery occasionally occurs by infection from the mother or the nurse, but outbreaks of gastro-enteritis in the newborn are most frequently due to Esch. coli of such serotypes as O111, O114 and O55. In some epidemics no agent can be isolated and a virus may be responsible. Gastro-enteritis is very infectious and spreads rapidly both through the air and by direct contact. The earliest sign of epidemic gastro-enteritis is anorexia. Frequent watery stools, rapid dehydration, a grey colour and shock soon follow in many, but not all, of the babies affected. Strict isolation should be enforced and arrangements made for the reception of the babies into a special ward away from the maternity hospital. It is wise to stop admitting new patients into the maternity ward until all the babies have been discharged home and the ward cleared and disinfected. The affected babies will require rapid restoration of lost fluid and electrolytes, correction of metabolic acidosis and administration of plasma if there is dehydration and shock. In slight cases, fluids can be given by mouth if there is no vomiting, but milk is withheld. In most cases and certainly when the infant is more than slightly affected, fluid and electrolytes will need to be given intravenously. Antibiotics are of limited use. Neomycin may suppress *Esch. coli* in the intestine, but the organisms often reappear when treatment is stopped.

Urinary infection

Urinary infection may occur with or without congenital malformation of the urinary tract and may be isolated or form part of a septic-aemia. In the newborn period it is commoner in boys than in girls. There are often general signs of infection such as refusal to feed, greyish pallor, fever and occasionally jaundice, but urinary infection in the newborn can be largely asymptomatic, or may simply cause failure to thrive. It is frequently unrecognized because the urine is not examined. To estab-lish the diagnosis, urine is obtained by supra-pubic aspiration from the bladder or, less satisfactorily, by clean catch or bag collection methods. It must be sent directly to the laboratory or refrigerated if a short delay is unavoidable. Urine obtained by bladder aspir-ation is normally sterile while in other speci-mens less than 10^4 organisms per ml can be accepted as evidence that the urine is not infected bacterially: since excretion of bacteria may be intermittent, however, several samples should be tested before this can confidently be assumed. Pus cells and more than 10^6 organ-isms per ml are usually found when urinary infection is present. Treatment should be instituted with kanamycin, or with sulphon-amide after the immediate newborn period, and continued for at least six weeks, with follow-up thereafter to make sure that relapse does not occur. It is wise to exclude the possi-bility of a major renal malformation by intra-venous pyelography: in the case of recurrent urinary infection, more extensive urological investigation may be necessary.

Osteomyelitis

Osteomyelitis is seen as a complication of a staphylococcal septicaemia, but the original focus of infection usually goes unnoticed. It may occur in the long bones, in the clavicle, and, characteristically in the newborn, in the maxilla. Sometimes multiple osteomyelitic foci are present.

With early and adequate antibiotic treat-ment the prognosis is good. Splinting of the affected part is needed in some cases, and occasionally pus has to be evacuated.

Syphilis

Congenital syphilis is now very rare in this country and does not occur if a syphilitic mother is adequately treated in the first half of pregnancy. The Wassermann test is not a reliable method of diagnosing syphilis in the newborn since a positive result can occur in a non-infected baby and not every pregnant woman with a positive test gives birth to a syphilitic baby. Signs may be slight or absent in the newborn period, but in the next two months a persistent purulent nasal discharge, a diffuse rash on buttocks, legs and trunk, enlarged spleen and liver, and desquamation of palms and soles are all suggestive of the disease.

Certain *virus diseases* may cause symptoms in the neonatal period. For example, the baby of a mother vaccinated during pregnancy may be born with generalized vaccinia; cytomegalo virus may cause jaundice and petechiae in the newborn and herpes simplex virus may also cause neonatal hepatitis: purpura and hepato-splenomegaly may occur in rubella virus infection.

THE INFANT OF THE DIABETIC MOTHER

In untreated diabetes, fertility is low and perinatal loss high, while the newborn baby is fat and has a florid complexion, the colour sometimes approaching that of a boiled lob-ster. When antenatal supervision is good and diabetes is carefully controlled, however, the infant may appear normal at birth and require little or no special treatment. Between these extremes there is a great variety of clinical presentation. The infant of the diabetic mother is generally larger and heavier than appropri-ate for gestational age, sometimes weighing 5kg or more at term. The excessive weight is mainly due to deposition of fat subcutaneously under the influence of fetal hyperinsulinism induced by maternal hyperglycaemia. The increased length of the baby suggests a pit-uitary effect, while there is an unexplained increase in the incidence of congenital mal-formations among these infants. The size and weight of the baby will be less if diabetes has been well managed during pregnancy, if labour is induced before term, ideally about 37–38 weeks, and perhaps if the mother has toxaemia of pregnancy, the vascular changes tending to restrict fetal growth.

In these infants the level of blood glucose

falls rapidly after birth, presumably as a result of the increased plasma insulin, and they are liable to all the disorders associated with pre-term birth, especially hyaline membrane disease.

Infants of diabetic mothers should always be born in hospital with special care facilities. At birth resuscitation is often required and the stomach should be emptied by tube. The baby will generally be cared for in an incubator and the level of blood glucose should be estimated at frequent intervals during the first few days. Intravenous infusion of glucose or fructose solution will usually be required to maintain the blood glucose at a satisfactory level and alkali may be needed to correct metabolic acidosis. Oral feeding is started as soon as possible and the quantity increased as rapidly as the infant will tolerate. At first, dried milk may be reconstituted with 10 per cent glucose water instead of plain water, in order to combat hypoglycaemia. As in other pre-term infants, hyperbilirubinaemia and hypocalcaemia may also require correction. Surviving children who are not malformed seem to grow normally, and have only a slightly increased liability to juvenile diabetes.

JAUNDICE, ANAEMIA AND OEDEMA

Jaundice, anaemia and oedema are common clinical features in the newborn period and have many causes. They may occur singly or in any combination.

Serological incompatibility of mother and baby —Red blood cell antigens inherited from the father and not present in the mother may pass from the fetus into the maternal circulation and stimulate the production of antibodies, which in turn pass into the fetal circulation and destroy the red cells. The result is haemolytic disease of the newborn, characterized by anaemia, oedema and jaundice. The Rhesus antigens are the most common cause of clinical incompatibility, the six principal antigens being C, D, E, c, d and e. The genetic inheritance of the individual determines his Rhesus constitution: possession of the D antigen by the fetus of a mother who is D-negative (i. e. possessing the dd genotype) is the most important cause of haemolytic disease. In the mating of a D-negative (Rhesus-

negative) mother and D-positive father, if the father is homozygous (DD) all his infants must have the D antigen but if the father is heterozygous (Dd) each infant has an equal chance of being D-positive or D-negative. In the latter case, of course, D-immunization cannot occur, though the mother and infant may still be incompatible in respect of other antigens, either of the Rhesus series or of other groups such as the ABO antigens.

In this country 17 per cent of mothers are Rhesus (D) negative. Incompatibility from this cause might therefore be expected in about 10 per cent of all pregnancies but clinical manifestations only occur in about 5 per 1000.

ABO incompatibility seems to confer some protection against Rhesus immunization. Three clinical pictures of haemolytic disease can be recognized, though these are not sharply separated and there is considerable overlap:

1. In *hydrops fetalis*, the most severe form of the disease, the fetus shows gross oedema, anaemia, enlargement of spleen and liver, and fluid in the serous cavities. The placenta is large and oedematous. Death usually occurs *in utero* or within a few hours of birth. The clinical picture of hydrops may rarely be due to other causes, including congenital haemoglobinopathies and congenital toxoplasmosis.

2. In *icterus gravis* the infant rapidly develops deep jaundice in the hours following delivery: occasionally slight jaundice may be present at birth. The spleen and liver are usually enlarged and anaemia may be present. The vernix caseosa and liquor amnii are sometimes stained yellow. If the deepening jaundice is not treated, bilirubin encephalopathy ensues, the infant showing signs of cerebral irritation or becoming very lethargic about the fifth day of life. At necropsy deep yellow staining of the basal nuclei of the brain (kernicterus) is seen. Prompt treatment of developing kernicterus can prevent death, but the infant may later develop athetoid cerebral palsy, with high tone deafness and mental subnormality in some cases.

3. *Haemolytic anaemia* occurs in both hydrops and icterus gravis, but it may present without oedema or jaundice as a late progressive anaemia when incompatibility of mild degree has not been recognized, or after treatment if there is continuing haemolysis.

Iso-immunization and haemolytic disease

of the newborn can be prevented in some cases by giving the mother an injection of anti-D globulin within 36 hours of delivery. The purpose is to destroy D-positive fetal red cells, which may have leaked into the maternal circulation during labour or delivery, before they can stimulate anti-D antibody formation. Such measures have reduced the number of babies affected by haemolytic disease but it is still important to recognize all 'at risk' pregnancies and to predict as accurately as possible the severity of haemolysis once antibodies have appeared in the maternal serum. It is important that all women who have developed immune antibodies should be delivered in a large unit where facilities for the immediate treatment of the baby at birth are constantly available. In order that they may be identified, all pregnant women should have their blood examined at the first antenatal visit in each pregnancy to determine the Rh and ABO blood groups. All who are Rh-negative, and all those who have had a previous blood transfusion, unexplained stillbirth or a baby who became jaundiced in the first 3 days of life should have blood tests for antibodies, repeated at around the 30th and 36th weeks of pregnancy and at delivery. Moreover, whether antibodies have been discovered in the maternal serum or not, umbilical cord blood from the babies of such women is tested at delivery for haemoglobin concentration and bilirubin content, for ABO and Rhesus groups, and for antibody adsorbed on the red cells by the direct anti-human globulin (Coombs') test.

Once antibody has been found in a pregnant woman's serum, the concentration or titre should be estimated at every antenatal visit, and weekly after the 32nd week. Each transfusion laboratory has established certain levels of antibody, below which serious haemolytic disease rarely, if ever, occurs. Once such a level has been reached an attempt is made to obtain confirmatory evidence of the severity of haemolysis by examination of a sample of liquor amnii obtained transabdominally through a fine needle. The concentration of certain pigments, principally bilirubin and oxyhaemoglobin, measured spectroscopically, has been found to bear a close relationship to the severity of the disease, although the test may have to be repeated at two to three weekly intervals in some women. (*See* Chapter 15.)

The husband's genotype is also ascertained in all affected pregnancies, and is one of the factors, together with the severity of haemolysis assessed on the basis of antibody titres, liquor examinations and the severity of the disease in any previously affected babies, on which a decision as to the optimum timing of induction of labour depends. Induction calls for nice judgment, the aim being to deliver a baby of good size before the haemolytic process has caused serious disease.

If the disease is so severe that the baby is likely to become hydropic and die *in utero* before completion of the 34th week of gestation, premature induction of labour has little to offer as the tiny infant is unlikely to survive. Transfusion of packed Rh-negative red cells into the fetal peritoneal cavity, a procedure first carried out successfully by Liley (1963), can combat severe anaemia in such cases. It is performed under X-ray control, and radiation dosage can be a problem, especially when it is carried out as early as the 22nd week. As the fetus can be damaged by the needle, intraperitoneal transfusion should be confined to the small minority of severe cases where the fetus is considered most unlikely to survive without it.

On the basis of the umbilical cord blood tests done at delivery, the clinical condition of the infant and the previous obstetric history, a decision is made whether exchange transfusion, immediate or delayed, should be carried out. Generally exchange transfusion is undertaken if the Coombs' test is positive, the cord blood haemoglobin is low and the bilirubin level high. Criteria widely used are a haemoglobin level below 14·8g per cent or a bilirubin level above 3mg per cent but practice varies in different centres. The principal objective of the initial exchange is to save life by correcting anaemia but additional aims are to remove bilirubin and antibody; subsequently exchange transfusion is carried out as often as necessary to prevent hyperbilirubinaemia. Exposure of the jaundiced infant to light helps to lower the level of bilirubin in the blood and may render further exchange unnecessary. In mildly affected infants, such phototherapy may obviate the need for exchange transfusion altogether. The risk of kernicterus increases rapidly if the unconjugated bilirubin in the plasma increases above 20mg per cent, however, and this level is usually taken as an indication for further exchange.

The technique of exchange transfusion is not difficult but it does require training and experience and should only be carried out in centres where the frequency of the disease ensures regular practice. Fresh compatible blood is usually exchanged through a plastic catheter in the umbilical vein and an exchange of 180ml/kg body weight will replace up to 90 per cent of the infant's blood by donor blood.

Even after exchange transfusion, the haemolytic process may continue for a few weeks and the infant's blood should be examined for anaemia at regular intervals for at least eight weeks so that a simple blood transfusion can be given if the haemoglobin level falls below about 8g per cent.

Other causes of jaundice. Jaundice may be seen in nearly half of all healthy infants during the first week of life and in a greater proportion of infants born before term. It is mainly due to relative hepatic inefficiency and is generally slight and transient, causing no clinical disturbance except occasionally a little drowsiness. If the infant becomes moderately jaundiced, e.g. with serum bilirubin in the range 8–15 mg per cent, phototherapy may help to reduce the level or prevent it from rising further. Hyperbilirubinaemia from this cause can result in kernicterus, however, so that exchange transfusion may be required, especially in pre-term infants. All infants who are jaundiced within the first 24 hours and all who are more than slightly jaundiced must be considered as possible cases of haemolytic disease and investigated accordingly.

Rare causes of jaundice appearing at or just after birth include infection with cytomegalovirus or toxoplasma gondii. Other infections may cause jaundice after the first few days, notably septicaemia, urinary infection and viral hepatitis. Galactosaemia, glucose-6-phosphate dehydrogenase deficiency and congenital anomalies of the red cells causing haemolytic jaundice are occasionally encountered. In congenital bile duct atresia the appearance of jaundice may be delayed for several weeks: as in other purely obstructive types of jaundice, there is little risk of kernicterus even when the jaundice becomes deep, because nearly all the bilirubin in the blood is in the conjugated form.

Rarely, severe jaundice may develop in a breast-fed infant presumably because human milk inhibits conjugation of bilirubin in the infant's liver. Cessation of breast feeding for a few days is usually sufficient to allow the bilirubin to fall to safe levels.

Other causes of anaemia. An infant who is pale and limp at birth may have sustained intracranial damage or may have haemolytic disease, but the possibility must not be overlooked that he may be severely anaemic due to acute haemorrhage, for prompt transfusion of 20ml blood/kg body weight into the umbilical vein may save his life. Such haemorrhage may follow damage to the placenta or umbilical cord or may have occurred transplacentally into the maternal circulation. In the latter case, fetal red cells and haemoglobin may be demonstrable in the mother's blood. Rarely, one twin may bleed into the other, if they share a common placental circulation.

Anaemia is the principal hazard of haemorrhagic disease of the newborn, which has become much less common. The reason for this decline in frequency is not clear, for the greater use of prophylactic vitamin K is only a partial explanation.

The haemorrhagic tendency is due to defects in the coagulation mechanism which are an accentuation of the normal state, for the coagulation time of the blood is usually prolonged in the first week of life. Bleeding occurs between the third and fifth post-natal days, and is usually from the gastro-intestinal tract. A sample of venous blood should be taken for laboratory investigation and the infant should be kept under close observation. When the bleeding is only slight, an injection of Phytomendione (vitamin K_1) is all the treatment required, but in more serious cases, a transfusion of fresh blood should be given without delay.

Anaemia developing later in the newborn period may be due to infection, anomalies of the red cells, marrow defects or continuing loss of blood from, for example, a Meckel's diverticulum. Blood disorders such as thrombocytopenic purpura and leukaemia occur in the newborn infant but the associated anaemia is usually overshadowed by other clinical features.

Other causes of oedema. Localized oedema is not uncommon in newborn infants, especially in those born before term. It is transitory and is seen on the backs of the hands and feet, the pubes and the eyelids. Oedema and petechiae of the face are seen when the cord has been twisted round the infant's neck but sometimes occur for no apparent reason. Rarely, oedema localized to the hands and feet may be a manifestation of gonadal dysgenesis (Turner's syndrome).

Generalized oedema not due to hydrops fetalis may occur in congenital malformation of the heart, in hypothermia and in severe infections. In extremely immature infants the oedema may be more generalized than localized. The cause will be obvious in many but not in all cases: generalized oedema sometimes occurs for no apparent reason and disappears without treatment.

Sclerema neonatorum has to be distinguished from oedema. An alteration in the subcutaneous fat seems to occur so that it hardens, producing a feeling of firmness in the thighs, calves and buttocks with no pitting on pressure and often livid mottling of the overlying skin. It affects infants enfeebled by immaturity or illness such as diarrhoea. Sclerema often spreads rapidly as the baby weakens, and death commonly occurs. Steroid therapy and general supportive measures are indicated.

Subcutaneous fat necrosis is sometimes seen on the face, shoulders or back when localized pressure has been applied during delivery. The discrete area of hardening appears in the second week after birth and disappears without treatment after a few months. The infant remains well throughout.

TWITCHING AND CONVULSIONS

Muscular twitching and convulsions during the first week after birth may be manifestations of disturbed cerebral function following perinatal hypoxia or birth trauma, or may indicate congenital malformation of the brain, in which case the birth may have been entirely normal. Often it proves impossible to determine which of these causes is the most likely, and indeed sometimes more than one may have been operative. Convulsions may herald the onset of meningitis or indicate a metabolic disturbance such as hypoglycaemia, hypocalcaemia or hypomagnesaemia: uraemia more commonly causes lethargy and refusal to feed. A hypothermic infant may develop convulsions if the process of re-warming is too rapid. Convulsions in a deeply jaundiced infant suggest that kernicterus has supervened.

Transient *hypoglycaemia* commonly occurs during the first 48 hours after birth, the level of blood glucose falling below 20mg per cent in about 2 per cent of infants, mainly those who are light-for-dates. Tremulous, jittery behaviour, transient apnoea and cyanosis, twitching and convulsions, and disinclination to feed are characteristic signs of hypoglycaemia but are not diagnostic, since they may be due to one of the other abnormalities listed above. Moreover, not all infants with low levels of blood glucose show such features, even when the level is 5mg/100ml or less.

All infants of low birth weight, infants of diabetic mothers and others at risk of hypoglycaemia should therefore be tested repeatedly during the first two days of life: the Dextrostix test may be used for screening but if it suggests that the blood glucose is low, a sample of blood should be sent to the laboratory for analysis.

Hypoglycaemia can be corrected promptly by the intravenous administration of glucose, 0·5g/kg, and if clinical signs disappear at the same time it is presumptive evidence that they were due to hypoglycaemia. In a small number of infants, continuous intravenous infusion of glucose will be required to maintain the blood glucose at a satisfactory level.

Convulsions due to *hypocalcaemia* occur most commonly towards the end of the first week of post-natal life, when the serum calcium may fall below 7·5mg/100ml. Feeding with cow's milk is probably an important aetiological factor, the neonatal kidneys being unable to excrete the excessive phosphate load. Transient hypocalcaemia of uncertain origin in the first 24 hours may also cause convulsions. When the serum calcium is low the tendency to convulse is increased by associated *hypomagnesaemia*: low levels of serum magnesium without hypocalcaemia can also cause convulsions. If the injection of calcium and/or magnesium results in immediate cessation of the convulsive movements, the diagnosis is confirmed.

The routine investigation of neonatal convulsions includes examination of the cerebrospinal fluid and subdural taps to rule out subdural haematoma. Serum levels of glucose, calcium and magnesium should be determined. If there are grounds for believing that hypoglycaemia is the cause, glucose should be injected intravenously as soon as the blood sample has been obtained, since the risk of hypoglycaemic brain damage is considerable. Depending on the clinical picture, other investigations may be indicated, such as electro-encephalography and X-ray of the skull, though the latter seldom proves rewarding. Treatment will depend on the cause but where this is not evident after investigation, every effort should be made to stop the seizures by the use of sedatives such as chloral hydrate, diazepam or phenobarbitone. Among the rare causes of convulsions, pyridoxine dependency should not be forgotten, since it is a simple matter to give an injection of 2mg of pyridoxine hydrochloride, which is immediately effective in such cases.

SEQUELAE AND OUTCOME

Close supervision during the weeks following birth will be required by some infants and will generally be undertaken by the paediatric staff of the maternity hospital, although sometimes the family doctor will assume responsibility. Infants requiring such follow-up include those with haemolytic anaemia, who will need frequent checks of haemoglobin for at least eight weeks after birth: those with major congenital malformations, especially when functional failure of heart or kidneys is a possibility: infants requiring continuing treatment for neonatal conditions such as convulsions: and infants with feeding and other management difficulties. In addition to treatment appropriate to the abnormality present, special attention must be paid to the infant's general progress and weight gain. Failure to thrive is generally an indication for thorough review, if necessary in hospital.

All infants, normal and abnormal alike, should be kept under surveillance at child health clinics and should undergo routine developmental tests at predetermined intervals during the first few years following birth. In addition, infants considered to be at increased risk of developmental abnormality should be examined more frequently by doctors experienced in developmental diagnosis in order to detect the earliest indications of retardation. Infants included in such special follow-up studies are commonly those of low birth weight, those with manifest cerebral abnormality in the perinatal period and those with family histories suggestive of increased risk: other categories of infant may be included depending on such factors as distance from clinics, resources in health care, special interest and parental anxiety.

Possible long-term sequelae of perinatal damage to the central nervous system are mental handicap, cerebral palsy, epilepsy, sensory defects and disorders of personality and emotion. While any of these may occur alone, several or all of them in varying degrees of severity commonly affect the same individual. Such neurological handicap was formerly common in children of very low birth weight but the incidence has been reduced, probably substantially, by recent improvements in neonatal care, especially the avoidance of hypoxia, hypoglycaemia and hyperbilirubinaemia. Children suspected of brain dysfunction by reason of developmental delay, abnormal physical signs or behaviour, or simply very high risk, should be fully assessed by a multi-disciplinary assessment team early in the pre-school years. Comprehensive assessment should be repeated after the age of school entry, since minor degrees of cerebral dysfunction can result in substantial disability which may go unrecognized unless special search is made for it. Nevertheless, many infants who seem to be seriously affected by perinatal hypoxia or birth trauma and manifest signs of cerebral irritation in the newborn period make excellent progress later and are apparently entirely normal children. It is thus almost impossible and certainly very unwise to give an opinion in the neonatal period about an infant's likely mental or physical state in later years.

CONGENITAL MALFORMATIONS

TELLING THE PARENTS
The birth of an infant with a major congenital malformation is always a great disappointment and may have disastrous consequences, especially if the situation is mishandled. When an abnormality is obvious or requires urgent surgery, the parents have to be given an immediate explanation: in other cases it is often wiser to wait until the mother has seen and handled her baby and recovered from the immediate effects of labour. While the parents should not be misled during this period into thinking the baby is normal and a direct question must not be answered untruthfully, it may be possible to evade the issue or simply to indicate that there is some concern about the baby, until the time seems ripe for a full discussion. This not only enables the doctor

to gather all the information for complete diagnosis but gives the mother time to form an attachment to her infant. Telling the mother very soon after birth can precipitate an extreme emotional crisis in a woman still upset by her ordeal and may lead to rejection of the infant. When survival is likely and the mother will have to care for the baby herself, perhaps for many years, a rejecting reaction makes the management of the family situation much more difficult.

When the matter is broached with the parents it must be done gently and with compassion, preferably by an experienced member of the hospital medical staff, although sometimes it is more appropriately done by the family doctor, who should always be kept fully in the picture. Both parents should be present if possible: the father should never be told long before the mother, since the knowledge is too much for him to bear alone and in any case he will seldom be able to hide his feelings from his wife. He may be told just beforehand, however, and asked if he would prefer to tell his wife himself rather than have the doctor do so.

At this stage the facts and implications of the abnormality should be fully and frankly explained, in language appropriate to the parents' education and intelligence. It may be useful in some cases to show photographs of other infants similarly malformed, especially if a photograph showing improvement after treatment is available, e.g. in the case of cleft lip. At this time parents seldom think of future infants and genetic counselling can usually be left until later, although the need for it must not be forgotten. Some of the anger and guilt often felt by parents may be shown by accusations directed at one another, and the doctor must try to diminish the sense of guilt by explaining the origin of malformations. Resentment may also be directed at the doctor himself, who must be prepared to accept and absorb it as part of his therapeutic role, recognizing that it is a natural reaction to such a calamity. The medical or psychiatric social worker can help greatly in the parents' further adjustment to their new circumstances. The special case of the illegitimate baby, whose malformation may have ruled out the possibility of adoption, will need particularly careful handling, usually by the social worker already involved in the case.

While the above are general guiding prin-ciples, there are no rules applicable to all situations, and the doctor must judge how and when to tell the parents according to the kind of people they are, the family and social circumstances and the nature of the abnormality.

MANAGEMENT OF THE MALFORMATION

Some malformations are incompatible with extra-uterine life and the parents must be prepared for the early death of the infant. Multiple gross abnormalities, renal agenesis, anencephaly, and some major cardiac malformations fall into this category. Others may allow survival if immediate surgical operation is carried out, e.g. complete atresia of some part of the alimentary canal, exomphalos or diaphragmatic hernia. In some conditions the likelihood of early death can be reduced by prompt treatment: examples are spina bifida, transposition of the great arteries and choanal atresia. In any of these cases a decision may have to be made whether to proceed with surgery or other treatment or to leave nature to take its course. Such judgments can be among the most difficult in medicine and depend on factors such as the probability of early death, the extent of disability should the infant survive, the family circumstances and the ethical views of the doctor himself. While the parents' own wishes should also be taken into consideration, the onus of deciding should never be placed on their shoulders, since the strain of passing sentence on their child and the remorse they may feel later are too great a burden for anyone to bear.

Most of these conditions present as pressing diagnostic and therapeutic problems in the neonatal period and brief clinical details of a few of the more important are therefore given below. Many other abnormalities are less urgent, can be successfully treated and leave little or no disability. Some of these may be evident on first inspection, e.g. cleft lip, hypospadias, others are discovered during routine examination, e.g. congenital dislocation of the hip, persistent ductus arteriosus, while yet others cause later symptoms, e.g. constipation in Hirschsprung's disease, vomiting in congenital hypertrophic pyloric stenosis. Some congenital malformations are compatible with life but are irremediable. They may be recognizable at birth, e.g. Down's syndrome (mongolism) and achondroplasia, on routine physical examination, e.g. certain cardiac abnormalities, or only after the passage of time, e.g. some malformations of the kidney, such as congenital bilateral hydronephrosis, only come to light when urinary infection indicates the need for urological investigation. In such cases the doctor's initial efforts must be directed towards helping the parents to accept the situation, while later on the secondary effects of the disability must be minimized by a planned team approach to the problems of the handicapped child and his family.

Oesophageal atresia

In the commonest type, the oesophagus ends blindly about the level of the third thoracic vertebra and the lower end has a fistulous connection with the trachea near its bifurcation. As soon as the infant begins to breathe, the contents of the upper oesophagus froth up and appear as bubbly mucus at the infant's mouth and nose. If this sign is overlooked or misinterpreted, the condition may not be recognized until the first feed is given: after a few sucks the feed fills the upper oesophagus and overflows into the trachea, causing coughing and cyanosis. Further attempts to feed are likely to cause fatal pneumonia, which may also be due to gastric contents forced up through the fistula into the trachea and bronchi. As soon as oesophageal atresia is suspected, an attempt should be made to pass a large firm tube into the stomach. In the presence of atresia, it will not pass more than 8–10cm: too soft and narrow a tube may curl up in the upper oesophageal segment, giving the illusion that it has passed into the stomach.

This malformation should be thought of whenever there is hydramnios, a family history or excessive frothy mucus at birth. Since it is more common in pre-term infants, a case can be made for passing a gastric tube routinely in all such infants, as well as on the indications mentioned above. Since reconstruction of the oesophagus is often difficult to achieve without tension leading to a leak of oesophageal contents into the mediastinum, many surgeons prefer to close the fistula, make a gastrostomy and exteriorize the upper segment of oesophagus in the neck. This allows the infant to be fed and to thrive, the definitive repair being made at a later date.

Diaphragmatic hernia

Congenital diaphragmatic hernia commonly occurs on the left side, the abdominal viscera within the thoracic cavity compressing the lungs and pushing the mediastinum over to the right. The infant may be difficult to resuscitate following birth or may show respiratory distress. Sometimes, however, he appears normal, although the astute observer may note flattening of the abdomen or may hear bowel sounds in the chest. The first indication of abnormality may be cyanosis, breathlessness or even sudden death, caused by progressive distension of the viscera with air and later with milk, consequent enlargement of the thoracic contents and further compression of the lungs. An endotracheal tube should be passed as soon as the condition is suspected, so that controlled inflation of the lungs can be maintained. Chest X-ray reveals the hernia, which should be repaired as soon as possible. Because the lungs are often hypoplastic, mortality is high even if surgery is technically successful.

Exomphalos

In severe degrees of exomphalos (omphalocele), the abdominal viscera of the newborn infant protrude as a large mass from the umbilicus. They may be covered only with a thin membrane or, if this has ruptured, they may lie freely on the abdomen. In the latter case, every effort must be made to replace the viscera in the abdominal cavity as quickly as possible and to obtain skin cover. Failing this, a cover of dacron sheeting may be used as a temporary expedient. If the covering membrane is intact, the defect may be repaired surgically or the sac may be painted daily with 1 per cent mercurochrome, which allows shrinkage and gradual epithelialization. Repair of the muscle of the abdominal wall is carried out at a later date.

Congenital intestinal obstruction

Congenital atresia or stenosis of the intestinal tract may occur at one or more points between the duodenum and the anus. Vomiting within the first few days of life, especially if the vomitus is green in colour, should always be considered obstructive until proven otherwise. The higher the obstruction, the earlier the onset of vomiting, the less the abdominal distension and the more quickly the infant becomes dehydrated and ill. Thus duodenal atresia causes bilious vomiting within a few hours of birth with rapid deterioration of the baby's condition, while atresia of the lower ileum may be associated with later onset of vomiting and progressive abdominal distension. The infant is usually constipated but even in complete atresia meconium may be passed, since it is formed below the site of obstruction. It is usually scanty and light in colour, however, in contrast to normal greenish-black meconium. A plain film of the abdomen taken in the upright position shows distended loops of bowel with fluid levels. Laparotomy is carried out and the obstruction relieved, not forgetting that the sites of atresia may be multiple. Duodenal atresia is commonly associated with Down's syndrome and the baby should be carefully inspected to rule this out.

The clinical features of stenosis are similar to those of atresia but less dramatic, since the obstruction is incomplete; diagnosis is correspondingly more difficult.

Hirschprüng's disease is a special form of obstruction of the large intestine, due to absence of ganglion cells of the myenteric plexus in a segment of the bowel. Delayed passage of meconium or constipation in the newborn period with abdominal distension and sometimes vomiting suggest the diagnosis, which is confirmed by radiological examination and by biopsy to show the lack of ganglion cells. Immediate relief is obtained by colostomy proximal to the aganglionic segment, recto-sigmoidectomy being carried out later as a planned procedure.

Cardiac malformations

The possible variations in malformation of the heart are almost infinite but the anomalies most frequently found in the newborn are septal defects, persistent ductus arteriosus, coarctation of the aorta, transposition of the great arteries and Fallot's tetralogy. Abnormality of the heart may be suspected in the newborn period if the infant is persistently cyanosed, if a cardiac murmur is heard or if the femoral pulses are absent on routine examination, if there are signs of cardiac failure such as feeding difficulty, breathlessness or enlargement of the liver, or if there is simply failure to thrive. Any of these are indications for further investigation and possible action. Among the more urgent situations are those of the cyanosed infant with transposition, when

interatrial septostomy by the Rashkind method may be lifesaving, and of the infant with a large ductus causing cardiac failure, which may be cured by surgical closure of the ductus.

Choanal atresia

Bilateral obstruction of the posterior nares (choanae) causes an acute crisis after birth, since the newborn baby does not open his mouth to breathe. Death is therefore likely unless the condition is rapidly diagnosed and the obstruction removed. Respiratory distress and cyanosis, relieved transitorily when the baby cries, suggest the possibility, while inability to pass a probe through the choanae confirms the diagnosis. The obstruction must be pierced and plastic tubes inserted to allow breathing: thereafter the openings are gradually enlarged by regular dilatation.

Spina bifida

Spina bifida cystica may occur at any level but is most common in the lumbosacral region. There may be a simple meningocele, covered only with meninges or with skin as well, or a myelocele, in which the spinal cord tissue is involved. A baby born with myelocele is liable to have in addition hydrocephalus, loss of motor power and sensation in the lower limbs, paralysis of urinary and anal sphincters with dribbling incontinence, talipes and possibly other malformations such as renal or skeletal anomalies. The extent of the abnormality should be assessed as fully as possible immediately after birth and if it seems incompatible with post-natal life or compatible only with a short life with very severe disability, there may be a case for withholding treatment. In most instances, however, the degree of abnormality will be less than this, while even in extensive malformation it is often difficult to give an accurate prognosis. In such cases the defect in the back should be quickly closed, usually within a few hours of birth, since this gives the best chance of survival with the least possible handicap. In the next few weeks, a Holter valve may have to be inserted for increasing hydrocephalus, treatment for talipes instituted, the urinary tract investigated and meningeal or urinary infection treated. With such vigorous treatment more than half the infants may be expected to survive: untreated, only about 15 per cent survive to later childhood, although by no means only those less severely affected. Whether the increased survival of these handicapped children is desirable and whether the quality of their lives justifies the effort to save them can be argued on ethical, social and eugenic grounds: the fact remains that some will survive whether treated or not, and the eventual handicap in such untreated survivors may be much worse than if they had been treated from the start. Since there is no unanimity of opinion on this complex problem, the decision whether to treat or not must rest with the individual clinician after making a full appraisal of all the circumstances of the case.

With more conservative management and the possibility of antenatal diagnosis by measuring alphafetoprotein in amniotic fluid (Chapt. 18), the number of children with spina bifida may be expected to diminish.

REFERENCES

Berman, P. H. & Banker, B. Q. (1966) Neonatal meningitis. *Pediatrics*, **38**, 6–24.

Casaer, P. & Akiyama, Y. (1970) Estimation of postmenstrual age. *Devl. Med. Child Neurol.*, **12**, 697–729.

Cross, K. W. & Dawes, G. S. (1966) The fetus and newborn: recent research. *Brit. med. Bull.*, **22**, 1–96.

Davies, P. A. (1971) Bacterial infection in the fetus and newborn. *Archs Dis. Childh.*, **46**, 1–27.

Dawkins, M. and MacGregor, W. G. (1965) Gestational Age, Size and Maturity. *Clinics in Developmental Medicine*, No. 19. London: Heinemann.

Department of Health and Social Security (1971) Report of the Expert Group on Special Care for Babies. *Rep. Publ. Hlth.* No. 127, London: HMSO.

Department of Health and Social Security (1974). Present-day Practice in Infant Feeding. *Rep. Hlth Soc. Subj.* No. 9, London: HMSO.

Drillien, C. M. (1964) *The Growth and Development of the Prematurely Born Infant*. Edinburgh: Livingstone.

Dubowitz, V. & Goldberg, C. (1970) Clinical assessment of gestational age in the newborn infant. *J. Pediat.*, **77**, 1–10.

Farquhar, J. W. (1969) Prognosis for babies born to diabetic mothers in Edinburgh. *Archs Dis. Childh.*, **44**, 36–47.

Farquhar, J. W. (1970) *The Newborn Infant*. In *Child Life and Health*. Ed. R. G. Mitchell, 5th edit. London: Churchill.

Farr, V., Mitchell, R. G., Neligan, G. A. & Parkin, J. M. (1966a) The definition of some external characteristics used in the assessment of gestational age in the newborn infant. *Devl. Med. Child Neurol.*, **8**, 507–511.

Farr, V., Kerridge, D. F. & Mitchell, R. G. (1966b) The value of some external characteristics in the assessment of gestational age at birth. *Devl. Med. Child Neurol.*, **8**, 657–660.

Finnström, O. (1972) Studies on maturity in newborn infants. *Acta paed. Scand.*, **61**, 33–41.

Hoffbrand, A. V. (1970) Folate deficiency in premature infants. *Archs Dis. Childh.*, **45**, 441–444.

Keen, J. H. (1969) Significance of hypocalcaemia in neonatal convulsions. *Archs Dis. Childh.*, **44**, 356–361.

Liley, A. W. (1963) Intra-uterine transfusion of foetus in haemolytic disease. *Brit. med. J.*, **ii**, 1107–1109.

Mitchell, R. G. (1970) *Nutrition and feeding*. In *Child Life and Health*. Ed. R. G. Mitchell, 5th edit. London: Churchill. *Principles of Infant Feeding*. (1970) Edinburgh: HMSO.

Robinson, R. J. (1966) Assessment of gestational age by neurological examination. *Archs Dis. Childh.*, **41**, 437–447.

Schaffer, A. J. & Avery, M. E. (1971) *Diseases of the Newborn*. 3rd edit. Philadelphia: Saunders.

Scopes, J. W. (1970) Idiopathic respiratory distress syndrome. *Brit. J. Hosp. Med.*, **3**, 579–584.

Smithells, R. W. (1964) *The Early Diagnosis of Congenital Abnormalities*. London: Cassell.

Tanner, J. M. & Thomson, A. M. (1970) Standards for birthweight at gestational periods from 32 to 42 weeks, allowing for maternal height and weight. *Archs Dis. Childh.*, **45**, 566–569.

World Health Organisation (1961) Public Health Aspects of Low Birth Weight. *Wld. Hlth. Org. Techn. Rep. Ser.* **217**. Geneva: WHO.

World Health Organization (1965) Effects of labour on the fetus and the newborn. *Wld. Hlth. Org. Techn. Rep. Ser.* **300**. Geneva: WHO.

24. Analgesia and Anaesthesia in Obstetrics and Gynaecology

ANALGESIA IN OBSTETRICS

The contractions of the uterus in labour are accompanied by sensations which are normally felt as discomfort or pain. These sensations warn the mother to prepare for childbirth. Mechanical factors such as stretching of tissues, ischaemia of contracting uterine muscle and compression of soft tissues between the fetus and hard maternal parts cause the sensations to arise.

The conduction of pain

The pain of uterine contractions is referred to the lower abdomen, low back area, hips and groins, and extends into the thighs. The pain may sometimes predominate in just one of these areas such as the hip or groin. Nerve fibres conducting pain sensation from the uterus and cervix accompany sympathetic fibres from the uterus. They join the spinal cord at segmental levels T11, T12, L1 and sometimes T10. The pain of the first stage of labour may be abolished by depositing local anaesthetic solution in the base of the broad ligament, i.e. paracervical nerve block, by pre-sacral neurectomy, i.e. removal of the superior hypogastric plexus (which is sometimes undertaken to relieve dysmenorrhoea), by blocking the sympathetic chain opposite the 2nd or 3rd lumbar vertebrae with local anaesthetic, i.e. lumbar sympathetic block, or by epidural nerve block at spinal segmental levels T11, T12 and L1.

In the second stage of labour there is stretching of the vagina and perineum causing pain in addition to that from the uterus. At delivery perineal and vulval pain dominates. Pain fibres from the lower two-thirds of the vagina, the vulva and the perineum are somatic afferents of spinal segmental levels S2, 3 and 4, travelling mostly in the pudendal nerve and its branches. Some terminal branches of the ilio-inguinal (L1), genito-femoral (L1, L2) and posterior femoral cutaneous nerve of thigh (S1, 2, 3) reach the labia.

Parasympathetic fibres S2, 3 and 4 via the inferior hypogastric plexus supply the uterus, cervix and upper part of the vagina. They do not appear to be important in the carriage of pain impulses.

The uterus can function independently of any of its sympathetic T5–10 or parasympathetic S2, 3, 4 motor nerve supply.

The reduction of pain

The pain of labour can be abolished; by rendering the mother unconscious, by the successful application of local analgesic techniques, or by applying certain psychological methods in suitable subjects. In practice, the majority of women do not have the pain of labour abolished. They have it reduced.

The attitude of women to their role in labour and to the amount of discomfort and pain involved differs in different societies. It varies from time to time inside one society and the reasons for change may be difficult to determine.

Many women still do not wish to have painless labours. In two analgesia surveys in the Aberdeen Maternity Hospital involving ordinary methods of pain relief, one in the early part of 1970 and one in mid-1971, the following question was asked on the day after delivery: 'Would you have liked to have had your baby without feeling any pain at all during labour?' Forty per cent of 82 mothers in the first survey, and 34 per cent of 191 mothers in the second said 'No'. Furthermore, 35 per cent of the first 68 mothers who had epidural analgesia in 1972 said the same. In this last group, presumably the experience of contractions before the pain was abolished by the epidural was in some way important to them.

THE IMPORTANCE OF MATERNAL CO-OPERATION The approach to the relief of pain in labour in this chapter will be better understood if it is appreciated that about 80 per cent of deliveries in the United Kingdom are undertaken by midwives without the presence of a doctor, whether it be in the hospital or in the patient's home. Most mothers share one important aim with the midwife, namely delivery in the conscious state, without undue manipulative or operative interference. To achieve this aim the midwife requires the co-operation of the mother. Next to the safety of the mother and child, this need for co-operation is the most important single factor which influences the way in which analgesic agents are utilized in labour.

The maintenance of maternal co-operation is the key to the pattern of pain relief which has evolved in the United Kingdom. The factors which cause a deterioration in maternal co-operation may be summarized as follows:

Pain
1. Pain threshhold lowered by adverse psychological factors, lack of preparation, etc.
2. Pain unendurable on account of pathological severity.
3. Pain unendurable on account of pathological duration.

Drugs
1. Excessive sedation or narcotization.
2. The use of too high a concentration of intermittent inhalational agent resulting in intermittent loss of orientation.
3. Prolonged use of an accumulative inhalational agent.

Exhaustion
1. Prolonged labour.
2. Lack of adequate sedation.

During labour the midwife attempts to keep a balance between enough sedation, for adequate relief of pain, and too much, which causes drug depression.

The pattern of pain relief in labour
In the early part of labour before the first stage is established, the patient may feel anxious and excited. To allay anxiety at this point it is customary to administer a sedative during the day-time and a hypnotic at night. Sleep at the normal time is a necessary preparation for a stressful event. Narcotic analgesics should not be given too early as they may prolong labour (Friedman, 1955).

The first stage of labour is said to be established when the contractions occur at regular intervals, when the contractions are palpable for 45 seconds or longer, or when they are felt to be moderate to strong on palpation. The cervix at this time has usually attained a dilatation of 3cm in the primiparous and 5cm in the multiparous.

When labour is established and there is a need for relief of pain a narcotic analgesic is necessary. Pethidine is the one most commonly used and it can be repeated in the first stage of labour at an interval of 3 to 4 hours. In the first stage of labour the mother has no active part to play. She needs relief of pain, quiet and reassurance if she is to remain relaxed and co-operative, and rest well between contractions. If she has chosen to prepare herself for labour by the use of psychological methods of pain relief she should be given encouragement to persist in her methods and pressure should not be put upon her to take analgesic drugs.

During the last one to two hours of the first stage of labour, the discomfort caused by uterine contractions reaches a peak. The mother's morale may approach breaking point. But the need for more relief at this time cannot be met safely by increasing the accepted dosage of narcotics. The administration of narcotic analgesics is restricted to a level below the point of causing undue drug depression of the baby at birth. The need for greater relief should therefore be met by the use of intermittent inhalational analgesia which is self-administered. This normally provides additional relief without the danger of increasing respiratory depression of the baby.

The second stage of labour requires willing co-operation and physical effort on the part of the mother. Fortunately, entry into the second stage is often a great relief to the mother because she realizes the baby will be born soon. There is often quite a reduction in the amount of suffering she feels irrespective of actual pain, and despite the intensity of the contractions and the stretching of the tissues of the pelvic floor. Some mothers discard the inhalational apparatus early in the second stage of labour so as to get on with their work unencumbered. Others cling to the apparatus and derive essential support and relief from its use.

At the crowning of the baby's head, the mother is usually asked to inhale deeply and frequently into the mask of the inhalational apparatus in an attempt to prevent precipitate expulsion of the baby and to provide maximum relief from the pain of the final stretching or tearing of the perineum at the moment of birth.

A tranquillizing drug has a definite place in certain labours. The word tranquillizer is applied to a drug which is able to produce mental dissociation from present suffering and which is able to calm the agitated and relieve the depressed without causing undue somnolence or gross impairment of faculties. Promazine and diazepam are tranquillizers which appear to be of help to the very tense and frightened patient and they make it easier for the midwife to control her. They potentiate the sedative and analgesic properties of narcotics. Tranquillizing drugs are often used in patients with pre-eclampsia or hypertension in labour with a view to diminishing the rise in blood pressure. There is, however, no place for the routine use of tranquillizers in labour. Many mothers bitterly resent the feeling of being unable to control their actions. This particular subjective sensation arises from heavy sedation with almost any drug.

Intensity of suffering during labour
Figure 24.1 portrays a concept of the intensity of suffering in labour in a primigravid patient.

Intensity of Suffering Diagram is a gross simplification of what occurs and takes no account of the great variation in individual response which ranges from naturally occurring painless labour to extreme suffering in labour. It should be noted that suffering is the word used to describe a complex which is made up of pain, exhaustion, loss of morale, fear, distress, etc.

In 1971, 70 per cent of a representative sample of Aberdeen mothers said the pain of labour was very bad towards the end of the first stage of labour. Thirty per cent did not admit this. Half of the mothers in each of these two groups said that pain was very bad in the second stage of labour. So at least 15 per cent of all mothers find the second stage of labour is more painful than the end of the first stage of labour. The darkened cross-hatched area in the Intensity of Suffering diagram indicates that a significant number of patients do not experience relief with the onset of the second stage.

Psychological methods of blocking pain impulses
Both the interpretation of painful stimuli and the reaction to painful stimuli are profoundly influenced by psychological factors.

Psychological methods that are taught and used for the relief of pain in labour have been

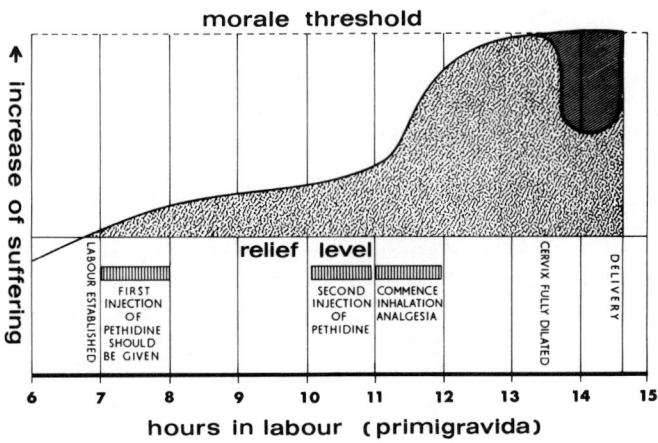

Fig. 24.1 Intensity of suffering during labour. The darkened area signifies the minority who do not experience any diminution of suffering in the second stage of labour.

The ideal times for administering pethidine and inhalational analgesia are indicated. In second and subsequent pregnancies the length of labour is usually shorter and the need for a second injection of pethidine is lessened. The

reviewed by Lee Buxton (1962). Examples of factors used in psychological methods are as follows:
Suggestion. When a contraction occurs you will feel only a tightening sensation.

Distraction. The endeavour to conform to a particular pattern of breathing during a contraction distracts the mother from the painfulness of a contraction.

Conditioning. The patient can be taught to palpate the Braxton-Hicks contractions of late pregnancy and say to herself—'I am feeling a contraction now and it is quite comfortable.' She becomes conditioned to contractions being painless.

Association. The words contraction, labour, etc. can be associated during training with pleasurable factors such as success, achievement, the arrival of a baby, etc.

It should be noted that the beneficial effect of such psychological preparation may be destroyed by ill-advised comments from relatives and friends. The attitude of uncertainty produced may make the suffering of childbirth worse than if no preparation had been undertaken.

Lee Buxton summarized psychological methods of pain relief under four headings—Natural Childbirth, Psychoprophylaxis, Autogene Training, and Hypnosis.

Psychological methods of preparation for childbirth require time, devoted and enthusiastic instructors, faith on the part of the patient and the co-operation of the hospital staff at all points of contact with the patient. Oversedation with drugs during labour is detrimental to the use of psychological methods.

Lack of information, misinformation and fear of the unknown may all increase the suffering of childbirth. Instruction and reassurance are basic functions of antenatal classes in preparation for childbirth for mothers. Some teachers stress the importance of neuromuscular self-awareness. This may help to overcome any tendency to resist relaxation of the muscular component of the pelvic floor in the second stage of labour.

The attitude of the mother towards her pregnancy and the approach of motherhood has an effect on the way she acts in labour, on the early mother-child relationship and possibly on the emotional development of the child.

It is readily understood that women in labour need to be treated with kindness, courtesy and common sense. These three attributes should be the natural possessions of all doctors and nurses. One point which needs to be stressed, however, is that most women in labour feel anxious when left alone.

Should it be necessary for the patient to be left alone even for a few minutes, she should be assured that it is only for a short time and that someone will respond instantly to the hand-bell attached to the bed.

The personality and experience of the attendant in the Labour Room can have a great influence on the behaviour of the patient in labour, and the variability of human interaction is such that the amount of pain relief in labour will vary greatly in individual cases.

DRUGS COMMONLY USED IN LABOUR

The barbiturates are used in the evening or at night to promote sleep in early labour. When barbiturates unaccompanied by analgesics are used in the presence of moderate to severe pain, restlessness and noisiness may be the result. Such barbiturates as quinalbarbitone (Seconal Sodium), or amylobarbitone sodium (Sodium Amytal), butobarbitone (Soneryl) are normally given in doses of 200mg by mouth.

Chloral Hydrate has proved itself to be a satisfactory day-time sedative for early labour. The dose is 2g and is given by mouth either as chloral mixture BPC or as triclofos (Trichloryl) 2g or dichloral-phenazone (Welldorm) 1·3g may be used.

Pethidine, since its introduction, has remained the most popular pain relieving drug in obstetrics. One hundred milligrams of pethidine corresponds to 10mg morphine. Pethidine has a relaxing action on smooth muscle but is less sedative than morphine. Its popularity in obstetrics is based on the general experience that, in the majority of patients, 100mg given intramuscularly at three to four-hourly intervals provides manifest relief from the suffering caused by uterine contractions, while at the same time the mother remains co-operative and the fetus is not unduly depressed. Midwives in Scotland are allowed to use a total of 200mg for their patient in labour before seeking medical advice for the administration of further doses. Where more than two separate injections of 100mg of pethidine are required, there is a greater likelihood of the fetus demonstrating some degree of depression at birth. If more than two injections are necessary the labour may be abnormal and an obstetrical opinion should be obtained. The peak respiratory depressant effect of pethidine on the baby is during the second and third hour after intramuscular injection in the mother (Shnider, 1970). Its respiratory depressant effect is potentiated by the use of phenothiazine drugs such as promazine and promethazine.

Morphine is the most suitable narcotic analgesic when labour is advancing slowly, the contractions causing undue distress and the morale of the patient low. It will relieve pain, cause sedation and mental detachment and promote sleep. Its unpopularity for routine use in labour is based on the view that if the mother arrives at the second stage of labour still under its influence, she will not co-operate so well in the second stage and in bearing down effectively. Further, the baby is likely to be more sleepy and difficult to stimulate than after an equivalent dose of pethidine.

Promazine is a phenothiazine derivative with tranquillizing, anti-emetic and narcotic potentiating properties. It is slightly analgesic. It will aggravate hypotension when this has been predisposed to by other agents or circumstances. It is given intramuscularly in a dose of 25–50mg, usually in conjunction with pethidine, to calm the tense, agitated and frightened patient in labour. The use of promazine in labour is also favoured when the patient is hypertensive or toxaemic.

Naloxone is a 'pure' narcotic antagonist which reverses respiratory depression only when caused by overdosage with narcotics such as pethidine. After resuscitation it is administered to the newborn via the umbilical vein in cases where there is delay in establishing respiration clearly due to depression of the respiratory centre by a narcotic. The dose is 0·005mg/kg body weight.

Levallorphan has been combined with pethidine under a trade name in ampoules containing 50mg pethidine and levallorphan 0·625mg in each ml. This drug combination was originally introduced into obstetrics in the belief that it would cause less depression of the fetus than pethidine alone. There is no acceptable scientific evidence to support the continued use of this drug combination in obstetrics. Except when used to counteract narcotic *overdosage*, levallorphan is a respiratory depressant.

Chlormethiazole is a sedative and anticonvulsant drug used to prevent and treat the convulsions of eclampsia. It is administered orally as tablets or capsules 1–2g four to six-hourly in pre-eclampsia. In situations where rapid control is required, or in labour, chlormethiazole is given by intravenous infusion as an 0·8 per cent solution. A maintenance infusion rate giving about 5–8mg/minute will keep the patient in a drowsy but communicative state. This level of depression will prevent eclampsia in almost all cases provided attention is paid to control of the blood pressure, if necessary, by specific hypotensive agents. During labour, pain must be controlled independently as chlormethiazole by itself has no analgesic properties. Epidural analgesia is ideal in this situation. If narcotic analgesics, phenothiazines or benzodiazepines, have been administered the dosage rate of chlormethiazole needs to be reduced. Deep sedation to the point of loss of consciousness with all its attendant dangers is not necessary and is to be avoided.

Newer drugs in obstetric analgesia
At the present time it is difficult to envisage the invention of any new oral or intramuscular preparation that could make an important reduction in the pain of labour unless normal maternal consciousness or awareness were significantly impaired, or the fetus unduly depressed.

Studies with diazepam represent the enormous amount of effort that is spent in looking for marginal advantages (Niswander, 1969; Friedman *et al.*, 1969; Flowers *et al.*, 1969). Diazepam, which is not an analgesic, reduced the requirement of pethidine; but diazepam produced hypoactivity and hypotonicity in the neonate.

The conclusion one can draw, from the extensive literature on the use of supplementary agents in labour, is that the *affective* component of pain is important and sometimes is all that requires to be treated.

It would still appear that if one gives the right amount of pethidine at the right times the use of supplementary agents should not often be required. Instead they should be reserved for specific purposes as agents for anti-emesis, tranquillization, mild pre-eclampsia, amnesia when indicated, etc.

Placental transfer of analgesic and anaesthetic drugs
All analgesic and sedative drugs cross the placental barrier and affect the fetus to a varying degree. Common usage is the compromise between maternal need and fetal depression. Nitrous oxide is the least depressant of analgesic and amnesic drugs and it is also rapidly

excreted. Neuromuscular blocking drugs do not affect the baby in normal clinical dosage as being highly dissociated they do not cross the placental barrier very easily.

Inhalational analgesia in childbirth

Self-administered inhalational analgesia has played a vital role in British obstetrics ever since Minnitt (1934) introduced his 'gas' and air apparatus. Seventy-eight per cent of mothers in England and Wales received some form of inhalational analgesia during labour in 1958 (Butler and Bonham, 1963). This figure probably still applies to the United Kingdom at the present time. Considering the effectiveness of the different forms of inhalational analgesia all together it has been shown that 50–75 per cent of mothers find the relief that is given is considerable or complete (McAneny and Doughty, 1963; *Report to the Medical Research Council*, 1970; Rosen *et al.*, 1969).

The widespread use of inhalational analgesia is explained by a number of factors. Firstly, in a situation where pain is not normally abolished, both the mother and the attendant feel that something is being done to help. Secondly, provided a few simple rules are followed the method is harmless to mother and child. Thirdly, it does provide reduction of pain in most cases.

The mechanism of relief is, in the first place, two-fold. The initial effect is due to distraction analgesia. Distraction is due to concentrating on the act of applying a mask to one's face and inhaling deeply. The subsequent effect is pharmacological analgesia. In the case of nitrous oxide there is a 30–45 second delay before an appreciable pharmacological reduction of pain occurs. In the second place, there is a cumulative effect if the volatile agents, e.g. trichloroethylene, are used.

INHALATIONAL ANALGESIA AND THE MIDWIFE

All the apparatus commonly used in British obstetrics is designed for safe use by a midwife acting on her own. The midwife has to follow the rules promulgated by the Central Midwives Board before she is able to administer inhalational analgesia on her own responsibility. This may be summarized as follows:

1. The midwife must have undergone a prescribed course of instruction and practical experience in analgesia.

2(a) The apparatus used must be one that is approved by the Board.
(b) A certificate is held signifying that the apparatus has been inspected and passed as fit for use, valid until a prescribed date.
3. The midwife has received special instruction in the essentials of obstetric analgesia and is proficient in the use of the apparatus (i.e. the particular type she is using).
4. A certificate concerning the mother has been issued by a registered medical practitioner that he finds no contra-indication to the administration of analgesia by a midwife.

Modifications and additions to the basic rules published in 1951 are announced in letters to various responsible authorities employing and teaching midwives.

The Rules for midwives in Scotland and Northern Ireland differ in minor detail from those for midwives in England and Wales.

The agents which midwives are allowed to use are 50 per cent nitrous oxide in oxygen (Entonox), 0·35–0·5 per cent trichloroethylene (trilene) in air, and 0·35 per cent methoxyflurane (penthrane) in air.

Entonox is a gas mixture of equal parts of nitrous oxide and oxygen stored compressed together under high pressure in steel cylinders. Trilene and penthrane are volatile sweet smelling liquids stored until use in darkened glass or opaque containers.

Apparatus

The essential features of apparatus for self-administered inhalational analgesia are as follows. There is a face mask, expiratory valve near the face mask, and a length of corrugated rubber breathing tube which is attached to the apparatus. The arrangement is shown in the illustration of the domiciliary model of the Entonox apparatus (Fig. 24.2). If the face mask is properly applied and if the expiratory valve closes firmly, all that the patient inhales must of necessity come from the apparatus via the breathing tube. The exhalation of the patient is vented via the expiratory valve. Reverse flow along the breathing tube is rendered impossible by the design of the apparatus.

The Entonox apparatus is similar to the demand regulators of aqua-lungs. The mechanism only releases the gas mixture when actuated by the negative pressure generated by inspiration. This is illustrated in a schematic diagram (Fig. 24.3). The Department of

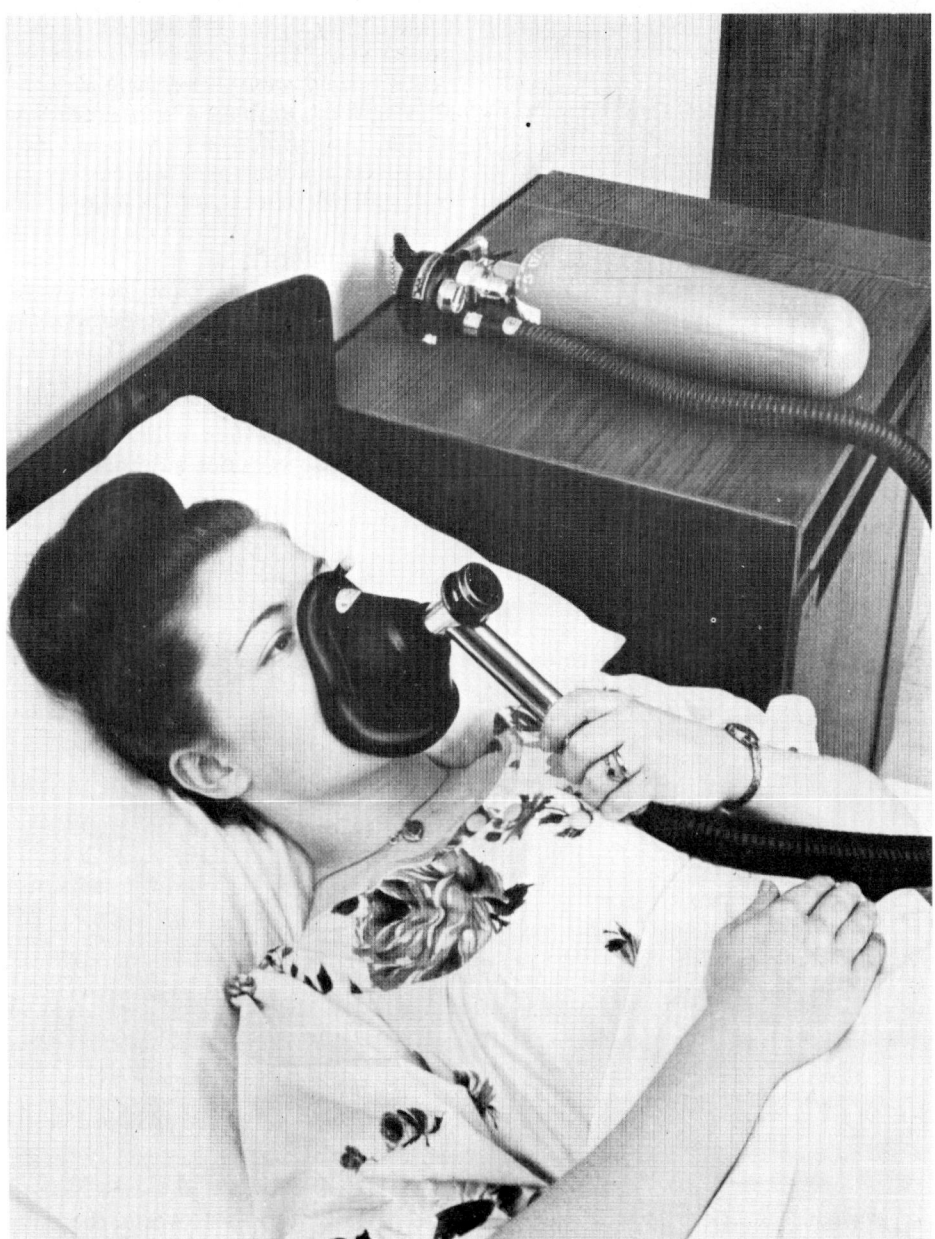

Fig. 24.2 Domiciliary Model of the Entonox Apparatus.

Health presently recommends that the Entonox apparatus is withdrawn from use every two years for factory reconditioning.

The apparatus used for vaporizing and administering a volatile agent such as trichloroethylene or methoxyflurane is called a drawover apparatus (Fig. 24.4). When the patient inspires via the face mask and tube, room air is drawn through the apparatus and part of the stream passes via a chamber containing the agent. Relative constancy of the vapour concentration is ensured by its design and a temperature compensating mechanism.

The apparatuses which are approved by the Central Midwives Board are for trichloroethylene, the Tecota Mk 6 (Fig. 24.5) and the Emotril, and for methoxyflurane the Cardiff inhaler. Each apparatus is required to be tested

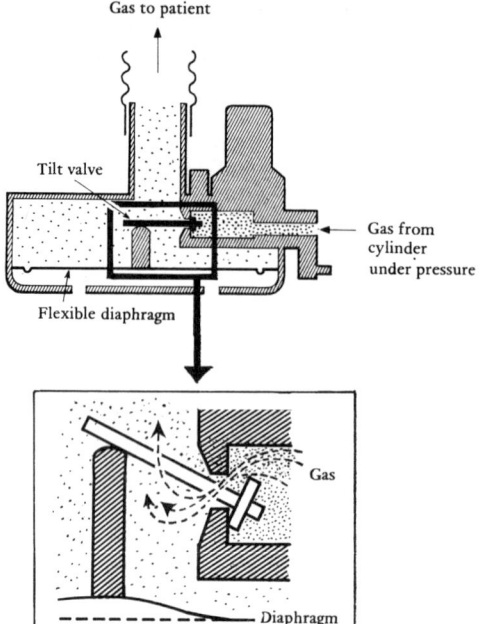

Fig. 24.3 Schematic diagram of Entonox demand regulator.

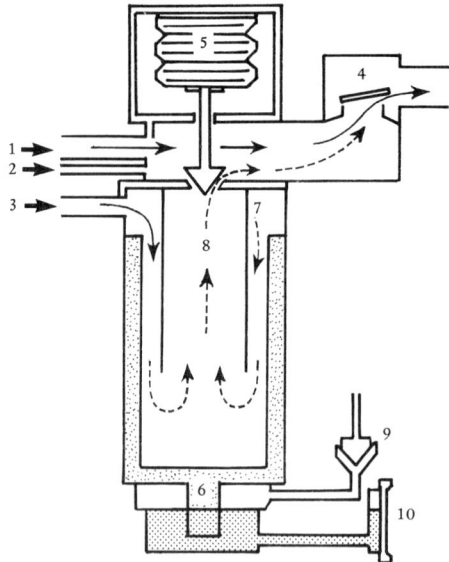

1. Bypass air inlet
2. Secondary air inlet. (It weakens the mixture when open)
3. Air inlet to vaporising chamber
4. Non-return valve and outlet to patient
5. Temperature compensating bellows
6. Wick
7. Baffle
8. Vaporising chamber
9. Filler cap for anaesthetic agent
10. Liquid level window

Fig. 24.4 Schematic diagram of a draw-over apparatus for a volatile inhalational agent.

for accuracy by the British Standards Institute once a year. This event is recorded on a small seal attached to the apparatus with the letters BST and the number of the month and year.

The Lucy Baldwin Apparatus, though not approved for unsupervised use by midwives in England, Wales and Scotland, is still in widespread use. It was introduced in 1958 (Spengler, 1961). It is a modified dental anaesthetic machine. The modifications are (1) nitrous oxide and oxygen mixtures are supplied only 'on demand'; (2) there is a choice of nitrous oxide concentration for the midwife from 0–70 per cent nitrous oxide in oxygen; (3) when the oxygen cylinder is empty the nitrous oxide cylinder automatically cuts out

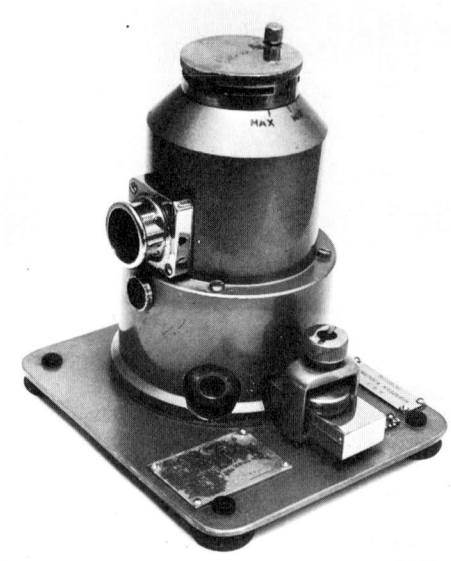

Fig. 24.5 The Tecota Mark VI Inhaler, for Trichloroethylene B.P. analgesia.

and the patient obtains only air. In the Aberdeen Maternity Hospital these machines are normally set at 50 per cent nitrous oxide. There is rarely a need for a higher concentration if initial sedation with pethidine has been efficiently undertaken.

Nitrous oxide gas is one of the most potent analgesics known to man. After ten minutes' continuous breathing of 25 per cent nitrous oxide there is more analgesia obtained than from either an injection of 10mg morphine or 100mg pethidine intravenously. In addition to superior analgesia there is no respiratory depression with nitrous oxide used in the above manner. The brain levels of nitrous oxide which provide optimum analgesia are within very narrow limits. The necessary levels vary from individual to individual. It is this difficulty of maintaining the correct level which restricts the wider use of this drug at the present.

If 50 per cent nitrous oxide is inhaled continuously for ten minutes, the majority of individuals are quite analgesic and amnesic. However, at this level of analgesia and amnesia these individuals are uncontrollable and liable to become overactive, especially on stimulation.

The success of 50 per cent nitrous oxide in labour is due, therefore, to the fact that contractions, and therefore inhalations, do not last long enough for the patient to become unco-operative. Though there are a small number of individuals who become inaccessible and unco-operative after inhaling 50 per cent nitrous oxide for as short a period as one minute.

The uptake and excretion of nitrous oxide is sufficiently rapid that for practical purposes there is no cumulative effect due to prolonged intermittent inhalation during labour.

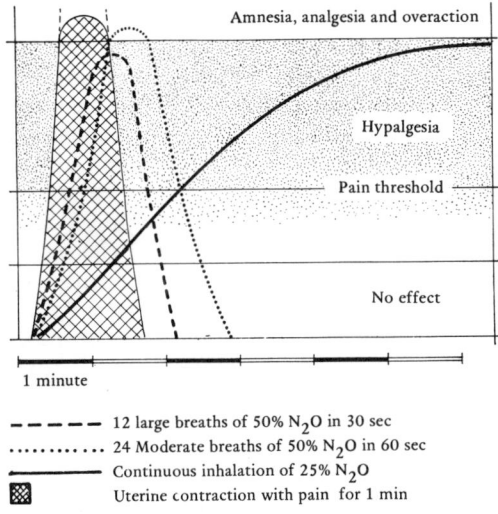

- - - - - 12 large breaths of 50% N_2O in 30 sec
· · · · · · · · · · · 24 Moderate breaths of 50% N_2O in 60 sec
————— Continuous inhalation of 25% N_2O
▨ Uterine contraction with pain for 1 min

Fig. 24.6 The Relationship of Pharmacological Analgesia due to Nitrous Oxide, to the Pain of a Uterine Contraction.

Figure 24.6 is a conceptual diagram which illustrates a lengthy uterine contraction drawn as the crossed area in the shape of a tower. The three other curves represent blood nitrous oxide levels due to inhalation commenced at the first warning of the contraction. Extension of the curves above the horizontal line in the middle of the diagram signifies both an increasing degree of painfulness of the contraction and an increasing degree of pain relief from the nitrous oxide. It can be seen that there is a 30-second delay before any pharmacological effect is appreciated. This does not match the amount of relief obtained in practice. One must assume, therefore, that the act of taking the mask and inhaling from it is a mental reaching-out for the relief which the gas ultimately gives if the contraction lasts long enough. This act provides distraction analgesia.

Owing to this delay in pharmacological relief for each contraction, it would seem logical to administer weak concentrations of nitrous oxide continuously where the intermittent relief was not enough. The patient could be rendered drowsy and hypoalgesic both between and during contractions but would remain co-operative. This has been tried in the past. The success of such a technique is dramatic in selected cases, especially under direct medical supervision. But there is no simple pharmacological answer for pain when it is severe. In practice it is simpler to allow the mother the refuge of a mask she can grasp herself for each contraction.

In the second stage of labour the warning period of a uterine contraction is shorter so that pharmacological relief from intermittent inhalation is relatively further delayed. The desire on the part of the mother to breath-hold and bear down is another factor which interferes with the amount of pharmacological relief obtained. But as it has already been stated, while some mothers readily dispense with the mask when they have the satisfaction of making expulsive efforts, many mothers continue to obtain great relief by holding on to the mask.

It is important to remember to time the use of inhalational analgesia correctly for delivery of the head. If the mother is asked to pant in and out of the mask for too long a period she may become inaccessible to command and explosive delivery may occur, especially when nitrous oxide is used.

Premixed gas. Premixed gas is the common usage term for a mixture of 50 per cent nitrous oxide, 50 per cent oxygen, v/v, which is stored under pressure in a cylinder. The cylinders are normally filled to 139·2kg f/cm^2 (kilogram force per square centimetre) gauge. At this pressure and above −7 °C this mixture remains in a single phase. The mixture does not obey the simple gas laws of Physics. Above a pressure of 52kg f/cm² at 20 °C the mixture may be described as a liquid-like gas or as a compressible liquid. It should be remembered that when nitrous oxide is compressed by itself it forms a liquid above 52kg f/cm² at room temperature. The point of all this information is that below −7 °C the nitrous oxide in premixed gas separates to form a liquid at the dependent portion of the cylinder. Furthermore, if the cylinder is rewarmed after separation has occurred and if the cylinder is kept upright and not agitated, reversion to a single phase may take several days. If the cylinder is kept in the horizontal position above 10 °C after rewarming, reversion to a single phase takes place in less than 24 hours. If, however, the cylinder is agitated after rewarming by the simple expedient of completely inverting the cylinder to and fro three times, even mixture is at once restored. This manoeuvre is convenient for the 500 litre domiciliary size cylinders.

For practical purposes cooling of a cylinder of premixed gas to below −7 °C may occur under two conditions. Firstly, there is open-air storage or transport of cylinders in the winter months. Secondly, there is the remote possibility that a cylinder already cool, say below +10 °C, being emptied by a patient so rapidly that the cooling effect of gas decompression causes a fall of the cylinder contents to below −7 °C.

The consequences of using a cylinder in the upright position when there is phase separation is obvious. If, however, in the presence of phase separation the cylinder is used lying on its side, the layer of gas between the upper oxygen-rich portion and the lower nitrous oxide-rich portion is withdrawn. This layer is approximately a half and half mixture. During withdrawal the oxygen percentages fluctuate widely on analysis, but with the Entonox apparatus hypoxic mixtures are not usually delivered in samples over 500ml in volume.

Premixed gas for home confinements. The safety of the mixture in winter is assured if:

1. The cylinder is sufficiently warm immediately before use.
2. The cylinder has been agitated by inversion three times after warming.
3. The cylinder is used lying in the horizontal position.

The cylinder is sufficiently warm after it has been placed in warm water, at baby's bath temperature (not exceeding 38 °C or 100 °F) for five minutes, or alternatively it has been lying in the delivery room for two hours or more. It is assumed that delivery room temperatures are always above 10 °C.

Premixed gas for hospital use. In the case of 2000 litre and 5000 litre cylinders, the storage temperature, bonded storage (e.g. overnight after delivery in freezing weather), local transport arrangements, etc., are the responsibility of the hospital authorities. The basic safety rule is simple. The large cylinder is safe to use if it has been lying horizontally for 24 hours in a room at 10 °C or more. During subsequent inter-hospital transport the cylinder must not be exposed to freezing temperatures for more than 10 minutes. With satisfactory arrangements it is not necessary for the hospital midwife to concern herself with the temperature problem except if frosting on the cylinder (not the regulator) occurs during use. Under such circumstances the cylinder is returned to the pharmacy for checking.

Trichloroethylene is a colourless volatile liquid with a characteristic odour, sold and known as Trilene. Trilene is dyed blue for ease of identification. Inhalation of the vapour produces drowsiness, sedation and amnesia, and eventually unconsciousness. It is analgesic. Uptake and excretion of trichloroethylene is slow. It accumulates in the patient during intermittent inhalation.

If a general anaesthetic is required for a mother who has been taking Trilene, the anaesthetist must be told. Trilene is decomposed by soda-lime and heat to form phosgene and neurotoxic substances. It promotes cardiac arrhythmias when adrenaline is injected. The drug is cheap. It is useful for rapidly progressing labours where the use of pethidine has been neglected and the second stage appears imminent. Because of its cumulative action, prolonged use may result in a drowsy and unco-operative mother as well as a sleepy baby. Pethidine may be used in conjunction with Trilene provided it has been given at least half an hour before Trilene is commenced. If the mother becomes too drowsy the inhalation can be discontinued. Pethidine, on the other hand, cannot be withdrawn once given. The mother who has become drowsy due to the accumulation of trichloroethylene may still be distressed in labour. The addition of pethidine might render her semi-conscious, disorientated or quite unco-operative.

Methoxyflurane, trade name Penthrane, is a colourless, sweet-smelling liquid. In low concentrations it is a potent analgesic. It is administered via the Cardiff inhaler at a concentration of 0·35 per cent in air. It is forty-five times more expensive than trichloro-ethylene.

The choice of inhalational agent for self-administered analgesia

There are two considerations; fetal welfare and maternal welfare. With regard to the fetus there is theoretically an advantage in raising maternal arterial oxygen tension just before and after the peak of a uterine contraction, the time when utero-placental blood flow is impaired. This is more so when there is fetal intrapartum hypoxia. The advantage of added oxygen is clinically significant in the second stage of labour. Breath-holding, when breathing air, and straining associated with involuntary bearing-down effort may bring maternal arterial oxygen to below 40mm/Hg. Phillips and MacDonald (1971) studied the maintenance of PO_2 in arterialized capillary blood before birth, the Apgar scores at birth, and the acid base status and oxygenation after birth, of three groups of higher-risk babies. Groups were derived according to whether the mothers, who during the contractions of the second stage of labour, breathed air, trichloroethylene in air, or Entonox (premixed 50 per cent nitrous oxide 50 per cent oxygen). The babies of the Entonox group fared better in the results of all three sets of measurements. All the mothers had received pethidine during the first stage of labour. After birth the babies' pH improved in the air only and Entonox groups, but in the trichloroethylene group there was a serious fall in pH accompanied by an increase in the base deficit.

With regard to maternal welfare the superiority of analgesia of one agent over another is at first sight important. In theory, during intermittent use as in labour, both trichloro-ethylene and methoxyflurane are, on the grounds of their cumulative property alone, superior to nitrous oxide. In practice, the careful studies of Rosen *et al.* (1969) have shown that there is no significant advantage of any one of the above three agents over the other. With regard to the mother's opinion of pain relief, when pethidine has not been previously administered the volatile agents appear to have a marginal superiority.

In view of (1) the reversibility of the effects of nitrous oxide within a few minutes of its withdrawal; (2) the marginal differences that have been shown in various trials between inhalational agents; and (3) the extra oxygen inspired with premixed nitrous oxide and oxygen (Entonox), it would appear that Entonox should be the agent that is made generally available for pain relief in labour. In situations where the cost and transportability of gases stored in cylinders poses problems, trichloro-ethylene is the obvious choice.

GENERAL ANAESTHESIA FOR OBSTETRICS

In the United Kingdom the above phrase refers to the production of unconsciousness for operative procedures. The induction of unconsciousness purely for the relief of pain in labour is unlikely ever to be widely adopted in this country.

General anaesthesia in obstetrics is the province of the trained anaesthetist. For it the essential criteria, apart from safety, are, that:

1. The mother should be unconscious.
2. The fetus should be unaffected by the drugs used.
3. The surgeon should have a quiet and relaxed field.
4. The drugs necessarily used to fulfil the first three criteria should leave the uterine musculature unaffected.

A standard anaesthetic technique

These criteria are to all intents and purposes met by a 'standard technique' of obstetric analgesia (Hodges *et al.* 1959; Hodges and Tunstall, 1961; Crawford, 1962). In this technique the mother, after an intravenous injection of 200–250mg of thiopentone, is maintained in the unconscious state by 60–70 per cent nitrous oxide which is administered with oxygen. It would be difficult to develop a technique of general anaesthesia less depressant to the fetus than one which depends almost solely on 60–70 per cent nitrous oxide to maintain maternal unconsciousness. The needs of the surgeon are met by paralysing the patient with suxamethonium. In clinical dosage suxamethonium does not reach the fetus (Moya and Kvisselgaard, 1961).

All drugs in current obstetric practice which affect the mother's central nervous system cross the placental barrier. Nitrous oxide up to 70 per cent in oxygen therefore holds a key place in obstetrics for both analgesia and anaesthesia. It crosses the placenta but it is not a respiratory or cardiovascular depressant of practical significance. It is rapidly excreted by the lungs.

The amnesic and analgesic function of nitrous oxide 60–70 per cent may be replaced either by nitrous oxide at a lower concentration combined with a low concentration of a volatile agent, e.g. 50 per cent nitrous oxide with 0·4 per cent halothane, or entirely by a volatile agent at equivalent concentration. This equivalent concentration must be sufficient to guarantee unconsciousness in the mother but not so great as to depress the baby at birth. Due to the differences in rates of uptake of different agents, there are technical problems of achieving this aim; but one of the objectives in reducing the concentration of nitrous oxide used is to allow a greater maternal inspired oxygen tension during the anaesthetic. Advantages are claimed, and work is being undertaken to see if the objectives are worthwhile in practice.

The standard technique makes it necessary to secure the airway by tracheal intubation.

With the standard technique in trained hands the hazard of aspiration of vomit by chance is reduced compared to that with purely inhalational techniques. However, the occasional anaesthetist subjects his patient to less hazard by using purely inhalational techniques than by attempting techniques involving intravenous injections, skill at intubation and the control of ventilation.

The standard technique is capable of providing satisfactory operating conditions within two minutes of the venepuncture by the anaesthetist. It is therefore ideal for emergencies. It also allows under conditions of maximum control the administration of drugs such as amyl-nitrite or halothane which are given to relax the uterus to assist intrauterine or extra-uterine manipulations. Uterine relaxants are only administered at the surgeon's request.

The inhalation of vomit

This hazard is liable to occur in association with general anaesthesia, heavy sedation or states of collapse. In all three situations there is impairment of consciousness and depression of the protective reflexes of the airway. Gastric contents reach the pharynx on account of vomiting or regurgitation. Regurgitation is permitted by muscular relaxation brought about either by the administration of relaxant drugs or by depression of the central nervous system. Substances in the pharynx may be drawn into the trachea by gravity or by inhalation.

Women in labour, even when fasting, are known sometimes to retain dangerous amounts of fluid in the stomach. This combined with the emergency nature of much of operative obstetrics accounts for the fact that the inhalation of vomit is an appreciable hazard in obstetrics. In the six-year period 1958–63 there were 33 maternal deaths in England and Wales alone attributed to the inhalation of vomit as a complication of general anaesthesia (Ministry of Health, 1963, 1966). In the six-year period 1964–69 there were 52 maternal deaths, and probably 5 others, attributed to this same cause (Department of Health and Social Security, 1969, 1972). In the last triennial report (1972) there were 50 maternal deaths altogether associated with anaesthesia. In 26 of these there was inhalation of stomach contents. There were factors such as inadequate preparation of the patient; failure to undertake preventive measures; difficulties of intubation; failure to deal with the inhalation of vomit as soon as it happened; lack of continuous attention to patients during and after the anaesthetic, etc.

Vomit in the trachea may cause death from respiratory obstruction. Small quantities of acid gastric contents in the lungs may result in the acid pulmonary aspiration syndrome (Mendelson, 1946) which is sometimes fatal. The critical pH is 2·5 or below.

The onset of the acid aspiration syndrome appears within minutes or hours of the inhalation of acid. The features of the syndrome are bronchospasm, respiratory distress, cyanosis and pulmonary oedema leading to cardiac failure. Following acid aspiration, prevention and treatment of the syndrome consists of the immediate intravenous administration of 500mg hydrocortisone and the giving of oxygen as required. If respiratory failure cannot be prevented by the above measures, endotracheal intubation and intermittent positive pressure ventilation is mandatory and may be required for several days.

In any event steroid therapy needs to be continued and antibiotics should be administered as a preventitive measure. Hydrocortisone, 250mg six-hourly by intramuscular injection for three days has currently been proved to be satisfactory.

The prophylaxis of acid aspiration in obstetrics
Several precautions should be taken.

1. There should be a planned regime of food and fluid administration during labour (Crawford, 1972a).
2. 15ml Magnesium Trisilicate Mixture (BPC) should be taken by mouth every two hours during established labour.
3. Whenever the mother is undergoing the following procedures—
   a. general anaesthesia,
   b. deep sedation, used sometimes, for example, in the treatment of severe pre-eclampsia or eclampsia.
   c. major local anaesthetic technique, she must be on a bed or table, which, in emergency, is capable of being tilted rapidly into a steep head-down and feet-up position.
4. Powerful suction apparatus always at the ready should be in association with 3 above.
5. The patient should be given 15ml magnesium trisilicate mixture less than half an hour before administration of any general anaesthetic (Taylor and Pryse-Davies, 1966).
6. A deeply sedated or unconscious patient should always be nursed on her side. In addition there should be an indwelling naso-gastric tube so that 15ml magnesium trisilicate mixture may be placed in the stomach every two hours.

A trained anaesthetist can greatly reduce the hazard of inhalation of vomit during general anaesthesia by exercising judgment in the selection of methods of avoiding aspiration during the induction, maintenance and recovery periods of anaesthesia (Inkster, 1963; Elliott, 1963).

Gastric emptying would appear to be the right preparatory procedure for all obstetric patients coming to general anaesthesia. To be reasonably effective either a wide-bore stomach tube passed by the mouth, or apomorphine up to 3mg diluted in 10ml water injected slowly intravenously (at 1mg per minute to the point of nausea) must be used. Neither aspiration by tube nor induced vomiting by apomorphine guarantee an empty stomach. Both procedures are disturbing and are relatively contra-indicated in the very situations where the danger of gastric aspiration is high, e.g. intrapartum haemorrhage and prolapsed umbilical cord during labour.

Cricoid pressure
In many centres gastric emptying is used only for cases who have recently ingested food and reliance is placed by the anaesthetist on a mechanical manoeuvre to prevent regurgitation during induction of anaesthesia. In the standard anaesthetic technique described the patient is paralysed by the relaxant drug almost immediately after losing consciousness from the intravenous barbiturate induction. Therefore active vomiting is not possible and the risk is one of regurgitation. As the patient is falling asleep, an assistant pushes back the cricoid cartilage against the cervical vertebrae (Sellick, 1961). This compresses the oesophagus at its narrowest part and regurgitation into the pharynx is prevented. Once the anaesthetist has placed the endotracheal tube in place and made a seal by inflating the cuff, Sellick's cricoid pressure manoeuvre may be discontinued.

Failed endotracheal intubation
Ten of the 50 deaths in the 1972 report, to which reference has been made above, were associated with difficulties of intubation. The anaesthetist should be sufficiently experienced to abandon attempts at difficult intubation before death from asphyxia or aspiration of vomit is initiated. Before returning the patient to the supine position and proceeding with the operation under a purely inhalational surgical anaesthetic administered by face mask, the stomach should be emptied. This is done with the patient in the head-down left lateral position and the residual gastric contents neutralized by the insertion of magnesium trisilicate.

Obstetrical anaesthesia and the occasional anaesthetist
In the United Kingdom there is no place for occasional anaesthesia for obstetrics. The Obstetric Anaesthetists' Association in Britain currently recommends that ideally no one should take sole responsibility for an obstetric

anaesthetic before the completion of one year of full time post-graduate training in anaesthetics.

Where the occasional anaesthetist is obliged to give an anaesthetic for an obstetrical emergency, the following is recommended.

1. The stomach must be emptied by one of the methods outlined under 'gastric emptying'.
2. A wide-bore intravenous cannula secured in place to meet the need for emergency blood volume expansion.
3. Atropine 0·6mg given intravenously.
4. Anaesthesia induced and maintained by inhalational means only.

Intravenous anaesthetic agents, muscle relaxants, and endotracheal tubes are all potentially lethal, especially in obstetrics, and should be avoided by the occasional anaesthetist.

Of inhalational techniques, diethyl ether carried by 50 per cent nitrous oxide in oxygen (total flow 8 litres per minute), is probably the safest. For induction, the ether is set to its maximum concentration and the face mask is held three feet clear above the patient's face. The face mask is then lowered at the maximum speed that the patient will tolerate. Anaesthesia once established should be maintained at a light level indicated by regular automatic breathing with the intercostal element maintained. The pupils should be small to medium, central and fixed. This level is Guedel Stage III Plane 1–2.

In the absence of an anaesthetic machine, open-drop ether is recommended. If oxygen is available it should be run by catheter at 3 litres per minute under the Schimmelbusch mask. The speed of patient acceptance of open-drop ether is greatly enhanced if trichloroethylene is dripped on to the gauze of the mask for three minutes beforehand. This is 'introduction' and is to be distinguished from 'induction' through to surgical anaesthesia with some agent other than ether. The other agent is first used because of its more rapid action and then the anaesthetic is maintained by ether.

As an alternative to general anaesthesia pudendal nerve block is obviously much safer from the mother's point of view for a forceps delivery. Some pain and discomfort all too often remains but it is a small price for one's life. Spinal anaesthesia for Caesarean section is hazardous unless the problem of caval compression and the need for anticipatory blood volume expansion is understood. This is referred to elsewhere in the chapter. The mother who collapses under a spinal anaesthetic may vomit, inhale and die a respiratory death.

Obstetric haemorrhage and anaesthesia

Blood should be available in the operating theatre for every examination in which placenta praevia is even remotely suspected, and for all elective Caesarean sections. Haemorrhage in obstetrics is potentially sudden and calamitous. Avoidable deaths from haemorrhage still occur (Department of Health and Social Security, 1972). Where there is no blood storage refrigerator inside the operating theatre, the blood is brought into the theatre in the standard pre-cooled insulated boxes containing a plastic bottle of ice in an adjacent compartment. If unused the blood may be safely returned to the blood storage refrigerator at the end of the operation.

Anaesthesia may be required for immediate exploration while a bleeding patient is still shocked. Basically, what is required is controlled ventilation, with a negative phase if necessary, with a gas mixture containing not less than 50 per cent oxygen. Very little inhalation agent, and in desperate cases none, will be required to obliterate the patient's memory; 10 per cent cyclopropane or 50 per cent nitrous oxide will suffice. No other agents except atropine and the muscle relaxant suxamethonium should be used.

Awareness during surgery
The obstetric patient is more at risk of being awake while paralysed by muscle relaxants during an operation than most other groups of patients coming to surgery. The anaesthetist, in order to avoid depressing the baby, is giving as little anaesthetic as possible. The experienced anaesthetist will find, and keep to, a strict routine for a standard technique, after which he finds none of his patients complain of being awake. Two points are to be borne in mind. In obstetric anaesthesia room for the smallest error of technique or fault in the apparatus is very small. Significant remarks in the presence of even relatively deeply anaesthetized subjects are recorded in their brains and can sometimes be recalled under deep hypnotic trance. Therefore conversation in the operating theatre should be guarded, and gloomy remarks about the mother or the baby should be avoided.

Caval compression

The gravid uterus normally compresses the inferior vena cava in the supine subject (Scott, 1968). This impairs venous return from the lower limbs and pelvic region. Of Aberdeen patients coming to elective Caesarean section, 8·7 per cent will, after a few minutes, demonstrate a fall of systolic pressure of 20mm/Hg or more if kept lying flat on an operating table, prior to induction of anaesthesia. Those who experience faintness, nausea and discomfort are said to have the supine hypotensive syndrome of pregnancy. Patients who only demonstrate supine hypotension when subjected to sedation, partial vasomotor blockade or a small haemorrhage are referred to by Crawford (1972b) as having concealed caval occlusion.

The supine posture during the last two months or so of pregnancy is undesirable. Goodlin (1971) has confirmed the importance of a lateral posture during labour and its advantages to the fetus. It has been suggested that all Caesarean sections be performed with a patient in a half lateral tilt.

Heavily sedated obstetric patients being sent into hospital by ambulance should be kept in a lateral position.

During labour compression of the aorta during a contraction may produce significant impairment of circulation to the uterus (Poseiro, 1967). This also is aggravated by the supine position.

Maternal blood pressure and the fetus

As a general working rule the mother's systolic blood pressure should not be allowed to fall below 100mm/Hg (Hon *et al.*, 1960). In the absence of vaso-constriction and in the presence of a good cardiac output, the normal placenta can be adequately perfused at 80mm/Hg. The placenta of a toxaemic or hypertensive mother may require a higher perfusion pressure. Following external cephalic version under general anaesthesia, the author once observed in a mother a systolic blood pressure just over 100mm/Hg and a pulse rate of 160. At the same time, the fetal heart rate was 100 beats per minute. When the mother was placed in the left lateral position, normal figures for mother and fetus returned. The need for qualifying general statements on maternal blood pressure and placental perfusion is clear.

Toxaemia and general anaesthesia

This disease affects many organs and systems.

The 'standard anaesthetic' described for Caesarean section is suitable. It depends mainly on two drugs which are readily eliminated after use and have no damaging effect on hepatic and renal functions. Nitrous oxide takes no part in metabolism and suxamethonium breaks down under alkaline hydrolysis accelerated by the enzyme plasma cholinesterase. If this enzyme is deficient the effect of a single dose of suxamethonium is prolonged. This causes no problems in experienced hands. In a patient heavily sedated the induction dose of thiopentone may be reduced or omitted. Where hypertension has been of long standing the anaesthetist has to make allowances for a compensatory reduction in circulating blood volume. The problem that remains is the possibility of hypertensive crises during anaesthesia. This is unlikely even in severe cases of toxaemia or hypertension, if the patient is well controlled by sedation and specific hypotensive therapy. In cases where dangerous rises of blood pressure are anticipated or have occurred, pentolinium 7·5mg or hydrallazine 15mg are suitable agents to use during anaesthesia. Lateral tilt, and blood volume expansion with dextran '70' in 5 per cent glucose (Macrodex) may be required to prevent hypotension, following their use. The aim is to prevent systolic blood pressure rising much above 180mm/Hg systolic. Ergometrine is a dangerous vasoconstrictor when its use is associated with hypertension or the use of vasopressors, and it must be avoided. The reader is referred to the chapter on toxaemia.

Heart disease and anaesthesia

The patient who is in failure, needing to sit up and breathe extra oxygen continuously, is further stressed by general anaesthesia owing to the vasomotor responses to intubation and surgery under light anaesthesia. If Caesarean section is required it is best performed by an experienced surgeon under local infiltration anaesthesia. In patients with compensated cardiac disease, general anaesthesia or epidural anaesthesia for operative delivery, or epidural analgesia for labour, is satisfactory.

ANAESTHESIA AND ANALGESIA IN SPECIAL OBSTETRIC SITUATIONS

Breech delivery

Conscious co-operation of the mother is required so that she can actively assist in the final descent of the breech. It is possible that bearing down on command is not quite so effective as spontaneous expulsive effort. Therefore lumbar or caudal epidural analgesia is not at present widely used in breech delivery. General anaesthesia may be required rapidly at the last minute if there is difficulty at delivery. A skilled anaesthetist should always be immediately available. In the event of a breech extraction being necessary, priority is given to the production of uterine and pelvic floor relaxation. It is less hazardous for the baby to be drug depressed than to have suffered a difficult extraction. Halothane can be used to relax the uterus within minutes. It must be discontinued as soon as possible in order to reduce post-partum bleeding due to uterine atony.

Twin delivery
The same principles apply as for breech delivery.

Prolapsed cord
In the first stage of labour this requires delivery by Caesarean section. Before and during induction of anaesthesia the patient should be in the left lateral position with 10–20° head-down tilt of the operating table. Endotracheal intubation is easier with the patient on her left side as most laryngoscopes are designed to displace the tongue to the left.

Analgesia for surgical induction of labour
Low rupture of the membranes with Kocher's forceps after digital examination of the cervical canal causes suffering in a variable proportion of women. In difficult cases hypoaesthesia or amnesic sedation may be used. The technique is described below. The patients must be prepared as for a general anaesthetic if there is any question of intravenous sedation being required. For the majority of cases all that is required is adequate reassurance and explanation beforehand, technical skill with gentleness and sympathy and kindness from the operator.

Hypoaesthesia
This is the term used by Crawford (1958) to describe a technique in which a mixture of narcotic analgesic and tranquillizing agent is injected by slow intravenous injection. It is used as a substitute for general anaesthesia. The subsequent analgesic sedation allows procedures such as manual removal of the placenta provided the cervix is not tightly closed. Hypotension and hypovolaemia, if present, must both be corrected beforehand. In this chapter in the section on gynaecology, this sort of technique is referred to as amnesic sedation and its dangers are indicated. The currently favoured sequence is pentazocine 30–60mg plus diazepam, 10–20mg. In spite of communication and resistance on the part of the patient during a painful procedure, amnesia, due to the diazepam, is usually complete.

Post-operative care
In the latest report of 50 maternal anaesthetic deaths associated with anaesthesia (Department of Health and Social Security, 1972), 10 patients died soon after operation. The deaths were attributed to such factors as respiratory obstruction, over-sedation, muscle weakness from the muscle relaxant drug, inhalation of vomit, and lack of continuous attention. In the immediate post-anaesthetic period, continuous supervision of the patient is required by a person capable of detecting the slightest degree of airway obstruction. Even after the patient is awake the lateral posture should be maintained when possible for a further two hours. Narcotic analgesics depress the reactivity of the airway to obstruction or foreign matter. All patients anaesthetized during labour should have their stomachs emptied and checked for alkalinity before endotracheal extubation at the end of the operation.

OTHER OBSTETRIC EMERGENCIES
Ruptured uterus and amniotic fluid embolism are referred to in the chapter on shock.

Most states of catastrophic collapse demand oxygenation and very often artificial respiration. The anaesthetist is the member of the obstetric team best equipped to deal with acute cardio-respiratory calamity and he should be called immediately.

LOCAL ANALGESIC TECHNIQUES

The drugs used in obstetrics for infiltration or nerve block local analgesia are lignocaine (Xylocaine) or prilocaine (Citanest). These two drugs are equipotent but prilocaine is less toxic. Lignocaine should be used as a $\frac{1}{2}$ per cent solution. Prilocaine is used as a 1 per cent solution. Bupivacaine (Marcain) 0·5 per cent, which is long-acting and a more toxic drug, is reserved for epidural analgesia.

Local infiltration

Local infiltration of the perineum is necessary prior to episiotomy. After an initial wheal at the fourchette the needle is passed sub-cutaneously along the line of the proposed episiotomy. Local anaesthetic is injected during withdrawal. Aspiration to check that the point is not in a blood vessel is unnecessary if

Such infiltration affects the fibres from the perineal branch of the posterior cutaneous nerve of thigh and those fibres from the inferior haemorrhoidal nerve which may have escaped the main injection.

The technique of pudendal nerve block is as follows (Fig. 24.7). The first and second fingers together are inserted into the vagina and the

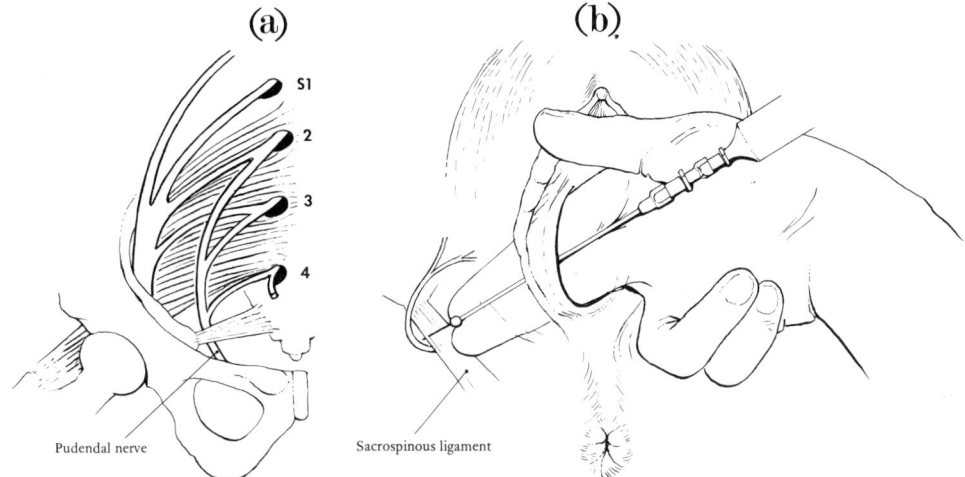

Fig. 24.7   Pudendal Nerve Block.   (a) Anatomical relations of pudendal nerve.   (b) Infiltrations of pudendal nerve.

the needle is moving during injection. It is unrealistic to hope that the patient without local anaesthesia will not be conscious of the additional pain if the incision coincides with a uterine contraction. Similarly, the edges of a torn perineum are not insensitive and local infiltration is required for suturing of the incised perineum or one that has been torn. Subcutaneous and submucosal injections may be made via the open surfaces of the tear; 10ml of 1 per cent prilocaine is adequate.

Pudendal nerve block

The pudendal nerve derives its fibres from the second, third and fourth sacral nerves. It passes behind and medial to the tip of the ischial spine and enters the anatomical perineum through the lesser sciatic foramen to traverse the pudendal canal in the lateral wall of the ischio-rectal fossa. The pudendal nerve supplies the vulva, perineum and anterior parts of the levator ani muscles. The nerve is blocked to provide pain relief for low forceps delivery. It is advisable to accompany pudendal nerve block by local infiltration of the perineum extending from the midline into the posterior portion of each labium majus.

ischial spine is palpated. The separate sheath of the pudendal block needle is passed down the trough, on the palmar aspect, formed by the first and second fingers and impinged against the vaginal mucous membrane 1cm medial to and below the tip of the ischial spine. The needle is then pushed down the sheath so that it penetrates the tissues to a depth of 1·5 to 2cm. When the needle is pushed through the sacro-spinous ligament near the tip of the ischial spine there is a characteristic 'give'. After aspirating to check that the needle is not in a blood vessel, 10ml of 1 per cent prilocaine (Citanest) is injected. The procedure is repeated on the other side. The left hand guides the needle in the left pudendal nerve block and the right hand in the right pudendal nerve block. The accompanying local infiltration, previously described, requires a further 10ml of local anaesthetic solution.

Paracervical nerve block

The pain of uterine contractions may be abolished by the infiltration of 5–10ml of local anaesthetic solution into the base of each broad ligament (Fig. 24.8). The sheath of the

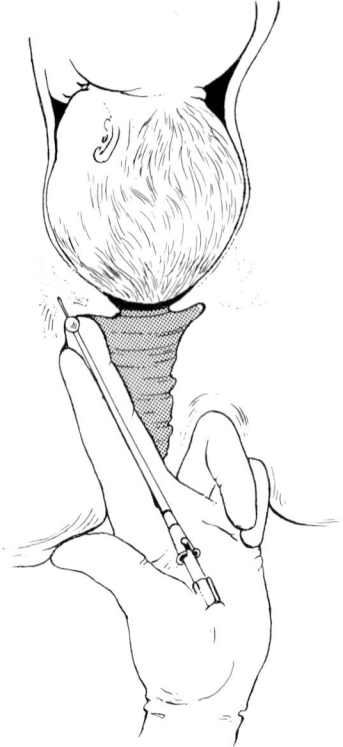

Fig. 24.8   Paracervical Nerve Block.

paracervical block needle is inserted in turn into each lateral fornix in the 3 o'clock and 9 o'clock position and the hub of the sheath is then held diagonally opposite so that on insertion of the needle in the sheath its point is directed away from the baby's head. Local anaesthetic solution deposited in the tissues deep to the lateral fornix spreads in the base of the broad ligament and blocks nerve fibres serving the uterus. The pain of uterine contractions is then relieved for one hour or more. The injection may be repeated. The value of paracervical block is greatest when the mother requires complete rest but is unable to obtain it, on account of severe continuous pain during the first stage of labour. One hour's respite during which labour progresses unimpeded is a relief both for the mother and her attendant and it helps to restore fortitude. On the other hand, there have been a sufficient number of associated and otherwise unexplained fetal deaths with paracervical nerve block to indicate that there is now little place for this technique in obstetrics, especially where epidural anaesthesia is available.

Vulval ring block

If in the second stage of labour the head is held up at the perineum and is too low down to permit pudendal nerve block, infiltration of the perineum and labia with a local anaesthetic will permit episiotomy and the application of outlet forceps.

Dosage of local anaesthetic

In the foregoing local anaesthetic techniques it is not necessary to exceed 30ml of lignocaine 0·5 per cent or prilocaine 1·0 per cent. Up to this amount may be used for pudendal block and the accompanying infiltration. With the above dosage toxic reactions should not occur. The serious toxic reactions to local anaesthetics are convulsions and/or vasomotor collapse accompanied by respiratory failure or cardiac arrest. Prompt action under these circumstances will avert disaster. In larger doses local anaesthetics should only be administered by those who are competent at preserving the airway, applying emergency intermittent positive pressure respiration (preferably with oxygen) and of giving an intravenous injection of a vasopressor and/or an anti-convulsant drug (barbiturate). If the administrator is a trained anaesthetist the injection of a relaxant drug is better for the control of convulsions than a central nervous depressant.

The complications of local analgesia

These are overdose, injury to mother or baby by the needle, intra-fetal, intra-neural or intravascular injection, injection of the wrong substance, and infection.

Extradural analgesia

The extradural or epidural space lies within the bony and ligamentous vertebral canal. It is external to the dural sac. The space is filled with a plexus of small vessels, fat, and loose areolar tissue and is traversed by spinal nerves. The spread of local anaesthetic injected into the space is up and down, but there is also some escape via the intervertebral foramina. The further away the site of injection is from the nerve roots that require to be blocked, the more local anaesthetic solution is required. Therefore, a greater volume of local anaesthetic solution is required when a caudal epidural injection as opposed to a lumbar

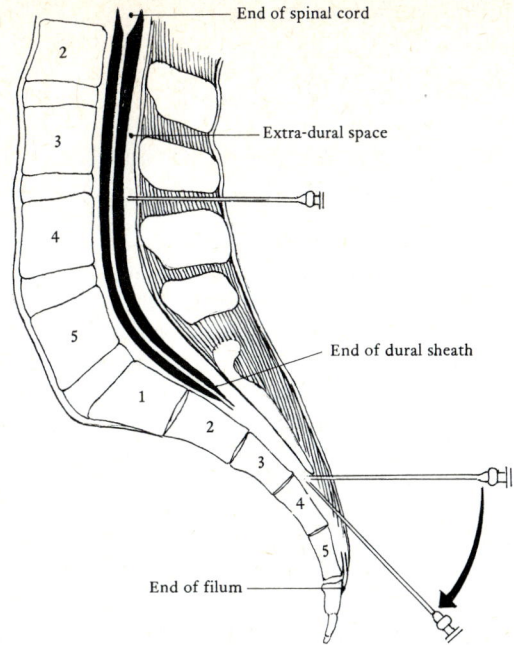

Fig. 24.9 Lumbar and Caudal Approaches to the Extra-dural or Epidural Space.

epidural injection is used. The two approaches are illustrated in the schematic diagram, figure 24.9.

The two methods are known in common parlance by the terms 'epidural' and 'caudal'. The needle which is used to enter the extradural space is also used for the passage of the fine indwelling plastic catheter used for repeat injections or 'top-ups' with local anaesthetic solutions.

It can be seen from Figure 24.9 that it would be much easier to perforate the dura mater by accident when the lumbar route is used. With the caudal route there is the possibility of perforating the rectum or the baby's head. The net consequence of these differences is that in the United Kingdom lumbar epidurals tend to be the province of anaesthetists and caudals the province of obstetricians. It should be pointed out that the normal incidence of bony abnormalities at the sacral hiatus produces a slightly higher failure rate in 'caudal' analgesia compared to the 5 per cent or less failure rate in lumbar epidurals.

Indications for epidural analgesia are:
1. Severe pain or distress.
2. Obstetric situations in which the use of parenteral analgesics might be harmful to the baby, as in moderate to severe pre-eclampsia, prematurity and diabetes.
3. Situations where maternal stress and effort should be avoided, as in cardiac and respiratory disease.
4. Dread of labour, possibly due to previous experience.
5. The request of the patient where epidural analgesia is normally an open commitment.

Contra-indications are:
1. Unwillingness on the part of the patient.
2. Infection near the site of puncture.
3. The presence of any likelihood of defect in control of bleeding such as in bleeding diseases, anticoagulant therapy, hypo-fibrinogenaemia; there is a risk of extradural haematoma.
4. Neurological disease; there may be medico-legal entanglement.
5. Orthopaedic problems in the lumbar region.
6. Blood volume deficit as in ante-partum haemorrhage.
7. Lack of 24-hour 'on the spot' cover by personnel trained in epidural anaesthesia, general anaesthesia and cardio-respiratory resuscitation.

Further contra-indications are obstetric. In breech and twin delivery it is considered that unimpaired maternal expulsive forces are necessary in order to reduce the need for an extraction. An epidural takes away the urge to push. Purely voluntary efforts are not considered to be so effective. Nor, on the other hand, are the efforts of a heavily sedated, exhausted or distressed and hysterical patient. Indeed the fully conscious and well rested mother does in fact bear down very well on command. Therefore some centres are using epidural analgesia for breech and twin delivery. Two advantages are claimed. The urge to bear down before full dilatation of the cervix is abolished. The obstetrician has perfect conditions for a controlled assisted delivery, as the perineum is relaxed and the mother is co-operative. In a case of previous Caesarean section, there would be no tenderness in the scar to warn of impending rupture of the uterus during labour. This problem of detecting undue thinning of the scar could be overcome by the technique of repeated intra-uterine digital examination advocated by Meehan et al. (1972).

Complications that are possible range from death, due for example to mismanaged accidental total spinal anaesthesia, or severe hypotension; to a permanent neurological deficit as a consequence of infection, trauma or chemotoxicity. In reality the complication rate from epidural analgesia is very low and Bonica (1967a) quotes 15 000 epidural anaesthetics in the departments with which he has been associated without serious neurological sequelae. Massey Dawkins (1972) records an incidence of permanent neurological damage of 0·02 per cent in a series of 32 718 cases (of all kinds and different circumstances of epidural analgesia).

Accidental puncture of the dura mater occurs from time to time, but it happens less often with the experienced operators. The patient should be kept lying flat on one or other side for 24 hours. This helps to prevent the occurrence of post-spinal headache. In severe cases epidural infusions of Hartmann's solution at 1ml per minute for 24 hours give good relief. Also the epidural injection, near the puncture sites, of 10ml of the patient's own fresh blood has been reported as being effective.

Hypotension occurs in a small proportion of cases and it is most commonly due to caval compression for which compensatory vasoconstriction of lower limb vessels has been blocked by the epidural. In a few cases in which the blood pressure does not recover after initial treatment, the rapid infusion of $\frac{1}{2}$–1 litre of Hartman's solution restores normality. In toxaemic patients dextran '70' in glucose is preferable. The initial treatment consists of placing the mother in the lateral position and giving the bed a 10° head-down tilt. The only vasopressor that is recommended is ephedrine 15–30mg intravenously, and even then it is only used if it is thought inadvisable to wait for the effect of other treatment. Ephedrine does not cause vasoconstriction of the uterine blood vessels.

No reference to the possibility of complications due to epidural analgesia is complete without reference to the neurological complications of obstetrics. There are many well documented cases of weakness and paraesthesia of the lower limbs, and retention of urine, following vaginal delivery without epidural analgesia (Edmonds, 1972).

If there is relaxation of the pelvic floor due to epidural analgesia it will increase the incidence of persistent occipito-posterior position. This is more than compensated for by the comfort of the patient and the relative ease of rotation, if necessary, in the second stage of labour.

The prevention of complications has been listed in detail by Tunstall (1972). The absolutely essential factors in the prevention and treatment of complications of epidural analgesia are as follows: (1) Technical ability of the operator or of his direct supervisor and instructor. (2a) Personnel and equipment for treating complications in continuous close proximity to the patient; (2b) An intravenous cannula indwelling in the patient. (3) Sterility of equipment, technique and puncture site. In this same paper thirteen other recommendations were made to which the interested reader is referred. Essentially the procedure should be standardized in all aspects and a strict routine followed.

Particular attention must be paid to the problem of caval compression due to the supine posture, discussed earlier in this chapter.

The technique of extradural analgesia should be studied in texts in the list of references and learned from an experienced operator. The epidural needle is inserted towards the ligamentum flavum using a paramedian oblique approach. This avoids damage to the interspinous ligament and the possibility of backache due to this cause. It also reduces the incidence of accidental dural puncture because the first real resistance to the advancement of the needle is only felt just before entry into the epidural space. When the tip of the needle is embedded in the ligamentum flavum a distended Macintosh balloon, or an air loaded syringe with continuous thumb pressure, is attached to the hub of the needle and it is slowly advanced. Sudden collapse of the balloon or syringe plunger indicates entry. Further advance has to be avoided to prevent dural puncture.

The present role of epidural analgesia in the United Kingdom as a whole is influenced by staffing resources. The use of this form of analgesia is expanding. It is a method capable of giving truly painless childbirth with a 95 per cent success rate. On the other hand, as it has been said earlier, 30–40 per cent of women do not want painless childbirth. Another 50 per cent appear to manage very well without epidural analgesia. In the light of experience to date, it would seem that it is 10–20 per cent of mothers who really do benefit from epidural analgesia in labour. In cases of toxaemia, prematurity and fetal distress, epidural analgesia eliminates the need for analgesic drugs which are harmful to the already jeopardized baby. It has been shown that fetuses at the end of the first stage of labour are less acidotic when an epidural is given to the mother (Pearson, 1972). In the case of toxaemia it blocks the part played by pain in aggravating hypertension. Epidural analgesia is indicated in cardiac and respiratory disease as it provides a quiet and restful labour. There is, finally, a small group of patients in whom labour appears to cause extreme suffering. They can harbour a memory of labour which fills them with a dread of childbirth. Without doubt these patients should be offered epidural analgesia.

Epidural analgesia for Caesarean section

If a patient with established epidural analgesia requires a Caesarean section, this may be done under the epidural alone. If, however, the mother wishes to be asleep there is no compromise over sedation. The full standardized general anaesthetic with endotracheal intubation should be used. Visceral traction reflexes can promote vomiting. Therefore, in order to avoid aspiration of vomit, the patient must either be completely awake or fully anaesthetized. Intermediate sedation would be dangerous.

OTHER LOCAL ANALGESIC TECHNIQUES FOR OPERATIVE OBSTETRICS

Spinal anaesthesia (subarachnoid block)
This technique provides good operating conditions for Caesarean section and for forceps delivery. The disadvantage is induced hypotension. This is due to the susceptibility of the unmyelinated sympathetic efferent fibres to low concentrations of the local anaesthetic solution which reach higher segmental levels by diffusion. On the other hand, it should be noted that vasoconstriction of the uterine arteries, resulting from the use of vasopressor substances, may be as harmful to the fetus as maternal hypotension. The best way to prevent severe hypotension associated with spinal anaesthesia is to load the circulation with a litre of Hartmann's solution shortly before and during induction of spinal anaesthesia. This will compensate for the increased accommodation of the vascular bed. If the use of a vasopressor appears to be obligatory, drugs of the ephedrine class should be used and direct acting vasoconstrictors such as methoxamine avoided. In addition to pre-loading the circulation, external left uterine displacement with the hand of an assistant reduces caval compression where this is a major factor in hypotension during spinal anaesthesia. Death due to 'spinal shock' should now be a thing of the past.

There are two causes of vomiting during spinal anaesthesia, unrelieved hypotension and visceral traction reflexes. The subject who is semi-conscious due to hypotension and who then vomits, may aspirate and die.

Local infiltration
A Caesarean section can be performed under the conditions provided if the obstetrician infiltrates the tissues layer by layer with dilute local anaesthetic solution. The patient who has had light premedication or none at all usually finds the operation most uncomfortable. On the other hand, heavy premedication is not advisable because of the risk of depression of the vital centres in the fetus. This method of local anaesthesia may be necessary in the absence of any facilities for spinal or general anaesthesia or in cases such as severe right-sided heart failure who have to remain sitting up and to breathe high oxygen concentrations. The main danger of the technique is overdosage with the local anaesthetic agent. One-quarter per cent lignocaine with 1:400 000 adrenaline allows the use of up to 200ml solution. The technique is described in detail by Bonica (1967b).

ANAESTHESIA IN GYNAECOLOGY

PREPARATION OF THE PATIENT
A written record of the patient's medical history and present state is of great value to the anaesthetist when he makes his pre-operative assessment. Special attention is paid to any treatment or medication within the previous two years. Steroid, anti-depressant, anti-hypertensive and maintenance therapies may have a significant influence on the course of an anaesthetic. Maintenance therapy may have to be modified in dose or route of administration. Medicines such as

insulin, anticoagulants and steroids are examples. Very few drugs need to be stopped pre-operatively, but it is advisable to terminate mono-amine oxidase inhibitors at least ten days before a general anaesthetic.

A history of bleeding tendency, allergy, adverse reaction to drugs or previous anaesthetics should be recorded.

Full information should be available on any concomitant disease and the results of recent investigations should be at hand, e.g. ECGs and radiographs. Associated diseases justify postponement of non-urgent gynaecological surgery, either if they require further investigation or if there is a possibility of improvement with rest and treatment. Examples are respiratory infection acute or chronic, asthma, hypertension, cardiac failure, anaemia and diabetes. Chronic bronchitics should be prepared with the help of physiotherapy and possibly antibiotics, especially for repair operations. Patients should be advised to give up smoking when first seen in the out-patient department.

The possibility of an early neurological condition simulating or resulting from a gynaecological disease should be borne in mind, especially if the anaesthetist is contemplating the use of spinal or epidural analgesia. An example of the former is incontinence due to multiple sclerosis, and of the latter, compression effects due to spinal metastases.

The haemoglobin and basic urinalysis are routine investigations. The blood count is important in anaemia even if it is considered that the gynaecological condition is the cause. A chest radiograph is essential in malignancy to exclude secondary involvement.

Cross-matched blood should be available in or adjacent to the operating theatre for all major pelvic surgery.

The anaesthetist should always be warned well in advance of any cases where there is likely to be technical difficulty in the surgery, where there is any complicating medical or surgical disease, or where the case is in any other way unusual.

PRE-ANAESTHETIC SEDATION
Ideally this should always be undertaken by the anaesthetist. Admission to hospital is a stressful experience and likely to produce insomnia. A hypnotic the night before in most cases should be considered an essential part of premedication. Sedative premedication an hour before the operation helps to dull the reality of transfer to theatre. Except for the frail and elderly, it is unlikely that any modern drug or combination of drugs can show a clear advantage from the patient's point of view over the time-honoured papaveretum (Omnopon) 20mg and hyoscine (Scopolamine) 0·4mg given intramuscularly, one hour pre-operatively. This dosage may have to be modified in the presence of low body weight or other drug therapy, etc. In other situations premedication which is a special precursor to a particular anaesthetic technique is ordered by the anaesthetist. For the ill and elderly, only atropine 0·4mg given intramuscularly three-quarters of an hour pre-operatively is suitable premedication unless the anaesthetist dictates that he requires none given.

PREMEDICATION FOR DAY-CASE SURGERY
This poses certain problems, depending on whether the patient is being admitted on the day of operation, discharged on the day of operation, or both. Contrary to instructions patients quite often drive themselves in a car to hospital and drive themselves away unaccompanied afterwards. It is simplest to avoid pre-operative sedation in day-cases and leave the administration of atropine to the anaesthetist in the anaesthetic room. The surgeon has a greater responsibility in recommending any cases other than fit subjects for day-case surgery.

Anaesthetic requirements of gynaecological surgery

Examination under anaesthesia
This is performed before all gynaecological operations and the essential requirement is good relaxation of the abdominal wall. Of the two methods of relaxing the abdominal wall, deep anaesthesia or the use of relaxant drugs, the latter is the most satisfactory. The depolarizing agent suxamethonium is the most convenient relaxant owing to its short duration of action, but it causes post-operative muscle pains especially in patients ambulant shortly afterwards. These muscle pains can be modified by the administration of a small dose of a non-depolarizing relaxant, such as 3mg d-Tubocurarine Chloride intravenously, two minutes before the suxamethonium is given.

Curettage and cauterization of cervix

Deep anaesthesia with volatile anaesthetic agents depresses the contractility of uterine muscle and promotes excessive bleeding. Halothane is notorious in this respect. As there are many alternative anaesthetic techniques there is no need to use the volatile compounds at all in this situation. Anaesthesia is essential for stretching of the cervix. The cervix is otherwise insensitive, and, for example, cauterization of the cervix is itself painless.

Termination of pregnancy

Again it is important to avoid volatile anaesthetic agents in high concentration. The conceptus in the first few weeks of pregnancy may be aspirated by a suction catheter through the cervix. It can be performed in the conscious subject more easily if associated with paracervical nerve block. Apprehensive and disturbed subjects require amnesic sedation in addition. This form of sedation is referred to later. When pregnancy has advanced to the point where cervical dilatation is necessary, a general anaesthetic is normally used. Prior to the insertion of the large bore metal vacuum aspirator or the curette, the patient is given 0·5mg ergometrine intravenously. This helps to maintain a firm uterine wall.

Repair of uterine prolapse

Where the surgeon proposes to infiltrate a solution containing adrenaline as a haemostat, the anaesthetist should be informed beforehand. There may be adverse cardiac reactions if certain anaesthetic agents are used.

Venous congestion produces troublesome bleeding in most gynaecological operations. It is avoided by smooth anaesthesia involving the absence of coughing, straining and movement. On the other hand, if this is achieved by deep anaesthesia without assisted or controlled ventilation, the resultant carbon dioxide retention will cause troublesome capillary oozing.

Radical hysterectomy

This operation requires perfect muscular relaxation and ideally a reduction of the patient's normal arterial blood pressure. There is much packing, exploration and retraction. Techniques which lower arterial blood pressure prevent classical shock. Maintenance of adequate blood volume during the operation becomes a primary function of the anaesthetist.

Vaginal hysterectomy

Some exponents of this operation depend on hypotensive spinal analgesia and heavy sedation for their good operative results. Such techniques are capable of producing a virtually bloodless operating field.

Laparoscopy

In this procedure the peritoneal cavity is distended with gas under pressure—oxygen, nitrous oxide and carbon dioxide have been used. Carbon dioxide is the preferred agent as it is the most rapidly dissolved in the event of intravascular injection. The anaesthetist should be prepared to deal with the consequences of rare complications such as haemorrhage due to puncture of a large vessel by the trocar of the laparoscope, and to deal with gas emboli. Gas embolus is treated by catheter aspiration of the right atrium with the patient lying on her left side.

The insufflating gas should be restricted to a maximum flow rate of 1 litre per minute and a maximum pressure of 25cm H_2O pressure. Three to five litres of gas usually provide sufficient distension. The anaesthetic technique of choice involves endotracheal intubation, controlled respiration with a relaxant drug, and avoidance of volatile anaesthetic agents with undesirable cardiovascular effects. Good abdominal wall relaxation reduces the amount of gas required to get adequate distension. The cardiovascular effects of the procedure, with useful references, are described by Smith and his colleagues (1971).

Ectopic gestation

This condition can be associated with internal haemorrhage and shock and is one of gynaecology's most urgent conditions. The anaesthetist may have to induce anaesthesia when the patient is virtually pulseless in spite of emergency transfusion. He needs to be experienced, as the patient may require artificial ventilation and 100 per cent oxygen via an endotracheal tube before it is safe to give her any anaesthetic drugs.

Pregnancy

The teratogenetic effects of drugs are greatest in the first few weeks of pregnancy. As the ultimate test of teratogenicity can only be made in human subjects, all new drugs, premedicant and anaesthetic, should be avoided if at all possible.

Certain anaesthetic techniques

Amnesic sedation defines a technique of depression of awareness, usually by an intravenously administered drug, to the point of amnesia. Ideally the depression is not taken as far as the point where there is loss of the airway. A drug commonly used for this purpose is diazepam. Ten to thirty milligrammes is injected slowly intravenously until the patient is very drowsy. The dosage is reduced in the presence of premedication with other sedative drugs. The technique is used for uncomfortable procedures such as therapeutic abortion by vacuum aspiration. At the amnesic level the operative field is not always immobile and there may be associated weeping and other forms of mental reaction. This is overcome by increased dosage or additive sedation with several different drugs. The belief that such a technique is safe because a full general anaesthetic has not been given is quite erroneous. The threat to life is progressive from the moment there is impairment of awareness. Loss of the airway, ventilatory embarrassment, inhalation of vomit, laryngeal spasm and hypotension are all possibilities. The temptation to overdose is great when the patient is reacting adversely. The patient must be prepared as for a full general anaesthetic. This includes pre-operative starvation.

Amnesic sedation is most helpful when it is used to cover procedures under local anaesthesia. When painful stimuli are blocked far less sedation is required.

Local anaesthesia. Dilatation of the cervix may be satisfactorily performed after paracervical nerve block with 10ml of 1 per cent lignocaine injected at 3 o'clock and 9 o'clock through the lateral fornices adjacent to the cervix. The addition of a bilateral pudendal nerve block is helpful if there is associated much stretching of the introitus and vagina.

Major local anaesthetic techniques such as spinal or epidural analgesia provide good operating conditions for major gynaecological surgery, provided there is no hypovolaemia such as that associated with severe chronic hypertension or blood loss; and provided that there is no contra-indication to spontaneous respiration such as gross obesity. These techniques give a quiet, relaxed operating field and bleeding appears to be reduced even in the absence of hypotension. Generally speaking, these techniques should be covered by a light general anaesthetic. This enables the anaesthetist to concentrate on the vital physiological needs of the patient. In any event, much intra-abdominal manipulation stimulates vagal afferents and causes retching and discomfort in the conscious subject.

Which anaesthetic technique?

The choice is so great that even textbooks of anaesthesia rarely describe in detail any particular technique for any particular operation. Anaesthesia for laparoscopy is an example where two greatly differing techniques have recently been advocated (Smith *et al.*, 1971; Scott and Julian, 1972). This has been followed by controversy in the correspondence columns of the journal concerned (Scott, 1972).

The anaesthetist depresses the central nervous system between the limits of two levels; the level of amnesia and analgesia and the level of surgical anaesthesia. At the former level the patients move on stimulation. At the latter they remain still. Relaxant drugs enable the anaesthetist to keep the patient still at the former level and with less depression. Therefore the relaxant drugs serve two functions. The first is to provide relaxation, the second is to permit light levels of anaesthesia. Relaxation of muscles can alternatively be provided by deep anaesthesia or by nerve block with local anaesthetics. Deep anaesthesia is harmful to the patient if prolonged. It can be useful if only short periods of moderate relaxation are required—as for bimanual pelvic examination. Here a rapidly given relatively large dose of thiopentone given on one occasion achieves the desired end without unduly prolonging recovery.

Major local anaesthetic techniques such as epidural and spinal analgesia are capable of providing very good operating conditions. Against this must be set the extra time and trouble that has to be taken with these methods.

Gynaecology and the occasional anaesthetist

General anaesthesia is best avoided altogether. Local infiltration or spinal anaesthesia, with amnesic sedation if necessary, should be used.

Posture on the operating table

Backache is a common enough complaint in parous women. Care and gentleness should be observed always when positioning the patient in dorsal lithotomy. The anaesthetized patient does not reflexly protect her lumbar and sacral ligaments by muscular contractions so both legs must be moved up and down together. The lumbar bolster should be more widely used on the operating table than it is. For operations which require a head-down tilt, shoulder rests should rarely be used, reliance being placed on a non-slip mattress. Shoulder rests must never be used with the arm outstretched on an arm-board with the patient in the Trendelenberg position, as this will greatly increase the chance of stretching and damaging the brachial plexus. With modern anaesthesia the steep Trendelenberg position is no longer required. It adversely affects the respiration and the circulation.

Post-operative care

Loss of the airway during recovery is a danger in all general anaesthetics. Patients should not be returned to the ward unless it is clear that they can protect their airways. The danger of aspiration of vomit persists if the patient remains heavily sedated and in these circumstances the patient should always be nursed on one or other side.

The problem of haemorrhage, internal or external, deserves special mention. If the anaesthetist has administered heavy sedation or shock-preventing drugs such as ganglion-blockers, phenothiazine or butyrophenones, the first obvious manifestation of internal bleeding may be a fall in blood pressure. Normally the rise in pulse rate is the first manifestation. The skin will remain warm and dry and the pulse full though easily obliterated. Pallor is variable. If this is understood and there is routine careful post-operative observation of the patient, the diagnosis should not be delayed and the urgency will be appreciated. The fall in blood pressure is treated by elevating the foot of the bed, administering oxygen, correction of the intravascular fluid volume deficit, relative or absolute, and treating the cause if it is still operative. Whenever there is a problem or doubt in connection with blood volume expansion, the measurement of central venous pressure, normally 9–12cm H_2O is invaluable. A raised central venous pressure suggests over-transfusion but if there is associated low blood pressure and poor tissue perfusion, heart failure should be considered. This may be due to cardiac disease or abnormality of electrolyte or acid base status.

Pre-operative and post-operative resuscitation is a responsibility shared by the anaesthetist. The anaesthetist is liable to have to appear before the Procurator Fiscal in Scotland and the Coroner in England on account of any death during or 24 hours after the operation. In cases of negligence the courts assess liability on a proportionate basis.

In intensive care situations there is rarely any problem in practice as to the division of responsibility. For example, if a central venous pressure line is required the most capable member of the team establishes it or allows someone else either to do it under supervision or to gain further experience. However, in spite of the team approach in modern medicine it is essential that the surgeon remains in charge of the case even though there may be considerable sharing or delegation of responsibility for specific matters.

REFERENCES

Bonica, J. J. (1967a & b) *Principles and Practice of Obstetric Analgesia and Anesthesia.* Vol. 1, pp. 618 and 531. Oxford: Blackwell.

Butler, N. R. & Bonham, D. G. (1963) *Perinatal Mortality*, p. 167. Edinburgh: Livingstone.

Buxton, C. L. (1962) *A Study of Psychophysical Methods for Relief of Childbirth Pain*, p. 116. Philadelphia: Saunders.

Crawford, J. S. (1958) Anaesthesia for Obstetrics, Recent Advances. *Brit. med. Bull.*, **14**, 34.

Crawford, J. S. (1962) Anaesthesia for Caesarean Section: Proposal for Evaluation with Analysis of a Method. *Brit. J. Anaesth.*, **34**, 179.

Crawford, J. S. (1972a & b) *Principles and Practice of Obstetric Anaesthesia*, 3rd Edition, pp. 193 & 8. Oxford: Blackwell.

Dawkins, C. J. M. (1972) Complications of Epidural Analgesia: Summing up. In *Proc. Symp. Epid. Analg. Obstet.*, p. 67. Edited by A. Doughty. London: Lewis.

Department of Health and Social Security (1969) Report on Confidential Enquiries into Maternal Deaths in England and Wales, 1964–1966. *Rep. publ. Hlth med. Subj.*, No. 119. London: H.M.S.O.

Department of Health and Social Security (1972) Report on Confidential Enquiries into Maternal Deaths in England and Wales, 1967–1969. *Rep. Hlth Soc. Subj.*, No. 1. London: H.M.S.O.

Edmonds, J. (1972) Complications of Epidural Analgesia: Neurological Complications. In *Proc. Symp. Epid. Analg. Obstet.*, p. 54. Edited by A. Doughty. London: Lewis.

Elliott, C. J. R. (1963) A Study in Regurgitation. *Anaesthesia*, **18**, 324.

Flowers, C. E., Rudolph, A. J. & Desmond, M. M. (1969) Diazepam (Valium) as an Adjunct in Obstetric Analgesia. *Obstet. Gynec.*, **34**, 68.

Friedman, E. A. (1955) Primigravid Labor. *Obstet. Gynec.*, **6**, 567.

Friedman, E. A., Niswander, K. R. & Sachtleben, M. R. (1969) Effect of Diazepam on Labor. *Obstet. Gynec.*, **34**, 82.

Goodlin, R. C. (1971) Importance of the lateral position during labor. *Obstet. Gynec.*, **37**, 698.

Hodges, R. J. H., Bennett, J. R., Tunstall, M. E. & Knight, R. F. (1959) General Anaesthesia for operative obstetrics. *Brit. J. Anaesth.*, **31**, 152.

Hodges, R. J. H. & Tunstall, M. E. (1961) The Choice of Anaesthesia and its Influence on Perinatal Mortality in Caesarean Section. *Brit. J. Anaesth.*, **33**, 572.

Hon, E. H., Reid, B. L. & Hehre, F. W. (1960) Electronic evaluation of fetal heart rate; Changes with maternal hypotension. *Amer. J. Obstet. Gynec.*, **79**, 209.

Inkster, J. S. (1963) The induction of anaesthesia in patients likely to vomit with special reference to intestinal obstruction. *Brit. J. Anaesth.*, **35**, 160.

McAneny, T. M. & Doughty, A. G. (1963) Self-administered nitrous oxide/oxygen analgesia in obstetrics. *Anaesthesia*, **18**, 488.

Meehan, F. P., Moolgaoker, A. S. & Stallworthy, J. (1972) Vaginal delivery under caudal analgesia after Caesarean Section and other major uterine surgery. *Brit. med. J.*, **ii**, 740.

Mendelson, C. L. (1946) Aspiration of stomach contents into the lungs during obstetric anaesthesia. *Am. J. of Obstet. and Gynec.*, **52**, 191.

Ministry of Health (1963) Report on Confidential Enquiries into Maternal Deaths in England and Wales, 1958–1960. *Rep. publ. Hlth med. Subj.*, No. 108. London: H.M.S.O.

Ministry of Health (1966) Report on Confidential Enquiries into Maternal Deaths in England and Wales, 1961–1963. *Rep. publ. Hlth med. Subj.*, No. 115. London: H.M.S.O.

Minnitt, R. J. (1934) A new technique for the self-administration of gas–air analgesia in labour. *Lancet*, **i**, 1278.

Moya, F. & Kvisselgaard, N. (1961) Placental Transmission of Succinylcholine. *Anesthesiology*, **22**, 1.

Niswander, K. R. (1969) Effect of Diazepam on Meperidine Requirements of Patients during Labor. *Obstet. Gynec.*, **34**, 62.

Pearson, J. F. (1972) The effect of continuous lumbar epidural block on maternal and fetal acid-base balance during labour and at delivery. In *Proc. Symp. Epid. Analg. Obstet.*, p. 16. Edited by A. Doughty. London: Lewis.

Phillips, T. J. & MacDonald, R. R. (1971) Comparative effect of pethidine, trichloroethylene and Entonox on fetal and neonatal acid-base and PO_2. *Brit. med. J.*, **iii**, 558.

Poseiro, J. J. (1967) Compression of the aorta or iliac arteries by the contracting human uterus during labour. In *Effects of Labor on Fetus and Newborn*. Edited by R. Caldeyro-Barcia. New York: Pergamon.

Report to the Medical Research Council (1970) Clinical trials of different concentrations of oxygen and nitrous oxide for obstetric analgesia. *Brit. med. J.*, **i**, 709.

Rosen, M., Mushin, W. W., Jones, P. L. & Jones, E. V. (1969) Field trial of methoxyflurane, nitrous oxide and trichloroethylene as obstetric analgesics. *Brit. med. J.*, **iii**, 263.

Scott, D. B. (1968) Inferior vena caval occlusion in late pregnancy and its importance in anaesthesia. *Brit. J. Anaesth.*, **40**, 120.

Scott, D. B. (1972) Cardiac arrythmias during laparoscopy. *Brit. med. J.*, **ii**, 49.

Scott, D. B. & Julian, D. G. (1972) Observations on cardiac arrythmias during laparoscopy. *Brit. med. J.*, **i**, 411.

Sellick, B. A. (1961) Cricoid pressure to control regurgitation of stomach contents during induction of anaesthesia. *Lancet*, **ii**, 404.

Shnider, S. M. (1970) *Obstetrical Anaesthesia*, p. 46. Baltimore: Williams and Williams.

Smith, I., Benzie, R. J., Gordon, N. L. M., Kelman, G. R. & Swapp, G. H. (1971) Cardiovascular effects of peritoneal insufflation of carbon dioxide for laparoscopy. *Brit. med. J.*, **iii**, 410.

Spengler, D. B. (1961) The Lucy Baldwin nitrous oxide and oxygen machine. *Nursing Times*, **57**, 1237.

Taylor, G. & Pryse-Davies, J. (1966) The prophylactic use of antacids in the prevention of the acid–pulmonary-aspiration syndrome (Mendelson's Syndrome). *Lancet*, **i**, 288.

Tunstall, M. E. (1972) Complications of Epidural Analgesia: Precautions against Complications. In *Proc. Symp. Epid. Analg. Obstet.*, p. 64. Edited by A. Doughty. London: Lewis.

FURTHER READING

Bonica, J. J. (1967) *Principles and Practice of Obstetric Analgesia and Anesthesia*, Vol. **1**. Oxford: Blackwell.

Crawford, J. S. (1972) *Principles and Practice of Obstetric Anaesthesia*, 3rd Edition. Oxford: Blackwell.

Doughty, A. Editor (1972) *Proc. Symp. Epid. Analg. Obstet.* London: Lewis.

Gray, T. C. & Nunn, J. F. Editors (1971) *General Anaesthesia*, Vol. **2**. London: Butterworths.

Moir, D. D. (1971) *Pain Relief in Labour: A Handbook for Midwives*. Edinburgh: Churchill.

Obstetric Anaesthesia and Analgesia (1971) Postgraduate Educational Number. *Brit. J. Anaesth.*, **43**, 823–902.

25. Risk to Mother and Child

Throughout the text risks to mother and child have been described in relation to the particular situation under discussion and the student should study completely the relevant chapter.

Environmental factors, in the broadest sense and the resulting epidemiology of maternal and perinatal death are very fully discussed and described in Chapters 1 and 2.

Lawson (1971) has emphasized that in the tropical situation factors of malnutrition, infection, infestation, hygiene, custom and taboo are almost the most important primary factors in maternal and fetal death. The developed countries also have, of course, malnutrition, poor hygiene, strange (mainly medical) taboos and often poorly organized services.

Proper care can, therefore, be given to any pregnant woman or to any group of pregnant women only if their total social environmental and medical situation can be considered and evaluated and the necessary preventative and corrective therapies instituted.

Various lay publications suggest that 80–90 per cent of women have normal pregnancy and labour. Total physiological normality is however seen in only some 30–50 per cent (depending entirely on the social structure of the community under study). Nearly 30 per cent of all pregnant women need hospital admission antenatally.

MATERNAL MORTALITY

Maternal death is viewed with significant horror in most communities but was, until very recently, relatively common and accepted as a known hazard of reproduction. Munro-Kerr, in 1933, published a text wherein he reviewed the problem of maternal mortality and morbidity as he saw it at that time. He stated then that the problem was largely one of organization, so that the extent of care required could be given to each woman. He suggested that the requirement for adequate results are the same in all countries and all areas.

1. Efficacious antenatal and intranatal care for all women.
2. Highly skilled and well trained midwives.
3. Medical practitioners thoroughly and specially trained for maternity care in general.
4. Adequate accommodation under highly skilled care in special hospitals when such care is required.
5. A highly trained, skilled and disciplined specialist group working preferably in the best possible conditions in a group or team.

The basic needs are unchanged. The problem is entirely one of organization so that each woman gets the standard and quality of care she needs.

It must be obvious that in countries where terrain makes communication difficult like Ethiopia, the North American Tundra or the rain forests of Central America, or where distance is great, or where education is non-existent as in the Indian village, that maternal death from haemorrhage, difficult labour and other serious maternal complications must be common and almost unpreventable. In those situations salvage or emergency is the best that can be offered. Conditions of malnutrition, fever, drought, epidemic and indigenous disease must make the mother less able to withstand pregnancy hazards. It is fascinating to note however, that in all tightly controlled areas even in the African developing countries how much can be done to improve quality of care, *see* Chapter 26.

As with all medical care frequent and careful analyses of results is essential. Unless results are constantly monitored no improvement can be possible.

In England and Wales confidential inquiry into maternal death has been reported at regular intervals since 1952, the last for the years 1967–69. In Scotland the first report covers the years 1965–71.

In the period 1855–1930 the maternal mortality in England and Wales was virtually unchanged at about 4–5 per 1000 births. In Scotland the rate was highest in the period 1915–30 and reached nearly 7 per 1000 total births. It was likely that improved registration and more clear recognition of puerperal causes increase the registration especially in Scotland and thus mask a true improvement but nevertheless the situation in the period 1927–30 particularly in Scotland was a serious cause for concern.

In Chapter 2 are outlined the causes of maternal death in England and Wales. In Scotland in 1965–71 the causes have been somewhat differently recorded.

In England and Wales abortion, pulmonary embolus, haemorrhage and toxaemia were the main causes with anaesthetic death, sepsis, ectopic pregnancy and amniotic fluid embolism of lesser numerical importance.

In Scotland, *pulmonary embolism* is by far the most common single cause (16·5 per cent of all deaths and 24·8 per cent of all deaths due to true obstetric causes). *Sepsis* is second (at 20·6 per cent of 'true' deaths) and haemorrhage (16·5 per cent).

Judgment by a panel of experts considers that at least 36 per cent of all cases had avoidable factors and in some groups at least half of the deaths were clearly preventable.

The reader is particularly referred to chapters on Puerperal Infections and Anaesthesia for a review of the risks and dangers.

The particular hazards created by the greatly increased incidence of therapeutic termination of pregnancy and induction and stimulation of labour merit very careful thought. All invasive techniques are dangerous and all techniques of pregnancy termination and all inductions should be conducted with due regard to asepsis and antisepsis with due surgical skill and in the proper surroundings.

MATERNAL MORBIDITY

The conditions responsible for maternal death are clearly also responsible for maternal morbidity. It is difficult to evaluate the immediate or long term maternal risk.

Puerperal. The immediate risk of the puerperium are discussed in Chapter 21 and Chapter 31.

In the textbooks of some twenty years ago it was stated that a fairly large area of gynaecology was due to post-obstetric morbidity. Particular reference was made to pelvic floor prolapse and to chronic pelvic sepsis. Little or no reference was made to psychological factors which are now emphasized.

DAMAGE TO SOFT TISSUES IN THE LONG TERM
Damage to maternal tissue in association with difficult labour or delivery may occur with permanent or semi-permanent effects.

Complete tear of the perineum into the rectum may, if not properly repaired at the time, leave a recto vaginal fistula or a permanently incontinent sphincter. Repeat repair is then necessary after three to six months and, while usually successful, dictates great care at the next delivery (wide episiotomy and forcep guided delivery) or even elective Caesarean section.

Trauma to bladder due to a direct tear or following a slough due to head pressure over a long period may lead to vesico vaginal fistula (*see* Chapter 26) with all the distressing difficulties social and technical.

Rupture of uterus may occur at termination of pregnancy, spontaneously in labour or secondary to manipulation. Frequently treated by hysterectomy or repair and sterilization there are, nevertheless, a few patients who are allowed to have subsequent pregnancy and the greatest care is necessary with late bed rest in hospital and elective Caesarean section.

Incompetence of the cervix secondary to vaginal termination of pregnancy leads to mid-trimester abortion or premature labour. If this probability is always remembered a 'Shirodkar' suture can be inserted at any time in pregnancy up to thirty weeks.

Prolapse of the organs of the pelvic floor is seen, rarely, in the nullipara because of congenital herniation (e.g. enterocele) or in the older women in association with extreme loss of supporting tissue tone.

All forms of herniation—cystocele, rectocele, urethrocele, enterocele and prolapse of the uterus itself, usually, however, occur only in women who have delivered a child through the vagina. They are all associated with tearing or overstretching of fibro muscular supporting tissue sheaths. Such tearing or overstretching may occur in a relatively simple delivery but are, of course, more likely when the later part of the first stage is prolonged and with mechanical difficulty in the second stage, especially if undue 'pushing' is encouraged with a slowly stretching pelvic floor or, of course, if relief is not given in an over stretched situation. Properly performed forcep delivery does not of itself cause tissue damage especially where episiotomy is carefully and correctly performed and sutured.

In many young primigravidae the pelvic floor stretches slowly and easily, if permitted to do so, to allow spontaneous delivery without damage, but after the age of 25, in primigravidae, such easy stretching is less likely and overstretching of tight tissues and tearing are more likely.

Prophylactic episiotomy, often midline, or low forceps are more often required.

Prolapse is not necessarily a greater problem after higher parity as most damage occurs in the first pregnancy and labour.

It is perhaps significant that in the Eastern States of America where prophylactic episiotomy and forceps are common that pelvic floor prolapse in the white population is relatively rare. In British women prolapse is certainly less often seen now in women before the menopause. This is due possibly to the improved obstetric care of the last 25 years.

There is no doubt also that in the black peoples of Africa, of the West Indies and of the eastern United States, prolapse is also uncommon and that episiotomy and forceps delivery are rarely required. Perhaps this can best be explained by youth at first delivery. Certainly in the West Indies the girls are tall and well nourished and disproportion is uncommon.

Inversion of the uterus. This rare condition presents usually acutely and dramatically and is described in Chapter 31. As a chronic or subacute cause of irregular menstruation it is very rare.

DAMAGE TO BONE AND JOINTS
Pregnancy is associated with softening of cartilaginous and fibrous tissues and there is lordosis as part of the normal postural change. Movement at the sacro iliac joints and some separation of the symphysis pubis are normally seen. It is not surprising, therefore, that backache, disc lesions, sacro iliac strain, are occasional long term sequelae of pregnancy and delivery, especially if the exaggerated lithotomy position is used.

Osteitis pubis as a long term sequela of symphyseal separation is a rare complication.

VARICOSE VEIN AND THROMBO EMBOLISM
Pregnancy exaggerates lower limb varicosity and frequent pregnancy produces a steady deteriorating situation. Low grade multiple thrombo embolism following puerperal sepsis is a relatively rare cause of chronic pulmonary incapacity.

OTHER CONDITIONS
The wide ranging physiological changes of pregnancy and the strain on the patient with associated disease has been discussed in the chapter concerned. It is not surprising that, especially where adequate care is not available or given, pregnancy and delivery can have permanent deleterious effects.

SEPSIS
Chronic pelvic sepsis following childbirth or abortion was extremely common in the first half of this century. Mostly such infection followed long and difficult labour or septic abortion and was due to anaerobic organisms to staphylococcus or E. coli. Lesion due to the haemolytic streptococcus was more usually acute and often fatal.

The risk of chronic sepsis is still present but is very much less often seen.

This is due firstly to hospitalization with less risk of low grade infection at delivery, with more frequent temperature recordings, with investigation of all pyrexia, with the frequent and early use of antibiotics where pyrexia occurs, with adequate blood transfusion where required, and with immediate action if there is suspicion of retained material. The new risks in association with induced abortion of damage and post-abortion sepsis must be very carefully looked for and actively treated.

Great care should be taken to ensure that the uterus is empty. Ultrasound studies show that incomplete emptying is not too uncommon and this is borne out clinically where re-admission with sepsis or bleeding occurs.

PSYCHOLOGICAL FACTORS
Pregnancy, labour and the post-natal period may by themselves have a devastating psychological effect on a susceptible person. However, difficulty in pregnancy (and nearly 30 per cent of women require antenatal admission), prolonged or difficult labour, a painful or anxious post delivery phase will affect some women often seriously and perman-

ently. Much of the effects are associated with pain, and the biochemical changes of a long labour. Loneliness, fear and frustration also are involved.

Walker and Dunn (1970) in a follow-up study of women who had suffered difficult labour or delivery found, at personal interview of women first delivered after the age of 25 years, that prolonged and distressing labour, especially ending in the frustration of operative delivery, prevented many women having a further child. This was not so in women delivered first under the age of 20, and less so from 20–25. It is claimed by some that the maternal/child relationship may be also affected but this is much more difficult to prove. It must, however, be remembered that many women seriously affected by pregnancy and childbirth are themselves unusual in their responses and need different and special care.

Women's organizations are now more articulate in expression of their needs and beliefs about childbirth and the dialogue should ensure better understanding and perhaps improved care.

PREGNANCY AND INDUSTRY

The present attitudes and legal guidance towards the employment of pregnant women is in Great Britain a mixture of minimal legislation, reasonable common sense and a great deal of ignorance and apathy. Traditionally in Britain women do not undertake dangerous employment so the problem is supposedly less than in other countries. Britain is not a signatory to the International Labour Convention 103 of 1952 which suggests that pregnant women should have:

1. Twelve weeks' leave of which six weeks post-partum was compulsory.
2. No night work and no overtime.
3. No employment likely to be prejudicial to pregnancy and not for at least three months after delivery.

In Britain the only legal protection is of women employed in Factories or Workshops, Factories Act (Scotland (1961)) and the Public Health Act 1936 (E & W) which precludes an employer 'knowledge of employing women within 4 weeks of the birth of a child'.

Attitudes to time vary: In any Civil Service employment a woman is entitled to two months' paid leave—most take one month before and one after. This is probably inadequate. It can be argued that in many instances work during pregnancy by increasing the income of the woman enables better food to be purchased and a better living standard to be obtained which reflects itself on the quality of the pregnancy.

In most studies where communities are matched for age and social class and for type of work undertaken, there is little evidence that work in the general sense during pregnancy has an adverse effect on the outcome of pregnancy. This is, however, a somewhat illogical finding and probably further detailed studies are essential.

There are however, occupations of risk where the employment of pregnant women should be limited severely, e.g. high level noise, whole body vibration and exposure to toxic chemicals.

With the new interest in equal pay and rights and privileges of the pregnant woman, new legislation is inevitable and necessary.

PROPHYLACTIC VACCINATION OR INOCULATION DURING PREGNANCY

Poliomyelitis

Although the risks of poliomyelitis are small in the pregnant woman, she is nevertheless particularly susceptible in epidemic situations. The use of vaccination with live polio virus (e.g. oral) in pregnancy is warranted after careful assessment of the relative risks, which are the risk that family contacts might be infected and fatal disease could occur. It should not be given in the first sixteen weeks.

Rubeola (*measles*)

Many female children are now immunized, but if a pregnant woman, not immune, is exposed to measles in a serious epidemic situation specific gamma globulin may be indicated during the incubation phase.

Influenza

In the presence of a virulent epidemic strain of influenza, vaccination in pregnancy may be advised in view of the serious maternal risk. It is, however, often extremely difficult in any epidemic to obtain readily a vaccine specific to the infecting strain.

Varicella

There is some evidence that γ-globulin given to the exposed mother may limit the extent and severity of her disease.

Variola (*Smallpox*)

Specific immune γ-globulin may be helpful in exposed mothers in epidemic situations.

Vaccination during pregnancy is *not* to be recommended unless in the presence of epidemic conditions. The risk to the fetus of maternal vaccination is, of course, greatest when she has not been previously vaccinated, or has had poor previous 'takes'.

Rubella

Ideally all pregnant women should be screened for rubella antibodies and vaccination given in the immediate puerperium to those found to be negative. Eighty per cent of adult women in this country are already immune and vaccination should not be offered to young women unless the immune status is known. Vaccination inadvertently given during pregnancy does obviously carry a risk to the fetus, and the virus has been recovered from the tissues of fetus aborted in such circumstances. There is as yet (1974) insufficient evidence to advocate continuation of a pregnancy where vaccination has been given although, apparently normal children have been born.

Yellow Fever

Vaccination is clearly contra-indicated in pregnancy.

TAB

There is no contra-indication to giving TAB vaccine in pregnancy. It is, of course, a killed vaccine which is not attended by the same risks as live vaccines.

PERINATAL MORTALITY

It has been stated in Chapter 2 that 'it is difficult to provide satisfactory statistical evidence of the extent to which perinatal mortality rates are affected by the nature of the maternity services available'. This is correct in a way but it should not encourage the student or practitioner to limit the range of quality of his care or to debit high rates entirely to the poor quality or high parity of the population from which his patients are drawn. In the United Kingdom maternity and neonatal care should be everywhere superb as there is little excuse for other levels of care. In the less privileged situation high risk or problem cases should be selected out on clinical or epidemiological grounds for special care.

Nevertheless, it is interesting to compare perinatal mortality in Glasgow and Dundee, two cities of roughly similar social and industrial backgrounds and similar obstetric cover. The perinatal mortality in Glasgow is at 27·6 (1970) much higher than that of Dundee 15·8 (1969–73), and this difference is seen in all parities. Glasgow has a relatively high rate in parity over four. However, analysis of the cause groups by the technique of Baird, Walker and Thomson (1954) demonstrates that the excess of Glasgow deaths is mostly in the antepartum haemorrhage and premature unknown groups, which very largely reflect the less good socio-economic and possibly nutritional state of the Glasgow mother— (only 12 per cent over 165cm in height compared with 17 per cent even in Dundee, a city also with a social history of poverty). There is also an excess, in Glasgow, of death associated with late pregnancy anoxia, the *mature unknown* group which should be largely preventable.

Prevention of perinatal death

If any community or country wishes to improve its perinatal death rate and coincidentally to improve the quality of its maternity care, and the ultimate quality of its children, it must firstly find out why babies are dying and the types and features of the mothers of these babies.

Analysis of perinatal death (stillbirth and first week death reported and analysed separately as well as together as 'perinatal death') should be made by all the standard parameters of maternal age, parity, height, social class, urban and rural etc. as far as possible. Then an expert group should study the actual clinical circumstances of each death by a system such as that discussed by Baird, Walker and Thomson (1954), so that the maternal and child aetiology of the death is clear. In addition, there should be if possible, information of the immediate cause of the death so that the role of deformity, infection or immaturity, etc. in the neonatal period can be assessed.

In any country the quality of the maternal health and nutrition is of immense importance and every corrective measure should be applied. Analysis by cause will show the conditions where there is unnecessary loss from poor obstetrics and where clinical action is necessary.

Fetal morbidity

There are certain hazards to the child in pregnancy and labour and in the post-natal period, which are preventable or where the damage can be mitigated. There are some very theoretical risks or risks with low statistical frequency—an outline is discussed.

Risks to the fetus *in utero*

The developing fetus is dependent on the efficiency of his mother's supply system, on his mother's and his own transport system, and on his own ability to utilize nutrients presented to him. He is capable of some defence against inadequate supply or noxious materials, but is sometimes highly susceptible to influences which have a minimum effect on his mother.

The mother who is seriously ill has much less ability to maintain and nourish a pregnancy. An intra-uterine death or abortion may occur for this reason only. The effects of many of those diseases have been discussed in Chapter 12. Where there is toxicity or high fever, maternal infection may cause abortion, premature labour, or long term damage to the child. In infections associated with viraemia, bacteraemia or septicaemia, there may be direct viral or bacterial transfer to the child itself. Alternatively exo toxins can be themselves damaging to the developing fetus.

Although for many years the toxic effect of chemicals (e.g. lead) has been known or suspected, the advent of the thalidomide era has raised new and interesting problems of fetal pharmacology. There is little doubt that any drug given to the mother and soluble in her serum must be transferred to the child. The effects in the child may be minimal, or lethal. Largely, the effects are dose related, e.g. with sedation, but with some drugs, like thalidomide, the mere presence of the drug is sufficient for serious effects to occur.

In Chapter 19, are discussed the possible adverse environmental situations of labour.

There is risk to the population of the poisonous effects of many chemical agents in the environment, ranging from chemicals in prescribed medicines, to chemicals in food, exhaust fumes, industrial waste or insecticides which may enter food or drink. In some situations evidence of damage to a fetus is immediate and positive like the deformity due to thalidomide or say rubella. In other situations damage occurring *in utero* or in labour may result in ultimate failure of normal development or the growth of malignant tumours and not, therefore, be manifest for months or years.

Especially with drugs the period of pregnancy at which exposure occurs to the noxious influence is important. In the pre-implantation period, for example, drugs or other traumas may kill but rarely deform, as toti potential cells can replace damaged cells.

After implantation each organ or tissue has a period of greatest risk when it is being actively differentiated—*see* Chapter 6, and the extent of damage, degree of damage, or the actual tissue damaged by the same external influence will vary.

INTRA-UTERINE RISKS TO THE FETUS

Viral infection

Viral infection of the mother and fetus has been very fully discussed by Monif (1969 & 1974). The effects of viral infection may be slight in the mother and lethal or seriously damaging to the child. While the placenta is probably involved when the child is involved, it is difficult often to prove or delineate the evidence of infection. Viraemia must exist in the mother first. Viral infection in the fetus may, as with rubella, vaccinia, variola and some others, persist in the fetal tissues up till the first year of life. Even an immune response determined by the presence of fetal IgM immunoglobulin and circulating maternally derived IgG immunoglobulin may not eliminate the infection or necessarily limit its activity. Elevation in the fetal blood of IgM antibodies specific to the virus may be considered presumptive evidence that fetal intra-uterine infection has occurred, but proof requires isolation of the virus or other infecting organism from fetal or abortus tissues.

POLIO VIRUS

In maternal poliomyelitis most fetal death is associated with prematurity associated with delivery in the acute phases of the disease, virus is sometimes isolated from these fetuses. Where poliomyelitis affects the mother early in pregnancy and abortion does not occur, the child may rarely have poor growth, some retarded development after birth and neurological disease. Specific IgM antibody may be isolated.

COCKSACKIE

Most maternal diseases are subclinical and fetal infection may result in subclinical disease with retarded development. However, congenital and neonatal infection with Cocksackie Group B virus can result in meningoencephalitis, myocarditis, and hepatitis.

Viral isolation or demonstration of specific IgM antibody in cord blood or evidence from special immunofluorescent stain e.g. of myocardium, are essential for diagnosis. Epidemics in nurseries may be serious and fulminating or totally subclinical with minor diarrhoea but with later evidence of damage to the child.

ECHO

Although infection can be proved no morbidity or mortality is to be expected.

MEASLES (*Rubeola*)

Abortion and premature labour may be associated with acute maternal disease and the fetus might show infection. Mild congenital measles does occur in the neonate but usually follows a benign course.

MUMPS (*Parotitis*)

It is doubtful if there is any specific fetal risk although congenital disease has been reported.

INFLUENZA

Fulminating pneumonia may occur in the pregnant woman who is exposed in epidemic conditions and fetal death may follow but due entirely to the effect of the disease on the mother. There is no real evidence of fetal deformity but some suspicion of later child leukaemia when pregnant women suffer influenza.

HERPES

Herpes hominis Type 2 is the likely infector in pregnancy (Type 1 naso-oral rarely). Pre-existing cervical infection may cause abortion. The fetus may be infected *in utero* rarely with microcephaly and retinal dysplasia and a rash at birth. Neonatal infection may follow delivery of the child through a vulvo vaginitis and is associated with splenomegaly, jaundice, skin lesions and encephalitis, etc. Active herpes vulvo vaginitis at the time of labour is an indication for Caesarean section within four hours of rupture of membranes (Tobin, 1975).

VARICELLA-ZOSTER (*Chickenpox*)

Infection of the fetus early in gestation may lead to abortion, later infection to prematurity or clinical disease. Acute maternal illness may itself, result in abortion or premature labour. Congenital herpes zoster has been reported but there is no evidence of a long term affect in mental development. There is, however, a statistical suggestion of some increase in leukaemia risk to the child (Adelstein and Donovan, 1972).

CYTOMEGALO VIRUS

Some 20–80 per cent of all pregnant women have had previous exposure to the virus and specific complement fixing antibodies can be demonstrated in their serum (*Brit. med. J.* (1974) **i** 341 and **ii** 593). The virus has been isolated from 2–10 per cent of abortuses and from newborn infant urine. Infant or adult infection with this virus results in latent infection with prolonged shedding of virus. It is, however, more likely that the fetus is infected from a maternal viraemia associated with a primary infection during gestation, and 2–3 per cent of susceptible women have such viraemia. The neonate can be infected from his mother's colostrum.

The infant born with cytomegalo virus infection is infective, and some 400 children born in England and Wales annually are mentally retarded from this cause and very many more are deaf or intellectually impaired.

VARIOLA (*Smallpox*)

The malignant disease may kill the mother or her serious illness may cause her to abort or go into premature labour. Transplacental infection arises during the pre-eruptive fever and may occur even in the previously immunized mother. Congenital disease occurs and is of course, highly infectious. Sometimes infants affected *in utero* survive and are immune to the disease.

VACCINIA

Almost all fetal vaccinia has resulted from maternal vaccination during pregnancy and usually where the mother has no previous successful vaccination. The child may be aborted or prematurely delivered dead or alive with clinical vaccinia. (Green, Reid & Rhaney, 1966.) For this reason maternal vaccination is contra-indicated in pregnancy.

Rubella is very fully discussed in Chapter 11.

The earlier the disease occurs in pregnancy, the greater the likelihood of abnormalities developing. Different systems are usually affected at different times by the virus. The incidence of defects is also dependent on the type of virus involved, as it appears that some epidemics have been associated with a higher incidence of malformations than others. The incidence of malformations is about 50 per cent if the infection occurs in the first four weeks, 40 per cent in the second four weeks, 30 per cent in the third four weeks and between 10 and 20 per cent between 12 and 16 weeks (Dudgeon, 1967).

Direct fetal damage may follow maternal infection up to the twentieth week. Congenital viral infection may persist and these infants are highly infective to their attendants.

The permanent stigmata of the syndrome are cataracts (Gregg, 1941) corneal clouding, chorioretinitis and other eye lesions, patent ductus, septal defects, myocardiopathy, microcephaly and leptomeningitis, inner ear damage, liver malfunction, interstitial pneumonia and nephritis, maldevelopment of bone growth.

The child born after an apparent maternal infection should be checked by attempted viral isolation techniques from throat swabs and urine.

'Reinfection' of the previously infected or vaccinated patient during pregnancy would be unlikely to damage the fetus, as there is no evidence that viraemia exists in the reinfected patient. The fetus would be at risk only if rubella specific IgM antibody could be demonstrated in the mother.

HEPATITIS

Infectious or serum hepatitis is transmissable to the fetus and both maternal and fetal hepatitis has been found after intra-uterine transfusion.

Transmission of the virus from the mother to her fetus with birth of one or several children with congenital giant cell hepatitis may occur. Skip phenomena may also occur due to inconstant viraemia.

When the infectious condition occurs the mother may abort or have premature delivery of a somewhat toxic infant which may or may not have hepatitis with later post-hepatic cirrhosis. Maternal preconception infective hepatitis has been reported to be associated with an increased incidence of mongolism in the children subsequently conceived, and there is some suggestion that mongolism may be associated with maternal infection at a previous delivery from contact with a mother recently delivered of an affected baby (Harlap, 1973).

Other infection

SYPHILIS

In the undetected untreated pregnant woman with syphilis, the infant may die *in utero* or be born with the disease. Recurring fetal death should always raise a suspicion of syphilis as a cause.—Routine check of *all* pregnant women and care of the detected case can virtually completely prevent the fetal or infant disease.— The condition is discussed in full in Chapter 36.

Bacterial infection

TUBERCULOSIS

Congenital tuberculosis is a rarity and occurs only when there is a blood spread to the uterus during the pregnancy. Caseous lesion are found primarily in the fetal liver.

INTRA-UTERINE PNEUMONIA

The fetus may be infected across the placenta from a maternal septicaemia, but it is more likely that intra-uterine pneumonia crosses from ascending infection after rupture of the membranes (Smith *et al.*, 1956). Infection is much more liable in very late pregnancy and at least 6 per cent are infected after the membranes have been ruptured for 48 hours. Other organisms e.g. B. welchi, E. coli, can similarly infect the fetus by ascending infection after membrane rupture. (Shubeck, F., Benson, R. C., Clark, W. W., Berendes, H., Weiss, W., Deutschberger, J., 1966.)

LISTERIOSIS

Listeria monocytogenes infection of the maternal vagina and cervix is said to predispose to abortion. Certainly intra-uterine infection with fetal meningoencephalitis can occur. Stillbirth may be due to hepatic necrosis.

Parasitic disease

TOXOPLASMOSIS

It is estimated that the incidence of maternal

toxoplasmosis in the United Kingdom is between 1:4000 and 14000. It is known that there are at least 1 in 14000 newborn children affected by congenital toxoplasmosis.

Therapy is impossible and prevention difficult. The disease is carried by cats and it has been suggested that the exposure of pre-pubertal girls to cats would result in likely immunity for their fetuses (Fleck, 1974).

The fetus is infected usually when a mother acquires the infection acutely during pregnancy but chronic toxoplasmosis endometritis has been blamed for recurrent stillbirth. Therapeutic abortion is probably indicated if a mother is known to have become infected but normal children have been born.

The earlier fetal infection occurs in pregnancy the worse the effects. In early pregnancy abortion occurs, and in later pregnancy, with the development of placental foci, stillbirth, or premature delivery of an infected baby. Severe congenital disease affects the eyes and the central nervous system, and may not fully develop for some months.

MALARIA is fully described in Chapter 26, but intra-uterine infection can occur and the child may be born with the disease, but this is rare in mothers with high immunity, since the placenta tends to be a barrier. Women entering epidemic areas must be protected since unprotected pregnant women may acquire **P.** falciparum infection with maternal anaemia, placental parasitization and fetal growth retardation, mostly in first pregnancies. The maternal anaemia secondary to malaria is largely responsible for the poor fetal growth which can, therefore, be prevented (Harrison, 1974).

TRYPANOSOMIASIS

Infection by **T** Cruzi (Americas) or **T** gardienise or rhodesiense (Africa) tends to cause infertility or abortion, prematurity and stillbirth due to the effect of the disease in the mother. Congenital infection can occur but is rare in the African, but more likely in the American (**T** Cruzi) infection.

PHARMACOLOGY

Anaesthetic agents, analgesics and sedatives

ANAESTHESIA

There is some evidence that prolonged exposure to operating room environment in-creases the risk of abortion: prematurity and deformity in the babies of nursing staff, female anaesthetists and the wives of male anaesthetists (Kaiser, I. H., 1973).

Volatile anaesthetic agents are rapidly transferred to the fetus. Parity of blood levels in nitrous oxide is reached in about 20 minutes and similar patterns apply to other agents. Depression of the child is inevitable when anaesthesia lasts any length of time. Accompanying high maternal ambient oxygen protects to some extent.

Drugs used in *epidural* spinal, pudendal and other blocks rapidly cleared by the mother, are normally at insufficient maternal blood level to affect the child, to any serious extent (except when paracervical anaesthesia is used with high dosage).

After lignocaine or maperocaine the drug is present in the fetal blood for some hours and the babies are floppy but alert.

Tubo-curarine and other paralysing agents may affect a child if used for a prolonged period but in normal practice the risk is small.

Atropine given as a premedication greatly increases fetal heart rate.

Morphine and *pethdine* especially in repeated dosage clearly depress the child's ability to respond at birth, but also have effects which last for some days. As with barbiturate withdrawal affects in the child may be quite severe.

Barbiturates have the effect of lowering the neonatal level of unconjugated bilirubin and are some protection against the risks of neonatal jaundice. However, withdrawal symptoms in the child may not appear for up to 10 days—*see* 'phenytoin'.

Diazoxide in heavy dosage e.g. in specific hypertensive disease may cause newborn alopecia.

Chloropromazine has an affinity for melanin containing tissues and eyes of the newborn should be checked.

Thalidomide the main effect of this drug on the fetus is to produce hypoplasia and interference with embryonic development and so phocomelia. It appears to have its effects between the 34th and 50th day after the first day of the last menstrual cycle or the 20th–36th day of fetal age.

Drugs taken to control epilepsy *phenytoin*, *phenobarbitone* and *primidone* singly or in combination are clearly responsible for some increase in hare lip and cleft palate and possibly deformities associated with chromosomal anomaly. The risk is low and not sufficient to justify stopping use where they are necessary to control epilepsy.

Magnesium sulphate used as a sedation in the mother may suppress acetylcholene release at the neuromuscular junction in the fetus and make the newborn less able to respond.

Diazepam in a total dose of 30mgm to the mother in the 15 hours before delivery has little effect on the fetus. Larger doses are, however, accompanied by apnoea, and hypotonic reluctance to feed. The drug may have an effect up to eight days. However, where used to control eclampsia the fetal risk may be well acceptable.

Antibacterials and antibiotics

Antibacterials and antibiotics used in pregnancy should be selected for the specificity of their action, or sometimes for their ability to cross to the fetus or into the amniotic cavity. They should however, be reviewed for possible adverse effects and the manufacturers literature studied.

Septrin and *Bactrim*. Because of the content of trimethoprim which is a mild anti-folate, these drugs are contra-indicated especially in early pregnancy.

Nitrofurantoin. The makers recommend certain caution in pregnancy use. It is known to produce haemolytic anaemia in glucose 6 phosphatase deficient infants.

Chloramphenicol should be used only in life saving situations when it is the drug of direct choice.

Terramycin: tetracycline given after 20 weeks, stains the milk and permanent teeth of the fetus, and may retard long bone development.

Streptomycin. Interferes with the inner ear, and should not be used in early pregnancy. Gentamycin is also ototoxic, both should be used only in life saving situations.

Clindamycin — must not be given
Lincomycin — in pregnancy or
Phthalyl sulphathiazole — to the newborn
Clofazimine. Used as an anti-leprosy drug is probably safe in pregnancy.

Drugs of addiction

Lysergic acid (LSD). There is no clear proof of danger but there is some evidence of deformity after maternal and paternal consumption in early pregnancy.

Marjuana does not appear to carry a risk.

Methadone however, while probably not a risk to the child interferes with pregnancy tests inhibiting latex particle agglutination (e.g. Gravindex).

Heroin—withdrawal symptoms in the neonate of the addicted mother can be quite severe.

Chronic maternal alcoholism has been reported to be associated with serious fetal defect.

Cytotoxic drugs, folic acid or folinic acid inhibitors

These drugs by their very nature are certain to interfere seriously with fetal development especially in the early months, and should be considered contra-indicated—*see* Septrin.

Hormones

There is some evidence that progestogens given in pregnancy may have an adverse effect on the child.

Progestogens used in pregnancy as diagnostic tests or taken mistakenly for contraceptive purposes have been reported to be associated with multiple fetal anomaly. They must not be used.

Androgenic steroids with a 17 HO group may cause masculinization of the female fetus if given before the 12th week.

Diethylstilboestrol given to the mother during pregnancy has been reported to be associated with teenage vaginal adenosis, vaginal adenocarcinoma and vaginal septal defect. By stimulation of fetal adrenal androgens there may be some masculining effects in the female fetus, or loss of masculinity in the male.

Progesterone given during pregnancy has been reported to be associated with the birth of highly intelligent and exceptional children, but all reports suggesting techniques of producing 'super' children should be in general viewed with caution.

Other drugs

Aspirin and *Promezathine* may interfere with neonatal platelet aggregation.

Cortisone to the mother has apparently little fetal effect where its use is essential to the mother. But the child may at delivery suffer from suppression of its own adrenal corticotropin output, and special supportive therapy may be necessary.

Iodides taken by mothers in expectorant mixtures can produce euthyroid goitres in the newborn. In the contrary situation gross iodide deficiency can produce cretinism and unfortunately iodized salt for the first time in pregnancy does not protect.

Tolbutamide and *Chlorpropamide* (Chapter 12) can be successfully used in the control of diabetic pregnancy but in excess dosage can produce deformity or profound neonatal hypoglycaemia.

Heparin is safe.

Warfarin and the dicoumoral drugs should be used with caution.

Stelazine. Transplacental passage of phenothiazone used in the treatment of late vomiting may adversely affect fetal liver function. This would show as excess bilirubin in the amniotic fluid.

Podophyllum. This drug is highly toxic if absorbed and can cause severe vomiting and peripheral neuropathy in pregnant women. It is also anti mitotic. It is therefore, clearly contra-indicated in pregnancy or in any situation where excessive dosage is likely to be necessary.

Lead causes abortion and low birth weight defective infants. Recently there has been much interest in chronic lead poisoning in children and adults in large urban centres. Perhaps we should think more often of lead as a fetal risk.

Lithium. There seems to be a minimal risk to the fetus where mothers are having lithium therapy for manic depressive states, although a risk has been shown in animal experiments. Lithium is excreted in the milk.

Transplacental carcinogens
The role of diethylstilboestrol in the possible aetiology of adolescent vaginal adenocarcinoma (latent period 14–22 years) has been mentioned earlier. This aetiology was noticed by discovery of a small cluster of cases in the Boston area (Herbst *et al.*, 1971), but has not yet been (1974) reported in Great Britain.

Many neonatal and infant cancers must arise *in utero* since infants can be born already with malignant tumours. Theoretically exposure to carcinogens like to nitroso ureas, immuno suppressives, phenytoin, chloramphenicol, etc., could produce intra-uterine cancer since fetal tissues in their embryonic state could easily go out of control. Substances which are embryonic early on could be teratogenic in the second quarter of pregnancy and carcinogenic in the latter half.

A high abortion rate in a given patient may signal later carcinomas in the siblings if a similar factor was at work.

Maternal phenylketonuria
Phenylketonuric infants adequately treated are now grown to adulthood and having pregnancies of their own. Their infants are at acute risk of the high circulating maternal phenylketons, as are also the infants of mothers heterozygous to the disease.

Other external factors

POTATO FUNGUS
Potato fungus of late blight type has been suggested as the direct cause of anencephaly in the British Isles. Epidemiological data is suggestive (Renwick, 1972). There are, however, two types of anencephaly, the first in primigravida and secunda gravida which tends to recur (and be related to neural tube defects in siblings) and the rather more general sporadic type found in any parity which does not recur. Perhaps the second type may be more closely associated with a fungal cause.— Research continues.

SONAR
Currently there is no evidence that diagnostic sonar is a danger to the mother or to the fetus at any stage of pregnancy. Sonar in early pregnancy may by damage to the fetal gonad produce a risk to the next again generation. Sonar in late pregnancy may produce a risk to special senses. Extensive research investigation will be necessary to prove absolutely freedom from risk. Like all special tests, sonar should be used only where the knowledge gained is of immediate benefit to the care of the patient and her child.

CIGARETTE SMOKING
Cigarette smoking is hazardous to the fetus during pregnancy and to the immediate and late development of the child.

The effects are due (1) to the direct action of nicotine on the vessels causing some vasoconstriction, (2) to the chemical effect on maternal B_{12} metabolism of cyanide secondary to the metabolism of nicotine and (3) to the interference by carboxy haemoglobin with the position of maternal and fetal disassociation curves for oxygen so altering the pO_2 at various oxygen saturations. The pCO_2

of fetal blood is double that of maternal and so the effect is enhanced in the fetus (Cole et al., 1972).

The mother already at some disadvantage with threatened abortion or antepartum haemorrhage, hypertensive disease or under-nutrition, whose fetus may be already some-what hypoxic is more likely to be at serious disadvantage if she smokes cigarettes.

It is interesting to note that, while some 25 per cent of pregnant women in the upper social group smoke cigarettes, the rate is at least doubled in the poorest social group and especially in young women of high parity. The most up-to-date evidence of the effect of maternal cigarette smoking during pregnancy is available from Andrews and McGarry (1972), who studied 18 631 maternities in women resident in Cardiff who had babies from 1965–68. Babies of mothers who smoked were lighter and more likely to be premature and the effect was greater with the increasing number of cigarettes smoked. National studies have shown that children of mothers who smoked during pregnancy are less intellectually developed and smaller and lighter at the age of seven (Davie et al., 1972).

The raised perinatal mortality is associated with some increase in antepartum haemor-rhage and respiratory distress syndrome in the new born. There is, however, a very much *lower* incidence of pre-eclampsia in mothers who smoke, not enough, however, to offset the bad effect of smoking on birth weight, prematurity or perinatal death. Detoxication of the cyanide to thiocyanide may reduce maternal blood pressure. There was in the babies a slightly increased risk of cleft palate and hare lip. All these effects are relatively slight but they are clearly significant.

BLOOD TRANSFUSION

Thymus dependent lymphocytes introduced by intra-uterine transfusion can respond to histo compatability antigens with a graft/host reaction. This theoretical and minimal hazard must not be allowed to detract from the value of blood transfusion to the newborn or prevent its use.

IRRADIATION AND RADIO CONTAMINATION

There is a danger that the pregnant woman and her fetus may be exposed to radiation as a result of diagnostic radiology or radiation therapy, and with the widespread use of nuclear energy in industry she may be acci-dentally exposed to environmental radio con-tamination.

Diagnostic radiology

X-radiology of the abdomen of the pregnant woman increases the risk of later juvenile malignant disease. Risk appears present even with very minimal radiation doses below 200 millrads.

Radiographs in pregnancy are advocated most in diagnosis of twins, in hydramnios, in malpresentation and in pelvimetry.—There is some evidence that the risk is dose related and that the cancers begin at the time of the radiation.—The lesion to be expected are the haemopoetic neoplasm, neuroblastomas, other intracerebral tumours and oesteogenic sar-comas, but it would appear that the carcinomas are more likely when X-radiology is before the 20th week and the leukaemias are the main risk in late pregnancy X-ray (Stewart, 1961).

It is now recommended that radiological examination of the area from the mid chest to the knees of *any female* within the child-bearing years (for all practical purposes 14–45) should not be undertaken in the second half of the menstrual cycle unless it is considered impossible for pregnancy to be present. Responsibility for the exclusion of pregnancy rests with the doctor requesting the examina-tion and all X-ray request forms should record the date of the last menstrual period. Radio-logical departments are expected to book examinations for the 10 days immediately post period.

Radiological examination of the pregnant woman should be required only where the result is essential to the health and welfare of mother or child. Examination before the 20th week should be done rarely. It is reported that where the radiation dose to the fetus is likely to be more than 5r fetal damage is likely.

Radioactive substances

During pregnancy radioisotopes should be used rarely. Radioactive I^{131} is for example, extremely dangerous to the thyroid, skeleton and central nervous system of the early fetus. The most important part is the ability of the carrier substance to cross the placenta and so take the radioactivity to the fetus. The fetus appears to be most susceptible to radiation induced deformity or death between the 30th and 60th days after first day of last menstrual period.

The widespread use of radioisotopes in diagnosis (thyroid, blood volume, brain, liver, Vit.B12, renal function, etc.) means that radiation of the unsuspected pregnancy may occur. Mineral iodine crosses the placenta rapidly and there is soon five times the concentration in the fetal plasma. The fetal thyroid is at acute risk in its early developing phase and the fetus actively stores thyroxine so that any radioactive material would be at increasing concentration in the gland.

If in pregnancy a radioactive iodine must be used for diagnostic purposes, then one of the short lived isotopes I^{132} or I^{123} is preferable and if possible after the 60th day.

Placentograph or blood flow studies with isotopes are commonly used in pregnancy. The minimal dose to the fetal gonads or thyroid is obtained with Iodine 132; Technitium 99 or Chromium 51. While Iodine 125 carries a minimal risk to the gonads it carries a very high risk to the fetal thyroid. Sodium injected into the chorio decidual space or myometrium carries a fairly high fetal risk.

Xenon 133 should probably be used for organ irradiation studies only in the first half of a menstrual cycle.

Krypton-85 has not been shown to be a risk.

Organ scans
Renal scan with I^{131} hippuran is probably safe in pregnancy especially after the 60th day and if the fetal thyroid is protected with lugols iodine to prevent radiolysis. The iodohippuran is bound to the maternal protein and is not transferred.

Mercurial compounds Hg^{203} or Hg^{197} in chlormerodrin used for brain scan are safe in the pregnant woman as they too are bound to the maternal protein and do not cross.

All scans using colloidal material are similarly safe but bone scan with Strontium 85 is very risky indeed. Calcium 47 or some such short lived isotope could be used if scan is clinically essential. Selenium 75 methionine is very dangerous indeed.

Radioactivity from the environment
Women pregnant when exposed to nuclear fallout or direct atom bomb effects in Hiroshima, Nagasaki and the Marshall Islands had a high perinatal mortality which was distance/dose related. The incidence of childhood leukaemia was very high and children did not grow well.

There is some radioactivity normally in the surroundings and in some parts of the world the natural radioactivity in the soil or rock is very high indeed. There is no clear evidence of a proven fetal risk even in these centres, e.g. Kerala, but studies are in hand.

Cosmic rays produce radiation, but the risk to a pregnant woman flying at altitude (where of course, the cosmic ray effect is higher) is minimal. Supersonic flight at very high altitudes should be compensated by the shorter duration of exposure and the risk should still be of little importance. (*See also* 'altitude', below.) General principles as outlined by Sternberg (1970) seem valid:

1. Any radiological or radioisotope procedures in a woman of childbearing age should be undertaken in the first 14 days of the menstrual cycle.
2. If a test must be done during pregnancy the isotope or procedure with minimal risk should be positively selected.
3. After extensive use of radioisotopes in a woman—pregnancy should be prevented for three months by ovulation suppressives. If the husband has received an isotope with a known risk of chromosomal damage e.g. Phosphorin 32, pregnancy should be prevented for six months.
4. If radioactive procedures can be proven to have produced fetal damage or damage is extremely likely, therapeutic abortion should be considered.

Altitude—Travel by air.
Risk to the unadapted pregnant women from altitude begins about 10 000 feet when the alveolar partial pressure of O_2 begins to fall. Travel by commercial aircraft pressurized at 5000–7000 feet is, therefore, safe even if flights are frequent and prolonged (air hostesses) (Cameron, 1973).

However, pregnant women unacclimatized to altitude should not fly in non-pressurized aircraft over 9000–10 000 feet. Nor should they consider crossing the high mountain passes many of which rise over 12 000 feet. Women who constantly live at altitude over 5000 feet (e.g. Denver) have, of course, a degree of acclimatization which allows them a little more freedom of movement at 10 000–12 000 feet, but not above.

Subsequent development of the child

The obstetricians must be concerned with the ultimate quality of the child. His concern must reflect not only his intelligent interest but also his concern with regard to events in pregnancy and labour which might influence that quality for the worse. He should consider whether he might by improved care or subsequent research prevent altogether pregnancy risk or counteract or minimize the effects.

It is very clear from the studies of the Newcastle school (Neligan, 1974) that the long term outcome for any child is very much determined by the home into which he goes and especially by the quality and attributes of his mother. In a statistical way social class is the best single determinant of the situation of possible childhood deprivation which will have serious effects on his development even if he is not handicapped at birth. If handicapped, the situation is worse.

Within each social class, of course, the quality of maternal care is variable. Poor growth leading even to apparent dwarfism may be due to poor maternal care, rejection and inadequate feeding. Growth, especially leg length will suffer more than weight or apparent nutritional state.

A child born in 1958 before the 37th week as a fifth or later child to a mother less than 155cm in height, of low social class, who smoked in her pregnancy, is not only likely to be up to 500g lighter at birth, but is, at 7 years old, some $5\frac{1}{4}$ inches less tall than the best children of his age (Davie, Butler and Goldstein, 1972). This reflects not only the poor intra-uterine and birth situation but the dreadful environment of upbringing.

Pringle, Butler and Davie (1966) and Davie, Butler and Goldstein (1972) report a follow-up of 11 000 children born in one week of March in 1958 throughout the United Kingdom. The first group report the range of behaviour ability and medical illness and anomaly discovered in the whole group and produce a base line of what should be expected. For example, a surprising proportion of children were unsettled and maladjusted at school. Some 5 per cent of children showed serious maladjustment resembling that seen in later delinquents and at least another 10 per cent had moderate difficulty. Some 5 per cent had hearing difficulty and 16 per cent speech difficulty. Twenty per cent had eight or more missing, filled or decayed teeth. It is against this type of background that the long term follow-up of obstetrically abnormal children needs to be judged.

Butler and Bonham (1963) confirmed that variation in birth weight, gestation (long or short) adverse social factors and high birth order substantially increased the risk of perinatal death, in addition, of course, to specific and individual causes. Davie *et al.* (1972) studied the long term effects at age 7 years and showed that educational handicap and clumsiness were more common in children born too early or too late. Both problems were as to be expected more serious in the children from the lower social group, of whom 3–5 per cent were seriously educationally handicapped.

Deafness, sight impairment, cerebral palsy and serious mental defect are partially predictable from birth order, type of delivery and the condition in the first week.

Mild mental difficulty, educational backwardness are more related to birth rank, social class, birth weight for gestation, and method of delivery.

The predictive value of condition in the first week has been studied by Brown, Purves, Forfar and Cockburn (1974), who found that in a series of 740 infants considered to have asphyxia at birth (half due to antepartum causes and 40 per cent due to difficult labour) those who showed hypotonia serious loss of flexor tone ($12\cdot4$ per cent) did on the whole badly but those who, in the neonatal period, had adequate muscle tone on the whole did well.

The effect of therapy

Authors of recent years from Drillien (1969) reporting children born before 1960, and Ambries, Weintraub, Niswander, Fischer, Fleshman, Brers and Ambries (1970) and many others have recorded that low birthweight (below 1500g) was by itself responsible for well over 50 per cent of the survivors having poor mental development at follow-up. The obstetrician was therefore concerned with prematurity and poor growth and considered that the conditions which led to such poor growth were primarily therefore causal.

Coyle (1970) however, showed for example that not only was it wise from the point of view of fetal survival to deliver before term those babies whose mothers had low urinary oestriols, but that the intellectual quality of the survivors born before term was much better than of those delivered at or after term, so that proper antenatal care and therapy based on this could improve the chance for the child.

In general newborn care has improved to such an extent that in the special nurseries in the Medical School in Dundee survival of babies born weighing less than 1500g is now over 50 per cent as also reported by Rawlings, Stewart, Reynolds and Strang (1971). These later authors however, have shown that not only has survival greatly improved but that subsequent development is equally good, and at a mean age of 2 years 3 months, 86·7 per cent were thought to be normal and only 7·4 per cent clearly abnormal.

Success of modern therapy is confirmed by a study of *head growth* of very low birth weight (1500g) infants studied by Davies and Davis (1970) showed that if such infants were not maintained in ideal conditions of temperature and feeding subsequent brain growth could be impaired. The results in babies cared for in the later years (1965–68) were much better.

Cross (1973) suggested that much of the poor survival and presumably the mental damage suffered in the babies under 1500g born in the period 1955–65 was due to grossly inadequate oxygen therapy in view of a quite unjustified scare of the risk of retro-lental fibroplasia. There is little doubt that in this period inadequate oxygen was given and that of course, neonatal hypoglycaemia was encouraged by refusal to feed small babies and that the need to keep them warm was not recognized.

Greatly improved knowledge of neonatal physiology and application to the care of the small newborn has greatly improved immediate and long term results (Chapter 23).

SUMMARY

It seems clear, therefore, that the obstetrician must continue to improve overall his techniques of care, must learn how to prevent poor growth, must improve the intra-uterine environment of the growing fetus, and must learn to know when it is in distress so that he can deliver it. The paediatrician is correspondingly greatly improving the intensity and quality of his care so that the child handicapped at birth by weight, prematurity or damage, may have a very much better chance of survival and normality.

However, the environment into which the child is born is highly significant for his ultimate wellbeing, but that is another story.

REFERENCES

Adelstein, A. N. & Donovan, J. W. (1972) Malignant Disease in Children whose mothers had chickenpox, mumps or rubella in pregnancy. *Brit. med. J.*, ii, 629.

Ambries, C. M., Weintraub, D. H., Niswander, K. R., Fischer, L., Fleshman, J., Brers, I. D. J. & Ambries, J. L. (1970) Evaluation of survivors of respiratory distress syndrome at 4 years of age. *Amer. J. Dis. Child.*, 120, 296.

Andrew, J. & McGarry, H. M. (1972) A community study of smoking during pregnancy. *J. Obstet. Gynaec. Brit. Cwlth.*, 79, 1057.

Baird, D., Walker, J. & Thomson, A. (1954) Cause and preventions of stillbirths and first week deaths. Part iii: A classification of deaths by clinical cause. *J. Obstet. Gynaec. Brit. Emp.*, 61, 433.

Brown, J. K., Purves, R. J., Forfar, J. Q. & Cockburn, F. (1974) Neurological Aspects of Perinatal Asphyxia. *Dev. Med. Child Neurol.*, 16, 567.

Bryant, G. M., Gray, O. P., Fraser, A. J. & Ackerman, A. (1970) Fate of surviving low birth weight infants with coagulation deficiencies in the first day of life. *Brit. med. J.*, ii, 707.

Butler, N. R. & Bonham, D. G. (1963) *Perinatal Mortality*. London: Livingstone.

Cameron, P. G. (1973) Should air hostesses continue flight duty during the first trimester of pregnancy. *Aerospace Med.*, 44, 552,

Cole, P. V., Hawkins, L. H. & Roberts, D. (1972) Smoking during pregnancy and its effects on the fetus. *J. Obstet. Gynaec. Brit. Cwlth.*, 79, 782.

Cross, K. W. (1973) Cost of preventing retrolental fibroplasia. *Lancet*, ii, 954.

Cytomelagic Virus Again (1974). *Brit. med. J.*, ii, 593.

Davie, R., Butler, N. R. & Goldstein, H. (1972) *From Birth to Seven*. London: Longman.

Davies, P. A. & Davies, J. P. (1970) Very low birth weight infants and subsequent head growth. *Lancet*, ii, 1216.

Drillien, C. M. (1969) School disposal and performance of children of different birth weights, 1953–60. *Arch. Dis. Child.*, 44, 562.

Dudgeon, J. A. (1967) Maternal rubella and its effects on the fetus. *Arch. Dis. Child.*, 42, 110.

Fleck, D. G. (1974) Toxoplasmosis and Embryopathy. *Brit. med. J.*, i, 244.

Green, D. M., Reid, S. M. & Rhaney, R. (1966) Generalised vaccinia in the human fetus. *Lancet*, **i**, 1296.

Gregg, N. M. (1941) Congenital cataract following German measles in the mother. *TR Ophthal. Soc. Austral.*, **3**, 35.

Harlap, S. (1973) Association between Downs Syndrome Births. *Lancet*, **ii**, 44.

Harrison, K. A. (1974) Malaria transmission and fetal growth. *Brit. med. J.*, **ii**, 229.

Herbst, A. L., Ulfelder, H. & Poskanzer, D. C. (1971) Adenocarcinoma of the vagina. *New Engl. med. J.*, **284**, 878.

Kaiser, I. H. (1973) Pregnancy wastage in operating room personnel. *Obstet. Gynec.*, **41**, 930.

Lawson, J. B. (1971) Maternity care in the Tropics. *Tropical Doctor*, **1**, 31.

Lubchenko, L. O., Bard, H., Goldman, A. L., Coyer, W. E., McIntyre, C. & Smith, D. M. (1974) Newborn Intensive Care and Long Term Prognosis. *Dev. Med. Child Neurol.*, **16**, 421.

Monif, G. R. G. (1969) *Viral infection of the Human Fetus*. London: Macmillan.

Neligan, G. (1974) The role of the paediatrician in the cycle of deprivation. *Proc. R. Soc. Med.*, **67**, 1055.

Pringle, N. L. K., Butler, N. R. & Davie, R. (1966) 11,000 Seven Year Olds. Edinburgh: Longman.

Rawlings, Grace, Reynolds, E. O. R., Stewart, Ann & Strang, L. B. (1971) Changing prognosis for infants of very low birth weight. *Lancet*, **i**, 576.

Renwick, J. H. (1972) Hypothesis—Anencephaly and spina bifida are usually preventable by avoidance of a specific but unidentified substance present in certain potato tubers. *Brit. J. Prev. Soc. Med.*, **26**, 67-68.

Shubeck, F., Benson, R. C., Clark, W. W., Berendes, H., Weiss, W. & Deutschberger, J. (1966) Fetal hazard after rupture of the membranes. *Obstet. Gynec.*, **28**, 1.

Unsuspected cytomegalic mononucleosis (1974) *Brit. med. J.*, **ii**, 341.

Smith, J. A. McC., Jennison, R. F. & Langley, F. A. (1956) Perinatal infection and perinatal death, clinical aspects. *Lancet*, **iii**, 1956.

Stewart, A., Webb, J. & Hewitt, D. (1958) A survey of childhood malignancies. *Brit. med. J.*, **i**, 1495.

Stewart, A. (1961) Aetiology of childhood malignancies congenitally determined leukaemias. *Brit. med. J.*, **i**, 452.

Stewart, A. M. & Kneale, G. W. (1970) Age distribution of cancers by obstetric X-ray and their relevance to cancer latent periods. *Lancet*, **ii**, 4.

Tobin, J. O'H. (1975) Herpes virus hominis infection in pregnancy. *Proc. roy. Soc. Med.*, **68**, 371.

Walker, J. & Henderson, J. L. (1967) A review of perinatal mortality in Dundee. *Scott. med. J.*, **12**, 37.

Walker, J. & Dunn, F. (1970) Obstetric sequelae of difficult labour in primigravidae. *Int. J. Gynaec. Obstet.*, **8**, 147.

FURTHER READING

Batstone, G. F., Blair, A. W., Slater, J. M. (1971) A handbook of prenatal paediatrics. *Med. Techn. Pub. Aylesbury.*

Bithell, J. F. & Stewart, A. M. (1975) Prenatal irradiation and childhood malignancy: A review of British data from the Oxford Survey. *Brit. J. Cancer*, **31**, 271.

Departmental Committee on Maternal Mortality and Morbidity. *Interim Report 1930, Final Report 1972.* London: HMSO.

Hurley, R. (1970) 'Microbiology' in *Scientific Foundations of Obstetrics and Gynaecology.* Ed. Philipp, E. E., Barnes, Josephine B. & Newton, M. London: Heinemann.

Immunisation against Infectious Disease (1972) DHSS. *Rep. stand. med. advis. Comm.*

Intrauterine Infections—Problems and Prevention (1973) Ed. *Lancet*, **i**, 868.

Intrauterine Infection (1973) (Ciba Fdn. Sym. 10) Ed. Elliot, K. & Knight, J. *Excerpta Med.* Amsterdam.

Intrauterine Infection—a symposium (1975) *Proc. roy. Soc. Med.*, **68**, 365.

Kerr, J. M. M. (1933) (Ed.) *Maternal Mortality and Morbidity.* Edinburgh: Livingstone.

Monif, G. R. S. (1974) *Infectious Diseases in Obstetrics & Gynecology.* London: Harper & Rowe.

Palmisano, P. A., Polhill, R. B. (1972) Fetal Pharmacology. *Paediat. Clin. North Amer.*, **19**, 3.

Pollution of the atmosphere of operating theatres. A statement of advice (1975). In *Anaesthesia*, **30**, 697.

Report on Confidential Enquiries into Maternal Deaths in England and Wales 1967-1969 (1972) HMSO.

Report on an Enquiry into Maternal Deaths in Scotland 1965-1971. (1974) HMSO.

Stern, J. (1973) Biochemical Hazards and the Developing Brain. *Dev. Med. Child Neurol.*, **15**, 521.

Sternberg, J. (1970) Irradiation and Radio Contamination during Pregnancy. *Amer. J. Obstet. Gynec.*, **108**, 490.

Tuchmann, D. H. (1970) The Influence of Certain Drugs in the Prenatal Development. *Int. J. Obstet. Gynec.*, **8**, 777.

26. Tropical Obstetrics

In most tropical countries childbirth is still accompanied by massive casualties. This is due basically to adverse social factors and not to exotic 'tropical' diseases. Indeed, the great killers are much the same as in the rest of the world: eclampsia, anaemia, difficult labour, haemorrhage and sepsis. In Britain maternal mortality has nearly disappeared and infant losses are declining steadily. However, the achievement of the same improvement in the underdeveloped tropics will not occur until effective prophylaxis and early treatment of complications becomes available for all mothers.

As well as inadequate maternity services, social and biological factors also have an adverse effect. Poor nutrition and uncontrolled infections in childhood stunt the growth of future mothers, leading to a high incidence of prematurity and contracted pelvis. Childbearing often starts too early, before the mother has stopped growing, and high parity is common. Poor nutrition and endemic infections during pregnancy produce social diseases such as prematurity and anaemia.

In all developing countries lack of confidence in modern medical facilities (even where they exist) keeps patients away from doctors and hospitals until their diseases are very advanced. This is especially true in obstetrics, the mysteries of birth resisting new ideas to the last. The traditional conduct of labour by unskilled attendants adds to this by causing delay in the presence of dystocia and haemorrhage, and intervention in the home may lead to severe infection.

However, economic development and education are beginning to be effective and the benefits of modern health care are now becoming available to mothers in the tropics who were previously denied them. The difficulty is to provide the midwives and doctors needed, and money to support them and to provide hospital and maternity centres in which to work.

Even if this difficulty can be overcome, the maternity care provided must be related to local needs and common clinical problems to be effective. Methods developed in very different circumstances in Britain may be inappropriate: old traditions and taboos have to be taken into consideration if the new maternity services are to be acceptable. All this means that careful study of the local clinical situation and social attitudes is essential if the introduction of modern maternity care is to make childbirth safer in a tropical community.

MATERNITY CARE

It is unfortunately not possible anywhere in the world to provide full specialist care for every pregnant woman, and in the under-doctored tropics the butter has to be spread very thinly on the bread. The intention should therefore be to provide minimum standards of maternity care for all pregnant women and to identify those at particular risk so that they can receive more specialized supervision.

It is not enough to make facilities available: a conscious effort must be made to win confidence in them, as otherwise the benefits of scientific maternal care will not reach beyond the enlightened minority, and amongst women whose lives still follow traditional patterns the morbidity and mortality of childbirth will remain unaltered.

Antenatal care in Britain is mainly concentrated on the detection of obstetric abnormalities such as pre-eclampsia, malpresentations, and so forth. Positive health measures are mostly limited to routine prophylactic therapy such as the administration of iron, and improvement of general health in pregnancy receives little emphasis. In the tropics, where ill-health is very much more prevalent, priority must be given to the correction of faulty nutrition and the prevention and treatment of endemic disease. Pregnancy provides a golden opportunity for successful health education, as the advice given is likely to be accepted because of the beneficial effect on the coming baby which can be promised. Instruction on diet is particularly important, but this must be practical so foods which are scarce or expensive or are forbidden by local custom or religious beliefs should not be advocated. Prepared demonstrations of specimen meals giving a balanced daily diet are very effective.

Instruction in the care of the coming baby is very important and should continue in the lying-in wards after delivery and later in the well-baby clinics. The importance of successful breast feeding must be strongly emphasized, in the hopes of countering the modern trend towards bottle feeding which has now reached the urban areas in the tropics with disastrous results.

Family planning is best introduced to a community through the maternity services. Too frequent pregnancies debilitate the mother and when birth intervals are short the loss of life in infancy and early childhood

local customs and attitudes is required to present the advice in an acceptable form. The emphasis, obviously, must be on preserving the health of the family rather than on nebulous concepts of population control.

The identification of high-risk cases can be achieved at the first visit to the antenatal clinic in many cases. The unusually old or the unusually young, the grande multiparae, those with a bad obstetric history, the very short and the very fat, all can be picked out easily for special care. Simple clinical examination by a midwife who is well trained will identify other high-risk cases. A battery of special tests may be impracticable but estimating the haemoglobin should not be omitted.

Unfortunately many women who attend antenatal clinics in the tropics have every intention of delivering themselves at home. Ultimately delivery under skilled supervision should be aimed at in all cases. Village or suburban maternity homes can provide an adequate service, provided the midwives are

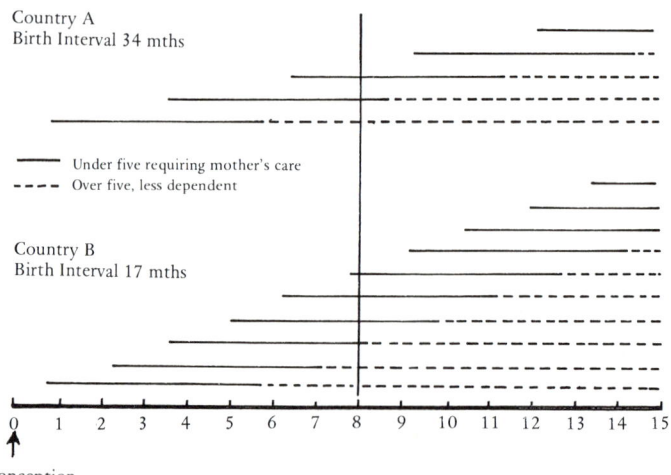

Fig. 26.1   In country A (Nigeria), birth interval 34 months, never more than two children under five for the mother to care for. In country B (Brazil), birth interval 17 months, four children under five at any one time.
(From *Paediatric Priorities in the Developing World* by David Morley.)

is high (Fig. 26.1). Women are usually most willing to accept the new idea of controlling their fertility when they are pregnant or just delivered, and this opportunity should not be missed. Here again an intimate knowledge of

supervised by frequent visitors from the nearest health centre or hospital and clear instructions for the referral of abnormal cases are carried out. Good communications are important in ensuring this, and arrangements for the transport of patients in labour must be secure should complications supervene.

Sending midwives to deliver patients in the home is uneconomic, and the trend is to concentrate women in labour in peripheral centres and in hospitals. However, cross-infection of babies can be a danger in these institutions in the tropics so discharge early in the puerperium is best in normal cases. In order to maintain breast feeding when an infant is premature the mother should stay as long as necessary and, for this, cheap hostel accommodation will be required nearby.

After discharge from the maternity unit all mothers and babies should be followed up by maternal and child health nurses to ensure that the effort during pregnancy and labour to produce a healthy baby is not set at naught by avoidable disorders in early infancy. This follow-up naturally merges into the work of the under-fives clinics which have been so successful in the tropics, and whenever possible the same personnel should be involved in providing family planning services.

The limitation of maternity care in Britain to antenatal, intrapartum and early puerperal care is inappropriate to tropical countries, where a continuum of care for the family unit from early pregnancy to the end of the vulnerable childhood is essential.

INTERCURRENT INFECTIONS

Serious infections of all sorts are far more common in tropical populations than in Britain, and pregnant women are more susceptible than others to many of them. For example, both the attack rate and the severity of smallpox, viral hepatitis, poliomyelitis, pneumococcal infections and amoebiasis are increased in pregnancy. In part this is certainly due to modification of the immune response by pregnancy.

Leprosy

This effect is dramatically exemplified in leprosy. Pregnancy precipitates the development of overt leprosy in a patient who is incubating the disease, and widespread initial lesions characterized by numerous active macules may appear quite suddenly. However, in women with established leprosy exacerbation of the condition more commonly occurs three to six months after delivery and may take the form of an acute reactive state, with oedematous erysipeloid swellings on the face, erythema nodosum leprosum or even progressive lepra reaction. These phenomena are not due to the organisms themselves but to immune responses to them which are modified during pregnancy and re-established after the puerperium.

Malaria

Of much greater importance is the effect of pregnancy on immunity to malaria. In endemic areas this immunity is acquired by repeated infections in childhood and by the age of 7 the survivors have acquired a high level of immunity which is maintained by further infection. In pregnancy the ability to limit parasitaemia is reduced from about the 14th week and becomes more obvious as pregnancy advances. The breakdown of immunity is most marked in first pregnancies, for reasons which are as yet obscure: the phenomena for which malaria is responsible are therefore most obvious in primigravidae, although they also occur in multigravidae.

P. falciparum infections are particularly serious, and in those parts of Asia where it is common, and in tropical Africa, chemoprophylaxis is essential throughout pregnancy and the puerperium. The most convenient regime is a weekly 25mg tablet of pyrimethamine, but if resistance to this drug appears in the locality a weekly dose of chloroquine (600mg) may be substituted. There need be no fear that preventing parasitaemia by this means for the short span of a pregnancy will cause a significant reduction in acquired immunity.

Malaria may alter the course of pregnancy both by affecting the health of the mother and by interrupting the pregnancy. The most important influence of the disease on maternal health in pregnancy is indirect, by causing anaemia which commonly develops about the 24th week (Fig. 26.2). An acute attack of malaria may cause abortion or premature labour, as pyrexia tends to activate the uterus (Fig. 26.3). This is a particular hazard in susceptible women unprotected by chemoprophylaxis.

The placenta in malarious pregnancies appears to act like the spleen. Particularly in *P. falciparum* infections, an intense cellular reaction is found in the intervillous spaces which slows the circulation of maternal blood through them. The growth and oxygenation of the fetus is impaired as a result, the mean birth weight of babies with placental infection being significantly lower than of those without.

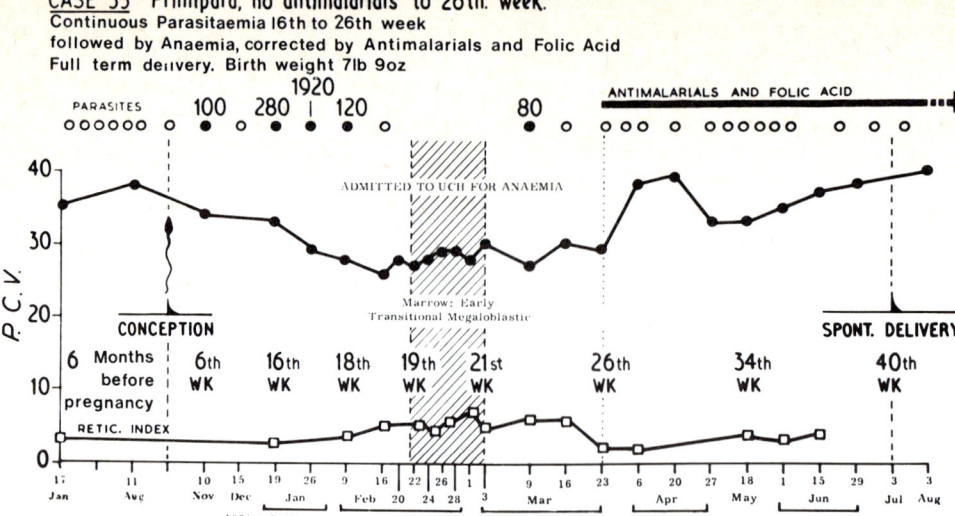

Fig. 26.2 Pregnancy without antimalarials. Parasitaemia followed by haemolytic anaemia, treated with antimalarials and folic acid.

In some cases this impaired placental function may contribute to perinatal loss from antepartum and intrapartum asphyxia.

Transplacental infection of the fetus can occur if the mother is susceptible to malaria and has not been adequately protected during pregnancy. However, an immune mother passes her antibody across the placenta, thus conferring passive immunity to the fetus which is thereby effectively protected for the first two to three months of extra-uterine life.

Tropical splenomegaly syndrome

In some areas where *P. falciparum* malaria is holoendemic sporadic cases of tropical splenomegaly syndrome are found, due to an abnormal immune response to recurrent malarial infection. Characterized by massive splenomegaly and hyperglobulinaemia, there is a chronic anaemia associated with shortened red cell survival, sequestration of red cells in the spleen and hypervolaemia.

Pregnancy precipitates acute haemolytic episodes, superimposed on the chronic hae-

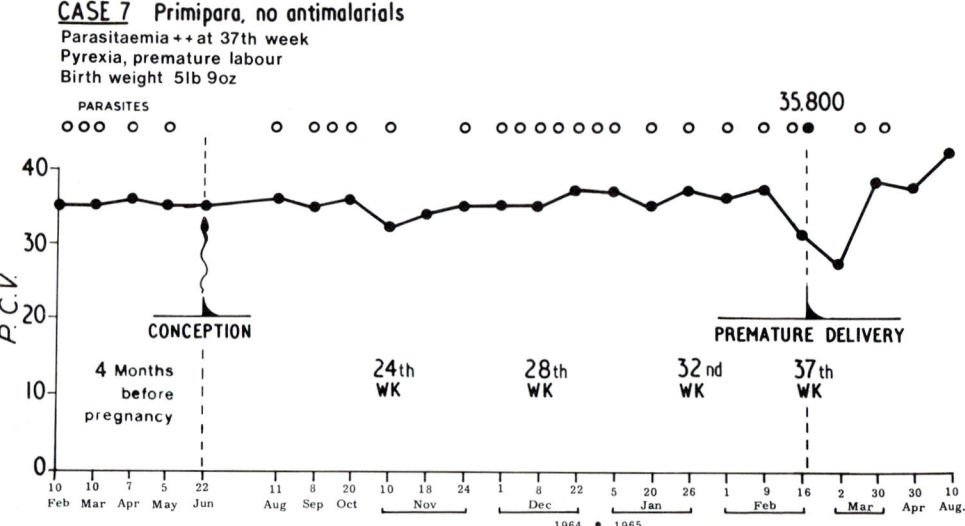

Fig. 26.3 Pregnancy without antimalarials. Heavy parasitaemia with pyrexia precipitates premature labour at 37th week.

molytic state. There is a high abortion rate and perinatal mortality from acute reduction in the oxygen-carrying power of the blood, and the enlargement of the spleen may itself contribute to premature expulsion of the fetus.

The condition can in many cases be improved or even cured by long-term antimalarial prophylaxis with proguanil for one to four years, but the prognosis for maternal and fetal survival in the untreated case is poor.

Diarrhoeal diseases
Most diarrhoeal diseases are caused by pathogens which gain entry to the body through contaminated food or water, and they are therefore particularly common in tropical communities where sanitation is poor.

These diseases include the enteric group caused by salmonellae, bacillary dysentery caused by shigellae, and amoebic dysentery due to infection of the large bowel by *E. histolytica*. In the food poisoning group the diarrhoea may be due to ingestion of food contaminated by *Cl. welchii* or staphylococcal enterotoxin. Other infections may be due to enteroviruses, and explosive epidemics of cholera have recently occurred in many tropical countries.

All these diarrhoeal diseases are liable to precipitate abortion or premature labour because intestinal hyperactivity may reflexly activate the uterus. In the understaffed and overcrowded hospitals of the tropics crossinfection is a serious problem. Patients with diarrhoea are particularly dangerous in obstetric wards because of the ease with which newborn babies may become infected, often with devastating results.

The first line of treatment of undiagnosed diarrhoea is sulphonamide but a special problem is posed by amoebiasis, which is unusually severe in pregnancy. Latent infections may flare up and overt infections may progress rapidly to a fatal outcome. Therefore in all cases of muco-sanguinous diarrhoea associated with abdominal pain a fresh stool should be examined microscopically to see whether free forms of *E. histolytica* are present, in which case treatment with metronidazole should be initiated immediately.

In bacillary dysentery and cholera the diarrhoea may be severe enough to produce disturbance of electrolyte and water balance very quickly. Correction by intravenous therapy is particularly urgent during pregnancy as labour may be imminent, precipitated by the diarrhoea.

Tuberculosis
Although pulmonary tuberculosis has now been effectively controlled in Britain it remains an important complication in pregnancy in most tropical countries. Since the advent of chemotherapy it is accepted that pregnancy does not alter the prognosis in tuberculosis, provided treatment is regular and efficient and the pregnancy and delivery are skilfully managed. Untreated tuberculosis, however, is likely to deteriorate in pregnancy, and particularly in the puerperium, especially if obstetric care is defective. Premature labour is common in toxic and cachectic patients and so is anaemia, which will not respond to routine haematinics until the tuberculous infection is brought under control.

Early detection of pulmonary tuberculosis in pregnancy is important in order to initiate effective treatment and render the patient sputum-negative by the time she is delivered. Unfortunately tuberculosis is more common amongst pregnant women admitted without previous antenatal care than amongst those who attend antenatal clinics, who are more likely to report for anti-tuberculous treatment. The yield from screening regular antenatal clinic attenders may therefore be disappointing: women who come to hospital only after a difficult labour or because of illness in the puerperium should be subjected to special scrutiny as unsuspected cases are particularly dangerous to other patients and their babies.

In the obstetric management of patients with pulmonary tuberculosis, pregnancy and labour should be conducted with the specific object of maintaining resistance to the disease. The patient should reach the puerperium in the best possible condition, with her resistance unimpaired by exhaustion, anaemia or sepsis.

If the mother is still infectious by the time she is delivered particular problems will arise over the management of her newborn baby. Unless it is protected from infection it is very likely to die in the first month of generalized tuberculosis. Immediate segregation is therefore desirable until the mother is no longer infectious or at least until BCG given at birth has achieved Mantoux conversion, which may take up to six weeks. However, this would necessitate bottle feeding, which may be as great a danger to the baby as acquiring tuberculosis.

A compromise may have to be adopted, by continuing to breast feed while protecting the baby from tuberculosis by prophylactic INAH and at the same time giving INAH-resistant BCG.

Viral hepatitis

Hepatitis in pregnancy usually runs a mild course in Britain, similar to that in males and non-pregnant females. In the tropics this is not so. Fulminating hepatitis, usually between the 28th and 34th week of pregnancy, not infrequently leads to massive hepatic necrosis with a high maternal and fetal mortality.

Any pregnant woman who develops jaundice therefore has to be taken seriously. If neurological evidence of impending portosystemic encephalopathy appears, such as tremor or diminished lucidity, all protein intake should be stopped and glucose given intravenously. Oral neomycin or tetracycline and daily saline purges are also indicated to reduce the absorption of protein breakdown products from the bowel.

Once hepatic coma develops the outlook is very grave, but if all cases are energetically treated some will survive.

Treponematoses

The distribution of syphilis in the tropics is patchy. As there appears to be cross-immunity between *T. pallidum* and *T. pertenue* infections, syphilis is rare in communities where yaws is endemic, although this picture is changing as a result of the WHO yaws eradication campaigns in the 1950s.

The non-venereal treponematoses (pinta— *T. carateum*, yaws—*T. pertenue*, bejel—*T. pallidum*) mainly cause disease in childhood and, since congenital transmission to the fetus does not occur, they do not affect the course of pregnancy. However, serological changes due to these childhood infections persist into adult life and may cause diagnostic confusion in pregnancy, as latent syphilis cannot be distinguished from yaws by the usual Kahn, VDRL and TPI tests. A decision on whether to give anti-syphilitic treatment during pregnancy to sero-positive reactors may therefore have to be made on probabilities, which frequently leads to unnecessary treatment to be on the safe side.

ANAEMIA

Anaemia is the most important complication in pregnancy in the tropics, not only because of its greatly increased incidence but also because of its severity. Both combine to make this condition a major cause of maternal and fetal loss. In almost all cases the anaemia is caused by multiple factors whose individual importance varies from area to area. This makes rational prophylaxis and treatment much more difficult.

Iron deficiency is prevalent throughout the tropics, and in many areas hookworms are an important contributory factor when parasite loads are heavy and the iron intake is low. Haemolytic anaemia secondary to *P. falciparum* infections has already been mentioned. This is particularly serious in pregnancy as the accelerated rate of haemopoiesis needed to keep abreast of the destruction of erythrocytes increases the folic acid requirements. These may not be satisfied during pregnancy, particularly if there is already a dietary deficiency of folic acid, owing to the competing demands of the developing fetus. Folic acid deficiency may therefore result, and in severe cases marrow activity changes to megaloblastic and erythropoiesis virtually ceases. In the Negro populations of tropical Africa and the Caribbean haemolytic anaemia due to sicklecell disease may similarly produce megaloblastic anaemia if prophylactic folic acid has not been given.

The geographical variation in the aetiology of pregnancy anaemia makes it necessary to identify the factors involved in each area, to ensure that prophylaxis is locally applicable. In most places supplementary iron will be indicated and usually folic acid as well: antimalarial chemoprophylaxis will also be required of course in areas where *P. falciparum* infections are endemic.

In the absence of effective treatment, anaemia develops insidiously as the pregnancy advances. It is therefore important to assess the haemoglobin level when patients first register for antenatal care, and if possible the tests should be repeated at the 28th and 36th weeks. When large numbers of patients need to be screened for anaemia, estimation of the packed-cell volume by the microhaematocrit method is quicker and more accurate.

Minor degrees of anaemia are so common in the tropics that the haemoglobin level below which the maternal and fetal prognosis is seriously impaired has to be selected, and every effort made to maintain it above this level throughout pregnancy. In most parts of Africa and the Indian subcontinent a level of 9g per cent will have to be accepted as the minimum level for safety. Below this, close supervision and energetic out-patient treatment is necessary unless the haemoglobin falls to another critical level at which life is endangered. Experience has shown this to be about 6·5g per cent, and at this level admission to hospital for investigation and urgent treatment is mandatory.

Local investigation of a large number of anaemias in pregnancy will indicate standard methods of treatment appropriate to the area. Where iron deficiency is the main problem intravenous preparations given by the total dose infusion technique may be best as they ensure that an adequate amount of iron is given to correct the anaemia and replenish the body stores, which cannot be ensured by long-continued follow-up oral treatment. A more rapid improvement is also achieved than with oral iron, and scarce hospital beds are saved.

Where the main aetiological factor is malarial haemolysis, initial treatment with a curative course of antimalarials and full doses of folic acid should secure rapid improvement. However, occasionally the haemolysis continues and has to be abated with prednisone.

There is little place for blood transfusion in the treatment of anaemia in pregnancy unless the haemoglobin has fallen to a very low level and more rapid correction of the anaemia is required than can be achieved by simple medical treatment.

Sometimes patients present for the first time with very profound anaemia, with haemoglobin levels below 4·5g per cent. This is particularly likely if the anaemia is haemolytic, recurrent episodes having produced rapid deterioration when folic acid deficiency has supervened. An acute attack of dysentery or, in the puerperium, genital sepsis may also produce sudden deterioration of a pre-existing mild anaemia.

In the end the patient may die, either undelivered or in the first two weeks of the puerperium. The main cause of death is congestive heart failure due to cardiac muscle oxygen lack. The worst danger period is during the first twelve hours after delivery, when the work of the hypoxic heart muscle is suddenly increased by the raising of the peripheral circulatory resistance when the arteriovenous shunt behind the placenta closes. It is at this time, incidentally, that a simple transfusion of whole blood is most hazardous, however small the volume and however slowly it is given.

This sombre picture of the effects of profound anaemia in pregnancy indicates that it is a major obstetric emergency which requires immediate and effective treatment if disaster is to be avoided. The problem is to augment the circulating red cell mass without increasing the total volume of blood and thus precipitating acute pulmonary oedema. The simplest emergency technique is to give a rapidly-acting diuretic intravenously just before starting a transfusion of 500ml of packed cells slowly over a period of about six hours. The diuretic rapidly reduces the plasma volume and thus makes room for the infused packed cells. Ethacrynic acid (50mg) is preferred, but frusemide (20mg) is also effective. The slower-acting diuretics like hydroflumethiazide are not effective as they only eliminate extravascular tissue fluid and do not reduce the plasma volume.

Severe anaemia in pregnancy also influences the maternal prognosis indirectly by making even small blood losses at delivery highly dangerous, and by diminishing resistance to infection during the puerperium.

It also adversely affects the fetal prognosis. Mid-trimester abortions and premature labours are common. When the haemoglobin is below about 7g per cent, intra-uterine growth is impaired which results in lowered birth weight at term. Severe maternal hypoxia may cause intra-uterine death before the onset of labour or stillbirth or early neonatal death from intrapartum asphyxia.

From what has been said, it is obvious that anaemia is a very serious problem in tropical obstetrics and every effort should therefore be made to prevent it. Patients who have been successfully treated for pregnancy anaemia should have the cause of their illness carefully explained to them so that a recurrence can be prevented in subsequent pregnancies by effective prophylaxis.

SICKLE-CELL DISEASE

In people of Negro origin in tropical Africa and the West Indies haemoglobinopathies are common and may cause serious problems in

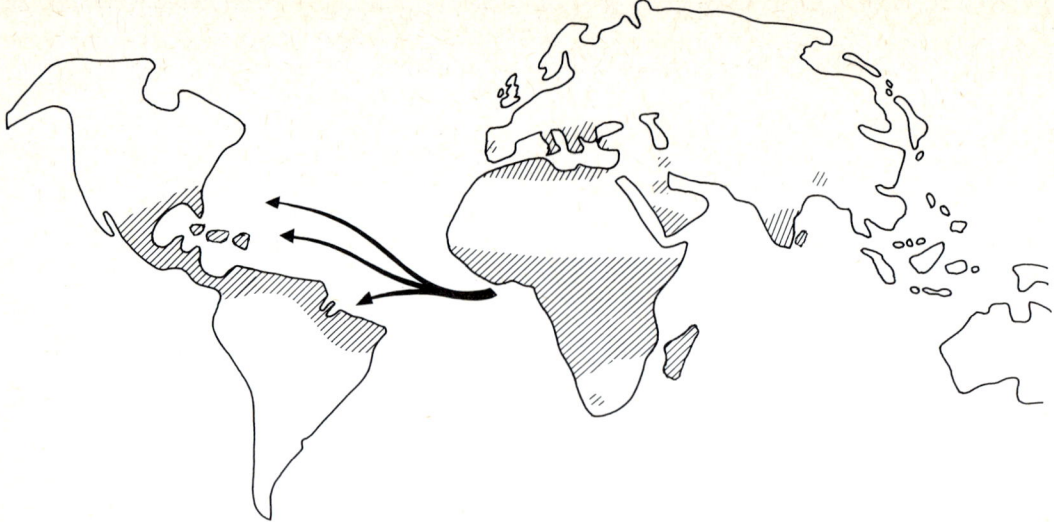

Fig. 26.4   The distribution of Haemoglobin S.

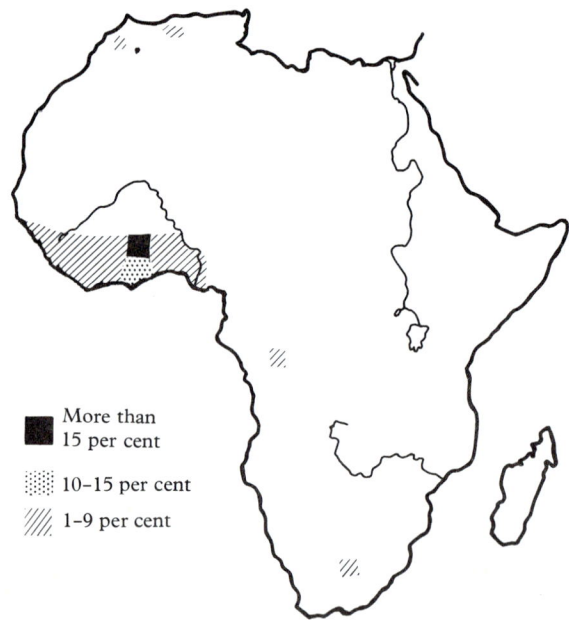

■ More than
  15 per cent

▦ 10–15 per cent

▨ 1–9 per cent

Fig. 26.5   The distribution of Haemoglobin C in Africa.

pregnancy (Figs 26.4 & 26.5). Genetically-determined abnormalities in the formation of the haemoglobin molecule occur because of amino-acid substitution in the globin moiety. The most important abnormal haemoglobins which result are haemoglobin S and haemoglobin C. These are transmitted in Mendelian fashion, and although heterozygotes (haemoglobin AS and AC) are symptomless trait-carriers, S homozygotes (haemoglobin SS) and double heterozygotes (haemoglobin SC) have

sickle-cell anaemia and sickle-cell haemoglobin C disease respectively, which are particularly dangerous in pregnancy.

Sickle-cell anaemia is inherited by one-fourth of the children if both parents carry the S trait.

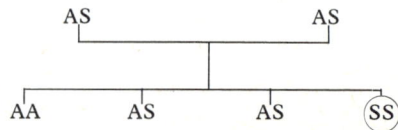

If one parent carries the S trait and the other the C trait, one in four of their children will inherit sickle-cell haemoglobin C disease.

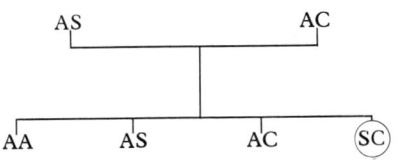

The clinical effects of sickle-cell disease are partly due to the fact that the red cells survive for a shorter time, resulting in chronic haemolytic anaemia. Also, reduced haemoglobin S has high viscosity so sludging leads to vascular obstruction, infarction (especially of the bone-marrow) and embolism. Sickling phenomena are produced by infection, acidosis and lowered oxygen tension (hence the need to avoid hypoxia during anaesthesia). All the effects of sickle-cell disease are worse in pregnancy and are therefore more likely to be fatal.

Sickle-cell anaemia is rare in adults because of the high mortality in childhood. It therefore seldom complicates pregnancy in tropical Africa but is less uncommon in the more favourable environment of the West Indies. Sickle-cell haemoglobin C disease follows a more benign course and seldom causes death in childhood, so it is quite common in pregnancy and may be unsuspected until it causes serious complications. In patients with sickle-cell anaemia who survive to adult life there will be a history of chronic ill-health with recurrent bone pains, anaemia and jaundice. Growth may be stunted and there may be skeletal deformities and chronic leg ulcers. In haemoglobin SC disease there is not always a history of recurrent bone pains: anaemia and jaundice are unusual except during pregnancy.

To detect sickle-cell disease, ideally all pregnant Negro women should be screened with a simple blood-test for sickling. Haemoglobin electrophoresis on those who are positive will distinguish the trait-carriers (AS) from those with sickle-cell disease (SS and SC). If electrophoresis is not available, careful examination of the blood film will usually identify the target cells typical of sickle-cell disease.

People with sickle-cell disease usually have surprisingly low haemoglobin levels while remaining quite well. In sickle-cell anaemia 8g per cent appears to be normal, and 10g per cent in haemoglobin SC disease: re-peated transfusions do not maintain the haemoglobin higher than this. However, during pregnancy the increased demand for folic acid by the growing fetus is superimposed on the high marrow requirements for continuous massive erythropoiesis. Folic acid supplementation is therefore essential throughout pregnancy if progressive anaemia is to be prevented. The severest degrees of anaemia ever seen in pregnancy result from a combination of malarial haemolysis and sickle-cell disease with secondary folate deficiency: this is often fatal.

Bone-pain crises due to marrow infarction are more frequent in the last four weeks of pregnancy, in labour and in the first four days of the puerperium than at any other time. Their frequency may be reduced by preventing acidosis and infections, so antimalarial prophylaxis is particularly important.

Patients in bone-pain crisis must be hospitalized and given analgesics and antibiotics: oral bicarbonate and magnesium salts are indicated on theoretical grounds, but appear to have little clinical effect. Fatal marrow embolism may supervene in these crises, particularly in the last four weeks of pregnancy and the puerperium. The risk of this appears to be reduced by heparinization which is therefore indicated at this time. The appearance of systolic hypertension and albuminuria during a bone-pain crisis is of particularly sinister significance as it indicates that embolism may be imminent. In these circumstances the effect of the heparin should be reversed with protamine, followed by emergency exchange blood transfusion and termination of the pregnancy by Caesarean section.

Another serious complication of sickle-cell disease in the last few weeks of pregnancy and the first week of the puerperium is acute sequestration crisis. This is due to an acute and massive episode of sickling which results in a rapidly progressive anaemia in which the haemoglobin may fall by as much as 4g per cent in 24 hours. The liver and spleen increase rapidly in size. Detection of this most lethal complication is only achieved by close observation of those at risk, so that a lifesaving exchange blood transfusion can be given without delay.

Another complication of sickle-cell disease in pregnancy is poor wound-healing. Caesarean section wounds and episiotomy repairs therefore commonly break down.

The perinatal mortality is raised in sickle-cell disease even with faultless management. Birth weights tend to be lower, which is probably related to the haemoglobin levels. When anaemia is profound intra-uterine death may occur from fetal hypoxia, and any obstetric factor which causes intrapartum asphyxia is more likely to diminish the chances of fetal survival.

The maternal mortality in undiagnosed or mismanaged cases of sickle-cell disease is very high, perhaps 20 per cent in sickle-cell anaemia and 10 per cent in sickle-cell haemoglobin C disease. Even those who receive impeccable care during pregnancy, labour and the puerperium are at substantial risk, so women with sickle-cell disease should be advised to limit their families to not more than two or three children.

PRE-ECLAMPSIA AND ECLAMPSIA

The incidence of pre-eclampsia and eclampsia varies widely throughout the world, as do the clinical features. For instance, pre-eclampsia is considerably less common during pregnancy in tropical Africa than in Britain, but it develops more readily during labour. However, when antepartum and intrapartum cases were added together in Ibadan, the incidence of pre-eclampsia in primigravidae was found to be comparable to that in Aberdeen.

In South India eclampsia is a greater contributor to maternal mortality than in tropical Africa, and in both areas fits occur at deceptively low blood-pressure levels. Pre-eclampsia appears to progress more rapidly to eclampsia, particularly in labour, in contrast to the more chronic course which is common in Europe. In tropical Africa the disease may progress rapidly from the earliest physical signs right through to eclampsia in the space of a 24-hour labour. The prognosis for the fetus is correspondingly better, because there is little time for placental damage to develop, but eclamptic fits are more difficult to prevent.

A special problem in rural areas in the tropics is the eclamptic who only reaches hospital after having had many fits. Comatose, exhausted and acidotic, these patients have a very different prognosis from women who have their first fit in hospital and are then immediately brought under control.

Hyperpyrexia is a very real danger and is usually due to anoxic damage to the temperature-regulating centre in the brain. It is worsened by the tradition that eclamptics should be cared for in darkened quiet rooms, which in the tropics are hot and stuffy unless they are air-conditioned.

If not corrected immediately, temperatures of 106 °F (41 °C) and over may cause irreversible brain damage. Hyperpyrexia also throws a considerable strain on the heart, and a very rapid pulse-rate coupled with a falling blood pressure foreshadows death from circulatory failure. The rectal temperature should therefore be recorded every half hour in eclamptic patients in the tropics. If the body temperature rises above 100·4 °F (38 °C) active steps to cool the patient are required. Clothes must be removed and tepid sponging and fanning commenced, and if necessary the patient should be covered with cracked ice.

OBSTETRIC HAEMORRHAGE

Antepartum, post-partum and post-abortal haemorrhage endanger life anywhere in the world, but their consequences are much more serious in the tropics for the following reasons:

Pre-existing anaemia in pregnancy is very common and if it is present even minor blood-loss may be disastrous.

If the haemorrhage takes place at home when far from help, poor transport facilities may cause long delay in reaching hospital.

The fatality rate is very high unless massive and safe transfusion can be provided immediately: unfortunately, stored blood is a rarity in the peripheral centres where such patients commonly present.

Where hospital facilities are inadequate, excessive pressure on overworked doctors and nurses may cause delay in emergency treatment to arrest haemorrhage.

The effect of these difficulties may be a degree of exsanguination unheard of nowadays in Britain, and very profound shock. In these circumstances, up to two litres of Ringer lactate (Hartmann's solution) may be given while blood is being prepared for transfusion. Fast infusion is indicated, but the volume of fluid and rate of administration must be carefully judged by observing the jugular venous pressure.

When there has been a long delay between the initial haemorrhage at home and arrival in hospital, oligaemia may have been corrected by haemodilution, restoring the venous pressure and cardiac output. The skin will be warm but very pale, and marked tachycardia will show that the circulation is in the hyperkinetic state. The jugular venous pressure may be raised.

In these circumstances rapid intravenous infusion of fluid may precipitate acute pulmonary oedema. Blood transfusion should therefore be cautious with the patient sitting up, with a close watch kept for the appearance of crepitations at the lung bases. Intravenous frusemide will be indicated if they appear, to reduce the plasma volume.

Prolonged hypotension and anoxia are occasionally followed by acute tubular necrosis. After severe and prolonged shock, therefore, an indwelling catheter is advisable in order to record the urinary output for the first 48 hours.

DIFFICULT LABOUR

Contracted pelvis
In developing countries in the tropics malnutrition and uncontrolled infections in childhood and adolescence commonly cause delayed development and stunting of growth of future mothers (Fig. 26.6). Many women therefore fail to achieve their genetically-determined stature. Contracted pelvis is accordingly much more common than in Britain.

Perhaps fortunately, birth weights are usually much lower in the peoples of Africa and Asia than in Europe: if they were not, the

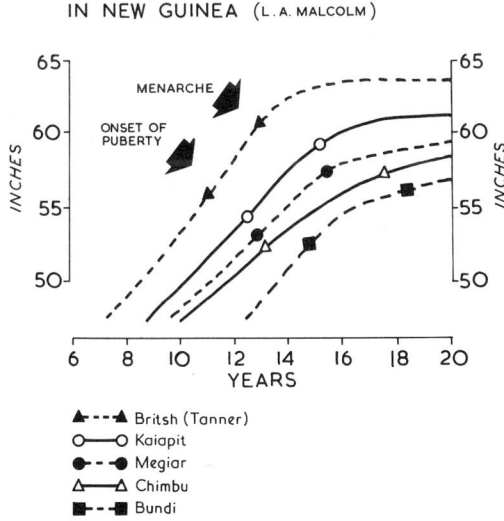

GROWTH & DEVELOPMENT OF GIRLS IN NEW GUINEA (L.A. MALCOLM)

Fig. 26.6 Malnutrition and untreated disease in childhood and adolescence retard growth and development in the New Guinea Highlands.

incidence of cephalopelvic disproportion would be even higher. It seems that in any society women usually have babies to match their pelvic capacity, except where the women are very stunted when even small babies cannot traverse their small pelves.

Although the antenatal diagnosis of contracted pelvis is not easy, it can be inferred from a woman's height as this is usually directly proportional to the size of her pelvic brim. Many racial groups are, of course, genetically short in stature. By analysing the outcome of a large number of labours it is possible to choose a critical height level for any group below which difficult labour becomes common. Simply measuring the heights of all pregnant women and selecting for special care those below the critical level is thus a valuable prophylactic measure.

A particular problem in Negro people is late engagement of the fetal head. This hardly ever occurs before the onset of labour and usually not until cervical dilatation has passed 6cm. It is thought to be due to the steep angle of inclination of the pelvic brim which is associated with the characteristic posture of exaggerated lumbar lordosis. Only when uterine action drives the fetal head firmly into the pelvis does it descend through the brim, whether there is disproportion or not. The implication of this is that all labours, except when the fetus is very small, are trials of labour.

The approach to Caesarean section should be much more conservative in the tropics than in Britain, where approximately 3·5 per cent of all babies are nowadays delivered by section. Most of these operations are performed to anticipate difficulty instead of to deal with impending disaster. Traumatic vaginal deliveries have thus been largely eliminated, so that perinatal deaths from birth injury are now relatively rare. The modern liberal approach to Caesarean section in Britain is not only adopted because of the proven safety of the procedure but also because of the change in the attitude to childbearing. An increasing proportion of pregnancies are deliberately planned with a view to producing a family of two or three children, so the fear that a Caesarean section might prejudice a woman's obstetric future by limiting the number of children she can have therefore no longer operates: sterilization at second or third section is readily accepted.

The position is entirely different in tropical

developing countries where losses in infancy and early childhood are high, and a woman may have to have six or seven babies to achieve three or four survivors. In these circumstances, Caesarean section in the first pregnancy may prevent a woman from achieving the size of family she desires. Apart from this, Caesarean section is much less safe, both in the small rural hospitals with limited facilities and in the overcrowded understaffed obstetric units in the cities. The operation itself may carry considerable risks when performed by the 'occasional surgeon', particularly from haemorrhage when there is no stored blood. The difficulties of anaesthesia for Caesarean section when the patient is in poor condition after a prolonged labour may defeat the anaesthetic skills available. Furthermore, Caesarean section late in labour when infection is already established carries grave danger of general peritonitis which even massive doses of broad-spectrum antibiotics may not control.

The later risk of rupture of the uterine scar in a subsequent labour is even more important, although less obvious. Caesarean section is particularly disliked by the unsophisticated, and the fear of another operation may keep a woman away from hospital in her next pregnancy. Apart from this, in scattered or nomadic communities a woman may live so far from the hospital that she cannot get there in her next labour even if she wishes.

The implications are that Caesarean section should be avoided when possible and operative vaginal delivery preferred if the patient is unlikely to return to hospital for delivery next time. In any case, it is vitally important to leave as sound a scar in the uterus as possible, and for this reason a classical operation through the upper segment should not be performed unless the tubes are to be tied at the same time.

OBSTRUCTED LABOUR

Disorders of feto-pelvic relationships commonly cause prolongation of labour which may end in obstruction when all progress ceases. The uterus reacts to obstruction by increasingly frequent and more violent contractions of the upper segment which may pass into a state of tonic contraction. The lower segment becomes progressively thinned and in the multipara ultimately ruptures. This may be the *coup de grâce* for a woman who is already exhausted, ketotic and infected.

Tonic uterine contraction in the primigravida seldom results in spontaneous rupture of the uterus. She may die undelivered from the effects of prolonged labour, but sometimes the obstruction is spontaneously relieved by the death of the fetus which, after days more of labour, becomes sufficiently macerated to be squeezed through the unyielding birth canal. It is these cases that are most commonly followed by vesico-vaginal fistula.

In obstructed labour four processes conspire to impair the chances of fetal survival. The preceding prolonged labour results in intrapartum infection, and placental respiratory exchange is impaired by the strong and continued uterine contraction and retraction. Excessive moulding of the fetal head in vertex presentations may result in a tentorial tear, and in shoulder and compound presentations there may be compression of prolapsed cord. All too often, therefore, the fetus dies, either before delivery or shortly afterwards, from a combination of asphyxia and infection.

If maternal and fetal disaster is to be avoided, the imminence of obstruction should be detected before it is actually established. Cessation of cervical dilatation in spite of strong uterine contractions is an important warning. Later, tonic uterine contraction supervenes. The firmly-contracted upper segment no longer relaxes, being bunched up like a cap on the tender distended lower segment: occasionally Bandl's retraction ring can be seen. Surprisingly, tonic contraction does not usually produce continuous pain: if this is not appreciated, a patient admitted in obstructed labour whose uterus is about to rupture may be thought to have 'gone out of labour', a disastrous mistake.

The vulva is often oedematous and the liquor frankly purulent. In vertex presentations extreme moulding and caput formation may so elongate the head that it becomes almost tubular, its lower end distending the perineum although its upper end has still not passed the pelvic brim. The urine is usually blood-stained, although if catheterization is impossible this sign may not be elicited until after delivery.

By the time obstruction is established the fetus has, more often than not, perished: if this has not yet happened, signs of severe fetal distress are usually evident.

It is important to decide whether the uterus has ruptured, which is often difficult when the fetus has not yet been extruded into the peritoneal cavity. Vaginal bleeding in a case of obstructed labour is very sinister. So is circulatory collapse, although this may occur before the uterus ruptures if intrapartum infection is severe.

The basis of management of obstructed labour is, of course, urgent delivery to prevent further distension and thus rupture of the lower segment, and to salvage the fetus if it is still alive. However, before embarking on any operation to relieve obstruction, correction of the effects of the preceding prolonged labour should be started. Dehydration and keto-acidosis indicate the rapid infusion of at least 1 litre of 5 per cent dextrose. To combat the inevitable intra-uterine infection, the circulation should be flooded with a broad-spectrum antibiotic, preferably intravenous ampicillin or tetracycline. Blood should be cross-matched. These measures should be initiated while preparations are being made for operative delivery, but they must not be allowed to cause undue delay.

If the fetus is still alive and labour is obstructed by only a moderate degree of cephalo-pelvic disproportion, symphysiotomy under local anaesthesia followed by Ventouse extraction after a generous episiotomy may be the best treatment (Fig. 26.7). If there is very gross disproportion, however, symphysiotomy is contra-indicated. The symphysis would have to be too widely separated to enlarge the pelvis sufficiently, and disabling sequelae such as severe stress incontinence and chronic back-ache due to sacro-iliac instability would follow.

When labour is obstructed by transverse lie or compound presentation and the fetus is still alive, Caesarean section is nearly always indicated. Internal version and breech extraction is not a safe alternative: when the uterus is firmly contracted round the fetus an attempt at version is almost certain to rupture the lower segment.

When the fetus is dead, obstruction due to cephalo-pelvic disproportion can be relieved by reducing the size of the head by craniotomy, provided the fetal head is firmly impacted in the pelvic brim (Fig. 26.8). However, if the head is high and mobile above the brim, craniotomy is difficult and dangerous and subsequent extraction may even be impossible. In these rare circumstances delivery of the dead fetus by Caesarean section, with all its risks, will be safer.

When labour is obstructed by a dead fetus lying transversely, vaginal delivery is best achieved by decapitating the fetus with a Blond-Heidler saw (Fig. 26.9).

Rupture of the uterus
When an obstructed labour has been relieved by any operative vaginal procedure, delivery should be followed immediately by manual exploration of the uterus to detect rupture. Delay in diagnosing rupture of the uterus is disastrous, as laparotomy must be quickly performed if the patient is to survive. Indeed, if a rupture is discovered during a vaginal operation before the fetus is delivered, the procedure must be abandoned immediately and delivery effected per abdomen without delay. Because of this, all obstetric operations to relieve obstructed labour must be performed

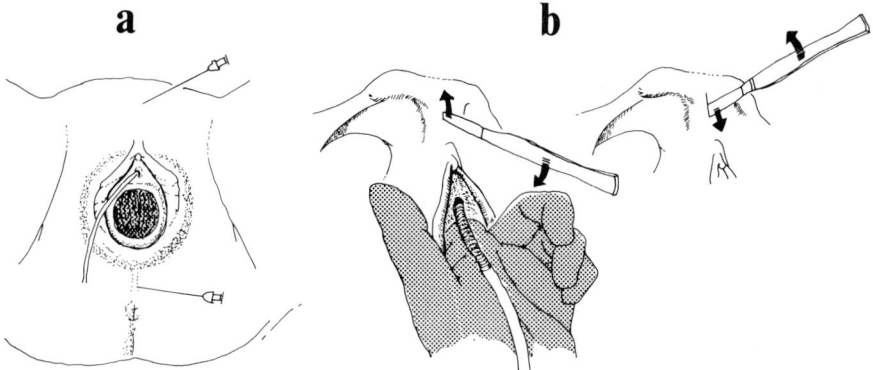

Fig. 26.7 Technique of symphysiotomy. (a) Infiltration with local anaesthetic over symphysis pubis: perineum infiltrated before episiotomy. Catheter in urethra. Angle of abduction of thighs less than 90°. (b) Division of the fibro-cartilaginous plate in the centre of the joint with a solid-bladed scalpel. A finger in the vagina displaces the urethra to one side.

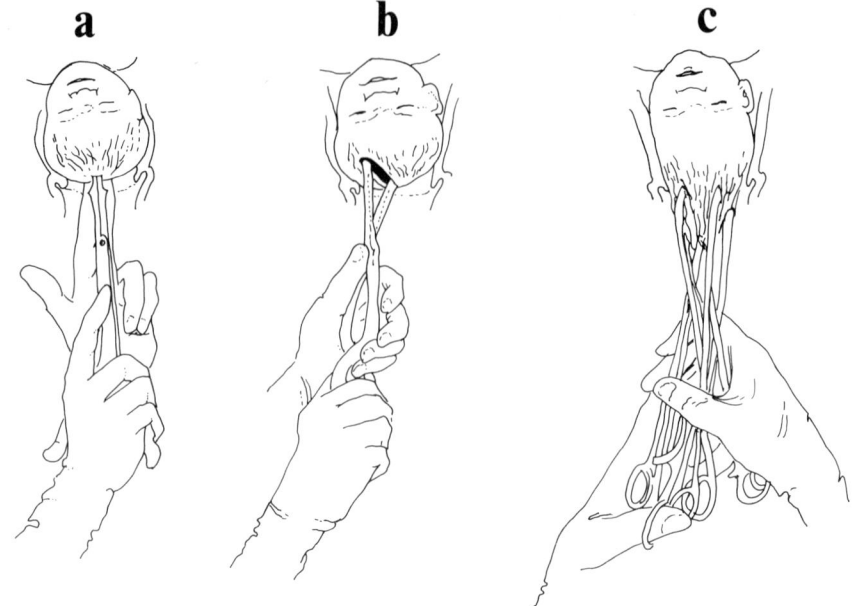

Fig. 26.8   Technique of craniotomy. (a) Perforator inserted into fetal skull. (b) Perforator is rotated with blades open to break up the septa. (c) Traction on the skull edges with Morris' craniotomy forceps.

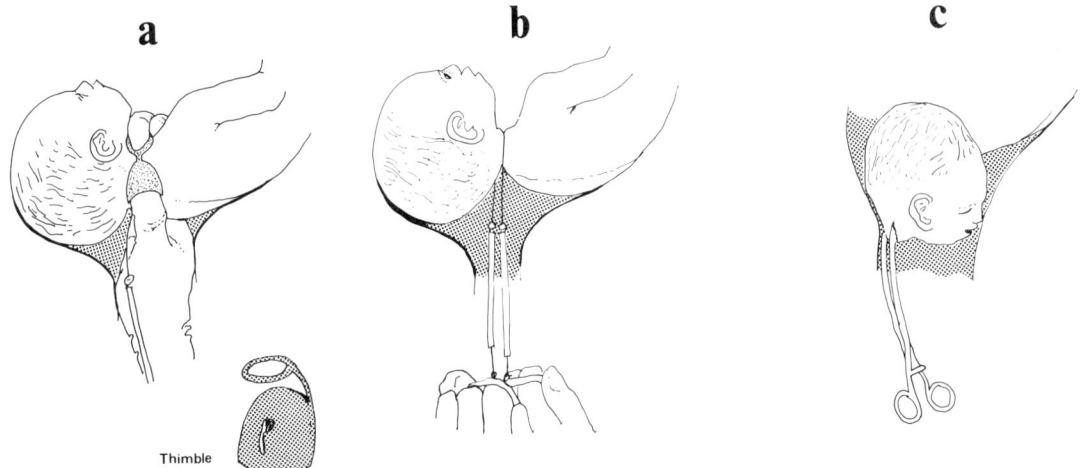

Fig. 26.9   Technique of decapitation. (a) Blond-Heidler decapitation saw is passed round fetal neck with the help of special thimble. (b) With a few firm strokes of the saw, the neck is severed. (c) The after-coming head is delivered by traction on the stump of the neck with volsellum forceps.

in an operating theatre where a tray of laparotomy instruments is ready for immediate use if a rupture is found.

The surgical treatment of rupture of the uterus aims to secure haemostasis and close off the infected birth canal from the peritoneal cavity as quickly as possible, producing the minimum shock in the process. As a rule, repairing the rent is easier and quicker than hysterectomy, except when the rupture is very extensive. The defect is closed rapidly with a continuous haemostatic suture, and since a sound scar cannot be produced in the battered and infected muscle the Fallopian tubes should usually be tied before closing the abdomen. Massive blood transfusion is essential for the successful management of rupture of the uterus.

After-treatment of obstructed labour

Whether the uterus is ruptured or not, intravenous therapy will be required for at least the first 24 hours post-partum to complete the correction of dehydration and keto-acidosis begun before delivery. Similarly, antibiotic therapy should be continued intravenously until the oral route can be substituted.

The bladder should be drained continuously by a self-retaining urethral catheter for at least 48 hours. If the fetal head has been impacted in the vagina for a long time before delivery, pressure necrosis of the bladder wall is likely. In these cases bladder drainage should be continued for at least ten days in the hopes of preventing full thickness sloughing which would otherwise be followed by a vesico-vaginal fistula.

When the patient has recovered, the cause of her traumatic experience must be fully explained both to her and to her relatives. That it could have been prevented by adequate obstetric care should be firmly emphasized, in the hopes of convincing her before she leaves hospital of the importance of receiving skilled obstetric care in all subsequent pregnancies and deliveries.

PUERPERAL SEPSIS

In the unhygienic home surroundings where most deliveries in the tropics still take place it is surprising that birth-canal infection is not more common. The most serious infections that occur follow prolonged and difficult labour, especially when there has been unskilled and unsterile interference.

By the time the patient reaches hospital peritonitis may be already established. A particularly fatal combination is anaemia pre-existing in pregnancy plus that due to blood loss at delivery, combined with birth-canal infection.

Tetanus

A special problem is posed by tetanus, which usually develops about the eighth day after delivery. The preceding labour has usually been prolonged, causing devitalization and necrosis of soft tissues, often contaminated by unsterile intervention in the home before admission to hospital.

Tetanus much more commonly affects the infant and the neonatal death rate is high. The infection enters through the umbilical cord stump which has been contaminated by an unsterile cutting instrument or a dirty dressing. Babies born at home without skilled care are therefore particularly at risk.

The incidence of tetanus neonatorum can be substantially reduced by actively immunizing mothers who intend to deliver themselves at home. At least two injections of toxoid should be given during pregnancy, and instructing traditional midwives to cut the cord with a new razor-blade and apply a clean dry dressing to the stump has also produced successful results.

FURTHER READING

Gebbie, D. A. M. (1974) Symphysiotomy. *Tropical Doctor*, **4**, 69.

Gilles, H. M., Lawson, J. B., Sibellas, M., Voller, A. & Allan, N. C. (1969) Malaria, anaemia and pregnancy. *Ann. trop. Med. Parasit.*, **63**, 245.

Gopalan, C. (1972) Nutrition in pregnancy. *Tropical Doctor*, **2**, 188.

Lawson, J. B. & Stewart, D. B. (1967) *Obstetrics and Gynaecology in the Tropics and Developing Countries*. London: Edward Arnold.

Lawson, J. B. (1971) Severe anaemia in pregnancy: a tropical obstetric emergency. *Tropical Doctor*, **1**, 77.

Lawson, J. B. (1972) The place of Caesarean section in developing countries. *Tropical Doctor*, **2**, 30.

Lawson, J. B. (1974) Embryotomy for obstructed labour. *Tropical Doctor*, **4**, 188.

27. Obstetric Operations

All obstetric operations should be carried out in a delivery room or theatre of a hospital, but if this is not possible every attempt should be made to simulate conditions in a hospital if the delivery is being carried out in the patient's home. Only minor procedures should be carried out in domiciliary practice unless the patient's condition is so critical that she cannot be moved to hospital. Usually with an adequate 'flying squad' it is possible to restore the patient's condition to a satisfactory state so that she can be transferred.

Suitable obstetric beds are usually provided in General Practitioner Maternity Units and in Maternity Hospitals in this country. There are many advantages in having custom built beds, which can serve as operating tables. Usually the beds can be folded or divided so that the woman's buttocks can be brought to the edge and her legs put up in stirrups. Many beds are now available which can be tilted into the 'head down' position or in the opposite direction. This is of considerable value when general anaesthesia is being applied or when the patient is in a state of shock. Formerly the left lateral position was preferred by British obstetricians, but now the dorsal or lithotomy position is preferred, particularly as so much regional anaesthesia by pudendal block or other methods is now employed in preference to general anaesthesia.

Pre-operative preparation

The vulval area is usually shaved and the vulva, upper thighs, lower abdomen and buttocks are swabbed with an antiseptic solution. A popular solution is 1 per cent Hibitane (Chlorhexidine). Although it is usually considered that it is not possible to sterilize the vagina it is customary to pour in some of the antiseptic solution into the vagina. A catheter should always be passed as a full bladder is liable to trauma during operative vaginal delivery. As the urethra is elongated it is necessary to use a long catheter, and in some cases it is necessary to displace the head upwards to allow passage of the catheter when the presenting part is low down in the pelvis. The vulva is swabbed again and the area is draped with sterile towels. A thorough vaginal examination is then carried out using a liberal amount of antiseptic cream (Hibitane or Dettol). If necessary the whole hand should be passed into the vagina to allow easier palpation.

EPISIOTOMY

This is one of the simplest yet one of the most effective obstetric operations. Manual stretching of the perineum is now considered to be outmoded. The perineum is incised to allow easier and quicker delivery of the baby, whether it is coming as a cephalic presentation or as a breech. Episiotomy also avoids over stretching and tearing of the maternal soft tissues. When the baby's head is distending the perineum the skin of the perineum becomes tense. This is almost always the case in a primigravida and an episiotomy is performed then or preferably earlier. An episiotomy should always be performed in a breech presentation before the buttocks are delivered. Most obstetricians perform an episiotomy for all forceps deliveries. If the perineum has not been distended by the presenting part bleeding can be troublesome when the perineum is incised, but bleeding can usually be controlled by pressure with a pad while traction is being exerted on the forceps.

An especially long and deep episiotomy is required if there is narrowing of the sub-pubic angle or if the position of the baby's head is occipito-posterior, or if it seems likely that there is going to be damage to the urethra. This occurs occasionally when the head begins to emerge with the occiput very far forward under the pubic arch, and the urethra may be driven downwards in front of the presenting part. This possibly predisposes to stress incontinence of urine.

Episiotomy is commonly used in primiparae but it may also be required in a multiparous patient if the perineum is rigid or scarred or if the baby is unusually large, and especially if performed correctly in earlier pregnancies.

Types of episiotomy

The medio- or postero-lateral episiotomy is the one most commonly performed. One blade of the episiotomy scissors is inserted into the vagina taking care to avoid the baby's scalp, and the skin and underlying muscles of the perineum are incised. A cut about 4cm long is usually sufficient. The skin is elastic and retracts but the vaginal epithelium is not elastic and usually requires more incision than the perineal skin. (*See* Fig. 27.1.)

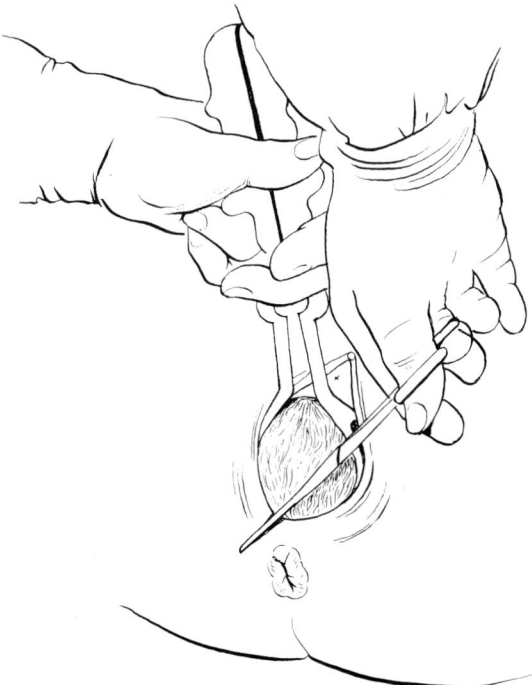

Fig. 27.1   Right postero-lateral episiotomy.

A median episiotomy is directed posteriorly in the middle line of the perineum towards the anus. Although suturing of this incision is easier than the medio-lateral episiotomy the disadvantage is that it may extend to involve the anus.

A 'J' shaped episiotomy is one in which a median episiotomy is extended by curving the excision to one side to avoid the anal sphincter. It is sometimes helpful in making an episio-

tomy to insert two fingers of one hand into the vagina, stretching the area of the perineum to be incised by separating the fingers.

Repair of episiotomies (Fig. 27.2)

The cut vaginal epithelium is drawn together with a continuous catgut suture (number 0 or number 1 chromicized catgut). The perineal muscles are united with interrupted catgut sutures tied without too much tension. The skin is then closed with nylon or mersilk sutures. A very satisfactory result can be obtained when the skin edges are closed with a subcuticular catgut suture.

The dangers of episiotomy are haemorrhage and extension of the incision to involve the rectum. Haemorrhage is liable to occur especially if the incision is made before the head has come down sufficiently far to distend the perineum. Direct pressure can control the bleeding, but if there is still free bleeding after the baby is born the episiotomy should be repaired as quickly as possible. Extension of the episiotomy towards the rectum is liable to occur in a breech or occipito-posterior delivery, and in such cases tearing should be anticipated by extending the incision. Pain in the episiotomy can cause retention of urine in the puerperium, but this can be usually relieved by analgesics. Persisting pain due to involvement of nerves in scar tissue occasionally occurs and this is more likely where the incision has been made at some distance from the mid-line.

SYMPHYSIOTOMY AND PUBIOTOMY

In this operation a partial division of the symphysis pubis is done through a small supra-pubic incision. The patient can either be allowed to continue in labour or a forceps delivery is performed. It is essential that the patient's legs should be supported by two assistants so that the separation of the divided joint can be controlled. This operation has never been popular in Great Britain, but in places like Eire and South Africa there has been an increasing interest in the operation in recent years. The operation is usually recommended where a woman·with a contracted pelvis is uncertain of receiving the necessary medical supervision in a subsequent pregnancy. The operation is, therefore, used in place of Caesarean section when there is slight brim disproportion and trial of labour

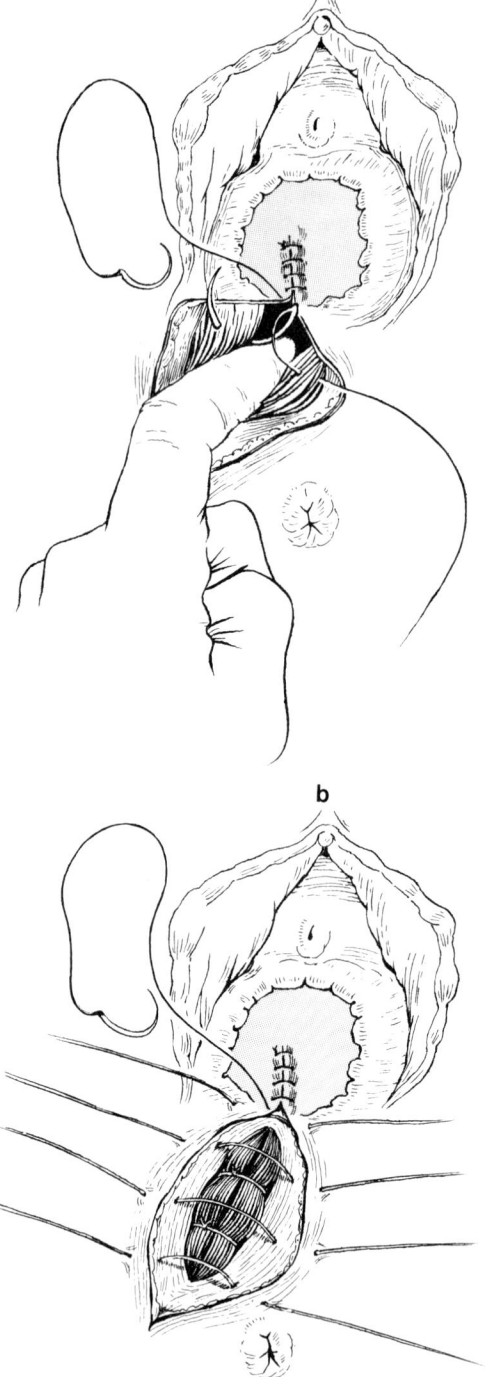

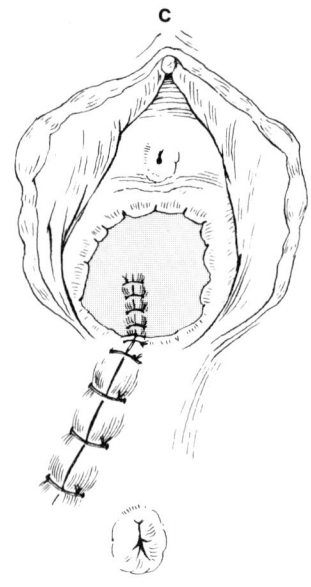

Fig. 27.2   Repair of Episiotomy—
(a) the vaginal epithelium is closed,
(b) the perineal muscles united with catgut and
skin sutures inserted,
(c) skin closed with interrupted sutures.

The operation of pubiotomy which involves division of the pubic bone is not nowadays performed.

INCISION OF THE CERVIX

Manual dilatation or incision of the cervix used to be performed in cases of uterine inertia when the head was so deeply impacted in the pelvis that delivery by Caesarean section would be difficult (Fig. 27.3). In such cases the vacuum extractor or ventouse is now used. Incision of the cervix may very rarely be

has failed or in severe disproportion at the outlet. It is said to be a very satisfactory operation in carefully selected cases, but the selection is difficult and highly undesirable complications such as vesico-vaginal fistula and locomotor difficulties can occur.

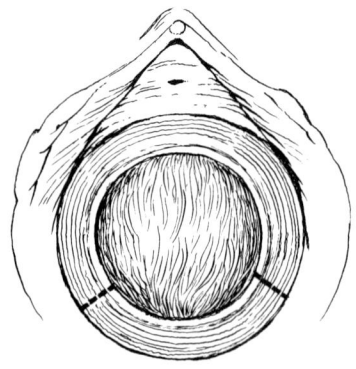

Fig. 27.3   Incision of cervix.

required nowadays if there is a true stenosis or scarring of the cervix and it seems likely that the cervix will tear if the ventouse is applied. The other indication for cervical incision is to facilitate the delivery of the aftercoming head of a premature breech delivery when the baby is small and the trunk has slipped through the partially dilated cervix. In such cases access to incise the cervix is difficult to obtain and great care must be exercised not to damage the baby with the scissors. Haemorrhage must be controlled as quickly as possible afterwards by suturing the cervix.

FORCEPS DELIVERY

The story of the invention of the obstetric forceps and their subsequent development makes fascinating reading. A French Huguenot refugee family by the name of Chamberlen arrived in England in 1569. The eldest and youngest of the children were both named Peter and they became obstetricians. One or possibly both of them was thought to have been the inventor of the obstetric forceps. Peter the elder was an obstetrician to the Royal Court and Peter the younger first suggested the creation of an incorporation of midwives. The secret of the obstetric forceps was kept in the family for over one hundred years. The forceps were simple in design and had only a cephalic curve. The pelvic curve of the forceps was introduced in 1747 by Levret in Paris, and Smellie, the famous Scottish obstetrician introduced the simplified 'English' lock. The axis traction forceps was invented by Tarnier in 1877 (Fig. 27.4).

Many improvements were made in the instrument in France, England and in other countries, but because of overenthusiastic use by unskilled operators the forceps operation fell into some disrepute. It was criticized by William Hunter, the Scottish anatomist and obstetrician who practised in London, and a cautious and conservative era followed. In the early 19th century, however, under the leadership of Sir James Young Simpson further improvements were made in the instrument and the introduction of general anaesthesia in 1847 renewed the interest in the operation. Tarnier's invention of the axis traction rods also increased the popularity of the forceps. These forceps allowed traction to be applied close to the fetal head and the direction of

traction could be determined by the axis of advance of the head as it entered the brim, descended through the pelvic cavity and swung upwards and forwards through the pelvic outlet.

Many modifications and improvements have been made in the obstetric forceps and Milne Murray's axis traction forceps were for many years the favourite in this country. However, the need for axis traction became less as Caesarean section became a popular operation. It is now never considered permissible to apply forceps to a head which is arrested above the pelvic brim, and mid-cavity forceps and pelvic outlet forceps only are performed. If the head is arrested in the transverse position in the cavity or in the occipito-posterior position Kjelland's forceps are used. In these the pelvic curve is almost eliminated and this allows a correct cephalic grip to be obtained, even if the head is arrested in the occipito-transverse position. The lock is sliding and this allows a better adjustment to the sides of the baby's head.

The main action of the obstetric forceps is traction and the amount of traction which can be exerted is enormous, so that great caution has to be exerted to ensure that undue force is not employed. The child's head may be compressed if the blades are not accurately employed. An oblique or antero-posterior application of the blades should be avoided as serious damage to the fetal head can occur with such grasps. It is possible to use a lateral lever action with the forceps, but this is seldom indicated. Rotation of the baby's head should be done only with the forceps which are specially designed for this, that is the Kjelland's forceps.

Indications for forceps delivery
Forceps delivery is indicated when it is considered desirable to terminate the second stage of pregnancy rapidly, provided that certain criteria can be fulfilled.

Conditions to be fulfilled if forceps are to be employed:

1. The cervical os should be fully dilated. If the cervix is not fully dilated there is a danger of laceration and haemorrhage occurring. If it is necessary in the interests of the mother to deliver the baby before the cervix has reached full dilatation the ventouse (*see* p. 534) should be employed or Caesarean section performed (*see* p. 540).

2. The membranes must be ruptured.

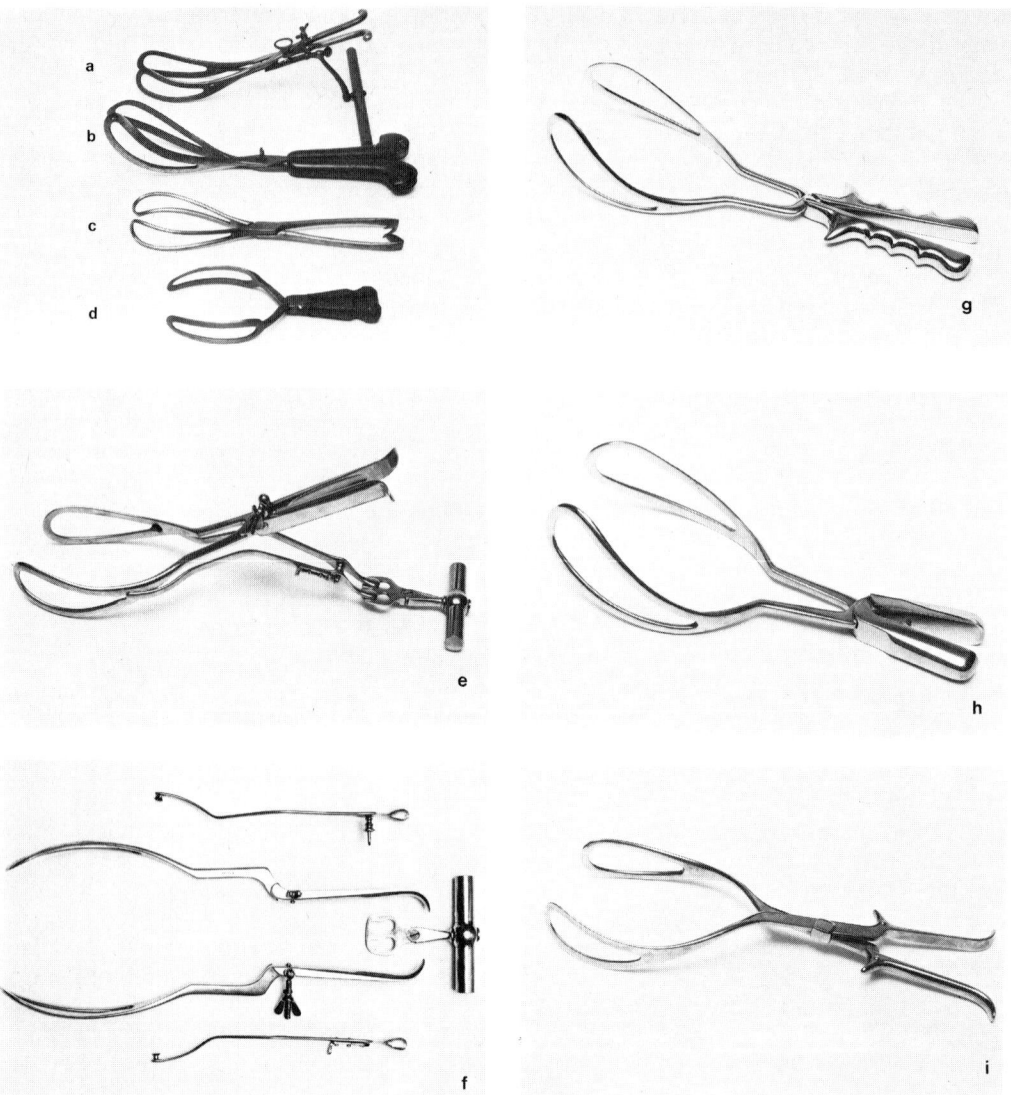

Fig. 27.4(a)   Tarnier's Axis Traction Forceps. Etienne Tarnier was born near Dijon, France in 1828. He developed the concept of traction being applied at the blades to direct the forceps through the pelvis.
(b)   Dubois Forceps. Antione Dubois was Professor of Midwifery at the Maternité in Paris and designed his forceps in 1791. They are a modification of Levret's forceps and have a marked pelvic curve. An unusual feature of these forceps is that the wooden muff covering the handle can be removed leaving a hook which could be used to remove a dead child.
(c)   Gregoire's Forceps, 1746. The Gregoires, father and son, practised midwifery in Paris. There is no pelvic curve and the blades are only 2¼ inches apart at their widest so that there is considerable compressive potential. Note the crochet hook on the handles.
(d)   Orme–Lowder Forceps, 1782. Orme was a graduate of Edinburgh and Lowder of Aberdeen University and they practised midwifery in London. These forceps are a modification of the forceps designed by William Smellie, the famous Scottish obstetrician, who was born in Lanark in 1697. Orme made the cephalic curve rounder and Lowder made the forceps an inch longer.
(e)   Milne-Murray forceps assembled.
(f)   Milne-Murray forceps separated.
(g)   Simpson's forceps.
(h)   Wrigley's forceps.
(i)   Kjelland's forceps.

3. The presentation must be suitable. Preferably the presentation should be a well flexed head, but in a face presentation forceps delivery is possible if the head is in the mento-anterior position. Forceps is particularly useful when applied to the aftercoming head in breech deliveries. Brow presentation is generally unsuitable for forceps delivery unless it is corrected or converted to a face presentation.

4. The head must be in the pelvic cavity (Fig. 27.5). Applications of the forceps is

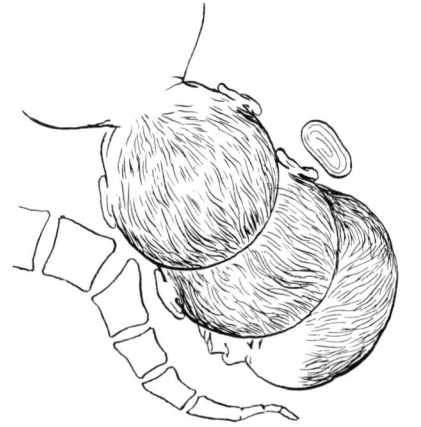

Fig. 27.5   High, mid-cavity and low positions of head as it descends and rotates from occipito-lateral to occipito-anterior position.

contra-indicated if the head is above the pelvic brim. Obviously the lower the head is in the cavity the easier is the forceps delivery provided there is no contraction of the pelvic outlet.

5. Pelvic cavity and outlet should not be contracted. Forceps must not be employed to pull the head past a bony resistance.

A trial of forceps operation may be carried out by an experienced obstetrician in selected cases. The forceps is applied in the operating theatre with preparation made for Caesarean section should it be thought that vaginal delivery would prove to be too difficult.

6. The bladder and rectum should be empty. Probably the commonest indication for forceps delivery is delay in the second stage of labour, and concern for the safety of the baby. If there is any uncertainty about the regularity, strength or rate of the fetal heart and all the conditions are otherwise suitable then forceps delivery should be undertaken. If the mother's condition is causing concern and particularly if there is a pre-existing maternal disease such as a

cardiac lesion, prophylactic forceps delivery at the time of full dilatation of the cervix is indicated. Generally speaking the indications for forceps delivery can be summarized as:

1. Faults in the forces.
2. Faults in the soft tissues of the passages.
3. Faults in the child.
4. Dangers threatening the life of the mother.
5. Dangers threatening the life of the child.

Dangers of forceps operation

The immediate danger to the mother is of laceration and haemorrhage. Lacerations can occur in the cervix, the anterior wall of the vagina, around the urethra or in the posterior part of the vagina. Careless and forceful application of the blades will cause trauma, but more commonly severe lacerations are due to rotation of the forceps. With the more general use of local anaesthesia and the greater care taken with general anaesthesia there is less likelihood of anaesthetic complications nowadays. If there has been laceration and bruising of the vagina, sepsis may occur.

The remote sequelae of forceps operations are those of utero-vaginal prolapse and of damage to the sphincters of the bladder and rectum. This is very unlikely to happen with a low forceps operation, because the head has already begun to leave the vagina and the only pressure which is being exerted is on the soft tissues of the perineum so that an episiotomy will avoid the possibility of residual damage. This is one reason for the prophylactic episiotomy which is usually done in primigravid patients. The mid-forceps delivery can sometimes cause the vagina to be pulled down in front of the head and this possibly predisposes to stress incontinence of urine in later life. Strong traction can also cause stretching of the transverse cervical ligaments and this will allow descent of the uterus later. Cervical lacerations can predispose to parametritis, and this will give rise to chronic pain in the pelvis and in the back. Low backache is a common sequel of childbearing and particularly after difficult forceps deliveries. This may be due to damage to the pelvic floor, but can also be due to damage to the sacrum or sacro-iliac joints.

The baby may be damaged by inaccurate application of the blades. An accurate cephalic grip with the blades over the sides of the fetal head lessens the risk of damage as the chief compression is on the cheeks and zygomatic

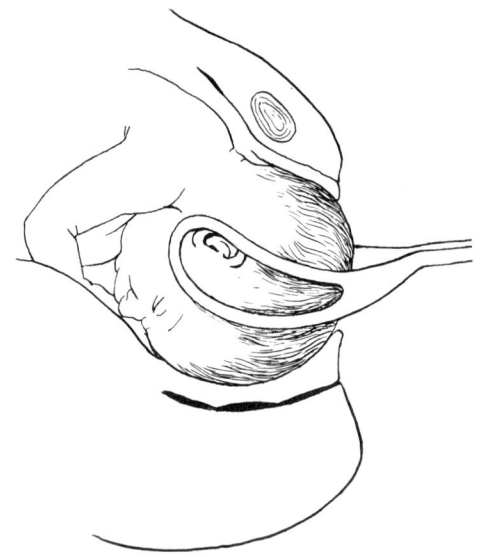

Fig. 27.6   Accurate application of forceps blades.

arches, and there is no direct pressure on the base of the skull (Fig. 27.6). If the application is oblique or antero-lateral there will be pressure on the base of the skull. Inaccurate application or very strong traction can cause abrasions to the scalp and face or more serious damage resulting in intra-cranial haemorrhage, particularly if an oblique or antero-lateral grip is obtained.

The low forceps operation

Regional anaesthesia is induced by pudendal

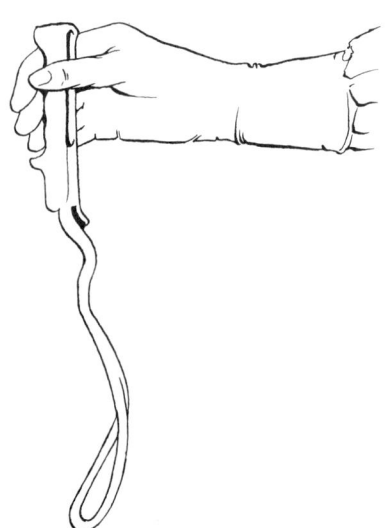

Fig. 27.7   (a) Left forceps blade.

block or epidural anaesthesia. If an inhalational anaesthetic is required precautions are taken against gastric regurgitation. The patient is prepared as previously described and a vaginal examination is made to check that conditions are suitable for forceps delivery.

The left blade is identified and held in the right hand (Fig. 27.7a). The fingers of the left hand are placed in the vagina. The blade is held with the fenestra perpendicular and the cavity of the cephalic curve directed towards the vulva. The fingers of the left hand in the vagina are curved round the baby's head and the blade is gently introduced and guided along the fingers of the left hand into the hollow of the sacrum keeping the blades close to the baby's head (Fig. 27.7b). The blade is then rotated to the left side of the pelvis and the handle of the forceps is pushed down towards the horizontal. When curving the blades out towards the mother's left side the handle of the forceps will describe a wide arc towards the mother's right. The left hand is kept in position in the vagina and the first blade is kept in position (Fig. 27.7c). The second blade is then introduced along the left hand into the hollow of the sacrum and rotated into the right side of the pelvis (Fig. 27.7d).

On no account should force be used to rotate the blades into the position on the sides of the baby's head. The blades are now brought together and locked. Usually in a low forceps operation there is no difficulty with the locking, but it may be necessary to depress the handles backwards. It should be noted that the left blade is always introduced first, because it forms the lower part of the lock and the right blade fits on top of it. If there is any real difficulty in locking the blades then they must be withdrawn and reintroduced.

The forceps are now grasped either by the traction handle or with one or more fingers applied between the shanks (Fig. 27.7e). Traction is exerted in a downwards and backwards direction. The traction should be only sufficient to produce slight descent of the fetal head, and should be applied intermittently for about fifteen seconds at a time. If a forceps with a locking device is being used the lock should be loosened after each rotation. If there is no descent of the head with moderate traction the position and size of the baby's head and application of the forceps should be carefully checked. It is important to emphasize that the line of traction should be downwards

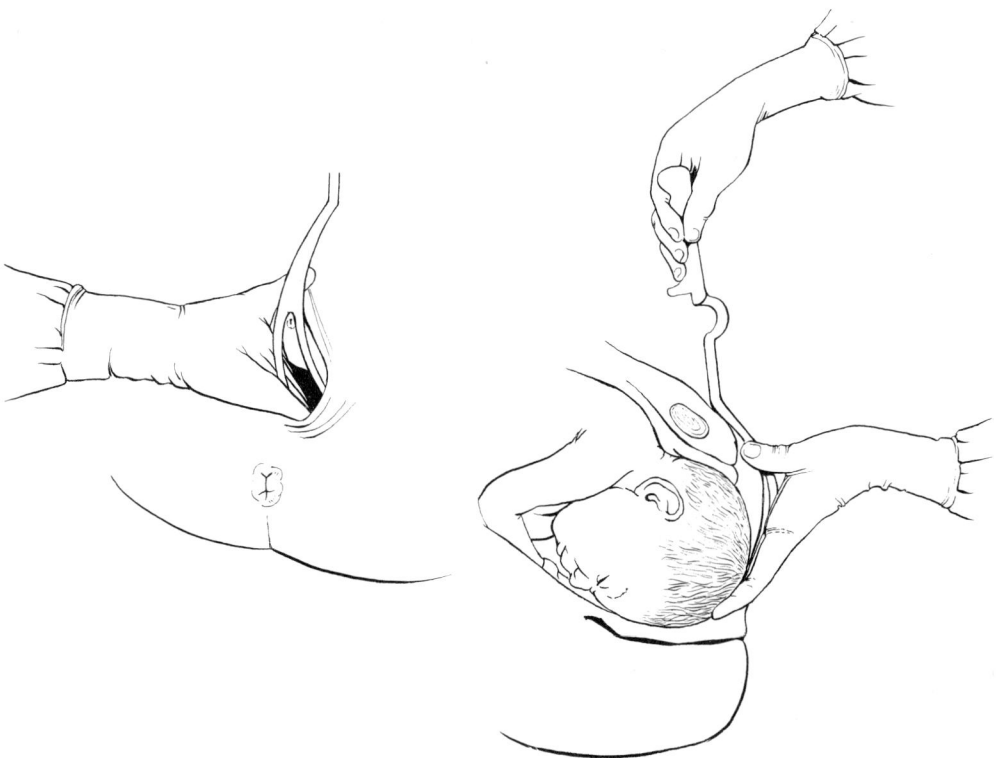

(b) Inserting left forceps blade.

and backwards until the occiput appears below the apex of the pubic arch (Fig. 27.7f). Thereafter the traction is brought more and more forwards until the handles of the forceps are pointing straight upwards (Fig. 27.7g). The forceps should only be used for traction and there should be no attempt to lever the head from side to side. When the head begins to distend the perineum an episiotomy should be performed (Fig. 27.7h). It is preferable not

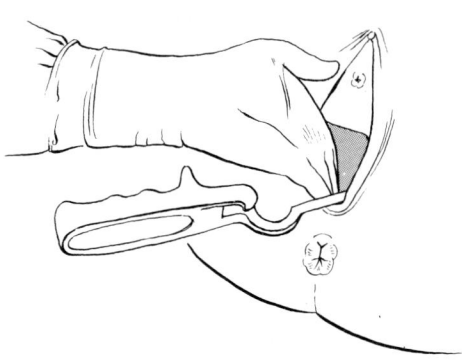

(c) Left forceps blades kept in position prior to inserting right forceps blade.

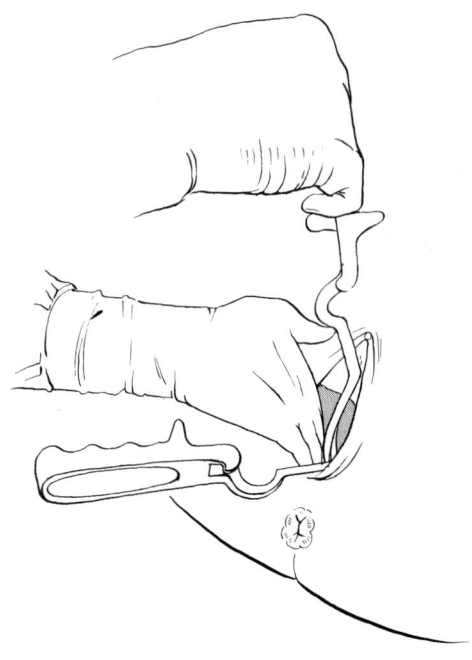

(d) Inserting right forceps blade.

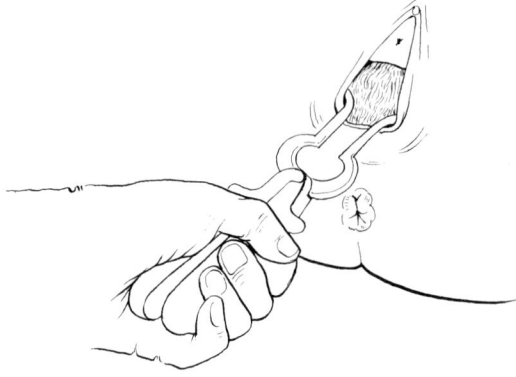

(e) Traction downwards and backwards.

to do this too soon otherwise needless bleeding occurs. The forceps are kept on until the head is delivered as the escape of the head can be readily controlled with the forceps. Some prefer to remove the forceps when the head is crowned and to complete the delivery by pressure made on either side of the anal region behind the perineum (Fig. 27.7i, j). There is the possibility that the forceps may be removed too soon, and would have to be reapplied.

Mid-forceps operation

This should not be undertaken outside a hospital unit unless in quite exceptional cir-

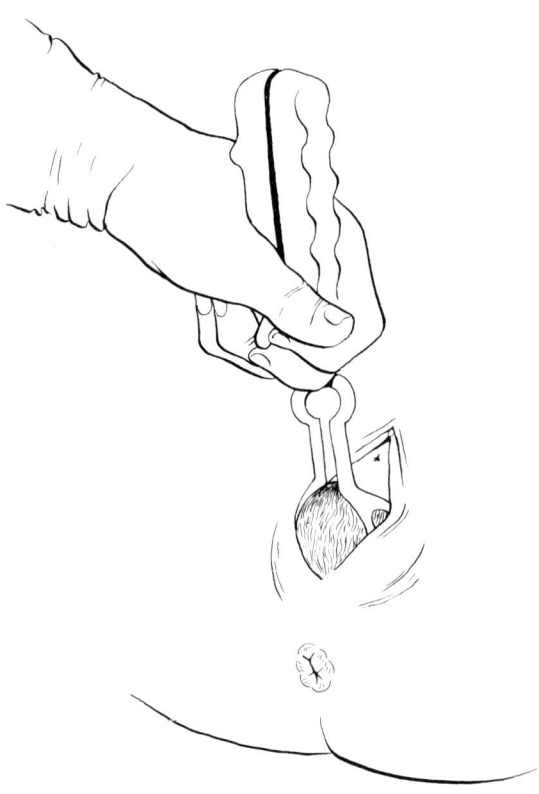

(g) Traction upwards as head emerges from vagina.

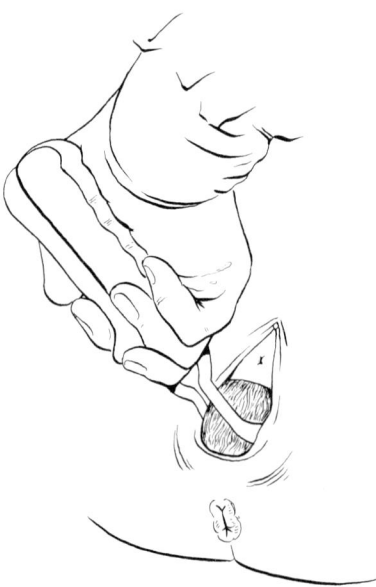

(f) Traction moving forwards and upwards as occiput appears.

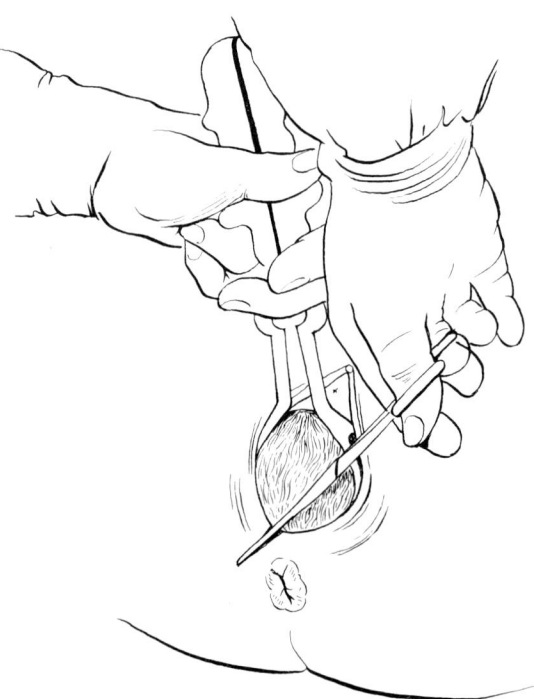

(h) Episiotomy performed when perineum begins to stretch.

To add to the difficulties it is usually necessary for a general or regional anaesthetic to be given. Local analgesia is seldom adequate for a manual rotation of an occipito-lateral or occipito-posterior position. Therefore, unless it is certain that the occiput is directly anterior a general, caudal or epidural anaesthetic is usually indicated. A medical colleague with experience in anaesthesia is essential if reasonable standards are to be maintained, even if this means some delay. After the usual preparation of the patient and catheterization the operator introduces a whole hand into the vagina to make a careful assessment to determine whether all the conditions necessary for safe forceps delivery exist. It is particularly important to ensure that the cervix is fully dilated and to determine whether rotation of the occiput will be required. It may be necessary to give a general anaesthetic before sufficient relaxation can be obtained to assess the pelvic conditions adequately. The leading part of the head should have reached the level of the ischial spines. When the occiput is directly anterior the forceps are applied as for a low forceps delivery, but a larger excursion of the blades is required, and it is essential that each blade is passed deeply into the posterior segment of the pelvis before rotating into position by the swinging movement which carries the blade across the baby's face.

A careful check is made to ensure that no part of the maternal soft tissues is caught between the blades and the baby's head. The handles should be depressed to ensure correct locking. If there is difficulty in locking the handles then the blades should be removed and the position of the head carefully checked. It is probable, in such cases, that the head has not rotated completely to the anterior position. If the head is lying in a transverse or oblique position then it should be manually rotated to the antero-posterior position (Fig. 27.8), or alternatively Kjelland's forceps should be applied. In doing a manual rotation to the anterior position it is usually desirable to overcorrect the head because it will tend to rotate back to its original position.

Once the blades are correctly applied intermittent traction is exerted, remembering that it is necessary in the mid-forceps operation to pull more downwards and backwards than in the low forceps operation. Usually more force is required to deliver the baby from the mid-cavity position than in the low forceps

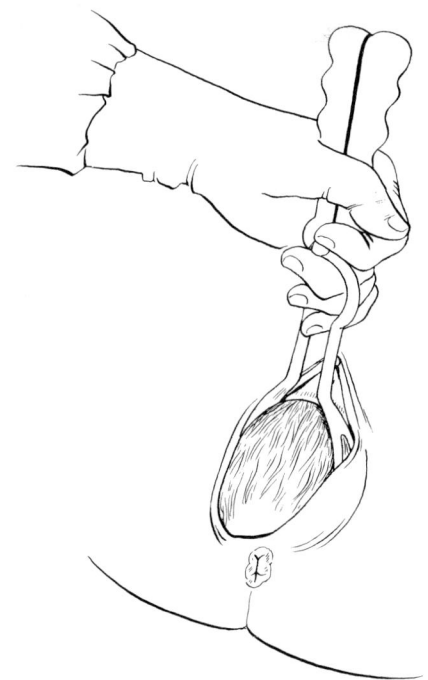

(i) Head being born.

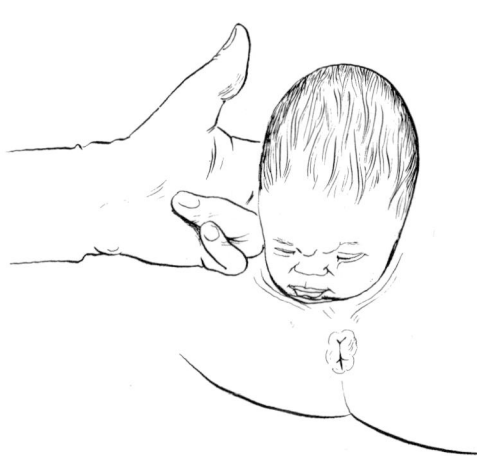

(j) Checking for cord round neck after birth of head.

cumstances. A country practitioner working in a General Practitioner Maternity Unit has to be more self reliant than a city doctor and he will have had post-graduate experience in a Maternity Hospital. If there is particular difficulty or if the general practitioner does not wish to undertake a mid-forceps operation then an obstetric specialist can usually be obtained. In a city practice the patient should be transferred to the specialist Maternity Hospital.

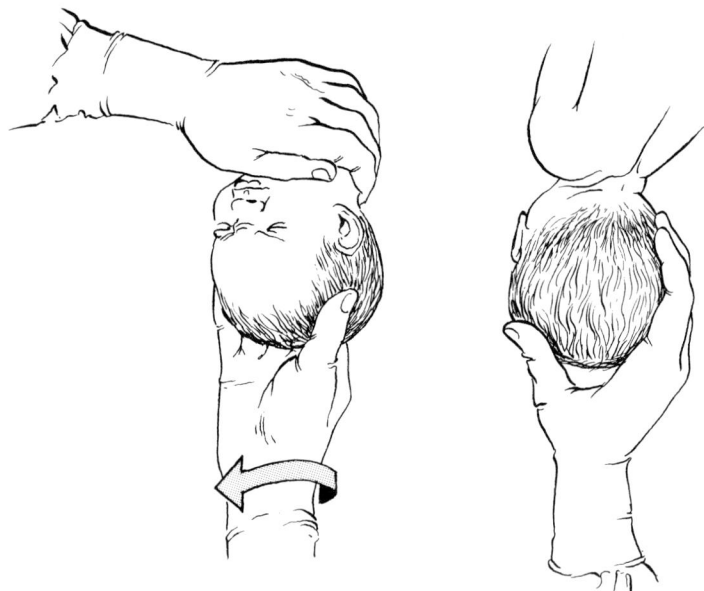

Fig. 27.8   Manual rotation of head. The external hand assists the rotation by pushing on the shoulder.

delivery, but very strong traction or any jerking or levering movements should be avoided. Once the head has been brought down to the low cavity the operation is completed as for a low forceps delivery.

Occipito-posterior position

When the head is in the mid-pelvis it is preferable to rotate it to an anterior position either by manual rotation or with the forceps before attempting to deliver the baby. It is not always possible to do so, however, and it may be necessary to deliver the head in the occipito-posterior position or as it is often termed 'face to pubis'. When the head has descended in the occipito-posterior position to the introitus it is considered preferable by many to apply the forceps directly and to deliver the baby in the occipito-posterior position without attempting to rotate (Fig. 27.9).

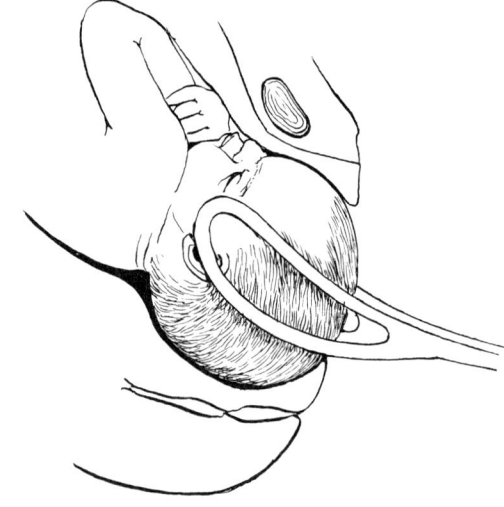

Fig. 27.9   Forceps delivery 'face-to-pubis'.

The blades are introduced over the fingers of the left hand into the hollow of the sacrum and the blade is swept over the baby's occiput towards the side of the baby's head and the side of the maternal pelvis as already described. Traction should be made downwards and backwards and more and more forwards until the occiput is born, and in this way stimulating the movements which the head makes in a spontaneous 'face to pubis' delivery. Once the occiput is born the face is brought down from behind the symphysis pubis. As the

biparietal diameter of the baby's head is distending the perineum instead of the narrower bitemporal diameter as in an occipito-anterior position it is essential to perform a wide episiotomy when delivering 'face to pubis', otherwise severe damage to the anal sphincter may result.

Face presentation

When the head is well extended and the chin is anterior the head can come well down in the

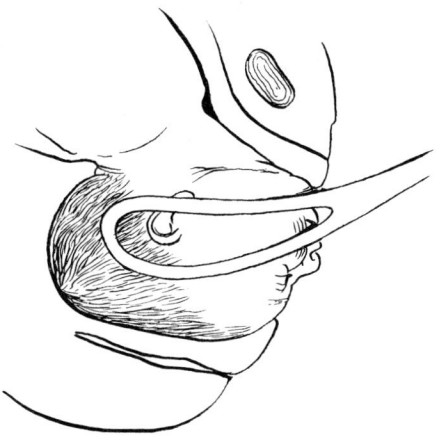

Fig. 27.10 Forceps delivery of mento-anterior. Traction is exerted downwards until the chin has cleared the symphysis pubis.

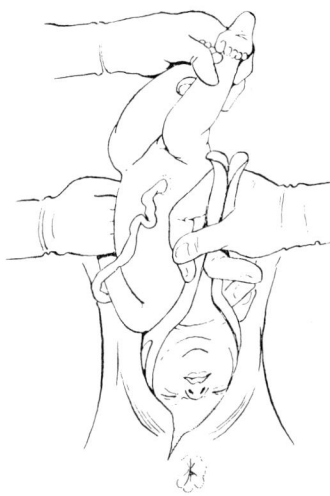

Fig. 27.11 Forceps delivery of aftercoming head.

pelvis and make forceps delivery possible. A mento-posterior position of the head is usually considered to be suitable for forceps delivery. For a mento-anterior position the blades are introduced in a similar fashion to that for an occipito-anterior position, and again care is taken not to injure the baby's face. The blades lie alongside the baby's head with the baby's ears usually coming through the fenestra (Fig. 27.10). Traction is again exerted downwards and backwards and it is important to ensure that the chin is delivered from under the symphysis pubis before the rest of the head is delivered. Rotation of a mento-posterior can be attempted with Kjelland's forceps. This should be done while traction is being exerted,

but it is not likely to be successful unless the baby's head is relatively small and the pelvis is roomy.

Brow presentation

Forceps should not be employed in brow presentation unless the brow can be converted either into a face or a vertex presentation, which is only possible in exceptional circumstances.

After coming head

Forceps should always be ready in breech presentations for use on the aftercoming head. The baby's trunk must be held upwards and well out of the way by an assistant so that the forceps can be introduced along the ventral aspect of the baby (Fig. 27.11). When the

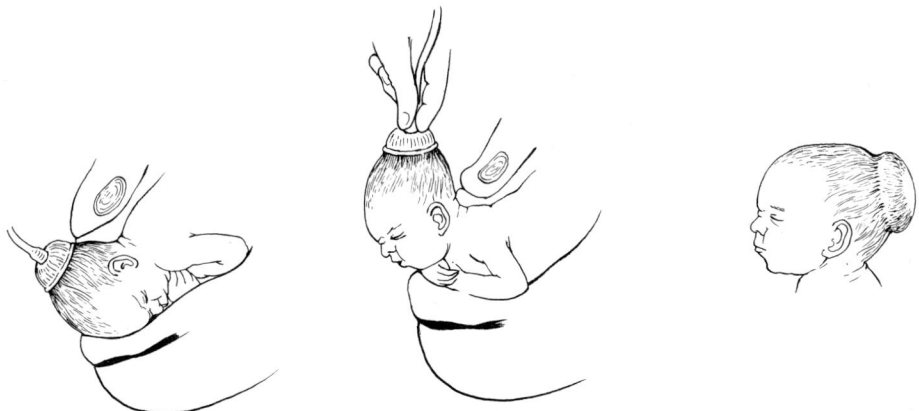

Fig. 27.12(a) Delivery by vacuum extractor (Ventouse). The cup is applied as far back on the occiput as possible. There is usually a marked caput succedaneum formed.

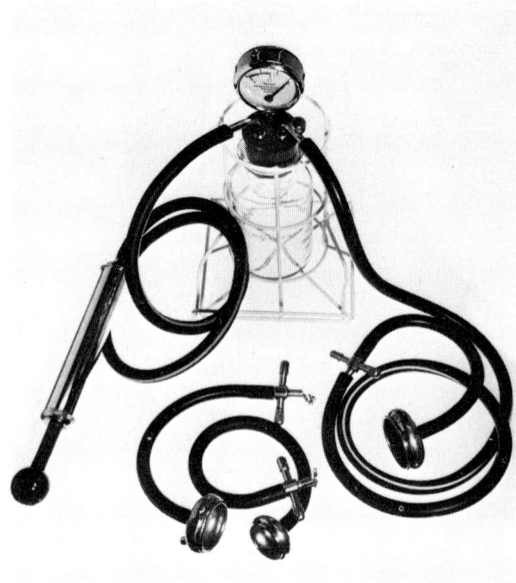

Fig. 27.12(b)   Vacuum extractor (Ventouse).

head is being extracted the trunk should be carried upwards towards the mother's abdomen.

THE VACUUM EXTRACTOR (VENTOUSE)
Although various attempts have been made in the past to devise a suitable suction apparatus to apply to the fetal head, no suitable instrument was devised until 1953 when Mälmstrom described the ventouse or vacuum extractor. This instrument is composed of a metal cap, made in three sizes, attached by a chain, enclosed in rubber tubing, to an air chamber to which a hand pump is attached (Fig. 27.12b). The suction is gradually increased until a negative pressure of not more than 0·8kg per square cm is reached. The vacuum extractor can be used instead of forceps, and is best used with pudendal block anaesthesia rather than general anaesthesia so that traction can be exerted when the patient is making bearing down efforts. The ventouse has an additional advantage over the forceps in that it is possible to apply the cup to the fetal head before the cervix is fully dilated.

The ventouse is, therefore, indicated in cases where it is desirable to achieve delivery within a fairly short time and the fetal head is in the pelvic cavity but the cervix is not fully dilated. It is possible with this instrument to avoid some Caesarean sections. Care must be

taken to ensure that there is no pelvic contraction in such cases and time must be taken to ensure that the cervix is not dilated too rapidly. When applying the cup care must also be taken to ensure that the cervix does not become caught between the cup and the fetal head (Fig. 27.12a).

If a caput succedaneum has formed the metal cup is placed over this, but if not a caput is gradually raised by slowly increasing the suction. This instrument now has an established placed in obstetrics, but over-enthusiasm in the use of the instrument in unsuitable cases can lead to damage, particularly to the baby. Injudicious use has caused the death of babies from intra-cranial haemorrhage and necrosis and abrasions of the scalp have occurred from prolonged suction being applied.

VERSION

Internal version
Internal podalic version means the turning of the baby to convert either a shoulder or a head presentation into a breech presentation. This can be a dangerous manoeuvre both for the mother and for the baby. It is associated with a high fetal mortality and there is a danger of rupture of the uterus in the mother. The manoeuvre is seldom used nowadays and is only used to correct a shoulder presentation, in the unlikely situation of the cervix being sufficiently dilated and the shoulder not being impacted or for the delivery of the second twin. It is very seldom, if ever, indicated for a placenta praevia or a prolapse of the cord except possibly where the baby has already died, but the uterus has not yet closed around the baby. The cervical os should be sufficiently dilated to allow the whole hand to pass into the uterus, and deep anaesthesia is usually required. A foot of the fetus is grasped and drawn down through the cervix into the vagina, at the same time the baby's head is pushed upwards towards the fundus by abdominal manipulation with the external hand (Fig. 27.13). The foot can be differentiated from the hand by the presence of the heel. Although some recommend bringing down both legs, the usual practice is to bring down only one leg and exert traction on it. The operation is not difficult if the membranes are still intact or have only recently ruptured, but gentle handling is required if damage to the baby or rupture of the uterus is to be avoided.

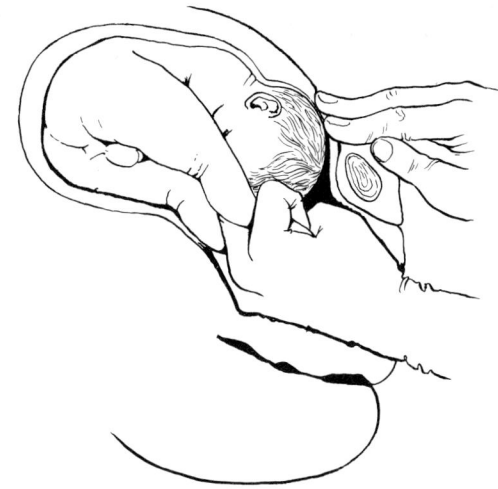

Fig. 27.13   Internal version. The head is pushed upwards with the external hand and a foot is pulled down through the cervix.

In all cases of version the uterus must be carefully palpated after delivery to ensure that a rupture has not occurred. Breech extraction should be proceeded with as soon as the version has been accomplished as placental separation not infrequently occurs and prompt delivery of the baby is desirable.

Bipolar version
This is really an elaboration of the technique of external podalic version. Most of the version is performed with the external hand while the fetus is pushed in the appropriate direction by pressure with one or two fingers through a partially dilated cervix. It differs from internal podalic version in that the whole hand is not introduced through the cervix. There are few indications for this manoeuvre nowadays as Caesarean section is preferable in cases of placenta praevia, for which bipolar podalic version used to be one of the main forms of treatment. Almost the only indication nowadays is for a shoulder presentation which is recognized very early in labour, before the whole hand can be introduced. Even in such cases, however, external version under anaesthesia is usually possible or a Caesarean section is performed. When the foot or feet are pulled down into the vagina the labour is allowed to proceed as in a breech delivery.

DESTRUCTIVE OPERATIONS

The operations of embryotomy or embryulcia are seldom performed nowadays even when the baby is dead as it is usually considered safer for the mother to have a Caesarean section.

Craniotomy

The only indication for this operation nowadays is in cases of hydrocephalus when the child's head is too large to allow delivery through the vagina. This is usually considered preferable to doing a Caesarean section and delivering a baby with such a gross degree of hydrocephaly that successful surgical treatment is impossible, and the child will be a paralysed idiot.

Although in modern obstetric practice there is no place for destructive operations on a normal and in particular a living baby, there are still parts of the world where obstetrics has to be practised differently. In some developing countries where women can be in labour for many days with contracted pelves, destructive operations may still be preferable to Caesarean section. The operation may be life-saving for the mother under such circumstances, but in such cases of protracted labour damage, especially of the bladder wall, is likely, resulting in vesico-vaginal fistula.

Craniotomy of the aftercoming head is sometimes required because of the impossibility of vaginal delivery without reducing the size of the head. This is particularly likely to happen if it is a hydrocephalic head. The perforation should be performed early in labour at 3–4cm dilatation of the cervix so that overstretching of the lower segment is avoided.

Craniotomy of the forecoming head is

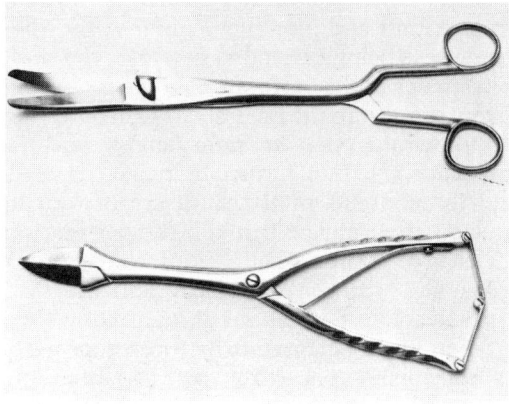

Fig. 27.14   (a) Cleidotomy scissors (*above*).
Simpson's perforator (*below*).

usually performed with special perforators (Simpson's or Oldham's) but if these are not available the operation can be carried out with a pair of large sharp-pointed scissors, although these are not so effective or easy to use as the perforators (Fig. 27.14a and b). The patient should be prepared in the same way as for a forceps operation, and indeed some obstetricians recommend the application of forceps to

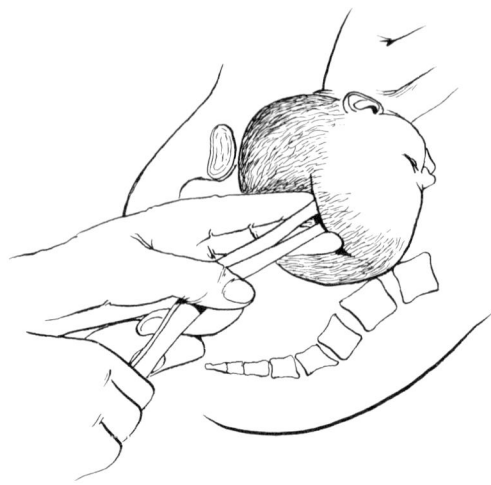

Fig. 27.14(b)   Perforation of head.

steady the head while the perforation is performed, but this is not usually necessary. The application of forceps in such cases may be difficult and traumatic because of the oedema of the vaginal tissues. The head can be kept quite satisfactorily in position by pressure from above. The perforator is carefully introduced into the vagina and carefully pushed into the skull, preferably between the bones in the line of the sutures. Care must be taken to ensure that the perforator blades do not slip off the skull and into the vaginal walls when pressure is being exerted to perforate the skull. The blades of the perforator should be pushed firmly down into the base of the skull and then withdrawn, turned at right angles and reintroduced, so that a cruciate incision is made and the contents of the skull are broken up to allow their escape through the perforation. If it is a hydrocephalic skull the cerebrospinal fluid drains off rapidly and the skull quickly collapses. Labour is then allowed to proceed. If the perforation has been done in the hydrocephalic at an early stage in labour, the labour is often stimulated and proceeds quite quickly and spontaneous delivery occurs. This also occurs when the cervix is fully or almost

fully dilated, but in some cases it may be necessary to attach pressure forceps to the edges of the skull and to gently extract the baby. If there has been impaction of the head and no hydrocephaly the woman will possibly be in an exhausted state and unable to bear down. Forceps are applied in such cases if it is thought that a reasonable grip can be obtained to allow delivery; if not, long pressure forceps are attached to the skull edges and traction is applied.

Craniotomy on the aftercoming head is performed in a similar fashion. The legs of the baby are grasped and traction exerted to bring down the base of the skull as far as possible so that the perforator can be introduced under direct vision. Care must again be taken to ensure that the vagina is not damaged by the sharp edges of the perforator, which is introduced through the skull just behind the baby's ear near to the postero-lateral fontanelle. When the perforator has been introduced the blades are opened and the brain contents broken up. The head is then extracted with a crotchet, which is introduced through the hole made by the perforator and traction is exerted on the bones at the base of the skull (*see also* Fig. 26.8).

Decapitation

This operation is performed when there is an impacted shoulder presentation and the baby is dead. If, however, the pelvis is contracted and the baby is large it may be less traumatic to do a Caesarean section with a vertical or classical incision than to do a decapitation. The operation consists of severing the head from the trunk and extracting the trunk and then the head. A variety of instruments can be used, but usually some form of decapitating hook is employed (Fig. 27.15a, b, c, d). If an arm has not already prolapsed then one should be brought down and by pulling on the arm the neck is brought within easier reach. The decapitating hook or Gigli saw is passed over the neck, usually from the front and by a backwards and forwards motion the neck is divided (Fig. 27.16). Further traction on the prolapsed arm causes delivery of the trunk. Difficulty sometimes arises in delivering the head and it is necessary to fix the head at the brim by suprapubic pressure and to perforate the head before it can be delivered. (*See* Fig. 26.9.)

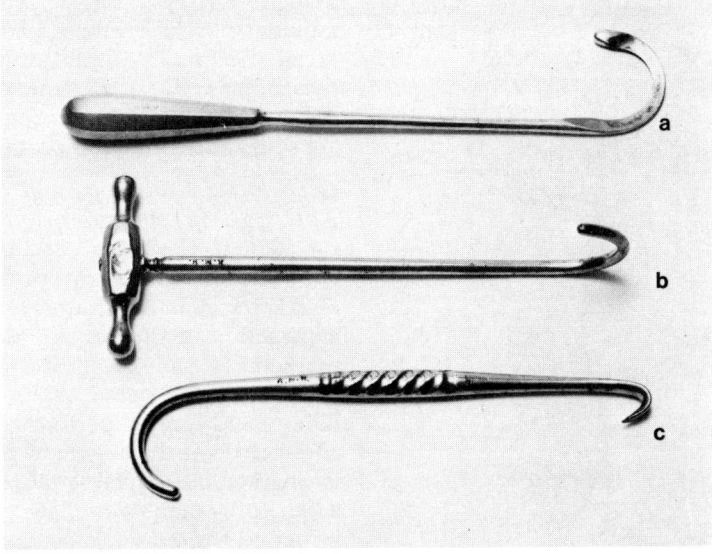

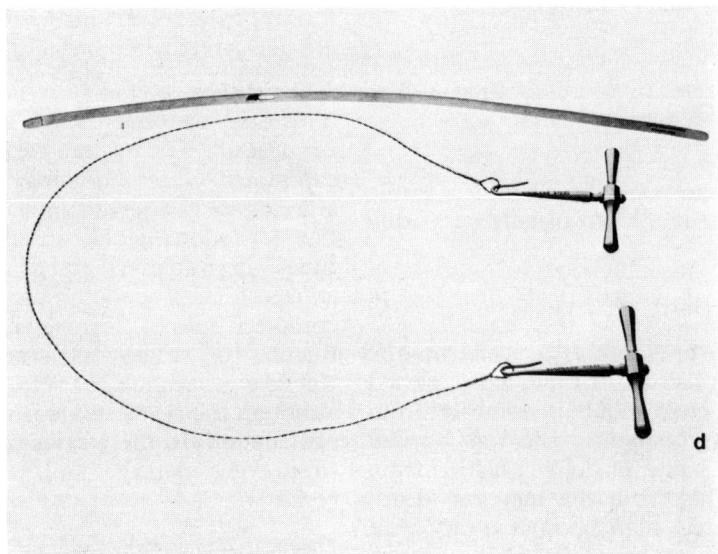

Fig. 27.15 (a) Decapitation knife.
          (b) Hook.
          (c) Combined hook and crotchet.
          (d) Gigli saw.

Evisceration

This operation consists in the removal of the abdominal or thoracic contents to diminish the bulk of the child. It is performed in cases where there is distention of the fetal abdomen by ascites, tumours or enlarged viscera. The perforator or scissors can be used to incise the abdomen or thorax and the contents can then be removed.

Cleidotomy

This is the operation for division of the clavicles and is employed when the shoulders become so impacted that they cannot be brought down. It is sometimes necessary to do this after a craniotomy has been performed. Special heavy scissors are used to divide the clavicles. They are passed along the fingers of the left hand and along the ventral aspect of the child until the

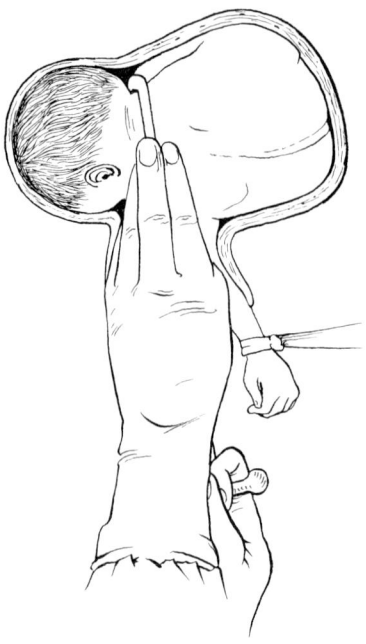

Fig. 27.16   Decapitation. The hook or saw is passed round the neck while traction is put on the arm.

clavicles are reached. The shoulder girdle collapses and the trunk can usually be readily extracted.

Caesarean section

The name of this operation is derived from the Lex Caesarii or Caesarean Law, which stated that the unborn child should be removed from the mother's womb before she was buried. Attempts were made to deliver babies from living mothers also, but the maternal death rate was extremely high because no attempt was made to suture the wound in the uterus. This was not done until towards the end of the 19th century, and in Britain much of the pioneer work in popularizing the operation was due to the Glasgow obstetrician Murdoch Cameron. The operation performed at that time was the classical Caesarean section in which a vertical incision is made in the upper uterine segment. Although it was technically easier the operation has been almost entirely replaced by the lower uterine segment Caesarean section, which has a better immediate and remote prognosis. The classical Caesarean operation is now only performed for special indications, such as, an impacted shoulder presentation.

INDICATIONS FOR CAESAREAN SECTION

It is not possible to give a comprehensive list of all the possible indications and indeed in most cases there are multiple reasons for doing the Caesarean section. The following are some of the more important indications:

Cephalo-pelvic disproportion

This was the commonest original indication for doing Caesarean sections and it still accounts for quite a large proportion of Caesarean sections in this country, but the degree of contraction of the pelvis nowadays is seldom marked. It may be indicated in either contraction of the pelvic inlet, cavity or outlet. The operation is performed before labour commences if the degree of pelvic contraction is marked. Frequently such contraction is seen in women who have sustained severe injury to the pelvis, most commonly because of road accidents. Most Caesarean sections for cephalo-pelvic disproportion nowadays are performed after a trial of labour has failed.

Soft tissue obstruction

This may be caused by tumours such as cervical fibroids, ovarian cysts or even cervical carcinoma. Obstruction may also be caused by scarring as in previous gynaecological operations or following difficult labours. It is sometimes desirable where there has been a gynaecological operation such as a repair of a complete perineal tear, repair of stress incontinence, or of a vesico-vaginal fistula that Caesarean section should be done even although the cicatrization is not likely to cause obstruction. In these cases the section is done to prevent damage and recurrence of the condition.

Disordered uterine action

When it is established that progress in labour has ceased or is so slow as to indicate that the mother would be exhausted before vaginal delivery could be achieved, it is now considered desirable to perform Caesarean section. Sometimes it can be very difficult to decide the optimum time to do the operation in such cases. Formerly the tendency was to allow the labours to go on too long before doing the section. There is now possibly a tendency to stimulate uterine activity and to perform Caesarean sections much earlier if there is not a sufficient response.

Malpresentation of the baby

Face, brow and shoulder presentations are

frequently dealt with by Caesarean section and occipito-posterior position above the brim of the pelvis is also an indication. A large baby giving rise to cephalo-pelvic disproportion has to be delivered by Caesarean section. Twin pregnancy is seldom an indication since the babies are usually small. Breech presentation is more frequently being dealt with by section now, particularly in the older primigravida.

Antepartum haemorrhage

Placenta praevia particularly of major degree is generally an indication for Caesarean section. In cases of suspected placenta praevia the usual practice is to examine the patient in theatre at the optimum time with preparations made for the operation.

Abruption of the placenta is occasionally treated by Caesarean section and this is usually indicated when the abruption has been of recent occurrence, and the baby is thought to have good prospect of surviving. The more usual treatment is to rupture the membranes and labour often proceeds quickly thereafter. If, however, there is delay in labour and there is continued bleeding the baby should be delivered by Caesarean section before there is severe fetal distress.

Fetal distress

This is one of the commonest indications for performing Caesarean section and it can arise from many causes. Where there is no obvious cause predisposing to fetal distress the need for the operation is less obvious and in such cases reliance must be placed on the methods for determining fetal distress. Nowadays there are modern methods for making a more precise diagnosis of fetal distress, and possibly some Caesarean sections can be avoided. Alternatively in some cases where the fetal distress would formerly have been considered to be of a transient or minor nature modern methods of monitoring the fetal heart would indicate that Caesarean section should be performed.

Pre-eclampsia and eclampsia

At one time the treatment of eclampsia was radical and Caesarean section was considered to be the best form of treatment. This has been replaced by a conservative approach and eclampsia is now rarely treated by Caesarean section. Caesarean section is only indicated in cases of eclampsia once the convulsions have been controlled, but labour cannot be induced or where labour is prolonged or there are factors present which might complicate labour. Much the same can be said of pre-eclampsia although there are some obstetricians who favour Caesarean section in severe pre-eclampsia in early pregnancy. Labour can usually be induced quite easily in these cases and is surprisingly rapid. However, if labour does not progress quickly in these cases Caesarean section is indicated. The operation in such cases is done in the maternal interest as the chances of fetal survival are usually small owing to immaturity.

Maternal diseases

Although Caesarean section is seldom justified for the treatment of patients with cardiac disease it is generally accepted that Caesarean section should be performed if there is some other factor which is likely to cause difficulty in labour, even though this factor in itself would not be sufficient to warrant Caesarean section.

Diabetes

Caesarean section used to be performed at about 36 weeks in cases of diabetes. With improved management of cases of diabetes delivery is now quite often carried out at 38 weeks, and if the labour is expected to be short then induction is carried out and a vaginal delivery can often be achieved.

Prolapse of the cord

Caesarean section is the best treatment for this condition if the mother can be conveyed to the operating theatre before the fetal heart stops.

Post-mortem Caesarean section

Living children have been delivered by Caesarean section from women who have died suddenly during the last weeks of pregnancy. There are obvious difficulties in determining precisely the time of death of the mother and in most cases by the time that it is possible to be certain that the mother has in fact died the fetal heart will have stopped. There is considerable doubt about the ethical justification for carrying out Caesarean section in such circumstances.

Previous Caesarean section

Many obstetricians particularly in North America believe in the adage 'once a section always a section' but this belief is not popular in the United Kingdom. It is essential, however, that any woman who has been previously delivered by Caesarean section should have all her future deliveries in a fully equipped maternity hospital. Repeat Caesarean section, of course, is necessary where the primary indication persists as in a contracted pelvis. The possibility of having to do Caesarean sections in all subsequent pregnancies should be borne in mind when deciding to do the first Caesarean section, particularly in a young primigravida.

INCIDENCE OF CAESAREAN SECTION

The Caesarean section rate for the city of Aberdeen rose from 2·2 per cent in 1948–52 to 5·4 per cent in 1963–66 (MacGillivray, 1968). The incidence is higher in small women, in primigravidae and in older women. The Caesarean section rate in the city primigravidae has remained at the same level of 6·3 per cent in the periods 1948–62 and 1963–66 and was 6·5 per cent in 1967–70.

OPERATIVE TECHNIQUE

There are some advantages in performing the operation early in labour while the membranes are still intact, such as the minimal risk of infection, the activity of the uterus reducing the likelihood of post-partum haemorrhage and the dilatation of the cervix allowing escape of blood; the disadvantage of operating at inconvenient times, and possibly operating in hurried circumstances outweigh the advantages, and this has led to the more frequent performance of elective Caesarean section at a set time before labour commences. Before performing the operation it is sometimes desirable to have an X-ray taken of the baby to exclude an abnormality. The anaesthetic for Caesarean section may be general inhalation anaesthetic with a relaxant, an epidural analgesic or local block analgesia. The anaesthetic methods are described in Chapter 24.

LOWER SEGMENT CAESAREAN SECTION (Fig. 27.17a–l)

A longitudinal incision about 15cm in length is made through the abdominal wall between the pubis and the umbilicus. Sometimes a transverse (Pfannenstiel) incision is preferred. The lower end of the wound is retracted with a broad-bladed Doyen retractor and packing is inserted at each side of the uterus to prevent blood and amniotic fluid from reaching the peritoneal cavity and to keep the bowel from coming into the wound. The loose peritoneum

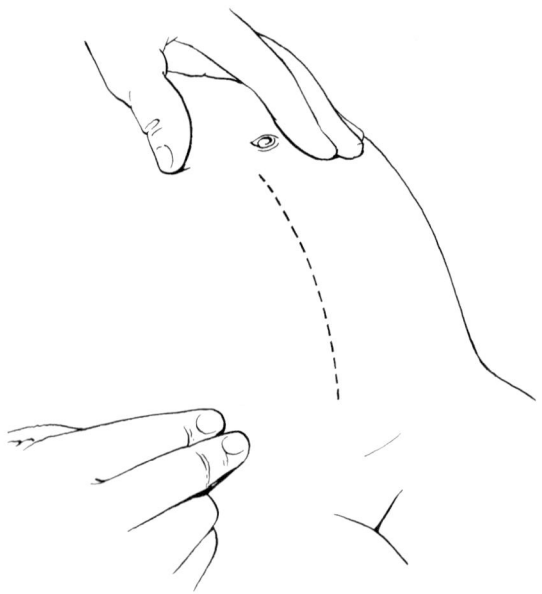

Fig. 27.17   (a) Right paramedian subumbilical incision.

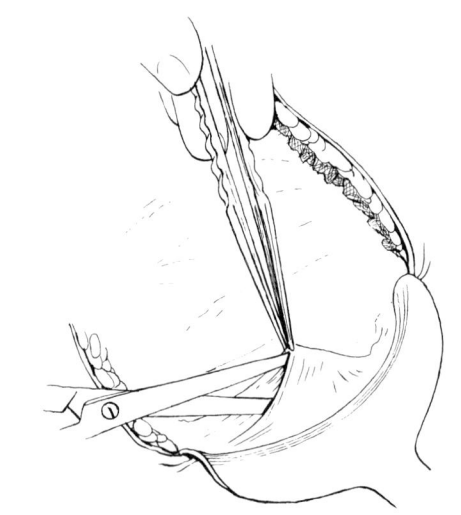

(b) Incision of loose peritoneum above bladder.

on the front of the lower uterine segment just above the bladder is then incised transversely and the incision is carried outwards on each side until the peritoneum leaves the uterus to become the anterior leaf of the broad ligament. The bladder is pressed gently downwards with a swab on a holder and the upper flap of the peritoneum is also mobilized. A shallow transverse incision is then made in the muscle of the lower uterine segment curving the ends upwards on both sides. This demarcates the length of the opening which will be

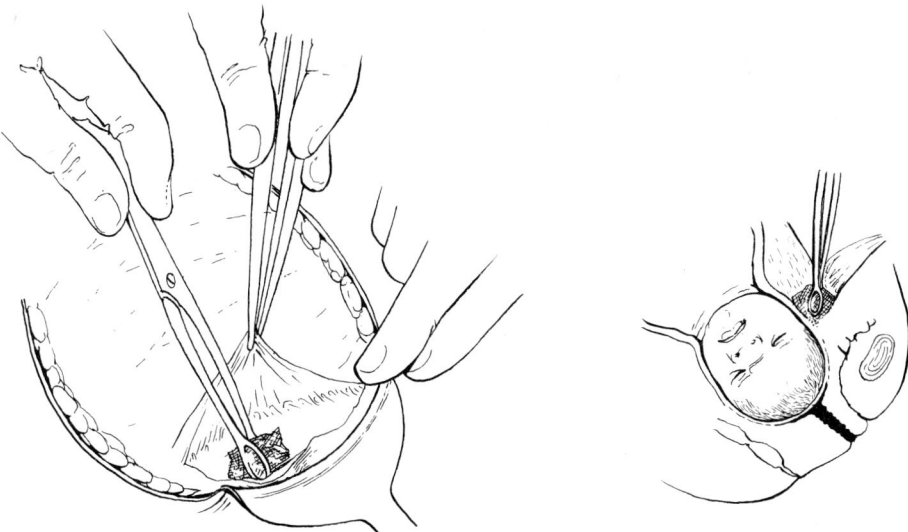

(c) The bladder being pushed downwards off the lower uterine segment.

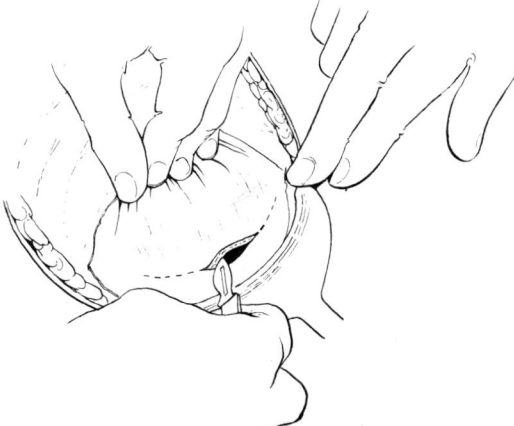

(d) The shallow transverse incision is curved upwards at both ends and deepened in the centre.

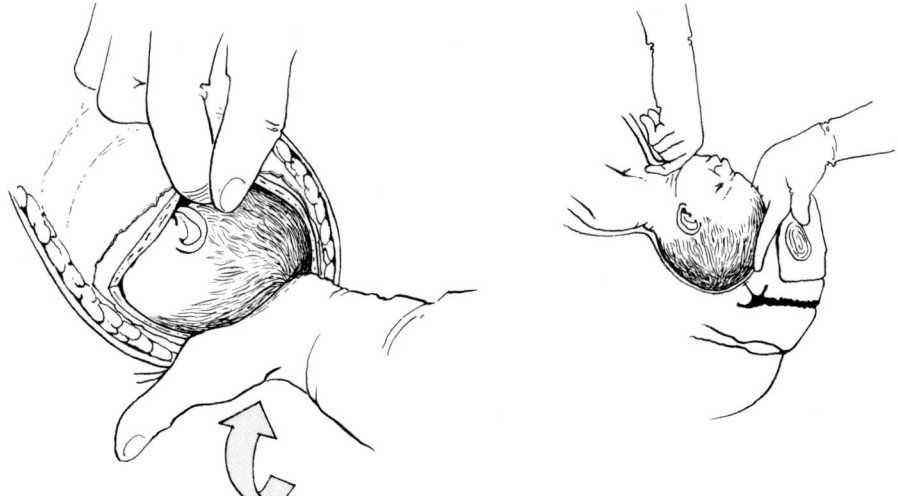

(e) The baby's head is rotated so that the face comes into the incision.

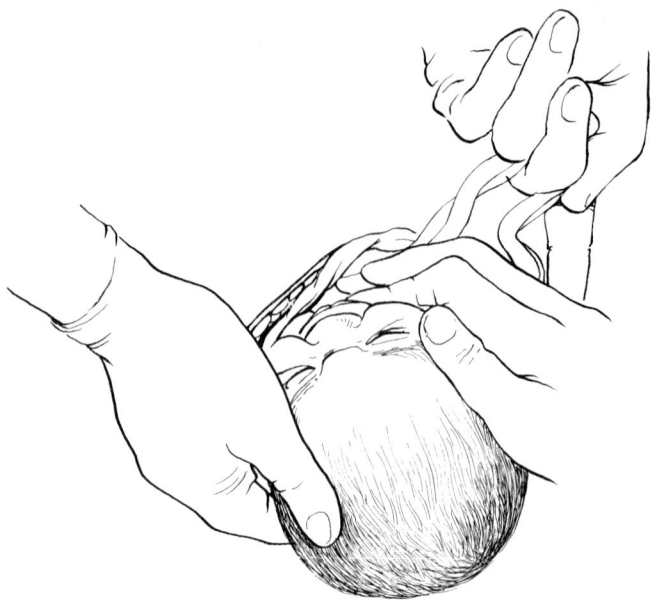

(f) The head is eased out of the incision.

made in the lower uterine segment. The centre of this incision in the mid-line is then gradually deepened until the presenting part comes into view. Care is taken to avoid cutting the child and if possible the membranes are kept intact. Once the fetus is visible the whole incision is opened up, either by inserting curved scissors and cutting outwards on each side, or doing this with a bistoury. An effective and quick method is simply to extend the

incision with the fingers. The incision should not be extended too far laterally otherwise the branches of the uterine vessels may be injured and give rise to troublesome bleeding.

The retractor is now removed and a hand is passed into the uterus through the incision below the baby's head and the presenting part is manipulated into the uterine opening. If the head is presenting, this manoeuvre can be facilitated by turning the baby's head so that

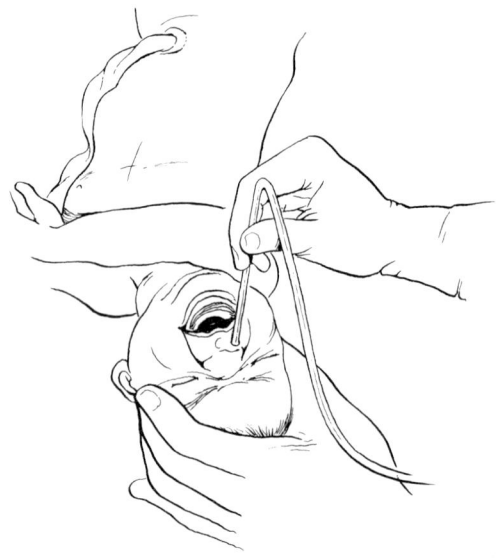

(g) Mucous is aspirated while the baby is held downwards.

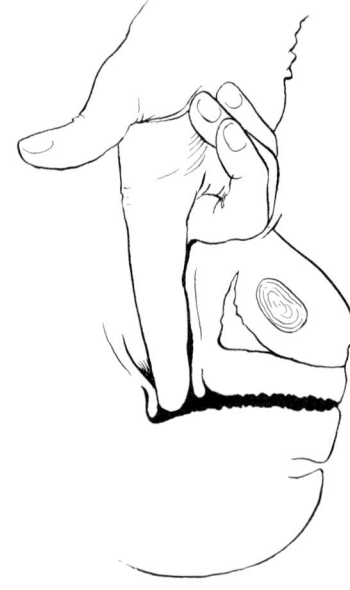

(h) The cervical canal is dilated from above.

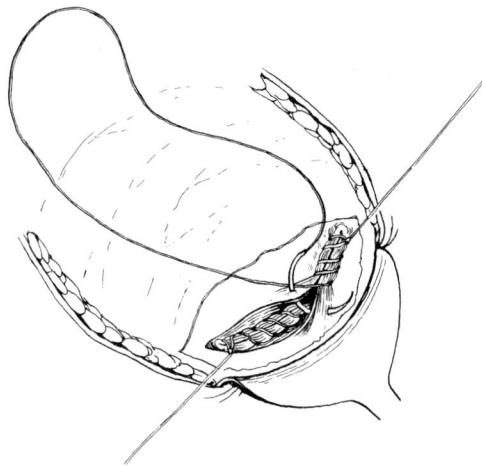

(i) The lower uterine segment is closed in two layers.

the face comes into the incision and is delivered
first. If the presenting part has descended into
the pelvis it is necessary to pass the hand deep
into the pelvis so that the head or breech can
be disengaged. This should be done gently
to avoid compression of the baby's head or
tears in the lower flap of the uterine muscle.

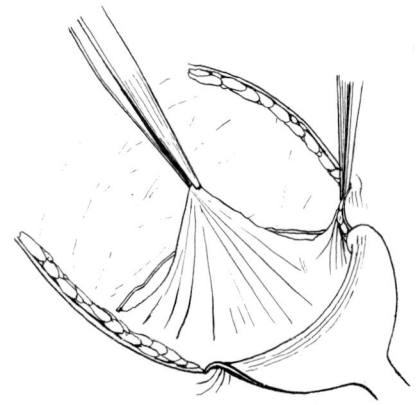

(j) The edges of the peritoneum are identified.

When the head or the breech has been
delivered through the incision pressure by the
assistant on the uterine fundus is exerted to
expel the rest of the baby. Some operators
prefer to apply obstetrical forceps to the head
to effect delivery. After delivery the baby's
airways are cleared by an assistant and this
usually stimulates the baby to take the first
gasp and the umbilical cord is then clamped
and divided. If the baby fails to breathe the

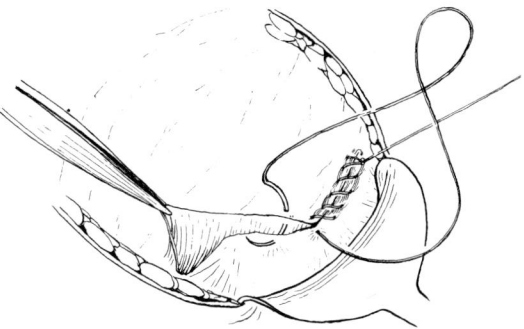

(k) The peritoneum over the lower segment is closed with
a continuous suture.

cord is 'milked' towards the baby before being
divided. The abdominal retractor is then re-
inserted and the edges of the uterine incision
are picked up with broad-bladed tissue forceps
preparatory to closing. Syntometrine is injected as the child is delivered so that bleeding will
be reduced. The placenta is delivered by cord
traction or manual extraction.

Before closing the incision in an elective
Caesarean section it may be necessary to ensure
that the cervical os is dilated. This can be done
with a finger. The uterine incision is repaired

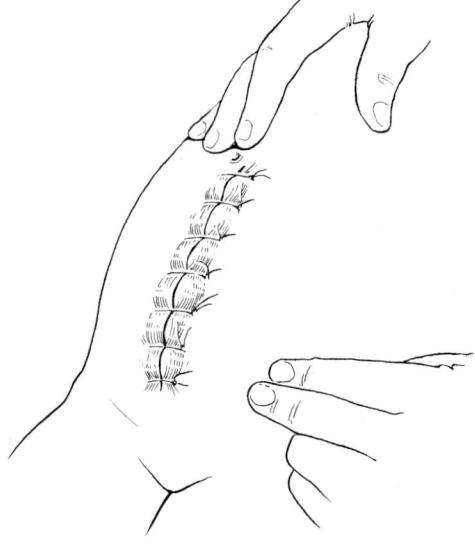

(l) The skin is closed with interrupted sutures.

in two layers using continuous catgut sutures.
Any oozing is controlled with mattress sutures.
The peritoneum is closed with a continuous
catgut suture. Blood and liquor are then
swabbed away, and once haemostasis has been

ensured the packs are removed and the abdominal wound is closed.

CLASSICAL CAESAREAN SECTION (Fig. 27.18a, b, c) This is now performed only in exceptional circumstances, as in an impacted shoulder presentation, fibroid tumours obscuring the lower uterine segment, carcinoma of the cervix or occasionally in cases of placenta praevia where an exceptionally large and widespread venous plexus is present. The operation is easier and quicker than the lower segment

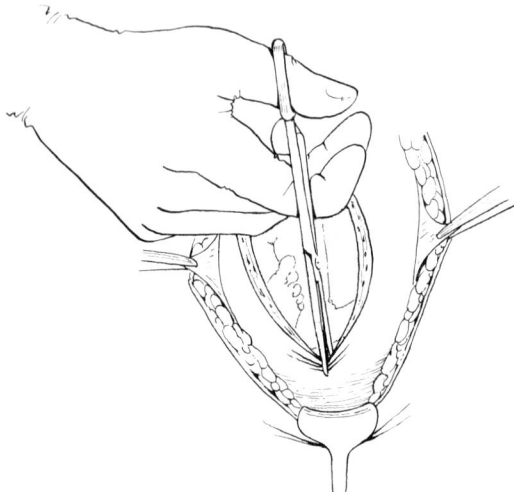

Fig. 27.18 (a) Longitudinal incision in upper segment for classical Caesarean section.

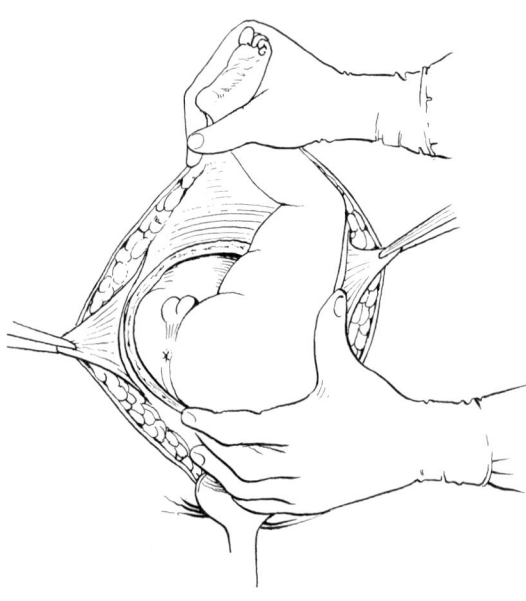

(b) Extracting the baby by the breech.

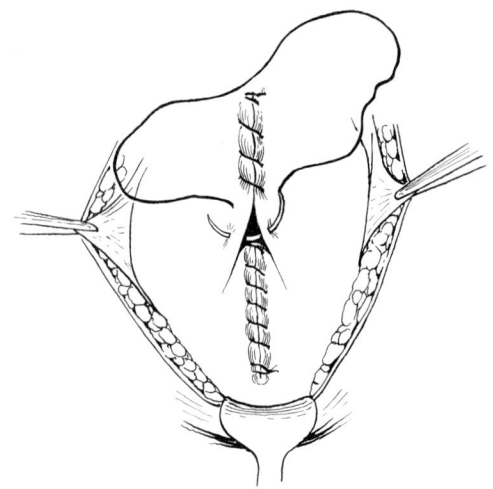

(c) Closing incision in upper segment with two layers of catgut.

operation, and may be performed where rapid emptying of the uterus is required in a very shocked patient. The incision in the abdomen is placed to the side and extends above and below the umbilicus, about $\frac{1}{3}$ above and $\frac{2}{3}$ below. The uterine incision is made in the mid-line of the anterior wall of the uterus after correcting the usual dextrarotation which is present (Fig. 27.18a). With a few rapid strokes of the scalpel in the mid-line the membranes are revealed. The hand is then introduced through the membranes and a foot of the fetus is grasped and drawn through the incision and the fetus is extracted as a breech through the uterine wound. Occasionally it is easier to bring the head out first. The placenta is then delivered and the uterine incision repaired in two layers.

DANGERS AND DISADVANTAGES OF CAESAREAN SECTION

Caesarean sections especially the classical operation can be performed quite easily, and may seem to be an easy way out of the difficulty, but there are certain disadvantages and dangers which must be emphasized.

Haemorrhage
Considerable blood loss can occur from the uterine incision and from the placental site. This can obscure the incision and make repair of it difficult.

Sepsis
Infection is less likely to occur in elective Caesarean sections than in cases where the patient has been in labour for some time with

the membranes ruptured. It is important to ensure adequate drainage of blood from the uterine cavity by dilating the cervix. If infection occurs it is less likely to cause widespread peritoneal infection if a lower segment Caesarean section has been performed rather than the classical operation.

Thrombosis and embolism are more likely to occur after Caesarean section than after vaginal delivery. Paralytic ileus is one of the most common complications of Caesarean section, but it usually responds to treatment and is unlikely to progress to complete paralytic obstruction. Paralytic ileus is more likely to occur in patients who have been in labour for a long time, as it is likely that there is already some gut distension in such cases, and this is aggravated by the abdominal operation.

Infection of the abdominal incision is more likely to occur if the Caesarean section has been done as an emergency operation. It is probably no more likely to occur following Caesarean section than after other abdominal operations, and careful suturing of the wound and avoidance of infection should ensure that complete breakdown of the wound does not occur. The remote consequences of Caesarean section may be rupture of the scar. A weak uterine scar is usually due to infection of the uterine wound. Usually a well healed Caesarean section scar cannot be recognized at the time of subsequent Caesarean section, but sometimes the lower uterine segment may be so thin that the decidua is almost protruding through the peritoneum. Infection at the time of the operation or during the puerperium may suggest that the wound may not be well healed. An uncomplicated course on the other hand does not necessarily indicate that good healing has occurred. Rupture of the scar usually takes place in labour, but may occur during pregnancy so that the patient must be carefully observed, particularly during the last four weeks of pregnancy. She must always be booked for delivery in subsequent labours in a specialist maternity hospital. She must be admitted to hospital about a week before term, and must be advised to report to the hospital if she has any symptoms suggesting that labour has begun, or if she has any symptoms suggestive of impending uterine rupture.

It is often said that many women who have had a Caesarean section never become pregnant again, but it is uncertain whether this is voluntary and how much is due to fear, or how far it is involuntary and due to complications of the operation. Walker (1970) however, has shown that primigravidae under twenty-five years having a Caesarean section are just as likely to have another baby in five years as women having vaginal deliveries.

Endometriosis of the abdominal scar is uncommon but it is easily recognized from the history of recurrent monthly pain and swelling. The area should be excised. Adhesions, ventral hernias and intestinal obstruction occasionally occur as late sequela of Caesarean section.

Caesarean hysterectomy

Hysterectomy is sometimes performed immediately after Caesarean section when the uterus contains multiple fibroids and the couple do not wish to have more children or when the uterus has ruptured. Very rarely a hysterectomy is required for placenta praevia because of bleeding from the placental site in the lower segment.

An extended or Wertheim's hysterectomy might very occasionally be performed for a carcinoma of the cervix diagnosed late in pregnancy. A hysterectomy performed after a Caesarean section is carried out in the same way as for removal of the non-gravid uterus. There is a greater likelihood of bleeding because of the distended vessels, but the tissues are more easily separated. Special care must be taken to avoid the ureters as they lie closer to the sides of the cervix than in the non-pregnant state.

Myomectomy after Caesarean section

It is usually considered best not to attempt removal of a large fibroid at the time of Caesarean section unless access to the baby is otherwise going to be too difficult. Haemorrhage can be profuse and it may be necessary to do a hysterectomy.

Sterilization with Caesarean section
It is usual to offer sterilization to a woman who is having a second or third Caesarean section. This is carried out in the same way as in the non-pregnant state, *see* Chapter 44.

INDUCTION OF LABOUR

It has become increasingly common to terminate pregnancy artificially as the methods have become easier and safer. Although it must be recognized that no method of inducing labour is entirely free from risk to the mother or child. The induction rate in the Aberdeen Maternity Hospital in 1970 was 37·5 per cent of cases. This figure includes many abnormal cases brought in from outside of the city. For the total city population the induction rate was 34 per cent.

Originally induction of labour was used to bring on labour prematurely in women with pelvic deformities, so that a smaller baby might be delivered vaginally. Nowadays the commonest indication is probably post-maturity and indeed many obstetricians now feel that labour should be induced at term if the woman is reasonably certain of her dates. This practice is more common in North America than in Britain, but it is becoming more prevalent on this side of the Atlantic. There is no great harm in this practice provided that the maturity is known with certainty and careful supervision of the use of oxytocics can be ensured, and also that the obstetrician is prepared to carry out a Caesarean section if the induction fails. These 'inductions for convenience' are most often indicated where the woman has to travel a considerable distance to the place of delivery, and when she would be occupying a hospital bed for several days awaiting the onset of labour, or when a policy of 'day-time deliveries' is in vogue.

INDICATIONS FOR INDUCTION OF LABOUR

1. *Post-maturity*
Fetal post-maturity is associated with a risk of perinatal death. In primigravidae and women of high parity there is an increasing risk from the 40th week onwards, and in second, third and fourth pregnancies, the perinatal mortality rises after the 42nd week (Perinatal Problems, 1969). A commonly accepted practice is to induce labour in the older primigravida (age 25 years or more) five days after the expected date of delivery to try to ensure delivery by the end of the 41st week, and in young primigravidae and parous women to induce at the end of 42 weeks.

2. *Antepartum haemorrhage*
In severe abruption of the placenta immediate induction of labour is indicated. In antepartum haemorrhage of unknown origin induction is often performed at 38 weeks, provided that the haemorrhage has not been too severe. If the haemorrhage is severe then immediate induction is indicated. Minor degrees of placenta praevia are treated by induction, usually at about 38 weeks.

3. *Hypertension of pregnancy*
The hypertension disorders of pregnancy are often treated by induction of premature labour. This is particularly true if there is proteinuria present.

4. *Rhesus iso-immunization*
Careful assessment of the severity of the condition by assessing the amounts of antibody present and by estimation of the bilirubin content of the liquor amnii obtained by amniocentesis will allow the selection of the optimum time for induction.

5. *Maternal diseases*
Both clinical and chemical gestational diabetes are indications for induction of labour before term. In well controlled clinical diabetes and in cases of chemical gestational diabetes induction is usually performed at 38 weeks, but in more severe cases, or ones which are difficult to control induction may have to be performed earlier. Chronic renal conditions such as nephritis or pyelonephritis may require induction. Jaundice occurring in pregnancy is usually considered to be an indication for induction, if the pregnancy has reached near to term but it may be considered undesirable to induce labour early on in pregnancy depending on the severity and cause of the jaundice.

6. *Cardiac disease*
Acute febrile conditions particularly occurring towards the end of pregnancy may sometimes necessitate induction of labour.

7. *Fetal death or malformation and hydramnios*
Labour very often starts spontaneously when the fetus dies, but in some cases the dead fetus can be retained *in utero* for many weeks. This is undesirable and induction is preferred usually with Syntocinon or prostaglandins rather than rupture of the membranes because of the risk of infection. When a major degree of malformation which is likely to be lethal is detected induction of labour is usually indicated. Hydramnios may cause such acute symptoms as to require induction of labour whether there is coexistent fetal abnormality or not. In cases of acute hydramnios occurring early in pregnancy repeated amniocentesis

may be successful in allowing the pregnancy to continue, but often such cases go into premature labour.

8. *Malpresentations and cephalo-pelvic disproportion*

Generally speaking malpresentations are not considered to be an indication for induction of premature labour, except by some obstetricians in breech presentations. When external version has failed they advocate induction of premature labour at the end of the 38th week. When an unstable lie has been corrected it is sometimes advisable to start labour and a 'stabilizing induction' is performed. This means that a Syntocinon infusion is started first to induce contractions before rupturing the membranes. Although induction of labour was first practised in cases of contracted pelves it is rarely performed for this reason nowadays. The difficulty is in deciding the optimum time for the induction and also the uncertainty of producing efficient contractions. If induction is performed too early the baby is likely to suffer, and if it is performed too late then cephalo-pelvic disproportion may still prevent delivery. The only place for induction for suspected cephalo-pelvic disproportion may be in multiparae with a slight degree of contracted pelvis, where the performance in previous labours is known. This also applies where excessive size of the fetus is suspected. Second and subsequent babies are on average about 0·5kg heavier than first babies. If a primigravida has produced a baby of excessive size induction of premature labour is justified in a subsequent pregnancy.

METHODS OF INDUCTION OF LABOUR

Many methods have been used in the past to induce labour and were either described as medical, which involved the use of castor oil and or enemas or the use of oxytocics and surgical inductions, which meant rupturing of the membranes, separation of the membranes by sweeping with the fore-finger, introduction of solid rubber bougies, stomach tubes or catheters into the lower pole of the uterus, or the introduction of balloons through the cervix. The use of oxytocics and rupture of the membranes are the only methods nowadays practised.

Rupture of the membranes

This has been practised from ancient times and is now the commonest method used. Some indication of the likelihood of success of this method is gained from assessing the state of the cervix. If the cervix is shortened and the canal is partially dilated and the cervix is soft then labour will usually begin sooner than when the cervix is long, firm and the canal is narrow. However 'unripeness' of the cervix should not be considered a contra-indication to rupture of the membranes. It does mean, however, that the procedure is made more difficult and a decision may be made to rupture the hindwaters with a Drew-Smythe catheter (Fig. 27.19) which can be slipped through the cervical canal and a stilette is used to rupture

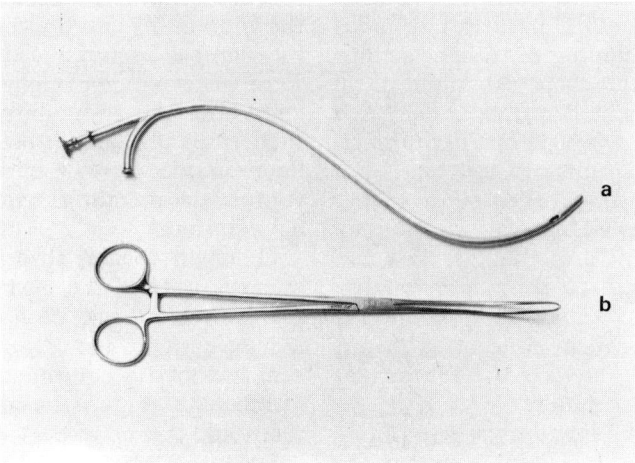

Fig. 27.19   (a) Drew-Smythe catheter.
            (b) Amniotomy forceps.

the membranes. This method of hind-water rupture is also sometimes recommended when the head is high, and it is claimed that there is less risk of prolapse of the cord, and less risk of infection of the fluid. There is, however, the risk of placental separation and it can also be argued that infection is more likely to be carried up inside the uterus by this method.

In the operation of fore-water rupture the fore-finger is introduced through the cervical canal and if possible the membranes are swept off the lower pole of the uterus, so that a bag of water forms. Amniotomy or Kocher's forceps are then introduced and the membranes are torn. If the cervical canal is closed the forceps can be introduced through the canal by direct vision. It is not usually necessary to use a general anaesthetic, but if the patient is nervous Pethidine 100mg and Chlorpromazine 25mg is given.

Oxytocin induction

Originally Oxytocin was administered intramuscularly in quite large doses with sometimes disastrous results, because the uterus responded so vigorously as to cause death of the fetus or rupture of the uterus. In recent years Oxytocin (Syntocinon) is given as a continuous infusion, so that the dosage can be carefully controlled. The infusion is given by the so-called titration method (Turnbull and Anderson, 1968), which is as follows:

The infusion is started with two 540ml bottles of 5 per cent dextrose both connected by separate sets via a disposable two-way tap to the cannula. A $\frac{1}{2}$ unit of Oxytocin is added to one of the bottles and the drip is commenced at 15 drops per minute. The drip rate is increased every 10 minutes until contractions begin, and thereafter every 20 minutes till they are adequate. The drip rate is increased from 15 to 30 and then 60 drops per minute. Next a bottle with 2 units of Oxytocin is put up at first 15, then 30 and then 60 drops per minute. This is followed by a bottle containing 8 units of Oxytocin, and the rate is again gradually increased to 60 drops per minute. If in some cases after careful assessment it is decided that the Oxytocin concentration can be increased, 32 units are given at 15, then 30 and then 60 drops per minute.

It is essential that a low dose is given initially if the patient is in labour to avoid the possibility of uterine spasm. It is possible to commence at 2 units in the 540ml of 5 per cent dextrose if the patient is not in labour. When a stronger solution is commenced it is important to run it through the whole giving set to the connection at the needle or the cannula. While this is being done the other bottle containing 5 per cent dextrose is switched on. It is worth noting that 2 units at 60 drops per minute delivers the same amount of Oxytocin as 8 units at 15 drops per minute. An automated system (The Cardiff Pump) is available.

After the baby is delivered the drip should be speeded up at the concentration then in use. Once the placenta is delivered and the uterus is firm the drip rate should be reduced gradually over a period of 30 minutes. If the uterus remains retracted the 5 per cent plain dextrose drip is switched over and run for 30 minutes. If everything remains satisfactory the drip can then be disconnected.

This titration method of doubling the Oxytocin dose every 10 or 15 minutes is usually very successful but it is sometimes necessary to use very large amounts of Oxytocin to produce strong regular contractions, and it is very important that the dose of Oxytocin is not increased once adequate regular contractions are established. Even then it sometimes happens that the uterus becomes over sensitive to the Oxytocin and it is necessary to reduce the dose which had previously been satisfactory. If there is any sign of fetal distress or if the uterus is not relaxing completely between contractions it is essential to switch the tap to the bottle containing no Oxytocin.

A Syntocinon infusion is usually started some hours after rupture of the membranes if labour has not commenced. The time between the amniotomy and the commencement of the infusion has been reduced to a few hours, and some believe in starting the infusion immediately after the amniotomy. Where the lie of the fetus is unstable or the head is high it may be desirable to start the infusion first and rupture the membranes once the contractions have started.

Oxytocin can be absorbed from the nasal mucosa or from the buccal membranes, and these routes have been used to stimulate uterine activity. However, the rate of absorption cannot be controlled precisely and the intravenous route is usually considered to be safer, and is preferred.

In cases where the fetus is dead intra-amniotic saline is injected or quinine may be used in some cases.

INDUCTION OF ABORTION

It is only in fairly recent years that much attention has been given to developing new effective methods of termination of pregnancy, because in this country gynaecologists performed small numbers of abortions and these were usually done by curettage or by hysterotomy. Many substances have been advocated as abortifacients which may be taken by mouth. The most common being apiol, pennyroyal, aloes, quinine and ergot. These substances are not likely to be effective except in dosages which would endanger the life of the women. Other methods which have been developed by the criminal abortionists involve the introduction of foreign bodies into the uterus. The crochet hook and other similar implements were commonly and possibly still are used. Rubber catheters, sounds, needles, slippery elm and even slivers of wood have been used in the past. Soap or antiseptic solutions introduced into the uterus by a syringe or douche are commonly used methods. The complications which may occur are haemorrhage, infection, renal failure, soap intoxication, air embolism and trauma of the vagina, cervix, uterus or bladder.

Substances introduced into the uterus, in particular Utus paste (medicated soft soaps), are fairly effective but there is a risk of infection, embolism or haemorrhage occurring. Laminaria tents (seatangle tents) are also used. These are introduced into the cervix and as they absorb water they become swollen and cause the cervix to dilate. Sepsis is again the problem and the abortion is often incomplete.

It is now recognized that there is no effective means of procuring abortion by any oral drug, and that any drug which is going to be effective must be given parenterally. Intramuscular or intravenous ergometrine or pitocin or syntocinon have been tried but are not effective in causing an abortion, although continuous syntocinon infusion intravenously can aid in the emptying of the uterus if another method, e.g. the intra-amniotic injection of a substance, has been employed.

It has been known for a long time that substances introduced into the amniotic cavity will cause the uterus to contract and expel the contents. This was found to be one of the disadvantages of using radio-opaque substances injected into the amniotic sac for the localization of the placenta. Various substances (dextrose, saline, inulin and formalin) have been used. These are quite effective in causing abortion, but there is a considerable risk of intra-uterine sepsis particularly if dextrose is used and fatalities have been reported with the use of saline due to intravascular injection causing cerebral infarction. These methods must be employed with considerable care, and obviously can only be employed if the uterus is enlarged to a sufficient size to allow the amniotic sac to be entered with assurance. Although the technique is usually employed after the uterus is enlarged to sixteen weeks' size or more through the trans-abdominal route the method has also been employed in earlier pregnancies using the trans-cervical route.

In pregnancies before about twelve weeks the usual method employed was to dilate up the cervix and remove the contents of the uterus with forceps and curette, but more recently the method has been introduced of evacuating with a suction aspirator. It is possible to evacuate a uterus by suction up to fourteen weeks' gestation, but generally at this stage or later a vaginal or abdominal hysterotomy is performed if an operative procedure is decided on. The vaginal operation is technically more difficult but leaves no abdominal scar. For the abdominal operation a vertical incision can be made or a low transverse incision which will be less visible. This might be considered to be of psychological importance because a woman might react badly to being constantly reminded by an abdominal scar of a termination of pregnancy.

This has been replaced recently by a new method which is very successful. This is the use of prostaglandin. There are several different prostaglandins, but the ones most commonly used are E and F. The results so far reported are encouraging and there are many reports now from a number of centres allowing a good assessment of their value.

The methods most commonly in use will now be considered in detail and on assessment made of their advantages and disadvantages and also the specific indications and contraindications for each method.

1. Dilatation and curettage

A general anaesthetic is usually given and the cervix is dilated with a graduated dilator sufficiently to allow an ovum forceps of sponge holding forceps to be passed through the cervical canal into the uterus. The conception is then grasped and removed piecemeal with the forceps. The small pieces remaining are then scraped out with a curette. It is usually recommended that a blunt curette is used. It is considered essential that an oxytocic preparation, either syntocinon or ergometrine or a combination of the two is given before the uterus is evacuated, otherwise haemorrhage can be considerable. There is a danger too that the uterus might be perforated either with the forceps or with the curette. Care must be taken to try to avoid tearing of the internal cervical os as this might lead to incompetence of the cervix and spontaneous abortion of a subsequent pregnancy. Dilatation of the cervix can often be facilitated by an injection of a local anaesthetic into the paracervical tissue. Sepsis can usually be avoided by attention to technique. This method is indicated in early pregnancy, but is contraindicated after the twelfth week of pregnancy. It was the method of choice in early pregnancy until the advent of the next method.

2. Vacuum aspiration

This method was used in China and then in Russia and Czechoslovakia before it was introduced to Britain. It has become increasingly popular here over the past five or six years. A general anaesthetic is required if the pregnancy is ten weeks or more but a paracervical block is sufficient before then. The procedure may be done in multigravidae without anaesthesia or dilatation up to six weeks as an out-patient using a plastic Karman curette. The cervix is dilated in the same way as for curettage after an oxytocic substance has been given. The metal or plastic aspirator is then introduced through the cervix. The size of the aspirator depends on the duration of pregnancy. A negative pressure of 0·4–0·6kg/ square cm is then applied and the uterine contents aspirated. Blood loss is usually slight if the uterus is firmly contracted. There is a danger of causing damage to the cervix in dilating it. This is particularly true the further on the pregnancy is and the more the cervix has to be dilated, but is minimized by using a paracervical block as an adjuvant. This method can be used up to fourteen weeks pregnancy size, but the dangers and complications increase the further on the pregnancy is.

3. Intra-amniotic injections

Hypertonic saline is at present the most commonly used substance. A not too wide needle is introduced into the abdomen about two or three finger-breadths above the symphysis pubis, after infiltrating the abdominal wall with a local anaesthetic. The technique is usually most effective when the fetus is 14–20 weeks' gestation. It is important that in this technique a general anaesthetic is not used so that the patient's reaction to the intra-amniotic injection can be observed. The amniotic fluid is then aspirated. Usually about 200ml are removed, and 200ml of 20 per cent saline are injected either through the needle or through a fine plastic catheter. Abortion usually occurs within 24 hours but may be delayed in some cases and have to be assisted by an oxytocin infusion. The method is effective and safe if great care is employed. The dangers are the introduction of infection, intravascular injections or the injection of too large a volume of saline causing cerebral infarction. In some cases the placenta is retained and has to be removed after dilatation of the cervix under general anaesthesia. The method is contraindicated in cases with severe medical conditions such as renal disease, cardiac disease or hypertension.

4. Utus paste

The utus paste is injected slowly at a rate of 2ml per minute in an amount of 1–2ml per week of gestation through a canula which is introduced into the uterus through the cervical canal. Pre-medication is given but it is usually not necessary to give a general anaesthetic. This method has the advantage that the procedure is easy and it is possible to cause abortion of advanced pregnancies. It is, however, not an infallible method and further stimulation with a Syntocinon drip or a further injection of utus paste is sometimes necessary, and complete evacuation of the uterus can only be achieved by curettage or suction. Other disadvantages of the methods are the risks of infection and trauma. The method is not popular in Britain.

5. Hysterotomy

This is done either by the abdominal or vaginal route. In the abdominal operation a vertical or low transverse incision is made. In the vaginal operation an incision is made high in the cervix and the isthmus of the uterus is opened after the bladder has been displaced upwards out of the way. The advantages of hysterotomy are that sepsis and haemorrhage are usually avoided and sterilization can be carried out while the abdomen is opened. The disadvantages, however, are a longer stay in hospital and scarring of the uterus. The operation was carried out in women where sterilization was also going to be performed and in other girls or women with pregnancies enlarged beyond fourteen weeks, but now the following method is preferred.

6. *Prostaglandins*
The continuous infusion of prostaglandins intravenously is a fairly effective method of emptying the pregnant uterus (Karim, 1968) but vomiting and diarrhoea are troublesome side effects. A more effective method is the infusion of prostaglandin between the amniotic membrane and the uterine wall. Injections into the amniotic sac do not seem to be so effective unless combined with urea. Results of the use of vaginal prostaglandins are encouraging. This method has proved successful and has rapidly taken the place of all others.

REFERENCES

Butler, N. R. & Alberman, E. D. (1969) *Perinatal Problems* (National Birthday Trust Fund) Edinburgh: Livingstone.
Karim, S. M. M. (1968) *Brit. Med. J.* **iv**, 618.
MacGillivray, I. (1968) Trends in the Incidence of Caesarean Sections in a Community. *J. Obstet. Gynaec. Brit.*
Turnbull, A. C. & Anderson, A. B. M. (1968) Results with Amniotomy and Oxytocin Titration. *J. Obstet. Gynaec. Brit. Cwlth.* **75**, 32.
Walker, J. (1970) Obstetric Sequelae of Difficult Labour in Primigravidae. *Proc. 6th Wld Cong. Gynaec. Obstet.*, No **147**. New York.

FURTHER READING

Munro Kerr's—*Operative Obstetrics*, 8th edn., Ed. Chasser Moir, J. & Myerscough, P. R. Bailey, Tindall & Castle, Great Britain: 1971.
Seedat, E. K., Crichton, D. (1962) Symphisiotomy, technique, indications, limitation. *Lancet* **i**, 554.

28. Sonar and X-rays in Obstetrics and Gynaecology

In this chapter X-rays and sonar are considered together. They are, however, completely different diagnostic dimensions and should not be regarded as competitive techniques but rather as complementary. Since the one can achieve results which are beyond the reach of the other. Both are capable of penetrating tissue and of producing pictorial representations of structures within the body but there is no other point of similarity between them.

The term 'sonar' is an abbreviation of 'sound navigation and ranging' and is related to the earlier term radar, developed during the last World War as RDF (radio direction and range finding). The term thus acknowledges its wartime origins and embraces all varieties of ultrasonic echo sounding. 'Sonar' has the additional merit of brevity, as well as euphony. Its uses are purely diagnostic and are to be distinguished from power ultrasound in which very high energies are employed, often to destructive levels.

Entirely different types of energy are used in the two diagnostic systems. The energy of X-rays is derived from the electromagnetic spectrum, whereas in the case of sonar the energy consists of sound waves of very high frequency above the range of animal hearing, hence the term 'ultrasonic'. The energy of the former is ionizing whereas of the latter it is purely mechanical. As might be expected therefore the biological effects, as well as the physical, are different.

An X-ray is a shadow picture in which the whole part of the body to be examined is simultaneously flooded with penetrating X-ray energy which is recorded on a photographic plate or fluorescent screen on the far side of the body. The resulting shadows depend on differing degrees of radio-opacity, a property which is much influenced by the heavy metal content, for example, calcium. However brief the exposure all tissues within the area come to be irradiated. This total energy bath is not applicable in the case of ultrasound although it was first attempted, unsuccessfully, by Dussik in Austria in 1941.[18] There are many technical reasons for this, not the least being that so far it has been difficult to produce a receptor plate of sufficient size on the far side of the patient. Furthermore the part of the body under examination would have to be totally immersed in a tank of degassed fluid since air/tissue interfaces will not transmit ultrasound. No piezo-electric plates have yet been built of such a size and capable of withstanding the necessary pressures. Nevertheless some success has been obtained with this shadow technique by Jacobs in the United States (1965)[29] who has been able to demonstrate, for example, the passage of blood through the heart chambers of small animals.

For these reasons, amongst others, sonar relies upon *echo* techniques in which both transmitter and receiver are on the same side of the patient. This is very convenient because it is possible to examine the patient without disturbing her, but the volume that can be examined at any one moment of time is only that which is included within the diameter of the exploring ultrasonic beam. This involves a search technique and a relatively lengthy recording process.[17]

Soft tissue differences can produce echo signals which X-rays could only indicate as a very undifferentiated shadow at best.

The subject of X-radiology has had more than half a century start over sonar. Furthermore its acceptance after Roentgen's earliest and rather obscurely published paper in 1895 was seized upon avidly by the whole civilized world and even as early as 1901 a society has been formed in England to exploit this new and marvellous method of 'seeing within the body.' In spite of greater technical sophistication today, clinical application and acceptance of sonar has been somewhat slower. We ourselves in Glasgow, for example, have been at work on the project for over seventeen years and we were by no means the first in the field. Paradoxically however the breakthrough in sonar has come in obstetrics and gynaecology more readily than in other fields of medicine, whereas the full exploitation of what radiology had to offer in obstetrics came more slowly in the course of the last thirty years.

RADIOLOGY IN OBSTETRICS

Female pelvis

In the days before the mechanist concept of labour had been superseded by the more modern functional approach, radiopelvimetry became a much used and even more abused part of the obstetrician's art. The irradiation doses inflicted are considerable. It was not until the dangers both to mother and fetus came to be recognized that routine X-ray of the pelvis in pregnant women gave place to a more rational approach restricting the use of X-ray to difficult labour requiring urgent radiological diagnosis, at all. Nevertheless, thanks to the excess radiology of a couple of decades ago we now know a very great deal about the varieties of pelvic shape which are dealt with elsewhere in this book. Pelvimetry is now very seldom carried out during pregnancy; except where it is necessary to investigate some obvious deformity, either congenital or traumatic, which might influence the safety of labour. It is common practice, however, still to carry out a full radiopelvimetry in the puerperium where the course of labour indicated a maternal source of mechanical difficulty. During labour itself radiology may be required at any hour of the day or night and particularly when the fetal head fails to progress in its descent through the pelvis. Even a single, lateral erect film very often answers the problem although commonly a single anteroposterior view is also taken. This may not only reveal possibly unsuspected disproportion but may show deflection attitudes of the baby, even an undiagnosed brow presentation. The degree of moulding is readily shown, also the presence of an undiagnosed fetal abnormality which may influence treatment and the method of delivery. The degree of rotation of the head including occipito-posterior position is readily demonstrated. All manner of sums and indices have been devised, often eponymous, to assist prognosis in labour, but are to a greater or less degree fallible. The features of all vagaries of pelvic shape and size are discussed in Chapter 3.

Twin pregnancy
The merit of diagnosing twins clinically, or by any other means including sonar, is completely negated if a triplet is missed. When dealing with multiple pregnancy such mistakes can have disastrous consequences.

Fetal abnormality
The diagnosis of fetal abnormality very frequently rests upon radiology which is far more precise than sonar. It is sometimes worth-

while to take a standard X-ray to exclude skeletal fetal abnormality before undertaking elective Caesarean section since fetal interests can be discounted when there is clearly an anomaly incompatible with reasonable chances of survival (Fig. 28.1). To subject a woman to

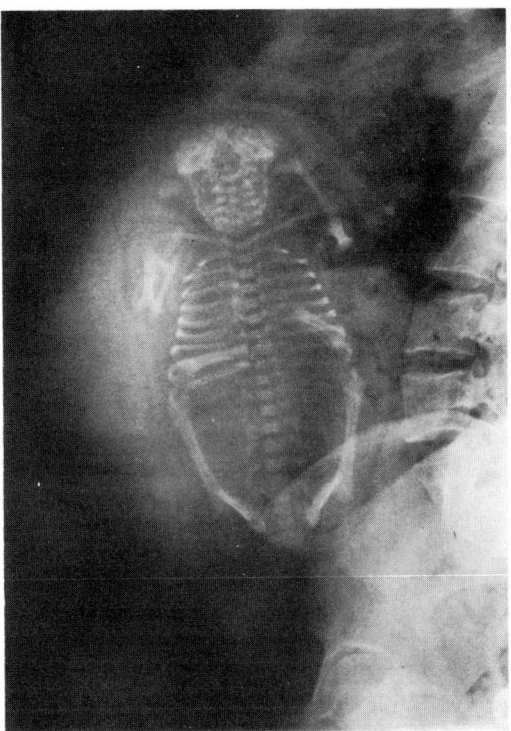

Fig. 28.1   Anencephaly and spina bifida.

Caesarean section simply to present her with an anencephalic monster is defensible only in cases of major degrees of placenta praevia and degrees of pelvic abnormality severe enough to prevent safe vaginal delivery.

Because of the known association of hydramnios with anencephaly and twins it is always as well to examine such a patient first by sonar which may answer the question straight away or by X-rays or by both. As a screening procedure sonar is adequate for anencephaly and hydrocephalus but not for minor degrees of the latter. In addition to these common abnormalities all types of maldevelopment, deformity, duplication or absence of the fetal skeleton can be revealed by radiology, ranging from spina bifida, anomalies of the fetal limbs and achondroplasia to a variety of double monsters. Many important diagnoses can be made or at least inferred radiologically by the attitude of the baby which may be abnormal due, for example, to a tumour of the fetal thyroid, or gross hepatomegaly. Likewise in severe degrees of Rh haemolytic disease the child may adopt a Buddha attitude (Fig. 28.2)

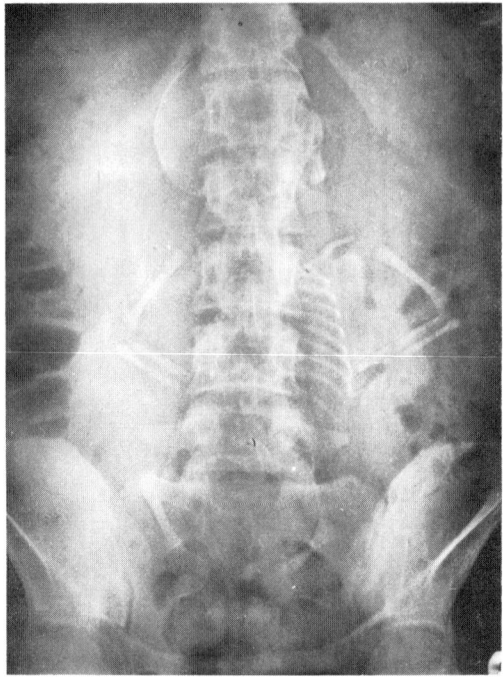

Fig. 28.2   Hydrops fetalis. 'Buddha' position.

because it is oedematous and the 'halo sign' may appear surrounding its outline because of oedema of the subcutaneous tissues. It commonly indicates fetal death.

Intra-uterine fetal death

Spalding's sign, which consists of over-riding of the sutures in the cranial vault because of cerebral shrinkage is considered pathognomonic of fetal death provided the patient is not in labour with moulding of the fetal skull. The sign may take as long as ten days or more to develop after fetal death. Another important X-ray sign of fetal death is the appearance of gas within the heart chambers and great vessels. This may appear within twelve to twenty-four hours and always within about two days. After that it may disappear. It is the earliest radiological sign of fetal death. Finally, due to a loss of tone following death, X-rays may reveal strange attitudes of spinal contortion (Fig. 28.3).

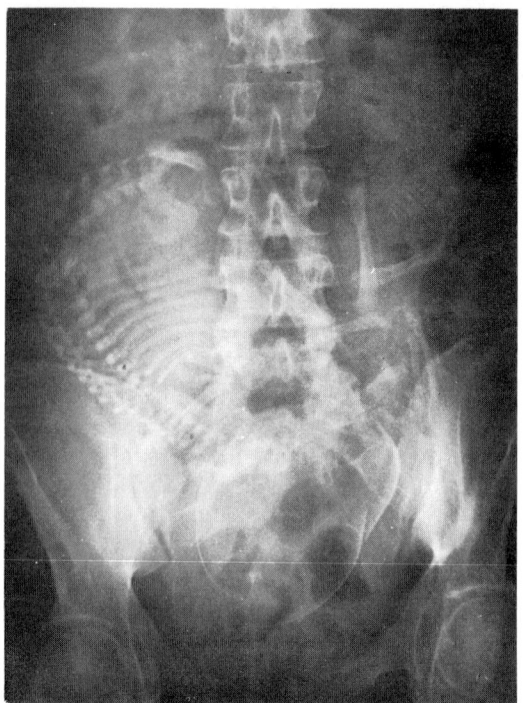

Fig. 28.3   Intra-uterine fetal death (IUD). Note gross Spalding sign of overlapping cranial vault bones, the hyperflexion of spine and gas shadows within the great vessels.

Figs. 28.1–28.3 by Courtesy of Dr E. Sweet, Glasgow.

Malpresentation and abnormal fetal attitudes

These are of less importance in pregnancy except in the more elderly and in high degrees of multiparity of uncertain maturity. It is usually sufficient to identify the baby's head by sonar if this cannot be done clinically but occasionally malpresentations which cannot be corrected by version may be associated with uterine deformity such as a subseptate uterus. Unfortunately accurate cephalometry by X-rays is not feasible for geometrical reasons because it is not possible to make accurate allowance for the distance of the fetal head from the photographic film.

Maturity

Estimate of maturity by X-rays is also less satisfactory than by sonar. Only a general impression of size can be obtained and the appearance of ossification centres is notoriously variable, often by as much as plus or minus two weeks which greatly reduces the usefulness of the examination. The centres most characteristically sought after the thirty-sixth week are those of the lower end of femur and upper end of tibia and at term the cuboid in the tarsus. Fetal radiography is useless before the sixteenth week at the earliest because there is not sufficient calcification of the fetal skeleton. In the obese or in cases of hydramnios an accurate X-ray diagnosis of pregnancy is even more difficult until later in pregnancy.

Associated pelvic tumours

Except for ovarian dermoid cysts containing teeth, X-rays are of very little help since, at best, all they can demonstrate is a vague and indefinite type of opacity. Nevertheless the sheer size of this and the presence of a very small fetus may arouse a suspicion of an associated cyst which is far better resolved by sonar.

X-rays in the management of Rh haemolytic disease

Here very sophisticated radiology is necessary in order to undertake intraperitoneal blood transfusion of the affected baby during pregnancy (see Chapter 15).

Placental localization

The most commonly employed method of placental localization by X-rays used after the thirty-fourth week is the soft tissue method, especially when combined with alterations in the posture of the patient to demonstrate or exclude some space occupying tissue preventing engagement of the presenting part in the pelvis. With good quality films and a very experienced eye it is possible to obtain a fair impression of the whereabouts of the placenta but the errors are high, in our experience of the order of 15 per cent, which is unacceptable in the exclusion of placenta praevia.

The use of amniography to show an alteration in the intra-amniotic outline due to the presence of the placenta has now been practically abandoned and outlining the bladder and rectum with contrast media has never enjoyed much popularity or success.

The identification of the maternal placental blood pool by the use of radioactive isotopes, nowadays usually 99 Technetium, is extensively used in certain centres but a description of it would not be appropriate in this chapter. The same may be said of infra-red thermography which is of doubtful value.[35]

The one definite X-ray method for identifying the placenta is by pelvic arteriography, usually by means of a catheter inserted via the femoral artery into the aorta above the level of its bifurcation and through which is rapidly injected a large bolus of radio-opaque dye.[38] This technique demands skill and radiological facilities of a very high order and is not wholly without risk and, because of the irradiation exposure, cannot be regularly repeated. Its use therefore is restricted to a very few enthusiastic centres.

It is in early pregnancy that pelvic arteriography comes into its own, particularly in the complications, e.g. ectopic pregnancy or hydatidiform mole.[20] Although the diagnosis can be more readily made by sonar, pelvic arteriography may produce a characteristic X-ray appearance with the multiple blood spaces within the tumour mass. The other contribution X-rays have to make to the diagnosis of hydatidiform mole, is the failure to demonstrate a fetal skeleton which is relevant only after the sixteenth week.

RADIOLOGY IN GYNAECOLOGY

If one excludes radiological examination for associated conditions such as pyelography, lymphography, venography, skeletal surveys for metastases and pulmonary conditions pre- and post-operatively which are discussed in relevant chapters and considers only purely gynaecological uses, X-rays have only one common and essential role, namely in hysterosalpingography.

Only two kinds of pelvic tumour show up with certainty on a plain film of the abdomen, calcified fibroids and dermoid cysts containing elements of teeth. It is surprising how little even quite large tumours will show on an X-ray apart from a general impression of opacity.

Hysterosalpingography comes into a category of its own because not only will it show the shape and capacity of the endometrial cavity but the competence of the internal os and, more important still, the site of occlusion or of deformity caused by certain diseases of the Fallopian tubes. It becomes therefore an almost indispensable part of the investigation of female infertility. Nevertheless the examination should be carried out only within the first half of the menstrual cycle for fear of disturbing a newly conceived and implanted pregnancy. Congenital abnormalities of the uterus are most readily shown up by this technique and deformity of the endometrial cavity by fibroids is often demonstrable, even sometimes intra-uterine adhesions which may follow repeated curettage. As a means of defining endometrial carcinoma the technique is not recommended, curettage and histology being more certain. Sometimes tuberculous endosalpingitis can be suggested by irregularities of the tubal lumen but this is nowadays an uncommon finding due to the progressive disappearance of this disease.

Defects in the healing of the uterine scar after Caesarean section can also be sometimes demonstrated by an appropriate view of the uterine cavity distended with radio-opaque dye.[36]

Gynecography

It is sometimes possible to outline the surface of a mass within the pelvis by pumping enough dye through the Fallopian tubes to coat its surface. Likewise the use of a pneumo-peritoneum to help outline a pelvic mass has been used but largely given up. These techniques have lost their importance with the advent of sonar and laparoscopy in which a direct view can be obtained very simply with the patient in a position already prepared and draped for laparotomy should the diagnosis be confirmed.

Pelvic arteriography

Again using the Seldinger catheterization technique,[38] help may be provided by X-rays not only in cases of hydatidiform mole but in studying trophoblastic tumours (see Chapter 9). X-ray arteriography may give an idea of the extension of the tumour which may not only influence treatment but also prognosis.

Venography and Lymphography are discussed more fully in relation to carcinoma of the pelvis in Chapter 38.

Limitations of X-rays

As will be shown many of the limitations of X-rays have been met by the applicability of sonar, although there still remain enormous gaps to be filled in visual diagnostic techniques. Whereas X-rays are at their most useful when dealing with tissues with a high mineral content, such as bone, their usefulness with soft tissues, particularly in gynaecological masses and early pregnancy is certainly limited.

The use of radio-opaque dyes is necessary to outline the interior surfaces of viscera such as kidneys and intestine, stomach and gall bladder but clearly these techniques are inappropriate in the case of the gravid uterus and pelvic tumours. The most serious limitations, however, are tied up with the question of safety. Many of the pioneers of radiology of only a few decades ago suffered terribly from the effects of over-exposure, often ultimately dying of metastases from epitheliomata of hands and fingers and what made the subject so treacherous was that the effects of X-irradiation were often long-delayed in making their appearance.

It is now reckoned that every X-ray exposure, however long ago, is cumulative with the whole exposure to ionizing radiation throughout the patient's life history and in the case of the sex cells, gene mutations may be handed on to later generations. Increasing care has been taken to limit the exposure of personnel in X-ray Departments but it was not until 1956 that Alice Stewart and her colleagues[40] in Oxford first drew attention to the damaging effects of maternal X-rays upon the human fetus in utero, initially demonstrated by a significant increase in childhood leukaemia.

It is difficult even with careful coning to avoid some exposure of the fetal gonads when X-raying the pregnant uterus and damage, latent or overt, may be done to the bone marrow and rapidly growing tissues if X-rays are indiscriminately employed in pregnancy. Yet the clinical value of X-rays may outmatch these dangers and one has to decide, in ordering an X-ray between a choice of evils, namely of the hazards thereof, actual and hypothetical, and the dangers of not making a correct diagnosis. It is this sober reflection which has made the advent of sonar in obstetrics so timely, although here too one must be on the look out for possible signs of damage. It would be safe, however, to assume that the damage, if any, would be of a totally different sort, since the energy is mechanical and non-ionizing.

The whole science of ultrasonic echo sounding dates back to the 1914/18 war when the French and British Admiralties, faced with the growing menace of the German U-boat campaign, formed a joint 'Anti-Submarine Detection and Investigation Committee' (Asdic) to counter it. The French scientist, Professor Langevin, developed this underwater technique of detection which is used to this day. After the war oceanographic studies of the depth and contour of the ocean bed were made by the technique and even quite small yachts, including my own, are now equipped with ultrasonic depth finders which are extraordinarily reliable and accurate. The presence of herring shoals within the sea can likewise be detected, but it was not until the last world war that Firestone in the United States[21, 22] developed the technique, in miniaturized form, for detecting flaws in metal structures. Thus grew up the present engineering subject of non-destructive testing. This work was classified as secret during the war but thereafter the engineering world took it up readily and metal flaw detectors, using pulsed ultrasonic energy and the echo principle, began to appear on the market.

It was not until some years later, in fact the early 1950s, that medicine, came to embrace the technique. One of the very earliest workers in this field was Wild from Minneapolis who sought to detect the presence of malignant ulcers of the stomach by passing probes down the oesophagus.[44] He then turned his efforts to scanning breasts for early carcinoma by dangling them face downwards in a tank of water through which a beam of ultrasound was passed. These techniques have not found general acceptance in clinical practice but were certainly an innovation. One of the most important contributors to this subject was the late Douglas Howry,[27, 28] also in the United States, who managed to produce some quite remarkable two-dimensional pictures by ultrasonic echo sounding but, in order to do so, he had to immerse the naked subject in a large tank of water which, for obvious reasons, is unsuitable in clinical practice. Howry's untimely death prevented him from seeing the present-day scope of ultrasonic usage but at least it is hoped that his genius will never be forgotten. We ourselves entered the field in the mid 1950s through engineering channels and it was in fact within a neighbouring, heavy engineering factory that we carried out our first experiments with a variety of pelvic tumours.

The technique with metals is to coat the surface with oil and apply an ultrasonic probe directly to it and to record any echoes which might be caused by discontinuities within that metal, such as, for example, a faulty weld, and we were fortunate in being able to borrow this industrial equipment with which even the crudest results were sufficient to convince us

of the future of the subject as applied to medicine.

It will now be seen why we have such marked preference for the term 'sonar' to cover diagnostic ultrasonic echo sounding, since its historical naval origins are thereby acknowledged.

ULTRASOUND

Ultrasound is vibrational energy of a mechanical nature. The frequency is above the range of human hearing which does not normally exceed 16 000 vibrations per second (Kiloherz), hence the term 'ultrasonic'. Bats use ultrasound in the 70KHz range and, although blind, can avoid a wire stretched across a room by the use of ultrasonic direction and range finding. It happens that when wavelength is less than about one-third of the diameter of the propagating source, energy can be propagated as a beam, as in the case of short wave radio and even more precisely with ultra high frequencies in radar. Herein lies the use of ultrasound whereas ordinary sound is emitted in all directions in concentric waves. Megaherz (millions of vibrations a second).

The ultrasonic beam is almost parallel and has minimal divergence. Since one has control of the direction of beam one can determine the direction from which an echo returns and the time taken for the echo to return will indicate the distance of its point of origin, provided that the speed of the ultrasonic wave through the tissue under examination is known, as is now the case.

The very high levels of energy used in power ultrasound are, as already stated, a different subject and are capable of generating intense heat, even sufficient for cooking, emulsifying liquids which would otherwise be immiscible, smashing up the envelopes of bacteria and liberating enzymes, degreasing and cleaning instruments and even, so it is said, producing a spurious maturation of spirits by altering the alcohol ester ratio, the liquid presumably intended for sale. In medical practice, power ultrasound has been limited almost entirely to the destruction of the semi-circular canals in Menière's disease by direct application at open operation and as a crude method of prefrontal leucotomy by a type of diathermy for which neurosurgeons have little enthusiasm, preferring the precision of a knife. In a cruder way power ultrasound can be used as a means of generating deep heat within the body in Departments of Physiotherapy.

The production of ultrasonic energy

In its simplest form this can be produced by a coil wound round a soft iron core through which a very high frequency alternating current is passed (magnetostriction). This causes the core to expand and contract at the given frequency usually however only within the kiloherz range. Modern practice involves the use of piezo-electric materials, that is to say substances which have the property of being able to convert mechanical energy into an electrical signal (the piezo-electric effect) and an electrical impulse into a mechanical distortion (the converse piezo-electric effect). There are a limited number of such substances. Those mainly used today are quartz or better still barium titanate, or lead zirconate. They are crystalline and have to be cut in a certain axis in order to have this property. The mechanical effect is at right angles to the electrical stimulus and vice versa. The piezo-electric effect is commonly employed in gramophone pick-ups.

So much for the recording system but the generating system depends upon the converse piezo-electric effect, namely the conversion of an electric stimulus to a mechanical pulse. The same crystal can act both as transmitter and receiver of mechanical vibrations and returning signals. Because of their ability to convert one type of energy into another these crystals are known as 'transducers.' They are cut along the appropriate axis into wafers whose diameter and thickness determine their natural resonance frequency. A thyratron-controlled electrical discharge starts the crystal wafer 'ringing' at this frequency and a beam of ultrasonic energy is thus driven into the body. Since the echoes from within return within a matter of microseconds it is important to silence the crystal almost immediately by suitable damping, otherwise it would still be resonating when the first signals arrived and this would confuse the diagnosis.

The electrical voltages employed to strike the crystal vary from 400 to 2000 volts but are of extremely low amperage. The whole process of transmission and reception takes considerably less than a kilosecond, so that pulse repetition frequencies of between 50 and 600 per second allow time for the echo process to complete itself before it is repeated and yet to occur often enough for a sustained image to be picked up without flicker.

The power used is calculated in watts per square centimetre of crystal face. In the case of power ultrasound this averages several watts but in sonar the average energies are in the microwatt range and even in continuous ultrasound techniques amount only to a few milliwatts. In the case of pulsed ultrasound it is very hard to estimate the energies employed because the pulse is of such brief duration, having usually a half life of about one to two microseconds only but it is believed that the actual pulse may have an energy of a few watts momentarily although the average energy may amount only to microwatts.

These are important points to consider when discussing the safety of ultrasound.

Physical properties of ultrasound

The ability to penetrate tissue has already been mentioned, together with the feature of directional control and minimal divergence of the beam. In its passage through the body the ultrasonic energy may not only be scattered by reflecting surfaces but is liable to become progressively attenuated. Different tissues transmit ultrasound at different speeds and provide varying degrees of absorption. For example water and other fluids, such as blood, pus and urine, transmit ultrasound well but bone absorbs it very heavily, a fact which has limited its usefulness in the diagnosis and localization of cerebral tumours.

Whereas X-rays penetrate tissues more readily the higher the frequency, in the case of ultrasound the reverse holds true and the frequency has to be lowered and the wavelength consequently coarsened to penetrate denser types of tumour masses. The degree of transparency to ultrasound or rather 'transonicity' as we prefer to call it, can to some extent be calculated and may give an indication of the type of tissue being insonated. What is more important, however, is the fact that whenever a beam of ultrasonic energy crosses a boundary, or interface, between two different types of tissue a number of events occur depending upon the difference in acoustic impedance which is specific for each tissue.

Acoustic impedance is defined as the product of the density of the tissue and the speed of the sound wave passing through it (ρc). Where, for example, the difference in acoustic impedance of tissues on either side of a given interface is small, the ultrasonic beam will pass straight through with very little interference or return echo signals, but where the difference is very great, as for example between the gas contained within the lumen of bowel and the bowel wall itself, the difference is so great that almost total reflection occurs. The first important event therefore at tissue interface is the phenomenon of reflection and the amount of energy reflected depends upon these differences in acoustic impedance in accordance with Rayleigh's Law.

$$E_R = E_I \left(\frac{\rho 1^c 1 - \rho 2^c 2}{\rho 1^c 1 + \rho 2^c 2} \right)^2 \times 100$$

When E_R is the reflected energy and E_I the incident energy at the interface.

The percentage of energy reflected at a given interface is therefore expressed as the square of the quotient of the difference in acoustic impedances divided by their sum, multiplied by one hundred. The direction of reflection is the same as in the case of light and only an interface presenting itself at right angles to the ultrasonic beam will return an echo to the transducer along a reciprocal path. Deviations from this perpendicular or normal incidence, even of as little as a few degrees, divert the echo away from the receiving system. It will therefore be seen that a search mechanism is necessary. Where the angle of incidence of the beam on the interface reaches the critical angle as in optical physics refraction occurs and can distort the picture too.

At each interface there is some loss of energy, probably in the form of heat although in medical sonar it has so far proved impossible to measure this even with the most sensitive apparatus. The residual part of the beam not reflected, nor scattered continues in attenuated form until it encounters the next interface, when the process is repeated and so on until its energy is spent and the echoes become progressively weaker. It is therefore necessary in handling the echo signals from depth within the body to use a compensatory mechanism of amplification in relation to depth, or in electronic parlance, to employ 'time-varied gain.'

In addition to the hypothetical conversion of the energy into heat, as yet not measurable, the phenomenon of cavitation is a possibility when the pressure of the ultrasonic wave exceeds the ambient pressure but this requires great power to achieve it. Cavitation can be likened to the apparent bubbles which appear round the blades of a motor boat's propellor starting up in still water and there is much argument about whether this is a vacuum phenomenon or is due to the release of dissolved gas. However it need not concern us in sonar, since it has never been observed, nor are the energies anywhere near sufficient. The phenomenon of microstreaming is also known to occur and this could hypothetically apply shear stresses to individual cells and tissues. Again these have not been measured nor directly demonstrated but their possible effect on cell membranes and internal cell structure requires fuller investigation.

Fields of application in medical diagnosis

The hopes of Wild and others to reveal early cancer have not been realized, partly because sonar can only provide a macroscopic, rather than a histological diagnosis and any suggestion of malignancy is purely inferential.

Early work on the brain has proved disappointing because the intact skull not only absorbs such a large proportion of ultrasound but the unpredictable unevenness of its outer and inner surfaces is liable to cause refraction and distortion of any echo picture obtained. Nevertheless, in spite of this, striking success has been achieved in studying shifts of the mid-line structures of the brain due to space occupying lesions on one side, such as, for example, tumour, or, in accident cases, subdural haematoma. This very simple examination which involves applying a probe directly to the unshaven head through a film of grease will show if there is any displacement to one side and may help in the differential diagnosis of unconsciousness due to head injury or drunkenness for example. Its use therefore in casualty departments is becoming fairly general.

The eyeball and the retro-orbital tissues are more accessible, however, and results are beginning to look promising.

The lungs have so far not proved a very profitable field, except where there is gross consolidation or effusion because the air contained within the alveoli tends to discourage the passage of ultrasound unless very low and coarse frequencies of $1-1\frac{1}{2}$MHz are used.

The investigation of abdominal tumour masses has proved much more rewarding and from the very first, being gynaecologists we concentrated on these.[17, 16] Success was almost immediate and we soon gravitated from gynaecology into the study of the pregnant uterus and its contents. The reasons for the success achieved in obstetrics and gynaecology are not far to seek. First of all there is not so much difference in physical principle between a fetus floating in liquor amnii and a submarine submerged in the ocean. It is simply a question of scale. Secondly, because patients come either to delivery or, in the case of gynaecology, to operation, confirmation of diagnosis is readily made and mistakes rapidly appreciated. In a variety of medical conditions, for example, in the liver, the patient may not come to laparotomy or may not die and undergo necropsy for a very long time after the ultrasonic examination, by which time the findings may have altered beyond all recognition.

Diagnostic expertise in obstetrics and gynaecology has been built up quickly by the instruction afforded by mistakes and the declared outcome of the case in a very short time. Further advantages are that most gynaecological tumour masses displace impenetrable bowel to a greater or lesser extent and are accessible to sonar through the anterior abdominal wall. The same applies to the gravid uterus after the tenth week. Retroperitoneal tumours are much more difficult although confidence is now being rapidly gained in the case of the kidneys which can, whenever necessary, be scanned from the posterior aspect of the patient. The liver is partly inaccessible because of the rib cage and lung margins above it while stomach and intestines contain gas and are more amenable to radiological diagnosis using radio-opaque dyes within their lumen.

There are two varieties of usage of sonar. The first is the pulse echo technique already referred to in which a silent, non-ringing transducer crystal picks up returning echoes successively from ever increasing depth within the abdomen and displays the signals in pictorial fashion on a cathode ray tube. The other main usage employs the Doppler effect in which a transmitting and receiving transducer are placed side by side. The transmitter emits a continuous ultrasonic beam at a fixed frequency and the echo from any moving structure as it approaches and recedes from the transducer will cause an apparent alteration in the frequency of the received echo, in other words the Doppler effect. This alteration in frequency can be processed as an auditory or light-flashing or even pen-recorded signal but is only applicable when studying moving structures such as the fetal heart[1, 30] the fetal chest wall or the flow of blood within the vessels.

Pulse echo apparatus
A piezo-electric transducer is made to act both as transmitter and receiver and is applied directly to the surface of the patient through a coupling film of some unobjectionable fluid such as olive oil since it is important not to let any air intervene between crystal face and skin. In the simplest apparatus this transducer can be held by hand but in the more sophisticated forms of apparatus to be described it has to be gantry mounted. The returning ultrasonic echoes are converted into electrical signals by the transducer and thereafter amplified. The information from such an amplified signal can then be applied either to the deflecting plates or to the cathode or grid of a cathode ray tube depending upon the type of display. There are three main types of display.

A-Scan. This uses the engineering principle for metal flaw detection in which a signal from a reflecting interface is applied to the vertically deflecting plates of a cathode ray tube whose time-base sweep is triggered by each individual pulse. The deflection of the time base sweep as a vertical blip therefore recurs with every pulse, for example, 300 per second, and its distance across the face of the tube is proportional to its depth within the structure examined.

When employing an A-scan technique in medicine one is often dismayed at the profusion of unidentifiable blips and the technique is only useful when one is measuring the position of a known structure, for example, the mid-line echo of the brain, usually accepted as the falx, and the parietal eminences of

the fetal skull on which is based the whole principle of biparietal cephalometry; in other words it will measure a diameter whose existence and location can be readily found with reflecting interfaces at right angles to the exploring beam.[16] The two sides of the fetal skull give very strong echoes with a clear space in between except for a small echo representing the mid-line (Fig. 28.4). If the ultrasonic beam does not

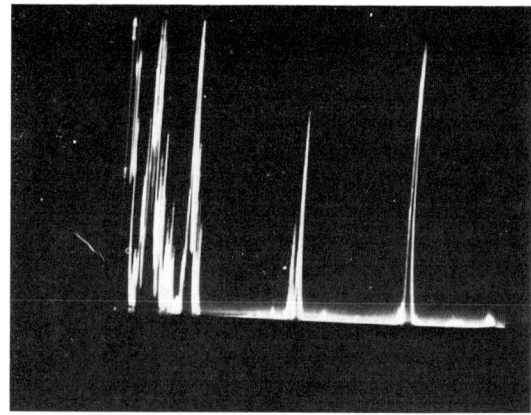

Fig. 28.4 Biparietal cephalometry by sonar, employing A-scan. Reading from left to right are the echoes from the superficial structures then finally two large isolated echo blips from the fetal parietal eminences with a smaller cerebral mid-line blip midway between them.

truly transverse the biparietal diameter but passes through the fetal head obliquely the reflected signals will not return on a reciprocal path to the probe and consequently the simultaneous appearance of these echoes on the cathode ray tube will be lost. Unless one can therefore be sure of the anatomical structure which one is looking at an A-scan unidimensional echo can be relatively meaningless, but when it comes to measuring the distance of these echoes very great degrees of accuracy can be achieved, especially with the use of electronic cursors as is now our practice.[2, 45, 46]

B-Scan. Here some form of gantry is necessary to hold the probe in a known position and a known attitude. It is thus possible to graduate from one dimension into two dimensional display. The technique is to arrange the time base sweep to correspond exactly with the height, traverse and inclination of the probe by the use of linear potentiometers for X and Y axis shifts and a sine/cosine potentiometer for the rotary movement of the probe.[17] Because of the need for a search technique it is now practically universal practice to employ what is called compound B-scanning in which a probe is rocked through an angle of anything up to 30 degrees as it traverses the body in a given plane, either longitudinal, transverse or oblique.[7] This calls for very definable mobility of the apparatus. Our own apparatus, the Diasono-

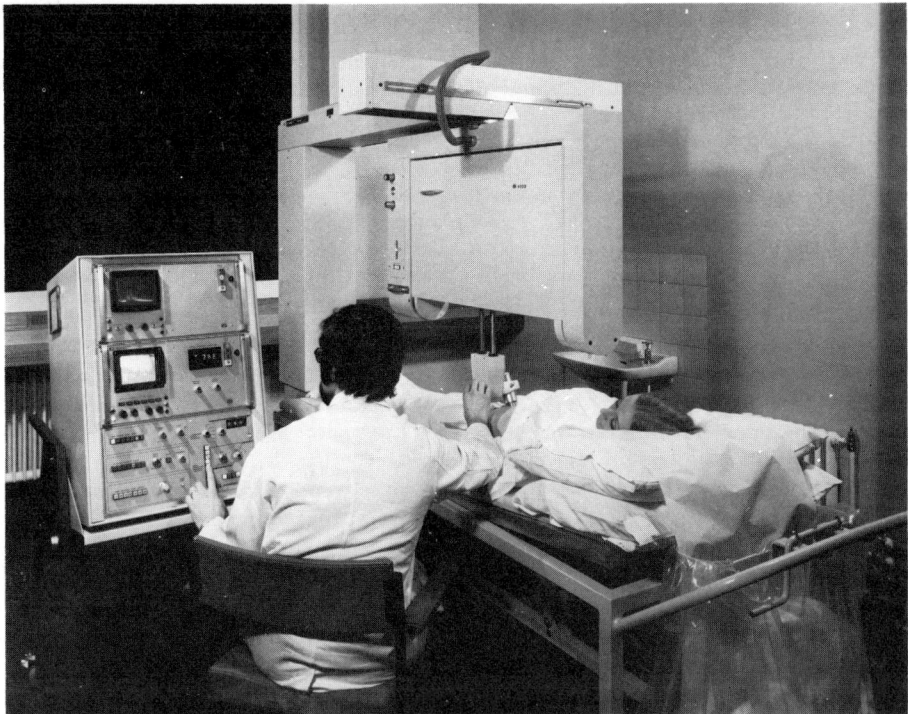

Fig. 28.5   Diasonograph apparatus NE4102 by Nuclear Enterprises Ltd, Edinburgh.

graph (Nuclear Enterprises Ltd) meets these requirements and allows for tilted sectional views as well with the minimum of manoeuvring of the gantry (Fig. 28.5).

In obstetrics and gynaecology one good longitudinal scan is worth half a dozen transverse scans and this point seems to be lost sight of by many manufacturers whose apparatus requires quite a palaver to convert from a transverse view to a longitudinal section.

The echoes within the field of search are limited to a single, two-dimensional plane at one time, rather like a 'slice' of the patient. The signals are processed by amplification and then applying them either to the grid or to the cathode of the electron gun, thereby accelerating or decelerating the flow of electrons towards the phosphor on the face of the cathode ray tube. This causes a dot of light whose brightness can be modulated to correspond to echo strength, whereas in the case of A-scan the height of the blip indicates the strength of the echo.

By suitable adjustment of power output and amplification of the received signals it is possible to accumulate a very large number of little dots of light scattered over the face of the cathode ray tube, each of whose position corresponds geometrically to the position of the point of origin within the body, thereby producing a sectional outline of all structures encountered and capable of reflecting (Fig. 28.6). A picture is thus gradually built up and either retained

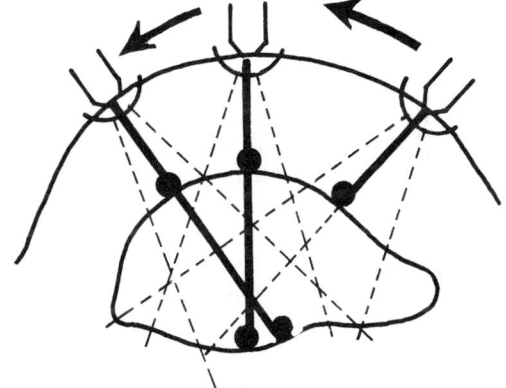

Fig. 28.6   Two-dimensional compound sector B-scanning technique. Echoes are located by search method of angular scanning and are represented as dots on cathode ray tube corresponding in position and intensity to site and nature of echo—thus making up a composite echogram.

Note: In all ultrasonograms in longitudinal section, cranialwards is to left of picture.

Patient in dorsal position unless otherwise stated.

Whenever the 'full bladder' technique has been used, arrows indicating points of interest are directed whenever appropriate through the echo free space caused by the quantity of urine in the bladder.

for inspection by time-exposure Polaroid photography with the shutter open during the process of scanning or by the use of a persistence cathode ray tube in which the picture remains on the face until deliberately cancelled.

Although very much more pictorial information can be obtained from a two-dimensional B-scan picture than from A-scan, nevertheless any sectional view may miss the main point of interest. Therefore before making a diagnosis it is usually necessary to make many scans at different levels and in different directions. We commonly make half a dozen or more. Each scan takes under half a minute to complete and less than half a minute for the development of the Polaroid photograph and it is possible, including documentation, to examine four patients to the hour. For example a given tumour mass may involve three or four longitudinal scans at different distances from the mid-line and as many transverse scans at different levels above and below the umbilicus.

Time-position scanning. The third method of signal processing which is less applicable to gynaecology is known as time-position scanning, or time-motion mode (T.M.), in which the time base sweep is made to travel directly across the face of the tube but at a steadily altering level. A structure such as the anterior leaf of the mitral valve is first identified and its movements to and fro will appear as signals moving from left to right and back again on the time base sweep. As the time base sweep is made to spread itself slowly upwards across the face of the tube the echoes now portrayed as dots of light trace a movement pattern which is readily identifiable. This technique is particularly useful in cardiology.

Patients' reactions

The only inconvenience to the patient is the need to smear the abdominal wall with olive oil. Any oil would suffice for the purpose and there are quite expensive jellies on the market but the main purpose is to secure acoustic coupling. Water would do but dries too quickly and we have found that olive oil is the easiest to remove and we usually supply it warmed from a thermos flask. Some units use a large paintbrush. The important matter is not to be stingy with the oil or the quality of the pictures immediately falls off.

Before we came on the scene seventeen years ago, water tanks had been thought necessary with the distance between transducer and body surface exceeding that of any distance between the patient's skin and an echo deep within her body in order to avoid the confusion of reverberations between transducer and body surface within the tank. Reverberations were also encountered from the side walls of the tank and the whole idea of immersing a naked patient in a tank of water, which had to be degassed to eliminate microbubbles, usually by boiling, was clinically so objectionable and impracticable that we tried first of all to use tanks with plastic membranes such as buckets with thin rubber bottoms perched precariously on the abdominal surface into which we dipped our transducers. Accidents and wet beds were frequent. With the help of Tom Brown, a research engineer and his colleagues of the firm of that time, namely Kelvin Hughes, a series of ever more sophisticated direct compound sector scanning machines were produced and these underly the principles of our work to this day.

The patient normally lies on a couch under the transducer gantry in the dorsal position although occasionally we have reason to examine her on her side and often when examining the kidneys in the prone position. Supine hypotension is sometimes troublesome in late pregnancy but can often be overcome by raising the feet with the knees extended, otherwise the examination has to be stopped and the patient turned on her side.

The patient experiences no discomfort whatsoever, not even a sensation of warmth and the rapidity of the examination is another commendable factor.

Unfortunately ultrasonic access to pelvic organs below the level of the symphysis pubis and which were not sufficiently enlarged to be accessible through the anterior abdominal wall could not be examined until I hit on the happy expedient of allowing or encouraging the patient's bladder to fill,[8] if necessary using a powerful diuretic to save time, in which case even the normal empty uterus, whether anteverted or retroverted, can be readily displayed as well as quite small distension cysts of the ovaries. The function of the bladder is to displace the impenetrable intestine out of the pelvis and to provide a built in transmitting tank since urine allows the passage of ultrasound practically without attenuation. The uterus being an immediate posterior relation of the full bladder is thus easily outlined and its contents, if any, even the earliest pregnancies can be depicted (Figs. 28.7a & b).

General principles of diagnosis

In two-dimensional scanning, such as we can at present achieve, one is still able to miss important tissue interfaces which lie at a bad angle of incidence in a third dimension. The limitations of two-dimensional scanning therefore must be to some extent compensated by multiple scans and at least some knowledge of

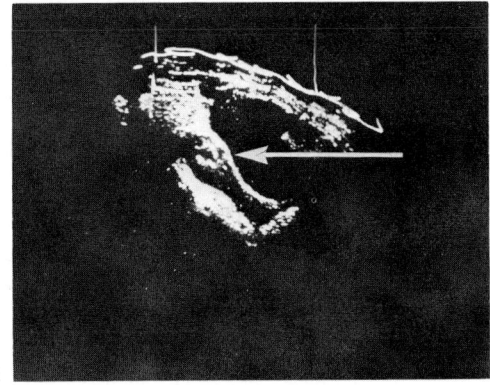
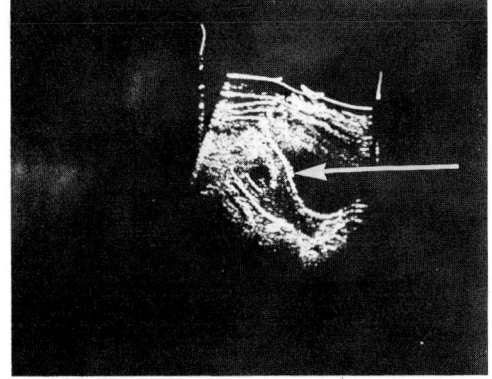

a   b

Fig. 28.7(a)   Early gestation sac, 6 weeks amenorrhoea. Uterus not yet appreciably enlarged. History of three abortions. No living children.
   (b)   Same case 3 weeks later (9 weeks amenorrhoea) following cerclage of cervix. Note very satisfactory growth, closed cervix and fetus seen as a small echo dot within gestation sac. Successful delivery near term.

the likely pathology to be encountered since, bearing in mind the principles of Rayleigh's Law, the strength of the echoes depends upon differences in adjacent tissues rather than the individual tissues themselves.

Some indication of the macroscopic texture of a tumour may be indicated by its transonicity. If one can 'see' the back wall of a tumour one can safely assume that the ultrasonic beam has reached that surface and returned and that the tissue of the tumour is capable of transmitting it. Since the penetrating power of ultrasound is inversely proportional to the frequency it may be noted in certain types of tumours, for example, uterine fibromyomata that penetration can only be fully achieved at $1\frac{1}{2}$MHz, indifferently at $2\frac{1}{2}$MHz and not at all at 5MHz, whereas a fluid-containing ovarian cyst will transmit sound well at all these frequencies. In other words transonicity is frequency-related. An ovarian fibroma because of its extreme density transmits even $1\frac{1}{2}$MHz ultrasound badly, as might be expected. Solid elements and septa within a tumour will be picked up and this may help to give some indication of diagnosis.

The next important point to bear in mind is that sensitivity of the apparatus, or as we prefer to call it, the gain, may render certain tissues visible which a lower gain setting would render undetectable. The gain is calibrated in decibels.

Decibels represent the logarithmic ratio, to the base 10, of the power delivered at the face of the crystal divided by the power of the system as a whole and must therefore always be a minus quantity. A gain setting therefore of -10dB is very much higher than one of -20dB and the difference furthermore is logarithmic.[13] This system of gain control was built into our apparatus deliberately in order to minimize the amount of ultrasonic energy used at a time. Other forms of apparatus deliver a given output of power and cut back on the sensitivity of the receiving system. In terms of decibel ratio the answer may be the same but in terms of energy received by the tissues there may be a very great difference.

Intestine always contains gas and even quite a thin film of gas can reflect ultrasound almost completely. This fact alone may help to differentiate between a pelvic mass due, for example, to diverticulosis of the colon and a left-sided ovarian tumour. An inflammatory phlegmon containing bowel is less readily penetrable than a haematocele within the pelvis.

Patients differ in the apparent transonicity of their abdominal walls and it is often useful to aim for some known reference point such as the sacral promontory and to adjust the gain setting of the apparatus accordingly. This compensates for obesity and unusually thick skins.

Signs of clinical importance in ultrasonic diagnosis are clarity, i.e. large black spaces indicating the likely presence of fluid (but only if the deeper outlines are visible), and the complexity of structure. In the case of ovarian tumours, or ascites, complex echo patterns strongly suggest malignancy.

Sonar in non-pregnant conditions

All palpable abdominal masses lend themselves to ultrasonic diagnosis since the following features can be readily ascertained, namely contour, size, transonicity, complexity and relation to bowel. Ovarian tumours may be partly solid and partly cystic, especially if malignant, or on the other hand may appear perfectly clear with an occasional septum as in mucinous cystadenomata (Fig. 28.8).

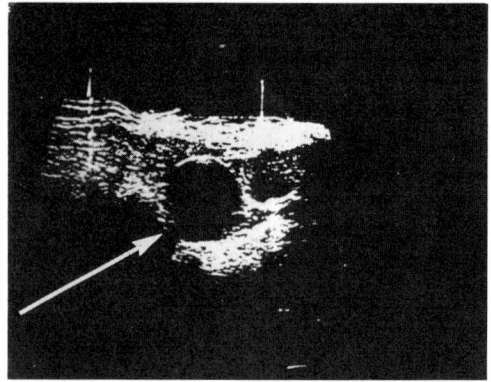

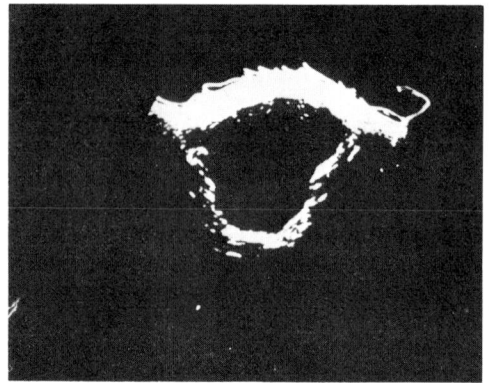

Fig. 28.8   Ovarian cyst. Clear and transonic right through to its posterior aspect even at the high frequency of 5MHz.

Fibromyomata are identified by their reluctance to transmit ultrasound at the higher frequencies of $2\frac{1}{2}$MHz and particularly 5MHz as compared with their ready outlining at the coarser $1\frac{1}{2}$MHz frequency (Fig. 28.9).

Ascites shows fluid which is not encysted and with strongly echoing bowel floating within it. The more bizarre the picture, the more certain is the diagnosis one of malignant ascites due to peritoneal carcinomatosis. Non-malignant ascites is nowadays becoming rather rare, thanks to efficient medical treatment of cardiac failure and the disappearance of abdominal tuberculosis, but fluid can be seen to collect in the flanks (as is demonstrable on clinical percussion), with the bowel floating up towards the centre. The pelvic viscera and particularly the uterus, whether retroverted or not can almost always be outlined using the full bladder technique.[8]

There are pitfalls in the diagnosis of ectopic pregnancy since the macroscopic signs may vary from those of an unruptured tube or a peritubal haematocele or a frankly liquid haemoperitoneum.[10] It is not surprising therefore that the diagnosis by sonar presents many

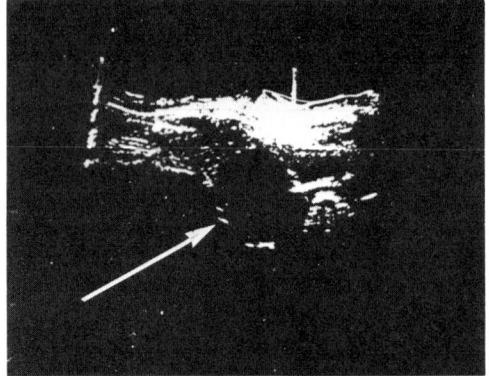

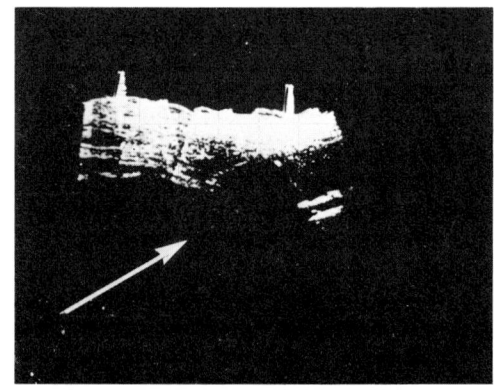

Fig. 28.9(a)   Fibromyoma—transonic at coarse frequency of $1\frac{1}{2}$MHz.
   (b)   Ditto at $2\frac{1}{2}$MHz, but less transonic.
   (c)   Ditto at 5MHz. Not transonic in spite of maximum gain settings.

difficulties, but at least the finding of a gestation sac definitely within the uterus may help to distinguish an intra-uterine from an extra-uterine pregnancy.

The bladder nearly always shows an apparently open-mouthed lower end to it. This is due to the fact that the trigone and internal meatus are hidden behind the shadow of the symphysis pubis. However, if retention of urine is acute due to incarceration of a pelvic tumour or gravid uterus within the pelvis, the bladder may become a totally abdominal organ in which the lower end is pointed, since it represents the trigone, a matter which serves to distinguish it immediately from a large ovarian cyst.

Obesity is no bar to ultrasonic examination and, in fact, sonar may be very useful in eliminating the presence of a tumour in a patient so grossly obese that clinical examination becomes almost impossible.

Papillomata of the bladder can be readily seen and vesical carcinoma is suggested by the projection of a mass with a wide and infiltrative base into the lumen of the bladder. (Barnett & Morley—*personal communication*)

The kidneys, if not enlarged, are best explored from the dorsal aspect of the patient. When they lie at different levels as is often the case, some oblique tilting of the scanning head may be necessary to reveal both simultaneously. Ultrasonic renography becomes useful in identifying kidneys with poor excretory function on X-ray pyelography. Hydronephrosis shows up as a cystic space, unilateral or bilateral in the region of the kidney. Polycystic kidneys show a trabeculated pattern and this has recently been demonstrated even in a fairly young child.[32] Perirenal extravasations being fluid in nature show the appropriate large, dark areas surrounding the kidney region.

An aneurism of the abdominal aorta is, of course, transonic since it contains blood but it will be observed that only the anterior wall pulsates but not the posterior, since it lies against the vertebral column. This helps to distinguish it from cysts lying in front of the aorta, e.g. pancreatic, which demonstrate transmitted pulsation in both the anterior and posterior walls.[16]

A spleen is not easy to demonstrate unless it is enlarged when it can be recognized in transverse section arising from the left side and having a pointed right hand border on its right side, unlike an ovarian or renal tumour. Splenic enlargement due for example to myelomatosis simply appears as an echo-free type of splenomegaly whereas we have demonstrated echoes within spleen containing lymphadenomatous deposits.[9]

The liver is a difficult organ and the limitations of access and of two-dimensional scanning are here very apparent. Nevertheless when combined with radio-isotope scintiscanning, much useful information can be obtained about the likelihood of hepatic metastases which show up as echoes within the liver substance. Hepatic cysts can be seen but the different varieties of cirrhosis are still very hard to distinguish and experience is only being rather slowly gathered.

The outline of the lower parts of the liver, however, may be important since deformity may indicate malignant infiltration.

A haematoma is always transonic, showing up simply as a black space-occupying area. A haematoma within the sheath of the rectus abdominis may present deceptively as a case of acute abdominal pain due to an apparently palpable and very tender ovarian cyst. We have occasionally made such a diagnosis by sonar and saved the patient an unnecessary laparotomy.

Sonar in early pregnancy

The applicability of sonar in pregnancy can be best considered under two headings, namely, early pregnancy and late.

Where the uterus has not yet risen out of the pelvis sufficiently to be palpable per abdomen it is necessary to employ the full bladder technique in order to display it but the gestation sac can be seen from the fifth week of amenorrhoea onwards and its rate of growth will be seen to be very rapid, approximately doubling in size every ten days.[12] It appears first as a small white ring and the site of implantation is of some importance since this should be definitely in the upper half of the uterine cavity. It should be possible to display it as an entire ring and we have now become familiar with normal growth rates (Figs. 28.7a & b). The ultrasonic signs of early pregnancy can be just as early and sometimes earlier than urine gonadotrophin tests. What is much more important is that an early assessment can be made of normality.

The fetus within the gestation sac 'ring' first appears as a small dot within it, sometimes at the seventh week, always at the eighth week, and with absolute certainty by the ninth week, provided scanning is sufficiently carefully carried out. It may require a combination of longitudinal and transverse sectional scanning to reveal it. Not only is the level of implantation important in as much as low levels signify a poor prognosis with a likelihood of early abortion, but the site of nidation and thereafter presumably early placental differentiation may become evident between the eighth and ninth week of amenorrhoea. This matter is still being followed up and the conclusion is no more than tentative at present.

The incidence of very early blighted ovum has never been fully estimated although early reports by Hertig & Rock[26] indicated something in the region of a quarter of all pregnancies. One of the difficulties in assessing the size of the problem is that there is usually a reason for examining a patient at this very early stage of pregnancy, such as, for example, a history of early recurrent abortion which loads the figures in favour of some abnormality. Nevertheless we are becoming increasingly convinced that not only is the condition extremely common but usually unrecognized, since it is passed off as a late and heavy period ultimately.[14]

Blighted ovum

Several signs suggest this diagnosis in early pregnancy. Firstly, the ring itself may be imperfectly formed and may have a speckled, blotchy appearance (Fig. 28.10). Next, it may

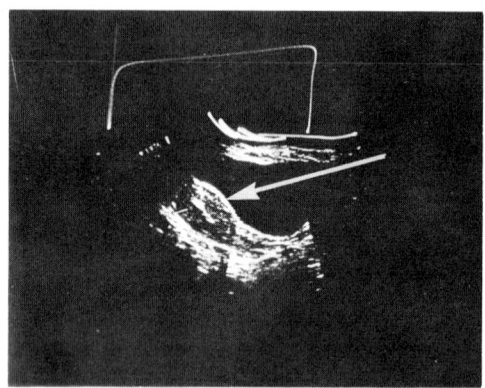

Fig. 28.10 Blighted ovum (speckled embryonic mass within uterus) 6½ weeks amenorrhoea. Aborted at home a few days later.

be impossible to delineate a complete ring which assumes the characteristics of a type of capital 'C'. Another unfavourable sign is a failure to grow at the normal rate and failure to demonstrate a fetal echo by the ninth week of amenorrhoea. When bleeding in early pregnancy occurs sonar can provide an estimate as to the normality of the pregnancy and to what lengths one ought to go to try and preserve the so-called threatened abortion from becoming inevitable.

Twins

We have frequently been able to demonstrate two gestation sacs at the eighth week of amenorrhoea but not earlier than the seventh.[14] The diagnosis of the famous Queen Charlotte quintuplets, made with a replica of our own apparatus, at the ninth week was a truly remarkable feat and must have contributed in

no small measure to their remarkable ultimate survival.[5]

Abortion

Sonar can be of the greatest assistance not only in distinguishing threatened from inevitable abortion but whether abortion is complete or incomplete. A normal-looking gestation sac ring which continues to grow at a normal rate in spite of a history of bleeding indicates a good prognosis. An opening cervix may be seen, low implantation of the ring, or frankly some echoes without proper ring formation may indicate that the abortion process is already inevitable and possibly incomplete. A narrowing or waisting of the intermediate area of the uterus almost certainly indicates a recent abortion whether the uterus is empty or not.

Retained products of conception show up as white echoes in the region of the uterine cavity and may indicate the need for evacuation (Fig. 28.11). It is now our practice, in the

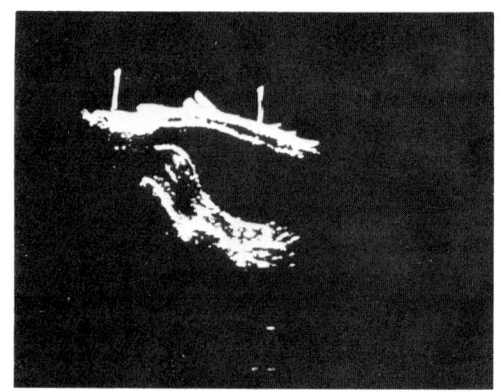

Fig. 28.11 Incomplete abortion. Retained products of conception. Evacuation.

absence of an emergency situation due to haemorrhage or infection, always to examine the uterus by sonar in cases of early abortion in order to determine whether the uterus is empty or not. Provided bleeding is not serious and the uterus appears to be empty we have no hesitation in sending the patient home without operation and without more ado and we have no reason to regret this policy.[37] It certainly saves unnecessary curettage and hospitalization.

In deciding whether a case of recurrent abortion is suitable for a Shirodkar operation for structural or functional cervical incompetence we always carry out an examination by sonar to determine, as far as possible the normality of the pregnancy, since there is little point in trying to salve a fetus already doomed.

Maturity

The assessment of maturity is very easy in early pregnancy since the growth rate is very rapid within the first twenty weeks. We are beginning to achieve an accuracy to within half a week or, at worst, a whole week. The first signs of placentation are demonstrable usually between the ninth and tenth weeks. At the eleventh week the gestation sac ring apparently appears to break up, presumably from the differentiation of chorion frondosum from chorion laeve. A difficult period around the eleventh and twelfth weeks follows in which one has to rely upon the presence of confusing echoes within the uterus and a suitable uterine size. Sometimes it is possible to see the fetal head late in the eleventh or twelfth weeks of amenorrhoea and nearly always by the thirteenth week. By the fourteenth week not only can the placenta be seen with certainty but the head may actually be outlined with a mid-line falx visible (Fig. 28.12). From then onwards the period of

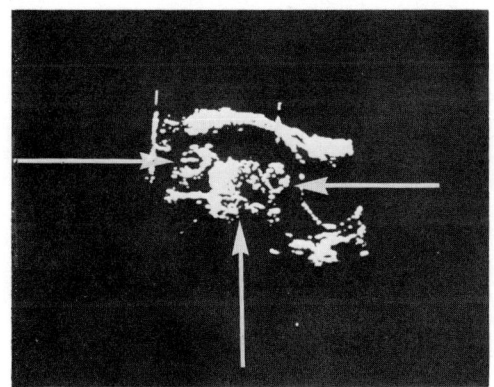

Fig. 28.12 Patient 'large for dates'—$14\frac{1}{2}$ weeks amenorrhoea. Twin heads (horizontal arrows). Posterior placenta (vertical arrow).

gestation is estimated from fetal head size which can be carried out by eye, and with experience, right up to the twentieth week, after which it is advisable to start measuring its diameter. Fortunately the head in early pregnancy is very nearly circular and the measurement does not have to be as critical as in later pregnancy.

Associated pelvic tumours

The suspicion that a pelvic swelling in a patient apparently large for dates, may be due to twins, mistaken maturity, hydramnios, or an associated tumour, is well worth investigating by sonar since each gives different and characteristic appearances. The matter is of clinical importance since fibromyomata can usually be managed conservatively whereas ovarian tumours require operation. During pregnancy, however, because of increased vascularity they are more transonic than they would be in the non-pregnant state and this factor has to be borne in mind in making this diagnosis. In addition, careful scanning may help to distinguish a tumour which is separate from the uterus or a part of its structure. The employment of different frequencies in order to assess transonicity is thus an important measure.

The uterus which is large for dates is a common clinical problem and whether the patient is obese or not, whether her menstrual history is reliable or not, these cases are a common reason for referral to the ultrasonic department.

Hydatidiform mole

The diagnosis of hydatidiform mole on clinical grounds is often difficult and is very often not made in spite of persistent bleeding and equivocal high gonadotrophin excretion rates until the passage of hydatidiform vesicles confirms clinical suspicion. To wait for the appearance of identifiable fetal bones with X-rays to exclude the diagnosis is often to wait dangerously long. We soon found that by altering the sensitivity of the apparatus, i.e. the gain, it was possible to demonstrate the speckled appearance of a hydatidiform mole within its cavity[16, 34] (Fig. 28.13a & b).

Mention was made earlier of the 'gain sensitivity' of certain tissues and hydatidiform mole and placental tissue certainly come into this category.

It is important to distinguish these appearances from artefacts due to over-amplification producing what is known in the electronic world as 'grass' and therefore we insist that the speckled appearance must disappear with a reduction of about 10–15 decibels in gain setting and yet the posterior wall of the uterus must still show up perfectly clearly. Furthermore to avoid confusion which has occurred in the past with a very degenerate fibromyoma[10]

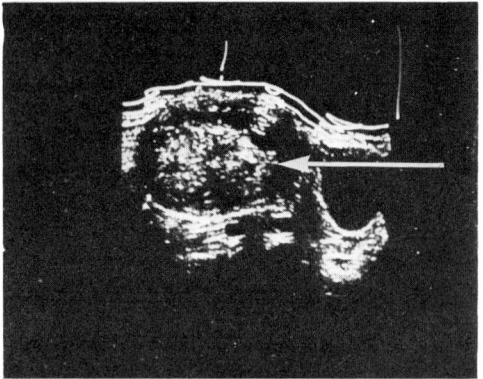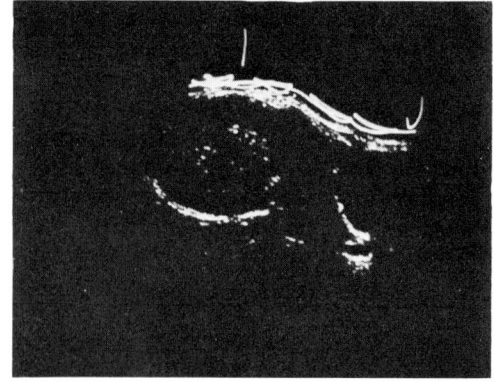

Fig. 28.13(a)   Hydatidiform mole. Moderately full bladder is to the right.
(b)   Same as above but at low gain sensitivity. Speckled mass has almost disappeared, but uterus is still 'transonic'.

we now insist on confirming the diagnosis at the very high frequency of 5MHz. Our experience now runs to many dozens of cases.

The diagnosis of hydatidiform mole by the use of Doppler ultrasound is somewhat suspect but the hearing of a fetal heart by this means makes the diagnosis very much less likely. The problem is particularly difficult when a fetus co-exists with a hydatidiform mole.

Sonar in second half of pregnancy

The head is very easily identified after the first trimester as a more or less complete circle and from this the presentation may be inferred. The identification of individual limbs is neither possible nor a profitable exercise.

Twins
Multiple pregnancy is best diagnosed in the second and third trimesters by counting heads.[41] It is fairly easy to mistake a sectional view of the fetal thorax for a fetal head but by suitable manipulation of the gantry and the position of the scanning probe one should always seek for the falx or mid-line equatorial echo which rules out the possibility of the structure being thoracic (Fig. 28.14).

Intra-uterine death
This may first be indicated by the absence of an ultrasonic Doppler signal from the fetal heart. Serial examination will also show that there has been no increase in the size of the head. Sometimes the shape looks characteristically abnormal, but X-radiology is more prompt and efficient than sonar in making this diagnosis.

Fetal abnormality
The only fetal abnormalities which can be diagnosed with certainty so far by sonar are hydrocephalus, in which biparietal diameters exceeding 11cm make the diagnosis definite and anencephaly in which a fetal skull vault cannot be found.

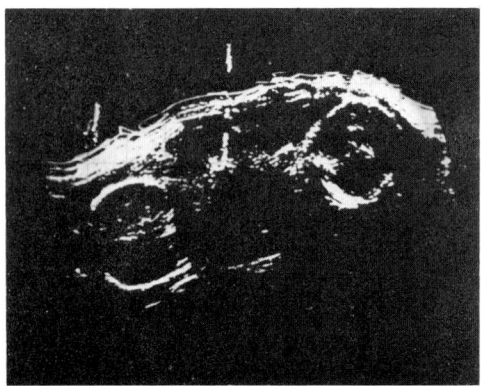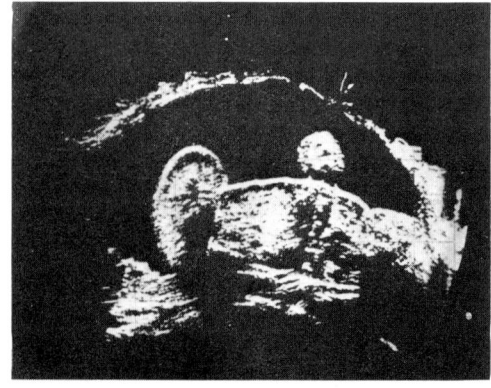

Fig. 28.14   Twin heads.

Fig. 28.15   Hydramnios and anencephaly.

Hydramnios

Not only is the uterus clinically large for dates but the ultrasonic appearances are quite definite and show large black, echo free areas with blob-like complexes believed to represent limbs floating within an excess of fluid. These characteristic appearances were first noted in Sweden[41] and have been amply confirmed by us (Fig. 28.15).

Associated tumours

Associated tumours whether renal such as hydronephrosis (*see back*), ovarian (Fig. 28.16), or uterine may be hard to distinguish on clinical examination alone and, as in the case of early pregnancy, the abdominal size which is apparently large for dates, is a common reason for referral.

BIPARIETAL CEPHALOMETRY

In about 1960 I started a series of tank experiments with a fetal skull since we had already observed that the head could be identified even by A-scan by recognizing two powerful echoes presumably from either side of it. The point at issue was to decide whether the biparietal diameter as such could be identified. It was soon clear that this was indeed possible, provided the ultrasonic beam was made to cross the true diameter of the fetal head and not a chord thereof. This could only happen in two situations, either the biparietal diameter or the occipito-frontal since in no other position were the walls of the skull parallel to each other and available to scanning at perpendicular incidence.[16] Within a matter of months we were beginning to achieve accuracies of the order of 2mm which we would now regard as unacceptable and Willocks applied the method to studying intra-uterine fetal growth.[45, 46] This technique has been further elaborated and refined by measuring the distance between the appropriate blips by electronic cursors which superimpose an additional brightness on the time base sweep which can be adjusted by manipulating the dials to coincide with the blips, the dials themselves being calibrated in centimetres and millimetres, thus giving a direct reading (Fig.

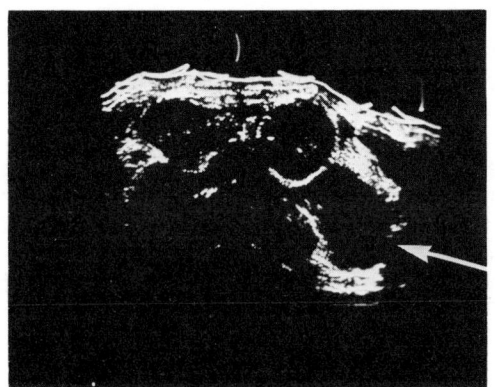

Fig. 28.16 Ovarian cyst deep in pelvis displacing fetal head upwards. Caesarean section.

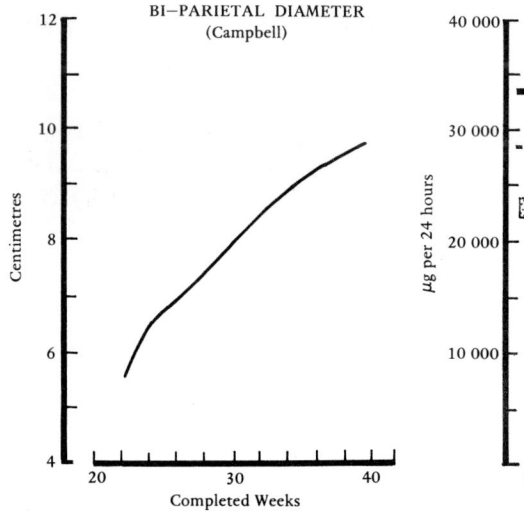

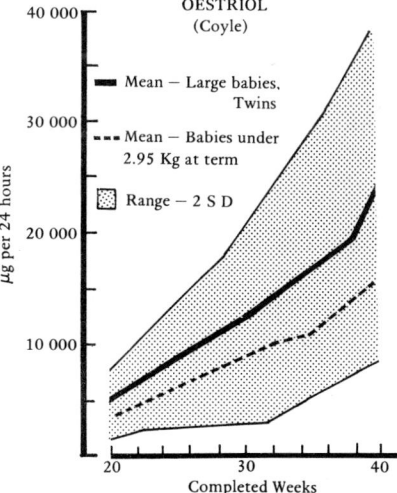

Fig. 28.17 Standard chart for simultaneously reviewing fetal head growth (Campbell) and maternal oestriol excretion levels (Coyle).

28.4). The technique was further refined by Campbell by identifying not only the fetal skull but its attitude and the mid-line echoes on B-scanning and then converting to A-scanning for the measurement of the biparietal diameter thus already visually identified.[2, 3, 4] Experience of this technique in a number of centres including Glasgow, London and Aberdeen has confirmed the use of this method.

Graphs have been produced indicating the normal growth rates of the biparietal diameter and relating these to maturity, which is far more closely associated than is actual fetal weight.[3, 14] In this way it is not only possible to assess the maturity of a fetus where the dates are in doubt but by taking the sequential readings to observe abnormal growth rates.[4, 42] It is now common practice to plot these biparietal growth rates alongside graphs of oestriol excretion (Fig. 28.17). A failure of either or both to rise at the appropriate rate as pregnancy advances may indicate intra-uterine malnutrition and a baby at risk from dysmaturity.[6] This kind of monitoring is extensively used for all cases in which the fetus is believed to be at risk either on the basis of maternal obstetrical history, clinical signs or associated diseases known to jeopardize placental nutrition.

In the case of twins it is also useful to know which of the two, whether the first or second, has the larger head.

Placental growth
Helman *et al.* (1970) have devised a technique of multiple longitudinal and transverse placental scans using the greatest diameter of the chorion plate for measurement. The technique, once fully established will measure placental growth and volume as part of early pregnancy growth studies.

Placental localization. Half of our work with sonar in obstetrics is concerned with biparietal cephalometry measurement. About a quarter is devoted to localization of the placenta. The great advantage in the case of sonar is that this can be carried out at an early stage of pregnancy, in fact, the earlier the easier. The same rules first worked out in the diagnosis of hydatidiform mole apply to the identification of the placenta. Time-varied gain is very necessary to reveal a posterior placenta which may be in shadow behind the fetus and wherever possible by suitable positioning an attempt should be made to show up the white

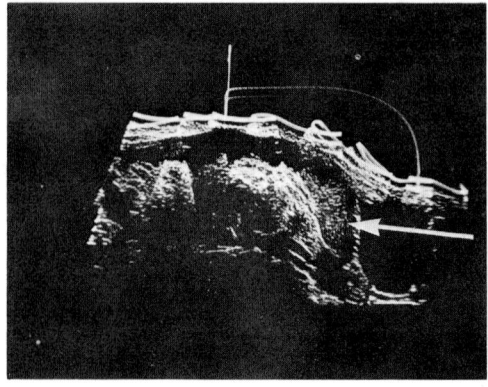

Fig. 28.18   Anterior type I. placenta praevia. Antepartum haemorrhage at 32 weeks' gestation. Confirmed at Caesarean section four weeks later.

line representing the feto/placental surface (Fig. 28.18). Alterations of about 15 decibels will convert a speckled placental mass into a dark area but will not submerge the fetal surface when it can be found. Again longitudinal and transverse scans may be necessary. It is a good plan to have at least some urine in the bladder in order to delineate the level of the lower uterine segment in making a diagnosis of placental praevia (Fig. 28.19).

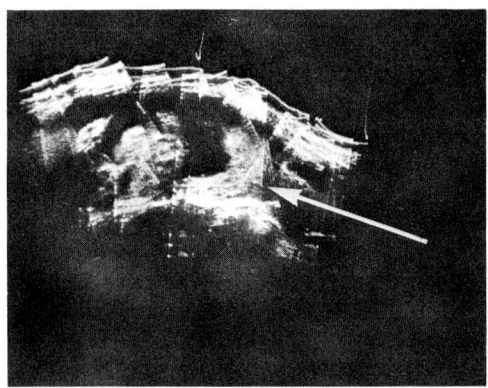

Fig. 28.19   Case of continual bleeding at 24 weeks' gestation. Posterior placenta praevia type 3–4. Eventual Caesarean section required at 32 weeks' gestation. Diagnosis confirmed.

It is now in our practice to employ placental localization by sonar whenever possible in all cases of antepartum bleeding in order to confirm or exclude the diagnosis of placenta praevia, in all cases of unstable lie for the same reason and always before amniocentesis, in order to prevent trauma to the placenta with its attendant risks of fetal bleeding into the amniotic cavity or into the maternal circulation. With regard to the latter it has now been observed by our Department of Haematology that the incidence of feto-maternal transfusion following amniocentesis has dropped dramatically since the practice became general in 1967.[47] The technique, however, is not yet sufficiently sophisticated to make as detailed an anatomical study of the placenta *in utero* as one would like but research is proceeding along these lines. We prefer ultrasonic localization of the placenta to all other methods because of its ready availability in a hospital such as ours at any hour of the day or night and because of the minimal disturbance involved for the patient, who may be bleeding, since the examination can be carried out even in her own bed. In our published series we indicated an overall accuracy of over 94 per cent which compares reasonably with other methods and is certainly an improvement upon soft tissue radiography.[15]

The placenta in cases of Rh haemolytic disease is a matter of some interest to us since it would appear to be larger and more opaque than normal, but we cannot yet claim to be able to assess the severity by the ultrasonic appearances, although that is certainly one of our objectives.

Puerperium

The main use for sonar in the puerperium is in cases of secondary post-partum haemorrhage in order to determine the presence of retained placental tissue (Fig. 28.20). This may help to swing the decision in favour of exploring the uterine cavity under anaesthesia in cases

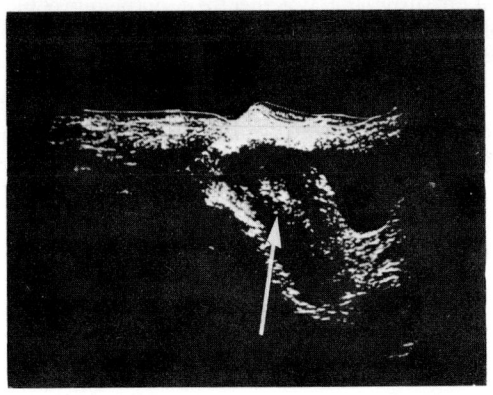

Fig. 28.20 Secondary post-partum haemorrhage. Retained placental remnants necessitating evacuation.

of doubt. A haematoma in association with a ruptured uterus or a lower segment uterine Caesarean section scar may also be revealed and help to indicate the reason for a patient's post-operative anaemia or shock. The rate of involution can likewise be studied.

DOPPLER EFFECT

There are a number of excellent machines on the market at a reasonable price measurable in hundreds of pounds, rather than in thousands, as in the case of B-scanning machines. They are simple to use, simply with an on/off switch and volume control. It is possible to pick up Doppler signals from the beating fetal heart as early as the eleventh week of amenorrhoea although this is often difficult but it should be possible, in all cases, by the thirteenth and certainly the fourteenth week. This gives a very reassuring indication of continuing fetal life.[1, 30]

The diagnosis of placenta praevia by listening for the sound of blood going through the suspected placental site, alleged to be of a swishing nature, is simply not to be trusted and claims by manufacturers to this effect should be treated with the greatest caution. The diagnosis of placenta praevia is too important to entrust to so imprecise a technique. Similar remarks have already been made about the diagnosis of hydatidiform mole. The diagnosis of twins is not easy to make unless two independent machines are employed simultaneously and there is appreciable disparity between the two fetal heart beats.

Recently, however, Doppler ultrasound has come into more extensive use as a method of continuous fetal heart rate monitoring in the course of labour. It is difficult if not impossible to use any method of direct auscultation for listening to a fetal heart at the height of a uterine contraction, especially late in labour and this is just the period when one is most anxious to know what effects uterine contractions are having upon the fetal heart. Fetal electrocardiography, using scalp electrodes, is only applicable after membrane rupture but of all external methods of auscultating the fetal heart and assessing its rate on a beat to beat basis sonar is vastly superior to phonocardiography which is sensitive to extraneous noise and interference. The ultrasonic transducer, nowadays usually consisting of a central transmitter and a ring of receiving transducers

(Sonicaid) in order to pick up the fetal heart movements from as wide an area as possible is quite simply applied to the abdominal wall with elastic bandaging and coupled to the maternal skin by jelly or grease. The subject of continuous fetal heart monitoring in labour, although it has a long history, is only now just beginning to come into its own and it is likely that the Doppler principle will be increasingly employed.

Safety of sonar

The profound difference between diagnostic sonar in medical practice and power ultrasound has already been stressed but, by analogy with hazards of X-rays, there is need for vigilance and a readiness to explore every suggestion that tissues, particularly developing fetal tissues, are in any way damaged by this mechanical form of energy. After all it took about half a century for the risks to the fetus by X-rays to be recognized[40] and it would be ironical, if by increasing the use of sonar, one were simply to substitute one risk for another. Since the types of energy used in ultrasonics are mechanical and not ionizing a completely different set of biological effects, if any, would be expected and evidence of these has, so far, been very hard to find.

There is indeed more need for careful experimentation and less for pure speculation.[23] Intensive studies are already in plan to establish the immediate or long term fetal risk if such a risk exists. One of the first difficulties is to know where to look and even then to know how to measure the power levels being employed. The electrical powers used can be calculated but the amount of energy reaching the target area within the body is much less easy to assess. Furthermore it is by no means yet certain to what extent continuous as distinct from pulsed ultrasound differ in their effects. One would expect continuous ultrasound to favour microstreaming and the relatively higher impact energies of pulsed ultrasound to be more instantaneously dramatic even allowing for the relatively long periods of recovery between each pulse. Much of the damage due to ultrasonic energy which has been recorded is due to heat and to cavitation, neither of which has been observed in animal tissues with the employment of present day sonar. This is not to deny that future machines may, by an increase in power and penetrating

capacity, exceed a threshold level of safety, even assuming that such a level exists.[31]

The possibility that the early growing fetus might be damaged by ultrasonic echo sounding was one of the earliest challenges and resulted in a pooling of results between New York, Glasgow and Sweden, which indicated no such effect, regardless of the period of gestation at which ultrasonic examination was first carried out or the number of exposures.[24] Animal experiments in the case of small rodents[39, 48] have failed to show any teratogenic effect, even through to the second generation. Then came a preliminary communication from South Africa suggesting chromosome damage in the case of insonated tissue cultures.[33] Much notice was taken of this suggestion and a number of centres including our own have tried hard to reproduce these results but without success and we are now confident that this preliminary communication cannot be substantiated.[43]

More recent conjecture applied to enzyme changes has stimulated experimental work at present in progress to demonstrate even temporary vacuolation within the cell in the lyzosomes. The possibility that microstreaming, especially with continuous ultrasound, may set up shear stresses on cell membranes thus influencing their permeability is another matter requiring investigation. Blood vessels running in a certain direction in chick embryos within a wide continuous ultrasonic field can demonstrate temporary conglomeration of red blood corpuscles at nodal points corresponding to the ultrasonic field.[19] This effect disappears as soon as the ultrasound is switched off and reappears immediately on switching on. Its significance is by no means certain and on the basis of ordinary physical considerations, in dealing with a fluid containing particulate matter like blood, it is not surprising. Whether the endothelium of blood vessels can be damaged by this phenomenon has yet to be further explored.

There is thus no lack of awareness of the possibility of hazard but none has yet revealed itself in clinical practice, although a number of units in the United Kingdom, including our own, have an experience running to many thousands of patients. Meanwhile the obvious diagnostic benefits conferred by sonar in facilitating diagnosis are becoming more and more apparent with ever-extending usage.

CONCLUSION

The scale of usage of sonar in obstetrics in

the Queen Mother's Hospital, Glasgow has already exceeded that of radiology and in fact about a quarter of all our maternity patients, for one reason or another, at one time of pregnancy or another, often repeatedly, undergo examination by these means (*see* Table 28.1). Already within the city of Glasgow six

sentation. (This has never been achieved—Donald, 1975 in press.)

Since sonar is now rapidly expanding in fields other than gynaecology, particularly cardiology and urology, it is likely that the subject will come increasingly under the wing of radiologists and X-ray departments al-

Table 28.1   Clinical functions of sonar and X-rays

Sonar	X-rays
Early pregnancy—	Fetal skeletal abnormality
Placenta	Multiple
Sac	Deflexion attitudes
Multiple	Ossification centres
Growth	Hydrops fetalis
Blighted ovum	Placental localization $\pm$
Bleeding—	Hydatidiform mole (only by exclusion and arteriography)
Retained products	Spalding sign ⎫
Placenta localization	Gas in major vessels ⎬ IUD
Intra-uterine death	Tooth in dermoid
Ectopic	Pelvimetry
Hydatidiform mole	Angiography
Later—	Lymphography
Cephalometry	Venography
Longbones	
Maturity	
Associated tumours	
Large for dates	
Pelvimetry	

major hospitals are equipped. It is suggested that we cannot do worse than already achieved and are likely in fact to do very much better. This is not to deny the existing limitations which apply particularly to the study of the brain and lungs.

There is a lack of resolution which gives grounds for discontent and restriction to two-dimensional scanning is a very real drawback. It is difficult to look into the future and see in which direction the subject is likely to develop. Had I done so seventeen years ago I would have dismissed my conjectures and the success of the subject has both surprised and delighted us. Rather than prophesy one would prefer to state desirable objectives for the future. First among these must come an improved method of information storage and subsequent retrieval after a standard examination of the patient has been carried out, enabling a diagnosis to be thoughtfully prepared in her absence.[13] This is already the case with angiocardiography. The need for three-dimensional presentation and storage of echo signals is urgent and to a lesser extent grey scaling, as is already possible in television, would increase the scope of pictorial repre-

though, without the primary clinical interest of those who have been in it from the beginning, it is doubtful whether the project would have got off the ground. These days are now past, however, and it can safely be predicted that every major diagnostic unit in the civilized world will find itself of necessity equipped with this new diagnostic method within the next ten years.

ACKNOWLEDGMENTS
The University of Glasgow has set up and staffed a department of Ultrasonic Technology at the Queen Mother's Hospital, which has made continuing progress possible. Financial help on a very generous scale is also acknowledged from the Medical Research Council, the Scottish Hospital Endowments Research Trust, the Department of Health for Scotland, the Western Regional Hospital Board and from the Board of Management of the Yorkhill Associated Hospitals which administers the Queen Mother's Hospital. On the technical front special mention must be made of Mr Tom Brown of Nuclear Enterprises, Mr John Fleming and Mr Angus Hall, of the University of Glasgow, Department of Ultrasonic Technology and to Mrs Ida Miller. The co-operation from my medical colleagues, even their forebearance with mistakes, are by no means taken for granted and deserve special acknowledgment.

REFERENCES

1. Bishop, E. H. (1966) *Amer. J. Obstet. Gynec.*, **96**, 563.
2. Campbell, S. (1968) *J. Obstet. Gynaec. Brit. Cwlth.*, **75**, 568.
3. Campbell, S. (1969) *J. Obstet. Gynaec. Brit. Cwlth.*, **76**, 603.
4. Campbell, S. (1970) *J. Obstet. Gynaec. Brit. Cwlth.*, **77**, 1057.
5. Campbell, S. & Dewhurst, C. J. (1970) *Lancet*, **i**, 101.
6. Campbell, S. & Dewhurst, C. J. (1971) *Lancet*, **ii**, 1002.
7. Donald, I. (1961) *Charles J. Barone Lecture*, University of Pittsburgh.
8. Donald. I. (1963) *Brit. med. J.*, **ii**, 1154.
9. Donald, I. (1965) *Amer. J. Obstet. Gynec.*, **93**, 935.
10. Donald, I. (1965) *J. Obstet. Gynaec. Brit. Cwlth.*, **72**, 907.
11. Donald, I. (1968) *Brit. med. Bull.*, **24**, 71.
12. Donald, I. (1969) *J. Pediatr.*, **75**, 326.
13. Donald, I. (1971) *Proc. R. Soc. Med.*, **64**, 991.
14. Donald, I. & Abdulla, U. (1967) *Brit. J. Radiol.*, **40**, 604.
15. Donald, I. & Abdulla, U. (1968) *J. Obstet. Gynaec. Brit. Cwlth.*, **75**, 993.
16. Donald, I. & Brown, T. G. (1961) *Brit. J. Radiol.*, **34**, 539.
17. Donald, I., MacVicar, J. & Brown, T. G. (1958) *Lancet*, **i**, 1188.
18. Dussik, K. T. (1942) *Ztscher. Neurol.*, **172**, 153.
19. Dyson, M., Woodward, B. & Pond, J. B. (1971) *Nature*, **232**, 572.
20. Fernstrom, I. (1955) *Acta radiol (Stockh.)*, Suppl., **122**.
21. Firestone, F. A. (1945) *Metal Progr.*, p. 505.
22. Firestone, F. A. (1946) *J. Acoustical Soc. Amer.*, **17**, 287.
23. German, J. (1968) *J. Pediatr.*, **72**, 440.
24. Hellman, L. M., Duffus, G. M., Donald, I. & Sunden, B. (1970) *Lancet*, **i**, 1133.
25. Hellman, L. M., Kobayashi, M., Tolles, W. E. & Cronb, E. (1970) Ultrasonic studies on the volumetric growth of the human placenta. *Amer. J. Obstet. Gynec.*, **108**, 740.
26. Hertig, A. T. & Rock, J. (1949) *Amer. J. Obstet. Gynec.*, **38**, 968.
27. Holmes, J. H., Howry, D. H., Posakony, G. I. & Cushman, C. R. (1954) *Trans. Amer. clin. climat. Assoc.*, **66**, 208.
28. Howry, D. H. & Bliss, W. R. (1952) *J. Lab. clin. med.*, **40**, 579.
29. Jacobs, J. E. (1965). In *Biomechanics & Related Bio-engineering Topics*. Edited by R. M. Kennedi, Oxford, p. 63.
30. Johnson, W. L., Stegall, H. F., Lein, J. N. & Rushmer, R. F. (1965) *Obstet. Gynec.*, **26**, 305.
31. *Lancet*. Editorial. Safety of Sonar in Obstetrics (1970), **1**, 1158.
32. Lyons, E. (1972) *Personal communication.*
33. MacIntosh, I. J. C. & Davey, D. A. (1970) *Brit. med. J.*, **iii**, 92.
34. MacVicar, J. & Donald, I. (1963) *J. Obstet. Gynaec. Brit. Cwlth.*, **70**, 387.
35. Millar, K. G. (1966) *Brit. med. J.*, **i**, 1571.
36. Poidevin, L. O. S. (1959) *Brit. med. J.*, **ii**, 1058.
37. Robinson, H. P. (1972) *J. Obstet. Gynaec. Brit. Cwlth.*, **79**, 90.
38. Seldinger, S. J. (1953) *Acta radiol. (Stockh.)*, **39**, 368.
39. Smyth, M. G. (1966). In *Diagnostic Ultrasound*. Edited by C. G. Grossman, J. H. Holmes, C. Joyner & E. W. Purnell, p. 296. New York: Plenum Press.
40. Stewart, A., Webb, J., Giles, D. & Hewitt, D. (1956) *Lancet*, **ii**, 447.
41. Sunden, B. (1964) *Acta Obstet. Gynec. Scand.* **43**, Suppl., 6.
42. Underhill, R. A., Beazley, J. M. & Campbell, S. (1971) *Brit. med. J.*, **iii**, 736.
43. Watts, P. L., Hall, A. J. & Fleming, J. E. E. (1972) *Brit. J. Radiol.* (In press.)
44. Wild, J. J. (1950) *Surgery*, **27**, 183.
45. Willocks, J., Donald, I., Duggan, T. C. & Day, N. (1964) *J. Obstet. Gynaec. Brit. Cwlth.*, **71**, 11.
46. Willocks, J., Donald, I., Campbell, S. & Dunsmore, I. R. (1967) *J. Obstet. Gynaec. Brit. Cwlth.*, **74**, 639.
47. Willoughby, M. L. N. (1971) *Personal communication.*
48. Woodward, B., Pond, J. B. & Warwick, R. (1970) *Brit. J. Radiol.*, **43**, 719.

29. Disturbances of the Reproductive System Complicating Pregnancy

Normally in early pregnancy the uterus is anteverted, slightly anteflexed and dextro-rotated. In certain cases, the anteversion and anteflexion may be exaggerated but this calls for no treatment. On examination, the uterus feels large, globular and soft, and can be readily palpated bimanually, with two fingers of one hand in the anterior fornix and the other hand placed over the abdomen and behind the uterus. With the fingers in this position it is possible to elicit Hegar's sign which is described fully in Chapter 3.

Occasionally, it may be difficult to differentiate an early pregnancy from a fibroid tumour in the anterior wall of the uterus, or less frequently from an ovarian tumour which has become lodged in the uterovesical pouch, and may be palpated through the anterior fornix. If there is doubt about the presence of a pregnancy an immunological pregnancy test will help in the diagnosis. A pregnancy at this stage may also be seen by sonar. This technique is fully described in Chapter 3.

In the later months of pregnancy anteversion may be greatly exaggerated if the abdominal muscles are overstretched and weak. This would be especially so in multipara or in plural pregnancy: the uterus may then project forwards and when the patient stands the abdomen becomes pendulous. A pendulous abdomen is particularly noticeable in women of short stature where there is contraction of the pelvic brim. It favours malpresentation of the fetus and interferes with the engagement of the presenting part. The patient may experience considerable abdominal discomfort and backache; she may have difficulty in walking. A corset or surgical belt may support the back and give comfort.

When a pregnancy occurs following operative correction of retroversion anteflexion of the uterus may be more marked than usual and some discomfort may be felt over the course of the shortened round ligaments. Rest and sedation is required in this instance.

Retroversion and retroflexion

Malposition of the pregnant uterus during the early weeks may give rise to no symptoms.

The aetiology of these displacements is fully considered in the gynaecological section. In the pregnant woman it is hardly necessary to distinguish between retroversion and retroflexion; both are associated with the same symptoms should the gravid fundus become incarcerated in the pelvis. This tended to occur following fixation of the retroverted uterus to the pelvic floor by inflammatory disease but due to the introduction of antibiotics this is now much less common and, therefore, incarceration of the gravid uterus is seldom encountered today. Retroversion may result also from pressure exerted by a tumour of the uterus or ovary.

The retroverted gravid uterus may be discovered during vaginal examination before 12 weeks and after this time may be suspected when the fundus is not felt on abdominal palpation after 12 weeks' gestation (*see* Fig. 29.1). If the uterus is found to be retroverted before 12 weeks of pregnancy it is probably

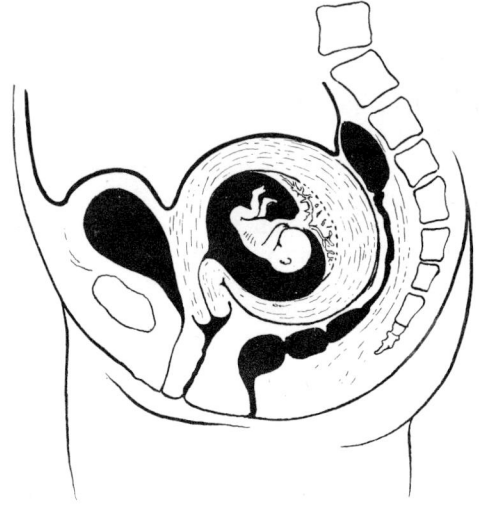

Fig. 29.1   Retroverted gravid uterus.

advantageous to insert a watch-spring pessary which will correct the retroversion. The pessary should be inserted without making a manual correction and the pressure of the device in the vagina will slowly correct the abnormal position of the uterus. The pessary can then be removed at about 16 weeks of gestation.

Incarceration of the retroverted gravid uterus

Severe symptoms may develop when the enlarged gravid uterus becomes incarcerated in the true pelvis usually about the 13th or 14th week of pregnancy.

The earliest and most characteristic symptom is dysuria which, if the displacement is not corrected, becomes more pronounced until there is complete retention with or without an overflow incontinence. The urinary disturbance is caused by pressure on the neck of the bladder and urethra by the cervix, which is displaced upwards and forwards. The obstruction is not entirely due to mechanical pressure on the urethra. Probably the cervix, pressing on the veins of the bladder, produces congestion and oedema. If pressure is prolonged there is a tendency for the bladder wall to become necrotic and infected and pus, blood and pieces of bladder mucosa may be passed or withdrawn by catheter. The increased intravesical pressure and the oedema of the ureteric orifices may predispose to ureteric reflux and pyelonephritis. This latter sequence of events should be very rare where antenatal care is adequate.

On bimanual examination an elastic swelling is found in the pouch of Douglas; the cervix may be very much drawn up behind the symphysis pubis and difficult to reach; there is an absence of the enlarged uterus above the symphysis pubis. The distended bladder may be mistaken for the pregnant uterus and the swelling in the pouch of Douglas for a tumour of uterus or ovary, or even an ectopic pregnancy. The overdistended bladder, however, is tender to palpation and the passage of a catheter will establish the diagnosis.

The diagnosis of retrodisplacement is not always easy, although it should be suspected if there is any difficulty in passing urine. It may be necessary to examine the patient under anaesthesia before a decision can be reached. Two conditions very closely resemble it: (1) tumour (ovarian or uterine) in the pouch of Douglas complicating pregnancy; (2) the sac of an ectopic pregnancy with pelvic haematocele. An ovarian cyst can usually be felt apart

from the uterus but in the case of a soft intramural fibromyoma this is more difficult.

Ectopic pregnancy with a pelvic haematocele may be very difficult to distinguish from a retrodisplaced gravid uterus. The differential diagnosis between these two conditions has been more fully considered in connection with ectopic pregnancy. It is most important that a correct diagnosis should be reached for if attempts are made to push up an ectopic sac in the pouch of Douglas, under the impression that it is a gravid uterus, the sac may be ruptured with serious consequences. In these cases, the use of the laparoscope will settle the diagnosis.

The bladder should be emptied before manipulation is attempted. If the urine is infected, an antibiotic should be commenced but the uterus should be replaced in anteversion as soon as possible. General anaesthesia will be required and the replacement can be effected by pressure upon the fundus by two fingers in the vagina with the patient in the lithotomy position, thereafter a watch-spring pessary should be inserted to keep the uterus in the correct position and this pessary should be removed at about 16 weeks of pregnancy when the uterus will be unable to fall back into the pouch of Douglas again. Only on very rare occasions should it be necessary to resort to abdominal operation to move the uterus from its incarcerated position in the pelvis.

Partial retroflexion or sacculation

This is a very rare condition in which part of the uterine body remains imprisoned in the pelvis. It may result from adhesions anchoring the fundus in the pouch of Douglas or tumours of the uterus or ovary preventing the fundus from rising.

Treatment. Where the impaction is due to tumours and especially where there are adhesions of the pouch of Douglas it may be impossible to reduce the sacculation during pregnancy. If it persists, Caesarean section is necessary at term unless symptoms are so severe as to necessitate operation sooner.

Prolapse of the uterus. The prolapse has usually existed prior to the pregnancy and, as a result of congestion brought about by the pregnancy, the symptoms may be aggravated. During the first three months of pregnancy, while the uterus is in the pelvis, the prolapse may become much worse so that the cervix projects beyond the vaginal orifice. It may become infected and this may spread to the uterine cavity and cause abortion. As the pregnancy advances and the uterus rises into the abdomen, the prolapse tends to become less marked and the cervix may be drawn up into the vagina again. Occasionally the prolapse may become very oedematous and impacted. If the patient lies flat in bed with the foot of the bed elevated, the oedema would usually become less and the cervix may then be replaced in the vagina and treated with packs soaked in flavine and glycerine or a saturated solution of magnesium sulphate. An antibiotic may be necessary if there is evidence of infection of the cervix. When the prolapse has been reduced, a plastic or watch-spring pessary will often help to maintain the uterus in good position.

In the later weeks of pregnancy the prolapse may again become more troublesome, due to the pressure exerted by the engagement of the presenting part of the fetus. In such cases bed rest may be essential. The condition gives surprisingly little trouble during labour and seldom impedes delivery.

The management of pregnancy and labour in a woman who has undergone a plastic vaginal operation for prolapse needs special care particularly if the operation has included amputation of the cervix. The membranes may rupture at any time in the third trimester of pregnancy followed soon afterwards by the onset of labour. In order to prevent this patients who have had the cervix amputated may be considered for insertion of a cervical suture early in a subsequent pregnancy. Where pregnancy proceeds to term there is much to be said for Caesarean section, this is especially so if stress incontinence was the main pre-operative symptom. Then again the cervical stump may be hard and cicatrized, and in such cases dilatation of the cervix may be slow with the eventual risk of a tear extending into the lower uterine segment.

As a rule, vaginal delivery should be planned only where the repair has been limited to the posterior vaginal wall. It may be reasonable to delay a repair operation where further child-bearing is soon intended.

OTHER COMPLICATIONS

Malformation of uterus
Extreme malformations such as uterus didelphys, in which there are two distinct uteri and vaginae, do not usually give rise to serious trouble during pregnancy. There are even cases on record where each half has become gravid and pregnancy has progressed undisturbed. Occasionally the non-gravid horn is displaced into the pouch of Douglas and interferes with the blood supply of the gravid horn, or with the passage of the child during delivery. Again fibroids of the non-gravid half may very occasionally cause complications.

The less-pronounced malformations, where there is a communication between the two halves, such as the subseptate uterus, are frequently associated with abortion or premature labour, and malpresentations are not infrequent at term. Occasionally, malformation of the fetus is encountered.

In the slightest deformity of all, the arcuate uterus, pregnancy usually progresses undisturbed but an oblique or transverse lie of the child may commonly occur.

Diagnosis. The diagnosis of malformations of the uterus complicating pregnancy is not always easy and may be overlooked. There is, of course, no difficulty in making a diagnosis if two vaginal orifices are visible. The presence of any vaginal abnormality, however, should suggest the possibility of deformity higher up the genital tract and possibly also a deformity in the urinary tract, e.g. double ureters. The presence of a second horn, normally developed or rudimentary, may simulate a single gravid uterus with a fibroid in its wall or an ovarian cyst. Malformations are apt to cause recurrent abortion, recurrent premature labour and recurrent retention of the placenta. The possibility of uterine abnormalities should be considered when any of these conditions obtain.

Treatment. No treatment is called for during pregnancy. Difficulties arise in connection with parturition and are referred to elsewhere.

A hernia of the gravid uterus between the rectus muscles or through a weak abdominal scar is very occasionally encountered. Cases have been described where the ring of the hernial sac has been so tight that there has been difficulty in replacing the uterus. Generally, however, it can be replaced and held in satisfactory position by an abdominal binder. The repair of the hernia should be postponed till a convenient time in the postnatal period.

TUMOURS COMPLICATING PREGNANCY

Tumours are not infrequent complications of pregnancy. The three commonest are:

1. Fibromyomata of the uterus,
2. Ovarian cysts,
3. Carcinoma of the cervix;
   Less commonly,
4. Solid and cystic tumours of the vagina,
5. Solid and cystic tumours of the vulva,
6. Tumours of the rectum,
7. Tumours of the bladder,
8. Tumours of bony pelvis and cellular tissue.

1. *Fibromyomata of the uterus* (*see* Fig. 29.2). The aetiology, symptomatology, diagnosis and treatment of this common neoplasm are fully

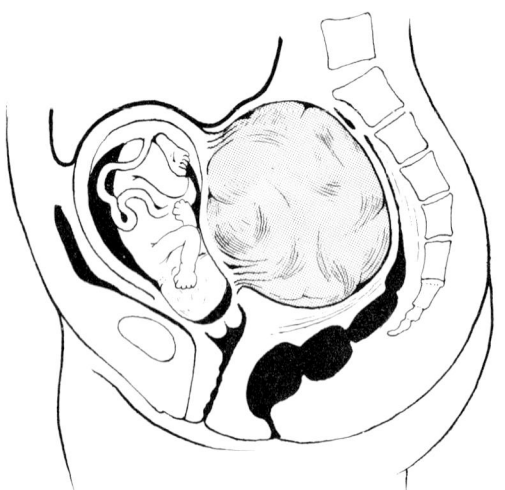

Fig. 29.2   Fibroid complicating pregnancy.

discussed in the gynaecological section. They are frequently associated with infertility but may be encountered in pregnancy. Estimates suggest that they are present in 5 per cent of pregnant women, but they are generally small and of little consequence. Larger tumours may prevent conception or predispose to abortion.

The tumours which interfere with pregnancy are generally situated in the lower part of the uterus and may project into the true pelvis. As enlargement of the uterus occurs, the tumours increase in size, partly due to hypertrophy of the muscle fibres but more especially from oedema. They, therefore, press on the surrounding parts causing dysuria,

constipation, occasional rectal tenesmus, haemorrhoids, sciatica, and unilateral oedema of the lower limbs and venous engorgement. The amount of enlargement which occurs is very variable. In pregnancy a fibroid itself may undergo degeneration. This is particularly of the red type of necrobiotic degeneration. When this occurs the tumour enlarges and becomes tender. Other symptoms are severe pain, nausea and vomiting, and frequently a rise of temperature and pulse rate. The tumour has a characteristic appearance, its cut surface resembling a raw beef steak, hence the term red degeneration. Some fibromyomata of the uterus in pregnancy are very large indeed and it is sometimes difficult to tell whether a pregnancy is present or not.

Treatment. When fibroids in the pregnant uterus cause no symptoms they should be left untreated. If pressure symptoms arise the treatment depends on the site of the fibroids. If they are only partially in the pelvis the enlarging uterus may draw them upwards into the abdominal cavity and the pressure symptoms will thus disappear. In this case, sedation and expectant treatment are all that is required. If a fibroid should become impacted in the pelvis and cause acute symptoms such as retention of urine, operation may be necessary. Every effort, however, should be made to avoid operating on the pregnant uterus. A myomectomy may be done in the early months but this is very likely to result in abortion and every effort should be made by expectant treatment to continue the pregnancy until the fetus is viable when Caesarean section may be performed in the later months.

If it is certain that pain is due to red degeneration of the fibroid in pregnancy, expectant treatment should be given even in the presence of acute symptoms. Diagnosis, however, may be difficult where the fibroid is situated in an area which makes the symptoms resemble appendicitis, cholecystitis, or torsion of an ovarian cyst or a strangulated hernia. Pyelitis of pregnancy and, in some cases, abruptio placenta may have to be excluded. When the diagnosis has been established, sedation may be required. This should be in the form of pethidine or omnopon. It is very important in these cases to avoid operation since frequently the patient is an older primigravida with a history of infertility in which the pregnancy will be likely to be her only one. If the acute symptoms do not settle, in spite of intensive palliative treatment, an operation becomes necessary, myomectomy or even hysterectomy may be required. The choice of operation will depend on the nature and extent of the tumours and such other considerations as the parity of the patient or her future desires as to further children. In the primigravidae, myomectomy is the operation of choice but there is a high incidence of abortion following this operation. The patient should, therefore, be kept well sedated in the post-operative phase in an effort to prevent this complication.

Fibroids may also complicate labour especially when they are situated in the lower part of the uterus when they will tend to impede the descent of the head and obstruct labour (see Fig. 29.2). In these cases, the incidence of retained placenta is greater and there is also an increased liability of post-partum haemorrhage due to interference in the mechanism of uterine contraction due to the presence of the fibroid.

When a fibroid is subject to undue pressure during the course of labour or at delivery necrosis and sometimes infection may result. It is also possible for infection to occur later in the puerperium. These complications should be anticipated and with the help of chemotherapy can often be prevented.

2. Ovarian and parovarian tumours (see Fig. 29.3).

All varieties of ovarian tumour may complicate pregnancy and labour. The most common,

however, are cystic in nature. They may be discovered accidentally or only after serious complications have arisen. The most frequent and serious complication of ovarian cysts is torsion. This usually occurs in the first trimester but the cyst may rupture and extrude its contents into the peritoneal cavity during labour. The most troublesome tumour is the dermoid which, being a heavy tumour, is usually situated in the pouch of Douglas and thus prevents descent of the head during labour. When rupture of a dermoid occurs this may be followed by peritonitis. Torsion causes symptoms such as sudden abdominal pain, sickness and collapse and this occurs in about 15 per cent of all ovarian tumours complicating pregnancy. The presence of an ovarian tumour in the pelvis should always be considered in differential diagnosis of failure of the head to descend in labour for no apparent reason.

When an ovarian tumour is diagnosed early in pregnancy it should be removed preferably about 16 weeks' gestation. Although the chances of abortion or premature labour may be increased by the operation this danger is small compared with that of possible torsion or rupture of the cyst. There is a relatively high incidence of abortion following excision of an ovarian cyst during the earlier part of pregnancy. If discovered in the later months of pregnancy it may be desirable to postpone operation until the child is mature. Caesarean section may then be performed and, immediately after this, removal of the cyst may be undertaken.

Malignant ovarian neoplasms are rare in pregnancy. If a tumour is discovered at the time of laparotomy or if disease is widespread the treatment is the same as in the non-pregnant patient. There is no place for allowing the pregnancy to continue in the suspected presence of a malignant ovarian tumour. Other growths which may resemble ovarian tumours are the pelvic ectopic kidney, a rare complication of pregnancy, an enlarged spleen or even an echinococcal cyst may occasionally be found in the pelvis.

3. Carcinoma of the cervix

The diagnosis and treatment of carcinoma of the cervix is considered in the gynaecological section. Here we are concerned with the tumour as it occurs during pregnancy.

Carcinoma in situ. Where carcinoma *in situ* is suspected during pregnancy the condition

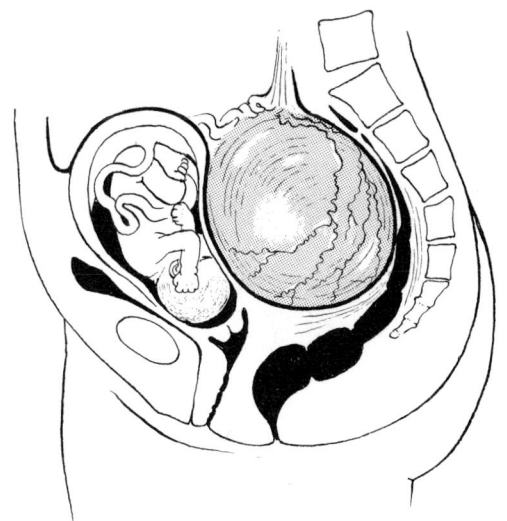

Fig. 29.3 Ovarian cyst complicating pregnancy.

should be treated expectantly until delivery has been completed. Such patients, however, should have cervical smears done regularly during their pregnancies. If the grading of the smear becomes more severe and the suspicion of invasion is strong a cone biopsy of the cervix may be necessary during the pregnancy to confirm that the lesion is non-invasive. If a cone biopsy is done in pregnancy it is of advantage to insert a cervical suture at the same time as the cone biopsy is performed.

Invasive cancer of the cervix. In many clinics, routine cervical smears are taken in the antenatal period. This is a procedure to be recommended rather than performing the smear at the post-natal clinic from which there are many defaulters. These patients are usually the very ones who would benefit most by having cytology performed. The diagnosis of invasive cancer of the cervix can be missed in pregnancy unless this possibility is always kept in mind as a cause of vaginal discharge or bleeding. The carcinoma of the cervix may cause bleeding in the later weeks of pregnancy and give rise to a diagnosis of placental praevia or abruptio placentae. It is, therefore, essential that in all cases of bleeding during pregnancy speculum examination and cervical cytology should be performed if this has not already been done when the patient is first seen.

Where the carcinoma is already invasive, the cervix will bleed when touched and may feel irregular and hard even when symptoms are of short duration. When the disease is advanced, portions of tissue may be detached by the examining finger.

Treatment. The treatment of carcinoma of the cervix in pregnancy is essentially the same as in the non-pregnant state. The disease should be treated without regard to the pregnancy unless it is first discovered in the later stages of pregnancy. If the infant is alive at the time of diagnosis the pregnancy can be prolonged for a few weeks without altering the prognosis, but treatment of the cancer should normally be given priority. Delay in pregnancy may lessen the chances of permanent cure.

Stage I carcinoma is probably best treated by radical hysterectomy and lymphadenectomy, the uterus having first been emptied by hysterotomy in the second trimester and by Caesarean section in the third. All other stages are probably best treated by radium and external radiation after uterine evacuation.

However, good results have also been reported when all cases were treated by radium and external radiation. The treatment of carcinoma of the cervix is fully described in a previous chapter.

4. *Solid and cystic tumours of the vagina*

These growths are relatively uncommon, but fibroids of the anterior and posterior walls and cystic tumours situated more laterally are occasionally encountered. These tumours are fully considered in Chapter 10. They are very easily recognized by vaginal examination as smooth growths projecting into the lumen of the vagina. They occasionally interfere with the descent of the fetal head. In general, it is better to remove them when they are recognized if it looks as if they are going to obstruct labour. If removed during parturition, the wound in the vagina may extend during descent of the child and become infected. If the tumour is diagnosed for the first time late in pregnancy or during labour, Caesarean section should be performed and the tumour removed as a cold procedure at a later date. When the tumour is situated on the anterior wall, special care must be exercised to avoid damage to the urethra or bladder and, in these cases, Caesarean section may be the optimum method of delivery.

5. *Solid and cystic tumours of the vulva*

The tumours of the vulva occasionally encountered in pregnancy are those described in Chapter 10. They cause very little disturbance to pregnancy but occasionally they may interfere with delivery. They should be removed when recognized.

Bartholin's gland, which is placed posterolaterally at the base of the labium majus, may

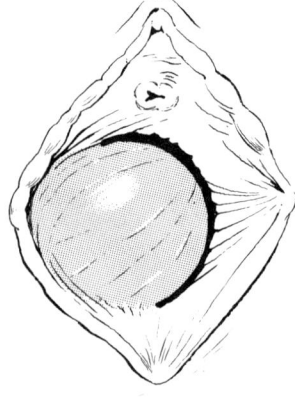

Fig. 29.4   Abscess of Bartholin's gland.

become infected and form a large abscess (*see* Fig. 29.4). It should be incised and chemotherapy given. Marsupialization or excision can then be performed later.

6. *Tumours of the colon and rectum*

This is a very rare complication. The tumour is generally a carcinoma, which may assume considerable dimensions before it is recognized. If the condition is operable, a radical operation should be performed: if it is inoperable, the pregnancy may be allowed to continue. There are a few cases now on record in which the pregnancy has continued undisturbed after a radical operation. If in doubt about the operability, it is probably best to perform laparotomy and attempt to remove the tumour.

7. *Tumours of the bladder*

Tumours and calculi in the bladder are very seldom seen in pregnant women. The principles of management are the same as those for other tumours described above.

8. *Tumours of the bony pelvis and cellular tissue*

Tumours arising from the pelvic bones and the pelvic cellular tissue are rare in pregnancy. Fibromas, osteomas, chondromas, carcinomas and sarcomas of the pelvis have been described. These sometimes grow large and become cystic. Chondromas are most common. The pelvis may also be deformed by bony outgrowths. These exostoses are usually found on the posterior surface of the symphysis, in front of the sacro-iliac joints and on the anterior surface of the sacrum.

Tumours and exostoses may obstruct the progress of labour and Caesarean section is usually necessary for delivery.

Carcinoma of the breast in pregnancy and lactation. Carcinoma of the breast is infrequent during pregnancy and lactation but when it does develop it is a much more malignant disease. Approximately one-third of patients who have mastectomy for carcinoma of the breast during pregnancy or lactation survive five years (Haagensen, 1967).

The accurate determination of the clinical stage of advancement of breast cancer is essential. If advanced disease is present—the majority—these patients all die whatever treatment is given. If axillary metastases are found at radical mastectomy, cure is unlikely.

The percentage of survivors in women whose carcinoma developed during pregnancy or lactation is less than half that in non-pregnant women of similar age.

Published data are inadequate to decide on the value of termination of pregnancy. If the disease is in the early stage with no axillary metastasis, it may not be necessary to interrupt the pregnancy if the child is much desired. Interruption may, however, have a palliative value and may prolong the life of the mother when cure seems unlikely.

If the disease is discovered in early pregnancy, it is reasonable to terminate as early as possible. If the pregnancy is far advanced and palliation is questionable the pregnancy might be allowed to continue but the decision must be determined by the circumstances of each case. Young patients with treated Stage I lesions need not avoid pregnancy (Cooper and Butterfield, 1970).

REFERENCES

Cooper, D. R. & Butterfield, J. (1971) *Ann. Surg.*, **171**, 429.
Haagensen, C. D. (1967) *Ann. J. Obstet. Gynaec.*, **98**, 141.

30. Psychological, Psychosomatic and Psychiatric Aspects

INTRODUCTION

It is generally agreed that psychological factors play an important part in health and disease and that they should always be taken into account in good medical practice. These factors must therefore be studied systematically and not set aside as simply 'common sense'. Emotions are among the factors most relevant in this context since these are always accompanied by manifest physical changes. Thus, even in these normal and natural situations encountered by most women—the menarche, marriage and the menopause—it is the emotional significance of the occasion that will make for healthy adjustment or a state of ill-health. (In like manner, in the everyday stresses that assail the average woman, emotional reactions may be shown primarily as disorders of genito-urinary function.)

The psychological approach goes beyond the objective facts of the case—the signs and symptoms, the past medical history, the family and social history—to the meaning of these facts for the individual patients. Thus the doctor must acquaint himself with the inner life of thought and feeling of his patient.

While the 'whole person' approach to the patient is the foundation to all good medical practice, nowhere is this more relevant than in obstetrics and gynaecology. It is, therefore, necessary not only to consider the pathology of particular tissues or the malfunctioning of organs, but to consider the human being as unique with a distinctive past experience living in a unique family situation and subject to the pressures and expectations of a certain culture.

This chapter focuses attention upon the patient as a person. It describes how to approach and understand the patient, how emotional stress affects bodily function and illustrates the commoner disorders encountered in this field. The reader should not regard the psychological approach as some-thing detached from the main theme of this book or requiring specialist experience, nor should it be imagined that there is any fundamental clash between the physical and the psychological approaches; in other words, the doctor must not try to make up his mind in any given case whether it is 'genuinely physical' or 'merely psychological'. A blend of the two gives, as it were, a stereoscopic view of the case.

The chapter is divided into three sections—Psychological, Psychosomatic and Psychiatric.

The psychological section attempts to sketch in the relevant background different types of women and the way in which healthy development may be brought about. This is essentially a brief study of personality and its development in the family and social setting.

It is hoped that the psychological section will enable the reader to appreciate in any given case how a woman is likely to face and react to the various stresses peculiar to women and the meaning attached to them. For example, each person tends to react in a characteristic way to these various life stresses. Just as homeostatic mechanisms come into play to cope with somatic change or injury, so psychological mechanisms operate to deal with alterations in the psycho-social environment. Many of these processes have been laid down in early life or are present at birth, depending on constitutional and hereditary factors. It is because so much is learned in the short period of infancy and in the intimate relationship with the mother or mother substitute that this period will be given detailed attention.

In the psychosomatic section more detailed attention is paid to the particular emotional states that are present in association with somatic dysfunctioning. It is in this section that a 'monistic' approach is most helpful. Here the terms 'psychological' and 'physical' are best regarded as two aspects of the same basic process. In other words, it is most helpful to think of emotional states and somatic dys-functioning as *correlated* and not to think of one state *causing* the other. Much confusion in theory and practice has arisen from a failure to keep this distinction clearly in mind.

The final section 'psychiatric' deals with overt psychiatric and personality disorders encountered in obstetric and gynaecological practice. There are few conditions that are unique to obstetrics and gynaecology but certain modifications, both in the clinical picture and in actual management, must be recognized.

PSYCHOLOGICAL ASPECTS

Personality and its development

For a proper understanding of psychological disturbances, it is necessary to have a sound knowledge of the way in which the individual person develops his particular characteristics through the interaction of biological, psychological and social factors. A study of this kind is essentially a study of biography. A good biography always takes into account the antecendents of the individual subject, his development through various stages of childhood, youth and adulthood and the particular environmental influences that have been brought to bear at different times in his life. It is sometimes the case that the life history of an individual is best understood from the point of view of his hereditary predisposition. It is as though some destiny determines the important events in his life, and that he had no chance, whatever the circumstances, of avoiding this destiny. Clearly in such cases inherited characteristics play a dominant part. In other cases the opportunities, or the lack of them, at critical moments play a more significant part. While, therefore, either heredity or environment may predominate in certain cases, it is most common to find an interplay of these two factors in most people.

The study of biography also implies a study of individual differences. Thus even at birth particular characteristics of babies can be recognized. For example, level of activity, irritability, sensory threshold, liability to boredom, sucking behaviour, sleep patterns and responsiveness to other humans. It is remarkable to observe that many of these distinguishing features seen at birth persist as behaviour patterns that can still be recognized several years later.

Compared with lower animals, human behaviour appears to be much more flexible and adaptable and less constrained by inbuilt patterns. However, these latter patterns can be most readily observed in certain particular respects. Intelligence, that is to say the capacity to learn, is one such aspect. This is particularly the case with those of low intellectual endowment and of poor general physique. For example, a woman of low intelligence may present several types of problem, such as an inability to observe simple hygienic principles leading to minor states of physical disability. There will be a lack of understanding of the aims and methods of contraception or the responsibilities of marriage and motherhood. There would also be the problem of co-operation, both in giving a clear history and in playing her part in treatment.

The studies of Gesell, Piaget and such psychoanalysts as Freud, Bowlby and Erikson, have shown that the individual passes through fairly clear-cut stages of intellectual, social and emotional development. They point out that certain factors aid this development and others may retard it.

For example *Gesell* has considered human development as basically an unfolding of those basic patterns present at birth allowing for progressively more complex patterns of functioning to occur as the brain and central nervous system grow and new events are experienced.

Jean *Piaget* also stresses the maturational aspects but concentrates greater attention on the organization of incoming sense data and comparing these data with those already accumulated in the memory store. Development is thus a continuous process of recognizing the familiar in that which appears to be new and adapting to this new information appropriately. It should be made clear that Piaget has concentrated more particularly on the development of thought processes and of understanding the external world at a conscious, intellectual level.

Learning theory approaches are by contrast concerned with the way in which the child responds to external situations by a series of processes having their origin in the classic conditioning of Pavlov. Thus learning takes place by a system of rewards and punishments. No attempt is made to understand what is happening within the individual and the central nervous system which is described as a 'black box'. This is an approach antipathetic to that of e.g. neurophysiology concerned almost wholly with these internal events but from the experimental point of view it has the advantage that the incoming information (input) can be measured in various ways and the response to this information (output) can be similarly measured. Learning theory at its present state of development seems to have established itself more securely in the study of animal behaviour, where inner experience and language play little or no part, than in humans where these factors are of the greatest importance.

The *psychoanalytic approach* has characteristically laid greater emphasis on emotional development and indeed on psychosexual development in its broadest sense. These approaches will, therefore, be dealt with later under the heading of the nature of sexuality.

A sound understanding of personality development is, therefore, essential in making a proper formulation of the problem in the individual patient.

A special feature of the psychological approach to the patient is that she is not seen in isolation. The whole person is seen as living within the context of a family and of society in general. This means that a study of *personal relationships* is essential. In any medical setting this study would, therefore, have to include a thorough understanding of the doctor/patient relationship and the meaning of ill-health on the part of the patient.

A pregnancy or physical illness can be regarded as a crisis in a woman's life, superimposed on the more gradual trends of the female life cycle. She is supported (and sometimes hindered) in this crisis by friends, relatives and also those in the medical sphere.

She also brings her own repertoire of coping mechanisms which are part of her distinctive personality pattern. It will, therefore, be seen that a knowledge of the more enduring patterns of reaction in the individual woman is of value not only in dealing with the present situation, but in predicting future behaviour and the outcome of any particular crisis. The questions that one should ask would include: 'What are her strengths?', 'What are her psychological weaknesses?' 'What are the special stresses playing upon her now?' 'Why has she made contact with the medical profession at this particular point in time and with these particular complaints?'

Answers to these and other similar questions will throw light on the way in which a woman will cope with a serious illness. One might react by a characteristic denial and repression of all feeling. Another may react with anger and hostility often directed at medical and nursing staff. Yet another may show an extreme degree of anxiety either for herself or for those close to her.

Psychosexual development

The most pertinent aspect of development so far as obstetrics and gynaecology is concerned is that within the psychosexual sphere. It is, therefore, necessary to go into this aspect in greater detail.

1. *Establishment of gender identity*
This aspect of development is best considered as a state of learning experience taking place against the background of hormonal and other physical effects. Most human societies place considerable emphasis on the sex of the individual. Being a female will carry certain obligations and prohibitions. In spite of movements towards a greater degree of opportunity for women in modern society, it still remains the case that more restraints and restrictions are placed on opportunities for women than is the case for men. Because of the different values placed on males and females, there is often psychological concern on the part of parents expecting a child whether that child will be male or female. For example an inadequate parent of either sex may wish the child to belong to his or her sex as a kind of fulfilment of lost opportunities and ambitions.

After the *social sex or gender* have been assigned to the individual, usually on the basis of the morphology of the external genitalia, it is officially registered and broadcast to friends and relatives. Thus from a very early age this assignment of social sex or gender exercises a profound effect on future development. It is probably the case that no individual is completely certain of his or her gender and particularly at a later stage such questions as 'Am I a proper woman?' are often posed.

Genetic sex is determined at fertilization by the chromosomes and the early embryo is basically female in morphology. Unless a specific embryonic organizer associated with the 'Y' chromosome begins to act and androgens are present, it will continue as a female even if gonadal tissue is removed. There is growing evidence from animal experiments that the presence of appropriate hormones at critical periods in embryonic life, possibly in infancy, affects brain functioning and both sexual attitudes and behaviour. For example, male patterns of pituitary functioning can be produced in female rats by testerone injections within four days of birth. Furthermore there is also evidence that patterns of sexual behaviour in the adult animal can be influenced by these early sensitizing injections of hormones. There is, therefore, understandable speculation that human sexual deviation, including homosexuality, might be due to anomalous hormonal sensitization in intra-uterine life.

Besides these manifest effects of hormones on sexual behaviour and attitude, sexual deviation in humans remains for the most part a baffling problem. For example, some individuals with clear-cut biological (including gonadal) sex which coincides with their assigned sex, nevertheless believe from an early age that they are members of the opposite sex. They may dress accordingly and request appropriate treatment, including operations to change their external genital characteristics. This is the condition of transsexualism.

In the case of the true hermaphrodite who possesses both male and female secondary sex characteristics, he will usually and consistently maintain the sexual attitudes and behaviour of those which have been assigned to him/her at birth. This strongly supports the view that social factors may be as important as biological factors in determining gender but Stoller has reported a number of cases which appeared to be transsexualists in early life (that is to say they believed they were members of the opposite sex) who in later life actually developed those secondary sex characteristics to which they had felt entitled from birth.

The gender assigned to an individual must, as already indicated, be assigned within an interpersonal and social context and particularly in western civilization the common factors between the sexes far outweigh the differences in daily life. In the areas of work, artistic achievement, sport, dress, language and so forth, it is often impossible to identify maleness or femaleness. Indeed there is to be found examples of 'role reversal' where men perform functions that formerly have been exclusively carried out by women and vice versa.

2. *The nature of sexuality*

From the psychological viewpoint, sexuality developing through its various stages to adulthood manifests itself in many ways and is experienced by the individual by a wide range of emotional responses, from the pleasurable to the unpleasurable, the good to the bad. In consequence it has now been generally accepted that the sex drive is present at birth and gradually develops throughout the first sixteen years or so of life until, in maturity, it assumes its appropriate role in mating. It is the drive which seeks temporary and repeated satisfactions in genital orgasm, less transient satisfactions in pregnancy and labour, and more enduring satisfactions in lactation and in parenthood.

But it is not only individual satisfaction that is sought: the sex drive establishes relationships between the individual and external objects—both human and non-human. The energy serving these functions is termed *libido*. In early life libido is diffused throughout the body so that sexual gratification may be achieved by stimulation applied to any bodily part. In the first year of life, the mouth zone is the most sensitive and later the anal region becomes erogenous. Gradually, libido becomes centred on the genital organs, for the adult the primary means of sexual expression. Correspondingly, libido at first seeks gratification in an indiscriminate relationship with any object in the environment, but later it becomes the more discriminating until only a single member of the opposite sex becomes the object of desire. The child, by nature promiscuous and fickle, develops into the mature, socially responsible adult.

Psychosexual development does not always proceed along a smooth and uncomplicated path. Most individuals in our culture are, in some degree, retarded and repressed sexually. The dictates of reality in the form of taboos, prohibitions and frustrations are such that libido is often prevented from natural expression. It becomes transformed into other kinds of energy, notably aggressiveness. It is probably true that every healthy adult is normally endowed with libidinal energy. Therefore if he has not attained the state in which this energy can have some degree of natural adult expression, it will be expressed in some less satisfactory ways. In women this will often take the form of physical symptoms, presenting commonly as dyspareunia, dysmenorrhoea, premenstrual tension and frigidity. When these symptoms are encountered, some significant interference with the normal and natural development of the sex instinct may be found.

The factors which most often retard the normal development of emotional and, in particular, psychosexual maturity are parental disharmony, parental deprivation, over-protection and traumatic experiences.

It follows, conversely, that unfavourable emotional attitudes in individuals whose psychosexual development has been retarded by adverse factors can be prevented when favourable circumstances operate in the child's life. Emotional development can be promoted most by a secure home life and by proper education in sexual matters.

Basic emotional attitudes laid down in early life are determined in large measure by the parents. The child's first love is the mother. All later loves derive their character from this experience. Where the relationship is unsatisfactory by reason of strain, anxiety, rejection, neglect or separation, the individual's capacity for love is reduced. Where the relationship is satisfactory and the bond of affection strong, the individual is able, as development proceeds, to make new contacts with confidence, gradually moving from a state of infantile dependence, characterized by an attitude of taking, to a state of mature dependence (but not of independence, which is an adolescent transitional state), characterized by an attitude of giving.

Sex education should be an integral part of general development and learning. It is not sufficient that the child should have a knowledge of sex—however acquired—but that attitudes towards sex are healthy and natural. While it is necessary to acquaint the child with the 'facts of life' it is also necessary to enlighten the child under the best emotional conditions. For this reason it is always best for the parents to be the educators. The child is naturally curious and wants to be let into parental sexual secrets. While it would be merely a routine procedure for a teacher or a doctor to give a sex lecture, it is an act of confidence for a mother to tell her daughter something of her own experience. Ideally, sex education should be a 'running commentary' throughout the child's life and right through adolescence. When curiosity is aroused and questions are asked the parent should answer fully, frankly and honestly, and in as much detail as it is thought the child will understand. In this way sex will be looked upon objectively as part of the serious business of living and a topic which requires thought, discussion and planning. As no sexual experience should be sudden, the child should be given ample preparation for coming events, such as the menarche. Parents who make a secret of sex and attempt to conceal from their children the fact that they have sexual experiences are in reality afraid of their own natures. This fear is communicated to the children and perpetuates distorted attitudes. The true foundations for sex education are to be found in a stable home life, in a positive love relationship between sexual partners and in a responsible attitude to living.

3. Puberty and menstruation

The period of development from the dependant infant to the young girl experiencing her first menstruation need not be detailed in this chapter since it is of less direct relevance to the understanding of individual gynaecological or obstetric problems. Undoubtedly the next most important period in the life of the girl is that of puberty.

At this stage there are fairly rapid bodily changes and heightened sexual awareness not only within the girl herself but in her relation to other people, particularly those of the opposite sex. These changes have taken place during the relative quiescence since childhood but evidence does not suggest that the so-called 'latency period' in the later phase of childhood before puberty is devoid of significant experiences of an emotional and sexual nature.

The menarche is best understood as occurring within the context of general adolescent experience. It is undoubtedly a period of general turbulence and change. Relationship with parents changes with the seeking of greater independence from them. Close identification with members of the same sex in peer groups play an important part in preparing the young girl for more direct relationships with members of the opposite sex. This is a period when the girl thinks deeply about her own identity and her place in the world. Problems concerning future career and marriage slowly assert themselves. It is the phase of mood swings, sudden enthusiasms and rebelliousness whether shown by behaviour unacceptable to the older generation or by private reflection upon parental and authority attitudes which may be rejected or radically modified.

The onset of the menses is one of life's normal crises. It indicates the onset of womanhood and heralds the capacity for childbearing. The kind of preparation for this crisis will play a crucial part in later sexual attitudes. In particular the way in which the mother relates to her daughter during this time is crucial.

In modern society it is probably the case that the majority of women are prepared for the menses. Shipman (1964) found that 65 per cent of 131 women studied were prepared for the menses but only 50 per cent were actually told about sex. However, it is almost certain that girls pick up this information (sometimes distorted) from various friends and acquaintances and from what she reads.

The menarche provides the opportunity for the mother to express her feelings about menstruation and of being a woman. This gives a clue to her own sexual attitudes and in particular her attitude to her own daughter. Negative attitudes may be implanted by the mother (or others) as 'a curse', 'being unwell', 'getting rid of bad blood' and so forth. Psychoanalysis has brought to light the close relation that exists in the phantasy life of women between menstruation and the other excretory functions of urination and defacation. This throws some light on feelings of disgust about sexual matters as 'dirty' or 'unclean'. Often this is the occasion for an over-anxious and over-protective mother to give repeated warnings about boys. It may be represented as a disability and a disadvantage that women suffer from compared to men.

That the menarche is for the most part looked on with disfavour is suggested by the fact that Shainess (1961) found only 15 per cent of mothers in the series she studied had reacted with pleasure to the daughter's menarche.

More healthy adjustment to sex is experienced if there is adequate preparation, factual information about hygiene and other practical details and that it is looked upon as part of normal growing up. It is a time when mother and daughter can come closer together as women though occasionally if their relationship has been negative or ambivalent, it may cause further deterioration with heightened feelings of envy on the part of the mother and a check in the daughter's normal development.

It should not be overlooked that the relationship with the father plays an important part at this stage. The daughter can no longer be easily regarded by him as a little girl. She may be seen as a sexually attractive woman, perhaps reminding him of his own wife when young. The menarche may, therefore, give rise to quite abrupt changes in the father's behaviour towards his daughter. He may become more distant, restrictive or over-protective as the defence against his own feelings.

It cannot at this stage be stated what is 'normal' throughout the menstrual cycle but while the study of sexual activity in lower animals indicates that this is closely controlled by hormones, in human subjects psychological and social factors play a much more important part.

4. *Adult sexuality*

The particular features of adult sexuality are that it is directed consistently towards members of the opposite sex and with time narrows down to the choice of a mate, thus bringing together the sex drive and those of home-building, child-bearing and rearing. It is, therefore, impossible to consider adult sexuality in isolation from these other inter-personal and social experiences. However, it would not be appropriate to expand on these latter topics in this chapter and, therefore, as far as possible only the sexual attitudes and behaviour will be described.

The relation between hormonal change and sexual behaviour has already been described. However, so far as experience of human coitus and orgasm are concerned, Udry and Morris have found that these are high at the mid-cycle, that there is a post-ovulatory trough followed by a further rise in the pre-menstrual period. Waxenberg found no change in responsiveness after ovariectomy or in the post-menopausal period associated with low oestrogen levels. Kinsey has described coitus and orgasm still occurring in elderly women some in their eighties and one in her nineties. However, Waxenberg describes women who have undergone adrenalectomy or hypophysectomy as having experienced complete loss of sexual desire and relates this to lack of androgens previously supplied by the adrenal cortex.

The meaning of sexuality in the adult woman has been strongly influenced by early experience and learning. For example, sexual curiosity or sexual display discovered by parents or authority figures may be punished strongly thus giving rise to sexual repression and the emergence of neurotic symptoms designed to defend the individual against any kind of sexual arousal. In extreme form this is manifested in a total taboo on sex.

Child victims of sexual assaults may also experience high anxiety levels, particularly if the parents have also reacted to this experience by undue anxiety and over-protection. The close connection between sexuality and feelings of disgust have already been described.

If the earlier life of the woman has been characterized by secure experiences of love and affection and if the male partner responds in a stable and appropriate manner, healthy responses would be expected and more understanding and tolerant attitudes will be displayed to the whole subject.

Masters and Johnson have in recent years carried out a series of intensive direct studies of sexual activity in human volunteers. These studies have been concerned both with coitus and with auto-stimulation. They describe the sexual response cycle both for males and females as passing through four different phases: (1) phase of excitement, (2) plateau phase, (3) phase of orgasm, (4) resolution.

The excitement phase can be produced fairly readily by a variety of physical and/or psychological stimuli. If the stimuli and the situation are acceptable to the individual and effective arousal continues, a marked rise in muscle tension and vasocongestion takes place, leading to a sustained high level of sexual tension in the plateau phase. Depending on both the nature of the stimuli and the person's individual characteristics, orgasm may supervene, and a rapid release of the heightened tension and vaso-congestion take place accompanied by a widespread discharge of neural impulses through the spinal cord and feelings of pleasure. A much more gradual reduction of the tension then takes place in the resolution phase associated with a tired but relaxed sensation. Following resolution there is a refractory period for the male which may last for some hours, but the female in contrast is capable of multiple orgasms in rapid succession.

The full sequence described above may be interrupted for the woman at several points. If the initial stimulation is unacceptable, the excitement phase may be short lived or move into a resolution phase without progressing to the plateau. In turn, orgasm can be prevented from developing from the plateau phase if sexual stimulation is not sufficiently prolonged or effective (as in premature ejaculation by the male) or if the situation is psychologically unacceptable. A very prolonged resolution phase with continuing vasocongestion and tension may then occur—possibly the basis of the so-called pelvic congestion syndrome.

It has long been thought that stimulation of the clitoris represented a different and probably more immature form of orgasm than stimulation of the vagina. However the observations of Masters and Johnson indicate that they represent essentially the same process. The various changes during sexual excitement are identical regardless of whether the clitoris or the vagina is stimulated. Here again psychological aspects must not be underemphasized since women vary markedly in their sexual knowledge and their expectations, particularly if clitoral stimulation has been regarded in the past with pain, disgust or excessive guilt.

Masters and Johnson also stress that the successful sexual cycle is dependent to a large extent on mutuality between male and female.

Sexual variations

As already indicated, patterns of sexual behaviour are determined to a considerable extent by culture and society. Ford and Beach have shown that there is variation by class, society and historical period. Even within the same class and at the same point in time there is considerable variation, thus confirming that there is no 'normal' or 'healthy' sexual relationship as such. It is as well to make this point clear in order to overcome the almost universal anxiety on the part of sexual partners that they may be in some respect failing in their proper performance. In a stable marital situation for example much is learned over a period of weeks or months from each partner by the other and 'experimenting' is possibly more common than undeviating repetition. During the early months of the sexual relationship each partner brings to the situation much that is immature or even irrelevant and there is a tendency towards self indulgence at this time. Later these earlier sexual patterns are incorporated in more mature activity with the aim of giving satisfaction and pleasure to the partner.

While it is true to say that there are considerable variations within everyday sexual behaviour, abnormal deviations do occur and these will be dealt with in the section concerned with psychiatric disorders. However it is sometimes difficult in the individual case to make a clear distinction between what is normal and acceptable and that which is abnormal and requires appropriate treatment.

Contraception and family planning

As indicated in other sections of this textbook contraceptive methods and family planning have brought about very considerable changes in sexual behaviour of women and attitudes towards intercourse and childbearing. Important issues related to a population control, pre-marital and extra-marital sex, avoidance of unwanted children and the precise economics of childbearing and rearing have all become involved.

Despite the introduction of many new and simple methods studies (for example those of McCance and Hall) have indicated wide variations in sex education even among those of above-average ability and formal education.

To some extent there has been failure on the part of girls and young women to learn about contraception. Equally there have been failures among parents and educators in providing the necessary knowledge but it is by no means clear as yet that those who are most knowledgeable are at the same time those who most consistently employ effective contraceptive methods. If sexual education is badly given (for example in the wrong circumstances or by the wrong person) difficulties are bound to arise. Similarly a young person learning about contraception for the first time when undergoing a period of personal instability may react with anxiety and denial of what she has learned. Even with an adequate amount of knowledge it has been shown that the intentions of women are not necessarily correlated with their contraceptive practice.

Many young unmarried women, despite their knowledge about contraception, reject it as artificial or as coming between them in a way that destroys the spontaneity of the relationship.

It is clear that both conscious and unconscious motives are involved in the use of contraceptives and for this reason a thorough understanding of the personality and psychology of the individual woman is necessary before offering appropriate advice or supplying the most suitable device.

In practice many women who start a course of contraception do not persist. For example Herzberg and Draper (1970) in a series of 218 women found that 25 per cent discontinued oral contraceptives due to their side effects. Thirteen per cent discontinued the use of the intra-uterine device because of breakthrough bleeding. A not uncommon side effect from the use of high progesterone content pills is that of depression, headaches, change in sleeping pattern, loss of libido and capacity for orgasm being the principal symptoms. A few instances of psychosis associated with the pill have been reported. The clincal picture is that of an acute schizophrenic like illness often with a previous history of post-partum disorder (Daly, Kane, Ewing, 1967). The interesting finding of Herzberg and Coppen (1970), is that women who stopped taking the pill tended to be those with previous psychiatric illness, pre-menstrual depression, who had been depressed in previous pregnancies, or who had had treatment with anti-depressants at some previous date. Rodgers and Ziegler (1968) by contrast showed that women who had always enjoyed sex and those used to controlling their own lives tended to continue with the pill. Many women appeared to make better sexual adaptation when on the pill than previously, that is to say their sex life was improved, there was less depression and irritability.

Another approach to contraception is that of *vasectomy* for the male. This has recently been permitted within the National Health Service. The main indication is that the man is happily married, is emotionally stable and that both he and his wife are satisfied that they have completed their family. It is as yet too early to make comparisons between this method employed by the male and those employed by the female but not unnaturally at the present time many women (and indeed men) entertain irrational fears of this method as being equated with castration or at the least the loss of masculine characteristics. At the present time some wives prefer their own sterilization to the husband having a vasectomy.

Pregnancy

Pregnancy is undoubtedly an important phase in a woman's life especially when it is the first. For the primigravida it represents a new experience and a transition to full womanhood. To some it is the fulfilment of a 'biological destiny'.

There are both positive and negative attitudes to an existing pregnancy: for some it is the means of a long desired end, for others, especially the unmarried, it may be seen as a personal tragedy.

Attitudes to pregnancy—as we have seen in the case of contraception—vary according to circumstances and the personality characteristics of the woman. Unconscious fears and phantasies play their part so too does the psychological mechanisms of identification in which the pregnant woman becomes almost totally involved with the experience of other women, such as her mother, elder sisters or friends.

A vivid contrast in attitudes is seen when some women wish only for the experience of pregnancy, but do not want to have a child, whereas others dread the prospects of pregnancy and labour wishing only for a child.

The physical manifestations of advanced pregnancy are accepted by some as normal, paraded in an exhibitionist manner by others and experienced as acute embarrassment by others again. In the last century, embarrassment among 'respectable' people led to the term 'confinement'.

A pregnancy may be *unwanted*, but it is often far from easy to be sure that the woman is single-minded on this subject. Most commonly she is ambivalent, at times wanting the child and at times rejecting it for fear of its appearance. Encouragement to the pregnant woman to talk freely about her thoughts and feelings will bring out the nature of these mixed motives and the negative feelings can be seen as set against more positive wishes to go through with the pregnancy. It is extremely important to establish the presence of consistent and serious feelings that the pregnancy is unwanted since the questions of termination and even sterilization arise.

It is important to recognize not only that motives may be mixed but that they may change throughout the course of pregnancy, usually towards a more positive attitude and resulting in constructive activities.

Stages of normal pregnancy

1. *First trimester*

Often the woman initially finds it difficult to accept that she is pregnant, and in the extreme case there is a total denial, especially if the child is unwanted. As indicated already, there will almost certainly be some degree of ambivalence and also some uncertainty about the reality that the child growing inside her is a separate entity. In a study by Cohen (1966) it was found that 85 per cent of lower and upper-lower class women were disturbed and upset when they became pregnant but by the end of the first trimester 90 per cent had accepted the pregnancy and found it to be of particular value in intensifying the relationship with the father of the child.

Morning sickness though common is for the most part transient and only a small minority need to be treated. Coppen (1959) in a random series of primiparae attending an antenatal clinic found that 58 per cent had vomited during their pregnancy which in other respects had been normal No significant difference was found in this group as regards psychological factors compared with those who had not vomited. Nor were unmarried pregnant women more likely to be affected than married women. During the first trimester the woman is often emotionally labile, irritable and easily fatigued. She becomes tearful with small arguments and trivial upsets. She feels separation from husband keenly and shows a wish to be protected and cared for.

Disturbances of food intake are well known. Dickens and Trethowan found food cravings in 51 per cent of their series of primigravidae, especially for fruit. Aversions to certain food stuffs are also common, especially to tea, coffee and fatty foods previously enjoyed. Craving and aversion tended to go together. These manifestations tended to diminish progressively during the rest of the pregnancy. No close relationship has been established between eating disturbances and vomiting. Cravings and aversion were found to be more common among those with a history of *Pica*, i.e. eating inedible material in childhood.

2. *Second trimester*

With the occurrence of quickening, the fetus becomes more real as a separate entity and the pregnancy is experienced as more enjoyable.

Many women saying that they are at their best at this time. There is a growth of confidence and apparent maturity and the earlier physical symptoms have remitted. Active preparation for the arrival of the baby begins, with knitting, buying a cot and pram, preparing a nursery and thinking about appropriate names.

For some, earlier conflicts and fears persist and may become more prominent, and in this group may be found those who are vulnerable to later breakdown.

Many women relate the presence of disturbing dreams; of catastrophy, harm to oneself or to husband, the birth of a deformed baby and so forth.

3. Third trimester

By now the body is more burdensome, distorted and embarrassing. Shopping, climbing stairs and housework become more difficult. Backache, haemorrhoids, constipation and other physical disabilities emerge.

During this time with delivery now approaching possibly with some apprehension, key figures in the woman's life are of importance to give support. The husband, the mother and elder sisters, together with mature female friends all have their part to play but it is not necessary for them to try and talk the patient into a more tranquil frame of mind.

It should not be forgotten that the husband may himself be going through a variety of stressful experiences. For example, some husbands look upon the addition to the family as an economic burden or as a threat to his exclusive love. Previously powerful, sexual drives have to be brought under control. Very close identification with the wife may produce the 'couvade' syndrome which is characterized by the husband apparently undergoing a pregnancy of his own complete with morning sickness, abdominal discomfort, fatigue to the point of prostration and a wish to be 'confined'. This identification may take place throughout the pregnancy, labour and puerperium or in only one of these phases. (*See* Trethowan and Conlon, 1965.)

LABOUR AND DELIVERY

It is important that a trusting relationship develop between the pregnant woman and her medical and nursing attendants. Ideally there should be continuity of care during the antenatal period and the opportunity for developing a supportive doctor-patient and midwife-patient relationship. Wherever possible, these same attendants should also be present at the birth. In general, involvement of the husband in his wife's pregnancy and antenatal care is beneficial to both parties. Interview with the husband or joint attendance at certain preparation classes are ways of extending this involvement.

Inevitably many women, especially those having their first baby, will harbour fears of the unknown though it may be difficult for them to express these openly. Some may have been conditioned by their mothers or sisters to expect the worst.

Clearly it is important to reassure the patient that she will not be left alone when the time comes for delivery and that insufferable pain will not be allowed to persist.

A wide variation in attitude will be found, ranging from those who have a 'do it yourself' attitude to those who are unduly passive and completely dependant upon the ministrations of doctors and midwives. A central problem is that of pain. As has already been indicated, it is always difficult to estimate the intensity of pain suffered by someone close and nowhere is this more clearly exemplified than in the case of labour pains. Women's accounts of the experience of labour vary from a virtually painless process to something so undesirable it could never be repeated. This poses special problems in the administration of pain killing drugs and anaesthetics. Some women feel cheated of a key experience if they are not fully conscious throughout the whole procedure, and there are others who want to be put to sleep until it is all over. In the absence of obvious mechanical conditions, it has been claimed (notably by Grantly Dick Read) that pain in labour is mainly the product of fear. This principle has formed the basis of various methods claimed to reduce or even abolish pain in childbirth. A wide variety of psychoprophylactic measures have been advocated, including muscle relaxation exercises and hypnosis (Chertok, Vellay 1969). This still remains an area of considerable controversy and no one method seems useful for all types of women.

Psychologically a programme of preparation where basic information about the events of pregnancy can be performed, where the part the woman can play in the process of labour can be explained, where doubts and fears can be tackled and morale sustained, seems advantageous.

In the midst of the clinical efficiency of the busy labour ward, it is vital that the woman, as a unique person who is going through a major psychological and physical crisis, should not be lost sight of. Her embarrassment at nudity or her feelings of indignity at being suspended in the lithotomy position should not be lightly brushed aside.

Attendance by the husband at the labour and delivery where this is requested by the woman, in general seems to be a beneficial arrangement and helps to promote understanding and mutual involvement of the couple.

One of the mother's first concerns is usually about the health of the child and its freedom from deformity. The early establishment of the bond between mother and child is an important priority. Placing the child shortly after birth for the mother to cuddle and examine helps in this process as well as probably hastening the expulsion of the placenta. Undue separation from the mother, for example where the baby has to be placed in an incubator or where severe post-partum haemorrhage has occurred may well disturb this bond formation.

A delicate psychological situation develops where the baby is deformed or has died. There is the problem of when the news should be broken to the mother. Though hard and fast rules cannot be laid down, in general the sooner this is done the better, consistent with the mother's physical state (Berg *et al.*, 1969). Special opportunities must be given to these women to talk about their disappointment and express their grief. Certain special arrangements might also have to be made such as not placing the mother of a stillborn child in a room with mothers who have given birth to normal healthy babies.

In the immediate post-partum period special attention should be given to relief of pain for episiotomies etc. and ensuring adequate sleep.

PUERPERIUM

Hitherto in this chapter psychosocial factors in the sexual and reproductive experiences of women have been considered as much more important than hormonal influences. In the puerperium, however, the balance is probably more in favour of physical factors determining the woman's emotional state. The labour itself has been associated with varying degrees of pain, sleep disturbance, possibly vaginal bleeding or discharge, painful breasts and so forth.

Even more significant appears to be the massive hormonal changes that take place before parturition and in association with the sudden loss of the hormone producing placenta. Increased levels of neuroticism have been noted in a general group of women at the puerperium (Kear-Colwell, 1965) and in addition the frequent occurrences of a sluggish, mildly confused mental state has also been reported (Treadway *et al.*, 1969).

The *post-partum* blues is a most interesting syndrome that is very common though mostly benign and transient. Unexpected spells of weeping, feelings of fatigue, irritability and insomnia occur almost exclusively during the first ten days post-partum, particularly between the fifth and tenth day. Often the reason for crying is inexplicable to the patient and there may be no obvious precipitant. According to Yalom *et al.* (1968) sustained mild post-partum depressions were especially likely with women who had an early menarche, menstrual difficulties such as dysmenorrhoea or premenstrual tension, low parity, a prolonged interval since the previous pregnancy and high distress in a previous pregnancy.

These findings are suggestive of endocrine influences though sometimes the onset is associated with insecurity in the relationship with husband or doubts about mothering capabilities.

The condition is mainly self limiting and no special treatment is called for. Its relationship to the more florid post-partum psychoses is still uncertain. Having commented on possible hormonal effects in the puerperium it is pertinent to discuss the particular psychological and social changes occurring at this period.

1. There is a new responsibility placed on the mother to look after her helpless infant.
2. New techniques such as feeding the baby and attending to the baby's toilet have to be learned and mastered.
3. Considerable changes in the mother's routine must take place and it is now the infant who will determine much of her own routines.
4. Conflict may well occur with her own parents or in-laws whose experiences and attitudes will be regarded as two or more decades out of date.
5. There will be concern over the particular mode and timing of feeding the baby.

Strong cultural and social pressures play

prominent parts in determining patterns of baby feeding. Fashions in breast and bottle feeding come and go. These are related to the role of the female in society where the woman is expected to adopt a purely 'feminine role', there is a tendency to expect her to breast feed. Differences with class and educational background are to be found even in the same society and at the same period. The individual convictions and prejudices of doctors and nurses may also be crucial in influencing practice.

The feeding process is a complex interaction between mother and child. While milk ejection is to be understood as a reflex caused by oxytocin production, this can be inhibited by emotional arousal, for example embarrassment. The primary stimulus is sucking but auditory, visual, olfactory and tactile stimuli from the infant also play their part. The reaction of the infant in turn either by over- or under-activity or by giving rise to pain and discomfort may affect the smooth functioning of the process. There is a close relationship between suckling and sexual excitement. It has been shown that in both situations nipple erection and uterine contractions take place.

If it appears that breast feeding is not only possible but desirable, then the mother should be given every encouragement but if she does not succeed she should not be castigated. Favourable circumstances for successful breast feeding are privacy, encouragement and contact with other breast-feeding mothers.

The time of weaning clearly varies according to the capacity of the mother, progress of the child and to certain cultural factors but whenever possible weaning should be a slow and not an abrupt process.

As was noted above, pregnancy and the puerperium requires adaptation to a whole series of new situations.

In the puerperium the new mother's main psychological task is to adjust to the presence of the baby as a separate individual rather than a fetus about whom phantasies and idealized images have been formed. Essentially the experience is a two-way process, often with extremely rapid interchange between mother and child. It is in these early days that stimulus and response on the part of mother and child are so rapid that they can hardly be systematically observed nor expressed verbally by the mother.

The mother must be prepared for considerable differences in the baby's activity and its response to cuddling and soothing. Striking differences may occur as between siblings in this respect. Because of these differences the mother may reject in some ways an unresponsive or alternatively a very demanding baby. Similarly rejection could occur if the baby is the 'wrong sex' or if obviously handicapped. In this time of possible rejection the mother may quite unconsciously and automatically over react by 'smothering'. Often a mother, especially a primiparous mother, may fail to interpret the baby's signals and cater for its needs in the proper way or at the right time. In the most severe form the mother, unable to tolerate infantile demands and ceaseless crying, may make physical assaults upon it, leading to the so-called battered-baby syndrome. This will be dealt with in the psychiatric section.

Particular care must, of course, be taken when it is found that the baby is in fact deformed or grossly handicapped mentally.

A simple principle that emerges is that the mother should be well prepared and helped in every possible way to become emotionally warm, self aware, understanding and consistent in her behaviour towards her child. The quality of this mothering will in all probability profoundly affect her own child's emotional responses to other people and his later attitude to life (Bowlby, 1971).

The menopause

The end of menstruation and childbearing is an important psychological and biological milestone in the female life cycle. Attitudes to 'the change of life' appear however to differ widely among women though many have been conditioned by their own mothers to expect problems at this time. For those who have invested much of their personality in reproduction, who have always taken a pride in being pregnant and have never been happier than when they are bearing or caring for their babies, the menopause may come as a great blow, a major loss of life satisfaction. Women who have placed great store by their physical attractiveness may recognize the menopause as marking the end of their precious youth and the first sign of old age. Spinsters or married women with childless marriages, who had entertained hopes of a full reproductive life with children of their own, must now give up the hope of what they regard as every woman's right. Not surprisingly such women will view 'the change' as an unhappy event and mourn their loss.

Others who have had unfortunate experiences with sex and childbearing, perhaps haunted by the fear of pregnancy may experience the menopause, by contrast, as a time of release and relief.

A large proportion of women apparently report symptoms such as 'hot flushes', sweating, depression and irritability, headache, vertigo, paraesthesiae, chronic fatigue and insomnia as being particularly prevalent at this epoch, though few are seriously incapacitated (Neugarten and Kraines, 1965).

The 'average' woman in our society, going through the menopause at about 48 years of age, will also have to cope around this time with the death of her mother, her children leaving home, and with the fact that her husband is perhaps engrossed in his work or spends a lot of time and energy at his club, pub or golf course. The term 'empty nest' syndrome has been coined to describe her feelings of uselessness and aimlessness. This is often a time for a reorganization of aims and activities, for a part-time job or some voluntary work, until the arrival of grand-children on the scene perhaps gives a new role and purpose.

She may then re-establish ties with her own daughter and re-live earlier child rearing satisfactions looking after her grand-children. An understanding husband and supportive friends and relatives may help her to surmount this period of readjustment, but for some women communication with husband may prove more distant with their sexual relationship proving less satisfactory.

There is a widespread belief that sexual interest declines considerably after the menopause for biological reasons, and in fact some women do report abrupt changes at this time.

Psychological attitudes rather than biological factors seem to be the main reasons for any such alterations in libido. Some women appear to equate fertility with sexuality and consider that they can be no longer attractive now that they cannot bear children. Others may even feel that sex without the possibility of conception is a joyless activity, that sex is only for younger women and rather obscene in middle age. Kinsey's researches have shown that female sexual responsiveness declines comparatively slowly with age from its peak in the 30's and that it was mainly lack of interest on the husband's part that led to a decrease in sexual activity in the later years of marriage. Those for whom sexual intercourse has proved to be a meaningful and pleasurable part of their marriage are most likely to continue, whereas for others, the menopause may prove a convenient excuse for stopping what they regard as a distasteful or uninspiring duty. It is important for the doctor to convey the idea that the menopause is a transitional period rather than a finale, that a normal, active sex life is possible for many years to come. Many women in this age-group can benefit greatly from talks with their doctors in which fears and worries about themselves and their families can be ventilated and accurate information about the 'change of life' conveyed. The presentation of many gynaecological symptoms can occur in the context of family difficulties at this time, but also they may not uncommonly be part of an underlying depressive illness requiring psychiatric treatment. (*See* section on Psychiatric Disorders.)

Involution and old age

Sexual aspects of old age have been relatively neglected in the literature and it is often assumed that they are irrelevant. However, given reasonable physical health and an interested partner, satisfactory sexual intercourse is possible for many women into the 70's and beyond according to Masters and Johnson. Oestrogen therapy was recommended to counteract certain ageing processes including atrophy of the vaginal mucosa, diminished vaginal lubrication and increased liability to clitoral and urethral irritation which predispose to coital and post-coital pain.

The correction and relief of comparatively minor physical disabilities can do much to improve the quality of life of older women. Such procedures as pelvic floor repair, the treatment of senile vaginitis and urinary infections, the prescription of spectacles and hearing aids can reduce discomfort considerably.

Psychological and social pressures on the elderly must always be borne in mind in gynaecological assessment and management. As well as having to adjust to her own failing bodily functions, the older woman must cope with her husband's retirement, having to manage on a reduced income, deaths of contemporaries and very often her own husband's death. Many of the older gynaecological patients will be widows or spinsters living with a degree of social isolation and feeling that life hasn't much more to offer. The doctor must, therefore, be alert to her feelings of depression and loneliness and must be able to elicit and listen to her fears about the future as well as current physical symptoms.

PSYCHOSOMATIC ASPECTS OF OBSTETRICS AND GYNAECOLOGY

The term 'psychosomatic' has come to have several meanings in medicine in recent years but perhaps the most generally accepted understanding deals essentially with the presence of both physical and emotional symptoms occurring in a patient at the same time.

Commonsense has established a close causal link between psychological changes and bodily changes. For example, even thinking about pleasant or unpleasant situations can give rise to appropriate bodily responses. Reading disturbing news or being a spectator to some tragedy can lead to physical shocks of grief, horror and the like. The sight of blood can lead to fainting in some cases. Physical changes such as pain, fatigue, bowel irregularities, amenorrhoea and so forth can lead to a variety of psychological states.

However, it has never been made clear precisely by what mechanisms a causal relationship is established. Can the mind control the body and vice versa?

Fortunately for the medical practitioner, he can make a most useful working approach simply by adopting a *monistic* view of mind and body: i.e. that for all practical purposes mind and body are basically one, that both are subject to the same natural laws, but that there are certain aspects and attributes of the one not present in the other. In other words, we are looking at two facets of the same phenomenon.

One reason why the doctor can adopt this fairly simple approach is that the interactions between mind and body with which he is most likely to come in contact have to do with such basic emotions as anger, fear, hunger and sex. It is almost impossible to think of these emotional states in any purely psychological or purely physical sense. It is, therefore, when there is some exaggeration or disturbance of the emotional life of the individual that certain attendant physical changes would be expected.

From the examples given, it will be seen that the commonly occurring interactions between mind and body are of short duration, e.g. fits of rage or fear, sexual excitement etc. Psychosomatic disorders, however, are of longer duration and often pursue a chronic course. This raises the question whether emotional disturbances can be associated with prolonged or even irreversible physical change. A further important question that is raised in this connection is whether these more prolonged physical conditions persist after the initial emotional stress has subsided or has been resolved. This has an important bearing on treatment since it may well be that attention to the emotional disturbances long since past might have little or no effect on the present physical state.

Although a monistic approach is recommended, it would be unwise at this stage of our knowledge to drive the theory too hard. It is still useful to use the terms 'psychological' and 'physical' at least for the time being until more sophisticated terminology is introduced.

But with the monistic concept remaining as a guide, a redefinition of the term 'psychological' is called for and in practice should prove valuable. In medical practice, therefore, it is suggested that psychological phenomena are simply the manifestations of the higher functions of the brain and central nervous system: sensations, perceptions, thoughts, memories, feelings, states of conflict, dreams, aspirations and so forth. It is possible to arrange these manifestations in a hierarchical manner from the simplest stimulus response phenomenon to the most abstract intellectual activity. As one passes from one level to the next a more complex and, therefore, more abstract set of phenomena are encountered. It is the sheer complexity of the very high functions of the central nervous system that gives rise to their intangible and abstract character. Here the analogy of the computer is not out of place.

Psychological events can, therefore, for our purposes, be regarded as 'brain events', i.e. those concerned primarily with the central and autonomic nervous systems at their most complex levels of organization. All parts of the body come under humoral or neuronal control or both. Much of humoral (including hormonal) function is controlled by sub-cortical centres mainly in the hypothalamic area. Neuronal function likewise is organized centrally, much of it in the rhinencephalic areas or the 'limbic system'. The cortex is concerned with the recognition and comparing of incoming stimuli or information from receptor systems throughout the body and from the sub-cortical areas. Thus the cerebral cortex becomes the conductor of so many somatic 'performers' that run, not in tens or hundreds, but into millions.

By using this schema, it can be seen how higher functions can become closely associated with such physical functions as heart rate, temperature regulation, blood pressure, digestion, elimination and so forth. Endocrine changes can also be bound up with events taking place at more complex and abstract levels of functioning and how the personal and social environment can indirectly play their part in bringing about these changes. Thus every bodily event, however, peripheral and limited—even to the life of a single cell—has its counterpart or representation at the highest level of central nervous system functioning. This is another way of saying that at all times the body affects the mind and the mind the body.

From the psychosomatic viewpoint, it is important to keep in mind that the 'stresses' affecting the individual and leading to physical change may vary not only in their intensity and duration but in their *meaning* for the particular person. For example, the 'stress' of pregnancy may be experienced as a longed-for fulfilment; an overwhelming burden, or a source of shame. Even the most discrete stimuli though identical, may be experienced in quite different ways. For example the same male figure may be seen as father, husband, lover or stranger, depending on previous private and personal experience.

Disorders of menstruation

From the foregoing introduction to psycho-somatic concepts, it will be seen that sexual functions lend themselves well to a monistic approach. Disorders of menstruation provide a good example.

It is well known that the menstrual cycle is particularly liable to disturbances in acute psychological stress. Young women leaving home for the first time, going into the Services or indeed taking up any new way of life often encounter menstrual irregularity, infrequent menstruation or amenorrhoea. The stress factor in these cases is probably that of separation.

Amenorrhoea has been noted among women in concentration camps, at an early stage and before the effects of malnutrition could have played their part. Fear of being pregnant may produce amenorrhoea (*see* Engels, Patee and Wittkower, 1964).

The menstrual cycle has been related to a multiplicity of symptoms appearing and disappearing in cyclical fashion.

The major patterns most commonly encountered are:
1. Dysmenorrhoea
2. Pre-menstrual tension

DYSMENORRHOEA

Some degree of discomfort is an inevitable accompaniment of the menses. The relationship between dysmenorrhoea and accompanying psychological symptoms is well documented from studies of special groups of the population such as schoolgirls (Dalton, 1968; Golub *et al.*, 1957), women students (Schuk, 1951), service women (Drillien, 1946) and factory workers (Bickers and Woods, 1951). Coppen (1965) in a study of the prevalence of menstrual disorders in psychiatric patients found that neurotics experienced much more menstrual pain than did patients with affective disorders, patients with schizophrenia and normal non-patient controls. High scores for neuroticism, the presence of sexual difficulties and emotional irritability characterized those with severe dysmennorrhoea.

A general population survey by Kessel and Coppen (1963) revealed that 13 per cent of women of menstrual age usually experience severe pain and that a further 32 per cent usually experience moderately severe pain. The prevalence of dysmenorrhoea is unaffected by marriage but is usually cured by pregnancy.

Clinical observations of patients with dysmenorrhoea provide only limited information on the nature of the psychological make-up of those who complain of this, but there is some evidence that those with severe pain have a pre-existing resentment of their feminine role. Also it is found that the more immature and neurotic the woman is, the more likely she is to experience unpleasant symptoms during menstruation. In patients with severe dysmenorrhoea, therefore, an appraisal of the psychological factors in their complaints should be thoroughly investigated.

Tension pain: psychogenic backache is often associated with dysmenorrhoea and for this reason is dealt with here. O'Neill (1958) defined tension pain as bodily pain associated with emotional tension appearing as a response to stress in a person predisposed to act in this way. Of 60 patients attending a gynaecological out-patient department, 22 gave pain apart from dysmenorrhoea as the presenting symptom, and 36 per cent complained of one or more of the following: fatigue, tension, depression, irritability, faintness, lack of energy and insomnia. The sites of pain were found to be in the back, the abdomen and the head, in that order of frequency. The pain in this condition is usually symmetrical, often continuous and without relief. The patient describes it as burning, aching or dull. It is found frequently that symptoms begin at moments of personal crisis.

Low back pain is one of the commonest complaints of women. In the absence of any sound organic reason for the pain an assessment of the woman's personality and environmental difficulties should always be made. Backache of psychogenic origin is analogous to the headache of the anxiety state, often described in vividly dramatic terms. It is frequently found that women with complaints of backache are tense and unable to relax; it is as if they were stiffening themselves in order to prevent the release of emotional tension or as if they were on guard against pain or the fear of pain.

A patient who reports pain always presents a special difficulty to the doctor since it is, of course, an entirely subjective phenomenon. Where an obvious lesion produced by trauma, infection, new growth, etc., can be demonstrated, it is easy for the doctor to accept the patient's word that she is in pain, but where no such clear-cut causes can be found, the patient is often led to believe that she is imagining her pain. This has most unfortunate effects, especially when it is almost impossible to discover what is meant by 'imaginary pain'. A sound and simple rule to observe here is to accept the patient's word as genuine initially (except in the case of transparent

lying) even if no obvious cause can be found. Muscle tension spasm etc. can clearly give rise to temporary or prolonged pain and functional disorders of the alimentary, genito-urinary and cardio-vascular systems can all lead to states that can induce pain of varying severity. It should also be borne in mind that individuals vary in their experience of pain intensity: some are extremely sensitive to quite minor noxious stimuli: others aim hardly to know what pain is. There are also variations in pain tolerance. Whatever the mechanism, therefore, it is essential to assure the patient that the complaint is accepted as genuine and that appropriate treatment will be forthcoming, whether this be the removal of the obvious cause, the administration of analgesics, the introduction of relaxation exercises or psychotherapy. In this connection it is as well to bear in mind that *hypnosis* which is essentially a psychological procedure affecting higher functions, can completely abolish pain from whatever cause, including severe organic pain during terminal illness.

PRE-MENSTRUAL TENSION SYNDROME

The pre-menstrual tension syndrome is another common condition which causes a good deal of distress to those affected by it. It is probably a group of conditions. Some workers prefer it renamed as the 'cyclical syndrome' since similar patterns can occur before the menarche, after the menopause or after hysterectomy (Sutherland and Stewart, 1965).

The condition usually begins two/twelve days before menstruation and remits soon after the menstrual flow begins.

Mental symptoms such as anxiety and depression may become so severe that active psychiatric treatment is indicated and even admission to hospital. In this connection it is of interest to note that various conditions not clearly associated with the menstrual cycle do seem to occur pre-menstrually. These include acute admissions to psychiatric and medical hospitals, suicidal attempts and suicides, accidents, criminal offences, misbehaviour in girls' schools and aggressive outbursts in psychotic patients, Dalton (1964).

Aetiology

A large number of theories exist but are as yet unproven. One set of theories concerns hormonal imbalance, another with water and sodium balance. A further set of theories has to do with unfavourable attitudes to menstruation, lack of acceptance of female psychosocial and psychosexual roles (Tonks, 1968).

Conditions described as psychosomatic or closely related to psychiatric syndromes have been reported as being exacerbated in the premenstrual period. These include eczema, migraine, vasomotor rhinitis.

FUNCTIONAL UTERINE BLEEDING

Irregular, excessive and frequent menstrual flow can all be associated with emotional disturbances. Dutton (1965) investigated the association between emotional disturbances and functional uterine bleeding, the nature and frequency of the association and the possible mechanisms involved in a series of 155 patients. He found that 83 per cent were psychologically disturbed, 70 per cent had acute or chronic anxiety and 64 per cent had other psychosomatic complaints, notably pylorospasm, chest wall pain and migrainous headaches. Most patients presented problems relating to sexual or reproductive difficulties. Dutton's findings support the view that functional uterine bleeding is often initiated by vascular changes due to abnormal autonomic nervous system activity brought on by adverse emotional dysfunction.

PSEUDOCYESIS

This is a condition of false pregnancy. The woman is convinced that she is pregnant and has several signs suggesting that this is so. The woman who has not experienced an actual pregnancy is more likely to develop pseudocyesis than one who has. It may occur before the menarche and after the menopause as well as in the child-bearing years. It is often reported after sterilization. An analogous condition is found in animals where there are signs of pregnancy after the period of heat and associated with persistent corpus luteum. It can be produced in female rats after mating with vasectomized males. The symptoms closely resemble those of true pregnancy including swelling, amenorrhoea, breast development and early morning sickness.

Psychologically it is found that there is an overwhelming desire for or alternatively fear of pregnancy. The woman may wish to please a disinterested husband, prove her youthfulness or feminity. A depressive mood is associated as a reaction to a recent loss. A celebrated case of pseudocyesis was that of Mary Tudor who wished to bear a child to her husband, Philip of Spain, at the time that he was already leaving her.

Despite the obvious psychological factors present, there is often an associated persistent corpus luteum. The possible chain of events would be suppression of ovarian activity by the anterior pituitary under the influence of the hypothalamus which in turn is controlled by the cortex, the control centre for all incoming information both from bodily sources and from the external environment. Emotional factors are presumed to alter hypothalamic function through this cortical activity giving rise to the syndrome (Brown and Barglow, 1971).

Disorders of sexuality

Disorders in the field of sexual relationships illustrate most convincingly the value of a monistic approach since love-making in all its varieties from its tentative and superficial beginnings to its denouement in orgasm invariably contains more a psychological than a physical component.

A further principle to keep in mind in this connection is that these disorders cannot be considered in isolation, that is to say within a single individual woman. They have to be regarded essentially as disorders of a fundamental psychological, physical and cultural relationship.

The most common of these sexual disorders are (1) frigidity, (2) vaginismus and (3) dyspareunia.

1. *Frigidity*

In this condition the achievement of orgasm by the woman during coitus is totally absent or very infrequent. Most patients who consult their doctor complaining of 'frigidity' are simply found to lack experience and sophistication in sexual matters or it may be that their husband lacks this experience or is inconsiderate. This problem is in most cases overcome during the period of general adjustment in the early months of marriage.

When the condition persists and is not amenable to these simple measures more detailed investigation is required. The associated emotional state ranges widely from simple passivity and lack of any feeling, whether positive or negative, to outright rejection, fear or revulsion towards sexual contact.

'Primary frigidity' occurs where this is the

only symptom while 'secondary frigidity' relates to diseases of the genito-urinary tract, organic diseases of the central nervous or endocrine systems. Similarly frigidity may be secondary to a psychiatric illness such as depression and can also be associated with drug addictions.

To illustrate the importance of the relationship aspect, frigidity may occur only with respect to a certain man but not with others. For example, a wife may complain to her doctor (and also to her husband) of frigidity but it is later learned that she is having a fully satisfying sexual affair with another man. Married women sometimes report that sexual relations were normal before marriage either with their present husband or with other men.

Just as fear of pregnancy, underlying conflicts or hostilities in the marriage may be associated with chronic gynaecological symptoms such as backache or pelvic pain, so these situations may inhibit the woman's full sexual response.

The frigid woman's personality has been described as frequently emotional, immature, egotistic and attention-seeking, i.e. the hysterical personality whose attitude to men is always ambivalent. Such a person while appearing superficially to be coquettish and sexually attractive, at a more superficial level will show deep hostility towards her male partner of a kind that is calculated to undermine his masculinity. Thus the woman uses her sexual attractiveness to lure men into a state of impotence. These are sometimes referred to as 'castrating' women. In this connection studies of prostitutes have shown that their personality structure involves a fundamental hatred for men: their underlying motive is to degrade men.

Other women of a fastidious and obsessional personality type have conflicts about the 'messiness' of sexual intercourse and in particular are afraid of the loss of emotional control that occurs in orgasm. Such individuals are 'tight' not in the purely physical sense, but also in the psychological sense.

Other possible factors giving rise to this condition centre round fears of being homosexual.

All these conditions reflect deep-seated personality problems which almost certainly are expressed in other ways, e.g. a deep dependence on parents and parent substitutes.

Intensive studies of women along psychoanalytic lines have shown specific difficulties in coming to terms with sexual fantasies related to the father.

Later learning experiences and cultural factors also play their part, for example young women may have been brought up to believe that everything connected with sex is sinful and dirty and she, therefore, comes into the marital situation with this fixed attitude which is not easy to change.

So far as treatment is concerned, almost invariably this requires specialized and intensive study of the whole history of emotional and sexual relationships from childhood onwards. It also implies an understanding of the relationship that is developing between husband and wife. If, therefore, simple measures are found to be ineffective after the first few months of marriage, then specialist referral is indicated.

Specifically designed behaviour modification therapy may prove effective in selected cases. Masters and Johnson (1970) have claimed 80 per cent success rate after a five year follow-up when both partners were required to have an intensive four day course of behaviour therapy. Each partner is taken separately by a therapist of the same sex in the initial sessions and then they are taken together with the male and female therapists. Straightforward counselling, together with advice on technique, are the main methods.

That the physical and emotional aspects of frigidity are inextricably related is illustrated by the report of the young frigid married woman who was ultimately treated by a handsome young gynaecologist by the use of graduated dilators. She reported subsequently complete success in intercourse with her husband but added that she was so grateful to the young gynaecologist that during intercourse she always kept him clearly in her imagination!

2. *Vaginismus*

Vaginismus is a condition which is not dissimilar from certain types of frigidity but with the more limited manifestation of vaginal spasm as the central symptom. It is an involuntary automatic response to penetration and is accompanied by pain. It may be linked with the initial experience of painful rupturing of the hymen but can occur at later stages.

In the early months of marriage the condition

responds very much as does frigidity in most cases, but where the condition is more persistent, the principles of treatment outlined for frigidity would apply (*see* Ellison, 1968).

3. *Dyspareunia*

Again this condition is very similar to frigidity. It is the experience of pain as a result of penetration during the sexual act. It does not seem to be associated with actual spasm but the patient may very well complain of the pain as being quite intolerable and certainly of such an intensity as precludes intercourse and may lead to complete cessation of sexual relations. Treatment for this condition is along similar lines to that for frigidity.

Infertility

Childlessness is still regarded with some stigma in our society and is of concern to many married women. It has been estimated that one-quarter of women attending infertility clinics are infertile from causes presumed to be psychogenic (Sandler, 1968). At least no physical causes in the woman or her husband are found to account for the childlessness.

A variety of mechanisms preventing conception have been postulated including tubal spasm, alteration of the characteristics of cervical mucus, rapid expulsion of semen from the vagina, all as responses to emotional stress. Psychotherapy has been recommended to deal with the stress and thereby remove the blocks to conception. These hypotheses have not so far been conclusively confirmed and the question remains open.

Though there are also many anecdotal stories about conception occurring in infertile women shortly after adoption, studies designed to demonstrate this effect have yielded conflicting results (Mai, 1971).

Disorders of pregnancy

A number of obstetric complications occur in which there is no clear-cut physical cause but where there is at least some evidence that emotional factors play their part. McDonald (1968) reviewed relevant articles over the previous fifteen years and concluded that while true cause and effect could not be established (and according to the monistic view this would not be expected in any case) there was support for the notion of a positive relationship between psychological and physiological functioning during pregnancy. This relationship appeared to be mediated through the autonomic nervous system at the physiological level and anxiety at the psychological level. Women who showed consistently high scores on anxiety tests were found also to have greater instability in autonomic functioning. Any stimuli which set off these vulnerable women into states of anxiety also mobilized autonomic activity which in turn triggered off a host of regulatory mechanisms appearing as distressing symptoms. As indicated previously, the stimuli themselves could vary both in intensity and in their significance for the individual person, i.e. their meaning. The selection of symptoms would, therefore, be partly determined by constitutional factors and partly by their meaning for the patient. Furthermore symptoms may serve some (albeit inefficient or distorted) purpose, e.g. to escape from a situation, attract attention or resolve some inner unconscious conflict.

It will be seen, therefore, that it is important to have a clear idea about the physiological functions that give rise to the symptoms in these complications of pregnancy and also to explore the psychological background of the individual patient to see in what way it makes sense for her.

The commoner complications are now described to illustrate in more detail the general points outlined above.

Hyperemesis gravidarum

Mild nausea and vomiting—'physiological vomiting' or 'morning sickness'—are not uncommon in the first trimester and are often the first symptoms of pregnancy. In more severe vomiting there is considerable controversy concerning the role of psychological factors. For some it has been equated with rejection of the child or rejection of feminity. Since vomiting is biologically an ancient protective device, ridding the body of noxious ingested material, it is thought that this mechanism is brought into play in an effort to get rid of the unwanted mass growing inside the womb. Chertok *et al.* (1963) however maintains that ambivalence rather than rejection is involved. Coppen (1959) could find no significant psychological difference between vomiters and non-vomiters but found that vomiters had a higher androgyny score, i.e. a more male-type physique. Brown (1964) comparing a group of patients with hyperemesis and a normal group of women described a significantly greater number of pregnancy worries and bodily symptoms in the patient group compared with the controls.

A general conclusion appeared to be that if vomiting continues throughout the day and persistently after the third month, emotional symptoms become increasingly common. Paradoxically unmarried pregnant women do not show a high incidence of hyperemesis.

If the vomiting becomes severe and there is some evidence of electrolyte imbalance or adverse home circumstances, hospital admission is indicated. The underlying psychological factors should be brought out in a series of interviews with the patient and a very strongly supportive and reassuring line should be taken to restore the patient's confidence in herself and her future. Punitive measures of any kind should be avoided. With this regime and appropriate physical treatment, it is rare to require any termination of the pregnancy.

Pre-eclampsia

This common condition is still of uncertain aetiology though it is probable that biochemical and toxic factors play a more important part than do psychological factors. It has been shown, however, that conditions of psychological stress can be associated with alterations in renal blood flow with accompanying vasospasm and transient hypertension.

If psychological factors play their part, they are of a deep-seated nature and are probably incorporated into the very texture of the patient's personality. For example, Coppen (1958) found that many toxemic patients had shown difficulty at every stage of feminine development, i.e. at the menarche, during menstruation, in relation to sexual activity and in attitudes to pregnancy. Psychiatric symptoms in pregnancy were common and there was a history of pre-menstrual tension. Psychological testing revealed a high neuroticism score in this group. Glick *et al.* (1965) found pre-eclampsic patients had a significantly high incidence of abnormal childhood experiences, of separations from husband during pregnancy and of previous history of abortions. Pilowsky and Sharp (1971) in a prospective study comparing those who developed toxemia with those who did not, found that those with toxemia were less verbally intelligent, had less

desire for pregnancy, were more introspective, depressed and uncommunicative. They also found that the husbands were more dependant and immature and, therefore, less likely to respond with support.

These studies suggest that such patients should be helped in their overall personality adjustment to life rather than that specific stresses or conflicts should be tackled as might be indicated in cases of hyperemesis.

Spontaneous abortion

There is some evidence that emotional disturbance is one of the factors encountered in this condition. Deeper investigation of unconscious attitudes towards pregnancy is, therefore, worth while in such cases. Tupper and his colleagues (1957) in a review of the problem pay considerable attention to emotional factors and in 100 patients threatening to abort described two main groups of women with definite personality features. One group was dependant, uncertain and anxious and the other an independent, career-type with mixed feelings about the female role.

Habitual abortion, i.e. abortion occurring on three or more successive pregnancies, is probably due to a series of recurrent causes. Grimm (1962) found on psychological testing that habitual aborters demonstrated poorer emotional controls and stronger dependancy needs than controls. They tended to be more conventional and conforming, and more prone to anxiety regarding hostility, with greater proneness to guilt feelings.

Popular and probably apocryphal stories abound, of abortions occurring after extreme stress, e.g. bereavement or physical assault. The mechanism here is obscure but Bardwick and Behrman (1967) have shown that anxiety and sexually arousing stimuli produce changes in uterine contractions.

It has been found that psychotherapy with close physical supervision and hormone treatment, if necessary, are highly successful. The psychotherapeutic approach includes the doctor identifying with the patient and her problems, taking on along with her the responsibility for the birth and giving her an opportunity to ventilate her fears. It is not possible to say how many of the successes claimed would have coped as well without treatment, but this condition establishes an important principle in overall management and treatment by psychotherapy, namely that regardless of the direct relation between the condition and the presence of emotional factors, these latter deserve attention in their own right. It should be the task of the doctor in all such circumstances to estimate the patient's psychological needs and to try and meet these even if they do not have a direct bearing on the physical symptoms which would require other forms of treatment.

Prematurity

In the few psychological studies of this condition women who have premature babies (i.e. with a birth weight of less than $5\frac{1}{2}$ lbs) appear to resemble those subject to spontaneous abortion. Blau et al. (1963) in comparing 30 mothers of premature infants with 30 mothers of normal infants matched on many criteria, found that the premature group showed more negative attitudes towards pregnancy and were more emotionally immature and narcissistic.

Dystocia

Cramond (1954) in a controlled study of patients with difficult labour found on psychological testing that this group showed little overt anxiety compared with normal controls. It was concluded that these patients employed the mechanism of denial of their feelings excessively, attempting to remain outwardly calm while in fact experiencing considerable inner turmoil. Other studies have confirmed this finding which would be expected in the more introspective, sensitive and apprehensive type of person. It should not be too difficult for the doctor to recognize this type and to give the patient every encouragement during pregnancy to relax and talk more freely about her feelings, particularly her fears. Too readily the doctor can fall into the error of treating an overcontrolled person as a very good patient who is so much in command of the situation that she needs no help. The reverse is, of course, the case.

Other psychosomatic disorders

PRURITUS VULVAE

The majority of cases of pruritus vulvae are due to organic causes. In some women, however, this condition is much influenced by psychological factors. This possibility should be considered especially when somatic remedies prove ineffective or of only transient therapeutic value. Clinical observations have shown that inquiry will reveal one of the following sources of emotional aggravation: heightened but frustrated sexual desire; frustrated sexual excitement in failing to achieve orgasm, especially if coitus interruptus is practised; masturbation accompanied by guilt feelings about it; desire of masturbation rationalized by the patient's justifiable need to relieve the pruritus by handling her genitalia. Where psychological factors are found to contribute to pruritus, excellent results can be obtained from a combined approach of topical therapy and psychotherapy.

URINARY RETENTION

This condition is generally of fairly clear-cut physical aetiology. In some instances it may occur after a particularly painful operation, e.g. prolapse repair. It can, however, occur in the presence of emotional disturbance, particularly in younger women. In these cases the symptom is hysterical in nature and requires careful case history and psychotherapy for its removal.

A very large number of people are now on tricyclic drugs administered by general practitioners and specialists for conditions thought to be depressive but which in many cases are not. They are often administered erroneously as simple tranquillizers. One of the more distressing occasional side effects of these drugs is urinary retention. Women who are actually depressed whether mildly or severely and women who use the word 'depressed' to cover almost any emotional disturbance, must be carefully assessed from the point of view of drug intake if retention is a symptom.

Psychological reactions to physical conditions

When the integrity of the reproductive system is affected, or even threatened, this invariably gives rise to special psychological reactions. In general, these reactions may be termed *defence mechanisms* brought into play to maintain personal balance. These mechanisms will vary according to constitutional factors and the particular significance of the condition for the patient. The most common reaction is one of generalized anxiety but other common patterns include denial, overt and covert hostility (i.e. lack of co-operation), hysterical bouts, dramatization and exaggeration, regression to passive and childish behaviour (this often potentiated by the attitude of doctor and staff who often prefer obedience, even subservience in their patients), and the intensification of such existing traits as obsessionalism, paranoid suspiciousness and depression.

It is commonly assumed that a given condition, e.g. pan-hysterectomy, will give rise to a standard pattern of reaction, say, initial apprehension and then compliance. But some women may react with horror and with extreme emotional outbursts while others in whom a concealed depressive state is present, may welcome the situation as a blessed relief from the cares of this world, or possibly a just punishment for past misdeeds.

It should be remembered that the common factor running through all diseases of the reproductive system is that a threat is perceived to the person's femininity. Again, it must not be assumed routinely that such a threat is invariably unwelcome. Some women throughout life yearn to be rid of any sign of their gender.

The conditions which warrant close psychological attention are as follows:

Hysterectomy
Sterilization
Mastectomy
Malignancy

Hysterectomy
This can usually be talked about among women and hence has come to be associated with many old wives' tales. These centre round the loss of womanhood, the exaggeration of menopausal symptoms and the disappearance of the sexual life and a threat to the marital relationship. Doctors should always try to remember that their patients often do not possess any realistic anatomical or physiological knowledge and this ignorance constitutes a vacuum into which these lurid stories are precipitated. Very simple, straightforward explanations here are of the greatest value and constitute the best psychotherapy. It is when such a talk is given that questions are stimulated leading on to a clearer understanding by the doctor of the patient's attitudes to hysterectomy. Barker (1968) found that the referral rate to the psychiatric services of patients who had undergone hysterectomy was three times that for the general population and two and a half times that of a control group of patients who had undergone cholecystectomy. However this seems to be a specially pre-disposed group since 57 per cent gave a history of previous psychiatric referral.

Sterilization
The indications for sterilization are mainly symptoms of debility, multiparity, physical disease or serious obstetric complications. Only a small number of patients are sterilized on psychiatric grounds.

Most series report considerable improvement in general health and marital relationships, expressing 'satisfaction at the result (Thomson & Baird, 1968, Black & Sclare, 1968).

Regrets tend to occur if the marriage has deteriorated or been broken up by the husband's death or desertion. There are also regrets if there is a question of re-marriage or if one or more existing children have died and a replacement is wished for.

A special problem arises in women under 30 since circumstances could change so radically that the woman may wish to change her mind about having more children in the new situation. Conflicting views about the desirability of sterilization can also lead to trouble, for example, if a doctor refuses to abort a patient unless she is at the same time sterilized. The husband's view may be completely opposed to that of the patient either pressing for sterilization or being strongly opposed to it.

Generally speaking, however, the majority of women who are sterilized having completed their families, find considerable economic relief and release from the fear of further and unwanted pregnancies.

Mastectomy
As with hysterectomy, mastectomy is viewed by many women as a mutilation and as the removal of part of her womanhood. The more self-conscious and narcissistic types of women will be most severely affected by this adverse change in their appearance. It is, therefore, essential to reassure these patients and also to pay careful attention to the psychological significance of prostheses.

Malignancy
Both cervical and mammary carcinoma are susceptible to secondary prevention, i.e. from early diagnosis at a time when treatment can be extremely favourable in its outcome. Cervical smears and regular palpation of the breasts can for the most part be regarded as everyday matter of fact procedures and it is because of the very high proportion of women who are prepared to undergo these simple

tests that early diagnosis has been made possible. However there is a proportion of patients whose anxieties and other defences postpone diagnosis until it may be too late. The patient may be fully aware of some slight abnormality but cannot bring herself to report it to her doctor, her husband or to others. On the other hand she may so completely deny the reality of the situation that she is blind not only to the significance of what is there but to its actual presence. Extreme cases of denial have been reported where, for example, gross ulceration of the breast has been present over a long period of time and the patient has gone to extraordinary irrational lengths to hide the fact from herself, e.g. by never completely undressing or never looking at herself in a mirror or undressing in the dark.

It may be difficult to understand these cases or to know how they could possibly have been encouraged to seek medical aid at an early stage. However studies have shown that one important reason for delay in reporting cancer is a poor relationship between the patient and her general practitioner. In some cases she may not have a regular doctor at all. This gives a clue to early diagnosis, namely that there should be some regular professional relationship between a patient and her general practitioner such that at any time she should feel free to consult him even about matters that give a rise to anxiety or for that matter which she may wish to dismiss as trivial.

PSYCHIATRIC DISORDERS IN OBSTETRICS AND GYNAECOLOGY

This section deals with those conditions that present with recognized psychotic/neurotic symptoms or severely disturbed behaviour. For the most part they conform to descriptions of these conditions in standard textbooks of psychiatry to which the reader is referred. The presence of obstetric or gynaecological conditions poses special problems in establishing causative factors and in overall management.

The reader should first be reminded that psychiatric disorder is common in the general population as a whole. General practitioner surveys, for example, have shown that up to 14 per cent of patients in a given practice will consult their doctor in the course of a year for psychiatric conditions. The rates for women are uniformly higher in all conditions and the age-group 25–45 show the highest prevalence. It is, therefore, hardly surprising that many patients in obstetric and gynaecological clinics have psychiatric problems.

Neurotic illness and pregnancy

Two broad types of neurotic conditions may be encountered in the course of pregnancy. (1) Neuroses which have preceded the pregnancy and may be intensified or modified by it; (2) Neuroses which arise in the course of pregnancy.

1. *Neuroses which have preceded pregnancy* will have been present in fairly typical form either as acute attacks or as fairly chronic conditions. The more acute and short-lasting conditions include anxiety states and neurotic or reactive depression. During the pregnancy anxiety may be intensified or it may be redirected towards pregnancy, labour and the prospect of having a child. Certain phobic anxiety states might also be specifically intensified, for example women who fear closed spaces, going to see a doctor, entering hospital or having such physical procedures applied to them as injections and anaesthetics may all show quite marked intensification of these fears which could interfere with management.

Patients who have previously reacted to stress situations with symptoms of depression may show some change in the content of their depressive thinking, for example a previous feeling of unworthiness in relation to other situations might now show itself as an inability to go through with the pregnancy and face all the new situations thereafter. These patients may develop a marked antipathy to the pregnancy and wish for abortion. The more chronic conditions are those of obsessive compulsive neuroses, hysterical reactions and psychopathic or character disorders. These are invariably the most difficult to deal with during the course of pregnancy and thereafter, and there is little chance that much can be done to modify them during the period of additional stress. It is sometimes difficult to distinguish between a chronic neurotic condition and a constitutionally unstable personality. In either case the principle to observe in their management is to establish clearly the nature of the condition and the type of personality encountered and make due allowances for them. For example, in the case of the obsessive compulsive individual, it should be understood that her symptoms are beyond her conscious control and that her ritual acts of hand-washing, cleaning, checking, etc. are as alien to her as they are to those looking after her. These patients sometimes have fears that they may lose control of themselves and attack others, perhaps their unborn child or give rise to contaminations and disease. They may be particularly fastidious in matters of bowel and bladder function in which case the apparently normal and everyday encouragement from the nurse to the woman in labour that she should bear down 'as though opening your bowels' will simply have the effect of intensifying anxiety and tension.

Similarly with the hysterical personality or one who has shown frequent hysterical attacks in the past, a tolerant but firm understanding is essential. These patients almost invariably arouse hostility and resentment in staff members because of their exaggerations and dramatizations. It is worse than useless to respond to their behaviour 'in kind' but calm determination can usually allay the symptoms and encourage the patient to co-operate.

Where there has been a significant previous history of neurotic illness, it could well be that the pregnancy itself is a symptom of the total neurotic process. For example, it may be simply unplanned as in the case with many of the important events in the life of a neurotic person or the pregnancy may have been conceived from neurotic motives. Again a detailed personal and psychological history will bring these points to light and it will be clear enough to the doctor how best to proceed with the case in the light of this knowledge.

2. *Neurotic illness and pregnancy.* There is some evidence that pregnancy itself can be the main causative factor in the onset of neurotic illness, usually of a mild and temporary nature. Approximately one in five pregnant women show a severe neurotic para-partum reaction and a further one in four have a moderate degree of symptoms, the content of the neurotic fears centering around the fetus, the baby or the husband. It will be seen that these rates are substantially higher than those for the general population for women in the childbearing age-group.

Worries about the fetus are concerned with whether it will be born deformed or stillborn or that it might soon die. The patient is lethargic, complains of tension headaches and is often tearful.

The irrational fears about the baby centre round her inability to cope with feeding, attention to toilet, protecting the baby from any harm. This harm could come from injury in letting the baby fall, interference by other siblings or strangers and, of course, unknown and dread disease.

Irrational fears about the husband have to do with his safety in her absence, his fidelity, or his attitude to the child.

In the immediate post-partum period there is often a mild transient neurotic reaction with tearfulness, irritability, feelings of inadequacy and generalized anxiety.

Actual breakdown may arise either directly or indirectly from the circumstances of the pregnancy. Factors that directly arise from the pregnancy would include the physiological changes taking place and changes in physical appearance. More indirect factors would include an unwanted pregnancy, especially in unmarried women, unfavourable economic or housing conditions, an irresponsible husband, the existence of a large family already and so forth.

The *prevention and treatment* of neurotic conditions must begin with adequate preparation and education of expectant mothers, together with their husbands if possible, the presence of encouraging and realistic support from husband, close relatives and dependable friends is essential. The prospect of a family addition is associated with a sufficient number of complications in itself without adding such further confusions as moving to a new home, the husband changing his job or taking any other decisions which alter the life situations substantially. So far as possible the normal routine of life should be maintained along with the usual outside interests but unnecessary external responsibilities should be cut down.

The doctor attending the patient during the pregnancy can play a most important part in heading off neurotic breakdown by giving the opportunity for the woman to talk freely about her pregnancy and in particular her inner thoughts and feelings about it. In short her fantasies. These often become quite frightening if they are allowed to remain bottled up within the individual but are soon seen as mere imaginings when talked about in a tolerant and understanding atmosphere. When seen in their proper light irrational fears can become the object of laughter and humour. It cannot be too strongly emphasized that laughter plays a vital biological part in conditions of stress. It is a natural release of tension and is one of the best ways in which the individual can regain a proper sense of proportion in life.

Psychoses in pregnancy

The major mental illnesses are uncommon in pregnancy and they are concentrated particularly in the post-partum period. Many women who have been suffering from mental illness show amelioration of symptoms during pregnancy.

The fact that pregnancy as such does not appear to give rise to any of the commoner psychotic conditions should be borne in mind when considering the question of therapeutic abortion.

In this section only *post-partum psychosis* will be considered in detail. This can be a most dramatic condition and quite bewildering to the husband and the family. It can cause severe disruption of family relationships.

Approximately two per thousand pregnancies are admitted to psychiatric hospitals with psychoses. There is a significant excess of psychoses, especially affective disorders, in the first three months post-partum. This is not due to the condition having been present before birth and hence delay in admission until after the birth (Pugh *et al.*, 1963). About two-thirds of all cases show onset in the first month with a peak at about the tenth day. It is perhaps significant that the onset is extremely rare before the third day post-partum suggesting that the condition is due to some specific factor arising after this point in time.

Many writers do not consider that post-partum psychosis is a distinct entity. This is supported by the observation that a large proportion of women with post-partum psychosis are likely to have at some time a non-puerperal psychotic illness and to give a family history of psychosis, resembling that of non-puerperal psychotics. A possible reason for supposing that there is such an entity as 'puerperal psychoses' is that before chemotherapy and the antibiotics puerperal fever, which was common enough, was often associated with psychotic confusion of an organic nature. The disappearance of puerperal fever has removed almost completely this type of

psychotic reaction leaving only conditions that closely resemble classic psychotic conditions.

Prodromal symptoms include sleep disturbance, headaches, restlessness, irritability, suspiciousness, concern over trivia, food refusal and labile mood.

Nevertheless the *onset* and course of the condition often differs from that of common psychotic conditions as follows:

1. The condition appears suddenly and dramatically, the symptoms being of a florid character.
2. There is marked fluctuation in the clinical picture with remissions and relapses occurring in unpredictable fashion.
3. The majority show transient confusional elements without any evidence of toxic or infective causes.
4. There is a marked variety in the symptom pattern suggesting a schizophrenic illness at one stage and a depressive illness at another (Hamilton, 1962).

Women over 30 and multiparae are reported to be at greater risk but puerperal psychosis may also occur after uneventful first pregnancies. Only about one in five of subsequent pregnancies are associated with psychoses. This finding should also be taken into account when considering therapeutic abortion and the risks of further pregnancies in a given case.

Paffenbarger (1964) has suggested that the psychotic reaction in the puerperium is brought about by a combination of constitutional and hereditary factors on the one hand and specific hormonal and biochemical factors arising in the puerperium on the other. He has shown that post-partum mental illness is associated with low birth weight, shorter gestation, low parity, more physical complications in pregnancy, a stormy pregnancy, older women and a longer gap since previous pregnancy.

Considerable hormonal changes do occur in the latter part of the pregnancy and after loss of the placenta. Thus the condition might be regarded as analogous to psychotic reactions occurring in association with heavy steroid medication which shows many of the unusual clinical features seen in post-partum psychoses.

Affective disorders are mainly of the depressive type with marked feelings of guilt, self-reproach, lack of interest and attention to self and the baby. There is restless sleep, poor appetite and retarded speech and movement. In severe cases there are delusions of guilt or of being persecuted, e.g. by the police or of the body being altered. Auditory hallucinations may occur, usually of a derogatory kind. It is in association with this clinical picture that infanticide or suicide is a danger but with careful and sensitive history-taking and discussions with the patient about her inner thoughts and feelings these possibilities can emerge and be realistically assessed.

Occasionally a fairly typical *manic state* may be seen with over activity, pressure of talk, infectious gaiety, grandiose ideas, etc.

Schizophrenia will be observed as a state of withdrawal, preoccupation with bizarre ideas, characteristic disturbances of thought processes, auditory and sometimes visual hallucinosis and thoughts of being controlled by outside agencies.

The confusional state is usually of a mild type but there may be frank delirium. The typical features of confusion include disorientation for time, place and person, grossly impaired judgment and memory and marked emotional disturbances, such as states of terror. Persecutory delusions of a poorly expressed kind will be elicited. The condition tends to fluctuate markedly usually becoming worse at night when management may prove impossible unless in a psychiatric unit.

The treatment will depend on the nature of the main psychotic picture. In severe *affective disorders* the early and intensive application of electro-convulsive therapy with sedation will bring the condition under control in a very short time in most cases. In the *schizophrenic conditions* the phenothiazines such as chlorpromazine and thioridazine will prove effective, often in association with electro-convulsive therapy. In *confusional states* bed-rest and sedation with phenothiazines will assist in management and attention should be paid also to correct electrolyte, fluid balances and giving vitamin supplements. Should any infection be present, this should be dealt with by appropriate antibiotics.

An important principle in management of such cases is that wherever feasible the mother and baby should be together. In severe cases they should be admitted to psychiatric units where appropriate facilities are usually provided. The *prognosis* in these cases is on the whole good with the best outlook for patients who show predominantly affective disorders.

Protheroe (1969) found that 90 per cent of these showed complete recovery. Confusional states invariably recover but there is some controversy over the later outcome for schizophrenic reactions which may persist long after puerperal period is over.

Therapeutic abortion

In considering abortion from the psychiatric point of view, three questions must be asked:
1. Does pregnancy cause or predispose to psychiatric illness?
2. Does an unwanted pregnancy in a woman increase the risk of subsequent mental ill-health which would interfere with her way of life or that of existing children?
3. Will abortion be expected to improve the present health of the patient or at least maintain it at its present level?
   Conversely, can abortion give rise to subsequent mental ill-health?

Although the 1967 Abortion Act has indicated under what conditions abortion is legal, there have been quite wide variations both in interpretation and practice throughout the country. Indications based on the mental health of the pregnant woman will certainly be open to such variations but with the passage of time a reasonable degree of uniformity has been established.

There are no absolute psychiatric indications, that is to say, any answer to the first main question; there is no evidence that mental illness arising during pregnancy is specifically caused by the pregnancy. Studies of the commoner major psychiatric syndromes bear out this contention. For example, schizophrenia and manic depressive psychosis are no more common during pregnancy than at other times. Writers such as Sim (1963) in adducing this type of evidence concludes that there is no case at all for terminating a pregnancy on psychiatric grounds. He considers that if a psychosis supervenes during pregnancy, it should be treated as it might under any other set of conditions. Depressive states occurring in the early weeks might be associated with a strong desire for termination but it could well be that with appropriate anti-depressant treatment (ECT) or drug treatment, this condition could quickly clear up leaving the patient in a much more positive frame of mind about continuing with the pregnancy. Similarly pregnant women who have a history of psychiatric breakdown during previous pregnancies or in the post-partum period in more than four cases out of five are likely to have a current pregnancy free from mental illness. Each case must, therefore, be very carefully assessed on its own merits and it could well be that informed psychiatric opinion would be to recommend that the pregnancy should continue and that active psychiatric treatment should be given where necessary.

Most patients whose mental health is in question fall into the category of neurotic reactions or personality disorders. These are women who are on the whole vulnerable to stresses of different kinds and it is certainly the case that pregnancy and the prospect of having a child may constitute severe stresses for them.

The single girl going through an illegitimate pregnancy illustrates the special mental health problems that have to be assessed. It has been shown that unmarried pregnant women have previously had a significantly higher sickness rate (as measured by the number of general practitioner consultations) than matched controls. Some are 'accident prone', others of low intellectual or educational standard and others again have poor control over their emotional life and behaviour. Almost invariably these pregnancies are unwanted and in many cases there are very real adverse factors which must be taken into account as having a bearing on mental health. In some there is no prospect of marriage with the partner who may be married already or have deserted the girl. There may be disruption of the career and this is of a particularly serious nature if the girl is at school or a student or in a particular job which if given up may make further employment difficult or impossible. Parents are often thought to be quite unable to face up to this crisis perhaps because of their religious and moral attitudes or their health; or there may be only one parent.

Adoption seems to be less feasible since many girls are against this possibility although they may have little realistic alternative. One clue to the basic instability of many of these single girls is that they have quite deliberately taken no contraceptive precautions. It is highly probable that in these cases a low grade and long term self-destructive drive is present. For them if the pregnancy continues and a child is born they have succeeded primarily in harming themselves. They have also created much unhappiness and disturbance for others.

The married person presents a different picture. She will often have an existing family which she has regarded as complete. Many will say that the previous pregnancy had also been unwanted and that since the birth of the last child life has been particularly difficult from the socio-economic point of view. In addition there will be a history of intermittent and often vague physical ill-health and a deteriorating relationship with the husband. Attitudes to the other children will have become increasingly hostile and rejecting. The woman may be approaching the end of the childbearing period and her physical and mental capacity will have already proved to be inadequate to cope with the duties and responsibilities of running a home with her existing family. Usually there has been some failure in contraception rather than carelessness and there may even have been the suggestion of sterilization at the time of the previous birth. Some more unstable women have either come off the pill because of side effects or have not been sufficiently conscientious and careful to ensure against conception.

A substantial group of married women have illegitimate pregnancies, i.e. to men other than their husbands. They may be living with their husband or divorced, separated or widowed. These women face a particularly severe social stigma and if living with their husband risk the breakdown of the existing marriage.

It will be seen from these accounts that complex situations present themselves in connection with unwanted pregnancies. These must be very fully investigated, not only with the woman herself, but with others who are directly involved. For example, in the case of the unmarried girl, it is most helpful to see the man concerned if he is willing and if it seems as though some solution other than termination might be found. In the case of the married woman whose pregnancy is legitimate, the husband should always be consulted and questions of sterilization should also be gone into.

The doctor in some cases is subjected to a certain amount of 'blackmail' which takes the form of suicidal threats, determination to seek abortion by any means, including illegal abortions and histrionic shows of emotion with shouting, tearfulness and so forth. These should not be taken too seriously but, of course, are generally symptomatic of the instability that will show itself in other ways as well.

Some women may be considered definite suicidal risks even if they do not bring up this topic at all. Suicidal attempts are not unknown in pregnancy. Whitlock and Edwards (1968) found that 7 per cent of women under the age of 45 who attempted suicide were in fact pregnant at the time, though about half of these wanted to continue the pregnancy. However even if it is established that a suicidal risk is present in association with a depressive illness, it may not follow that termination should be recommended. As has already been pointed out, active treatment of the depressive illness may bring about a totally different situation in which the pregnancy should be continued.

Many studies on long-term effects of abortion have been carried out on too small a scale or for too short a period of time for valid conclusions to be drawn. Other studies have been carried out by those who have taken an explicitly partisan view either for or against abortion with results that might be expected. A number of Scandinavian studies are of better quality. Ekblad (1955) studied 479 Swedish women terminated on psychiatric grounds which included social indications. After a follow-up period of between 22 and 50 months, he found that 25 per cent had experienced some guilt and 11 per cent severe guilt. One per cent were severely incapacitated with psychiatric disorder but all these had a previous history of severe neurosis. Jannsson (1965) found that 1·92 per cent of women who had had legal abortions were later admitted to psychiatric hospitals compared with 0·27 per cent of women with histories of spontaneous or illegal abortions. Aren (1958) has reported that 48 of his series of 100 women experienced guilt feelings, 23 being severe enough to interfere with work or sleep. However a number of more recent British studies indicate that the majority of women are satisfied with termination and only a very small number suffer from psychiatric disturbance.

In general unfavourable results were found in women who were uncertain whether they wanted abortion or were under pressure from others to have it. Women with long term psychiatric problems were unlikely to have these in any way solved by termination but are not made worse by it.

A number of studies have been carried out in cases where an unwanted pregnancy has been continued to term. Höök (1963) in studying 249 Swedish women 7½–11 years after refused termination, reported a large proportion of serious problems connected with the pregnancy. Fifty-three per cent had symptoms of marked instability for several years which eventually cleared up, but a further 24 per cent still exhibited pathological symptoms that had originated in the pregnancy. An illegal abortion had been sought in 11 per cent.

Also to be taken into consideration is the effect on the child who was 'unwanted'. Forssman and Thuwe (1966) in a 21 year follow up of 120 children born after abortion application had been refused found an increased incidence in the children of delinquency and psychiatric disturbance. Compared with a matched control group they were underachieved, were more insecure and needed more public assistance. Infants killed within the first 24 hours after birth in most cases were killed by the mother and were unwanted (Resnick, 1970). There is a close association between the 'battered baby' syndrome, unwanted pregnancy and severe rejection after birth.

The most recent work carried out in Aberdeen by McCance, Olley and Edward (1973) with a group of 303 abortion applicants has shown that approximately 6 per cent of both single and ever married who aborted had severe regrets at eighteen months follow up. A further 15 per cent approximately had mixed feelings or mild regrets. Only about 2 per cent were found to be clinically depressed.

Severe regrets at the continuation of an unwanted pregnancy were found in 20 per cent of single and about 10 per cent of the ever married at follow up. Significantly more regrets at continuing the pregnancy were found among single women and slightly more regrets among ever married women compared with the aborted groups. Again about 2 per cent of those going to term were severely depressed clinically though it was the aborted group who were the most psychiatrically disturbed at the time of referral.

Adoption was found to be commonly associated with severe regrets. The most satisfactory general outcome in ever married women occurred for those in whom sterilization was also carried out at the time of abortion. A better relationship with the husband was reported, together with improved sexual adjustment.

Psychiatric illness and gynaecology

Major mental illness can occur as a sequel to gynaecological operations. A confusional state may develop perhaps in association with post-operative complications, such as infection, electrolyte imbalance or blood loss. On occasion a depressive or a schizophrenic illness may be precipitated, usually in predisposed women with a clear individual or family history of such breakdowns.

The possible presence of psychiatric illness must also be taken into account in the assessment of gynaecological out-patients. In this connection depressive illness, particularly in middle-aged or older women may present essentially with somatic symptoms which mask the underlying disturbance of mood. Thus, complaints such as pelvic or abdominal pain, menstrual disturbance, lack of sexual interest, may be part of a depressive condition. Many patients are unable to describe their feelings clearly and will instead talk about a loss of energy or a loss of interest in their family or their housework, rather than about being gloomy or depressed.

On inquiry intensification of symptoms in the earlier part of the day, improvement later in the day and a restless insomnia with early morning waking may be found. The onset of these difficulties may be related to a bereavement or a major disappointment or change connected with the family.

The risk of suicide in severe depressive states must be borne in mind and prompt psychiatric assessment and anti-depressant treatment are indicated in this situation.

Neurotic illness should be considered when evaluating states of prolonged disability, e.g. after operation. The sympathy and attention of relatives may invest the 'sick' role with considerable secondary gain for the individual.

Women presenting with persistent somatic complaints, e.g. burning sensations in the vagina, without organic cause being discovered despite numerous investigations, may have a grossly disordered personality rather than an illness.

Physical symptoms can for some women be a preferred way of expressing conflicts and dissatisfaction with their life situation. Often only supportive psychiatric measures and tranquillizers can be offered, as interpretations of underlying emotional problems are rejected.

Rarely a patient with schizophrenia may seek gynaecological help. In this case the physical symptoms often have a bizarre quality and are possibly ascribed to outside influences.

Disorders of personality

In gynaecological and obstetric practice women with disorders of personality will present special problems in assessment and management. For example, those who are mildly or severely subnormal mentally may be unaware of their condition or be unable to give a coherent account of it. High grade mentally subnormal girls are vulnerable sexually. Some drift into prostitution. Others may become pregnant. Special care may be required particularly from Social Work Departments in such cases and abortion may have to be considered if there is a pregnancy.

Psychopathic disorders may also be associated with unlooked for pregnancy and in general psychopathic women present difficulty in their management. They are often unreliable and unco-operative.

One of the most difficult conditions to identify is that of lesbianism which may occur both in single and in married women. There are many more lesbians in the population than might be supposed since it is in the majority of cases successfully concealed. The woman herself may not be fully aware that she is homosexual. Well meaning advice offered to such women on the assumption that they are heterosexual is clearly misplaced. Only skilled and sympathetic interviewing will bring the true situation to light but only in a very small proportion of cases would there be any question of the woman considering herself in need of treatment. Thus for the most part she should be considered as a normal person in her own right but with rather special problems by reason of her homosexual attitudes.

SOME GENERAL PRINCIPLES OF TREATMENT
The basic principle that underlies the management of patients suffering from emotional distress or psychiatric illness is to alleviate suffering as soon as possible by firm friendly support and reassurance. No special skills are required for this—only an informed awareness of the part played by psychological factors in each condition as it presents itself. It cannot be too strongly emphasized that this principle obtains where the condition has been diagnosed as psychiatric illness or where it is an emotional upset associated with obstetric or gynae-

cological conditions. Even when it appears that there are two unrelated disorders, one physical and the other psychological, it is still essential to tackle the psychological illness in its own right.

It is well established that patients with emotional troubles find it easier to report some physical symptom than to report their anxieties. It is still commonly assumed that if they are diagnosed as 'neurotic' they are wasting the doctor's time and that they should solve their own neurotic problems. However, although it may be time-consuming, one or two sessions in which the patient is positively encouraged to talk about her fears can be extremely rewarding and effective. Indeed one continuous hour given over exclusively to the anxious patient may be time-saving, if set against the much more frequent and frustrating attendances made by the patient with increasing demands for relief of her repertoire of seemingly physical complaints. Even if the doctor is only attentive and silent, he will have done much to help his patient by his support.

In 'talking it out' the doctor takes a more active part and encourages the patient to talk about problems some of which may be very distressing to bring out into the open. His sincere interest in his patient will help her to unfold her story to him and as her difficulties emerge, solutions will usually suggest themselves. In such cases it is always necessary to move towards a practical decision when the patient will feel that she has to take some active step—a frank talk with her husband or her mother, the giving up of an undesirable relationship, decision to have a family, to adopt a child or to change her occupation.

Symptoms related to anxiety are always intensified if they are not expressed and worked out in practical action. A vicious circle is thereby established and can only be broken if the patient has confidence in her doctor and feels secure in approaching him about what others might regard as stupid and childish.

Patients are particularly sensitive to the possibility that they will be told that they are imagining or exaggerating their symptoms or that they are malingering. The fact that she has little to show for her distress and indeed may successfully conceal it even from those close to her, lends support to her fear of being misunderstood.

It should be a matter of routine for the doctor to make tactful inquiries about how the patient is feeling within herself when she comes to see the doctor. Often very little encouragement is needed to let her open up about inner thoughts and feelings but a few leading questions are not out of place. For example, in the case of a pregnant women, she could be asked specifically if she has any particular worries about the pregnancy. Questions about the home situation, how she is getting on with her husband, her children and other relatives, how she is coping with her work and so forth all elicit sufficient information. Again systematic inquiry about pain and other discomfort including headaches, digestive upsets, indeed any symptom of autonomic instability, such as tachycardia and sweating can all lead into the patient's psychological problems.

In many cases, particularly those arising in obstetrics, the husband is usually seen, in which case he can be a most useful informant on psychological problems that the patient herself wishes to conceal. Joint consultations can be most beneficial in many such cases.

To return to the monistic theme followed out in this chapter, it will now be appreciated that this theme is well illustrated by a comprehensive approach to the patient's condition as at all times both psychological and physical in its nature.

In recent years drug treatment for both minor and major psychiatric and psychotic conditions has proved effective but there is evidence that their use is often indiscriminate. One reason for this is that doctors obviously find it easier and much less personally demanding to write a prescription than to become involved in his patient's inner conflicts and background life situation.

Over-prescribing of this kind leads to a total misunderstanding on the part of the patient about the nature of her trouble and does nothing to remove the basic causes. The more potent drugs can also be taken as overdoses.

A less common but equally serious error arises from mis-diagnosis as between anxiety states and depressive illness, two conditions for which potent drugs are very frequently prescribed. In cases of anxiety, it may be necessary to prescribe one of the phenothiazine drugs, such as chlorpromazine, or a minor tranquillizer, such as diazapam, to take the edge off the patient's symptoms while the psychotherapeutic approach outlined above is being pursued. Similarly if a patient is depressed one of the tricyclic compounds, such as imipramine, amitriptyline or chlorimipramine can be justifiably prescribed. However, particularly when the symptoms are present with minor severity, the anxious patient may be diagnosed as 'depressed' because she may actually say that this is how she feels, while the depressed patient may give the superficial appearance of apprehension. Anti-depressants are, therefore, prescribed for anxiety and tranquillizers for depression, with the results that are predictably unsatisfactory.

Generally speaking, patients with minor transient anxiety states do not respond to drug therapy, except temporarily. They should, therefore, be given infrequently and with caution. Anti-depressants on the other hand can give most effective relief provided a valid diagnosis has been made. These drugs do not have an anti-depressant effect for a week to ten days. The patient should be told of this and also warned of side effects, particularly somnolence which should clear up once the anti-depressant effect has become established.

Night sedation again should be prescribed with some caution. Often a patient's complaint of sleeplessness, particularly in the presence of anxiety, is transient and during a period of personal difficulty or even crisis. There may be even positive benefits to the patient to lie awake for a night or two to enable her to work out a solution for herself, albeit with a good deal of attendant personal discomfort. It is only if the insomnia is persistent and is clearly undermining the patient's general state of health and wellbeing throughout the waking period that sedation is indicated. The barbiturates which have for so long held pride of place should nowadays be avoided if at all possible. There are always risks of drug dependence arising and in some cases overdoses may occur. Nitrazepam sometimes in combination with a tranquillizer is usually adequate, particularly in depressive states when anti-depressants are also given. Amitriptyline, for example, may be used for its sedation effect in addition to its anti-depressant effect by being taken before retiring in a dose sufficient for 24 hours.

The special susceptibility of the fetus to damage in the early weeks of pregnancy should always be borne in mind when prescribing drugs during the first trimester.

In summary the therapeutic approach to the woman with obstetric or gynaecological problems must take into account both her physical and her psychological needs, together with the special circumstances in which these needs arise. It is often said that a careful history is sufficient to establish a diagnosis in most cases, without the need for physical examination and special investigations. By the same token the same history is sufficient to provide most of the psychological treatment or at least suggest how best to proceed with more detailed therapy. The most effective therapy is that which at all times considers the whole person.

Anorexia Nervosa

This rare disorder is characterized by gross loss of weight to the point of emaciation, failure to eat with avoidance of calorific foods and menstrual disturbance, usually amenorrhoea.

The patient is usually a young woman who has had an early menarche, had previously been well nourished or even over-nourished as a child. There may be some history of concern over her weight and her figure.

Although her condition is most painfully obvious to all, she persistently denies that she is hungry, tired or thin. The superficial impression is of an over-active, bright-eyed, often intelligent young person protesting her health and vigour.

The patient becomes so emaciated and so stubbornly opposed to any form of food intake that life saving physical measures may be required. Close observation is usually indicated since the patient may hide food, throw it out of the window or down the WC or surreptitiously vomit. The implacable denial of her symptoms, her refusal to co-operate and indeed her persistent and ingenious deceptions all make treatment extremely difficult, unless she is admitted to hospital with special nursing observation.

The physical consequences of the condition include emaciation, atrophy of breasts and buttocks, the growth of downy hair on face, limbs and back, bradycardia, hypotension, constipation and poor peripheral circulation. Investigations reveal a depletion of body potassium and there is evidence that release of gonadotrophic hormones from the pituitary is impaired though there is no global failure of anterior pituitary function.

The literature abounds in psychiatric speculation about this condition which has been variously diagnosed as depressive, schizophrenic, obsessive compulsive, phobic and hysterical. All treatments appropriate to these conditions have been tried but with only limited success.

Though no clear-cut causes can be found in the psychological sphere, nevertheless grossly abnormal inner psychological states are found almost invariably. These include a morbid fear of fatness, a distorted body image, a fear of adult sexuality, abnormal reactions to puberty and the presence of bizarre sexual fantasies, for example, that conception takes place through the oral intake of semen. Often there are serious doubts about sexual identity. The girl fearing that she may in fact be a boy or should have the body of a male.

Spontaneous recovery can be expected but only after a period of two or three years. Many cases continue through adult life and death occurs in 2·5 per cent of cases. Consider-able personality disorder may persist after the main symptoms have subsided. These include some disturbances of appetite, fluctuation of weight and menstrual disturbance.

The most successful form of treatment involves a total regime of management on an in-patient basis. The strictest observation in the early days actually with bed-rest is essential and various psychotropic drugs may be tried. However the most important element in the regime is that there should be at least one person in charge of the total management of the case who can act as a firm and ever-present parent figure. It is perhaps because of the non-specific nature of this last factor in the treatment regime that there have been so many apparently contradictory claims about the efficacy of some more specific drug treatment.

REFERENCES

Aren, P. (1958–59) *Account in Year Book of Obstetrics and Gynaecology*, p. 64. Chicago: Year Book Medical Publishers.

Bardwick, J. M. & Behrman, S. J. (1967) Investigation into the effects of anxiety, sexual arousal and menstrual cycle phase on uterine contractions. *Psychosom. Med.*, **29**, 468–482.

Barker, M. G. (1968) Psychiatric illness after hysterectomy. *Brit. med. J.*, **ii**, 91–95.

Berg, J. M., Gilderdale, S. & Way, J. (1969) On telling of parents of a diagnosis of mongolism. *Brit. J. Psychiat.*, **115**, 1195–1196.

Bickers, W. & Woods, M. (1951) The effects of certain antibiotics, anti-malarial drugs and Amoebicides on candida albicans. *Tex. Rep. Biol. Med.*, **9**, 406.

Black, W. P. & Sclare, A. B. (1968) Sterilization by tubal ligation—a follow-up study. *J. Obstet. Gynaec. Brit. Cwlth.*, **75**, 219–224.

Blau, A., Slaff, B., Easton, K., Welkowitz, J., Springarn, J. & Cohen, J. (1963) The psychogenic etiology of premature births. *Psychosom. Med.*, **25**, 201–211.

Bowlby, J. (1971) *Attachment*, Vol. 1. London: Penguin Books.

Brown, E. & Barglow, P. (1971) Pseudocyesis a paradigm for psycho-physiological interactions. *Arch. Gen. Psychiat.*, **24**, 221.

Brown, L. B. (1964) Anxiety in Pregnancy. *Brit. J. med. Psychol.*, **37**, 47–58.

Chertok, L. (1969) *Motherhood and Personality*. Psychosomatic Aspects. London: Tavistock.

Chertok, L., Mondzain, M. L. & Bonnaud, M. (1963) Vomiting and the wish to have a child. *Psychosom. Med.*, **25**, 13.

Cohen, R. L. (1966) Some maladaptive syndromes of pregnancy and the puerperium. *Obstet. Gynaec.*, **27**, 562–570.

Cooper, A. J. (1970) Frigidity, treatment and short-term prognosis. *J. psychosom. Res.*, **14**, 133–147.

Coppen, A. J. (1958) Psychosomatic aspects of pre-eclamptic toxaemia. *J. psychosom. Res.*, **2**, 241.

Coppen, A. J. (1959) Vomiting of early pregnancy: psychological factors and body build. *Lancet*, **i**, 172.

Coppen, A. J. (1965) The prevalence of menstrual disorders in psychiatric patients. *Brit. J. Psychiat.*, **3**, 155–167.

Coppen, A. J. & Kessel, N. (1963) Menstruation and personality. *Brit. J. Psychiat.*, **119**, 711–721.

Cramond, W. A. (1954) Psychological aspects of uterine dysfunction. *Lancet*, **ii**, 1241–1245.

Dalton, K. (1964) *The premenstrual syndrome*. London: Heinemann.

Dalton, K. (1968) Menstruation and examinations. *Lancet*, **i**, 386.

Daly, R. J., Kane, F. J. & Ewing, J. A. (1967) Psychosis associated with the use of a sequential oral contraceptive. *Lancet*, **ii**, 444–445.

Dickens, G. & Trethowan, W. H. (1972) Cravings and aversions during pregnancy. *J. psychosom. Res.*, **15**, 259–268.

Drillien, C. M. (1946) A study of normal and abnormal menstrual function in the auxiliary territorial service. *J. Obstet. Gynaec. Brit. Emp.*, **53**, 228.

Dutton, W. A. (1965) Functional uterine bleeding. *Canad. med. Ass. J.*, **92**, 398.

Ekblad, M. (1955) Induced abortion on psychiatric grounds. A follow-up of 479 women. *Acta. psychiat. Scand.*, Supplement 99.

Ellison, C. (1968) Psychosomatic factors in the unconsummated marriage. *J. psychosom. Res.*, **12**, 61–65.

Engles, W. D., Patee, C. J. & Wittkower, E. D. (1964) Emotional Settings of Functional Amenorrhoea. *Psychosom. Med.*, **26**, 682–700.

Ford, C. S. & Beach, F. A. (1965) *Patterns of sexual behaviour*. London: Methuen.

Forssman, H. & Thuwe, I. (1966) One hundred and twenty children born after application for therapeutic abortion refused. Their mental health, social adjustment and educational level up to the age of 21. *Acta. psychiat. Scand.*, **42**, 71–88.

Glick, I. D., Salerno, L. J. & Royce, J. R. (1965) Psychophysiologic factors in the etiology of pre-eclampsia. *Arch. Gen. Psychiat.*, **12**, 260–266.

Golub, L. J., Lang, W., Menduke, H. & Gordon, H. (1957) Teenage dysmenorrhoea. *Amer. J. Obstet. Gynec.*, **74**, 591.

Grimm, E. (1962) Psychological investigation of habitual abortion. *Psychosom. Med.*, **24**, 369.

Hamilton, J. A. (1962) *Post-partum psychiatric problems.* St. Louis: C. V. Mosby.

Herzberg, B. & Coppen, A. (1970) Changes in psychological symptoms in women taking oral contraceptives. *Brit. J. Psychiat.*, **116**, 161–164.

Herzberg, B. N., Draper, K. C., Johnson, A. L. & Nicol, G. C. (1971) Oral contraceptives, Depression and Libido. *Brit. med. J.*, **iii**, 495–500.

Höök, K. (1963) Refused abortion. A follow-up study of 249 women whose applications were refused by the National Board of Health in Sweden. *Acta. psychiat. Scand.*, Supplement, 168.

Jannsson, B. (1965) Mental disorders after abortion. *Acta. psychiat. Scand.*, **40**, 87–110.

Kear-Colwell, J. J. (1965) Neuroticism in the early puerperium. *Brit. J. Psychiat.*, **3**, 1189–1192.

Kessel, N. & Coppen, A. (1963) The prevalence of common menstrual symptoms. *Lancet*, **ii**, 61.

Kinsey, A. C., Pomeroy, W. B., Martin, C. E. & Gebhard, P. H. (1953) *Sexual behaviour in the human female.* Philadelphia: Saunders.

Mai, F. M. (1971) Conception after adoption: An open question. *Psychosom. Med.*, **33**, 509–514.

Masters, W. H. & Johnson, V. E. (1966) *Human sexual response.* London: Churchill.

Masters, W. & Johnson, V. (1970) *Human sexual inadequacy.* London: Churchill.

McCance, C. & Hall, D. J. (1972) Sexual behaviour and contraceptive practice of unmarried female undergraduates at Aberdeen University. *Brit. med. J.*, **ii**, 694–700.

McCance, C., Olley, P. C. & Edward, V. (1973) In *Experience with abortion.* A case study of N. E. Scotland. Ed. G. Horobin, Cambridge University Press.

McDonald, R. L. (1968) The role of emotional factors in obstetric complications: A review. *Psychosom. Med.*, **30**, 222.

Neugarten, B. & Kraines, R. (1965) Menopausal symptoms in women of various ages. *Psychosom. Med.*, **27**, 266–273.

O'Neill, D. F. (1958) Out-patient Gynaecology. *Brit. med. J.*, **i**, 1038–1039.

Paffenbarger, R. (1964) Epidemiological aspects of para-partum mental illness. *Brit. J. Prev. Soc. Med.*, **18**, 189–195.

Pilowsky, I. & Sharp, J. (1971) Psychological aspects of pre-eclamptic toxaemias: A prospective study. *J. psychosom. Res.*, **15**, 193–197.

Protheroe, C. (1969) Puerperal psychoses: a long-term study, 1927–1961. *Brit. J. Psychiat.*, **115**, 9–30.

Pugh, T. F., Jerath, B. K., Schmidt, W. M. & Reed, R. B. (1963) Rates of mental illness related to childbearing. *New Engl. J. Med.*, **268**, 1224–1228.

Resnick, R. J. (1970) Murder of the newborn: a psychiatric review of neonaticide. *Amer. J. Psychiat.*, **126**, 1414.

Rodgers, D. A. & Ziegler, F. J. (1968) Changes in sexual behaviour consequent to use of non-coital procedures of contraception. *Psychosom. Med.*, **30**, 495–505.

Sandler, B. (1968) Emotional Stress and Infertility. *J. psychosom. Res.*, **12**, 51–59.

Schuck, F. (1951) Pain and pain relief in essential dysmenorrhoea. *Amer. J. Obstet. Gynec.*, **62**, 559.

Shainess, N. (1961) A Re-evaluation of some aspects of femininity through a study of menstruation: A preliminary report. *Compr. Psychiat.*, **2**, 20.

Shipman, W. G. (1964) Age of menarche and adult personality. *Arch. Gen. Psychiat.*, **10**, 155–159.

Sim, M. (1963) Abortion and the psychiatrist. *Brit. med. J.*, **ii**, 1061.

Stoller, J. R. (1968) *Sex and Gender.* London: Hogarth Press.

Sutherland, H. & Stewart, I. (1965) A critical analysis of the premenstrual syndrome. *Lancet*, **i**, 1180.

Thomson, B. & Baird, D. (1968) Follow-up of 186 sterilized women. *Lancet*, **i**, 1023–1027.

Tonks, C. M. (1968) Premenstrual tension. *Brit. J. Hosp. Med.*, **1**, 383.

Treadway, C. R., Kane, F. J., Jarrahi-Zadeh, A. & Lipton, M. A. (1969) A psychoendocrine study of pregnancy and puerperium. *Amer. J. Psychiat.*, **125**, 1380–1386.

Trethowan, W. H. & Conlon, M. F. (1965) The Couvade Syndrome. *Brit. J. Psychiat.*, **3**, 57.

Tupper, C., Maya, F., Stewart, L. C., Weil, R. J. & Gray, J. D. (1957) The problem of spontaneous abortion. 1. A combined approach. *Amer. J. Obstet. Gynec.*, **50**, 353.

Udry, J. R. & Morris, N. M. (1968) Distribution of Coitus in the menstrual cycle. *Nature*, **220**, 593–596.

Vellay, P. (1972) Painless labour—a French method: In *Modern perspectives in psycho-obstetrics.* Ed. J. Howells. Edinburgh: Oliver & Boyd.

Waxenberg, S. E. (1963) Some biologic correlates of sexual behaviour. In Winokur, G. (Ed.) *Determinates of sexual behaviour.* Illinois: Charles C. Thomas.

Whitlock, F. A. & Edwards, J. E. (1968) Pregnancy and attempted suicide. *Comprehens. Psychiat.*, **9**, 1–12.

Yalom, I. D., Lunde, D. T., Moos, R. H. & Hamburg, D. A. (1968) 'Post partum blues' syndrome. A description and related variables. *Arch. Gen. Psychiat.*, **18**, 16–27.

31. Shock and Maternal Injury

Shock is a condition characterized by a failure of the circulation to adequately perfuse the tissues of the body. Four main factors contribute to the maintenance of perfusion, namely, the circulating blood volume, the cardiac pump, vascular tone and the viscosity of the blood. By far the commonest cause of shock in obstetric practice is a reduction in the circulating blood volume due to haemorrhage. In the event of haemorrhage, venous return to the heart becomes insufficient to maintain an adequate cardiac output, and in an attempt to compensate there is intense vasoconstriction in the skin and other less vital organs. This accounts for the typical appearance of the 'shocked' patient who is pale, sweating, anxious, restless and collapsed. The pulse is rapid and thready and the blood pressure is low. If the state of impaired perfusion is allowed to continue over too long a period, then changes due to anoxia will take place in the tissues at the cellular level. These changes include severe metabolic acidosis and, when they occur, the patient will enter the phase of 'refractory' shock when resuscitation will become increasingly difficult. It is clearly seen, therefore, that haemorrhagic shock requires early, rapid and adequate replacement of the circulating blood volume while, at the same time, steps must be taken to diagnose and remove the source of blood loss.

In contrast to the clinical picture described above is the one of bacteraemic shock. In this condition, a process of overwhelming infection causes generalized vasodilatation and, although the patient may look and feel well in the initial stages, the problem of inadequate tissue perfusion remains. By the time such a patient enters the phase of vasoconstriction, the prognosis has become extremely poor.

Classification

The commonest causes of shock encountered in obstetric practice can be classified as follows:

HAEMORRHAGIC SHOCK
Incomplete Abortion
Ectopic Pregnancy
Placenta Praevia
Abruptio Placenta
Atonic Post-partum Haemorrhage

BACTERAEMIC OR ENDOTOXIC SHOCK

TRAUMATIC SHOCK
Acute Inversion of the Uterus
Uterine Rupture
Maternal Injuries

OTHER CAUSES
Amniotic Fluid Embolism
Pulmonary Thromboembolism
Inhaled Gastric Contents
Myocardial Infarction
Previous Corticosteroid Therapy

MANAGEMENT OF HAEMORRHAGIC SHOCK

The clinical features of the various causes of haemorrhagic shock have been discussed in the chapters dealing with bleeding in early and late pregnancy but certain common principles apply to the treatment of the circulatory problem.

Blood transfusion
When shock is the result of haemorrhage, there is no truly satisfactory alternative to the use of blood transfusion. In the shocked patient, a blood sample is sent for cross-matching and, by emergency methods, compatible blood should be available within 30 minutes. In severe shock, it will be necessary to replace blood before compatible cross-matched blood is available, and screened group O Rhesus negative blood should be given. An alternative is to infuse plasma or a blood volume expander such as low molecular weight dextran and, although less satisfactory than blood, these substitutes can be valuable in emergency

circumstances. Since dextrans can interfere with cross-matching methods, it is important that blood is withdrawn before the infusion is started. If difficulties are encountered in setting-up an intravenous infusion in the collapsed peripheral veins of a shocked patient, there should be no hesitation in cutting down on a vessel in the leg or the forearm under local anaesthesia.

Central venous pressure monitoring
When large volumes of blood are required to resuscitate a patient, it is essential to monitor the central venous pressure. This can be done through a wide-bore cannula which is introduced through a forearm vein until its tip comes to lie in the subclavian vein or superior vena cava. In practical terms, a low central venous pressure indicates poor venous return due to inadequate blood replacement and a high reading suggests cardiac failure from overloading of the circulation. The objective of blood transfusion is, therefore, to maintain the central venous pressure between 2 and 10cm of water and the systemic arterial pressure at normal levels. Banked blood is stored at low temperatures, and when more than four pints of blood are required, it is important to raise the blood to body temperature by passing it through a blood-warming apparatus before transfusion. Citrate is used as the anticoagulant in blood and can exert a toxic effect on the myocardium if given in large amounts. These toxic effects are reversed by calcium and if more than 2 litres of blood are transfused it is recommended that 10ml of 10 per cent calcium gluconate should be injected for every litre of citrated blood.

Monitoring of fluid balance and urinary output
Shock occurs more readily in patients who are dehydrated and acidotic following prolonged labour. Dehydration increases blood viscosity and further impairs tissue perfusion so that infusion of adequate volumes of Ringer lactate solution will be of benefit. The acidosis following prolonged labour will be worsened by prolonged shock and an infusion of 100mEq sodium bicarbonate should be given to correct this. The need for fluid and electrolyte therapy is dictated by the changes in the blood urea, electrolyte and acid-base balance which should be measured at regular intervals.

Acute renal failure is a risk in any patient who has been shocked and its earliest warning comes from measuring hourly urinary output through an indwelling catheter. The aim should be to maintain urinary output between 20–30ml per hour. If the output of urine should fall, 100ml of 20–25 per cent mannitol can be given intravenously over a 30 minute period. It is necessary to maintain adequate fluid input to achieve the osmotic effect of mannitol. If the first dose of mannitol achieves a flow of 50ml of urine, it can be repeated but in the absence of urinary response, further doses should be withheld. When acute renal failure becomes established, renal dialysis may be life-saving and the opinion of a renal physician should be obtained without delay.

OTHER GENERAL MEASURES
In the immediate treatment of shock, the end of the patient's bed should be raised to encourage venous return from the legs and to maintain essential blood flow to the brain. Before delivery the patient should be nursed in the lateral position to prevent the pregnant uterus from further impeding venous return and to help maintain a satisfactory airway. It can be helpful to give the shocked patient oxygen by face-mask and a clear airway must be maintained using intubation or tracheostomy if necessary.

Prevention is always better than cure, and the effects of haemorrhagic shock can be minimized by ensuring that every patient approaches labour with a satisfactory haemoglobin level. It is also important that dehydration in labour should have early and adequate treatment by intravenous fluid replacement and that labour should not be allowed to be unduly prolonged.

Flying squad
When haemorrhage occurs outside hospital, the obstetric flying squad should be summoned so that facilities for resuscitation can be brought to the patient with the least possible delay. It is always better to resuscitate a patient in her own home than to transfer her to hospital in a shocked condition. It should be the aim of every hospital to have the flying squad on its way within seven minutes of receiving a call and this requires a fully equipped team being constantly ready to answer the emergency.

On reaching the patient, the flying squad should first assess the condition of the patient by taking the pulse and blood pressure. An estimate of the blood loss is also made and depending on the severity of the shock, fluid replacement will be commenced with either saline, a blood volume expander or screened O Rhesus negative blood. If the patient is still bleeding when the flying squad arrives, appropriate steps should be taken to minimize or arrest the haemorrhage. An intravenous infusion must be set up in all cases so that, in the event of haemorrhage during the journey to hospital, fluid replacement can be given at once.

There is controversy about the advisability of giving analgesics to the shocked patient. If the patient is in severe pain it may be necessary to give pain relief, but it is generally advisable to withhold morphia until the patient has rallied from her shock. It is worth remembering that a drug given intramuscularly is unlikely to be absorbed until the peripheral circulation is properly restored. If analgesia is urgently needed in a shocked patient, a small intravenous dose of morphia may be the best method of achieving the desired effect.

As antenatal care has improved and as more patients have been delivered in hospital, the flying squad has been called out less frequently but its proper use will continue to be life-saving in patients who develop shock outside the confines of a hospital.

BACTERAEMIC OR ENDOTOXIC SHOCK

Bacteraemic shock is shock occurring in patients with bacteria in their blood. Many of the clinical features are due to the liberation of endotoxins from the bacteria, giving the alternative name of 'endotoxic shock'. Since this syndrome can complicate any infection it is sometimes seen in obstetric patients following intra-uterine infection, wound abscess, infected pelvic haematoma, severe pyelonephritis or pneumonia. Bacteraemic shock has been more commonly associated with Gram negative bacteria although Gram positive organisms are sometimes responsible. In obstetric practice, an anaerobic infection with clostridium welchii following intra-uterine death or criminal abortion may also be responsible for bacteraemic shock. The syndrome is thought to be due to the effect of bacterial endotoxins on peripheral blood vessels which dilate and impair tissue perfusion. A wide-spread intravascular coagulation may develop which will further impede blood flow and result in organ tissue damage.

CLINICAL FEATURES
In the initial stages, the patient has a low blood pressure and a poor thready pulse, but looks pink and well due to peripheral vasodilatation. This is, however, misleading as her general condition is serious and will deteriorate when the phase of vasoconstriction supervenes. The patient then may become confused and lethargic with rigors, vomiting and diarrhoea. Oliguria due to renal failure will supervene and the condition carries a high mortality.

Diagnosis
The syndrome of bacteraemic shock should be suspected in any patient with a severe infection who becomes hypotensive. Blood cultures should be taken but these may be negative since the effects are due to the endotoxins rather than the bacteria themselves and treatment must be started before the blood culture results are available.

Treatment
Antibiotics should be given and the choice of drug will depend on the prevalent infections at any particular time. Ampicillin and cephaloridine will be effective against most organisms although gentamycin is a currently fashionable choice with a further antibiotic such as lincomycin given to cover the possibility of a bacteroides infection. The antibiotic should be given parenterally and in large doses, although the choice may be changed when the results of blood cultures become available.

Corticosteroid therapy is also given and it is necessary to give very large doses to achieve maximum benefit. Hydrocortisone given intravenously in a dose of 1Gm initially and a further 3–4Gm in 24 hours will be required. If there is any evidence of dehydration, fluid replacement may be required but any associated renal failure may dictate the needs of fluid balance. The general view is that vasoconstrictors are contra-indicated in bacteraemic shock because they worsen the underlying problem of impaired tissue perfusion. Alternatively, in the phase of vasoconstriction, a vasodilator such as phenoxybenzamine may be used to improve the perfusion of vital organs. Caution must be exercised in the use of vasodilators because, in a patient with reduced circulating blood volume, they may impair venous return to the heart to such an extent that cardiac asystole results. If patients with bacteraemic shock have bled, then the appropriate loss should be replaced with blood, but transfusion will not by itself restore a normal blood pressure. The management of seriously ill patients with bacteraemic shock has become increasingly specialized and the best results will be achieved by referring patients to intensive care units with experience in this type of condition.

TRAUMATIC SHOCK

Traumatic shock following obstetric procedures used to be given the old name of 'obstetric shock' but it was no different from shock encountered in other branches of medical practice. The causes of shock in these circumstances may be multifactorial with haemorrhage, neurological stimulation, tissue damage, anaesthesia and dehydration all playing a part. When traumatic shock is severe, the acute circulatory collapse may lead to cardiac arrest and sudden death. Such catastrophies may occur after severe emergencies such as rupture of the uterus, amniotic fluid embolism or inversion of the uterus. Some of the obstetric causes of traumatic shock will now be discussed.

Acute inversion of the uterus

This condition is now rarely seen but may occur when cord traction is applied while the uterus remains atonic. When inversion of the uterus is complete, the inverted fundus of the uterus will be outside the vulva and the placenta may still be attached. Incomplete inversion of the uterus should be suspected in a patient who becomes shocked after delivery with no evidence of blood loss. There will be a 'dimple' in the fundus of the uterus which may be suspected on abdominal examination and confirmed at examination under anaesthesia.

Treatment of inversion of the uterus
When the uterus has inverted, venous return is impaired by the constriction of the cervix and the tissues become congested and oedematous so that it may be difficult to replace the uterus to its normal position. It is imperative to correct the inversion as soon as possible and too much time should not be wasted on resusci-

tation which is unlikely to succeed until the inversion is reduced.

Two methods have been described for the reduction of uterine inversion. The first is to replace the uterus by manual manipulation under anaesthesia, starting with the tissues which prolapsed last and finishing the manœuvre by replacing the fundus. If the placenta is still attached, it is best to leave manual removal until after the uterus has been replaced, since the removal of the placenta may open the sinuses and encourage further bleeding. The second method is the hydrostatic technique described by O'Sullivan. In this method, the uterus is replaced in the vagina, and the lips of the vulva are held tightly round the examining hand by an assistant. Warm saline is then introduced into the vagina through a rubber tube and the hydrostatic pressure reduces the uterine inversion.

Inversion of the uterus is a highly dangerous condition and it is important that it should be diagnosed and treated without delay.

Rupture of the uterus

The signs and symptoms of uterine rupture can vary from acute abdominal pain with severe shock to mild abdominal discomfort with minimal constitutional upset. The severity of the clinical condition depends on the amount of bleeding provoked by the uterine rupture. A rupture in the highly vascular upper segment of the uterus is usually associated with severe shock in contrast to the almost 'silent' rupture encountered in some avascular lower Caesarean section scars. Rupture of the uterus can present before, during or immediately after labour and must be included in the differential diagnosis of any shocked obstetrical patient.

PREDISPOSING FACTORS
The most common factor predisposing to uterine rupture is a previous Caesarean section scar. Dewhurst (1957) found an incidence of scar rupture of 2·2 per cent following classical Caesarean section and of 0·51 per cent following the lower segment operation. These incidences rose to 8·9 per cent and 1·2 per cent respectively, when patients were allowed to deliver vaginally. If the placenta is implanted anteriorly over the site of a previous classical Caesarean section this may serve to undermine the integrity of the scar. Post-operative wound infection has also been blamed for weakening the strength of a uterine scar although the

importance of this factor has never been fully established. Myomectomy scars are said to rupture less frequently than Caesarean section scars, although any operation on the uterus must be regarded as a source of potential weakness. Uterine rupture may also take place in a patient who has had a previous operation on her cervix, such as a Manchester repair or a cone biopsy, because scar tissue on the cervix may split during labour with the tear extending into the uterine vessels.

Rupture of the intact uterus is less common but may occur in a highly parous patient whose uterine wall has been weakened by recurrent childbearing. Paradoxically, multiparous patients may also have hypertonic uterine activity and, for this reason, oxytocin should be used sparingly in such women especially if they give a history of very rapid labours. In countries where patients can labour without trained supervision uterine rupture may follow obstructed labour even in an intact uterus. When labour has continued for several days the lower uterine segment becomes very thin and rupture of the uterus may be provoked by intra-uterine manipulations designed to achieve delivery of the child.

SIGNS AND SYMPTOMS

Rupture of an upper segment scar usually causes severe abdominal pain and shock. The labour stops abruptly and the fetus may be palpated outside the uterine cavity. In these circumstances, the baby will be dead and there will be abdominal guarding and tenderness. Vaginal bleeding may also be present and sometimes ruptured uterus may be confused with abruptio placentae. The diagnosis will not be difficult in most cases, however, and laparotomy will be required at once.

The signs and symptoms of a ruptured lower segment are often much less obvious. Patients who are labouring with a previous lower segment scar must be delivered in a specialized obstetric unit under close supervision. Pain and tenderness over the lower segment scar may indicate a dehiscence but the significance of the pain can be difficult to interpret. Many repeat Caesarean sections are done because of pain only to demonstrate a healthy and intact scar. On the other hand, patients without pain have been found with large, but avascular, deficiencies in their lower segment scars at the time of repeat Caesarean section. Signs which raise suspicion of scar dehiscence are a rising maternal pulse rate, vaginal bleeding, haematuria and fetal distress. If, at any time there is any doubt about the integrity of a Caesarean section scar, it is safer to deliver the patient by repeat section than to wait and see.

MANAGEMENT OF PATIENTS WITH A PREVIOUS CAESAREAN SECTION

The incidence of scar rupture after classical section is so high that in modern practice these patients should be delivered by elective section in all subsequent pregnancies. In the case of previous lower segment section, the decision is more complex and several factors must be considered before deciding whether to allow labour or not. If the previous section was performed for a recurrent indication such as contracted pelvis, then a repeat section is clearly required. When the operation was for a non-recurrent condition such as placenta praevia, vaginal delivery can be contemplated and will be achieved safely in many cases. On the other hand, maternal age over 30 years, a history of infertility, a history of technical difficulty at the previous operation, placental failure or hypertension are all factors which might suggest repeat section as a more favourable alternative to a trial of vaginal delivery. As women are now tending to wish smaller families the trend is towards an increasing incidence of elective repeat sections and this pattern is likely to continue. After two sections, all patients should be delivered by repeat section and, although there is no absolute limit to the number of sections that are possible, sterilization should be offered to the patient after the third operation.

Treatment of ruptured uterus

In the event of ruptured uterus, the patient should be resuscitated with blood transfusion and taken to theatre for laparotomy without delay. The decision whether to repair the uterus or to perform hysterectomy will depend on the extent of the tear and the patient's desire for further children. In some ruptures of the lower segment, the bladder may be involved making the surgical treatment difficult. In such cases, the bladder must be repaired and then drained continuously by catheter for ten days. Any patient who becomes pregnant after a successful repair of a ruptured uterus will be most safely delivered by elective Caesarean section.

Maternal injuries

EPISIOTOMY

Bleeding can take place from injuries to the maternal soft tissues following delivery and even a clean episiotomy can lose a considerable volume of blood and should be repaired as soon as possible after delivery.

When a blood vessel continues to bleed in a repaired episiotomy, a perineal haematoma will form which may reach enormous proportions. Up to two litres of blood may be lost in the tissues and the patient will be shocked. Blood should be transfused, the haematoma evacuated and the bleeding point secured.

THIRD DEGREE TEAR

If the perineum is allowed to tear at delivery, this may extend to involve the anal sphincter and rectum causing a third degree tear. An episiotomy may also extend into the rectum but, if made properly, this is less likely to happen than with an uncontrolled tear. It is important that a third degree tear should be recognized and repaired at once under general anaesthesia. The mucosa and the muscular coat of the rectal wall are repaired in layers from above downwards using atraumatic buried catgut sutures. Care must also be taken to identify and approximate the cut ends of the anal sphincter because an inadequate repair of these may lead to incontinence of faeces or flatus. Post-operatively, a low residue diet followed by liquid paraffin may encourage healing by permitting the easy passage of motions. Following repair of a third degree tear, it is essential that an elective episiotomy is performed in all subsequent vaginal deliveries.

VAGINAL AND CERVICAL TEARS

When vaginal bleeding persists after delivery despite a well contracted uterus, then injuries to the vagina or cervix should be suspected. It is important that examination should be carried out under anaesthesia with a good light so that an adequate inspection can be made. Injuries to the maternal tissues are particularly liable to occur during forceps delivery or vacuum extraction before full dilatation of the cervix. Such procedures may also cause damage to the baby and their place in modern obstetric practice is doubtful. Caesarean section is probably safer for the child in these circumstances. Vaginal and cervical injuries must be sutured and, if the injuries are very severe, firm vaginal packing may be required to control the haemorrhage.

BROAD LIGAMENT HAEMATOMA

An uncommon cause of shock after delivery is bleeding from the spontaneous rupture of a blood vessel in the broad ligament. This may occur due to cervical damage extending upward to the uterine vessels or may be due to spontaneous rupture of veins in the base of the broad ligament, the uterus being intact. When this happens, the patient will complain of abdominal pain and a pelvic haematoma lateral to the uterus will be palpable on abdominal and pelvic examinations. The decision whether to operate or to treat the patient conservatively will depend on the size of the haematoma, its rate of growth and the degree of shock in the patient.

Risk to the fetus from direct maternal injuries
The fetus is extremely well protected within the pregnant uterus. The amniotic fluid seems to act as an effective cushion and it is rare for the fetus to suffer from direct injuries. When a pregnant woman receives severe injuries, as for example in a car accident, it is usual to find that the baby survives unharmed. Many women are anxious about the effect of a minor accident, such as a fall, upon the baby and it is important to give them the appropriate reassurance. The exception to this rule is a penetrating injury which enters the uterus itself. Such injuries must be rare and treatment will depend on the depth of the injury and the extent of any bleeding. An injury causing fracture of the pelvis could involve damage to the pregnant uterus and can lead to distortion of pelvic shape. This factor has to be carefully assessed before and during labour when deciding whether to allow vaginal delivery or not.

OTHER CAUSES OF SHOCK

Amniotic fluid embolism

This syndrome is one of the gravest encountered in obstetric practice because its outcome is frequently fatal. Its true incidence is impossible to determine because the diagnosis can only be finally established by demonstrating squames from the amniotic cavity in the lung at post-mortem. Amniotic fluid embolism was responsible for seven deaths in Scotland between 1965 and 1971 but it is probable that patients survived in some of the less severe cases.

CLINICAL FEATURES

Amniotic fluid embolism can occur during labour, following artificial rupture of the membranes or during Caesarean section. The patient is profoundly shocked immediately after the infusion of amniotic fluid into the maternal circulation and this may lead to cardiac arrest and sudden death. If the patient survives the shock, acute pulmonary oedema soon follows causing severe dyspnoea, cyanosis and tachycardia. The other major complicating factor is a severe coagulation defect which develops in many cases. The amniotic fluid contains thromboplastins which will establish a widespread micro-intravascular coagulation in the lungs. This results in a reduction of fibrinogen, platelets and the other blood clotting factors which are consumed in the clotting process. The body reacts to the intravascular coagulation by activation of the fibrinolytic system which attempts to resolve the coagulation and restore the patency of the vascular tree. The end point of the fibrinolytic system is the proteolytic enzyme plasmin which, under physiological conditions, has the role of digesting localized deposits of fibrin within the vascular bed. Normally, plasmin has no systemic effect because of the efficient action of the antiplasmins circulating freely in the peripheral blood. In amniotic fluid embolism, however, the generation of plasmin is so explosive that the antiplasmins are overwhelmed and plasmin can freely digest, not only fibrin, but fibrinogen and other plasma proteins as well. In this acute fibrinolytic or 'plasminaemic' state, blood clotting factors are rapidly depleted and the patient develops a haemorrhagic diathesis. She may have haemoptysis, vaginal bleeding and haematuria and will bleed from venipuncture sites. The bleeding problem is responsible for several of the deaths following amniotic fluid embolism.

Treatment of amniotic fluid embolism

The objectives of treatment are to correct the initial stages of shock, to maintain adequate oxygenation and to correct the coagulation defect. In the successful treatment of a case of probable amniotic fluid embolism, Willocks *et al.* (1966) employed the following measures.

1. Intermittent positive pressure ventilation with 100 per cent oxygen.
2. Tracheal aspiration and intravenous frusemide to reduce pulmonary oedema.
3. Aminophylline and low-molecular weight dextran to reduce bronchospasm and increase pulmonary blood flow.
4. Sodium bicarbonate to correct metabolic acidosis.
5. Hydrocortisone to protect against the effect of stress.
6. Digoxin to strengthen the action of the myocardium.

The correction of the coagulation defect is frequently difficult. Replacement of fibrinogen is not helpful because it will be rapidly lysed by the action of plasmin. This will lead to production of fibrinolytic degradation products which, by virtue of their antithrombin properties, may further worsen the coagulation problem. In cases where the fibrinolytic inhibitor ε-amino-caproic acid (EACA) has been given it has allowed the pulmonary intravascular coagulation to proceed unchecked. An increase in the intravascular coagulation will exacerbate the problem of pulmonary ventilation and may hasten the death of the patient. Paradoxically, the optimum treatment may be heparin which can attack the primary problem of the intravascular coagulation. It takes courage to give anticoagulants to a patient who is already bleeding but it may be the treatment of choice. More reports of successful treatment with heparin in amniotic fluid embolism will be required, however, before its place can be fully established.

Pulmonary embolism

Pulmonary embolism was found to be the most common cause of maternal death in Scotland between 1965 and 1971 (Report on an Enquiry into Maternal Deaths in Scotland, 1965 to 1971). Most of the blood coagulation factors rise during pregnancy and it is possible that this represents a 'hypercoagulable' state. It is during the puerperium that the incidence of pulmonary embolism is greatest and it is highest in older women of high parity who have had an operative delivery.

SIGNS AND SYMPTOMS

Many patients develop a pulmonary embolism without any previous indication of a deep-vein thrombosis in the leg. The main features of embolism are chest pain which is worse on inspiration, haemoptysis and dyspnoea. The patient may be shocked but this will depend upon the size of the embolism. Chest X-ray may be normal initially but evidence of pulmonary infarction usually appears within 24 hours. When the diagnosis is in doubt, pulmonary angiography is the most accurate diagnostic method but the large amount of radiation involved may not be suitable for a pregnant patient.

Treatment

Where there is good evidence of pulmonary embolism, the patient should be treated with anticoagulants. Initially continuous intravenous heparin is given in a dose of 10,000 units six hourly and then maintained to keep the whole blood clotting time at $2\frac{1}{2}$ times the pretreatment value. Warfarin can be started at the same time and used to maintain the patient once it has taken effect. After 36 weeks of pregnancy, warfarin should not be given because it crosses the placental barrier and may cause haemorrhage in the baby. At this stage, patients should be transferred to heparin and maintained on it until delivery. It seems sensible to stop heparin during labour and to re-commence therapy after completion of the third stage although some authorities say that anticoagulants can be maintained during delivery.

If a patient is desperately ill from massive pulmonary embolism there may be a case for embolectomy, although such a procedure would carry substantial risks. Fibrinolytic therapy has also been used to treat pulmonary embolism but such treatment would have to be used with great caution in pregnancy for fear of causing intra-uterine haemorrhage.

Prevention of pulmonary embolism

Early ambulation after delivery is of paramount importance to prevent stasis of blood in the leg veins. When patients are confined to bed, active leg exercises should be encouraged under the supervision of a physiotherapist. There is now evidence to show that oestrogens, given to suppress lactation, increase the incidence of puerperal thrombo-embolism and it is doubtful if their continued use for this purpose is justifiable.

A problem arises regarding the need for anticoagulants in patients with superficial thrombo-phlebitis. Only a very small number of these patients will develop pulmonary embolism, and it is debatable whether the potential benefits of anticoagulants would outweigh the risks of haemorrhage. As a general rule, it is probably reasonable to withhold anticoagulants when the phlebitis is confined to superficial veins below the knee and is not causing oedema; crepe bandaging and elevation of the limb is usually sufficient therapy. On the other hand, when there is generalized leg swelling extending into the thigh, anticoagulants should be given to reduce the risk of embolism and should be maintained for three to four months after the resolution of clinical signs.

Inhaled gastric contents

Acute collapse during or after general anaesthesia may be the sign of inhaled gastric contents. The inhaled material may be solid, leading to obstruction of a main bronchus and collapse of that segment of lung. Alternatively, Mendelson's syndrome may develop which is the reaction of the lung tissue to highly acid gastric juice. This causes acute pulmonary oedema, usually after a latent period, and presents as acute dyspnoea and cyanosis. The pulmonary oedema may be complicated by infection and can lead to maternal death.

The risk of gastric aspiration can be minimized by using general anaesthesia only when absolutely necessary. Forceps delivery can usually be done under pudendal block analgesia and epidural anaesthesia is a safe and effective anaesthetic for many obstetric procedures, including some cases of Caesarean section. The stomach should be kept as empty as possible by not giving solid food during labour and regular oral alkaline solutions will neutralize gastric acidity. Possibly the most important factor is that all anaesthetics should be given by properly trained anaesthetists who are available to give a 24 hour service to the obstetric unit.

Myocardial infarction

This diagnosis is rare in pregnancy, but should be kept in mind, particularly in an older patient who complains of chest pain.

Diagnosis and treatment are the same as for myocardial infarction in the non-pregnant patient.

Previous corticosteroid therapy

Patients who have been receiving corticosteroid therapy will be more prone to shock in the event of exposure to some form of stress. It is probably wise, therefore, to give prophylactic doses of intravenous hydrocortise to any patient in labour who has been on corticosteroid therapy in the previous two years. In this, as in all other forms of shock, it is best to anticipate possible problems and to take steps to avoid or minimize the worst side-effects before they occur.

REFERENCES

Dewhurst, C. J. (1957) The Ruptured Caesarean Section Scar. *J. Obstet. Gynaec. Brit. Cwlth.*, **64**, 113.

O'Sullivan, J. V. (1945) Acute inversion of the Uterus. *Brit. med J.*, **ii**, 282.

Willocks, J., Mone, J. G. & Thomson, W. J. (1966) Amniotic Fluid Embolism. Case with biochemical findings. *Brit. med. J.*, **ii**, 1131.

FURTHER READING

Shoemaker, W. C. & Walker, W. F. (1970) *Fluid—Electrolyte Therapy in Acute Illness.* Chicago: Year Book Medical Publishers.

A report on an Enquiry into Maternal Deaths in Scotland, 1965–71. Edinburgh: HMSO.

Shock. *Brit. J. Hosp. Med.* (1968), vol. **1**, No. 3.

32. An Approach to Gynaecology

There is scarcely need to emphasize the importance of reproduction and sexuality in human affairs. They are literally fundamental to everything else in society. Not surprisingly therefore all societies regulate the overt expressions of sexuality and their consequences. Such regulation may be formal, as in legislation, and in the United Kingdom there have been recent large swings in opinion in the matters of homosexuality and abortion, which have been incorporated into the law. At another level there has been, in some African and Latin countries, legislation about female dress, banning short skirts or long skirts or trousers, because they may be found to be sexually exciting. Rather less formally, churches of all kinds have felt it necessary to promulgate their ideas of appropriate expressions of sexuality. Among their adherents the views of the church have immense moral power in such matters as modesty, dress, courtship, chastity, promiscuity, pre-marital intercourse, forms of marriage, the place of women in society, pleasure in sexual intercourse, contraception, abortion, sterilization, the number of children which a family should have, monogamy, bigamy and so on. This list is enough to show the immense interest which these subjects engender in formalized society. But in an even less formal way there are ill-defined cultural attitudes determining the forms of sexual expression which a given group of people deem to be appropriate or inappropriate. 'Culture consists of everything which has ever been accepted as a way of doing or thinking, and so taught by one person to another' (Howells, 1965). It is important to recognize that the 'teaching' implied in this definition is both formal and informal. The child in his growth learns what is done and what is not done partly by being told explicitly, but more importantly, by observing for himself what actions of himself and others appear to receive approval or disapproval. It is these cultural attitudes which in large measure mould his thinking, and which determine his values and philosophy of life.

In simple communities where members remain within their cultures for the whole of their lives, attitudes tend to change little with time. But in our own mobile society and with increasing education requiring the entertainment of new ideas, attitudes may change quite quickly. Such changes are fed by the spate of views pouring forth from the mass communication media. There can be no complete consensus of opinion about what is right or wrong sexual expression, except within the very smallest groups or sects. So it is inevitable that attitudes will vary as between remote villages and large cities, and within cities between social classes and between groups based on schools, churches, clubs and neighbourhoods. At the present time this variability is most easily seen in attitudes to legal abortion, the spectrum of opinion ranging from complete acceptance to complete rejection.

Doctors, of course, deal with individual patients one at a time and the aim is to help the patient to the maximum degree possible; that is to restore the person to health if that can be achieved. But health is a nebulous concept and the requirements needed for a sense of well-being are different in the young professional footballer from those of the middle-aged businessman and from those of the lonely widow. This emphasizes that health is a variable phenomenon, differing between people and varying at different times of life in the same person. People vary and so do their environments. Health is attained when the individual shows the best possible adjustment to his complex environment; and even this definition begs the question for it involves a value judgment as to what is best. But it does emphasize that health must be a dynamic concept, since the changing person is moving within a changing environment.

The lesson for the good doctor is clear. He must, within the limits imposed upon him, especially those of time, try to help the patient as a whole person. A pathological diagnosis alone is not enough. Every disorder has some psychological components (the word 'dis-ease' implies this) and these together with physical limitations inevitably affect society. As soon as a person becomes a patient his role changes. If he is an in-patient he is withdrawn from his family, his work and his friends and plays a different part within the society of the hospital. Diagnosis is important and so is treatment. But even more important is management, for this includes diagnosis and treatment and yet adds a dimension of its own, which is a recognition of the need to try to adjust the patient's attitudes and/or to adjust his environment. Before this can be done a full appraisal of patient and environment is required. Knowledge must be gained of the physical symptom, of the psychological attitude to it and of the social background. In gynaecology pelvic symptoms may be the cause of altered behaviour and so affect all relationships within the family; or the social circumstances, as in bad housing, poverty or an uncongenial job, may cause emotional upsets resulting in a pelvic symptom.

Diagnosis

All medical diagnosis depends upon evidence obtained from the history, from the physical examination and from a variety of special investigations. Physical diagnosis is dealt with elsewhere in this book. Psycho-social diagnosis, which is the emphasis of this chapter, can only be made from the history and from observation of the patient's reactions.

In the doctor–patient relationship the attitudes of the doctor are too often ignored, as if he could maintain complete objectivity. But this is certainly not possible for he brings a received set of ideas to the interview. The range of attitudes among doctors to matters of sexuality and reproduction are almost as wide as they would be among any other group of people of like backgrounds and education. It is true that since they have received a somewhat similar education to one another they will tend to be moulded in the same patterns of thought. But each doctor brings his own individuality to his formal education, and this individuality conditions his thinking according to his age, social class, family attitudes, school education, his friends, the literature he reads and all the nuances which shape a personality. This means that the doctor must throughout his career be constantly subjecting himself to self-analysis. In gynaecology this is particularly necessary, for prejudices in relation to matters of sex and reproduction are inevitable in all of us. As far as it is ever possible the gynaecologist must attempt to recognize his prejudices so that they shall affect his advice to the patient as little as may be. Full objectivity is never attainable, but it should be aimed at, and self-knowledge is the first step to it.

The patient is inevitably less objective than the doctor. Going to him with any complaint is worrying for what it may portend. A gynaecological complaint often carries even more overtones of anxiety, for pelvic function is frequently less well understood by the lay public than other functions, and failure in sexual and reproductive function may bite more deeply into the personality than failure in other systems. In addition the patient knows that investigation will involve a pelvic examination, a matter which few women can view with equanimity. At the first interview therefore most women will show some signs of anxiety. It is essential that the doctor should recognize this and do his best to lower the emotional tone. A factual history taken largely without comment is best, with the doctor showing no other emotion than interest. It must be remembered that communication between people is not only verbal. We communicate through gestures, tidiness and untidiness and facial expressions and in innumerable other ways, and these often tell more of our thoughts than the words we use. And care in the use of words is also important for the doctor. It is vital that the patient should understand what is being said to her. Medical jargon in particular must be avoided as being very liable to misinterpretation by the patient. The doctor is making an appraisal of the patient but she is also watching him and his reactions and making decisions as to whether he is the one to help her and just how much of herself she will reveal. Sensitivity to the patient is required.

Diagnosis begins as the patient comes into view. Her age, her dress, use of cosmetics or no, her walk and deportment and her diffidence or self-assurance are all indices of the kind of person she is and of the image of herself that she holds. First impressions can be wrong so they should not be too influential and they should be capable of modification as the acquaintance proceeds. The life-style of the poor unkempt woman from the slums must differ from that of the well set-up woman from a fine residential neighbourhood, and so must their attitudes to pelvic function, even if they complain of the same symptom. The point needs no emphasis. Everything about them has differed from the moment of fertilization, which started them on their lives.

The age of the patient has significance. The sexual and reproductive expectations of a young woman of twenty are obviously different from those of the forty year old, which are different again from the post-menopausal woman. Moreover the physical diseases from which they are likely to suffer vary also, as later chapters show. It is especially important to realize that sexual activity can be as important to the old as the young. Quick assumptions about sexual ability and appetite in relation to age are out of place.

People do not take jobs purely for money. They try to find work which is congenial to their personalities, education and attainments. Schoolteacher working with young children, and nursery nurses, may be immature and shrinking from adult contacts. Nurses and doctors may be people who wish to dominate others and be held in high esteem. Physiotherapists may relish the bodily contacts which their work gives. Factory girls may need the companionship of working with others. Waitresses and barmaids may like the contacts and flirtations with men. Housewives may love or hate their work. Hairdressers may be unduly concerned with personal appearance. Such evidence is tentative but all sorts of women doing all sorts of jobs may be demonstrating something of themselves, their hopes and aspirations.

The accent and the way in which language is used may give clues to education and upbringing and especially of comprehension of bodily images and medical concepts. It is much easier for a middle-class doctor to understand and communicate with a woman of similar background than it is for him to understand a poorly educated woman, or for her to understand him. Moreover the middle-class woman has more power to influence the doctor in his decisions than the inarticulate. The ill-educated frequently suffer nameless fears of authority, for they have not learned how human societies work. The doctor and the nurse wield great authority within the hospital and may unwittingly intimidate the patient. The patient's mute appeal for help may go unheeded because she may be unable to communicate properly, unless the doctor is particularly willing to listen and try to understand. The problem is often even more complex with foreign nationals, since they may be unable to speak the language and in addition they may have such a different set of values that full understanding between patient and doctor is almost impossible.

During the history further non-verbal communication by the patient may be helpful. Many women clutch a handkerchief in the hand at the medical interview. It may be held tightly with the knuckles clenched, twisted nervously in the hands, passed from one hand to the other or used to wipe perspiration away. Involuntary hesitations in reply to questions about sexual intercourse, e.g. dyspareunia, may suggest attitudes to sexuality or to deep-seated marital difficulties which may perhaps need exploration later.

Religion is a major part of many people's culture. There will be obvious differences in attitude between Moslems and Roman Catholics or Plymouth Brethren on many aspects of sexuality. In many countries too the relative position of women is that of subjection so that they will make no decisions about themselves without consultation with their husbands, who are the final arbiters. Attitudinal differences will be found in connection with such matters as infertility, sterilization, abortion, myomectomy and hysterectomy. Birth control may be ardently desired by some women when their religion regards it as sinful. They may be quite unable to broach the subject, so that it may be kind to raise the subject unemotionally at some point, so that they may be able to discuss it.

The foregoing discussion can only give hints about the kind of things to look for. Patients are so variable in their outlook that details cannot be fully considered. Only constant talking to them can bring the required experience for better understanding. But the doctor can do much to increase his comprehension of social backgrounds and attitudes by seeing patients in their own homes and by asking them about their homes, specifically finding out the number of rooms they have, whether they have bathrooms and sole use of lavatories and water supplies. The husband's occupation will often give a hint of his income, and the rent and other outgoings on accommodation can be directly asked. Housing is such an important part of a woman's environment that some questions about it should always be included. If the place is damp or cold, if there is friction with her neighbours, if there is overcrowding—these may be the determining factors in her illness. Her symptomatology may be an expression of her despair of ever improving her lot and that of the family. A string of symptoms such as headaches, palpitations, breathlessness, black-outs, irregular periods, dysmenorrhoea, dyspareunia and discharge should especially awaken interest in the environment. Overt depression may be obvious in the patient's retardation, amenorrhoea, poor appetite and waking in the early morning. In circumstances such as these the patient may be more in need of psychiatric or social help than of gynaecological care. Only the really alert clinician will recognize the significance of some of these symptoms.

Insight into social factors and attitudes can be gleaned by the doctor from wide reading and from attention to the mass media. Newspapers, novels, plays, television and radio, advertisements and especially their picture content, all demonstrate attitudes which may be worth heeding. Women's magazines, and their correspondence columns will often show the sorts of problems which worry their readers. The attitudes of the modern teenage magazines to sexual problems is particularly revealing.

Specific symptoms

There are comparatively few gynaecological symptoms. They may be combined in different ways in various disorders and the mixture of physical, psychological and social factors in their genesis obviously varies from person to person. Allowing for the fact that many symptoms will have a pathological basis which needs treatment by medical or surgical means, it is essential to note that upset periods, pain with the periods, vaginal discharge, difficulties with intercourse, pain in the breasts before a period, premenstrual headaches, irritability and depression, and even infertility and recurrent abortion may all have a predominantly psychological basis. It must be the aim of the history to uncover this basis as well as any pathological one. Suggestions as to how to do this have been made.

Physical examination

Gynaecological investigation deals with very private areas both of the mind and body. This may inhibit communication between doctor and patient. The clinic may become commonplace for the doctor, but it never is for the patient. This is especially true of the pelvic examination and the doctor must always therefore approach it with due understanding of its emotional overtones. A woman has to develop a very special trust in her doctor, which he must try to foster by his whole demeanour. As emphasized before this may be more non-verbal than verbal. The build-up of trust begins with the appraisal of the doctor by the patient as he takes the history and as he proceeds with the physical examination.

Feeling the pulse is a good way of establishing the first physical contact, and its rate may suggest the degree of tension of the patient. The breasts should always be examined and palpated because of the prevalence of carcinoma. For some women the size of the breasts, if small or large, may be a source of embarrassment and this may show in the reaction to examination. It may give a clue to the person's body image of herself and her sexual attitudes, which may or may not be of importance.

Abdominal palpation is not usually associated with much emotion for the patient though resistance to pressure and undue tenderness may be a further index of nervousness.

The pelvic examination, digital, by speculum and per rectum, is obviously the most delicate for the woman. The reactions to it can be of great significance. Those whose adductor muscles of the thigh and levatores go into spasm are obviously very different from those who can relax completely and allow easy palpation of the internal genitalia. But even those who can relax may have problems of frigidity and sexual anaesthesia, unless they are gymnasts, ballet dancers or physiotherapists who have learned great muscular control. Certainly some types of reaction suggest that the sexual history should be further explored.

Deep tenderness in the pelvis without palpable lesions is a sign that is difficult to interpret. It is often diagnosed as being due to salpingitis or endometriosis which may not be borne out even by laparoscopy. When one is certain of the essential normality of the physical pelvis, then it may be worth pursuing the notion of sexual maladjustment as the underlying cause.

Talking to the patient

After the history and examination comes the moment for making the diagnosis and communicating its import to the patient. This may not be immediately possible since it may be necessary to have further investigations done, but these should be arranged with all possible expedition to minimize the suspense. When the time comes to explain to the patient it is then that the importance of the psychological and social approach comes to the fore. It will immediately suggest the way in which to talk to the patient. The educated woman will need full explanations, though it is necessary to avoid medical jargon or to explain in simple terms, for even the educated will not always understand the meanings of words they do not often use. The non-verbal communication may have suggested areas needing delicate exploration. Many patients come to gynaecological clinics with an overt symptom which may not in fact be the one that is worrying them. They may be suffering from some sexual maladjustment or cancerphobia or depression, which they may not recognize as the essential problem and so they may complain of pruritus, discharge or upset periods or something else. The symptom must be taken seriously and investigated, but a psychological or social genesis must be considered and much of this is best done when the physical examination is completed, for it is then when *rapport* may have been established.

Some patients may need only simple reassurance. This may vary from a full explanation of reproductive physiology, to an authoritarian statement that all is well. Patients without verbal facility may be confused and be made apprehensive by too much explanation, and over-elaboration must be avoided. Fitting the assurance to the patient is quite a difficult art and can come only with practice. The form of the explanation is dictated largely by the personality of the doctor which inevitably colours his assessment of psycho-social factors and therefore his suggested management of the disorder.

Where further investigation or operation is required then the doctor must explain why it is necessary and what it involves. In the case of operations the patient will want to know when she will be admitted, how long she will be in hospital and how long her convalescence will be and what the results of the operation may be expected to be. She needs all this information so that she can talk the matter over with her husband and make arrangements for him and any children whilst she is away from the family. In many of these difficulties the Medical Social Worker can often be of great help, and it should often be offered.

Husbands can be notoriously unwilling to discuss their wives' gynaecological illnesses. There is then perhaps no point in pressing unwelcome explanations upon them. But some women want their husbands involved and then it is well worth spending time with them. In modern jargon gynaecological complaints involve the marital unit, so the husband should more often be seen than is usually the case; especially is this so where there is infertility. Where there are sexual difficulties it may be that the doctor should insist on seeing the husband.

Many patients, particularly in the later age-groups, have a dread of cancer. Where one can be sure that there is no evidence of this disease it is frequently kind to say so to the patient. This is often repaid by an obvious sense of relief.★

After operations women should be told what has been done. In particular, unspoken questions should be answered. For instance after hysterectomy they will want to know if they will continue to menstruate, whether they will be able to have and enjoy sexual intercourse and when they may begin again and whether they will have hot flushes. Also some women get obese after hysterectomy and this should be discussed. It may be due to depression causing overeating, and the depression may be pre-existing or come on as a result of hysterectomy. Pelvic floor repair operations too may cause women anxieties about their ability to continue with sexual relations and these anxieties should be relieved before they leave hospital.

Conclusion

Gynaecology is an area of medical practice with a large cultural involvement. Cultural

---

★ Modern permission slips for operation insist that the reasons for, and nature of, the operation have been explained to the patient. She signs agreeing to the operation the surgeon has said he will do. Full and careful explanation is good manners, good doctoring and legally necessary.

clashes of opinion over matters of sex, reproduction and pelvic pathology are inevitable. Many of these opinions are irreconcilable. In his dealings with patients the doctor must try to recognize attitudes of the patient and those aspects of culture which have affected him. Only then can he be knowledgeable and tolerant of the vagaries of the human condition and so help all his patients to the maximum possible.

REFERENCE

Howells, W. (1956) *Man in The Beginning*, p. 46. London: Bell & Sons Ltd.

33. Signs and Symptoms in Gynaecology

Techniques such as laparoscopy, ovarian cystectomy, myomectomy and other surgical procedures in the operating theatre have their place in gynaecology but the essential primary unit in gynaecological practice is the occasion when a woman who is ill or thinks she is ill seeks the advice of a doctor whom she trusts. This is a consultation and all else in the clinical care of the patient derives from it. This concept stresses the professional relationship and is especially applicable to gynaecology, for great care and tact are required in dealing with patients whose complaints are so often of a personal and intimate nature. As the patient presents herself there is invariably a sense of hesitation, nervousness and modesty together with some anxiety as to the outcome of the consultation. It is important that receptionist, nurse and doctor be friendly and manifestly concerned with the patient's problems, emotional as well as physical. The patient's confidence is secured by a courteous, professional atmosphere. There are, however, certain medico-legal restrictions which apply.

MEDICAL LEGAL ASPECTS

All forms of medical examination are governed by legal restrictions, which are in general as protective to the practitioner as to the patient, but the intimate nature of a gynaecological examination emphasizes their importance to the physician. Except under conditions of military law, no person can be *compelled*, even by a Court of Law or police authority, to submit to a medical examination, and any attempt to make such an examination without the free consent of the subject is technically an assault. A vaginal examination could easily be represented and described as an indecent assault by a neurotic or unscrupulous woman motivated by malice or blackmail. The physician should therefore take steps to protect himself by some simple routine against such a possibility by having always a reliable third person (nurse, secretary or maid) present, or at least within easy call, during the consultation and examination. In ninety-nine cases out of a hundred such precautions are unnecessary, but the special features of the hundredth case or the dubious morality of the patient concerned may not be recognized until after the examination has been completed, when it is too late to organize precautions.

Particular care should be taken not to examine a child or minor without the specific consent of her parent or guardian; and an employee should never be examined at her employer's behest without the employee's free consent given in the presence of a reliable third person. Moreover, it is important to realize that in all the circumstances indicated the patient's consent should not be inferred simply from an absence of protestation at the time of examination. She should be made aware of her right to decline examination if she wishes, and consent should be formally expressed.

HISTORY

The first requirement is a searching history and it is preferable that this should be taken in a methodical way so that nothing of importance or relevance is omitted. With increasing experience it is possible for the doctor to pay more attention to some points of the history than to others without losing essential information. The following general format is offered for guidance:

GENERAL ENQUIRY
The patient's name, her age, where she lives and whether married, single or a widow. If a married woman, the duration of marriage. Her husband's occupation, if applicable, whether she herself is working, and her actual job.

The present complaint

A description of the primary complaint including its duration. A description of any subsidiary problems including their duration.

The menstrual history

The age of the menarche and the pattern of her menstrual cycle. The character of the menstrual flow. The date of the last normal menstrual period. Whether there are any abnormal associations such as pain, tension, diarrhoea, etc. Some idea of the nature and duration of the flow can be obtained from a question of the number of tampons used in the normal period. Inquiry ought to be made as to whether tampons or towels are used.

Past obstetric history

An account of previous pregnancies including all abortions in chronological order. For each pregnancy: any antenatal complication should be noted, the duration of the pregnancy, the duration of labour, the method of delivery, the place of delivery (so that official notes can be obtained), the sex of the child and the weight at birth and whether the child is alive and well at the present time.

Past medical history

Any medical or surgical illness, operation or accident at any time in the life of the patient should be recorded. Where there has been a previous operation, especially abdominal, full details should be sought if necessary from the hospital where the operation was performed.

Personal and social history

Information about her smoking and drinking habits. Tactful inquiries about her sex life including libido, frequency of intercourse, presence or absence of dyspareunia, achievement of orgasm and use of contraceptive techniques.

Family history

Inquiry about any significant or relevant illness in close members of her family, with special reference to diseases of hereditary or familial tendency.

SYSTEMATIC INQUIRY

The presence of symptoms or signs relating to any of the special systems but especially the urinary tract or gastro-intestinal tract. Urinary frequency, dysuria or incontinence and any alteration in bowel habit. It may be necessary to inquire fully into respiratory, cardiac or endocrine function if there is apparently any history of such disease or any symptoms suggestive of such disease.

General health

An account of the patient's general well-being, appetite, weight over the past few months and sleep and exercise habits.

The clinical history is all important and provided it is taken with care and in sufficient depth the diagnosis may be largely evident before the patient is examined.

Physical examination

The physical examination of the patient should include a systematic general examination as well as examination of the abdomen and pelvis. Details of the methods of examining the pelvic organs are given on page 636. The significance of many gynaecological symptoms and signs varies depending upon the age and parity of the patient and, where relevant, these are considered in the following account:

Primary amenorrhoea
In the United Kingdom the average age of the menarche is $13\frac{1}{2}$ years and if the onset of menstruation is delayed beyond the age of 16 or possibly 17 years, a diagnosis of primary amenorrhoea is made. Mostly these adolescents are suffering from delay in the onset of menstruation and the need is for reassurance rather than for concern. But this knowledge should not keep the doctor from seeing the young girl and using his clinical judgment as to whether a fuller investigation is called for at any time. Pregnancy is most unusual under these circumstances but must be kept in mind. Increasing lower abdominal discomfort at monthly intervals could raise the possibility of some congenital blockage to the outflow of menstrual blood (Cryptomenorrhoea). Simple inspection of the vulva should clearly demonstrate the bulging membrane. In others there may be clinical evidence of some endocrine dysfunction and investigation should not be delayed.

Secondary amenorrhoea

Amenorrhoea following previously normal regular periods has pregnancy as its most obvious and frequent cause. This diagnosis should always be kept in mind and carefully excluded by pelvic examination and, if necessary, by a pregnancy test before any other diagnosis is considered. The clinical history is helpful. When the patient's periods have previously been regular and the possibility of pregnancy is admitted then this is the most likely diagnosis. In younger women where periods, previously regular, gradually become less heavy and less frequent and finally cease altogether, the possibility of a serious alteration in pituitary ovarian function should be considered. Stein Leventhal amongst other syndromes is a possibility.

At the two extremes of the reproductive years—in adolescence and towards the menopause—it is not unusual for there to be some upset in the finely balanced endocrine control of menstruation. Where the influence of oestrogen is dominant there is steady proliferation of the endometrium with hyperplasia of the stroma and dilatation of the glands (cystic glandular hyperplasia) and a period of amenorrhoea lasting several weeks is not uncommon, before the hyperplastic endometrium is shed. The irregular pattern of bleeding which ensues is known as metropathia haemorrhagica. In other patients chronic illness or a period of anxiety or tension may well be associated with secondary amenorrhoea. An unusual cause of cessation of menstruation is a functioning ovarian tumour such as an arrhenoblastoma which first causes defeminization then masculinization.

Other alterations in menstrual function

Apart from total absence of the menstrual flow, which is amenorrhoea, menstrual function may be disturbed in other ways. It is often better to describe the abnormality rather than put a single term to it. In other words, the periods are either heavy and regular, or they may be heavy and irregular, they may occur too frequently or not frequently enough, or there may be episodes of bleeding independently of the normal periods. It has been customary, however, to apply certain titles to aberrations of bleeding but they are not as useful as the simple descriptive terms outlined above.

Menorrhagia. Prolonged or excessively heavy, though regular, menstruation is an important cause of anaemia and general debility. But menorrhagia is a difficult term to define in so much as what is regarded as normal and acceptable by one woman may be thought to be excessive by another. A patient's account of heavy menstrual loss should be checked against her haemoglobin level. In the absence of significant anaemia it is difficult to believe that a woman's periods are unduly heavy. Menorrhagia may be functional and related to some imbalance in the endocrine control of menstruation and there may be some underlying organic cause such as fibroids, chronic pelvic infection or endometriosis. In some instances the periods gradually become heavier but last no longer whilst in others the duration of menstruation increases from four or five days to six, eight or ten days with resulting heavier loss of blood. Regular, heavy or prolonged, menstrual loss is socially inconvenient and debilitating but in the sense of underlying pathology is less likely to be associated with malignancy than irregular bleeding.

Metrorrhagia. Here the bleeding has lost its cyclical pattern and is irregular. Although more frequent at puberty and near the menopause irregular bleeding can occur at any time during the reproductive years. In general, the older the patient the more likely will the underlying pathology be malignant rather than benign. In some there is no recognizable periodicity, episodes of bleeding lasting from a few days to several weeks with days or weeks between one episode and the next—the sort of history associated with metropathia haemorrhagica. When associated with other pelvic pathology, for example an ovarian cyst, metrorrhagia has a sinister connotation and malignancy should be suspected. In general at or around the menopause irregular and too frequent bleeding should always be suspected to arise in a neoplastic lesion and be carefully investigated.

Intermenstrual bleeding. This is a separate entity where bleeding occurs between what are relatively normal recognizable periods. Slight intermenstrual bleeding in mid-cycle at the time of ovulation and accompanied by some abdominal pain, is said to be associated with the follicle rupture, the so called Mittelschmerz. However, intermenstrual bleeding in the nature of contact bleeding, like post coital bleeding is highly significant. A submucous fibroid polyp typically causes irregular intermenstrual bleeding as does carcinoma of the body of the uterus in the pre-menopausal woman. Any intermenstrual bleeding should be looked upon with real suspicion. Menstruation which is cyclical but too frequent, for example, where the periods are less than three weeks apart is sometimes given the term 'polymenorrhoea' but this is not in general use.

Haemorrhage before puberty. Vaginal bleeding, usually in small amounts, occurs not infrequently in the newborn female. In intra-uterine life the fetal endometrium is stimulated by maternal oestrogen and after birth, once the oestrogen stimulus has gone, withdrawal bleeding takes place. There is no cause for alarm.

Precocious puberty. The average age of the menarche in the United Kingdom is somewhere between 13 and 14 years and is generally accepted to be precocious if it occurs before the age of 10 years. The subject is dealt with elsewhere.

Vaginal discharge. A common symptom of varying significance. In the young child it may represent no more than lack of local cleanliness but a foreign body in the vagina is equally likely. During the reproductive years the natural barrier in the vagina against infection is upset by periodic menstruation and by the inevitable cervical and vaginal trauma associated with childbirth. Various infections occur—mixed coccal, trichomonas, monilia and others. Depending upon the underlying cause the discharge may be clear and mucoid, white or yellow or brown and can be offensive and irritating. In the mature woman a bloodstained discharge is always ominous, for it may be an early feature of cervical malignancy; occasionally one of the earliest features of cervical or body cancer is a clear vaginal discharge. Beyond the menopause the vaginal epithelium becomes thin and the pH of the vagina rises. A low grade infection in the vagina gives rise to an atrophic 'punctate' vaginitis with associated thin, sometimes irritating discharge, which may be slightly bloodstained. At this age any bloodstained discharge should be thoroughly investigated and malignancy of the cervix or body of the uterus excluded. The subject is discussed fully elsewhere.

Pruritus vulvae. There are many causes of vulval itching and these, together with treatment, are fully discussed in another section of the book. It is sufficient here to say that the symptom may indicate a lack of personal cleanliness, especially in children and in elderly women; an irritation secondary to vaginal discharge; a local vulval skin disease such as lichen sclerosus et atrophicus or leukoplakia or furunculosis; a perianal lesion such as infected haemorrhoids or secondary infection associated with threadworms or a candida infection. Where there is no obvious cause for pruritis it is most important that a thorough examination be made to exclude diabetes.

Pain

Among women, as well as men, there is considerable variation in the pain threshold and what is distressing and unacceptable to one may hardly trouble the next. It is important to keep this in mind, for pain is a common symptom and it is for the gynaecologist to decide, after careful assessment, just how much investigation and treatment is required in the individual case. Mostly there is an underlying organic cause for pelvic pain but it is not uncommon for there to be a functional overlay, and it does take an experienced clinician to decide the relative proportions. Indeed the proper evaluation of pelvic pain can be one of the most difficult aspects of gynaecological diagnosis. One reason for this is that visceral pain is seldom precisely localized and the pain which brings a patient to her doctor may well be due to one of several causes. A further complication is that many extra genital conditions can give rise to pelvic pain or backache.

Non-gynaecological causes of pelvic pain or backache

Chronic *constipation*, not unusual in women, can give rise to pelvic congestion and discomfort. It is a diagnosis always to be kept in mind when the patient complains of rather vague lower abdominal 'heaviness' or pain. Following previous surgery, and associated with adhesions, small loops of bowel may be bound down in the pelvis and periodically become distended and give rise to quite acute, sometimes colicky, pain. The symptoms may last for several hours and be suddenly relieved as peristalsis is restored and the gas passes down the bowel.

The clinical features of *appendicitis* are well known and hardly need further description here—very often peri-umbilical pain slowly settling down into the right iliac fossa with increasing tenderness over McBurney's point. Acute *diverticulitis* produces symptoms very like those of appendicitis but with a tendency to localize on the left side of the abdomen and as the lesion becomes more chronic a mass may appear usually in the left iliac fossa. With this condition there is frequently some bowel distension associated with subacute obstruction. Diverticulitis tends to be a chronic lesion and in time constipation is likely to alternate with diarrhoea and bouts of colicky lower abdominal pain occur.

Any alteration of bowel habit complicating lower abdominal pain should raise the suspicion that bowel rather than genital tract is the cause. And these symptoms, especially if there is melaena, may be due to malignancy of the sigmoid colon or rectum.

Pain may arise in the urinary tract. Renal disease—*pyelitis,* and *renal calculi,* for example, may give rise to shooting pains passing down the ureters into the bladder. Acute *cystitis* is associated with suprapubic discomfort and pain and urethritis, either acute or chronic, is likely to lead to dull aching pain deep in the pelvis. Acute retention of urine and distension of the bladder with severe, colicky, lower abdominal pain, may be a direct complication of certain gynaecological conditions such as fibroids, ovarian cysts or acute pelvic inflammatory disease.

Chronic backache in the lumbo-sacral region is common among women but this is very rarely related to gynaecological disease. It may occasionally be a legacy from childbearing and this has already been discussed. This symptom is much more likely to arise from some orthopaedic disability such as bad posture, osteoarthritis, lordosis, scoliosis, kyphosis, sacro-iliac strain largely due to the patient being overweight or occasionally to some congenital defect such as spina bifida. At one time it was believed that a retroverted uterus could account for backache and many unnecessary uterine suspension operations were performed. But in some instances a retroverted uterus associated with such diseases as chronic pelvic infection or endometriosis where there is pelvic congestion can result in a downbearing feeling and some low sacral backache.

Pelvic pain originating in the genital tract. One of the commonest types of pain directly due to disease or malformation of the genital tract is *dysmenorrhoea.* In the young, single girl suffering from primary or spasmodic dysmenorrhoea the distribution of the pain is typically that associated with the autonomic nervous system—ill defined lower abdominal pain passing through to the patient's back and down into the thighs. A miserable, sickening, cramping pain that begins with the onset of menstruation and lasts for around 24 hours leaving the patient with a dull aching pain for another two, possibly three days. By contrast, secondary dysmenorrhoea arising as a complication of such diseases as chronic pelvic infection, endometriosis or fibroids begin a few days before the expected period, gradually reaches a climax and diminishes with the onset of menstruation.

Endometriosis, which is fully described in Chapter 39 is a relatively common condition in the United Kingdom and it may be associated with several different types of pelvic pain. Typically it results in increasingly severe premenstrual lower abdominal pain, relieved by the onset of menstruation. Acute, deep-seated, pain at the time of intercourse leaving the patient with a dull ache in the pelvis for several hours afterwards is also quite common. An endometriotic cyst may rupture spilling small quantities of blood into the peritoneal cavity; this results in peritonism with symptoms of an acute abdominal crisis. A plaque of endometriosis in the wall of the rectum or sigmoid colon gives rise to deep-seated pelvic pain as the lower bowel fills with faeces; this pain is relieved by defaecation. Similarly, a plaque in the bladder wall gives rise to suprapubic pain as the bladder distends. Isolated deposits of ectopic endometriosis, for example around the umbilicus and in a Caesarean section or episiotomy scar, give rise to regular, monthly discomfort as a little blood is shed each month into the ectopic lesion. These external deposits appear as small bluish areas, generally painless until the approach of the period when they distend and become tender.

As a *fibroid or ovarian cyst* enlarges and occupies more space in the pelvis, pressure is exerted on nearby organs and the patient may complain of frequency of micturition or occasionally of difficulty in passing urine. Bowel symptoms are less common but increasing constipation may be a feature. As the tumour enlarges there is congestion and a feeling of heaviness in the pelvis and lower abdomen. At any time a cyst or a pedunculated fibroid may twist; mostly this gives rise to an acute abdominal crisis with the patient complaining of severe 'twisting', abdominal pain and vomiting. In some the symptoms are less severe with occasional bouts of niggling abdominal pain; in time the pedicle of the cyst or fibroid necroses and the tumour becomes free and may become attached to omentum from which it can receive a new, limited, blood supply. Bleeding into an ovarian cyst provided it is fairly sudden and of reasonable amount, gives rise to sharp lower abdominal pain which settles down to a more continuous dull ache. In the same way, bleeding into a fibroid (and this is most likely to happen when there is an associated pregnancy) results in acute pain followed by a continuous ache. This complication, known as red degeneration, is described more fully elsewhere. *Ectopic pregnancies* and ruptured corpus luteum cysts produce varying degrees of pain depending upon how much blood is spilled into the abdominal cavity, for the peritoneum is very sensitive to the irritation caused by blood. With small amounts of blood the pain is pelvic but with larger amounts, as may happen in ectopic pregnancy, the blood tracks up under the diaphragm giving rise to pain between the shoulders or in one or other shoulder tip due to irritation of phrenic nerve endings.

It has already been mentioned that deep-seated, *acute dyspareunia* may be caused by the penis touching an endometriotic nodule in the Pouch of Douglas. Similar deep dyspareunia, though not so acute, may be due to chronic infection in the cervix or paracervical tissues or in the adnexa. Local vulval lesions such as a urethral caruncle, kraurosis, leukoplakia, lichen sclerosis and vulval or vaginal infection result in more superficial pain at the introitus and may prevent penetration.

The fundus of the uterus is poorly supplied with nerve endings but large sympathetic and parasympathetic nerve plexuses surround the cervix which is sensitive to trauma and infection. *Dilatation of the cervix*, whether attempted in theatre without anaesthesia or when the uterus is trying to extrude a polyp or a foreign body such as an intra-uterine device, causes pelvic and suprapubic pain. The pain becomes colicky when the uterus is trying to extrude something from its cavity.

Gynaecological malignancy and pain

Cancer of the cervix, body of uterus, ovary, vagina or vulva very rarely produce pain in the early stages. Pain is a late feature related to extension of the malignancy to other struc-tures and organs. Extension within the pelvis will, in time, involve lymphatic channels, nodes and nerve roots. A dull ache deep in the iliac fossa or hip gradually becomes worse and passes down into the thigh with paraesthesia of the overlying skin. As the malignancy advances the pain tends to become central and more severe and is precisely localized if there are bony metastases.

Urinary symptoms. It has already been noted that pelvic tumours such as fibroids or ovarian cysts, through pressure on the bladder, may be the cause of urinary frequency or lead to progressive difficulty in emptying of the bladder and occasionally to acute retention of urine. The same symptoms may be associated with acute pelvic inflammatory disease. Again, acute retention of urine may follow surgical procedures like hysterectomy or pelvic floor repair where there has been a good deal of handling of the bladder during the operation. Urgency, frequency and stress incontinence are clinical features associated with urethro-cele and cystocele. Dysuria is usually due to some degree of infection—trigonitis, urethritis, vaginitis. Incontinence may be associated with fistula due to anatomical abnormality or secondary to operative or obstetric trauma or malignant disease. Overflow incontinence from a grossly distended bladder may be due to undue age, or be secondary to a retroverted gravid uterus, a retroverted uterus with a fundal fibroid, or sometimes to an ovarian cyst jammed in the Pouch of Douglas.

The climacteric. The cessation of periods and the other clinical features which together amount to the climacteric are considered in detail in a later section of this book. It is sufficient here to emphasize that these various symptoms arising from the gradual reduction in output of oestrogen by the ovary take place over a period of several months or more. Common complaints at this time are hot flushes, headaches, nervousness, inability to concentrate, irritability and even depression. To a greater or lesser extent most women as they approach fifty years of age experience some of these symptoms.

Hirsuitism. Excess growth of hair is a male rather than a female attribute and hirsuitism is a source of embarrassment to most women. In a significant proportion the hirsuitism is determined more by racial and family factors than by any endocrine upset. One difficulty is a decision about whether hair growth is excessive or not. In practical terms it is for the patient herself to decide and if she is dark rather than fair then the hair on her upper lip, chin, arms and legs will be more noticeable and bring her more quickly to seek advice from her doctor.

Gynaecological signs

The clinical history is helpful in drawing attention to the sort of signs that should be specially looked for but every patient should have a complete systematic examination, for disorders in other systems may affect the reproductive tract. As already suggested, the examination of the patient should be carried out with due respect for her comfort and modesty. No more of the patient should be exposed than is necessary. Her general condition may be relevant—her stature, nutritional status and weight. Inspection of mucous membranes and nail beds will give some indication as to whether or not the patient is anaemic but the impression gained is notoriously unreliable and routine haemoglobin estimations ought to be done in all gynaecological patients where the test would seem at all relevant. Where indicated a specimen of blood should be sent to the laboratory for examination. Such matters as her build, breast development and hair distribution are noted. After the general physical examination attention is directed to the abdomen, pelvis, vulva and perineum.

The abdomen is first inspected and note taken of any obesity, of previous operation scars and whether they have healed soundly, the presence or absence of striae from childbearing, the state of the abdominal muscles and whether there is any weakness or divarication of the recti muscles. The femoral, inguinal and umbilical areas are inspected and palpated for evidence of herniation of abdominal contents. Any abdominal mass should be carefully palpated and its size, consistency and mobility noted. Tenderness or rigidity are of special importance if acute and of recent origin. If the patient suffers from chronic constipation a slightly tender, fusiform swelling will likely be felt in the left iliac fossa. A distended abdomen should be percussed gently, in order to establish whether the distension is gaseous or due to ascites or possibly to a large ovarian cyst or fibroid. With a large tumour, percussion is dull in the mid-line and often resonant in the flanks, due to displacement of loops of bowel.

Next the vulva and perineum are inspected. Any lack of personal hygiene is self evident. The anus is carefully inspected for evidence of external haemorrhoids, fissures or worm infestation. The state of the perineum and the perineal body is established by inspection and palpation and any scars, whether the result of tears or vaginal repair, are described. The vulval skin may show evidence of any one of a number of skin disorders—lichen sclerosus et atrophicus, leukoplakia, furunculosis, diabetes, vulvitis, etc.—and the appearance should be noted and described. Vaginal discharge, trickling over the introitus, out on to the vulva can set up a sensitivity reaction as in candida infections, giving rise to marked vulvitis. Any atrophy, hypertrophy, oedema or ulceration of the vulval skin or labia is noted. Ulceration of the vulva in older women is seriously abnormal with a strong likelihood of malignancy. Biopsy should be taken immediately.

Bartholin's gland lying deeply in the posterior part of the labium majus on either side of the vaginal introitus, is not normally enlarged but when the duct is blocked, usually the result of chronic infection, the swelling is seen and easily palpable between thumb and forefinger. The infection may go on to abscess formation with an acutely tender swelling, usually unilateral, just behind and to one or other side of the introitus.

In its virginal state the hymen is intact and admits one finger but following coitus the hymen is lacerated and the introitus more roomy. Small condylomata acuminata, or genital warts, may be seen in some women round the introitus and over the perineum. Occasionally these warts are more extensive and coalesce to form large, warty, masses. A flat, firm, greyish ulcer on the vulva is quite likely to be a primary, syphilitic chancre and should not be touched with the bare fingers. Yellow or creamy discharge, easily milked from the urethra or Skene's ducts suggests a gonococcal infection. A small mulberry, red swelling at the urethral meatus suggests a urethral caruncle, not to be confused with prolapse of the urethral mucosa. Small sebaceous cysts, generally multiple, and infection of hair follicles (furunculosis) are not uncommon and may affect the skin over any part of the vulva.

Inspection of the vagina, using a speculum, will reveal any excessive or abnormal discharge. A profuse mucoid discharge suggests chronic hypertrophy of the cervical glands with over-production of alkaline mucus. The clear discharge in the upper vagina tends to become yellow near the introitus due to superadded infection in the lower vagina. The typical, thin, frothy yellow discharge associated with Trichomonas infection is readily recognized as in the white, sometimes curdy, discharge in monilial infections. In these cases the vaginal walls are likely to be red and tender. Microscopic examination of a fresh drop of vaginal discharge in normal saline is helpful in diagnosis. Normally there will be numbers of healthy epithelial cells with no pus cells, though organisms, especially Doderlein's bacilli, can be seen actively moving about. Where there is infection with Trichomonas Vaginalis the protozoal organisms can be seen jerkily moving among pus cells. In monilial infection it is possible, on careful examination, to see transparent mycelia and spores among the epithelial cells. Small cysts on the antero-lateral aspects of the vaginal wall are most likely to arise from Gartner's ducts—remnants of the lower part of the Wolffian ducts. Although uncommon in the United Kingdom urethral diverticuli are now quite frequently seen in certain tropical countries where infection is more widespread. This diagnosis should be kept in mind when there is thickening and distortion of the urethra associated with an anterior, mid-line, cystic swelling. Solid tumours of the vagina such as fibromata and fibroids are uncommon and may be sited anywhere in the wall.

At the apex of the vagina the cervix is visualized. Normally it points backwards into the posterior fornix. With a retroverted uterus the cervix points forwards into the anterior fornix. Fibroids, particularly when sited in the lower part of the uterus, can cause considerable distortion and make it difficult to visualize the cervix. Common local cervical lesions such as erosion, polypus, eversion, Nabothian follicles, cicatrization, endocervicitis and hypertrophy of the glands are described later. Any congenital anomaly such as imperforate hymen, a vaginal septum or a double cervix is noted when an attempt is made to pass a vaginal speculum.

Vaginal examination with the index and second finger of the right hand whilst the patient strains down or coughs, will reveal any laxity of the anterior or posterior vaginal walls and whether there is descent of the cervix. These signs, when present, indicate prolapse of the urethra, bladder or rectum. On bimanual examination the cervix is palpated. It is generally possible to identify an erosion by its soft, velvety feel, though many cervical polyps are more easily seen than felt. The irregular, hard feel of a lacerated, cicatrized cervix or one with Nabothian follicles should not be confused with the irregular, friable cervix of malignancy. Tenderness on moving the cervix points to significant pathology in the pelvis. The tenderness is likely to be very acute in ectopic pregnancy and in certain forms of endometriosis where small nodules of endometrium are scattered over the peritoneum in the Pouch of Douglas.

The size, position and shape of the uterus is established. Retroversion is a common finding and of little relevance unless there is associated pathology such as endometriosis or chronic pelvic infection when the uterus will be fixed in the position of retroversion and tenderness is likely to be a feature. Symmetrical enlargement of the uterus can be caused by a single fibroid, by endometriosis affecting the myometrium, by pyometra or simply by a rapid sequence of pregnancies. Irregular firm enlargement suggests multiple fibroids. Gentle examination in the fornices and simultaneous palpation in one or other iliac fossae permits assessment of the appendages. Chronic infection is evidenced by thickening and tenderness of the appendages with, in some cases, a brawny swelling spreading out from the cervix to the pelvic wall on one or both sides. In ectopic pregnancy there is frequently exquisite tenderness and it may be possible to feel between the vaginal and abdominal fingers a fusiform, pulsatile swelling; this particular examination should be made with the greatest care and gentleness for it is very easy to rupture an ectopic pregnancy with immediate and heavy blood loss.

Enlargement of the ovary is detected on bimanual examination. Benign cysts are mostly freely mobile, well defined, unilateral and cystic. Malignant tumours are more likely to be firm in parts and soft in others, attached to surrounding structures, irregular in outline, bilateral, and secondary deposits may be felt in the Pouch of Douglas. If the cyst is large enough it will be felt abdominally as well as on bimanual examination.

It is important always to carry out a rectovaginal examination to establish that there is no pathology in the rectum or in the recto-vaginal septum.

CONCLUSION

Once the symptoms and signs have been elicited, the gynaecologist must consider whether anything has been missed before he makes his final diagnosis. Especially he should ask himself whether the patient's initial complaint is the real reason for her coming to seek his advice and help. It is not unusual for a woman to come to her doctor with a complaint of vaginal discharge or dysmenorrhoea or irregular menstruation and for him to elicit, after discreet questioning, that it is some other matter that is concerning her deeply. For example, her real concern may be fear of becoming pregnant again or she may be convinced that she has pelvic cancer, or frigidity or dyspareunia may be leading to the break up of her marriage. It takes an experienced clinician to elicit this sort of information and make the correct diagnosis but it helps if the possibility of such an oblique approach by the patient to her doctor is kept in mind.

34. Abnormalities of Menstruation

1. ABNORMALITIES OF MENSTRUATION

These may vary from no menstruation at all to frequent, heavy, irregular bleeding. In this chapter, the abnormalities dealt with in detail are related essentially to dysfunction of the endocrine system and more especially to abnormalities of the hypothalamo-pituitary-ovarian axis, the changes in the genital tract being secondary manifestations. Many organic lesions are only noted here since they are fully dealt with in other chapters.

THE MENARCHE

The normal age at menarche is a very individual matter and depends on the woman's genes and life history. In normal girls, signs of sexual maturation usually appear between 8 and 12 years of age and the first menstrual period occurs a little later than this. At first, menstruation may be irregular and the initial cycles are frequently anovular. Eventually the cycle becomes ovular and menstruation regular. Socio-economic factors play a part in the age of menarche and nutritional deprivation may be associated with delay (Ellis, 1945). The size of the family in which a girl grows up may be another factor, there being a delay in onset in families with many siblings (Roberts *et al.*, 1971). It is possible that this delay might be explained on nutritional and other factors since it has been shown that children brought up in a large family group may individually get less to eat than those in small families.

Vicarious menstruation

This is an uncommon condition, the term being applied to cyclical bleeding from extra-genital areas during the reproductive period. Bleeding may precede or coincide with normal menstruation or may occur cyclically in amenorrhoeic women. The nasal mucous membrane is the commonest site of extra-genital bleeding; other sites are the lungs, stomach, intestines, kidneys, lips, gums and eyes. The bleeding is not associated with the disintegration of tissue and is therefore not true menstruation. The aetiology of this type of bleeding is obscure but its occurrence only during reproductive life suggests that it may be related to the vascular changes which occur in response to hormonal stimuli. The oestrogenic and luteal hormones increase capillary permeability in extra-genital tissue. There may be, in addition, some local vascular defect due to trauma or local pathology. The haemorrhage as a rule is scanty and of short duration but at times may be so severe as to require blood transfusion.

Treatment

No treatment is necessary where the bleeding is scanty and of short duration but cauterization of the vascular area will control bleeding from the nasal mucosa.

Amenorrhoea and oligomenorrhoea

OLIGOMENORRHOEA

Oligomenorrhoea is the term used to describe a reduction in the length or duration of the menstrual flow although the cycle is usually, though not always, regular. The cycle may also be prolonged so that the interval between the menstrual periods may be seven or more weeks. The increased interval between the periods in ovulatory cycles is usually associated with a long proliferative phase but occasionally the luteal phase may also be prolonged. Bleeding from a proliferative endometrium—anovulatory bleeding—indicates abnormal ovarian activity. If ovulation is occurring then no treatment is indicated but if ovulation is not taking place and the patient desires a family then treatment should be instituted as described later in this chapter.

If a patient has oligomenorrhoea oral contraception may not be suitable for her as it may result in amenorrhoea.

Hypomenorrhoea, which is a reduction in the amount rather than the duration of periods, also occurs. Unless found with oligo-menorrhoea it is of no clinical significance.

AMENORRHOEA

Amenorrhoea means the absence of menstruation. It is physiological before the menarche, after the menopause and during pregnancy and lactation. Primary amenorrhoea denotes that the onset of menstruation has not occurred by the age of 16 years. Secondary amenorrhoea occurs when menstruation ceases after having been normal for many years. Mention has been made of the menarche and menopause as causes of physiological amenorrhoea. Amenorrhoea is present throughout the pregnancy and is due to suppression of pituitary function by the high concentration of oestrogens and progestational hormones present at this time. Scanty periodic bleeding may occur in the early months commonly before 12 weeks when there is a potential cavity between the decidua capsularis and the decidua vera. In the majority of cases it is symptomatic of a threatened miscarriage but may be associated with a polyp, erosion or neoplasm of the cervix.

After parturition the menses recur spontaneously within 6–12 weeks in the absence of breast feeding. In the nursing mother, however, menstruation does not usually return until lactation has stopped but occasionally may come as early as 6 weeks after delivery. The first few periods after parturition are frequently anovular but ovulation may occur even during the period of lactational amenorrhoea so that a nursing mother may conceive without having had a period.

Cryptomenorrhoea

Cryptomenorrhoea or concealed menstruation is the condition where there is an obstruction to the outflow of menstrual blood and this accumulates in the vagina. It is generally congenital and the commonest cause is incomplete canalization of the lower end of the Mullerian ducts but it may also be caused by complete absence of the vagina. It may rarely be due to cervical stenosis following amputation, cautery or a cone biopsy.

The menstrual discharge held up behind the obstruction causes distension of the vagina known as haematocolpos. The vagina may become very distended and fill the whole pelvis. Gradually the uterus, tubes, ovaries and bladder are displaced upwards on top of the swelling and may be felt on abdominal pal-pation. The tension in the anterior vaginal wall and vaginal fornices causes upward displacement of the bladder and elongation of the urethra leading eventually to retention which may be followed by incontinence of urine. Occasionally the intravaginal tension becomes so great that the cervix opens and blood is retained in the uterus-haematometra. If the condition is not treated, blood may be forced into and even through the Fallopian tubes causing peritoneal irritation with adhesion formation: later the abdominal ostia become occluded and accumulation of blood takes place in the tube—haematosalpinx.

Clinical features—the menarche is delayed but menstrual symptoms such as malaise, headache, sickness and abdominal discomfort occur from the age at which the menarche should have occurred. The abdominal pain tends to recur regularly each month. Gradual enlargement of the abdomen is noted. Such symptoms as perineal discomfort, frequency of micturition and later retention of urine or overflow may supervene.

Abdominal examination reveals a swelling arising from the pelvis. It may be uterus or a distended bladder. On vaginal examination the intact hymen is found and when a rectal examination is performed the pelvis is found to be filled by a large tense cystic swelling.

Treatment—the intact membrane should be excised by a cruciate incision and the pent-up blood allowed to escape. This treatment is usually adequate. When the uterus and tubes are involved antibiotic therapy should be given since there is a considerable risk of infection with possible subsequent sterility.

PRIMARY AMENORRHOEA

The differential diagnosis of primary amenorrhoea presents a complicated problem. With proper management it should be possible for the great majority of these patients to lead a normal life although many of them will be infertile.

Although the menarche may begin apparently normally as late as the age of 18 or even 20 years, 18 is usually the age at which investigation should be done if menstruation has not started. This is reasonable when the patient has developed normal secondary sexual characteristics and where cryptomenorrhoea has been excluded. If, however, there is evidence of sexual infantilism or stigmata of

Turner's syndrome or virilism, investigations should be performed earlier.

The aetiological factors in this condition may be grouped under four main headings: (1) General systemic disturbances, (2) Endocrine disorders, (3) Chromosomal abnormalities, (4) Genital abnormalities.

1. General systemic disorders

Debilitating diseases and poor nutrition in infancy and childhood which adversely influence general metabolism may delay puberty and the onset of menstruation. Delayed puberty from such causes was more common when the level of nutrition in certain socioeconomic groups was low. Debilitating diseases such as tuberculosis, severe renal disease, anaemia and cardiac disease can influence anterior pituitary function so that amenorrhoea results. In these cases the symptoms of the primary disease are paramount and amenorrhoea only a secondary phenomenon.

2. Endocrine disorders

a. *Pituitary*. Tumour formation, embolism and inflammation of the anterior pituitary gland in childhood disturb the normal functioning of the hypophysis and lead to retardation in the somatic and genital development.

Pituitary dwarfism—If the patient is less than 4ft 10in (147cm) tall then one or other of the chromosomal abnormalities leading to gonadal dysgenesis may be present but less frequently the diagnosis will be panhypopituitarism. Some of these conditions will have been diagnosed long before puberty and the amenorrhoea in these women will be inconsequential, e.g. the Laurence–Moon–Biedl syndrome when the classical features of retinitis pigmentosa, polydactylism or syndactylism and mental retardation will be evident in infancy.

Frohlich's syndrome (dystrophia adiposogenitalis) is primarily a hypothalamic disturbance which results in amenorrhoea, obesity, genital hypoplasia and hirsutism. Slow mental reactions are also a feature of this condition. It may also arise in later life.

b. *Ovary*. Absence of the ovaries is rare. Occasionally pelvic inflammatory processes such as tuberculosis or peritonitis in childhood may cause destruction of the ovaries but there are more common conditions which may cause failure of menstruation to occur.

Gonadal dysgenesis or congenital aplasia of the ovaries—the ovaries in this syndrome are represented by white streaks of tissue—streak gonads. Clinically the syndrome is characterized by normal stature, which may sometimes be increased, failure of mammary development, sexual infantilism and scanty or absent pubic hair. The diagnosis is usually between gonadal agenesis and hypogonadotrophic eunuchoidism. The karyotype is 46/-XX. There is no clinical way of differentiating these two conditions. If primordial follicles are present in the ovary the condition is gonadal dysgenesis but if absent it is hypogonadotrophic eunuchoidism. The latter patient will also show undetectable levels of urinary gonadotrophins but the oestrogen response can be stimulated by gonadotrophin treatment. This is not true of gonadal dysgenesis.

Bilateral polycystic ovaries—this may occur in the young girl the features being primary amenorrhoea, with normal development of the breasts and secondary sex characteristics. The uterus is smaller than normal and the ovaries may or may not be enlarged but there may be some degree of virilism. This condition will be more fully discussed under secondary amenorrhoea.

c. *Adrenal*. The adrenogenital syndrome in which adrenal hyperplasia occurs is usually present from birth and the condition should be suspected in any infant born with abnormal external genitalia. Occasionally adrenal hyperplasia may not become obvious until after puberty and in these cases amenorrhoea is usual although menstruation may be normal. Hirsutism is usually a feature of the condition.

d. *Thyroid*. Primary amenorrhoea may be present in cretinism and childhood myxoedema.

e. *Pancreas*. In some girls with juvenile diabetes of severe character, primary amenorrhoea may be present but in the well controlled case, menstruation should be normal.

3. Chromosomal disturbances

The description of true intersex is given in Chapter 40. Fuller discussion on this subject can be obtained by consulting Dewhurst and Gordon (1969).

Turner's syndrome. This syndrome includes short stature, sexual infantilism, cubitus valgus and webbing of the neck. The nipples are widely spaced and congenital cardiac lesions, especially coarctation of the aorta, may be present. The uterus, vagina and vulva are infantile and the ovaries are represented by the characteristic streaks of fibrous tissue resembling ovarian stroma. Buccal smears are chromatin negative. Most of the cases of Turner's syndrome have a karyotype of 45/-XO but sometimes mosaics such as XO/-XX are found. Most of these mosaics have amenorrhoea but some have menstruated. Subjects with karyotype XO/-XY may show variable degrees of virilism. Diagnosis of the fully developed Turner's syndrome is usually easily made. Karyotyping is interesting but not essential for clinical management. Laparoscopy or laparotomy are only indicated when there are differences between the clinical and laboratory findings.

Treatment of Turner's syndrome

The only treatment is to obtain sexual maturation with exogenous oestrogen. A dose of 0·01mg of ethinyl oestradiol twice daily in three weekly cycles will cause primary breast development. This should be given for several months and then cyclical oestrogen and progestin therapy can be continued indefinitely. A progestin such as Norethisterone can be added for the last ten days of each treatment cycle.

SECONDARY AMENORRHOEA

There are various definitions of this condition but it is most usually defined as the secondary absence of menstruation for more than twelve months and excluding causes such as pregnancy, lactation and the normal menopause. Secondary amenorrhoea is a symptom not a disease and may be due to many causes. It is frequently a symptom of a systemic disease and this must always be considered when such a case presents.

Normal menstrual cyclical activity necessitates an intact hypothalamic pituitary axis not suppressed by higher centres, a normal ovary which will ovulate and is capable of normal steroidogenesis and a uterus that will respond to the normal hormonal stimulus. Amenorrhoea results from faults in any of these organs. The uterus may be unresponsive to normally functioning ovaries, the ovary may not function normally due to abnormal development or in the case of secondary amenorrhoea, be unresponsive because of a premature menopause. If ovarian hormonal function is abnormal as in the case of the Stein–Leventhal syndrome, in cystic glandular hyperplasia or with functioning ovarian tumours, excessive hormones will be produced. Frequently the hypothalamo-pituitary axis is at fault and there is an isolated deficiency in gonadotrophin secretion either due to failure of the hypothalamus to produce releasing factors or of the anterior pituitary to respond to stimulation by these factors.

Aetiological factors in secondary amenorrhoea are very numerous and lists of conditions would be tedious. The causes can be subdivided for practical purposes into the same four main groups as suggested for primary amenorrhoea.

1. General systemic disorders

a. *General illness, acute or chronic.* Any acute or chronic severe illness can have amenorrhoea as a symptom—it may be of comparatively short duration. In these cases the amenorrhoea is usually irrelevant since the periods are likely to return when the primary condition is treated. Sometimes, however, the menstrual cycle does not return to normal and further treatment directed particularly to the amenorrhoea is required. Genital tuberculosis may present with amenorrhoea as the sole symptom and is a relatively frequent cause in some countries (Jeffcoate, 1967). Toxic drugs and alcohol may also be causal factors in amenorrhoea.

b. *Psychosomatic.* Such disturbances as changes in surroundings or work, disappointment in love or various degrees of emotional tension of personal grief or severe nervous tension may cause amenorrhoea. The mechanism here is probably the higher centres acting on the hypothalamus and causing a deficiency in the production of releasing factors. Psychosomatic factors are important and amenorrhoea may be a symptom of mental disease such as depression. In this context anorexia nervosa may be encountered, and most frequently occurs in the adolescent. The patient loses any inclination for food and may become greatly emaciated. These girls have a low blood pressure, slow pulse, low metabolic rate and often marked uterine hypoplasia. Treatment may be difficult and the patient often swears she is eating a normal diet. Psychiatric help with underlying emotional problems may be required and when weight improves, normal menstruation can return spontaneously.

Obesity, which may also be psychosomatic in origin is frequently associated with oligomenorrhoea and amenorrhoea. Reduction in weight will often result in the return of normal menstruation.

2. Endocrine disorders

a. *Pituitary and hypothalamus.* Deficiency of gonadotrophin secretion may occur without there being any deficiency of other pituitary trophic hormones. Very often there seems to be no cause for this and the period of amenorrhoea is of relatively short term. It may be emotionally determined but it is frequently difficult to find an emotional cause.

Pituitary insufficiency due to necrosis of the anterior lobe following severe post-partum haemorrhage or shock (Sheehan's syndrome) is becoming a rarer cause of amenorrhoea as obstetric techniques improve and severe trauma and haemorrhage at delivery is now properly and rapidly treated. If this abnormality is present, atrophy of the uterus and vagina, sterility, loss of libido, loss of weight, loss of axillary and pubic hair and low blood pressure will occur. Such patients are susceptible to infections and other forms of stress and live in a precarious state. Partial or total destruction of the anterior pituitary may also result from metastatic tumours, tuberculosis, trauma or thrombus of the main artery of the anterior lobe. Destruction of 50 per cent of the active gland tissue is compatible with normal function. Slight symptoms arise when 60 per cent of the gland is destroyed. Moderate symptoms develop when 75 per cent is involved and severe symptoms when 95 per cent of the gland does not function.

Any type of pituitary tumour can produce amenorrhoea. Most common is the chromophobe adenoma which produces amenorrhoea through gross destruction of pituitary tissue. The Forbes–Albright syndrome which is characterized by lactation in the absence of a previous pregnancy, atrophy of the uterus and vagina, small ovaries and a milky secretion from both breasts is due to a prolactin producing chromophobe adenoma.

Amenorrhoea which develops after childbirth and is associated with persistent galactorrhoea persisting after breast feeding has ceased, is known as the Chiari–Frommel syndrome.

Basophil adenoma is associated with Cushing's syndrome which will be described more appropriately under the section on the adrenal. The acidophil adenoma is associated with signs and symptoms of acromegaly and amenorrhoea may be part of the symptom complex. There is excessive growth of hands and feet and an increase in coarseness of all the features. Frohlich's syndrome, which has been described under primary amenorrhoea, may develop in later life giving rise to secondary rather than primary amenorrhoea.

Secondary amenorrhoea may develop after taking oral contraceptives. This is seen in under 4 per cent of cycles. Menstruation will usually return within 12 months but in some women ovulation has to be induced with clomiphene or gonadotrophins.

b. *Ovary.* Stein-Leventhal syndrome. The classical features of this syndrome are obesity, hirsutism with amenorrhoea or oligomenorrhoea and bilateral enlarged polycystic ovaries. In fact, obesity is not common and hirsutism not necessarily a feature. The diagnosis is made by the symptoms and by laparoscopy with ovarian biopsy. Diagnosis of the condition may be very difficult as the microscopic diagnosis may not readily include any unique features.

The capsule of the ovary is usually but not always thickened. There are numerous subcapsular follicular cysts and corpora atretica and the theca interna is often hyperplastic and may be luteinized. The stoma does not usually show much change but hyperplasia and luteinization have been reported. In this condition the ovaries produce an excessive amount of androgens mainly androstenedione, and plasma testosterone may also be elevated. An enzyme deficiency can be demonstrated in the ovary *in vitro* and there is also evidence of adrenocortical abnormality. It is highly likely that the basic abnormality is hypothalamic.

Persistent follicle cysts, provided the oestrogen level remains high, will prevent the usual menstrual disintegration of the endometrium with the result that amenorrhoea may result but is usually of short duration.

Granulosa cell tumours which synthesize large amounts of oestrogen may cause amenorrhoea during reproductive life for similar reasons.

Bilateral ovarian tumours rarely destroy all active ovarian tissue and will seldom cause amenorrhoea. Arrhenoblastoma—a masculinizing tumour of the ovary—causes amenorrhoea because of its high production of androgenic hormones.

Early senescence of the ovaries is a not uncommon cause of amenorrhoea. The cause of the ovarian failure is not known but it represents an early menopause, the ovaries becoming small and atrophic.

The same effect is caused by irradiation of the ovaries.

c. *Adrenal.* Cushing's syndrome. Adreno-cortical hyperplasia may be associated with a basophil adenoma of the pituitary which in turn causes over-activity of the adrenal cortex but may also be due to hyperplasia or a tumour of the adrenal cortex itself. The syndrome may arise at any age but occurs most frequently in adult life. The main characteristics are male type of hirsutism, 'buffalo' type of obesity, deepening of the voice, enlargement of the clitoris and regressive changes in other genital organs leading to amenorrhoea. In addition there is hypertension, glycosuria and osteoporosis. A differential diagnosis between adrenal hyperplasia and a pituitary tumour is very difficult. The classical manifestations are not always present but plasma cortisol levels are of value in screening these patients.

d. *Thyroid gland.* Secondary amenorrhoea is not commonly the presenting symptom in patients with thyroid dysfunction as other signs and symptoms of the hyper and hypothyroid states are more prominent. Measurement of the basal metabolic rate is of little value in assessing thyroid function in patients where disease is not obvious clinically. Useful information may be obtained in these patients by means of protein bound iodine, triiodothyronine and I^{131} uptake.

e. *Pancreatic lesions.* Amenorrhoea may be a symptom of untreated diabetes mellitus; controlled patients may show glycosuria only during menstruation. With good diabetic supervision, amenorrhoea is rare and even fertility is little altered.

3. *Local causes*

a. *Uterus.* Damage to the endometrium by radium, tuberculosis or puerperal infection may cause temporary or permanent amenorrhoea depending on the degree of destruction. Traumatic uterine amenorrhoea—Asherman's syndrome—is due to over-enthusiastic curettage with the resultant formation of intra-uterine adhesions. The breaking down of intra-uterine adhesions will sometimes cure this condition and after this has been done, insertion of an intra-uterine device may help endometrial regeneration. There is always the risk of placenta accreta should a pregnancy result after treatment of this condition.

Trauma at parturition or operations such as amputation and conization or cautery of the cervix may cause obstruction to the flow of menstrual blood and this may accumulate in the uterus with resultant apparent amenorrhoea. If untreated, blood may be forced back into the Fallopian tubes and may eventually escape into the peritoneal cavity giving rise to abdominal pain.

INVESTIGATION OF AMENORRHOEA

The amount of investigation given to each patient will largely depend on the circumstances. If there is any suspicion of organic disease, full investigation is necessary and the type of investigation done will depend on the clinical problem. As far as the gynaecologist is concerned, the most common type of amenorrhoea seen is that in which a woman stops menstruating but has no other symptoms at all.

The majority of conditions mentioned above are relatively uncommon and those where the amenorrhoea is secondary to a fully developed disease do not normally present to the gynaecologist since the amenorrhoea is not of consequence compared with the main disease. The investigation will therefore be discussed mainly from the point of view of the gynaecologist seeing the patient referred because of amenorrhoea this being the main symptom of which the patient complains.

In general terms, if a patient is otherwise well but has secondary amenorrhoea of under 12 months' duration as her main complaint, there is no indication for immediate investigation. There is a high spontaneous cure rate where the amenorrhoea is of short duration. Investigations, however, may be justified in some of these cases where infertility is of major worry.

In all instances at the clinic a meticulous history is essential. Factors occurring at the time of onset, such as a major environmental change, should be asked about. The time of last pregnancy and the nature of the delivery should be determined; the question of trauma or post-partum haemorrhage should be particularly asked about. In cases of primary amenorrhoea it is necessary to obtain information regarding any injuries at birth, injuries in infancy and childhood and in the pre-pubertal period. Questions of weight change, hot flushes, galactorrhoea, change in hair growth, menstrual molimena, etc. should all be asked.

Physical examination

It is important in all cases to exclude pregnancy.

A careful physical examination is essential. Particular attention should be paid to the general appearance of the patient, the breast development, the distribution of scalp and body hair and the presence of virilism and hirsutes. The height and weight should be measured.

Once a general assessment of the patient's appearance has been performed a decision then has to be made as to how far further investigations should be carried. If there is any suspicion of organic disease in a patient with secondary amenorrhoea or even primary amenorrhoea then full investigation is necessary. If from the history and physical examination this seems very unlikely, then some judgment requires to be exercised as to how far the investigations should be taken.

When secondary amenorrhoea has been present for over a year then full investigation is advisable but under this time, provided there is no obvious abnormality, observation of the patient for a further period is indicated. It is perhaps reasonable to perform radiological examination of the chest and the skull to eliminate the possibility of a pituitary tumour or a chest infection. It is also necessary to take into consideration whether the patient is wishing to become pregnant or not since much fuller investigation is required if this is the case. Generally, the investigations need to be tailored to the clinical problem and the patient's wishes as regards pregnancy.

If full investigation is necessary then the patient should be admitted to hospital when proper examination of the reproductive tract under general anaesthesia can be performed. Under anaesthesia the size of the uterus and length of the cavity should be assessed. Diagnostic curettage and histological examination of the endometrium should be performed. This will give information about tuberculosis and about the endometrial response to any ovarian activity which is present. Examination of vaginal smears may give further information. Full investigation under anaesthesia now includes laparoscopic examination. With this technique the condition of the tubes and ovaries can be assessed and their patency ascertained. Biopsy of the ovary can be undertaken and an assessment made of the histological appearance of the ovary.

The sella turcica should be X-rayed in all cases to detect the presence or absence of pituitary neoplasm and the presence or absence of congenital abnormalities of the genital tract can also be assessed during the laparoscopic and pelvic examination.

In all cases of primary amenorrhoea, karyotypic examination should be performed to diagnose chromosome abnormalities. This examination is only necessary in patients with secondary amenorrhoea if the ovaries are small.

Special hormonal investigations

Sensitive and specific radioimmunoassays for the determination of steroid and gonadotrophic hormones in small amounts of blood have allowed a better understanding of the endocrine status of patients with amenorrhoea. These examinations, however, require sophisticated laboratory techniques which are only available in some centres. Daily samples of blood for a period of four weeks and the measurement of FSH, LH, oestradiol and progesterone will give absolute information about the function of the pituitary-ovarian axis. This is not a very practical proposition for routine clinical practice and therefore it is usual to track patients over a period of four weeks with a sample twice a week. It is then possible to discover what hormones are being produced and what the levels are. This will give some indication of whether the pituitary or the ovaries are non-functioning. Recently more dynamic tests of hypothalamo-pituitary function have been evolved and also tests have been introduced using the releasing hormones from the hypothalamus. FSH/LH releasing hormones can be given by intravenous injection and the response in respect of LH and FSH measured. This will give some idea of the ability of the pituitary to respond to the releasing hormones. Similarly injections of gonadotrophic hormones and the measurement of oestrogen response either by plasma oestradiol or urinary oestrogen excretion will give information about the response of the ovary to gonadotrophin. The response of the endometrium to increased levels of steroid hormones is easily assessed by giving the patient a dose of oestrogen and noting whether withdrawal bleeding takes place. Investigations such as these will help to answer the patient's questions about pregnancy and the return of her periods. It is probably also valuable to assay plasma cortisol and perform thyroid function studies to assess the proper functioning or otherwise of the thyroid and adrenal glands, but amenorrhoea usually only occurs in these conditions when there is marked change in the patient and she is usually already under surveillance by a physician. The tests will also help to plan the treatment of patients who wish to become pregnant.

Treatment of amenorrhoea

Primary amenorrhoea. The object of the treatment of primary amenorrhoea should be to attain the maximum physiological function of which the individual is capable. No attempt should be made to treat these patients until a diagnosis has been made. In the case of delayed menarche provided some secondary sex characteristics have developed and are progressing, and provided all other causes of amenorrhoea have been excluded, no treatment is necessary in these girls. It is likely that spontaneous menstruation will occur by the age of 20 and only if pregnancy is desired will therapy be necessary.

Pituitary tumours are generally operated on. Pituitary dwarfism with deficiency of human growth hormones will undergo spontaneous puberty. Those who have panhypopituitarism will require treatment with human growth hormone and then pituitary gonadotrophins to induce ovulation when pregnancy is desired. Steroidal ovarian hormones should not be given in view of their depressing action on pituitary activity.

In Turner's syndrome, oestrogen in the form of ethinyl oestradiol 0·01mg bd will cause development of the breasts but only rarely withdrawal bleeding. In cases of gonadal dysgenesis there is a risk of the gonadal streaks developing malignant tumours and it is best to remove them. In the feminizing testis syndrome the testes should be removed because of the high risk of development of malignant tumours. If the testes are removed before puberty there will be no breast development and surgery should be considered after sexual maturation.

Adequate investigation of patients with primary amenorrhoea will lead to a more precise diagnosis and it is then possible to treat these patients more rationally. Most should be able to live a normal life but fertility may not be a possibility for many.

Secondary amenorrhoea. Here again treatment should not be undertaken until a proper diagnosis has been reached. Those patients who have some systemic disease causing the amenorrhoea will require to have this disease treated. For the remainder the treatment depends on whether they wish to conceive or not. The treatment for those who wish to conceive is to induce ovulation and the methods of doing this are described in the section on 'Infertility'. Women who do not wish to become pregnant have to be handled in a different way. If no organic disease has been discovered then the patient should be reassured that the amenorrhoea will cause her no harm. Many patients will accept this if they can be persuaded that lack of the menstrual period itself is harmless. However, there are some women who feel that their femininity is diminished by the absence of menstruation. This depends on their cultural and social mores. If these women do not desire children then they can be treated by sequential hormone therapy. Probably the best way of doing this now is to use an oral contraceptive preparation which will cause regular withdrawal bleeding. This should only be used where there is no question of the patient desiring pregnancy in the future as, of course, it results in further depression of the hypothalamo-pituitary-ovarian axis.

Other problems such as the lack of oestrogen being responsible for athero-sclerosis and coronary artery disease require further evaluation. The use of hormonal treatment in these conditions must be weighed against the possibility of a thrombo-embolic phenomenon. However, if the patient is suffering from a premature menopause then it may be necessary to give oestrogen therapy for symptoms such as hot flushes. It is probably best to treat the symptoms of these patients and not to lay down any routine therapy.

It is most important to discuss with these patients the stresses and strains of their lives and this plus the investigations often relieves their anxiety so that in a proportion menstruation will be restored. If depression should be present active treatment will be required. The attitude, therefore, of the modern gynaecologist to amenorrhoea depends very much on the individual patient but it should be stressed that an accurate diagnosis is essential before the decision is made as to the correct treatment and this mainly depends on whether the patient is anxious to conceive or not.

Abnormal uterine bleeding

Abnormal bleeding, at some time in a woman's life, is very common. Probably the most usual cause is some disturbance of the hypothalamo-pituitary-ovarian axis but it also may commonly be indicative of a pathological lesion in the reproductive tract. In some cases it may be symptomatic of a general systemic disturbance although, as in the case of amenorrhoea, if this general systemic disturbance is severe enough to cause menstrual irregularity, then the gynaecologist will only become involved secondarily to the doctor treating the primary disturbance. Abnormal bleeding may occur before or at puberty, during the reproductive period of life or after the menopause.

Haemorrhage before puberty. A bloodstained vaginal discharge which varies in amount may quite commonly occur within a few days of birth. Ten to fifteen per cent of babies may have a bloodstained loss of this type during the first few weeks of life. Oestrogen levels are high in the fetal circulation, concomitant on the high maternal levels, but these fall after delivery causing a form of withdrawal bleeding when there is insufficient hormone to sustain the uterine endometrium. Engorgement of the breasts, which may also be a manifestation of this oestrogen stimulation, can occur coincidentally with the vaginal bleeding. The amount of bleeding is in itself insufficient to cause concern but relatives may become alarmed if they are not aware of its nature.

Precocious puberty. Generally speaking, a girl in Britain can be expected to have her first period between the ages of 10 and 16 years. About half the number of girls menstruate by the time they are 13 or $13\frac{1}{2}$ years old. Puberty is said to be precocious when menstruation occurs before the age of 10 years. This precocity may be 'constitutional' or due to a pathological lesion. The most common cause is the premature function of the anterior pituitary gland without any organic lesion being present. Here the signs of puberty appear in their correct order and menstruation commences. Sometimes these girls have cystic ovaries, due to premature ovarian stimulation but these are the result and not a cause of the condition. The second most common cause of precocious puberty is the presence of some intracranial lesion such as tumour of the hypothalamus and encephalitis or meningitis. Pineal tumours rarely cause precocity in girls.

BLEEDING AT PUBERTY AND ADOLESCENCE

The normal menstrual cycle is regulated by a balance between the secretions of the hypophysis and ovaries and the cyclical endometrial response to stimulation by the ovarian hormone. It is quite common for the early menstrual cycles to occur irregularly. The interval between the periods, the amount of bleeding and the duration of bleeding are often variable for some months or even years in some girls. Regular menstruation may be established from the onset. Periods of amenorrhoea are common. Alternatively, profuse bleeding may occur at the first period and the menstruation may thereafter be prolonged and profuse.

Severe bleeding at this time usually occurs from a hyperplastic endometrium resulting from either a deficient anterior pituitary stimulus which causes only partial follicular development or a subnormal response of the ovaries to the hypophyseal stimulus. Ovulation does not occur in these early cycles and the endometrium is continuously stimulated by oestrogen, becoming hyperplastic. The endometrium eventually breaks down, due to the temporary lowering of the oestrogen level, or because it has reached a point of maximum growth which cannot be sustained. These irregular or heavy periods frequently alarm the parents who then take their daughter to see the doctor.

A general examination should be performed to exclude any important abnormality but a pelvic examination can seldom be performed. The vulva can be inspected and a bimanual rectal examination is usually possible. These are helpful in excluding gross lesions. The blood should also be examined in case anaemia is present.

Mild cases may be treated by firm reassurance to the mother and child telling them that this is not uncommon at the onset of menstrual life. It is a good idea to ask the patient to keep a close record of bleeding for three months so that proper evidence can be obtained of the amount and duration of bleeding. Admission to hospital may be necessary and curettage be performed. Bleeding can usually be controlled by a progestogen preparation such as norethisterone 5mg tds or by injection. The oral contraceptive pill may also be used satisfactorily. These drugs, however, interfere with the establishment of normal pituitary ovarian function and should only be prescribed when bleeding is heavy and causing anaemia. This type of bleeding is usually self limiting and drug or surgical treatment should be delayed as long as possible to allow spontaneous recovery to take place. Rarely it is severe and requires blood transfusion.

ABNORMAL BLEEDING DURING REPRODUCTIVE
    LIFE

Bleeding may occur cyclically so that the normal rhythm is maintained or it may be acyclical when the rhythm is completely distorted. Excessive bleeding from the uterus is a symptom not a disease and various bleeding patterns may be present. It is necessary to take a correct history since misunderstandings occur as a result of the physician and patient talking about different things. Various terms are used to describe abnormal uterine bleeding.

Menorrhagia means cyclical, excessive or prolonged menstrual loss.

Metrorrhagia refers to acyclical or arrhythmic uterine bleeding which may take the form of intermenstrual bleeding or may occur at such irregular intervals that the periodicity of menstruation disappears.

Epimenorrhoea or polymenorrhoea are synonymous terms and describe normal or profuse bleeding occurring at regular intervals of 21 days or less.

Ovular bleeding refers to bleeding which occurs regularly midway between the two periods at the time of ovulation.

Dysfunctional uterine bleeding may be diagnosed when all investigations fail to find an organic cause for abnormal bleeding.

In clinical practice the term menorrhagia is usually taken to mean irregular or heavy bleeding and the other terms are less used in practice.

Aetiology of abnormal uterine bleeding

Although abnormal bleeding from the reproductive tract may be due to general systemic disease such as pulmonary disease, cardiac disease or chronic nephritis, the gynaecologist usually sees this condition either related to pathological conditions of the reproductive tract or associated with endocrine dysfunction. However, cases are often referred with general systemic diseases or various blood dyscrasias and psychiatric disturbances which cause abnormal uterine bleeding but the main lesion is then under treatment from other sources.

Hypophyseal disturbances influence pituitary activity and include such conditions as malnutrition and chronic wasting disease as well as psychological trauma which probably acts via the cerebral cortex and the hypothalamus on the anterior pituitary gland.

The pathological conditions of the reproductive tract which cause abnormal bleeding include lesions of the uterus, tubes or ovaries. Complications of pregnancy are a common group and pregnancy should always be thought of in this situation. The bleeding may be from a spontaneous abortion, an ectopic gestation or retained products. In this case there is usually, but not always, a history of amenorrhoea. Tumours of the genital tract such as cervical polyps, carcinoma of cervix, endometrial polyps, carcinoma of the body of the uterus, sarcoma of the uterus and myomata of the uterus may occur. Choriocarcinoma is a rare cause of bleeding of this type. Tumours of the tube may rarely cause irregular bleeding and pelvic inflammatory lesions are also possible factors. Ovarian tumours, particularly those malignant neoplasms and others which secrete oestrogens, may cause menorrhagia and metrorrhagia. Endometriosis and torsion of an ovarian cyst can also give rise to irregular bleeding. The diagnosis of these conditions is usually made by full pelvic examination including curettage and sometimes laparoscopy and the appropriate treatment can then be carried out.

More commonly, however, the abnormal bleeding seen by the gynaecologist is due to some endocrine dysfunction. This so-called dysfunctional uterine bleeding occurs with no apparent organic disease and appears to be related to upset in the pituitary-ovarian axis. Bleeding may be anovulatory or associated with ovulation.

Anovulatory bleeding. This is the most common type of dysfunctional uterine bleeding. It is characterized by the absence of corpus luteum formation with the result that oestrogenic hormones are secreted continuously and are unopposed by progesterone. This unopposed oestrogen results in uterine hyperplasia and the endometrium eventually breaks down with resultant prolonged, heavy or irregular uterine bleeding. In this condition very variable patterns of oestrogen excretion are found and very high readings are frequently seen. The ovaries may be normal and then the endometrium frequently shows a normal proliferative appearance in the second half of the cycle. If, however, the ovaries are enlarged as a result of multiple follicles in various stages of maturation then fully developed cystic glandular hyperplasia may be a result. In this case the uterus may be enlarged due to thickening of the muscle wall and the endometrium may be overgrown and polypoidal. On micro-

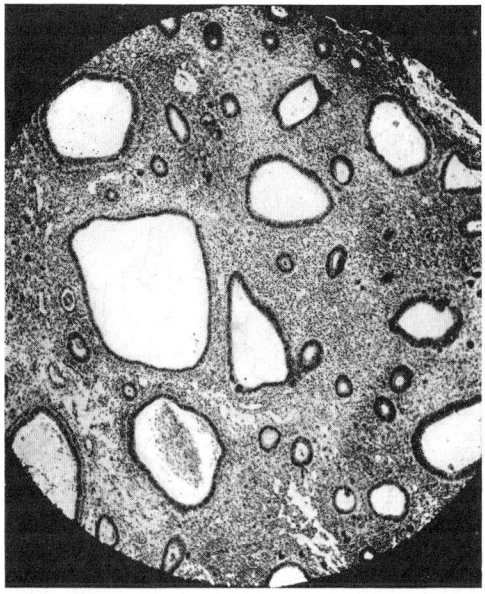

Fig. 34.1   Endometrium from a case of cystic glandular hyperplasia (low power).

scopic examination there are great variations in the size and shape of the endometrial glands which are scattered throughout the mucosa in a disorderly manner some being cystic and enlarged and others small. This disparity in size and distribution gives rise to the characteristic 'Swiss cheese' pattern (Fig. 34.1). The larger glands are usually lined by a single layer of low cuboidal epithelium while the smaller ones may show some stratification (Fig. 34.2). The endometrial stroma is abundant, cellular and compact, numerous dilated and thick-walled blood vessels extending throughout; active proliferation is evidenced by numerous mitotic figures. The degree of hyperplasia depends on the stage of the cycle when the tissue is examined.

The ovarian changes may be accounted for as a result of diminished reactivity of the ovaries to the normal pituitary stimulus. There seems to be two patterns of oestrogen output in these individuals. These were described by Brown et al. (1959) (Figs. 34.3 and 34.4) who found that some subjects had reasonably constant oestrogen levels over long periods of time while in others the levels varied markedly from day to day. Pituitary function in these patients may not be apparently abnormal as measured by FSH and LH patterns. The onset of bleeding is probably caused by a reduction in oestrogen secretion. In these patients the endometrium becomes so highly developed that the oestrogen production eventually becomes inadequate to main-

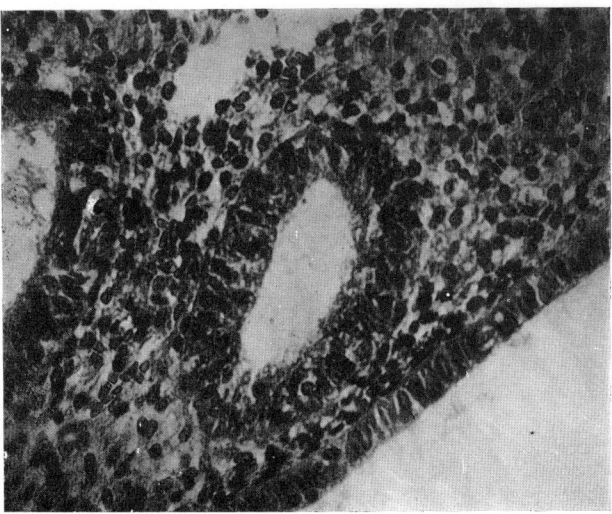

Fig. 34.2   Large gland lined by a single layer of cuboidal epithelium in juxtaposition to a small gland showing pseudostratification (high power).

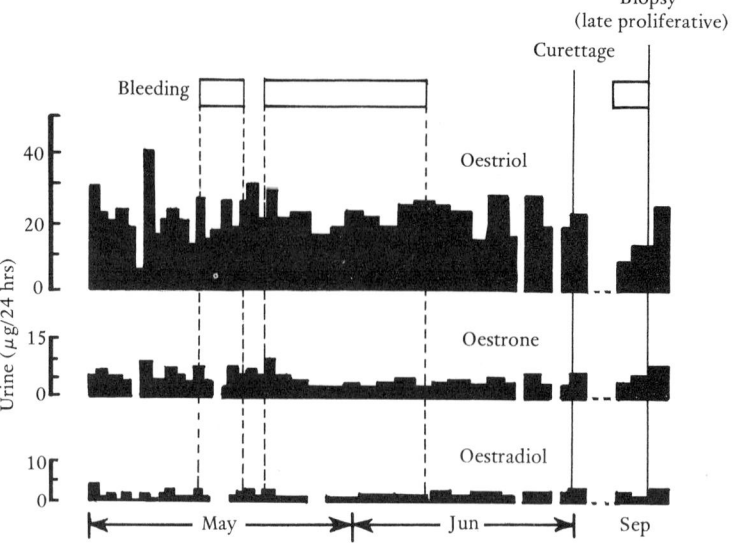

Fig. 34.3   Varying oestrogen levels in irregular uterine bleeding.

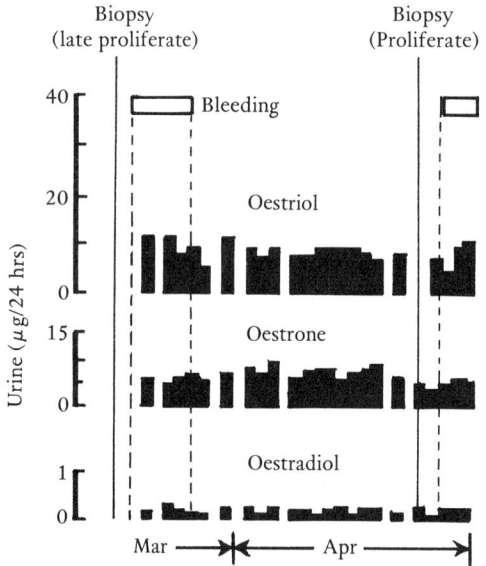

Fig. 34.4   Constant oestrogen levels in irregular uterine bleeding.

tain it and disintegration follows. Protracted bleeding may be due to sustained oestrogen stimulation at a lower level of concentration and results in patchy and irregular shedding of the endometrium at the time of menstruation.

The clinical features of cystic glandular hyperplasia may occur at any phase of reproductive life although it is most common at puberty and during the pre-menopausal years.

The main symptom is prolonged and irregular bleeding which is frequently preceded by a period of amenorrhoea. The bleeding may bear little relationship to the development of the endometrium and varies in amount from day to day continuing for as long as 5 or 6 weeks at a time. Occasionally the cycles may be regular like normal menstruation. The patient may become very anaemic and require blood transfusion. Spontaneous cure, especially in the young, is likely.

The diagnosis is usually made by examination of the curettings but a history of amenorrhoea followed by prolonged and excessive uterine bleeding indicates the likelihood of this condition.

Investigation of these patients includes a curettage and in some cases laparoscopy, to detect the ovarian abnormality, may be required. Curettage may be curative but if this is not so then hormonal therapy may be indicated. The aim of treatment is to control the bleeding and to prevent its occurrence. In severely anaemic women blood transfusion may be necessary but iron therapy is always indicated. Various endocrine preparations have been advocated in the past for management of dysfunctional uterine bleeding. Thyroid has been used since it was supposed that some of these cases were due to a mild degree of hypothyroidism. Progesterone preparations alone have been recommended. Combinations of oestrogen and progestogen have been used and androgens alone or in combination have been suggested. Oestrogen therapy, gonadotrophin therapy and clomiphene therapy have all been used for this condition. However, the optimum results are obtained by the use of an oestrogen/gestogen preparation such as is used in oral contraception. These preparations have really superseded other treatments and are the most effective way of stopping dysfunctional uterine bleeding. Such preparations as Metrulen (ethynodiol diacetate 2mg, ethinyloestradiol 0·05mg), or Enovid (norethynodrel 5mg) given in doses of 1–3 tablets daily for 24 days is the best treatment. Bleeding usually ceases within 48–72 hours and will recur a few days after the tablets have stopped. The tablets should be started on the day menstruation begins and stopped on day 24 resulting in bleeding on day 28 or so. This should be continued for three cycles and then stopped to see what the effect has been. This therapy may be continued indefinitely and if the dose is increased and the pills not stopped at all, complete amenorrhoea can be achieved. Although gonadotrophic hormones and clomiphene have been used for restoring a normal hormone balance, these drugs require sophisticated monitoring facilities and are best reserved for those women who desire a pregnancy. The method of giving gonadotrophins is similar to that described in the 'Infertility' section of this chapter.

Surgical methods, such as curettage, are indicated for diagnostic purposes and may also control bleeding in an emergency. If, however, this type of bleeding continues and the patient does not wish to have further children, total hysterectomy is the operation of choice. This may be done either by the abdominal or vaginal route.

X-rays and radium to produce an artificial menopause should only be used when hysterectomy is too great a risk. In general the treatment of dysfunctional uterine bleeding has become much easier in recent years due to the introduction of the oestrogen/gestogen preparations and the increasing safety of hysterectomy.

Excessive menstrual loss, particularly in younger women who have not responded to hormonal therapy and in whom hysterectomy is not desirable, may be given ε-aminocaproic acid.

Menstrual blood usually clots within the uterus and undergoes fibrinolysis under the influence of the fibrinolytic enzyme plasmin. This enzyme is formed from plasminogen under the influence of fibrinolytic activator released from the endometrium. Some women with heavy periods have a high concentration of endometrial plasminogen activator on the first day of the period. This may be a factor in causing the menorrhagia (Rybo, 1966).

ε-aminocaproic acid inhibits endometrial fibrinolytic activator and may thus reduce the excessive menstrual loss. The dose is 3·0g ε-aminocaproic acid 4–6 times daily until the period has finished.

2. FEMALE INFERTILITY

Introduction

The problem of infertility is an important one, both to the individual husband and wife and also to the State. Inability to beget children brings extreme unhappiness to many individuals whose whole quality of life is dependent on having a child. Many show great perseverance in their quest and turn to their doctors for advice and treatment of this complaint.

Although there are strong pressures throughout society at the present time to limit family size in the context of the overall world population problem, it is important for the individual doctor to consider the needs of the individual patient. The drive of individuals to reproduce is a very basic one. In most social groups the fertility of an individual is a matter of general concern. The psychological aspects of infertility are most important. A doctor must realize that whatever kind of therapy is instituted, proper psychological support is essential and in this the husband should be included. Each menstrual period that arrives, especially after treatment, is considered a disaster by the patient. The treatment must therefore be on a personal basis and one doctor or preferably a small team, should try to supervise the patient. The happiness of the infertile woman successfully treated is great and the contribution that these successes make to world population numbers is so small that it can be ignored. Work, however, on the problem of infertility contributes much to the general area of reproductive knowledge. This itself, in another way, is important in helping to deal with the major problem of world population growth.

There are two main types of female infertility. In the first, known as relative infertility, pregnancies do occur but are not carried to viability. In the second type, no pregnancy is achieved.

The incidence of infertility is not easy to assess. A statistical survey based on women recorded as childless in the 1911 British census gives a figure of 8 per cent. Davies (1967) in the report to the Committee on Human Reproduction reported a figure of 10 per cent. He suggested that another 10 per cent of couples suffer from absolute infertility, where no pregnancy has occurred at all and another 10 per cent suffer from relative infertility where a pregnancy does occur but is not carried to viability. Although in many couples it is possible to identify aetiological factors, in many it is also impossible to detect any lesion after detailed investigation of both partners. However, with recent advances in laboratory techniques of measurement of hormones concerned with the ovulatory process, other abnormalities are being detected which may be factors in the infertility problem. Emotional factors are also thought to be responsible in some cases and the action of the higher centres on the hypothalamus and its releasing factors has been suggested as the cause of this. Conception can occur for the first time after many years of normal married life and it is also not uncommon for a woman complaining of infertility having adopted an infant to become pregnant a few months later.

Any consideration of infertility in a couple must of course include the male as well as the female partner and it is thought that approximately 35–40 per cent of barren marriages are due to a male factor. The investigations on the female, which are expensive and time consuming are pointless if the male partner has, for example, azoospermia.

The essential requirements of the female in reproduction are that the ovaries should produce healthy ova and also an adequate hormonal secretion to prepare the uterus for implantation of the fertilized ova. The Fallopian tubes should offer no obstruction to the passage of the ovum and no obstruction to the spermatozoa. The cervical secretion should provide a favourable medium for spermatozoa during their passage from the cervix to the tube.

Aetiology of female infertility

Age. The period of maximum fertility in women is before 25 years of age. Thereafter there is a slow decline to the age of 35 and a more rapid fall to 45 years. Age must therefore be taken into consideration when assessing the cause of infertility in women.

Medical conditions

General medical conditions are not often seen by the gynaecologist as a causal factor in infertility, since, if these are severe enough to result in infertility, in most cases the patient is already being treated for the primary condition by the physician. General medical conditions, however, should be eliminated before specific gynaecological investigations and treatment are performed. Such diseases as tuberculosis, diabetes and renal lesions may lower fertility. The role of psychological factors in causing infertility is difficult to assess. There is much suggestive clinical observation and impression but little hard data on the subject. Vaginismus and coital difficulties due to psychosomatic factors may be responsible for infertility in a number of patients and in taking a history from a patient complaining of infertility the possible relevance of psychogenic factors should be remembered.

Nutrition

Severe underfeeding may result in infertility usually associated with amenorrhoea and anovulation. The nutritional defects require to be severe as countries where nutrition is poor at present still have high birth rates. Contrariwise, reproductive capacity may also be affected by obesity which is frequently part of a general endocrine or metabolic disturbance which interferes with the hypothalamic-pituitary function and results in amenorrhoea and anovulation.

Specific lesions causing infertility

Vulva and vagina. The main lesions of the vulva and vagina associated with infertility are those due to congenital abnormality such as the intact hymen which prevents intromission of the penis. It is true, however, that pregnancy may result without vaginal penetration so that unless the hymen is completely imperforate, pregnancy is possible. Severe vaginal infection may cause infertility although there are numerous patients with bad infections who seem to become pregnant. The infection, however, may cause severe vaginal irritation which may prevent the couple from having intercourse and therefore cause infertility. Local ulcerative lesions round the introitus may also prevent intercourse due to pain and result in failure to conceive from that cause.

The cervix. For fertilization to occur the spermatozoa must penetrate the cervical canal and the importance of the cervix in sperm transmission has been recognized more and more. The position of the cervix in the genital tract or abnormalities of the cervix itself may both cause infertility. If the cervix is displaced in cases of retroverted uterus it may not dip into the seminal pool in the posterior fornix and this will reduce the likelihood of sperm entering the cervical canal. Similarly, cases of genital prolapse may result in the cervix interfering with intercourse. Retroversions should be corrected and the uterus held in the correct position by a Hodge pessary, or a ventro-suspension operation may be required to hold the uterus in permanent anteversion. In the case of genital prolapse it is best to avoid an operation since this might further reduce fertility but advice on the depth of penetration during intercourse so that ejaculation takes place just inside the introitus is often helpful. Amputation of the cervix is an important association with infertility probably due to removal of a large part of the mucus secreting tissue. Fibrosis due to cervical cautery may also be a factor. Most cervical erosions do not interfere with fertility although, if the erosions are grossly infected and there are other signs of pelvic inflammatory disease, treatment should be instituted.

Cervical mucus. This secretion from the cervix is important in transmission of the spermatozoa and also in protection of the sperm from the hostile environment of the vagina. Cervical mucus increases in quantity during the proliferative phase and becomes profuse, watery and stretchable at the time of ovulation. In the secretory phase the mucus is scanty, thick and opaque. Cervical mucus taken just before ovulation and smeared on to a glass slide shows the typical fern pattern due to oestrogen stimulation. After ovulation, under the influence of progesterone, the ferning pattern disappears. If a fern pattern is found in the second half of the cycle this is suggestive of anovulation. Cervical mucus can therefore be used as a biological parameter of ovarian function and in some centres, combined with vaginal cytology, endometrial biopsy

and basal temperature charts, is used in monitoring patients undergoing ovulation stimulation with gonadotrophins. This is not such an accurate method as the use of urinary or plasma oestrogen assays but these may not be available in all centres. In some women cervical mucus appears to be hostile to sperm in that it exerts a noxious effect and prevents their transmission to the upper genital tract. Insufficient mucus may be present in which case a daily dose of 0·01mg of ethinyl oestradiol on days 9, 10 and 11 of the cycle may result in the improvement of postcoital findings and a resultant pregnancy. In other cases where the mucus appears to be lethal to the spermatozoa, artificial insemination with husband's sperm inserted directly into the cervical canal may be a practical solution. Sperm antibodies have been sought in the serum of infertile women and have been found in a varying percentage, and while sperm agglutinins may delay fertilization in some women these women seem to have the same capacity to conceive as women without serum sperm agglutinin activity (Pacheco-Romero et al., 1973).

The body of the uterus. The endometrium of the uterus is the target on which the ovarian hormones act. The endocrine aspects of infertility will be considered separately. Tuberculosis of the endometrium is an important aetiological factor although this is lessening as the incidence of tuberculosis decreases.

Hypoplasia of the uterus is a possible cause although its significance is in some doubt.

Retroversion of the uterus has already been mentioned in the discussion on the cervix and where this is due to an inflammatory process the uterus may be fixed in the retroverted position.

Uterine fibroids may also be responsible for infertility particularly where they interfere with implantation or with the uterine end of the Fallopian tubes. Myomectomy may be indicated when fibroids appear to be associated with infertility.

Fallopian tubes. Normal pregnancy is preceded by transfer of the ovum from the ruptured follicle in the ovary to the Fallopian tube where fertilization occurs. The blastocyst then remains in the tubal lumen for about three days before finally arriving in the uterine cavity. The condition of the Fallopian tube is therefore important for successful fertilization, ovum transport and implantation.

Parameters of tubal physiology are difficult to measure and are not done in clinical practice although some of these may be important in infertility.

Congenital abnormality, such as absence of one or both tubes, is responsible for only a small proportion of cases of infertility. The most common cause of tubal blockage appears to be the inflammatory lesion. These may follow infection with the gonococcus which produces great destruction by involving the mucous membrane and causing obstructive adhesions, tuberculous lesions which are equally destructive but less frequent, puerperal infection and those following abortion may also result in tubal blockage. In some cases partial obstruction may occur with an increased incidence of ectopic pregnancy. Inflammatory lesions may be associated with other intra-abdominal conditions such as appendicitis. Tubal neoplasms are rare but the tubal lumen may be distorted by ovarian or uterine tumours.

Ovary. Endometriosis adversely affects the function of the ovaries especially if a chocolate cyst has formed. Absence of the ovaries or streak ovaries such as may be found in some genetic abnormality, e.g. Turner's syndrome may also be associated with infertility. The polycystic ovarian syndrome already mentioned is another important ovarian cause of infertility.

Sexual disturbances

Some women believe that their inability to conceive is due to the lack of sexual feeling. This may be true in that lack of feeling may result in more infrequent intercourse and difficulty with penetration. The basis of these complaints is usually psychosomatic. The commonest one is severe vaginismus. Some indication that this may be a factor can be obtained during the examination of the patient when she resists vaginal examination. Some women also state that there is a considerable leakage of seminal fluid from the vagina following intercourse. However, only a small amount of seminal fluid is required for fertilization and it is unlikely that this is of much significance. The suggestion that the buttocks should be elevated to retain the seminal fluid after intercourse may be of psychological help to the patient. Sexual disharmony and ignorance of the sexual relationship are occasional causes of sterility and indication of this should be obtained during the history taking.

DISORDERS OF OVULATION

Anovulatory infertility. This group are the infertile women who persistently fail to ovulate or only ovulate infrequently. Occasional anovulatory cycles are not uncommon in women but it is only when this occurs persistently that infertility results. Anovulation may be associated with regular menstruation or with amenorrhoea. The bleeding is associated with a proliferative endometrium and may occur as often as 15 per cent in sterile women. The failure of ovulation may be due to a temporary ovarian defect or to a deficient hypothalamic-pituitary stimulus. Amenorrhoea and cystic glandular hyperplasia have already been considered. Anovulation may be due to failure of synthesis or release of the hypothalamic releasing hormones or the pituitary gonadotrophic hormones and will result in the failure of ovulation with or without cessation of the menses.

More recently defined endocrine abnormalities resulting in infertility are those in women who, by all the normal methods of detection, seem to be ovulating regularly. Only when intensive studies using newer hormonal assay methods such as radioimmunoassay for oestradiol and progesterone are done does it become evident that the hormone profiles in these women are abnormal. It can be shown that the follicular phase in some women is short and that the amount of oestradiol produced is low due to poor development of the follicle. These women frequently also have a resultant defective luteal phase in which the secondary rise in oestrogen or progesterone is low. The length of the luteal phase may also be reduced. Stimulation of women who have these defective cycles with either clomiphene or gonadotrophin may result in normal hormone profiles being produced.

Investigation of female infertility

At the first interview a detailed personal history should be taken, the age of the patient, duration of marriage and information as to past contraceptive techniques should be obtained, the menstrual history inquired into and in relative infertility information regarding previous pregnancies etc. should be documented. Previous illnesses and operations such as appendicectomy should be noted and the patient's knowledge of time and frequency of coitus relative to the menstrual cycle have to be obtained. Any sexual maladjustment or difficulties and abnormalities such as dyspareunia have to be noted. A general examination should be made to assess the patient's general state of health and to exclude specific diseases. During this examination the presence of abnormal distribution of hair should be particularly looked for. Pelvic examination at this stage will detect any lesion of the reproductive tract such as an intact hymen, cervical or uterine abnormality. If no abnormality is found it is usual to place the patient's name on the list for admission and allow several months to pass before conducting any further investigation. During this time the patient should take her early morning temperature and try to determine whether ovulation is occurring or not by this method. At the initial interview the name of the husband should be obtained and arrangements should also be made to investigate him at the same time.

The timing of further investigations depends on a number of factors such as the age of the patient, duration of marriage etc. Approximately 50 per cent of fertile couples achieve pregnancy within one month of commencing regular coitus and more than 70 per cent are successful by the end of six months. Before admission to hospital for further investigation it is important that the timing of the menstrual cycle should be ascertained so that the patient can be investigated further in the luteal phase of the cycle. The important aspects to be covered are: the occurrence of ovulation, patency and condition of the Fallopian tubes and the development of the endometrium and and presence of adequate cervical mucus which does not inactivate sperm.

Detection of ovulation. Numerous presumptive tests of ovulation are available but the only two final parameters which definitely indicate that ovulation has occurred are visualization of the ovum or pregnancy. Visualization of the ovum is possible by laparoscopy (Steptoe and Edwards, 1970) but arrangements for this are not realistic on a routine basis. Presumptive methods therefore have to be used. These are: (1) The biphasic basal body temperature graph, (2) Secretory changes in the endometrium, (3) Changes in the plasma levels of oestradiol and progesterone and 17-α-hydroxyprogesterone, (4) The cornification index of the vaginal smear, and (5) The increased amount and liquidity of the cervical mucus

followed by decreased amounts of mucus and the absence of ferning. It is only with relatively sophisticated laboratory facilities that the steroid hormone levels can be observed. The method used for detecting ovulation will depend on the facilities which are available to the clinician.

Patency of the Fallopian tubes. The condition of the tube is of importance for successful fertilization, ovum transport and implantation. The only tests done in the clinical investigation of fertility are those which test tubal patency and anatomical appearance. Three methods of testing tubal patency are available: (1) Insufflation using carbon dioxide, (2) Hysterosalpingography, and (3) Instillation of dye during laparoscopy. Tubal insufflation with carbon dioxide is probably the simplest and oldest method of assessing tubal patency. The cannula is inserted into the cervical canal and an airtight junction formed. The cannula is then connected to a kymograph and gas is passed through the cannula. With normal tubal patency gas begins to pass through the tubes at a pressure of 60–100mm. Variations in pressure recorded on the machine may be due to contractions of the tube and the amplitude of these may vary from 10–30mm. Tubal spasm may occur with this method and the initial pressure may rise as high as 200mm or more. When, however, the spasm is overcome the pressure rapidly falls to 40 or 50mm. Where bilateral tubal occlusion is present the tracing rises steadily until a pressure of 200 or more is reached and remains at this level.

Hysterosalpingography involves the insufflation of a radiopaque material into the cervical canal in a way similar to the gas insufflation. An aqueous solution such as Endographin is now used and in addition to demonstrating the shape of the uterine cavity (Fig. 34.5) and tubal patency or obstruction, this technique will also demonstrate uterine abnormalities such as subseptate uterus and submucous myomas. It will also outline damaged tubes such as hydrosalpinx.

Recently, laparoscopy has been used more and more in the investigation of infertility and will probably supersede tubal insufflation since this method gives a direct visualization of the tubes and ovaries. To test the patency of the Fallopian tubes, methylene blue dye can be injected into the uterine cavity via the cervix and can be seen to spill from the fimbriated ends into the peritoneal cavity if the tubes are

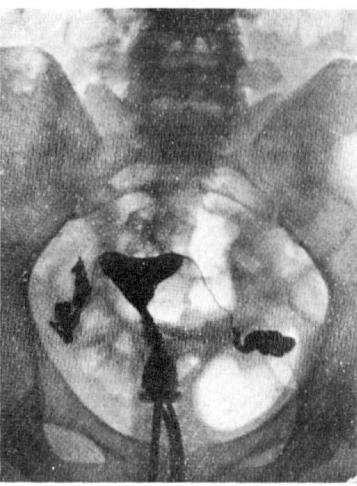

Fig. 34.5 Hysterosalpingogram showing normal bilateral tubal patency.

patent. If they are blocked, the site of the blockage may be established. If no dye is seen to enter the tube, cornual blockage is present. It is also possible to see the extent of any damage to the fimbriated ends of the tubes and in some cases to divide fimbriated adhesions which may be a factor in some women complaining of infertility.

Laparoscopy is now the method of choice for assessing tubal patency and should certainly be preferred where there is doubt about the condition of the Fallopian tubes. Laparoscopy can also be used to assess the condition of the tubes prior to tubal surgery and also to assess the results of operations on the tubes. An ovarian biopsy can also be made at the time of laparoscopy and therefore the diagnosis of such conditions as the Stein–Leventhal syndrome can be confirmed. The method of laparoscopy has been popularized by Steptoe (1967) whose monograph on this subject should be consulted by those wishing to use the technique.

Post-coital test

Sims–Huhner test. This should be performed on all women who complain of infertility. The cervical mucus should be collected as soon as possible after intercourse but periods as long as 24 hours after intercourse can give acceptable results. Cervical mucus should be taken from the endocervix but a specimen should also be taken from the posterior vaginal pool. The test should be performed in mid-cycle when the cervical mucus is receptive to sperm. The total number of sperm and the number of motile sperms are determined per high power field. An adequate number of approximately 10 or more sperm per high power field is usually considered satisfactory. A satisfactory post-coital test with a large number of actively motile sperm present in the mucus may in fact obviate the necessity for analysing the semen but in general terms a properly performed semen analysis should also be done. A single negative test should not be accepted and only repeated negative tests indicate some abnormality in the husband. The hostility of the cervical mucus to spermatozoa can also be investigated by the Kurzrok–Miller test. The method consists of placing one drop of seminal fluid and cervical mucus on a glass slide, a cover glass being pressed on to both drops so that they just come into contact. The test is positive when, on microscopic examination, the spermatozoae are seen to penetrate the mucus. Oestrogen therapy may increase the permeability of cervical mucus to sperm and 0·01mg of ethinyl oestradiol daily on day 9, 10 and 11 of the cycle has been proved to be of some help in these patients.

Treatment of infertility

The treatment of infertility depends on the cause. As mentioned before, infertility can be broadly divided into two main groups—*absolute*, where no previous pregnancy has occurred and *relative*, where the patient has had a previous pregnancy which has been unsuccessful or has failed to achieve a pregnancy following a successful one.

RELATIVE INFERTILITY

The major causes of this condition are three—uterine abnormality, incompetent cervix and possible corpus luteum abnormality. The conditions may all cause abortion and it is on these grounds that most of these patients attend for investigation and treatment.

Uterine abnormality. Most of the abnormalities result from incomplete fusion of the Mullerian ducts the commonest being bicornuate or subseptate uterus which is a cause of recurrent abortion and premature labour. This is first suspected by the history of recurrent abortions and should be investigated by hysterosalpingography. The treatment of bicornuate uterus is surgical and the details are given in the chapter on surgical operations.

The treatment is very successful and should be offered to patients with uterine abnormality who have had two or more abortions and have no living children.

Incompetent cervix. The history of a patient with cervical incompetence is characteristic and usually includes two or more mid-trimester abortions which frequently occur painlessly after the membranes rupture. There may be a history of cervical damage due to previous curettage or dilatation or a history of induced abortion. The diagnosis is difficult to make definitively and the history is usually the most satisfactory way of making a diagnosis. The cervical suture which should be inserted round the cervix should be done preferably early in pregnancy.

Possible deficient corpus luteum. As mentioned in the chapter on abortion it has been suggested that in habitual abortion there may be a deficiency of progesterone about the time the production of this hormone from the corpus luteum of pregnancy decreases and before progesterone from the trophoblast becomes adequate. Corpus luteal activity during pregnancy may be estimated by measuring the production of 17-α-hydroxy-progesterone since unlike progesterone, this substance is not manufactured by the trophoblast. This makes it possible to differentiate the production of the luteal hormone from the corpus luteum alone. In gonadotrophin induced pregnancy it has been found that the corpus luteum was functionally active for about 8–10 weeks.

It has been suggested, therefore, that if abortion was to be caused by deficiency of progesterone it would be expected to occur around the stage of 6–8 weeks. It is known, however, that human pregnancy can continue even if the corpus luteum is removed as early as 35 days of gestation. The role of the deficient corpus luteum in the production of recurrent abortion is therefore not yet established.

ABSOLUTE INFERTILITY

Medical conditions causing absolute infertility are not often seen by the gynaecologist in the first instance since if they are severe enough to result in infertility then in most cases the patient is already being treated for the primary condition. However, it has to be remembered that general medical conditions can cause infertility and have to be thought about in this context during initial examination. The commoner conditions associated with infertility are uterine and tubal disease which interfere with fertilization and implantation, abnormalities of menstruation such as amenorrhoea, oligomenorrhoea and anovulatory menstruation, the Stein–Leventhal or polycystic ovarian syndrome, which has been already mentioned, and genetic abnormalities such as Turner's syndrome.

Tubal blockage. This may result from a variety of causes such as pelvic inflammatory disease, tuberculosis or post-partum infections and a history of these conditions may be obtained from the patient. Diagnosis of tubal abnormality may either be made by hysterosalpingography or preferably laparoscopy. At laparoscopy it may also be possible to decide whether treatment is likely to be successful. Salpingostomy, the operation of opening the tubes, is described in the chapter on operations. Pregnancy rates varying from 11–30 per cent have been reported. Following the operation hydrotubation may be of value and both hydrocortisone and antibiotics have been used. In some instances the abnormality is a blockage at the cornua of the uterus. This is diagnosed by hysterosalpingogram which shows only the uterine outline with no evidence of dye entering the tubes (Fig. 34.6). The operation

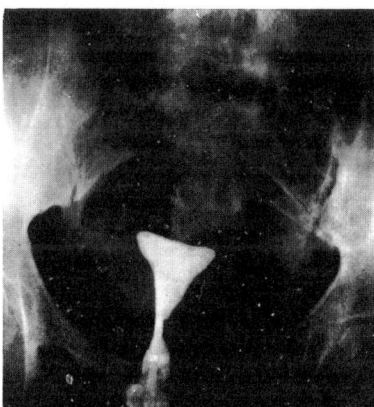

Fig. 34.6   Hysterosalpingogram showing bilateral cornual block.

in these cases is tubal re-implantation. This operation is marginally more successful than some others on the tubes and the success rate is 25–30 per cent or more. Any pregnancy following these operations should be terminated by Caesarean section since the risk of rupture of the weakened cornua is considerable.

In spite of the rather poor success rate, gynaecologists are frequently pressed to perform these operations so that the patient can feel that everything has been done. It is important to discuss the procedure fully with the patient and her husband to ensure that they understand all the aspects. Only when the patient insists upon the operation should it be performed. Abnormalities of menstruation such as amenorrhoea, oligomenorrhoea and anovulatory menstruation have already been described but when the patient presents with these conditions and is anxious to become pregnant, then some form of therapy has to be considered.

Induction of ovulation in infertile patients

At the present time two drugs are commonly used for induction of ovulation. The choice lies between clomiphene and human gonadotrophins. Clomiphene will induce ovulation in approximately 70 per cent of patients and is simpler to use than gonadotrophin therapy. The only contra-indication is the presence of ovarian cysts or tumours and in cases in whom pituitary ablation has been carried out for a pituitary tumour. Clomiphene is the drug of choice where polycystic ovaries are present. The classical type of patient suitable for clomiphene therapy is one with anovulatory cycles or secondary amenorrhoea with an intact pituitary gland. In these patients the amount of endogenous gonadotrophin produced is insufficient to result in ovulation. It is possible for clomiphene to induce hyperstimulation and multiple pregnancy but the risks of these occurring are much less than with gonadotrophin therapy.

The initial dose of clomiphene should be 50mg daily for 5 days. If the patient is menstruating the treatment should start on day 1 of the cycle as this will stimulate the pituitary and help to produce gonadotrophin at the early stage resulting in stimulation of follicular growth in the ovary. In many cases treatment has been started on day 5 but this is probably rather late in the cycle although well controlled series assessing the value of the two different types of treatment have not been performed to date. If ovulation does not occur the dose can be increased up to a level of 250mg daily for 5 days. If no response is achieved at this level of treatment the drug should be stopped and the patient treated with

gonadotrophins. Sometimes chorionic gonadotrophin has been added to clomiphene therapy but if this substance is given the likelihood of hyperstimulation is much greater and proper daily monitoring is necessary. Monitoring by hormone assay of patients on clomiphene therapy is not mandatory but it is difficult to know exactly what is happening unless some type of monitoring is done and the minimum necessary is monitoring by basal body temperature graphs or vaginal cytology. The pregnancy rate with clomiphene treatment is unfortunately much less than the ovulatory rate and estimations of 12 per cent or so have been given by various authors. Other substances like clomiphene such as tamoxifen, cyclofenil have also been used more recently and are still undergoing clinical evaluation. The clinical role of these substances compared with clomiphene has yet to be established.

Gonadotrophin therapy. The material most commonly used in clinical practice at the present time is human menopausal gonadotrophin (HMG). This material is extracted from human menopausal urine and is effective in inducing ovulation.

These preparations do not constitute pure FSH and all substances used so far have a significant LH component. The preparations are administered by intramuscular injection and the material most widely available is human menopausal gonadotrophin (Pergonal-Searle). Although dosage control may be by indirect methods such as vaginal smears or cervical mucus changes, it is really mandatory to control gonadotrophin therapy by steroid assays. There are various ways of administering the drug. Probably the best method is that suggested by Townsend *et al.* (1966). In this method the daily dose may range between 75 and 400 International Units of HMG given for 8–10 days. At the start a low dose is given and this is increased until an adequate response is obtained. The response is measured by daily assays of oestrogens and pregnandiol in the urine or by plasma oestradiol or plasma progesterone in the blood. It is necessary to have the result rapidly so that the next day's dose can be calculated. It is probably easier for routine use to have a urinary method of hormone assay for this treatment.

The object of the regime is to achieve a physiological level of oestrogen excretion, the level aimed at being between 50 and 100μg of total urinary oestrogen—the level approximating that found in the cycles of normal ovulating women. When this has been reached ovulation is then induced by a single injection of HCG usually 5000–10 000 International Units. It may be necessary to give additional doses of HCG if the luteal level of progesterone does not rise sufficiently. Other regimes of treatment are also used. Perhaps a more practical scheme is the 1, 3, 5 regime described by Butler (1972). In this method HMG is given in equal doses on alternate days if the patient is amenorrhoeic. If she has had a period the regime may start at day 1, 3, 5 of the cycle. HCG in this regime is given on day 8 of the cycle. Urinary assays of oestrogen are necessary before the HCG is given otherwise hyperstimulation may occur. Taking the various results achieved into account it is probable that the ovulation rate of selected patients is in the region of 70 per cent.

The two main complications of gonadotrophin therapy are hyperstimulation and multiple pregnancy. Hyperstimulation is potentially a lethal condition and is likely to occur if the urinary total oestrogen level is more than $150 \mu g/24$ hours. If this level should be obtained then HCG should be withheld in that particular cycle. Mild hyperstimulation presents slightly enlarged tender ovaries which can be felt on palpation and vaginal examination should be performed in women having gonadotrophin therapy before HCG is given. If the ovaries feel enlarged the drug should be withheld.

Even with careful monitoring the risk of multiple pregnancy is somewhere about 20 per cent and the patient should know about this risk before starting therapy. The overall pregnancy rate is probably somewhere around 30 per cent although Brown *et al.* (1972) achieved an overall pregnancy rate of 68 and 73 per cent using the technique of Townsend *et al.* already mentioned.

It is essential that gonadotrophin treatment should only be carried out in centres where adequate laboratory facilities are available to provide the proper assay control that is necessary to prevent complications. Gonadotrophin therapy is tedious for the patient and her husband, especially so if she lives at some distance from the laboratory or hospital since frequent visits, often daily, are required for proper control. It also requires determination and some degree of intelligence to carry through the treatment. It is therefore advisable

before embarking on therapy to explain the implications fully to the patient and her husband so that they can decide whether or not they wish to undertake this form of therapy.

The apparently normal woman who is infertile

There are a number of women who, after the usual routine investigations for infertility, appear to be normal. If daily hormone assays are performed on such subjects, abnormalities in levels are found at different stages of the cycle. Levels of oestradiol are low in the follicular phase of the cycle and the height of the luteal peak of progesterone is lower than that found in normal ovulatory cycles. It seems likely that the abnormal ovarian cycle is an important factor in these women. This well illustrates the point that when more intensive investigations are performed in women suffering from infertility, abnormalities of function can be found and treated (Fig. 34.7). It does seem important that

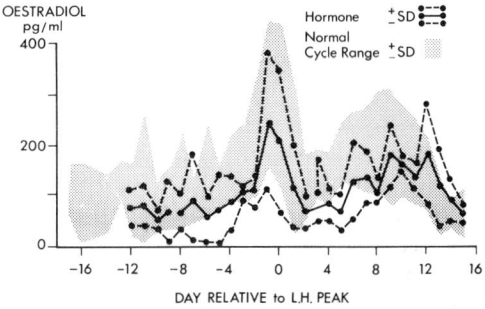

Fig. 34.7 Comparison of the mean levels ± one S.D. for plasma oestradiol in six ovulatory infertile patients with the normal cycle range for oestradiol. Note low follicular levels and poor secondary peak of oestradiol.
(Dodson, Macnaughton & Coutts, 1975.) Courtesy of the Editor, *British Journal of Obstetrics & Gynaecology.*

adequate follicular growth should occur in order to obtain satisfactory corpus luteum function. If follicle growth is poor then corpus luteum activity may also be abnormal. Rational therapy in these patients requires adequate stimulation of follicular growth by the use of either clomiphene or gonadotrophin therapy as described.

Artificial insemination

Some couples who are disappointed at their continued infertility where the husband is at fault, seek advice with regard to artificial insemination. The insemination can either be performed with the husband's semen—Artificial Insemination Husband (AIH)—or with the seminal fluid of a suitable donor—Artificial Insemination Donor (AID). It must only be undertaken when all the possible circumstances have been fully discussed with both partners.

Artificial insemination husband should be considered when there is some difficulty with intercourse due to a mechanical, developmental, or psychogenic defect in the husband but he is producing spermatozoa, the only difficulty being his inability to place them in the correct site. This type of artificial insemination may also be considered when the cervical mucus, in spite of treatment, is persistently hostile to spermatozoa or when the sperm count after treatment remains at a low level.

Before any type of artificial insemination is performed it is necessary to determine that the female reproductive tract is normal, that ovulation is occurring and the approximate time of this. The timing of ovulation is usually gauged by asking the patient to take daily temperature records for three months or so. In the normally ovulating patient this will be indicated by a rise in basal body temperature at the time of ovulation. On the day in which ovulation is expected the husband is asked to collect a specimen of seminal fluid by masturbation. The specimen should be used within one hour of its production. The sperm may be injected into the cervix and fornices with a cannula. It is usual to ask the patient to lie supine for 30 minutes after the insemination. A repeat insemination should be performed 48 hours following the first and it is usual to repeat this during several ovulatory cycles. The general results of this procedure are poor.

Artificial insemination donor is becoming much more common and frozen human semen is now in use in several centres. There are many problems about artificial insemination by donor and several interviews may be necessary with the couple to discuss their attitude to this before a decision can be made as to its suitability in the individual circumstances. It is true in general terms that the results in properly selected couples are good as far as psychogenic difficulties are concerned. Artificial insemination donor is particularly indicated when the husband is sterile

and the wife potentially fertile. The subject is one of considerable controversy since there are many legal, moral and other objections to this type of procedure. However, there is considerable demand for this now in suitable couples and it seems probable that some of these problems will be resolved in the foreseeable future. The donor material for artificial insemination must be carefully selected. The general health, genetic constitution and racial background must be carefully considered and it is usual to record the height, hair and eye colour of the donor. It is important that anonymity be preserved.

The use of 'sperm banks' to preserve seminal fluid in a frozen condition for insemination is being developed more widely. This has been used for many years in the case of farm animals with good results and there is now considerable experience of the use of frozen human semen in human infertility. For this technique semen is stored in liquid nitrogen at $-196\,^{\circ}$C and there is no evidence so far that storage produces genetic damage. It has the added advantage of making available supplies of donor material without the necessity of donor attendance at the time of ovulation of the recipient. It seems likely that this method will be more widely used in the future. The future of frozen human semen, however, depends on current acceptance and practice and changes in moral and legal attitudes may be necessary before widespread use of this technique becomes possible.

Male infertility

Male infertility is now recognized as an increasing factor in infertile marriages. It has been estimated that an identifiable male factor contributes to about 35–40 per cent of infertile marriages. Until recently the husband was not usually considered adequately until full assessment for fertility status and investigation had been performed on the wife. It is now good practice to assess both partners at the same time and indeed since the husband is much more easily assessed he should be evaluated before the wife is subjected to detailed investigation. While the majority of men are usually willing to share the responsibility with their wives and are prepared to be examined and investigated some consider the suggestion that they may be responsible for the infertility of their marriage as a slur on their physical vigour and so refuse. Others are hesitant lest any past indiscretions are exposed or any lesion discovered which might reflect on their virility.

CLINICAL ASSESSMENT OF THE HUSBAND

The inquiry requires careful, tactful and detailed assessment of many factors. The general health of the patient should be evaluated and the patient's habits studied; these including leisure and exercise, mental stress or indulgence in alcohol. Information should be obtained regarding sexual life, difficulty in performing coitus and its frequency. The patient's libido should be assessed, the adequacy of potency and ejaculation with particular reference to the presence of premature ejaculation. Knowledge of the timing of intercourse in relation to the wife's menstrual cycle must be considered. The main aetiological factors are listed in Table 34.1.

Table 34.1   Aetiological factors in male infertility (De Kretser, 1974)

1. *Defects in technique :*
   Infrequent intercourse
   Use of lubricants
   Impotence

2. *Testicular factors :*

Idiopathic	Chromosomal
Chronic illness	Trauma, torsion
Infection	Immunological
Cryptorchidism	Heat
Varicocoele	Endocrine
Irradiation	Toxic chemical

3. *Obstructive*

4. *Accessory glands :*
   Prostato-vesiculitis
   Congenital absence of vas and seminal vesicles
   Immunological

A complete history of the patient's development should be obtained with a past history of any venereal infection or mumps orchitis. Past history of renal failure or the use of cytoxic agents is also important. The environment in which the patient works may be significant and environmental heat or toxic chemicals may affect the seminiferous tubules. Details of any children from past marriages should be obtained.

General physical examination should be performed with particular reference to the patient's general state of health, hair growth and body hair and the sense of smell should be tested to detect the presence of hyposmia or anosmia which may be found in hypogonadotrophic hypogonadism.

Examination of the genital tract includes examination of the penis to exclude epispadias or hypospadias and phimosis, inspection and palpation of the testes and epididymes and measurement with calipers. In this way, atrophy, displacement, tumour formation, inflammation, varicocele and hydrocele can be detected. A rectal examination should be performed to exclude diseases of the prostate and seminal vesicles.

Semen analysis

The most important laboratory test in the infertile male is the analysis of his semen and this should be carried out by someone trained in this type of work to ensure that a reliable estimate of fertility is made. In addition to the sperm count, other parameters such as sperm morphology and motility are also important. If a low count is demonstrated then further investigations including chromosomal analysis, hormonal investigation and testicular biopsy may be necessary.

Semen should be collected by masturbation into a clean glass or plastic container. Masturbation is better than collection by coitus interruptus and collection by condom is unsatisfactory as many condoms contain spermicidal compounds. A normal ejaculate consists of 3–5ml of a white opalescent whitish/yellow gelatinous fluid which becomes watery and translucent on standing at room temperature for 30 minutes. It has a pH of 7.4 and contains over 60 million spermatozoa per ml, 90 per cent of which show activity and not more than 20 per cent abnormal forms. Certain biochemical estimations may also be added. The measurement of these parameters has been described by Eliason (1971) and his paper on this can be referred to for further details. The normal sperm count varies between 60 and 100 million/ml, the former figure being considered the lower limit of normality. However, the chances of conception do not apparently decrease significantly until the concentration falls below 20 million/ml (McLeod, 1971). At least three samples of sperm should be examined before a final evaluation is made. The diagnosis of azoospermia (the absence of spermatozoa) should not be made until the examination of three ejaculates has been completed. The

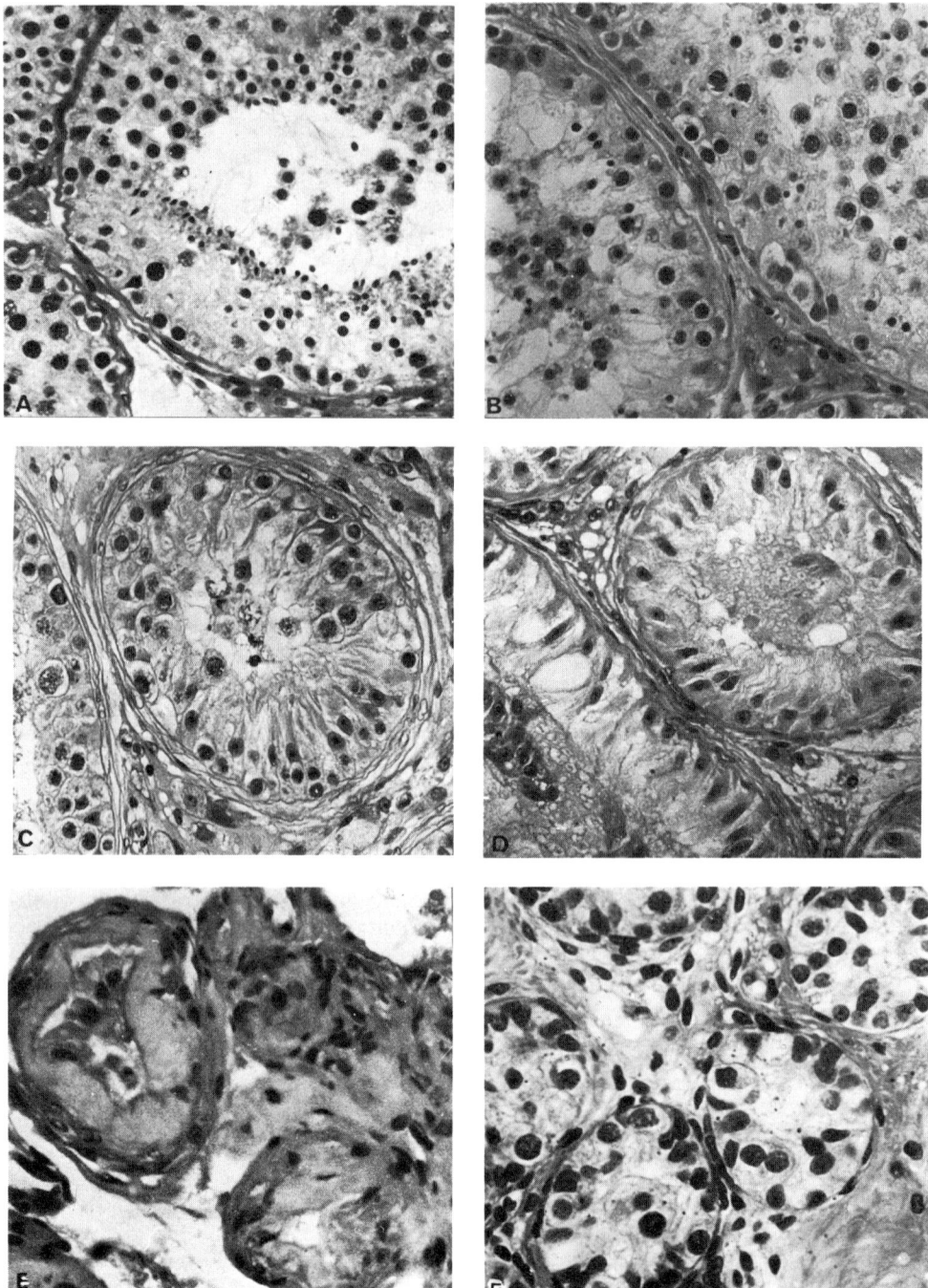

Fig. 34.8   The histological appearance of testicular biopsies is shown.

(A) Mild hypospermatogenesis.
(B) Severe hypospermatogenesis.
(C) Germinal cell arrest.
(D) Sertoli cell only syndrome.
(E) Seminiferous tubule hyalinization.
(F) Immature testis (hypogonadotrophic hypogonadism).

Courtesy of Dr D. M. de Kretser. Reproduced from *Clinics in Obstetrics & Gynaecology*, Vol. 1, No. 2, 1974. Edited by I. D. Cooke, London. W. B. Saunders Co. Ltd.

azoospermia may be due to an obstructive lesion in the ductus deferens or epididymis or to defective spermatogenesis. The presence of immature cells, such as primary spermatocytes and early spermatids should be assessed. If associated with azoospermia this may indicate patency of the duct system. Infection may also be assessed by a Gram's stain. Biochemical assessments such as estimation of fructose and acid phosphatase indicate seminal vesicle and prostate gland function may also be performed.

Testicular biopsy

Histological examination of testicular tissue removed by biopsy is a valuable method of assessment. It is only indicated in patients with a sperm count less than 15 million/ml. Changes in the epithelium with greater counts than this are difficult to assess. The histological appearances of testicular biopsies are shown in figure 34.8. Various types of testicular biopsy are illustrated.

Hormonal analysis

The measurement of levels of FSH and LH have not been particularly helpful in male infertility work but recently De Kretser (1974) has suggested that if a patient with azoospermia has an elevated serum FSH level his testicular biopsy will fall into one of three categories, viz. germinal cell arrest, Sertoli's cell only syndrome or seminiferous tubule hyalinization, all of which are associated with permanent sterility.

Low levels of testosterone and serum LH levels may be found in 30 per cent of males with testicular disorders. It is possible in the future that stimulatory tests for the evaluation of the pituitary-testicular axis may be helpful but further work is required on this aspect. The use of clomiphene and gonadotrophins in the treatment of male infertility has not so far proved as valuable as had been hoped.

Chromosomal studies

About 21 per cent of azoospermic patients have detectable cytogenetic abnormalities. It is important that Karyotypic analysis in males with infertility should be performed. The main abnormalities are related to sex chromosomes and again further work on this subject is required.

Treatment of male infertility

The treatment of male infertility is difficult and the results in general are disappointing both when the pathway of transmission of the seminal fluid is defective and when spermatogenesis is faulty.

Infections of the genital tract should be treated, as prostatic infection can cause decrease in sperm viability. Treatment of a proven infection may result in an increase in the sperm count.

Bilateral occlusion of the epididymis or ductus deferens may be helped in a small percentage of cases by vaso-epididymal anastomosis. The success rate of this procedure is not high due to changes in the epithelium which result from the cause of the obstruction, usually infection. Varicocele in men with subnormal seminal evaluation is an indication for treatment of the varicocele. Improvement in the seminal fluid in about 50 per cent of men so treated can be expected.

Factors associated with the patient's environment such as high temperatures, drugs or irradiation should also be eliminated.

Gonadotrophin therapy in general has not been successful unless there is some abnormality of the pituitary or in post-pituitary tumour ablation states where there are defects of FSH and LH secretion. Treatment of these men for up to 12 months with FSH and LH has resulted in increased sperm production. Some patients with oligospermia do respond to treatment with FSH and LH although levels of endogenous gonadotrophic hormones seem adequate and a therapeutic trial of at least 100 days is necessary to test this in the individual case. This is still a treatment that should be reserved for evaluation in specially equipped centres as the treatment is tedious, expensive and so far has not been associated with good results. Clomiphene has also been unsatisfactory in the treatment of infertile men. Further evaluation of the use of this compound and like compounds is awaited.

Regimes using testosterone have been in vogue for many years. Testosterone propionate in a dose of 25mg daily will suppress spermatogenesis but some investigators have found that improved spermatogenesis occurred 12 months later. However, the accuracy of these claims is in dispute.

Various other hormonal measures have been advocated and small doses of thyroid, for example, have been stated to have a beneficial effect. Properly controlled trials of these have not been performed.

Hirsutism

Hair follicles are distributed in approximately equal amount over the whole body surface except for the scalp where the number is increased. Sexual hair is found on the scalp, eyebrows and also on the forearms and legs. Sexual hair which appears at puberty is found on the pubis and in the axilla in equal amounts in both sexes. Hair appearing on the face and body is also present in both sexes but there are marked differences in amount between the two. Facial and body hair on a woman are regarded as unsightly. Significant hair growth in women is difficult to define and what may be unbearable to one woman would be unnoticed in another. Practically, therefore, any complaint from a woman of 'too much hair' should be considered significant. There are also variations in hair growth according to race.

Attempts have been made to relate various parameters of hirsutism to the production and levels of androgens and to consider the production of the ovary and the adrenal in this context, but expensive endocrine screening except in a few cases is unlikely to be clinically helpful. It is usual to think that hair present at any time is the result of the action of a biologically active androgenic compound on an end organ and the sensitivity of the particular end organ. Androgens are produced in women in the ovary and the adrenal. The adrenal produces most of the circulating androgens but ovarian production contains a higher proportion of the more active compounds. The liver and skin can also produce active androgens from precursors. Skin has recently been shown to be very active endocrinologically and to be capable of extracting precursors from the circulation to form androgens which will produce a biological effect at the site of formation.

Aetiology
Most women, complaining of excessive hair growth, who are seen by the gynaecologist, do not have organic disease of the ovary or adrenal. Ovarian causes of hirsutism are—masculinizing ovarian tumours, such as the arrhenoblastoma and hilar cell tumour which are believed to arise from remnants of the fetal gonad and may produce testosterone. The Stein–Leventhal or polycystic ovarian syndrome is another ovarian cause of hirsutism. Adrenal causes such as Cushing's syndrome

due to tumours or bilateral hyperplasia of the adrenal cortex may be associated with the overproduction of androgens. Tumours of the adrenal cortex with overproduction of androgen, the so-called adrenogenital syndrome, are also liable to produce hirsutism. Most cases of congenital adrenal hyperplasia present in childhood, but milder cases may not present until puberty when the stimulus of the menarche makes them manifest. Cushing's syndrome due to a basophil adenoma of the pituitary is also recognized. Iatrogenic causes may follow the use of androgen or anabolic steroid therapy given for a variety of therapeutic purposes.

Most patients with hirsutism suffer from a primary disorder. It is not possible to submit them all to a complete battery of tests to exclude all secondary causes and clinical examination and history is of great importance. Age of onset is significant as primary types of hirsutism usually begin at puberty and develop gradually thereafter. Most often there is an associated history of amenorrhoea, oligomenorrhoea or menstrual irregularity and frequently the patient is over weight. These patients are usually well feminized and there is no evidence of virilism. Virilization, which means masculinization of an individual by excessive hair growth, clitoral enlargement, deepening of the voice, failure of breast development and amenorrhoea or oligomenorrhoea, strongly points to a secondary cause of the hirsutism. If palpable tumours of the adrenal or ovary are present or gross signs of Cushing's syndrome apparent then the diagnosis becomes fairly obvious. As far as primary hirsutism is concerned the aetiology is very uncertain but it is usually advisable to examine these patients carefully under an anaesthetic and perform laparoscopy with ovarian inspection and biopsy. In this way, masculinizing ovarian tumours, hilar cell hyperplasia and Stein–Leventhal syndrome will be diagnosed. Hyperplasia of the adrenal gland will record high levels of plasma cortisol and ultrasonic studies may detect the enlarged adrenal gland. If organic disease is suggested by the sudden appearance of symptoms or by associated virilism then proper work up is necessary. Hormonal evaluation measuring 17 ketosteroids, urinary dehydroepiandrosterone excretion, pregnanetriol levels and adrenal suppression may help to localize the disease to the ovary or adrenal.

Hirsutism may also occur in pregnancy. Some of these patients have luteomas of pregnancy and a few are due to ovarian tumours. Some have no obvious cause and may be due to individual changes in steroid metabolism. If the hirsuitism occurs late in gestation it is wise to postpone the investigations until after delivery but if they occur early then further examination is necessary to eliminate the possibility of ovarian or adrenal tumours. Virilization of a female fetus is unlikely to occur if the development of the condition occurs after 16 weeks of pregnancy when organogenesis is complete.

Treatment of hirsutism

If the cause of the hirsutism is organic then this should be treated directly. For patients with hirsutism without virilization hormonal therapy is best. The oral contraceptives are useful and will decrease the amount of hair in these patients. Oestrogens and progestogens have been used alone it being possible that the synthetic progestogens displace active androgens at the skin binding site where they exert no effect themselves. It is also possible, however, that in a few women the synthetic progestogen may be metabolized to an active androgen. It is therefore difficult sometimes to prognosticate what will happen with treatment. Cyproterone acetate, a compound which competes with active androgens for their target organ binding sites, has also been used and although initial results of this therapy have been good, more studies are required. Patients who have the polycystic ovarian syndrome should be treated by wedge resection or clomiphene therapy as already discussed.

Treatment of the symptoms is very important. The longer the hirsutism exists the more refractory it is to treatment. Shaving or removing the hair with depilatories may be helpful but may result in unsightly effects. Chemical depilatories are often irritating and electrolysis, although expensive, is often helpful.

Reassurance and support are important since further stress will stimulate the adrenal with resultant increase of androgen production.

The treatment of hirsutism is difficult because the aetiology is obscure but in the future better understanding of the basic nature of the abnormalities in metabolism may lead to more satisfactory modes of treatment.

Dysmenorrhoea

Dysmenorrhoea means painful menstruation. Most women have some discomfort or upset prior to or during menstruation. When this pain or discomfort at the time of menstruation is of such severity as to require some form of treatment this is known as dysmenorrhoea.

Premenstrual tension. In this condition the main complaints are a feeling of fullness in the lower abdomen and pelvis, painful and tingling breasts which may feel tight, excessive gain in weight, intestinal distension and constipation, migrainous headaches and emotional instability. These discomforts although troublesome do not as a rule interfere with normal everyday activities. The aetiology of this is obscure but it is likely that emotional factors acting from the higher centres in the brain on the hypothalamus and through that on the pituitary and ovary are responsible. It seems likely that some abnormal tissue sensitivity to progesterone or androgen may also be a factor. Fluid retention occurs at this time, the fluid being retained within the tissue cells and also in the extra-cellular compartment of the body. This may be an additional cause of the symptoms. Management of the premenstrual tension syndrome requires sympathy in listening to the patient's story and a simple explanation of fluid retention being the cause of her many symptoms may give her some insight into her complaint. Diuretics such as thiazide derivatives or frusemide given on alternate days for the last week of the cycle may be helpful and mild sedatives or tranquillizers may be required. Headaches may be treated by analgesics or if severely migrainous, ergotamine tartrate may be necessary. A gestagen preparation such as Norethisterone 10mg daily may be given for 7 days before the period.

PRIMARY DYSMENORRHOEA

Primary dysmenorrhoea is indicated by painful menstruation arising at, or shortly after the menarche. This is sometimes known as spasmodic dysmenorrhoea and is maximal between the ages of 15 and 25 usually decreasing after that time and particularly likely to disappear after marriage, especially after childbirth, although in a few cases it may become more severe and can continue throughout menstrual life. Primary dysmenorrhoea is more a symptom complex than a disease and has important economic disadvantages involving loss of working hours by a great many women. There is a wide variation in the type of pain experienced and in the relationship of pain to the menstrual flow. The most characteristic pain is intermittent, spasmodic and cramp-like, situated in the lower abdomen. Pain usually starts a few hours before menstrual bleeding begins and ceases within twenty-four hours of menstruation, usually lasting not more than twelve hours in total duration. The pain is usually most marked in the middle of the lower abdomen but may radiate to the iliac fossa and extend down the thighs. It may also be accompanied by nausea and vomiting and even collapse if the pain is severe. The causation and mechanism of the production of pain in primary dysmenorrhoea is still unknown. Spasmodic contractions of the uterus are probably the immediate cause of the pain induced either by disturbance in the uterus itself or by some extrinsic factor.

Causative factors in primary dysmenorrhoea. A number of theories have been advanced to explain the aetiology of primary dysmenorrhoea. It is probably true that many factors are involved but the exact pathophysiology is not understood.

Obstructive or mechanical theory. One of the earliest theories for the explanation of dysmenorrhoea was that it was due to obstructive lesions of the cervix, narrowing of the internal os due to spasm, or a thick endometrium, acute anteflexion of the uterus, cochleate uterus, or congenital retroflexion or retroversion of the uterus. This theory does not now find much favour as a possible cause of dysmenorrhoea though pedunculated submucous fibroids or endometrial polyps can cause dysmenorrhoea because the uterine muscle contracts to expel these lesions. A similar mechanism is probably responsible for the dysmenorrhoea which is sometimes associated with the intra-uterine contraceptive device.

Psychological factors. It has already been stated that a moderate amount of pelvic heaviness and occasional cramp with menstruation is almost normal but in certain individuals this will be expressed as more severe discomfort and in a highly strung supersensitive patient as severe and, perhaps, incapacitating pain. Good results are obtained by reassurance and this suggests that psychological factors may play an important role in some patients. It is felt by some that these factors are so important as to be almost invariably the cause

of primary dysmenorrhoea but this seems an exaggeration. The response to menstruation is probably related to the patient's knowledge or lack of knowledge of the significance and normality of the menstrual function. Lack of explanation about menstruation and sex and the appearances of the first menstrual period without any prior warning or explanation may cause alarm and distress. Mothers who have failed to inform their daughters about menstruation, however, show great concern and anxiety when it does begin. They may view it as an illness more than a normal process and treat their daughters accordingly. When one hears of girls referring to menstruation as the 'monthly illness' or 'the curse', one gets some inkling of the kind of upbringing they have had with respect to menstrual function. The physician faced with this must take the trouble to review the history of the disorder and with tactful questioning can soon learn the problems of the psychogenic factor in the individual case.

Changes in environment or occupation may have an untoward psychological effect. This is seen in girls who experience dysmenorrhoea for the first time when they leave their home for a different environment. A nervous, emotional, apprehensive and introspective type of woman is always more likely to have primary dysmenorrhoea than her more stable level-headed sister.

Constitutional factors. Dysmenorrhoea is more common among those in sedentary occupations and is not common in those whose occupation involves hard, physical work. Patients who suffer from anaemia or a debilitating disease often suffer a lowering of the threshold of pain, primarily because of the physical factors, but often with a mixture of nervous and psychogenic factors as well. These women who normally have little or no menstrual discomfort experience severe pain when their general state of health and vitality is impaired. The persistence of this hypersensitivity to pain after the menopause suggests that the lowered threshold to pain is a constitutional factor. It is part of the treatment in every case of dysmenorrhoea to outline a way of living calculated to raise the patient's general health in every way and some times these measures are sufficient to mitigate the pain.

Endocrine factors. In this category various endocrine aberrations are suggested as possible aetiological factors. The crampy character of the pain in primary dysmenorrhoea has been accepted by some as due to exaggerated uterine contractions. The acme of pain in dysmenorrhoea has been shown to coincide with the peak of the contraction and during this phase the pulsation in the uterine artery disappears. This suggests that the menstrual pain might be due to ischaemia of the uterine muscle caused by temporary obliteration of the blood supply to the myometrium but it seems more likely that, in view of later work on the effect of the relative amounts of oestrogen and progesterone on the uterine muscle, some imbalance of these hormones at the cellular level in the uterine muscle in certain patients may be responsible. It has been found that pain was most apparent shortly after the height of contractions and disappeared after expulsion of a bolus of blood. Elevated myometrial tone between contractions has also been found and considered to be an important factor in both primary and secondary dysmenorrhoea. One cause of the pain may be uterine ischaemia associated with uterine hypercontractility and a sustained elevation of uterine tone. Uterine irritability caused by a bolus of blood backed up in the uterus behind a small cervical exit may be a second cause. Changes in hormone environment such as the giving of gestagens may relax the myometrium and decrease the resting tone in the secretory and early menstrual phases. They may also create a smoother shedding of the endometrium so that a larger volume of blood is not presented to the cervical canal at any one time. The possible imbalance of hormones at the cellular level is not yet possible to characterize. There are, however, many different factors which are not easily reconciled. For example, in some women with dysfunctional bleeding which may be associated with an excess of oestrogen and no evidence of corpus luteum formation menstrual pain may be absent. In contra-distinction, menstrual pain does not usually start until some time after the menarche when regular ovulatory cycles should have become established. It is frequently present when menstruation begins and when anovulation is common.

It is possible that prostaglandins may be involved in dysmenorrhoea. Under the influence of progesterone the secretory endometrium synthesizes prostaglandin $F_{2\alpha}$, a substance which causes contraction of smooth muscle. This substance is released when the endometrium disintegrates at menstruation and it acts on the uterine muscle and vasculature causing contraction and pain. If the amount of prostaglandins was excessive then exaggeration of pain could be possible. Abnormalities of menstrual discharge, innervation of the uterus and allergic manifestations have all been suggested as possible aetiological factors in dysmenorrhoea. The fact that so many aetiological factors are suggested only indicates that the true aetiology is unknown at the present time.

THE MANAGEMENT OF PRIMARY DYSMENORRHOEA

It is very important that full information should be obtained about the patient. The age of onset, the incidence, location, duration and apparent severity of the pain, the nature of the flow and any related discomfort such as headache and vomiting which precedes or accompanies the severe pain have to be ascertained. It is also important to inquire into the patient's general health, diet, environment, working hours, type of work, bowel action and the amount of exercise taken. The patient's personality should be assessed and the family situation, especially relationships, ascertained. It is usually undesirable to make a pelvic examination at this juncture as this is usually painful and contributes little to the helpful management.

Prophylaxis. It is important first of all to allay anxiety and ensure that the patient knows something about menstruation. She should be encouraged to regard menstruation as a normal function which should interfere very little with work, study or even physical activity such as games. Regular meals and daily movement of the bowels may help to relieve the pain.

These measures are usually combined with the use of simple analgesics in the first instance. These may give the patient enough relief to enable her to continue with her work during the time of the pain. The usual preparations, such as paracetamol, can be used and particularly helpful is a compound preparation such as Edrisal (amphetamine and phenacetin) which relieves the pain without making the patient too lethargic. Various mixtures including paracetamol and codeine or some of their derivatives are also used. When the pain is severe, rest in bed for a few hours and the application of heat to the lower abdomen may be necessary. Antispasmodic drugs are sometimes efficacious in relieving menstrual pain. Such preparations such as Bellergal (ergotamine and phenobarbitone) may be helpful while promazine in the form of Sparine may help to potentiate analgesics. Alcohol in the form of whisky, brandy or gin is frequently used but this has to be carefully watched because of the risk of habit formation. Stronger analgesics and hypnotics such as pethidine and opiates are very effective in controlling menstrual pain but should not be used because of the great risk of addiction.

In some women anti-allergic drugs such as promethazine (Phenergan) or trimeprazine (Vallergan) may be used. If these drugs prove to be effective the search for and desensitization to the offending allergic factors may give permanent relief.

Endocrine therapy. There are several endocrine approaches to the treatment of dysmenorrhoea. The most usual method nowadays is the suppression of ovulation which in many cases is followed by painless menstruation. The modern way to suppress ovulation is by prescribing one of the contraceptive pills of which there is a large variety and this is the optimum way of doing this at present. In former days oestrogen alone has been prescribed for suppression of ovulation but this tends to result in nausea and prolonged bleeding and these effects make it difficult for many patients to use. It is now not used for the treatment of dysmenorrhoea. Various attempts have been made to restore the suspected steroid imbalance. This seems at first sight to be a rational thought, but, difficulty in knowing what the imbalance is makes it impossible to be rational about this therapy. Various amounts of oestrogen and progestational substances such as 17 hydroxyprogesterone have been prescribed at various times in the menstrual cycle in the hope that a correct balance of steroids might be achieved. This may be helpful in some patients but the difficulty of knowing what in fact the imbalance is makes it almost impossible to use this type of treatment successfully. The use of androgens has been popular in dysmenorrhoea. They probably act by depressing pituitary activity thus inhibiting ovulation but this can now be done more effectively with the oral contraceptive preparations; provided a dose of no more than 200mg/cycle is given the virilizing effects are rarely induced.

Surgical treatment may be successful in making it possible at least for the patient to obtain enough relief to continue her daily tasks. If the dysmenorrhoea is severe the patient is admitted for examination under anaesthesia and dilatation of the cervix and curettage of the uterine cavity in case a polyp or other abnormality might be present. Dilatation of the cervix helps dysmenorrhoea in about 20 per cent of cases. The rationale of this procedure is uncertain but its therapeutic effect has been alleged to be due to disruption of the cervical sympathetic nerve fibres at the internal os or a change in polarity of the uterus. This treatment is not so commonly used nowadays because it is necessary to dilate the cervix to more than a number 10 size dilator in order to effect a cure and damage may be done to the internal os. Permanent widening of the canal may result and the os may become incompetent with resultant abortion or premature labour in subsequent pregnancy. Sometimes correction of a retroversion of the uterus and insertion of a Hodge pessary may be of value. If this correction is successful in helping the pain the pessary should be left in the vagina for about three months and then removed. If the retro-displacement returns and the pain occurs again then, some permanent method of fixing the uterus in anteversion should be considered.

Another procedure is to inject local anaesthetic into the paracervical tissue where Frankenhauser's plexus lies and this treatment has been successful in a number of cases. This can be done just prior to menstruation. One is tempted to think, however, since the action of the analgesic does not continue for more than four hours and yet menstruation, which occurs many hours later, may be helped, that the treatment may produce a psychological rather than a physical effect.

Presacral neurectomy was introduced by Cotte in 1923 for severe intractable cases of primary dysmenorrhoea. In this treatment the abdomen is opened by a mid-line paramedian incision and division of the superior hypogastric plexus or so-called presacral nerve, which is the pathway of sensation from the genital organs to the higher centres of pain perception and may also contain parasympathetic fibres which convey motor impulses to the uterus, is divided. The results of this treatment are very varied, some claiming almost 100 per cent success while others find failure frequently occurs. The operation is usually performed as a last resort.

Hysterectomy, which is very effective, is another drastic treatment and should only be considered in very special cases when all other methods of treatment have proved unsuccessful. It should be reserved particularly for those patients where the pain is so severe as to undermine the patient's physical and mental health.

Other procedures using X-rays are not now indicated as damage may be done to the ovarian cells by the treatment.

SECONDARY DYSMENORRHOEA

Secondary dysmenorrhoea is pain at the time of menstruation, occurring after years of painless menstruation and is usually associated with some kind of pelvic pathology. Secondary dysmenorrhoea is unusual before the age of 25 years and not common before the age of 30.

Uterine conditions

Perhaps the most common uterine condition causing dysmenorrhoea is adenomyosis where there is an increased tension in the uterine muscles due to the accumulation of blood in the cystic spaces. Interstitial or submucous fibromyomata and fibroid polypi interfere with normal rhythmic contractions of the uterus and may also cause these contractions to become spasmodic in attempts to expel a tumour. Fixed retroversion may cause considerable dysmenorrhoea and erosion of the cervix, especially if associated with a low grade pelvic infection or partial stenosis of the cervix following cautery or cone biopsy, may be a cause of secondary dysmenorrhoea.

Extra-uterine conditions

Dysmenorrhoea is one of the most characteristic symptoms of pelvic endometriosis. The pain is due to tension in the cystic spaces in the ovary and other sites coincident with the disintegration of uterine endometrium. Pelvic inflammatory disease, whether tubal, ovarian or peritoneal, causes increased pelvic congestion. The pain from these conditions usually starts two or more days before menstruation and increases in severity later on in menstruation when it reaches its peak, then taking some days to subside. This type of pain is in marked contra-distinction to the pain of primary dysmenorrhoea which usually begins just before or at the start of menstruation and begins to wear off fairly soon after the flow starts.

Extragenital factors

A chronically inflamed pelvic appendix may cause considerable right-sided premenstrual pain.

The ureter in its pelvic portion becomes congested at menstruation and narrowing due to spasmodic stricture is accentuated and may give rise to colicky abdominal pain simulating spasmodic dysmenorrhoea. A ureteric lesion should be suspected and a detailed investigation of the urinary tract performed, especially if urinary disturbances are evident or more marked at menstruation.

Treatment of secondary dysmenorrhoea

Since secondary dysmenorrhoea is usually a symptom of some organic lesion, the causal lesion should be treated. The management of the various conditions is discussed in the appropriate chapters.

Midmenstrual pain

The term 'mid-menstrual pain' or 'mittelschmerz' means lower abdominal pain experienced by some women during the period of the menstrual cycle corresponding exactly to the time of ovulation. The pain is usually intermittent in character and varies in intensity from a slight ache to severe cramp-like abdominal discomfort which may be present in either quadrant of the lower abdomen. The pain is almost certainly ovarian in origin and associated with ovulation. The discomfort is slight and transient in the majority of cases so that no treatment is indicated. However, if the pain is severe, analgesics may be required. The possibility, if the pain is very severe, of acute appendicitis or ruptured ectopic pregnancy should be borne in mind.

REFERENCES

Brown, J. B., Evans, J. H., Adey, F. D., Taft, H. P. & Townsend, S. L. (1972) Clinical induction of ovulation using gonadotrophins. *Proc. 4th Int. Congr. End.* Edited by R. O. Scow, F. J. G. Ebling & I. Henderson.

Butler, J. K. (1972) Clinical results with human gonadotrophin in anovulation using two alternative dosage schemes. *Postgrad. med. J.* **48**, 23–32.

Davies, M. E. (1967) Management of infertility. *J. Amer. med. Ass.*, **201**, 1030–1037.

De Kretser, D. M. (1974) The management of infertility. *Clin. Obstet. Gynaec.*, 409–427, August 1974. Edited by I. D. Cooke. London: Saunders.

Dewhurst, C. J. & Gordon, R. R. (1969) *The Intersexual Disorders.* London: Bailliere, Tindall & Cassell.

Dodson, K. S., Macnaughton, M. C. & Coutts, J. R. T. (1975) Infertility in women with apparently ovulatory cycles. I. Comparison of their plasma sex steroid and gonadotrophin profiles. *Brit. J. Obstet. Gynaec.*, **82**, 615–624.

Eliason, R. (1971) Standards for investigation of human semen. *Andrologie*, **3**, 49–64.

Ellis, R. W. B. (1945) Growth & Health of Belgian Children: during and after German Occupation (1940–1944). *Arch. Dis. Child.*, **20**, 97.

Jeffcoate, T. N. A. (1967) *Principles of Gynaecology.* 3rd edn. London: Butterworths.

McLeod, J. (1971) Human male infertility. *Obstet. Gynec. Surv.*, **76**, 335–351.

Pacheco-Romero, J. C., Gleich, G. J., Loegering, D. A. & Johnson, C. E. (1973) Sperm-Agglutinating Activity and Female Infertility: Study of Serum and Genital Tract Secretions. *J. Amer. med. Ass.*, **224**, 849–852.

Roberts, D. F., Rozner, L. M. & Swann, A. V. (1971) Age at menarche, physique and environment in industrial N. E. England. *Acta. Paediat. Scand.*, **60**, 158.

Rybo, G. (1966) Clinical and Experimental Studies in Menstrual Blood Loss. *Acta. Obstet. Gynec. Scand.*, **XLV**, Suppl. 7.

Steptoe, P. C. (1967) *Laparoscopy in Gynaecology.* Edinburgh: Livingstone.

Steptoe, P. C. & Edwards, R. G. (1970) Laparoscopic recovery of pre-ovulatory human oocytes after priming of ovaries with gonadotrophins. *Lancet*, **i**, 683–689.

Townsend, S. L., Brown, J. B., Johnstone, J. W., Adey, F. D., Evans, J. H. & Taft, H. P. (1966) Induction of ovulation. *J. Obstet. Gynaec. Brit. Cwlth.*, **73**, 529–543.

FURTHER READING

Ferriman, D. (1969) *Anovulatory Infertility.* London: Heinemann.

Karp, L. & Herrman, W. L. (1973) Diagnosis and treatment of hirsutism in women. *Obstet. Gynaec.*, **41**, 283, 294.

Sherman, J. (1963) Synopsis of use of frozen human semen since 1964. State of the art of Human Semen banking. *Fertil. Steril.*, **24**, 397–412.

Steinberger, C. E. & Smith, K. D. (1973) Artificial Insemination with Fresher Frozen Semen: Comparative Study. *J. Amer. med. Ass.*, **223**, 778–783.

35. The Menopause and Post-Menopause

The menopause denotes the final cessation of menstruation and therefore the end of reproductive life. The term 'climacteric' is also used in this context and more properly refers to the whole complex of changes which occur at the end of the reproductive period of a woman's life. These two terms are often used synonymously. Correctly used, the term menopause has much the same relationship to the climacteric as the menarche has to puberty.

The average age at which the menopause occurs in women in the United Kingdom is 50 years. Suggestions have been made that over the past 100 years in the United Kingdom, the median age of the menopause has increased by about four years. However, a recent British study did not confirm this suggestion (McKinley, Geffrey and Thomson, 1972). There are, however, wide individual variations.

Socio-demographic factors such as marital state, social class, parity and number of persons catered for in the home are also independent of menopausal status and symptoms (Thomson, Hart and Durno, 1973). Certain conditions such as pelvic infection, endometriosis and hereditary factors may influence menopausal age especially towards an earlier time. Other diseases such as myomata or carcinoma of the endometrium may be associated with a late menopause.

The climacteric, like pre-puberty, is a series of inter-related changes and it is doubtful if it is due to any one factor. The precipitating events of the climacteric appear to be primary ovarian failure, but why the ovaries should fail at this stage is not clear. It has been suggested that this is simply because of the exhaustion of available primordial follicles. This hypothesis does not explain why exhaustion should occur invariably and at roughly the same time in the human female, while many other mammals retain reproductive capacity until they die.

ANATOMICAL CHANGES OCCURRING AT THE MENOPAUSE

The size of the ovaries begins to decrease after 30 years of age and the quality of the ovum declines during the premenopausal stage. As a result developmental abnormalities and spontaneous abortion become more frequent. At the menopause no corpora lutea are found and the size of the ovary decreases further so that in the post-menopausal phase it is about half the size of the ovary found during reproductive life. Primary follicles are present until the menopause and some may be found in the deep layers of the ovary even after the menopause. The myometrium atrophies in the post-menopausal era and hyaline degeneration and arterio-sclerosis are found in the myometrium at this time. The endometrium is frequently hyperactive prior to the menopause and cystic glandular hyperplasia is not uncommon due to anovulatory cycles. In the post-menopause endometrial atrophy occurs. The vaginal skin becomes thin and smooth and the rugae, which are prominent during reproductive life, disappear. The pH of the vagina changes to neutral or alkaline thus making it less resistant to infection. The labia decrease in size and leukoplakia is more common in the post-menopausal woman.

Cessation of menstruation

The manner of onset of the menopause is important and abnormalities of this may have serious portent. Most frequently the periods become scanty and occur at longer and longer intervals before finally stopping altogether. Sometimes the periods stop abruptly and no further menstruation occurs. These types of cessation can be considered normal and any deviation from these patterns is abnormal, however commonly it may occur. In many women the menopause is signalled by irregular bleeding—the so-called menopausal menorrhagia. Although common, this must be considered abnormal since it is impossible to differentiate the bleeding from that caused by more serious pelvic pathology such as carcinoma of the endometrium, and curettage is necessary in these women to eliminate this possibility. This bleeding is in fact one manifestation of the endocrine changes which occur at the menopause. As the menopause approaches there is an increasing incidence of anovular cycles. When this occurs the bleeding takes place from a non-secretory endometrium. This bleeding, from a proliferative endometrium, due to oestrogen withdrawal, is heavier and more prolonged than that which occurs following involution of a corpus luteum during a normal ovulatory cycle.

ENDOCRINE CHANGES

The basic cause of the menopause is the decline in steroid production by the ovary. As a result of the lowered blood oestrogen, the feed-back mechanism to the pituitary is brought into operation and more and more gonadotrophin, especially luteinizing hormone, is produced. These two changes—low oestrogen and high gonadotrophin—bring about the series of circulatory and metabolic events which constitute the climacteric. It is difficult to demonstrate a direct connection between raised gonadotrophin production and any phenomenon of the climacteric and the lowered oestrogen production seems the likely basis for most of the changes.

As the menopause approaches, very high levels of luteinizing hormone are found in the urine. Follicle stimulating hormone excretion is also raised but less than LH. In general, oestrogen excretion is low but occasionally quite high levels are found and in some women oestrogens is cyclic for 3 to 12 months. After (Loraine and Bell, 1971).

During the menopause the excretion of oestrogens is cyclic for 3 to 12 months. After this the oestrogen decreases gradually to about $\frac{1}{6}$th of its excretion in a young fertile woman. As age increases the excretion of oestrone and oestradiol is more decreased than that of oestriol (Pincus, 1956). After the menopause the secretion of oestrogen decreases with age; the decrease being about 10 per cent in every five years. The amount of oestrogen secreted by the ovaries in the post-menopausal

era is insignificant and extirpation of the ovaries after the menopause has no effect upon the excretion of the oestrogens. Vaginal cytology can be useful in the post-menopausal woman to give some indication of her oestrogen status.

It had been thought that the main source of post-menopausal oestrogen secretion was the adrenal. This was based on the fact that, after oophorectomy in the post-menopausal women, there was no change in urinary oestrogen excretion and that dexamethazone reduced the urinary oestrogen excretion by suppressing adrenal function in post-menopausal women (Procope and Adlercreutz, 1969).

However, more recent work on androgen and oestrogen secretion (McDonald, 1971) throws some doubt on this and suggests that, in the post-menopausal woman following cessation of follicular maturation, oestrogen production is accounted for primarily via the conversion of circulating androstenedione to oestrone and suggests that there is no direct secretion of oestrone or oestradiol by the ovary or the adrenal in post-menopausal women. The site of this conversion is not known but it appears that aromatization of androgen to oestrogen may occur in many sites at the same time. Sites such as the liver and the endometrium may each contribute to the conversion but other sites may also be involved.

As has already been noted, the cycles tend to become anovular as the menopause approaches and there is some evidence that when all bleeding has ceased, a slow rise and fall in oestrogen production continues for some time.

One of the consequences of the decline in oestrogen production at the menopause is that the small quantities of androstenedione circulating are no longer opposed and slight virilization is common. This is usually shown by an increase in facial hair. This is usually slight in amount but may on occasion be severe.

CIRCULATORY CHANGES

These are mainly tachycardia, hypertension, ECG changes (ST depression) and hot flushes. In these changes oestrogen deficiency seems to be involved. The ST depression can be abolished by giving oestrogen. The most notable of these symptoms are hot flushes often accompanied by sweating. Although these seldom last more than a few minutes, they may occur with great frequency and sufficiently often at night to cause insomnia. The frequency and severity are very variable; they are almost absent in some women and severe in only a minority of women. In some patients a definite rhythm is noted corresponding to the time when a period would normally occur. As well as hot flushes the circulatory phenomena such as dizzy spells, palpitations and disturbances of cardiac rhythm or of blood pressure occur.

The mechanism of the circulatory changes at the menopause is not understood. There is good reason to suppose that the basic cause is oestrogen withdrawal. The circulatory disturbances can generally be controlled by the administration of oestrogen and the connection between oestrogen levels and vascular responses is an established one. On the other hand these symptoms may be related to the temporary rise in the output of gonadotrophin which takes place at this time. Although gonadotrophins given to induce ovulation in amenorrhoeic women do not cause hot flushes, neither do they occur in women with Turner's syndrome where there is an excess production of gonadotrophin. It seems unlikely that the circulatory phenomena are due to a direct effect of oestrogen on the vessel wall and the view that these effects are brought about by nerve centres sensitive to oestrogen levels has much to recommend it.

Coronary artery disease is rare in premenopausal women unless there is a family history or a predisposing cause such as diabetes mellitus. The sex difference between men and women in relation to coronary artery disease disappears slowly after the age of 55 years. Studies on the influence of the menopause on coronary atherosclerosis have not all agreed but there is an increased incidence in women after this time. It may be the result of the ageing process and lack of oestrogens and emotional stability may alter lipid and carbohydrate metabolism so that the rate of atherosclerotic changes is increased.

POST-MENOPAUSAL OSTEOPOROSIS

Osteoporosis is a condition where the bone mass is reduced in relation to the volume. This condition occurs in both sexes and is part of the ageing process. It does seem, however, that the menopause does have a specific influence upon bone loss. The development of premature osteoporosis following an artificial menopause suggests that ovarian function or non-function is related to the onset of post-menopausal osteoporosis. Dietary deficiency of calcium and physical inactivity do seem to play a minor role in the development of post-menopausal osteoporosis but hormonal factors are probably most important. Oestrogen seems to depress bone resorption without influencing bone formation and causes a reduction in the urinary excretion of calcium and hydroxyproline and reduces the level of serum calcium (Harris and Heaney, 1969). If oestrogen treatment is given, a new equilibrium is reached in which bone resorption remains suppressed but the accretion is reduced to correspond to the resorption. It is evident therefore that a lack of oestrogen is at least one factor involved in osteoporosis but the mechanism is so far poorly understood.

Symptoms of the menopause

Most women nowadays live 20–30 years past the menopause—a unique state of affairs in mammals. Decreased oestrogen production is the basic endocrine event at the menopause although gonadotrophin production is also increased. However, the symptoms which occur at the time of the climacteric and the metabolic changes which take place at this time do not seem to be simply a consequence of these hormonal changes. In the post-menopause the production of oestrogenic steroids from sources other than the ovary is very significant.

The symptoms of the menopause may broadly be divided into two groups: psychological and physical and the two groups are inter-related.

Psychological
Many women fear the menopause. They feel that it is the beginning of old age with loss of youth and beauty; that they are losing something of their femininity with cessation of menses and that the sexual partner may leave. Childbirth and care of her children have been the main part of the woman's life for the previous 25 years. She is no longer capable of bearing children, her existing family is grown up and no longer depend on her and she is liable to be selfconscious about the changes in

her appearance. Her husband is not undergoing the same sort of changes. He is probably at the peak of involvement with his career and hobbies. Under these circumstances depression is common and the hormonal changes produce an emotional liability which often results in weeping without apparent reason.

These psychological problems may manifest themselves in a variety of vague physical complaints such as tiredness, headaches, abdominal distension, insomnia, backache and lack of appetite. In the supportive psychotherapy of the menopause the doctor's understanding, tactful reassuring and sympathetic attitude is of great help to the patient. Libido may not necessarily decline with cessation of the menses and may indeed increase, possibly due to the relative predominance of androgen. Sexual intercourse usually continues to take place after the menopause and may persist for a surprisingly long time. It is therefore important to inquire about this before undertaking vaginal surgery in elderly women.

The emancipation of women in Western society has led to a reduction of the emphasis by women on their reproductive function. Women are more and more coming to realize that the menopause does not signify the end of their life's purpose but a change of roles, a reduction in domestic commitments which enables them to play a larger part in the affairs of the outside world.

Physical symptoms
Flushings are the most common presenting complaint as they affect a part of the woman which is seen by everyone she meets. The hot feeling and vasodilatation which occurs can include palpitation and cardiac arrhythmia. In a severe case flushings may occur as often as every 15 minutes day and night and treatment for this is definitely necessary.

Many women complain of symptoms of prolapse at or soon after the menopause. The symptoms may become worse at this time as withdrawal of the ovarian hormones causes slackening of the uterine supportive tissues. Perhaps the prolapse may have been present for years with symptoms but the patient may have been unwilling to ask for treatment because of her family commitments. Other contributing factors may be constipation and increasing weight which are common at the climacteric.

Dyspareunia in a patient in this age is nearly always due to an atrophic vaginitis perhaps with superadded infection but other causes should be excluded by manual and speculum examination. Many of the symptoms mentioned may seem minor to all but the woman who suffers from them. The patient requires support and treatment from her doctor and has to be handled with care and sympathy.

Therapy of the menopause

Not surprisingly, such a stressful situation has an impact on medical practice. The menorrhagia of the menopause may be severe enough to warrant a hysterectomy. Nowadays such bleeding can be controlled by the cyclical administration of synthetic progestational steroids and hysterectomy should less often be necessary. However, it is frequently done because the patient is anxious to be finished with her periods and not have to take any pills. The argument that by doing a hysterectomy one is removing potential sites of cancer such as the cervix, the endometrium and the ovaries (if pan hysterectomy is done) is a specious one. Logically it should lead to the removal of any organ whose function has been fulfilled or was not vital in the first place.

In many ways the treatment of a menopausal patient can be a searching test of the ability of a doctor. The more able a physician is and the more experienced he becomes, the more of his time does he spend listening to and talking to his patients. The capacity to make a woman understand the events of her menopause and give her reassurance and confidence is as important a measure of a doctor's skill as is his dexterity in removing her uterus.

A new view of the therapy of the menopause has come to the fore in recent years. If the basis of the menopause is a decline in oestrogen production, it is possible to make this good indefinitely by the administration of synthetic oestrogen. In the past the objection to such prolonged oestrogen treatment has been that it invariably led to irregular, sometimes severe, vaginal bleeding. By the addition of a synthetic progestational compound and by deliberately stopping the mixture for a week at three weekly intervals, it is possible to secure a regular succession of monthly bleeding indistinguishable from the normal cycle. Indeed this is the very regime to which millions of married women are exposed for the purpose of contraception. It is therefore possible to postpone the menopause almost indefinitely and in doing so to ameliorate or altogether avoid the ills which it brings in its train. This course of action has been embarked upon with notable enthusiasm, particularly in the United States. By arguing the case largely in the lay press its more ardent advocates have not recommended themselves to the conservative section of the medical profession but clearly this is a problem which requires thoughtful consideration and critical investigation of its long term social, physiological and psychological effects. It is now becoming evident that in this country a more active management of the menopause is indeed becoming common practice. Often contraceptive action as well as relief or prevention of menopausal symptoms may be needed. A sequential contraceptive might be a good compromise.

Therapeutic measures for the menopause have become established and are entirely acceptable. Oestrogen substitution therapy with synthetic compounds such as Stilboestrol 0·5mg or ethinyl oestradiol 0·05mg/day will effect great improvement in hot flushes or senile vaginitis. Such treatment should not be continued for more than three months at a time. Troublesome bleeding often results after withdrawal or even during treatment so that it is advisable to try first with a less potent compound. Oestriol in doses of 0·25mg twice or thrice daily has been used with great success. Investigations in Germany (Puck, 1957; Prill, 1970) recommend oestriol preparations for the treatment of menopausal symptoms. Wilson (1966) recommends treatment with conjugated oestrogens (Premarin) in slightly hypo-oestrogenic conditions as 1·25mg daily for 14 consecutive days starting on the first day of the menstrual period. If the menstrual period is irregular 1·25mg of conjugated oestrogen on days 5 to 25 of the cycle and 5mg of medroxy-progesterone acetate on days 15 to 24 of the cycle may be given. For the treatment of menopausal symptoms when menstruation has ceased for one year or more, 1·25mg of conjugated oestrogen daily for 42 consecutive days and 10mg medroxyprogesterone daily during the last 12 days of oestrogen treatment can be used. In the post-menopause where menstruation has been absent for many years and a vaginal smear shows atrophy, there are many different ways to handle the situation. Most of the women do not wish any medical treatment. If the patient is more than 60 years of age 0·0125mg of ethinyl oestradiol on 16 consecutive days and then a combination of this and 0·25mg megestrol acetate may suffice. Oral oestrogen treatment makes local treatment unnecessary but sometimes patients have benefited from the use of locally applied oestrogen in the form of pessary or cream. The investigations in Germany have brought to light the possibility that the cervix, vagina and vascular system may be particularly sensitive to oestriol while the more potent natural oestrogen, oestradiol, particularly stimulates the endometrium. There is a cogent argument in favour of prescribing oestriol in the menopause when one wishes to avoid endometrial effects. Many of the proprietary mixtures for the treatment of menopausal symptoms also include a barbiturate for the accompanying restlessness and irritability. Barbiturates should be given for specific symptoms such as insomnia and not as an ingredient of shotgun therapy. Testosterone in the form of testosterone propionate injections or tablets of methyl testosterone are sometimes used. They are often very effective in controlling menopausal symptoms. Androgens are protein anabolics, improve appetite and have a general tonic effect. They occasionally stimulate libido. They should, however, be used with discretion in view of their tendency to stimulate the growth of facial hair, already a natural propensity of the menopause. The total dose of testosterone should not exceed 200mg per month and all androgens are best kept in reserve for obstinate cases whose symptoms are not ameliorated by oestrogens or oestrogen-progestogen mixtures.

POST-MENOPAUSAL BLEEDING

The occurrence of vaginal bleeding, however slight, after menstruation has been in abeyance for a period of six months or more, must always be considered to be of serious clinical significance until it has been proved otherwise. Probably the commonest cause is oestrogen withdrawal bleeding associated with indiscriminate and long continued oestrogen therapy. It is important, therefore, to inquire in all cases as to whether or not the patient has been taking hormone preparations. Other benign causes are senile vaginitis, cervicitis and endometritis or a cervical or intra-uterine polypus. Not infrequently, the bleeding is associated with hyperplastic endometrium which may show the histological features of metropathia haemorrhagica. This may be due to the reactivation of some dormant ovarian follicles or to the presence in the ovary of an oestrogen producing tumour such as granulosa or theca cell tumour. Less common causes are urethral caruncle, vaginal ulceration associated with long standing uterine prolapse or a badly fitted or neglected pessary. Hypertension is a rare cause of bleeding.

Malignant disease of the reproductive tract, particularly carcinoma of the cervix and body of the uterus accounts for some 30 per cent of cases. Cervical cancer is not often found in nulliparae while body carcinoma is about equally common in parous and nulliparous women. Carcinoma of the body may occur before the menopause but its highest incidence is after the menopause. Other malignant conditions which give rise to post-menopausal bleeding are carcinoma of the vulva or vagina, sarcoma of the genital tract and malignant ovarian tumours.

Investigation and treatment
Immediate investigation is called for no matter how slight the bleeding. Detailed examination under anaesthesia and curettage of the uterus are necessary in every case. This is the only way that carcinoma of the corpus, which may co-exist with otherwise adequate causes such as senile vaginitis or cervical polypus, can be excluded. The treatment varies according to the cause found. Not infrequently, no cause can be found and only a little mucus is removed at curettage. An expectant attitude should be adopted in these cases. The recurrence or persistence of the bleeding necessitates further investigation and if bleeding recurs following a curettage then possibly hysterectomy is indicated. This may be the only way of detecting serious pelvic pathology at a stage when cure is possible.

REFERENCES

Harris, W. H. & Heaney, R. P. (1969) *New Engl. J. Med.*, **280**, 193.
Loraine, J. A. & Bell, E. J. (1971) *Hormone assays and their clinical application*. Edinburgh: Churchill Livingstone.
McDonald, P. C. (1971) In Control of Gonodal Steroid Secretion. Edited by Baird & Strong. *Pfizer med. Mono.*, **6**, p. 158. Edinburgh: University Press.
McKinley, S., Geffrey, M. & Thomson, B. (1972) *J. Biosoc. Sci.*, **4**, 161.
Pincus, G. (1956) *In hormones and the Ageing Process*, p. 1. New York: Academic Press.
Prill, H. J. (1970) In Klinik der Freuenheilkunde und Geburtshilfe, *ein Handbuch fur die Praxis*, Bd. 8, p. 398. Munchen: Urban and Scwarzenberg.
Procope, B. J. & Aldercreutz, H. (1969) *Acta Endocr. (Kbh.)*, **62**, 46.
Puck, A. (1957) *Munch. med. Wschr.*, **99**, 1505.
Thomson, B., Hart, S. A. & Durno, D. (1973) *J. Biosoc. Sci.*, **5**, 71.

FURTHER READING

Achte, K. (1970) *Acta. Obstet. Gynec. scand.*, **49**, Suppl. 1.
Pelkonen, R. (1971) *Acta. Obstet. Gynec. scand.*, **50**, Suppl. 9.
Vara, P. (1970) *Acta. Obstet. Gynec. scand.*, **49**, Suppl. 1.
Wilson, B. A. (1966) *Feminine Forever*. London: W. H. Allen.

36. Infections of the Reproductive Organs

Infection of the external parts of the genital tract, although quite common is not usually serious. On the other hand when the infection spreads upwards it tends to be much more severe with more serious consequences. Upwards spread of infection is surprisingly uncommon except during or just after pregnancy, even though the female genital tract forms a canal from the exterior to the peritoneal cavity. The vulva with its sebaceous glands, urethral opening, Skene's tubules and the orifices of Bartholin's ducts can easily become infected, as it has no special protective mechanism. The vagina on the other hand is relatively well protected and is much more resistant to infection so long as the pH remains low. The vaginal canal has no glands opening on its surface and it is covered with stratified squamous epithelium which extends from the vulva to the external cervical os. The endocervix is plugged usually by mucous and the endocervical, uterine and tubal mucous membranes are normally sterile. They are only likely to become infected during or after pregnancy.

PHYSIOLOGICAL PROTECTION OF GENITAL TRACT

There are usually large varieties and numbers of organisms on the vulva and adjacent perianal skin, but, in spite of this, infection of the vagina is less common than might be expected between puberty and the menopause. During reproductive life under normal conditions the organisms are quickly killed or made harmless because the vaginal reaction is acid. Amongst the organisms in the vagina the Gram+, anaerobic, Döderlein's bacillus predominates and causes the acidity. It is a large rod shaped organism which produces lactic acid by the fermentation of glycogen. The Döderlein's bacilli convert glycogen to lactic acid and keep the pH of the vagina between 4 and 5. The blood oestrogens regulate the amount of glycogen deposited in the vaginal epithelial cells. The vagina is sterile at birth, but within a few hours the Döderlein's bacilli and other commensals invade the tract as far as the external os. For two or three weeks after birth the oestrogens which have been produced in the feto-placental unit circulate in the baby's blood causing the vaginal epithelium to be fairly thick and rich in glycogen with numerous Döderlein's bacilli and an acid reaction. As the maternal oestrogens disappear from the baby the vaginal epithelium becomes thin, the bacilli disappear and the reaction becomes alkaline.

Similarly after the menopause when the level of oestrogen falls the epithelium of the vagina reverts to the pre-pubertal state. Much less oestrogen is necessary to cause the acidity of the vagina than is required to initiate menstruation. In the adolescent Döderlein's bacilli reappear in the vagina sometimes before the first menstrual period. In some women after the menopause the vaginal epithelium becomes very thin, the glycogen scanty and the reaction alkaline, but in other women after the menopause the Döderlein's bacilli persist for many years and there is little change in the reaction. In the latter cases it is likely that the oestrogens are still acting but they probably come from the adrenals rather than the ovaries. The risk of vaginitis after the menopause depends largely on the extent to which the oestrogens have fallen.

During the reproductive phase the vaginal pH can sometimes rise and this predisposes to infection. The pH can be altered by the presence of blood from the uterus either during menstruation, in the puerperium or after an abortion. The pH may rise so much in such circumstances as to become alkaline. In pregnancy the acidity increases and the uterine cavity is further protected by the plug of mucous or operculum which closes the cervical canal completely, especially in the primigravida. The outer third of the plug contains a variety of organisms, the middle third very few and the inner or upper third is sterile. In the non-pregnant the mucous secreted by the cervical glands fills the canal and also acts as a barrier.

The common method of infection is by spread from below upwards. In a healthy woman the genital tract above the external os of the cervix contains virtually no organisms. If, however, the protective mechanism is lacking or is overcome direct infection is possible. Lack of oestrogens either because of the age of the patient or in younger women because of deficiency in ovarian function will cause the vagina to be susceptible to infection. Infection may be introduced directly from below, for example, by the wearing of a pessary, injudicious douching or a forgotten tampon.

Lymphatic spread usually occurs where there has been laceration of the vagina or the cervix. Spread by the blood stream is not common except in the case of the tubercle bacillus which reaches the Fallopian tubes from a primary focus on the lungs or elsewhere by means of the blood stream. Direct spread from adjacent viscera may occur. On the right side the Fallopian tube may be infected from the appendix and on the left side from diverticulitis. Most of the common or pathogenic organisms may cause lesions of the reproductive tract. Some of the lesions are characteristic of the particular organism and these specific infections are considered later (page 700). Apart from such specific infections and the venereal diseases the majority of infections originate at childbirth or abortion. In these cases Gram+ cocci and coliform organisms are the commonest types.

Relatively few women with gonococcal lesions are seen at gynaecological clinics as most women with acute gonorrhoea attend special clinics. It is extremely difficult to isolate the gonococcus after the acute stage is past and women, especially those with poor personal hygiene, may never know that they have been infected and so may not seek advice at the time. Most of the cases of acute or chronic genital infection seen at gynaecological clinics are acquired at the time of parturition or abortion. A few are tuberculous and others are protozoal or fungal infections. In chronic infections it is often difficult to establish the causal organism.

VULVITIS

Non-specific vulvitis

This is quite common and is usually due to lack of personal hygiene or to a chronic vaginal discharge. It can be caused by the wearing of unhygienic underclothing or sanitary towels, or by incontinence of urine. This can cause an intertrigo as well as the vulvitis. Washing powders, particularly 'biological', can cause a sensitivity vulvitis. Nylon tights can give rise to vulvitis by causing increased moistness or by possible allergic responses. Open crotch tights have been advised. The vulval hair follicles may become infected causing folliculitis and furunculosis. The vulva becomes swollen, reddened, tender and may be excoriated. The predisposing cause should be removed and hexachlorophene or hibitane bathing instituted. A systemic antibiotic may be prescribed and hydrocortisone sprays and ointments may be used.

Vulvo-vaginitis in children

This is fairly common and is usually due either to *E. coli* or staphylococcus, but it is important to exclude the presence of a foreign body or threadworm infestation. Gonorrhoeal infection is uncommon. A foreign body may be detected by rectal or X-ray examination but if necessary vaginal examination may be done under anaesthesia. Systemic antibiotic therapy may be indicated if there is a pyogenic infection. Gonorrhoeal vulvitis is described later (page 703).

Diabetic vulvitis

This is nearly always due to infection with candida albicans. In diabetic patients, especially when untreated, glycosuria allows the fungus to grow very readily. The vulva becomes sodden and oedematous and has a characteristic dull red colour. The inflammation is widespread and involves the surrounding skin. There is a very marked pruritus and secondary infection is common as a result of scratching.

Aphthous vulvitis

The candida albicans also causes this less common type of vulvitis which occurs in debilitated patients, particularly at extremes of age. It may also develop during pregnancy if there is glycosuria. The treatment of diabetic and aphthous vulvitis is the same. Nystatin tablets 500,000 units are given orally tid or Nystatin pessaries inserted into the vagina and Nystatin cream over the vulva. Chlorphenesin powder can also be used for monilial infections.

Membranous vulvitis

This is a rare condition which may be due to diphtheritic or streptococcal infection. The lesion consists of large yellow sloughs. The diagnosis is made by bacteriological examination and the appropriate antibiotic treatment is given.

Gangrenous vulvitis

This is also very rare and is very similar to cancrum oris and noma. In this condition no specific organism has been established, but clostridium welchii, Vincent's spirilla and the Klebs-Löffler bacillus have sometimes been found.

Lipschütz ulcers

These ulcers come in crops and affect particularly the inner aspects of the labia. They vary in size but are usually deep and have ragged edges and a small sloughing base. The bacillus crassus can usually be isolated and may be the causative organism. The ulcers are very painful and this differentiates them from a gumma which has a similar appearance. The ulcers sometimes heal quickly but in some cases are more persistent. There is no specific treatment but antibiotics may be curative. Cortisone ointment may also be tried.

Behcet's syndrome

In this syndrome vulvar ulcers are associated with ulcers in the mouth and occasionally in the conjunctiva and cornea. The cause is unknown and the treatment is empirical.

Vulval warts

Warts and condylomata are probably due to viral infections in most cases but they are predisposed to by moisture and are thus quite common in women with vaginal discharge. They occur around the vulva and sometimes extend to the skin around the anus (Fig. 36.1). At one time gonorrhoea was probably a fairly common cause of vulval warts, but they are now more likely to be predisposed to by other types of discharge. The warts can be tiny and small in number or large and sessile and covering a wide area. The simple sessile type of wart is readily recognized but the vegetative type, which forms a rapidly growing mass extending over the vulva may be confused with a

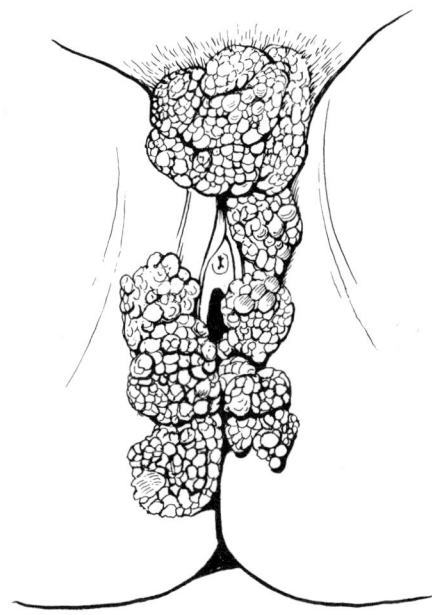

Fig. 36.1 Condylomata or warts around the vulva and extending around the anus.

cauliflower type of carcinoma. These forms of warts or condylomata acuminata are unlikely to be confused with the greyish, flattened, moist condylomata lata of secondary syphilis. The best treatment for these warts is to paint them with 25 per cent Podophyllin in alcohol or liquid paraffin. It is important not to use too much because of the dangers of absorption and also to protect the surrounding skin. The patient washes the emulsion off after about eight hours by sitting in a bath. If the vegetative type has become fungating it may be necessary to precede this with antiseptic baths. It is sometimes necessary to repeat the treatment with Podophyllin after an interval of two or three weeks. If this treatment fails the warts are excised by diathermy under general anaesthesia. It is important that any vaginal discharge should be cleared up to prevent recurrence of the warts.

Herpes vulvitis

This is a very painful condition of the vulva due to the herpes virus. It is fortunately uncommon and few cases have been reported because they have been misdiagnosed or have remained undiagnosed. The lesions start as vesicular eruptions on the vulva but rapidly go on to stage of inflammation and it is usually during this stage that the patient is seen. The ulcers are small and painful and occur along the labia majora and minora but do not spread to the vagina or the skin over the mons pubis. The ulcers spread and coalesce until the whole of the labia is involved. The ulcers are small erosions with a membranous, greyish yellow exudate covering the base. Clinicians should be alerted to the possible diagnosis by the severity of the pain in the ulcers. The lesions gradually heal and there is no residual scarring.

The diagnosis can be made by examining cytological smears from the lesions. Multinucleated giant cells, typical of herpes infection, can be identified. If facilities are available the virus should be isolated and identified or the serum complement fixation antibody is measured.

There is no specific treatment for herpes vulvitis but local treatment to give relief should be started as soon as swabs have been taken of the lesions. The vulva is bathed with an antiseptic solution such as Savlon and a local anaesthetic such as Novocaine is applied. Dressings soaked in adrenaline solution are then applied to the labia majora and minora to cause superficial vasoconstriction. A solution of 5–iodo–2–deoxyuridine is applied at frequent intervals to the dressing to keep it moist. Cortisone creams were used but are now considered to be detrimental. As the lesions are very painful analgesics are given liberally.

If herpes vulvitis occurs at the end of pregnancy, there is a high fetal mortality rate due to fetal viraemia. Even though large doses of gamma globulin are given and Caesarean section is performed there is still a high infant mortality rate.

Bartholinitis

Cysts of Bartholin's gland duct are common and quite often they become infected. In the past gonorrhoea was thought to be the common cause, but the gonococcus is now seldom isolated. Blockage of the ducts pre-disposes to the infections which may be unilateral or occasionally bilateral. In the early acute phase the orifices of the ducts appear as raised red spots near the fourchette and sometimes pus can be expressed from them. Later the glands can be palpated as tender swellings in the labia majora (Fig. 36.2).

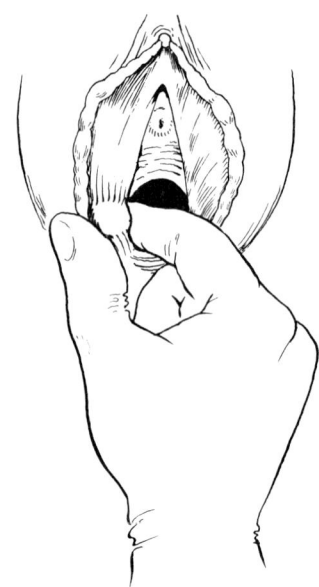

Fig. 36.2   A cyst of Bartholin's duct being palpated.

If the ducts become blocked an abscess develops which may either drain through the partially blocked duct or point and burst generally on the medial aspect. The abscess appears as a tender red fluctuant swelling situated on the posterior part of the labium majus, but sometimes extends forwards as far as the vestibule. The labium minus is displaced on the surface of the swelling and the skin is tense and glistening. Pain may be very severe and inguinal adenitis may occur. Treatment in the acute phase consists of antibiotic therapy and incision, marsupialization and drainage of the abscess. In this the incised edge of the cyst or abscess is sutured to the skin edge so that it is kept open and closes up from within outwards to the surface of the skin. This is the form of treatment commonly adopted for both the infected and non-infected Bartholin cyst. The alternative treatment of the cyst is to dissect it out, but this can mean an extensive dissection upwards along the pubic rami with sometimes extensive bleeding.

Tuberculous vulvitis

This is extremely rare. There are two forms the ulcerative and the hypertrophic. In the ulcerative form there can be marked destruction of the labia and the surrounding tissues are very oedematous. In the hypertrophic type there is gross oedema of the labia majora.

Actinomycosis of the vulva

This is extremely rare and it is characterized by an indurated brawny lesion in which multiple sinuses may develop.

Chronic vulval lesions and pruritus vulvae

The nomenclature of the chronic lesions of the vulva has presented a great deal of difficulty and there is still controversy over the terms used. The terms commonly used are kraurosis vulvae, lichen sclerosus and leukoplakia. These names have been given to various types of vulvitis both atrophic and hypertrophic. Much of the confusion arises because gynaecologists and dermatologists use different terminology, and also in different countries one term is used for conditions with differing prognosis, e.g. kraurosis vulvae is considered in the United Kingdom to be something different from leukoplakia and lichen sclerosus, while on the continent of Europe it is thought to be the same as leukoplakia and in the United States it is considered to be a possible end result of leukoplakia. The vulvar lesion can vary from time to time in the same woman so that different conditions under the old nomenclature can appear to be present at different times. The vulva particularly in obese and older women is subject to chafing, the effects of moisture and scratching so that the original condition causing the pruritus is masked by secondary changes. The old terminology, however, tends to persist and the popular terms are still kraurosis, leukoplakia and lichen sclerosus.

Kraurosis vulvae

This is considered to be a primary atrophy of the vulva. There is excessive shrinkage of the vaginal introitus which eventually leads to stenosis. The skin of the affected areas is thin and shiny, and the colour varies from white or yellow to bright red patches. There is a reduction in the amount of keratin and the dis-

appearance of the collagen there, associated with a sub-epithelial infiltration with leucocytes. The term kraurosis in Britain is a condition regarded as an exaggeration of the normal post-menopausal atrophy and shrinkage of the vulva. The condition can arise after an artificial menopause by radiotherapy, or in young patients in whom both ovaries have been removed at operation. Because of this it is thought that oestrogen deficiency is the cause, but the condition is sometimes seen before the menopause.

LEUKOPLAKIA

This as its name suggests is a condition characterized by white plaques of thickened skin on the vulva. The labia majora are affected and sometimes the labia minora, but the condition rarely extends beyond the perineum. *The vaginal orifice and vestibule are not* involved. The characteristic histological appearance in leukoplakia is the excessive keratinization of the superficial layers of the epidermis (Fig. 36.3).

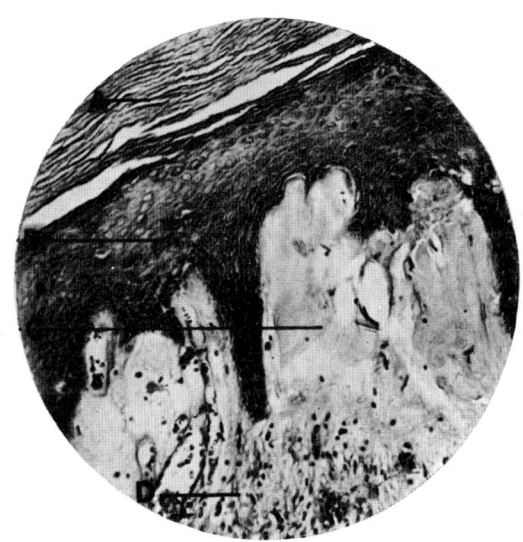

Fig. 36.3   Vulva: Leucoplakia. (A) Layer of keratin. (B) Squamous epithelium. (C) Collagenous layer. (D) Cutis vera with round cells.

The rete pegs become irregular and pointed as they dip into the adjacent connective tissue. There is infiltration of the upper layers of the corium with inflammatory cells and there is an absence of elastic tissue. The collagen layer is replaced by hyaline degeneration. The epithelial hyperplasia sometimes borders on the picture of carcinoma-*in situ*. Leukoplakia is generally considered to be the hypertrophic form of vulval dystrophy and kraurosis is the atrophic form, but the two forms can appear in the same patient at different times. It seems that the old idea that leukoplakia was premalignant but kraurosis was not is no longer tenable, as both forms of dystrophy can become malignant.

LICHEN SCLEROSUS

This is an atrophic form of scleroderma which can occur in various parts of the body apart from the vulva. The primary lesion presents as small flat white pustules which become confluent to form white sheets with clear cut edges, which spread over the perineal region and into the genito-crural folds. This is unlike leukoplakia which does not extend around the anus.

Histologically the epithelium is thin and atrophic with absence of rete pegs and loss of elastic tissue. There is hyalinization of the collagen layer and subepithelial infiltration with leucocytes.

The histological features of lichen sclerosus are very similar to those of kraurosis and leukoplakia, but the distribution of the lesion is different. Because of this Jeffcoate suggests that the terms leukoplakia, kraurosis and lichen sclerosus should be dropped and the term vulval dystrophy should be applied to all lesions. This seems quite a reasonable suggestion as the cause of these conditions is unknown and a diagnosis cannot be made until histological examination has been carried out. The most important consideration is the detection of any precancerous cells. These are most likely to be seen in the hypertrophic form of the disease. The suggestion was also reasonable as the conditions seemed to be interchangeable and the atrophic and hypertrophic forms can alternate in the same patient.

While it has been suggested that leukoplakia is frequently a precancerous condition it is on the other hand considered that kraurosis is seldom if ever precancerous. Both these observations are probably wrong and it is better that the terms should not be used, and that the histological appearance should be considered on biopsy.

Symptomology

The patient with a dystrophic condition of the vulva usually presents with pruritus or itching which may be associated with pain, dysuria and dyspareunia. In the early stages, however, or in periods of remission the condition may be asymptomatic. In severe cases the pruritus may, however, be intractable and cause great distress to the woman. On inspection the appearance of the vulva can vary very much from being purely white to red or purple. The skin may be hypertrophic and thick or atrophic, thin and glistening. In the severe hypertrophic cases the colour may be like white enamel with red fissures between, or the fissures may be white and sodden in appearance. The skin may be affected in only one or two localized areas of the vulva or the whole region may be involved. As there is such a wide variation in the appearance of the vulvar lesions and there can be so much secondary change because of scratching it is best that in all such cases a biopsy is performed.

Treatment of dystrophic conditions of the vulva
The vulva should be kept clean and as free from sweat as possible. Light, loose clothing is, therefore, recommended. If the condition is causing severe pruritus a local anaesthetic ointment containing procaine is useful for giving temporary relief. The inflammatory reaction of the skin can usually be temporarily arrested by a hydrocortisone ointment or spray. Emollient applications such as zinc oxide ointment can also give some temporary relief. Oestrogen cream or oral oestrogens in small doses can sometimes effect a cure, particularly in the atrophic forms and are well worth trying. Vitamin D ointment is also valuable in some cases. If the initial biopsy shows a carcinoma—*in situ* or severe atypia a local vulvectomy should be performed. Vulvectomy should be avoided if there is no suspicion of carcinoma developing, except where the dystrophy is very localized and in such cases a partial vulvectomy can be performed. It is essential that in all cases of chronic vulval dystrophy a careful supervision of the patients is carried out until such time as it is quite clear that there has been a complete remission of the condition and consultation with a dermatologist colleague is desirable if there is any doubt about the diagnosis or if the lesions are difficult to heal.

Other causes of pruritus vulvae
This very distressing symptom can be caused by a great variety of conditions and in many cases no definite underlying pathology can be found. Prompt investigation and treat-

ment is very important because of further irritation from scratching and infection. This can set up a vicious cycle which is often difficult to break. Only one localized part of the vulva may be affected or the whole area including the mons pubis and the perianal region may be involved. The itch tends to be worse at night while the patient is hot. Because of the perpetual desire to scratch insomnia and depression and even mental derangement may develop.

Apart from the vulval dystrophy already mentioned there are several other causes of pruritus vulvae.

Metabolic. Hypothyroidism, jaundice, uraemia, anaemia and Hodgkin's disease can all be associated with general pruritus which also affects the vulva. Adiposity particularly where it is associated with poor hygiene and where friction plays a part predisposes to itching. Malnutrition is another cause and may be due either to poor diet or deficient absorption which may possibly be caused by achlorhydria or hypochlorhydria. Glycosuria with or without associated fungal infection may cause pruritus whether it is due to diabetes or not.

Gynaecological. These causes are mainly due to vaginal discharges either caused by an erosion of the cervix or more likely from vaginitis due to trichomonas or candida albicans. The latter may be present without much discharge and should be searched for in all cases of pruritus. Vaginal wall prolapse can cause pruritus as can any form of vulvitis.

Anal. Although pruritus vulvae may spread to involve the anus the converse is also true and in taking a history the point of origin should be determined. Anal parasites, threadworms, haemorrhoids or fissures may all initiate irritation.

Dermatological. Neuro-dermatitis, scabies, psoriasis, seborrhoeic and contact dermatitis which may be due to nylon tights, washing powders, so-called anti-feminine sprays, cosmetics or contraceptives and other lesions may cause pruritus vulvae alone, or a more generalized pruritus. Where there is any doubt a dermatologist should be consulted.

Drug sensitivity. This may be due to laxatives, premedicated toilet paper or to topical applications, particularly if the patient increases the strength of a douche or lotion where weaker solutions have not relieved the symptoms.

Functional Pruritus. When all the above conditions have as far as possible been excluded there still remain quite a large number of cases which have to be treated empirically. Many of the patients are at or about the menopause and the aetiology of such cases is obscure. It must be emphasized that all other possible conditions are to be excluded before a diagnosis of functional pruritus is made, and it is important that any psychological disturbance should be detected and if possible treated.

Sexual frustration, erotic habits, marital troubles leading to avoidance of coitus may be the reason for pruritus. The diagnosis can be further complicated by the secondary changes due to scratching and various forms of treatment which might have been tried.

Management

As pruritus is only a symptom the first step is to find the cause and a complete history both gynaecological and general is essential. A thorough examination is also necessary so that any metabolic disease can be recognized. Evidence of skin disease elsewhere should be looked for and the hands and feet, in particular, should be examined for evidence of fungus infection. If there is a vaginal discharge this should be examined. Examination of the anus should also be carried out.

Where there is any evidence of vulval dystrophy a biopsy should be taken so that an exact diagnosis can be made. The treatment of pruritus without a recognizable cause is empirical and tends to be unsatisfactory. Hydrocortisone sprays and ointments because of their anti-inflammatory action are widely used. Although they are not specific and relief is transitory they nevertheless are valuable in breaking any scratch reflex which has developed. Antihistamines are also sometimes of value. As far as possible douching should be avoided as should any agent which might cause sensitization. Local analgesic agents such as benzocaine or amethocaine will give temporary relief but it is preferable not to use such preparations for a prolonged time, but rather try to effect a cure.

Oestrogen therapy may be of value, particularly in cases of secondary infection of the vulva in post-menopausal women. Division of the cutaneous nerves of the vulva can usually effect a relief for some months and can occasionally cause a permanent cure. Simpler local treatment is, however, usually effective and this radical form of treatment is usually unnecessary. The same applies to radiotherapy which was used in low dosage for pruritus. The results, however, were not good and this form of treatment has been abandoned. Where there is some psychological element to the condition a sedative or tranquillizer should be prescribed. If it is thought necessary the patient should be seen by a psychiatrist. It is important that the patient should have a deep sleep at night as there is a tendency to involuntary scratching if the sleep is light.

URETHRAL CARUNCLE

This is a painful small, bright red swelling arising from the mucous membrane of the urethra. Most of them arise from chronic infection of the urethra and occur on the posterior part. They are usually granulomatous in type and may be diffuse but are usually pedunculated (Fig. 36.4a, b). The swelling is

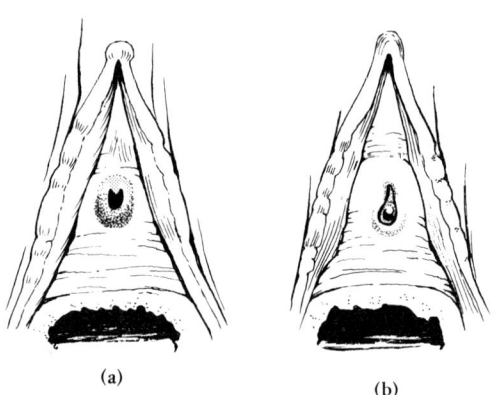

(a)

(b)

Fig. 36.4   Urethral caruncle. (a) Diffuse granulomatous type. (b) Pedunculated type.

composed of granulation tissue covered with a transitional epithelium. Adenomatous and angiomatous caruncles are less common than the granulomatous type. They give rise to dysuria, dyspareunia and sometimes to a feeling of a swelling in the vagina. Bleeding may be a feature particularly in the angiomatous type. They usually arise in post-menopausal women who are parous.

A prolapse of the urethral mucous membrane can be confused with a caruncle but the caruncle is brighter red in colour and is tender to touch. A carcinoma of the urethra rarely occurs and unless a large friable mass is present a diagnosis cannot be made without taking a biopsy. When symptoms are present the

caruncle should be excised and the base treated with diathermy. Any underlying urinary infection or urethritis could also be treated. Recurrence is due to infection of the cauterized area and it is sometimes necessary to apply an antibiotic cream to the area which has been cauterized to avoid recurrence of the infection. Recurring caruncles should always be examined for malignancy, although this is a rare development.

VAGINITIS AND VAGINAL DISCHARGE

In a healthy woman there is normally just enough moisture in the vagina to lubricate the surface of the walls. As there are no glands in the vagina this moisture comes partly as a transudate of fluid through the epithelium and partly from the mucoid secretion of the cervical glands. Theoretically the scant serous, non-mucoid secretion of the endometrium may pass down through the cervical canal, but in health this plays no great part in the production of moisture in the vagina. In addition Bartholin's glands and probably Skene's tubules and the other periurethral glands produce mucoid secretions. Their function is to lubricate the vulva during intercourse. The vaginal transudate together with the cervical mucous and the epithelial cells which are constantly being shed from the vagina produce a thin, white, curdy discharge. Even the shed cells have a high glycogen content and the lactobacilli thrive and keep the reaction strongly acid. Under certain circumstances, such as pregnancy, repeated erotic stimulation and congestion from other causes, this normal vaginal transudate is increased in amount and the patient accordingly complains of vaginal discharge. This discharge is white and non-purulent and strictly speaking it is only this type of discharge which should be called leucorrhoea, but the term has come to be accepted as including any non-haemorrhagic vaginal discharge. All vaginal discharges should be carefully investigated. The cause may be anything from poor hygiene on the one hand to malignant disease on the other. Unfortunately women are sometimes treated, without pelvic inspection or examination, with medicated pessaries for vaginal discharges which are later found to be due to carcinoma, particularly of the cervix. A vaginal examination is made eventually when the discharge becomes offensive and blood stained, but by this time the disease will be far advanced. A full bacteriological examination is not necessary in every case, but a bimanual and speculum examination are essential to find out from which part of the tract the discharge is coming. The vaginal discharge may be due to vaginitis or cervical lesions and these will be described in turn.

Vaginitis

In the normal vaginal discharge even though it is excessive there is usually a large number of epithelial cells, very few pus cells and large numbers of large Gram+ Döderlein's bacilli. When there is an infected vaginitis the discharge is composed of large numbers of pus cells, bacteria and very few epithelial cells. The common infections of the vagina are due to trichomonas and monilial infections or to senile vaginitis in which there is a loss of the protective Döderlein's bacilli (Fig. 36.5). Nonspecific vaginitis with different infecting organisms can also occur.

TRICHOMONAS VAGINITIS
This is one of the commonest forms of vaginitis and is due to infection with the

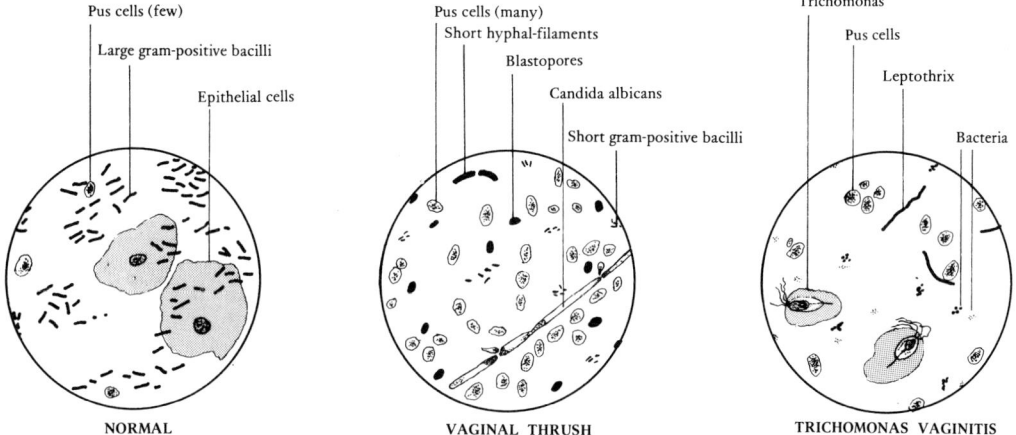

Fig. 36.5 Diagrammatic representation of microscopic picture from abnormal vaginal discharge, vaginal thrush and trichomonas vaginitis.

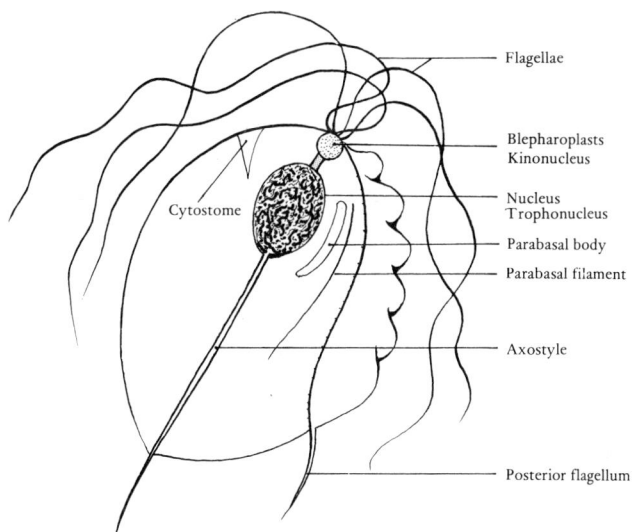

Fig. 36.6 Trichomonas vaginalis.

trichomonas vaginalis. It is an ovoid, motile, flagellated protozoan slightly larger than a leucocyte (Fig. 36.6). In a stained, dried film the flagellae are not readily seen unless special precautions are taken, and the organism is difficult to distinguish from a pus cell. For this reason the organism is best identified when a drop of discharge is mixed with several drops of normal saline and the preparation is examined at once. The organism can then be recognized as a lashing of the flagellae and the jerky movement of the body which seems to push aside adjacent pus cells. The organism can be cultured but special methods are necessary and for immediate diagnosis direct examination is the most reliable. If the wet film is negative, however, the parasite can be cultured in a special medium to which antibiotics have been added to inhibit the growth of contaminants. The trichomonas can be identified in smears stained for cytological examination. The trichomonas requires glycogen as a food and the infection is, therefore, not seen before puberty. The pH of the vagina in infected cases is usually between 5 and 7 and lacto-bacilli are rarely seen. It is not certain whether it is the absence of lacto-bacilli and the altered pH which allows the trichomonas infection, or the infection which deters the growth of the lacto-bacilli. About 20 per cent of adult women and up to 10 per cent of adult males are thought to carry the organisms in the urogenital tract. In men the parasite rarely causes symptoms but sometimes urethritis is a manifestation. Trichomonads can also be found in the lower genital and urinary tracts of women without symptoms. The method of infection is uncertain. It is not classified as a venereal disease, but it can undoubtedly be transmitted by coitus. The organism has been found under the prepuce in males and may cause urethritis or balanitis. A combined infection with trichomonas and gonorrhoea is not uncommon. There is a large group of trichomonads, one species is found in the bowel where it appears to cause no symptoms, but it is believed by some that vaginal infection sometimes comes from the rectum, the organisms undergoing certain changes in its new environment. Otherwise infection may be from infected persons or carriers by means of towels, bath water, instruments, gloves or infected clothing. Spread of the infection beyond the vagina or lower urethra is very unusual. Eradication of the infection is sometimes made difficult because the organism can penetrate into the deeper layers of the epithelium of the vagina. The discharge caused by the trichomonas is yellowish-green and is said to be characteristically frothy. The vagina is reddened and there are lesions particularly around the cervix and the external urethral meatus. There is pruritus, dyspareunia and sometimes dysuria.

Treatment
The easiest and most effective form of treatment is by metronidazole (Flagyl) in tablets of 200mg each, three tablets daily being given for one week, and a single course of treatment is usually sufficient. Oral medication alone is curative in 85–90 per cent of cases. If there is a recurrence then the patient's consort is treated simultaneously with metronidazole. Side effects are unusual but occasionally nausea, dizziness, headache and minor skin eruptions may occur. In the resistant cases of trichomonas vaginitis local treatment may be required. Local treatment may be either Stovarsol Vaginal Compound (SVC) pessaries each containing 150mg or Carbarsone (BPC) pessaries each containing 2gm or Penotrane pessaries. Tampovagan PSS pessaries or Terramycin pessaries combined with an anti-monilial preparation such as nystatin can also be used. The latter is used for one week but the other pessaries require to be used for at least six weeks including the time of menstruation. Intercourse should be avoided for the first month of treatment. Any associated erosion of the cervix should be cauterized.

MONILIAL VAGINITIS
This is due to an infection with candida albicans. The main predisposing factor is glycosuria and is very common in diabetics, and in pregnancy where the renal threshold for sugar is usually lowered. The discharge is typically thick, curdy, white and occurs as plaques on the vaginal walls. It gives rise to an intense pruritus. The fungus is easily recognized on films stained by Grams method provided a smear has been taken from a white patch. Otherwise the organism may be missed and repeated films may be necessary. In cases with transitory glycosuria the symptoms may vary from day to day and smears taken at a quiescent phase may fail to show the fungus. In positive cases the septate pseudomycelial filaments and the shorter hyphal filaments with budding blastospores are characteristic (Fig. 36.5).

Treatment

This is most conveniently carried out by giving nystatin tablets containing 500 000 units two or three times daily for ten days. Alternatively nystatin pessaries can be inserted nightly for ten days. Mycil pessaries or pessaries containing gentian violet can also be used. If there is an underlying cause for the glycosuria this should be treated. During pregnancy it may be necessary to give repeated courses of treatment. Recognition and thorough treatment during pregnancy are particularly important because of the danger of the child contracting oral thrush during delivery. When the mother is known to have been infected the child's mouth should be painted with gentian violet.

NON-SPECIFIC VAGINITIS

A variety of organisms including staphylococci, streptococci, coliform bacilli and haemophilus vaginalis can give rise to vaginitis. There is sometimes an underlying cause such as douches, pessaries, tampons, trauma, drugs and chemicals, ring pessaries and contraceptives. A non-specific vaginitis can also occur in debilitated patients and in those with poor personal hygiene.

The treatment is directed towards removing any cause and to improving the general health and hygiene. Pessaries of chemical origin, Floraquin, Penotrane, Betadine, or various forms of antibiotics and mixed chemical pessaries or creams are used. Prolonged treatment is often required and it is necessary to alternate the various forms of therapy. There is, however, a danger of drug reactions to make this situation worse and sometimes minimum emolument is all that can be used until the drug reaction settles.

SENILE VAGINITIS

This is a non-specific vaginitis which occurs in women after the menopause and is due to the diminished resistance to infection of the vaginal wall which has become atrophic as a result of the fall in the oestrogen level. The chief symptom is a slight watery discharge which may become blood stained. On examination the epithelium appears thin and haemorrhagic. There may be areas of ulcerations and sometimes adhesions occur between the walls of the vagina giving rise to constriction. There is sometimes an associated endometritis. Most of these cases present as post-menopausal bleeding and it is necessary to exclude carcinoma of the genital tract. Once this has been done treatment consists of replacement of the oestrogens by giving Stilboestrol 0·2mg twice daily for three weeks in every four. Other oestrogen preparations such as oestriol or conjugated oestrogens can also be used, or alternatively oestrogen pessaries or creams can be given as this is equally effective and there is less risk of uterine bleeding.

VULVO-VAGINITIS IN CHILDREN

This may be caused by a foreign body in the vagina, by threadworms, occasionally by trichomonas or monilial infection and also by the gonococcus. It is sometimes necessary to carry out an investigation under anaesthesia to exclude a foreign body. A swab is taken of the vagina to identify the possible cause and the appropriate treatment is given.

RARE CAUSES OF VAGINITIS

Granular vaginitis and emphysematous vaginitis are special names given to rare forms sometimes seen in pregnancy and usually associated with chronic gonorrhoea. In the former the vagina is covered with numerous small, hard, red coloured nodules and in the latter with small bullae containing gas due to superadded anaerobic infection. The aetiology is unknown but the condition usually resolves spontaneously. Membranous vaginitis may occur as an extension of membranous vulvitis.

CERVICITIS

Although the term cervicitis is very commonly used it is probable that it is only in the acute form that the condition is due to infection and most of the cases of chronic cervicitis are due to hormonal or chemical changes which occur with pregnancy. The rarer causes of cervicitis and vaginitis such as amoebiasis and lesions associated with bilharzia are discussed in Chapter 40.

Acute Cervicitis

An acute infection of the cervix can arise from direct infection or be secondary to inflammatory lesions in the endometrium or vagina. Simultaneous infection of the cervix and vagina are often found in cases of gonorrhoea, trichomonas, monilial or non-specific infections. Staphylococcal, enterococcal and streptococcal infections are likely to occur in the puerperium or when the cervix is injured.

Acute cervicitis may also occur in cases of measles, scarlet fever or diphtheria. A common cause of combined vaginitis and cervicitis is the presence of foreign bodies such as a pessary or a neglected tampon. Acute cervicitis is also caused by venereal infections such as chancroid and lymphogranuloma venereum.

In acute infection of the cervix there is a purulent discharge and palpation or movement of the cervix causes great pain. The cervix is seen to be red, congested and swollen on speculum examination.

result of a true inflammatory process due to organisms, in many cases it is probably due to hormonal changes and possibly a reaction to chemical changes. So-called chronic cervicitis can take many forms. Chronic cervicitis is a term which is given to a cervix which is lacerated or hypertrophied, or has an eversion of the endocervical mucosa (ectropion), or has the squamous epithelium replaced by endo-cervical columnar epithelium (erosion), or shows retention cysts (Nabothian follicles) (Fig. 36.7).

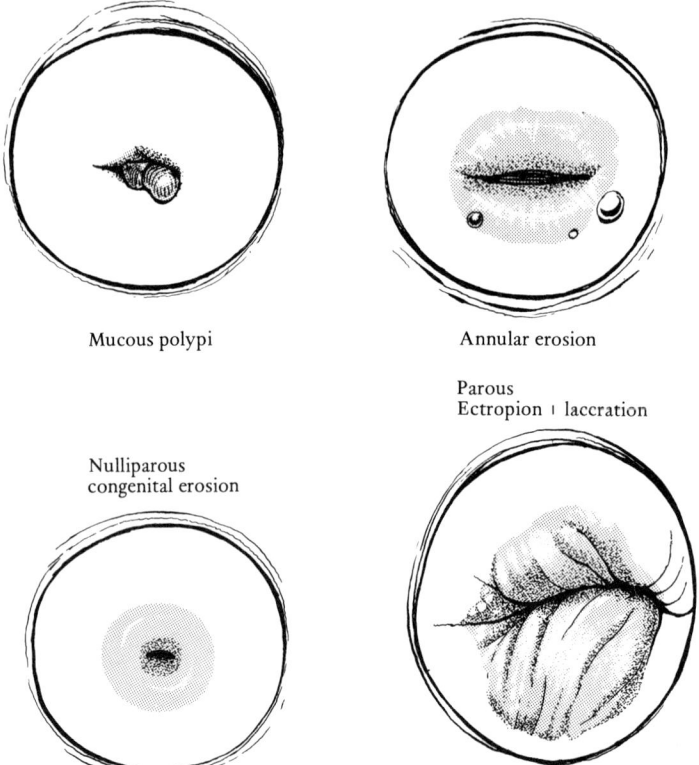

Mucous polypi

Annular erosion

Nulliparous congenital erosion

Parous Ectropion I laccration

Fig. 36.7   Cervical lesions.

Swabs are taken from the cervical canal to identify the organism and the appropriate antibiotic treatment is given. Cauterization or incision of the cervix is contra-indicated in acute cervicitis.

Chronic cervicitis

A sub-acute or chronic form of cervicitis may follow on the acute phase of the disease, but it may arise as a low grade infection or most commonly it follows after pregnancy or an abortion. Although in some cases this is the

These terms are all used for conditions which may occasionally be due to infection, but most often are the results of pregnancy or abortion or of hormonal imbalance.

Erosion

This is the commonest cervical lesion. The term is a misnomer as it suggests loss of tissue or ulceration and there is none. The erosion may be circular or annular or may only affect one lip of the cervix. The term erosion was originally used because it was believed that the appearances were due to superficial layers of squamous epithelium being eroded or eaten away leaving only the basal or cuboidal cells. Meyer pointed out that quite early in fetal life there is a differentiation between the columnar epithelium of the cervical canal and the squamous epithelium of the vaginal portion of the cervix. The line of demarcation, however, is not at first at the external os but well within the canal. According to Meyer the columnar epithelium begins to secrete about the sixth to the seventh month of intra-uterine life, and the effect of this secretion is to push back the squamous epithelium to the region of the external os and the circular area outside the os is covered with columnar instead of squamous epithelium. This gives the congenital erosion, not infrequently seen in virgins where there is no infection. The base of an erosion is very vascular and has a characteristic deep red colour. If there are numerous Nabothian follicles under the erosion then it gives rise to what is called a follicular erosion. Acquired erosions arising in later life usually occur after parturition or abortion. Meyer's view that acquired erosion is always the result of inflammation which causes destruction of the squamous epithelium which is then followed by an outward growth of the columnar epithelium is now questioned. Fluhmann for example concludes (1) that an acquired erosion is not accompanied by a loss of surface epithelium, (2) in its early stage the erosion is covered by columnar epithelium which arises from an ectropian or eversion of the cervical mucosa. This lesion may be of congenital origin, persisting into adult life, or results from cervical laceration in pregnancy, or a prolapse of the cervical mucosa, (3) an acquired erosion is not primarily caused by infection, but is usually although not always accompanied by some inflammatory reaction. (4) The base of an acquired erosion is variously composed of areas of columnar epithelium, squamous epithelium and transitional phases of the process called squamous prosoplasia or epidermidization. (5) An erosion is healed either spontaneously or as the result of treatment when it is covered by normal squamous epithelium. This is brought about by epidermidization. Erosions have been classified into different types—simple, papillary and follicular, but they are all stages of the same process and vary only with the size of the glands and the presence or absence of Nabothian follicles. The division is unnecessary so long as it is

realized that slight differences may occur both to the naked eye and histological appearances. The base of an acquired erosion is composed histologically of three types of epithelium (Fig. 36.8). There is first the columnar epithelium which is continuous with the cervical canal.

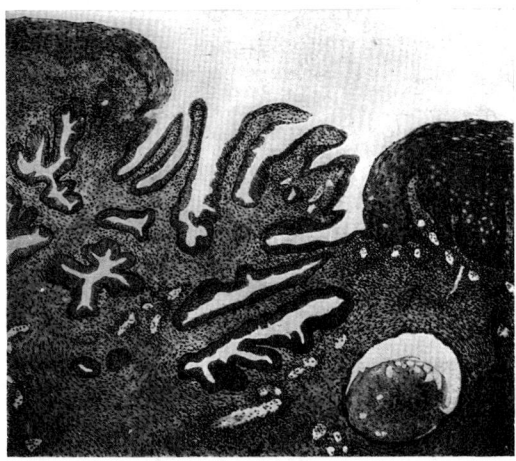

Fig. 36.8 Histological appearance of erosion of cervix showing also a cystic space.

Secondly the edges on the portio are composed of squamous epithelium which sends protrusions into the eroded areas in an attempt at healing. Finally, there are leucocytes, plasma cells and giant cells which extend into the submucosal tissues. These findings are characteristic of the erosions seen during post-natal life, but their inflammatory reaction may be completely absent. The congenital erosion before birth and the early months of life is covered with columnar epithelium and does not have the dense cellular infiltration until later years when transitions from columnar to squamous epithelium are making their appearance.

Ectropion
This occurs when there is bilateral laceration of the cervix allowing the two lips of the cervix to evert leaving the mucosa of the cervical canal exposed to the acid vaginal secretions.

Mucous polypi of the cervix
These are often seen in association with erosion of chronic cervicitis. The mucosa of the canal becomes thickened and when the thickening is localized and accompanied by cystic dilatation polyp formation results. Polypi are bright red pedunculated swellings pro-

truding through the external os (Fig. 36.7). They may be single or multiple and are very vascular.

Pathology of chronic cervicitis

Usually the only evidence of inflammation is a slight sub-mucosal accumulation of leucocytes in the region of the transitional zone, but if there is a marked inflammatory change then there is intense infiltration with leucocytes along the clefts and tunnels under the squamous epithelium and extension down it along the lymphatics to the whole substance of the cervix (Fig. 36.9). In almost all parous women the

Clinical features

The typical symptom of chronic cervicitis is the thick mucoid and occasionally frankly purulent discharge. General symptoms such as fatigue, headaches and arthritis have been attributed to chronic cervicitis, but this is doubtful, except in cases where there is a true chronic inflammatory lesion and these are rare. Pain is not a feature of chronic cervicitis and if there is pain on moving the cervix in such cases it is probably due to an associated parametritis, which may have resulted from infection spreading up usually along lacerations

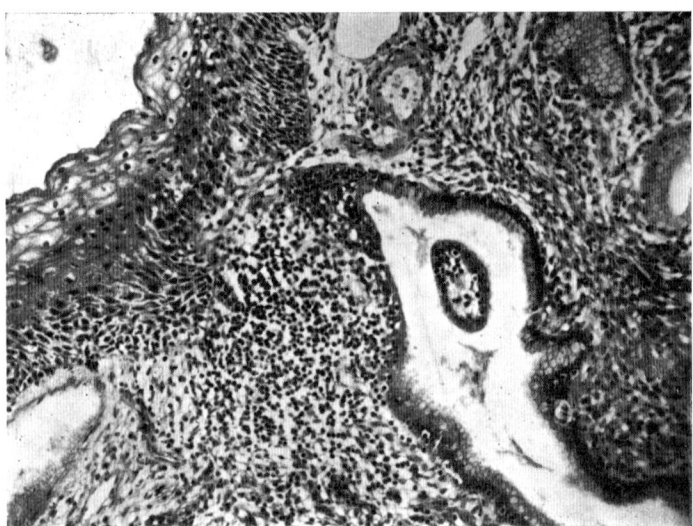

Fig. 36.9   Chronic cervicitis showing inflammatory iaction and distended glands.

cervix will show some small nests of leucocytes or lymph follicles in layers immediately beneath the mucosa, but it is doubtful if this should be classified as a true inflammatory process. When the change, whether it is inflammatory or endocrine, affects the endocervix giving rise to endocervicitis the glands of the endocervix are hypertrophied and enlarged producing an excessive amount of secretion. The cervix may be enlarged because of this, but enlargement may be due also to hypertrophy in the stroma or to blockage of the ducts of the glands with consequent distension with mucous. When the distended glands lie just under the squamous epithelium the collections of mucous cause small round white elevations on the cervix. These are called Nabothian follicles. Lacerations of the cervix very commonly occur at parturition and sometimes they can extend up into the vaginal vault.

which have extended up from the cervix. In some cases there may be an associated urinary tract infection and it is important if there is a complaint of frequency and dysuria that the urine is examined. Bleeding either intermenstrual or post-coital may be a feature of vascular erosions or of polypi. Dysmenorrhoea and dyspareunia may occasionally be associated with chronic cervicitis. Inflammation of the cervix may produce so-called hostile secretions which can be the cause of infertility.

Diagnosis

If an erosion is present then on digital examination the cervix may feel slightly granular and like wet velvet. The cervix may be lacerated or irregular and in some cases it is bulky. If there has been an extension of infection to the cellular tissues with resulting thickening of the pelvic ligaments the cervix may be relatively immobile and movement of the cervix may elicit pain. On speculum examination the red raw-looking erosion is easily identified and Nabothian follicles are seen as small raised areas which may have a bluish tinge. Polypi of the cervix are easily missed on digital examination but are readily seen on speculum examination. In cases of infected endocervicitis pus and mucous can be seen coming from the external os. If there is an associated pelvic cellulitis the diagnosis may be difficult from ovarian or tubal lesions or from pelvic floor endometriosis, but in doubtful cases examination under anaesthesia should make the diagnosis clear or if still in doubt laparoscopy or laparotomy should be performed. Early cervical carcinoma can be confused with chronic cervicitis but a cervical smear should be done routinely or histological examination of a biopsy specimen if necessary.

Treatment

This depends on the type and extent of the lesion. If there is an extensive laceration and ectropion of the cervix an operation is required to reconstruct the cervix (trachelorrhaphy). Alternatively amputation of the cervix may be necessary. Erosions and chronic cervicitis with Nabothian follicles are treated either with diathermy or electric cautery. If the erosion is small and extensive cauterization or diathermy is not required superficial cauterization can be done without anaesthesia. Superficial cauterization is all that is required and the erosion can be treated without dilatation of the cervix. If more extensive cauterization is required the cervix is dilated and cauterization is carried out radially from the external os. The cervical canal is also cauterized if it is thought that there is some endocervicitis, but this should not be done extensively as there is the risk that cicatrization may be produced. This can cause dysmenorrhoea, haematometra or, if pregnancy occurs, rigidity of the cervix during labour. Any Nabothian follicles are punctured and coagulated. It is common to find an erosion of the cervix at post-natal examination. No treatment is required at this time, but the patient should be asked to return in three months' time, and if she still has the discharge then cauterization should be carried out. This can generally be done without anaesthesia. Although the cervix is insensitive to pain it is important that the heat from the cautery should not cause discomfort of the

vagina. Erosions of the cervix frequently occur in women on a contraceptive pill containing oestrogen. It is unnecessary to treat them unless there is a discharge giving rise to discomfort. It is always important to ensure that a cervical smear has been taken to exclude malignancy of the cervix before cauterizing. The treatment of an erosion causes little general disturbance and requires only a very short stay in hospital. The results are generally satisfactory. The patient should be warned that the discharge will continue for a week or two after the cauterization until the cauterized tissues have separated and the area has completely healed. Very rarely about the tenth or twelfth day when the slough separates bleeding may occur, but this is seldom excessive. Cryosurgery is now proving useful for treatment of chronic cervicitis.

INVESTIGATION OF THE PATIENT WITH
VAGINAL DISCHARGE

The age of the patient may suggest the type of infection or lesion which might be expected. Before puberty vaginal infection such as monilial vaginitis may be present and after the menopause it is important to exclude malignant disease as the cause. The previous obstetric history may be informative particularly if there have been difficult deliveries, puerperal fever or abortions. The menstrual history may be relevant particularly if irregularity or variation in the amount of menstrual loss or the recent onset of pain with menstruation. It should be ascertained whether the patient is taking a contraceptive pill and if so whether the time of starting this method of contraception coincided with the onset of the discharge.

Prolapse of the uterus or vaginal walls often gives rise to discharge, especially if the cervix projects beyond the introitus or if a pessary is worn. The woman should be asked if she uses internal sanitary tampons, as they sometimes can be forgotten or a part of one can be unknowingly left in the vagina. Urinary symptoms may point to an associated urethritis which suggests a gonococcal lesion or to cystitis which might be secondary to a cervicitis. If there is parametrial involvement there may be pelvic pain, backache or dyspareunia, but the latter can occur with vaginitis alone. A discharge dating from delivery is usually due to cervicitis, and if it dates from marriage or sexual intercourse venereal infection is more usual. A discharge dating from puberty or soon after is most likely to be non-infective in nature. Cervical discharges and fungal infections of the vagina tend to be worse before menstruation, whereas trichomonas vaginitis is nearly always worse after the menstrual period, because the reaction of the vagina is less acid at that time. There may be a history of emotional upsets which sometimes seem to cause an excess amount of cervical discharge.

The patient's description of the discharge may be misleading because the fastidious patient may complain of a profuse discharge when it is only slightly in excess of normal. Whereas others with poorer standards of hygiene may not complain even though the discharge is very heavy and purulent. Quite a good guide is the necessity or otherwise for wearing a pad. Discharges which are described as thick and stringy are usually of cervical origin, whereas thinner discharges are more likely to be due to vaginitis. Purulent and offensive discharges are usually due to vaginitis and blood stained discharges suggest malignant disease, although it may also occur in such simple conditions as cervical polyp, severe cervicitis and senile vaginitis. The patient should be asked if she douches the vagina as a hygienic measure and if so with what agents and in what solution.

EXAMINATION OF THE PATIENT

The urethra and surrounding areas should be examined carefully before the patient is asked to void urine in case the stream washes away any urethral discharge. The urine should be tested for sugar, pus cells and organisms, and a Wassermann test should be done routinely. The patient is examined in the dorsal position and good light is essential. No lubricants or antiseptics should be used on the examining fingers or specula before swabs have been taken for bacteriological examination. Examination of the genital organs is carried out in the usual way as described in Chapter 32. When inspecting, particularly for the cause of the vaginal discharge the following procedure is adopted. The vulva is inspected for evidence of inflammation, warts or other abnormalities. The presence of smegma in the folds of the labia is indicative of faulty personal hygiene and is commonly associated with non-specific vaginitis. The labia are separated and any discharge mopped away from the urinary meatus. Vaginal discharge often collects in the meatus and gives a false impression of

urethritis. The uretha is then 'milked' and a smear is taken from just inside the meatus. A fine metal loop is best for this purpose but a throat swab can be used if the smear is made on a slide immediately. The Bartholin's glands are then palpated with a finger inside the introitus and thumb outside. A normal gland is not palpable so that any thickening or swelling is indicative of disease. In some cases pus may be seen coming from the opening of the ducts which may be inflamed, if so smears should also be taken from these. These and urethral smears should be stained by Gram's method and examined for the presence of gonococci. A speculum of the bivalve type is then inserted with the patient in the dorsal position. The character and the amount of discharge are noted. Gonococcal pus is typically yellow and creamy. The discharge from trichomonas vaginitis is very similar except that it is often more frothy. The discharge from cervical infection is usually mucopurulent and that from fungal infection of the vagina is white and curdy, while that caused by an excess of normal transudate is opalescent. While these are useful pointers the exact diagnosis depends on microscopic examination. A drop of normal saline is put on a slide and the discharge is mixed with this and examined for trichomonas. A smear should also be made on a slide treated with Gram's stain. Any excess of discharge is now mopped away to give a good view of the vaginal walls. In chronic vaginitis there may not be much obvious change, but in the acute or sub-acute cases the vaginal walls are reddened and sometimes oedematous. Often there are punctate petechial haemorrhages giving a strawberry appearance, and in such cases the vaginal walls are very tender. When the infection is due to a fungus characteristic white patches are seen either adherent to the wall, and are very similar to the 'thrush' patches in a baby's mouth. In senile vaginitis the epithelium is very thin, the vagina appears raw and in severe cases there may be areas of ulceration or haemorrhage. Adhesions may occur between the walls of the vagina and the vault tends to be constricted. The vaginitis can spread to the vaginal portion of the cervix and present the same appearances as in the vagina. The cervix, however, may be inflamed in the absence of any vaginitis. The common lesions of the cervix which may give rise to discharge are acute cervicitis, chronic cervicitis, cervical erosion and carcinoma. The appearances and pathology of these are described in later sections. The character of any discharge coming through the os is noted.

Mucopurulent discharge usually indicates infection of the racemose glands of the cervical canal (endocervicitis). A frankly purulent discharge suggests inflammation of the genital tract higher up. Pure mucous is sometimes excreted in excess as a result of excitement due to the examination or to excess of oestrogens, such as in women on the contraceptive pill. If a gonococcal infection is suspected a further smear is taken from the cervical canal after swabbing away any discharge from the external os. During the course of this examination any other obvious cause of discharge will have been noted, for example, a forgotten pessary or tampon, friction ulceration of a prolapse of the cervix or vagina, a sloughing fibroid polypus coming through the os or any tumour of the vaginal wall. A bimanual examination is then made to determine whether the body of the uterus, appendages or other tissues in the pelvis are involved in the infection. Tenderness, swelling in the fornices, thickening in the ligaments and cellular tissues around the cervix and impairment of mobility are particularly noted. Where these are present pain is usually the main symptom and the discharge is a subsidiary complaint.

A wet unstained preparation and a Gram's stained smear from the vagina, urethra and cervix are sent for bacteriological examination. If gonococcal infection is suspected then the cervical, urethral and Bartholin's ducts smears are taken and put into Stuart's transport medium. The main primary organisms of vaginitis are candida albicans, trichomonas vaginalis and in children, the gonococcus. In non-specific vaginitis a host of organisms, both Gram positive and Gram negative, coccobacilli, coliforms, Gram positive bacilli and others are found. These are also the type of organisms found in senile vaginitis. When a severe infection occurs there are many pus cells, a few epithelial cells and no Döderlein's bacilli, and many secondary invading organisms. The pH is usually above six. Trichomonas and candida albicans can be cultured with special media. For trichomonas Kupferberg's medium can be used and for candida albicans Sabouraud's broth or Nickerson's medium can be used, but by using Feinberg-Whittington medium it is possible to detect both candida and trichomonas reliably in one specimen. It

is highly desirable that the correct diagnosis is made before treatment is prescribed, and unless the diagnosis seems clear from vaginal examination it is preferable to take a smear for bacteriological examination, however, there is no point in sending a dry swab to the laboratory as it is probable that trichomonas will not be identified and secondary invaders will not be detected because the organisms stop growing once they are removed from the vagina. It is better to either send the swab in a special medium or send it in a tube with normal saline to keep the swab moist. If there is any suspicion of gonorrhoea swabs must be taken from the urethra and the patient should be referred direct to a venereal diseases clinic if the swabs are positive.

ENDOMETRITIS

Acute endometritis

This occurs most commonly from infection of the decidua following childbirth or abortion and is described in Chapter 21.

Acute endometritis may also occur following dilatation and curettage of the uterus or cauterization of the cervix. There is an increased pulse rate, lower abdominal pain and tenderness of the uterus. As the cervix has recently been dilated the drainage is good and the infection usually settles within a few days without any special treatment, but it is advisable to take bacteriological swabs and to give chemotherapy. A degenerating mucous fibroid or endometrial carcinoma can also occasionally cause endometritis. When gonococcal infection spreads from the cervix to the tubes the involvement of the endometrium is nearly always transitory and symptomless. Intra-uterine contraceptive devices can cause acute endometritis, but removal of a device quickly effects a cure. Radium used to produce a radium menopause or for the treatment of endometrial carcinoma can also cause acute endometritis, but again removal quickly relieves the infective condition. Before the cyclical changes in the endometrium were fully understood it was thought that oedema, small round cell infiltration and the presence of some polymorphonuclear cells found in the second half of the normal menstrual cycle were indicative of infection. In the cases of endometritis which are still seen the stroma is principally involved and as a rule the other pelvic organs are also infected. In order to establish the diagnosis histologically polymorphonuclear leucocytes must be seen in large groups and not scattered as in the normal premenstrual phase. Some workers claim that the finding of plasma cells is the only definite criterion of a subacute or chronic lesion. Chronic endometritis other than senile endometritis is almost always due to tuberculosis and a thorough search must be made for evidence of this. In the absence of tuberculosis it is usual that curettage will be sufficient to relieve the symptoms, but if menorrhagia persists, or if the other pelvic organs are affected hysterectomy will be required.

SENILE ENDOMETRITIS

This is an infection of the endometrium occurring after the menopause. The endometrium is thin and atrophic and there is loss of the glands. In severe conditions the stroma may be replaced by granulation tissue. Plasma and round cells are numerous both in the endometrium and in the myometrium. There is a thin watery irritant discharge from the uterus and there is often an associated senile vaginitis and even a vulvitis. Post-menopausal bleeding is the usual presenting sign. The treatment consists of dilatation of the cervix and curettage to confirm the diagnosis and to establish drainage followed by a course of oestrogens. This is usually given in the form of 2mg of Stilboestrol daily for seven to ten days and then gradually decreasing the dosage over a period of two months. If larger doses are given there is the risk that endometrial hyperplasia may be produced and this will give rise to bleeding on cessation of treatment.

TUBERCULOUS ENDOMETRITIS

This will be discussed later (page 701).

Pyometra

This condition is usually found in elderly women after the menopause but it can also occur when the cervix is stenosed, for example after cone biopsy or amputation of the cervix, in cases of carcinoma of the cervix or in cases where there has been excessive cauterization of the endocervix, or in cases of tuberculous endometritis. There is an accumulation of pus in the cavity of the uterus. Often the condition is unsuspected and it is only when the cervix is being dilated that pus is observed to escape through the os. In such cases the uterus may be soft, cystic, enlarged and tender. Carcinoma should always be suspected in such cases and after drainage of the pus a gentle curettage is performed. It is also essential to look for any evidence of carcinoma of the endocervix. If tuberculous infection and carcinoma have been excluded then the condition is treated by dilatation of the cervix and oestrogen therapy.

SALPINGITIS AND SALPINGO-OOPHORITIS

It is unusual for infections of either the tubes or the ovaries to occur alone. Usually both organs are involved and the condition is commonly bilateral. The infection may spread from the uterus, cervix or vagina either directly or by lymphatic spread. Tuberculous infection usually occurs by the blood stream. Infection can occur directly from appendicitis or diverticulitis. In the latter cases the infection may be unilateral but if a pelvic abscess forms then the tubes and ovaries on both sides may be affected.

Acute salpingitis

This is usually either gonococcal or puerperal. Occasionally it may be seen as a complication of carcinoma of the cervix or a sloughing fibroid of the uterus. It may also follow curettage of the uterus, cauterization of the cervix, hysterosalpingography, insertion of an intra-uterine contraceptive device or any other operative or diagnostic procedures involving the uterus. Acute salpingo-oophoritis may be seen alone or it may be part of a more extensive infection involving the uterus, connective tissues and peritoneum. In the acute phase of infection both tubes are markedly inflamed and swollen and can be seen to be congested and red on laparotomy. Pus can sometimes be seen exuding from the fimbriated ends of the tubes. There may be serous exudate over the tubes and in the Pouch of Douglas. The surrounding pelvic peritoneum may be reddened. The abdomen should be closed again when the diagnosis is made and chemotherapy instituted. If the condition has been present for some time and the diagnosis has not been made the tubes may become very distended and blocked. Adhesions form in the surrounding structures and the tube may become filled with pus forming an *acute pyosalpinx*. The pus may escape from the tube into the peritoneal cavity giving rise to a pelvic abscess or an abscess may involve both the tube and the ovary, giving rise to a *tubo-ovarian abscess*. In puerperal or post-abortal infections the spread is along the lymphatics, but in cases of gonorrhoea the spread is along the mucous membrane. In gonococcal salpingitis there is not much thickening of the wall of the tube, but the plicae are very oedematous and they tend to become adherent causing blockage of the lumen (Fig. 36.10a). In the puerperal type the tubes are greatly thickened and the main lesion is in the muscle, which shows marked inflammatory change. The lumen on the other hand is much less affected and may appear even normal (Fig. 36.10b).

Clinical features

The onset is usually rapid and is characterized by acute pain and rigidity in the lower abdomen, a rapid pulse and marked pyrexia possibly with rigors. The symptoms can simulate acute appendicitis if the right tube is mainly affected. With appendicitis there may be a history of previous attacks of abdominal pain or chronic intestinal disturbance of long standing, but the most important differential point is that the pain of appendicitis starts around the umbilicus and moves to the right iliac fossa. In gonorrhoeal salpingitis there may be a history of purulent vaginal discharge and bladder irritation, but such history is not always obtained. In the puerperium or

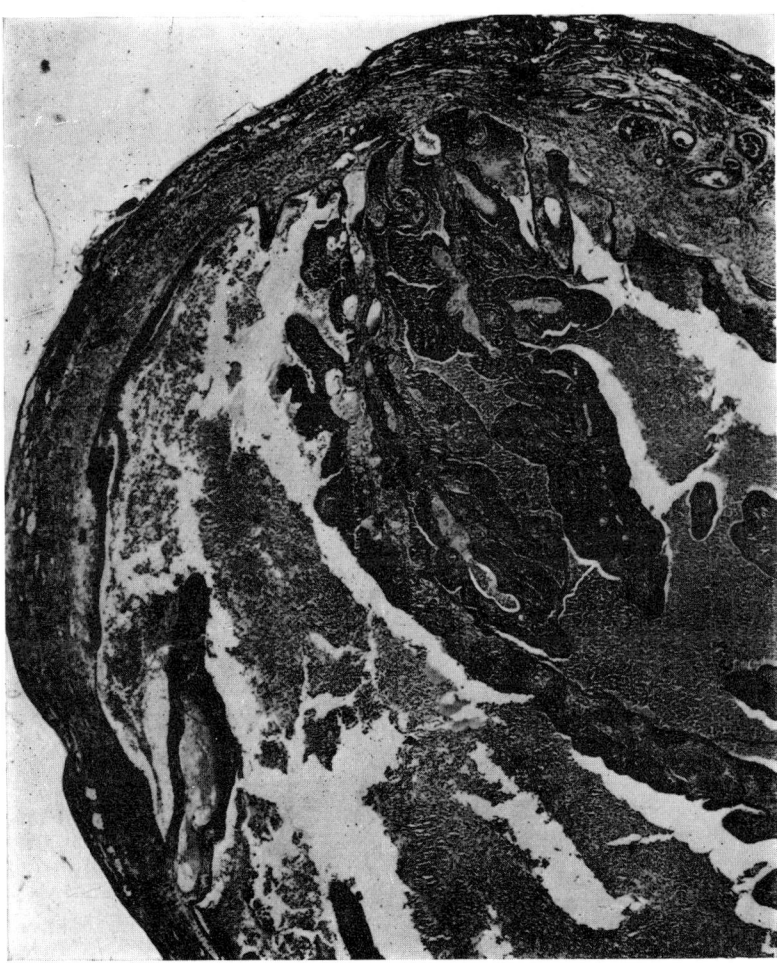

Fig. 36.10(a) and (b)   Photomicrographs of sections of Fallopian tube illustrating the striking difference in histology between the two types of salpingitis. The gonorrhoeal type (above) shows relatively normal muscle wall and distended lumen with oedematous inflamed rugae and purulent exudate. Here the infection originates from within the lumen.

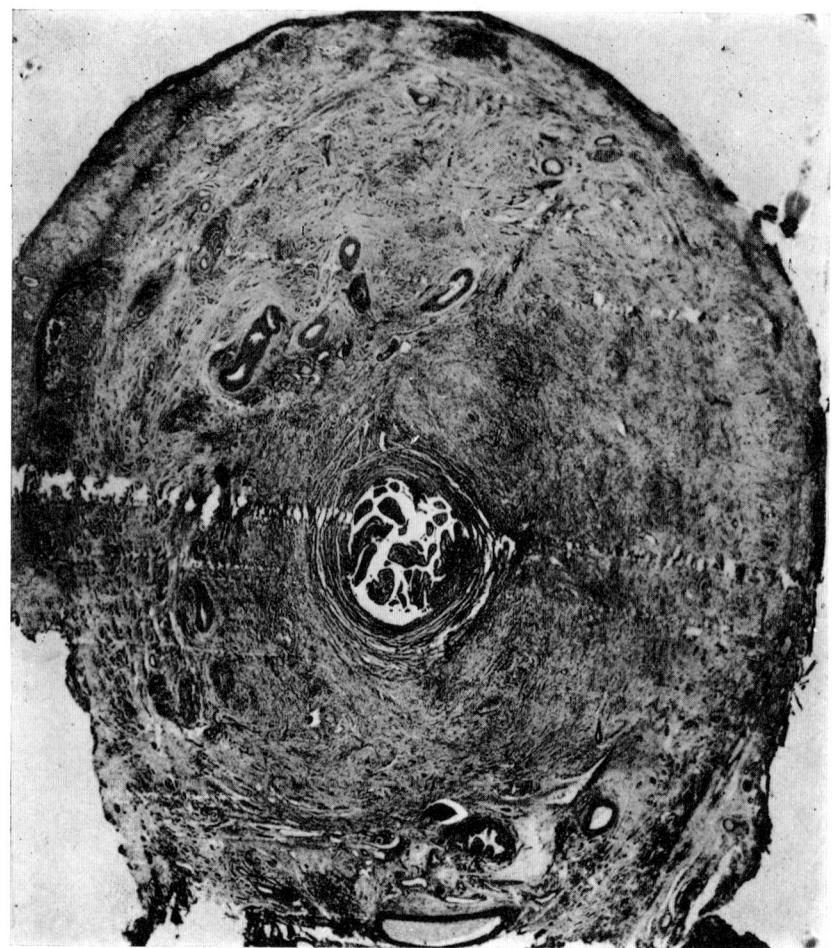

Fig. 36.10(a) and (b)   Photomicrographs of sections of Fallopian tubes illustrating the striking difference in histology between the two types of salpingitis. The puerperal type (above), where infection originates from without by means of the lymphatics, shows a relatively normal lumen but a greatly thickened muscle wall with cellular infiltration.

after an abortion the diagnosis of salpingitis is usually easy because of the history, but appendicitis does occasionally occur in the puerperium and the diagnosis may again be very difficult. Occasionally acute diverticulitis can cause difficulty in diagnosis, but usually there is a history of bowel trouble. It may sometimes be difficult to differentiate from an ectopic pregnancy, but the high pyrexia of salpingitis usually resolves the difficulty. The treatment of acute salpingitis is always conservative, but in cases of doubt about the diagnosis a laparoscopy or laporotomy is performed. The management of puerperal cases has already been described (p. 407). In gonococcal and non-puerperal cases dramatic

improvement occurs with chemotherapy. The only surgical treatment which should be necessary is the drainage of a pelvic abscess through the posterior fornix. Acutely inflamed tubes should rarely be removed and attempts to do so can be dangerous, even a pyosalpinx is best not removed in the acute stage because of the risk of spread of the infection. In time the pus is sealed off and becomes sterile. Antibiotic therapy should be instituted as quickly as possible. High vaginal or cervical swabs are taken and the organisms are typed, but while waiting for this to be done Penicillin and Streptomycin are recommended. If a gonococcal infection is suspected a urethral swab should be taken. Pain is relieved by giving Paracetomol (Panadol) or Pentazocine (Fortral), but if the pain is more severe and the diagnosis is definitely established then Pethidine can be given. If treatment is started promptly blockage and reduced mobility of the tubes can be prevented.

Chronic salpingitis

If an acute salpingo-oophoritis is treated early and adequately then there may be little or no residual damage, but in other cases chronic inflammatory lesions are formed. This late sequel of acute salpingitis can take the form of hydrosalpinx or pyosalpinx or chronic salpingo-oophoritis.

Chronic salpingo-oophoritis

The tubes and ovaries are thickened and sclerosed, but they may not be blocked. The walls are thickened but the tubes are not distended and the lumen is narrowed. The tubes and ovaries are covered with adhesions and are matted together in irregular masses. If there is nodular thickening in the tube wall then tuberculous salpingitis should be suspected.

PYOSALPINX
In this condition the tubes are filled with pus and both ends of the tubes are blocked. Because the ampullary portion can distend more than the isthmus the tube assumes a retort shape (Fig. 36.11). The fimbriae may be retracted or can be

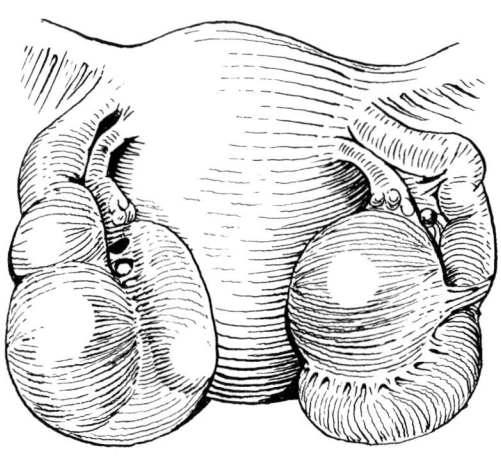

Fig. 36.11 Pyosalpinx showing the retort shape of the tubes due to the ampullary portion being more distended than the isthmus.

identified in the adhesions but sometimes only a dimple mark on the outer end of the tube marks the original ostium. The lesion is usually bilateral as the infection spreads from the uterus, but one tube is usually larger than the other. Dense adhesions may involve the reproductive organs, bowel, omentum and bladder. Because of the adhesions torsion of the tube cannot occur and they also help to prevent rupture of the tubes. Peritubal collections of pus sometimes form into large abscesses which can rupture into the bowel or into the general peritoneal cavity. The pus in the puerperal and gonorrhoeal types is usually thick and is odourless except in *B coli* infection. The pus becomes sterile in about two weeks, but organisms may survive for a longer time in the cellular tissues around the tubes.

HYDROSALPINX
This occurs either when the pus in a pyosalpinx changes to a watery fluid or can be the result of an infection of low virulence. Both tubes are generally affected and assume a retort shape like that of a pyosalpinx, but it is usually larger than a pyosalpinx. The distended tube may be large enough to be felt on abdominal palpation. The tubal epithelium becomes flattened and the plicae are reduced to small irregular ridges. Small retention cysts may be formed in the tube wall by adhesions between the plicae. The fluid in the tube is usually clear but occasionally it can be blood stained. It is almost always sterile. There is very little muscle tissue left in the thinned out tube wall. Usually there are fewer adhesions than are found with a pyosalpinx and the distended tubes are fairly mobile. Torsion can occur in a hydrosalpinx and cause the same symptoms as a twisted ovarian cyst. In a few cases the fluid from the distended tube escapes through the uterine ostium and passes out through the uterine cavity into the vagina. Infection of a hydrosalpinx from the bowel seldom occurs, and rupture of a hydrosalpinx is also rare.

Clinical features of chronic salpingo-oophoritis
The most characteristic feature of chronic salpingitis is recurrent attacks of abdominal pain. The pain can vary from pelvic discomfort to severe abdominal pain. Backache is also associated with the pelvic discomfort. In the early stages of the disease the recurrent attacks of pain are often associated with a rise of temperature to as high as 39·5 °C (103 °F). In more long standing conditions the fever may

be less marked or even absent. The attacks vary in intensity and in frequency. The pain is usually distributed over the whole of the lower abdomen, but it may be more acute on one side than on the other. The pain tends to be worse pre-menstrually. Irregular bleeding and menorrhagia are usually present and in long standing cases there is often general malaise and chronic ill health. The symptoms may be noted after a febrile puerperium, or shortly after marriage when a gonococcal lesion is suspected, particularly if there is a history of dysuria.

Physical examination
In severe cases there is marked abdominal tenderness with rebound pain. This may be more marked in one iliac fossa than the other. Pelvic examination may not be possible because of the acute pain. The uterus tends to be fixed and it is often retroverted. Irregular tender masses of variable size are found on each side of the uterus and often behind it. It is not usually possible to define the extent of the swelling because of the tenderness and the omentum or bowel might be adherent to the matted tubes and ovaries. During a quiescent phase, however, the swellings are much less tender and the matted tubes and ovaries can be outlined. A digital examination with the index finger in the vagina and the middle finger in the rectum sometimes makes the definition of the uterus and the tubes and ovaries easier. The white count is raised as is the ESR and anaemia may be present in long standing cases.

Differential diagnosis
During an acute exacerbation the chronic salpingitis may be confused with an acute appendicitis but in this condition the onset is usually more sudden and the pain and rigidity are more localized in the right iliac fossa. It is important to differentiate the two conditions because it is preferable not to operate on the tubes during the acute exacerbation and preferably a pyosalpinx should not be removed in the acute phase. Torsion of an ovarian cyst, hydrosalpinx or pedunculated fibroid will cause acute pain, but the onset is usually dramatic and the swelling is better defined in outline than an acute-or-chronic salpingitis and is unilateral. Pyrexia in such cases is usually slight. An ectopic pregnancy will also give unilateral signs, but may be difficult to differentiate particularly if the menstrual history is not characteristic. A unilateral hydrosalpinx will be difficult to differentiate, but the pyrexia, leucocytosis and raised ESR of acute salpingitis will help to differentiate. If there is no pyrexia it is justifiable to do a laparoscopic examination to try to determine the diagnosis.

Other acute intestinal lesions such as diverticulitis may resemble the acute phase of chronic salpingitis. If the diagnosis is still in doubt it is preferable to perform a laparotomy.

During the quiescent phase chronic salpingitis is likely to be confused with ovarian cysts if there are few or no adhesions. If on the other hand the chronic salpingo-oophoritis is associated with adhesions or the pelvic organs are bound down and fixed then the condition is very difficult to differentiate from pelvic endometriosis on examination. The history is usually of considerable help as symptoms following pregnancy or a gonorrhoeal infection point to an infective process while in endometriosis there is the history of pain of increasing severity associated with the periods. In both conditions the pain is related to the periods, but in endometriosis there is a gradual worsening of the pain over a period of months or years, whereas in salpingo-oophoritis the pain usually starts off severe and tends if anything to improve rather than worsen. Menorrhagia can be associated with both conditions. The degree of fixation of the pelvic tissues can be very much the same in the two conditions. If there are palpable nodules in the recto-vaginal septum however this is very suggestive of endometriosis. Often, however, neither history nor bimanual examination can differentiate between the two and this can only be done at the time of operation. An ectopic pregnancy is unlikely to be confused with chronic salpingo-oophoritis, but a partially absorbed pelvic haematocele with irregular thickenings particularly in the Pouch of Douglas may resemble chronic salpingitis. Ovarian tumours are not usually difficult to differentiate from chronic salpingitis, but an ovarian cyst may become infected, however, and it may be difficult to differentiate from a pyosalpinx.

In regional ileitis the thickened and oedematous bowel may become adherent to the pelvic organs and can closely simulate chronic salpingitis.

Treatment
During an acute exacerbation the case is

treated as for acute salpingo-oophoritis. Provided that there have not been frequent exacerbations conservative treatment should be carried out, but it is seldom completely effective. Treatment is by rest, antibiotic therapy and possibly short wave diathermy. This may allow the patient to carry on in satisfactory health without operation. If chronic salpingitis is causing persistent discomfort or pain or menorrhagia, or if there are recurring attacks of chronic salpingitis then permanent relief can only be obtained by operation. It is doubtful whether hysterosalpingography is justifiable in cases of chronic salpingo-oophoritis with thickening of the tubes because the procedure may cause an exacerbation of infection and even though the tubes are open it is doubtful whether they are functional and in any case salpingostomy is very unlikely to give good results in such cases. If attacks of acute inflammation recur it may be worth while combining corticosteroid therapy with antibiotic therapy, although the results in the long term are not very satisfactory. The adhesions of the tubes to the surrounding structures become more dense with each recurrence of inflammation and the patient's general health tends to become worse. Operation should not be unduly delayed in such cases as there is nothing to be gained, but it is important that the operation should be done during a quiescent phase. The best procedure is to carry out a total hysterectomy and bilateral salpingo-oophorectomy. If, however, some ovarian tissue appears healthy it should be conserved.

The various operations for this condition are described in Chapter 44.

PELVIC CELLULITIS

Acute cellulitis

Pelvic cellulitis can result from injury to the upper vagina and cervix during parturition or it can occur after pelvic surgery. This may occur in cases of lower segment Caesarean section or in gynaecological operations where the cellular tissues have been opened up and complete haemostasis has not been achieved. The infection usually remains confined or practically confined to the tissues of the pelvic floor, but occasionally cellulitis and salpingo-oophoritis occur concurrently. The cellular tissues may be damaged when dilatation of the

cervix is being carried out, particularly if there is difficulty in identifying the canal. The organisms usually found are varieties of anaerobic streptococci, staphylococci or B coli. The infection usually involves the paracervical tissues at the base of the broad ligament on each side of the cervix and also the cellular tissue in the space of Retzius between the anterior wall of the bladder and the symphysis pubis. The pelvic cellular tissues become increased in amount and more vascular during pregnancy. Infections in the puerperium can, therefore, spread very rapidly in the pelvic cellular tissues. The cellulitis may be limited to one side but usually it extends to the other side. Pelvic cellulitis seldom goes on to abscess formation with modern chemotherapy. Cicatrization may result causing fixity of the uterus. If an abscess should form it may point into the rectum or the vagina.

Clinical features
In the early stages before the condition becomes localized it may be difficult to distinguish from other infective conditions. In the puerperium there may be mild pyrexia which slowly worsens and the patient may have a rigor several days after delivery. There is usually pain on the affected side and the pulse is rapid. On vaginal examination the uterus is felt to be larger than normal for the stage of the puerperium and movement of the cervix causes pain. Fullness may be felt in the lateral fornices in the base of the broad ligament on the affected side, but it may be some days before definite induration can be detected. In cellulitis the fullness is usually felt in the anterior part of the pelvis. This is unlike a peritoneal infection where the fullness is likely to be in the posterior part of the pelvis.

Cellulitis following operations

This usually comes on early and there is a rise in temperature and pulse with pelvic pain. Examination at this time will reveal an effusion on the affected side. An infected haematoma of the vault following abdominal or vaginal hysterectomy is a common form of cellulitis. Drainage of the infected haematoma will readily relieve the condition. If pus forms then the temperature is high and of a swinging type and there may be constipation with painful defaecation and cystitis. The pelvic veins may become thrombosed. Extensive cellulitis is not likely to occur if adequate antibiotic therapy is started early, and if any pus formation is drained. If symptoms persist then it is likely that other organs have become involved. Antibiotic therapy usually prevents the formation of an abscess but if one forms, an incision should be made at its most dependant part and the best site may be the posterior vaginal fornix. When the abscess is larger and points above Poupart's ligament incision there is preferable. After the pus has been evacuated a rubber drainage tube is inserted.

Chronic pelvic cellulitis

There is a chronic inflammatory thickening of the transverse cervical and utero-sacral ligaments which may be the end result of acute cellulitis. This may have been sub-clinical or even unrecognized. There may be considerable scarring with displacement of the uterus which is usually rather fixed. Most cases of chronic pelvic cellulitis result from a spread of infection from the cervix and in such cases there is merely a thickening of the cellular tissue with congestion oedema and infiltration with leucocytes and plasma cells. The chief symptoms are pelvic pain, backache and dyspareunia. On examination thickening is felt on either side of the cervix or medially in the utero-sacral ligaments. The cervix may be thickened and lacerated and movement of it reproduces the pain of which the patient complains. If the utero-sacral ligaments are involved then they can be felt as two thickened ridges running backwards from the cervix, which may be displaced either backwards or to one side. Treatment is by antibiotic therapy, fucidic acid (Fucidin) 500mg tid is particularly useful; cauterization or repair of the cervix is carried out if necessary. A course of shortwave diathermy can be tried, but is not often successful and in many cases hysterectomy has to be performed.

INFECTIONS BY SPECIFIC ORGANISMS

Tuberculosis of the genital tract

With the fall in the incidence of tuberculosis in Britain and in many other parts of the world, genital tuberculosis has also become less common. It is still fairly common, however, in some tropical countries and amongst immigrants to this country, and it is important to bear this condition in mind, especially when dealing with cases of infertility. Most of the cases of pelvic tuberculosis were discovered in women complaining of infertility, indeed, even ten years ago the incidence was between 2 per cent and 5 per cent in women attending infertility clinics. The source of infection is either pulmonary or abdominal but in many cases the primary lesion is quiescent and may have been healed for some years. Other rare primary sites are bone and joint, neck, kidney or bladder and the infection may even be spread from a consort suffering from tuberculous epididymitis. In the great majority of cases genital tuberculosis is due to the human organism and only in a few to the bovine. The spread is either by the blood stream or from the peritoneum by direct spread or lymphatics from infected mesenteric glands.

The commonest pelvic sites are in the tubes or endometrium and it is very rare in the vulva, vagina or cervix. The Fallopian tubes are involved in about 90 per cent of cases and the endometrium is involved in about 50 per cent of cases, usually secondary to infection of the tubes.

TUBERCULOUS VULVITIS

There are two forms of this rare condition, the more common being the ulcerative and the other the hypertrophic form. Initially the vulva is indurated and swollen and then becomes ulcerated. The ulcers are usually multiple with yellowish bases and undermined edges. While the disease progresses in some areas there is healing in others with marked scarring. The inguinal glands may become involved and sinuses and fistulas may form. The rare hypertrophic condition occurs in adults and resembles elephantiasis but ulceration may also occur. Both the ulcerative and hypertrophic types of tuberculous vulvitis may be confused with carcinoma or venereal sores and a biopsy is necessary for diagnosis. Guinea pig inoculation and culture of the biopsy material should be performed as well as sensitivity tests and Wassermann reaction. The treatment is by chemotherapy as for tuberculous endometritis and salpingitis (see page 702).

TUBERCULOUS VAGINITIS

This can occur as a spread of infection from the vulva but is most commonly from the uterus or tubes. In addition to the ulcerative and hypertrophic type of lesions which occur on the vulva, there is also a miliary variety which is usually found in terminal cases. The ulcerative type can give rise to recto-vaginal or vesico-vaginal fistulas and the hypertrophic form resembles condylomata. Treatment is with prolonged chemotherapy.

TUBERCULOUS CERVICITIS

This can occur as a primary lesion but is usually secondary to tuberculosis of the uterus or tubes. Lesions may be either the typical ulcers or the hypertrophic type with papillary masses. Very rarely the tuberculous infection may be within the interstitial tissues of the cervix so that it becomes enlarged and swollen and ulceration does not occur until later.

There is usually an offensive discharge which may be blood stained and is very likely to be confused with a carcinoma of the cervix. The diagnosis is made on biopsy and treatment is again with prolonged chemotherapy.

TUBERCULOUS ENDOMETRITIS

Tuberculous infection of the uterus is usually associated with a tubal lesion.

As many of the cases are discovered in the course of infertility investigations, the lesion is often minimal with no abnormality found on pelvic examination. The pathological lesions in such cases are limited to the endometrium. The gland pattern appears normal and only a few tubercles may be found scattered in the stroma. As the disease advances in the uterus, giant cell systems form and may undergo caseation. The myometrium is involved and becomes thickened. As caseation progresses a pyometra may form.

Clinical features

About half of the cases of genital tuberculosis have no symptoms and patients complain only of infertility (Sutherland, 1966). The women are usually fit and young but in some cases there is a past history suggestive of pulmonary tuberculosis. No abnormality is found on pelvic examination and it is very important that such women should have an endometrial biopsy with negative results before any tests for tubal patency are performed.

Menstruation is usually normal but in some cases there is menorrhagia and in a few cases of advanced disease there is amenorrhoea. Pain is not a feature of tuberculous endometritis and it is only when the disease has spread to involve the tubes or other structures that pain develops. Pelvic examination is negative unless the infection has spread from the uterus. The

treatment of tuberculous endometritis, whether it is asymptomatic or not, is a full course of chemotherapy as described on page 702.

TUBERCULOUS SALPINGITIS

As already stated this is usually associated with tuberculosis of the endometrium and may present no clinical features but in advanced cases, there is gross distortion and distention of the tubes with adhesions and involvement of the ovaries.

Pathology

The tubes may show no gross abnormality and it is only on careful microscopic examination that the typical tubercles and giant cell systems and possibly acid fast bacilli will be found. In the grosser forms of the disease the lesions are of two types but in both as in other tubal infections, the condition is usually bilateral. In the first type, which is the most common, the mucosa of the tubes is first affected either from a blood or lymph borne infection. Initially the tubal lumen may remain patent but later becomes occluded. The walls of the tubes become thickened and the tubes become distended with caseous material. The swellings may become large and a tubo-ovarian abscess may form. Dense adhesions similar to those of endometriosis develop so that the bladder omentum, uterus, tubes and ovaries may become fixed together in a fibrous mass. In the second type the infection has spread from tuberculous peritonitis and the serous coat of the tube is affected first. There are typical tubercles studded over the peritoneal surface of the tubes and sometimes also of the ovaries, uterus and Pouch of Douglas.

Clinical features

The onset of the disease is usually insidious and there may be a history of lassitude, loss of appetite and perhaps night sweats for some time before more precise localizing symptoms of pelvic disease appear. As previously mentioned tuberculous salpingitis may be found on infertility investigation. The symptoms are similar to those of endometriosis with menorrhagia, vague lower abdominal pain and backache and dysmenorrhoea. As both conditions tend to be associated with infertility and occur in that same age-groups, the diagnosis can be difficult. Pyrexia, leucocytosis and a raised sedimentation rate, if present, are indicative of tuberculosis. On examination, there may be no abnormality found in the pelvis or at the other extreme, there may be a tender fixed mass filling the whole pelvis. In between there may be cases in which there are free adnexal masses suggesting ovarian cysts but in most cases with distended tubes there will be some fixity of the organs. Curettage of the endometrium with histological examination and guinea-pig inoculation will often clinch the diagnosis.

Treatment

Wherever possible surgery is avoided and is only employed when there has been a failure of chemotherapy or where the symptoms persist because of gross distortion of the pelvic organs and adhesions. If there are fistulas or sinuses it may be necessary to excise them surgically. If

are other sexually transmitted diseases due to viral, bacterial, fungal protozoal or parasitic infections, These give rise to non-specific urethritis, herpes genitalis, condyloma accuminata, trichomoniasis, scabies, pediculosis pubis, lymphogranuloma venereum, molluscum contagiosum, chancroid and granuloma inguinale. Lymphogranuloma venereum, chancroid and granuloma inguinale are rarely seen in the United Kingdom and are dealt with in the chapter on tropical gynaecology.

The incidence of sexually transmitted diseases has been increasing throughout the world in recent years and this is reflected in the figures from the Registrar General's Statistical Reviews for England and Wales from 1966 to 1971 (Table 36.1) showing a marked increase

Table 36.1 New Cases of Post-Pubertal Gonorrhoea from the Registrar General's Statistical Review for England and Wales

1966	1967	1968	1969	1970	1971
37 378	41 711	44 873	51 132	54 671	57 469

the ovaries are involved they must also be removed as well as the uterus and tubes. Fortunately most cases of pelvic tuberculosis respond to chemotherapy but the treatment must be continued for at least one year. The sensitivity of the organism is determined but the usual course which is given is streptomycin 1g and paraaminosalicylic acid 15g daily and isoniazide 100g thrice daily for one year, followed by PAS and INAH for a further year. The patient is then followed up for at least another two years and repeated histological and bacteriological examinations are made on the endometrium. This treatment is successful in over 90 per cent of cases and the adnexal masses are found to resolve or diminish greatly in size. A few successful pregnancies have been reported following such treatment but although some have reached full term the incidence of ectopic pregnancy and abortion is high. For at least the initial month of treatment the patient should be in a sanatorium.

Gonococcal infection

There is a large number of diseases which are spread during sexual intercourse and are rarely transmitted by other means. In addition to gonorrhoea due to *Neisseria gonorrhoeae* and syphilis due to *Treponema pallidum*, there

in gonorrhoea. The reason for this increase appears to be due to changes in sexual behaviour. There has been an increase in sexual intercourse at an early age, more pre-marital intercourse and possibly more promiscuity. Possibly, too, the use of the contraceptive pill rather than barrier methods of contraception with condoms, diaphragms or spermicides has also contributed to the increase in the incidence. The condom is particularly useful in preventing infection and should probably be recommended where casual sexual relationships are likely. Spermicidal agents are also of value as it has been shown that they are effective *in vitro* against T. Pallidum and N. gonorrhoea.

Clinical features

Gonorrhoea is the commonest of the sexually transmitted diseases and has a short incubation period. The symptoms appear in the male between two and ten days after intercourse with an infected person but it may take longer for symptoms to appear in the female. It must be remembered, however, that 30 per cent of women with gonorrhoea have no symptoms at all. They, of course, are the ones who are likely to affect other partners before they are traced and treated themselves.

When the organisms are introduced into

the genital tract by intercourse, they rapidly penetrate the columnar epithelium and become lodged in the submucous tissues. As squamous epithelium is much more resistant to the organisms, vulvitis and vaginitis are uncommon except in children. Infection may remain localized in the original site; this is usually in the Bartholin's or Skene's ducts, the urethra or the glands of the cervix. The infection may spread to the upper genital tract and involve the tubes. Mucous membranes elsewhere in the body, with the exception of the conjunctiva are rarely affected but occasionally cystitis, proctitis or pyelitis may occur. If the gonococcus invades the blood stream, distant lesions may develop particularly in the joints.

In the genital tract there is nearly always secondary invasion by streptococci, staphylococci or coliform organisms and these are responsible for most of the permanent tissue damage which occurs. Most infections remain localized to the vulva and cervix. The acute stage is overcome by local tissue reaction but some organisms may survive and lie dormant for a time particularly if there is inadequate drainage from the glandular tissue because of inflammatory oedema. There may be a flare-up of local infection in the infected gland and there can be a sudden spread to the upper genital tract. It is unusual for the infection to spread up to the Fallopian tubes at the time of the initial infection and gonococcal endometritis is uncommon. When acute infection occurs in the Fallopian tubes there is marked inflammatory reaction in the lining epithelium and spread into the stroma. The plicae of the tubes become adherent and pus is exuded into the lumen of the tubes. Acute salpingitis may subside with or without blockage of the lumen or else both ends of the tube may become blocked and give rise to a pyosalpinx. Peritoneal irritation and congestion occur in all these cases but tubo-ovarian abscesses or pelvic peritonitis develop only occasionally. Initially the gonococci multiply very rapidly and form considerable collections of pus. They are soon killed, however, by the products of their own metabolism and the pus becomes sterile in a few weeks.

Symptoms and signs

Urethritis is present in about 80 per cent of acute cases and there is frequency and dysuria but often this is quite slight. Initially it may be

severe and the urethra is tender on pressure. On inspection the mucous membrane of the urethra is pouting at the external meatus and is swollen and congested. Pus may be exuding from the canal and pressure on the urethra will cause pus to exude from the meatus.

Cervicitis occurs in most cases. It is often symptomless but patients may complain of lower abdominal discomfort or backache. A low grade pyrexia is not uncommon. On inspection the epithelium over the vaginal part of the cervix appears tense and congested. A muco-purulent discharge usually appears from the external os. When the condition becomes more chronic, the squamous epithelium may desquamate. There may be tenderness on palpation of the oedematous cervix.

Vulvitis is relatively rare in the adult but the vulva may become oedematous and congested as a result of purulent discharge from the cervix and urethra. Acute vulvo-vaginitis may occur in children. The infection may be transmitted by infected towels or may be transferred from an infected parent through handling. There is a profuse purulent discharge sometimes blood stained and the whole vulva is oedematous and inflamed. The labia minora may be excoriated or ulcerated, the urethra is usually involved and there is an acute vaginitis. Sometimes there is a general upset with pyrexia, malaise and inguinal adenitis but particularly in older girls discharge may be the only symptom. Organisms other than the gonococcus may cause similar clinical features although the gonococcal cases are the most severe.

Bartholinitis may occur in association with the urethritis and cervicitis at an early stage in the disease or it may occur in a more chronic form after the other local lesions have cleared up. The glands in the posterior third of the labia majora become markedly swollen and tender and abscesses form. The duct of the gland becomes blocked but in some cases a small bead of pus can be expressed on palpation of the gland. Bartholin's abscesses can be due to organisms other than the gonococcus.

Skene's ducts which open at the urinary meatus are often infected in association with the infection of the urethra.

Gonococcal salpingitis does not usually occur at the time of the initial acute infection, so that it usually presents in the same way as other cases of salpingitis due to other infecting organisms. Likewise chronic salpingo-oophoritis due to the gonococcus may not be distinguished from other causes of chronic salpingo-oophoritis because the organisms in such chronic cases have usually died off and the pus, on culture, is found to be sterile.

Diagnosis of gonorrhoea

Smears are collected from the sites of infection, preferably with a fine metal loop and the material spread on a glass slide and fixed by gentle heating. The slide is then stained with Gram's stain and the typical kidney-shaped Gram negative diplococci can be identified in the polymorphonuclear leucocytes. There are four types of Neisseria and sugar fermentation reactions are necessary to identify the N. gonorrhoeae. Other Gram negative organisms may cause confusion with the gonococcus so that examination by culture is essential. Specimens are collected on charcoal swabs and put into Stuart's medium for transporting and the cultures are set up on chocolate or blood agar.

The Gonococcal Complement Fixation Test is used to detect the presence of antibodies to the gonococcus. It is of most value in the chronic cases; it may be negative in the early acute cases. The test may remain positive for some time after treatment has been completed.

Fluorescent tests have recently been developed and may be of great value in the diagnosis of gonorrhoeal infection.

Treatment of gonorrhoea

Penicillin has, for many years, been the favourite antibiotic because of its effectiveness and lack of toxicity. The emergence of strains of gonococci which are relatively insensitive have necessitated the use of larger doses and also the use of substances to delay excretion. Oral penicillin preparations with slow release should not be used to treat gonorrhoea. Good results have been obtained with a single injection of 1·2 mega units of Procaine penicillin given in conjunction with 2g Probenecid orally which enhances the blood level by delaying excretion. Alternatively, a single injection of 1·25 mega units of Triplopen with cotrimoxazole or single doses of 2–4g of spectinomycin dihydrochloride or of 400mg of doxycycline can be used. As many as 30 per cent of patients suffering from gonorrhoea fail to come back to venereal diseases clinics after their first visit. The advantages of single dose treatment is therefore considerable, ensuring that as effective a cure rate as possible is achieved.

Syphilis

This is the most serious of the sexually transmitted diseases and its effect is much more general than in gonorrhoea where the principle effect is on the reproductive organs. The effects of syphilis are often much milder in females than in the male and as a result, as in gonorrhoea, the woman may be infected without having symptoms and the diagnosis is readily missed.

PRIMARY SORE

The primary sore or chancre may appear on the vulva, vagina or cervix. It is often missed either because its situation prevents it being seen or more often because it has disappeared before the patient comes for advice. It is typically circular and indurated with an eroded base and there is usually marked oedema of the surrounding tissues. It is usually single but multiple sores are more common in women than in men. It has a raised edge and there may be secondary infection. The primary lesion appears after an incubation period which ranges from 9 to 90 days. Although it appears ulcerated and swollen, it is quite painless. In most cases there is associated swelling of the regional lymph glands. The chancre may appear on the labia majora or minora at the base of the clitoris or on the vaginal walls where it usually takes the form of a fissure on the posterior wall. It may occur on the cervix and there it resembles a squamous carcinoma. The primary lesion heals spontaneously within two months and it may be overlooked if its significance is not realized and particularly if it occurs on the cervix.

Diagnosis

The characteristic chancre forms about three weeks after infection but as it is painless the patient may not consult the doctor until the inguinal glands become enlarged about two weeks later. The glands are discrete and rubbery in consistency and sometimes uncomfortable and tender. At this stage the most important diagnostic feature is the identification of the Treponema pallidum in the fluid expressed from the sore after cleansing the surface of the sore with saline solution. The serum from this sore is examined by the method of dark ground illumination.

If the specimen has to be sent to a laboratory, the serum should be drawn into a capillary tube which is then sealed at both ends. The spirochaetes have a characteristic appearance and remain motile for some hours after collection. Antibody tests such as the Wassermann reaction do not become positive until the sore has been present for two or three weeks and antibodies have formed.

SECONDARY LESIONS

Some six to eight weeks after the primary chancre appears the secondary changes occur. These changes take the form of papular lesions which involve the vulva and neighbouring skin. They take the form of condylomata lata and are raised, greyish white or livid growths with flattened surfaces. As the lesions become moistened with serous exudate the surfaces are rubbed off and shallow ulcers appear. On the inner surface of the vulva the usual secondary lesion is the mucous patch which appears as a sodden white area. There may be several patches present at the one time. They are also found on the vaginal wall and on the cervix. The typical hypertrophic flat-topped condylomata lata may spread extensively to cover the area around the vulva, the thighs and the perianal region to form large plaques.

Diagnosis

The lesions are highly infective and the Treponema pallidum can be identified on dark ground illumination of the exudate from the moist secondary lesions. The Wassermann test is positive in these cases. Newer tests such as the Reiter Protein Complement Fixation (RPCF) test and the Fluorescent Treponema Antibody (FTA) test are specific for antibodies from the Treponema pallidum, unlike the Wassermann test which is not so specific. Tertiary lesions, gummata and other lesions of tertiary syphilis have been reported in the vulva and uterus but they are extremely rare. The diagnosis is made by the specific antibody tests.

Treatment of syphilis

Both the primary and secondary stages of the disease can be cured by penicillin and other antibiotics. The latent stage of syphilis can last anything from two to twenty years and is symptomless. Routine blood testing may detect the disease in the latent stage and treatment then can cure or at least arrest the disease. Routine testing in Antenatal Clinics has led to the treatment of pregnant women and the reduction in the incidence of congenital syphilis. In early primary or secondary lesions the treatment is usually with procaine penicillin 600 000 units intramuscularly, daily for two weeks. Surveillance and serological testing is continued for two years after completion of the treatment and the serological tests should become negative in two to four months after beginning the treatment. It is usually recommended that a course of penicillin should be given during any subsequent pregnancy.

REFERENCES

Fluhmann, C. F. (1961) *The Cervix and its Diseases.* Philadelphia and London: Sanders.
Sutherland, A. M. (1966) Results of Treatment of Genital Tuberculosis in Women. In *Latent Female Genital Tuberculosis.* Basle: Karger, **196**.

FURTHER READING

Dickie, E. G. (1969) Herpes Vulvitis. *Obstet. Gynaec.*, **34**, 434.
Jeffcoate, T. N. A. (1966) Chronic Vulval Dystrophies. *Amer. J. Obstet. Gynec.*, **95**, 61.
Marshall, J. (1972) Sexually Transmitted Diseases. In *Mother and Child*, **44**, 65.
Nichol C. S. (1971) Venereal Disease in Women. *Brit. Med. J.*, **ii**, 328.

37. Displacements of the Uterus

The uterus normally lies in the pelvis with the corpus uteri bent forward on the cervix at a wide angle. In the erect posture, with the bladder empty, this anteflexion brings the body of the uterus almost horizontal and about one finger's breadth below the upper border of the symphysis pubis; it lies at an angle of about 60° to the vagina which runs in a direction parallel to the pelvic brim. The external os lies laterally in the pelvis, a little above the level of the ischial spines.

A line joining two points 1 inch above the ischial spines will be found to pass through the uterus at the isthmus. Round this transverse axis the uterus has freedom of movement, more particularly antero-posteriorly. Lateral movement is limited, as is also descent.

The term 'displacement' should refer only to an abnormal position of the whole organ. The uterus may be displaced upwards, downwards, backwards, forwards or laterally. Variations of the uterus are, however, usually included under the term 'displacement'. These are versions or departures from a normal direction of the uterine axis and flexions, or abnormal degrees or directions of the curvature of the axis. These may be forwards, backwards or lateral. Inversion is a turning inside-out of the uterus, which obviously involves downward displacement of the body of the uterus.

In some cases the displacement is primary and in others secondary; for example, the uterus may be displaced forward without alteration of its axis or curvature by a swelling in the Pouch of Douglas, such as a haematocele, a collection of encysted fluid or a new growth, or it may be wholly displaced backwards by a tumour in front of it, e.g. a dermoid or other cyst of the ovary, or a fibroid (Fig. 37.1), or it may be dragged backwards by the shrinkage of posterior adhesions. The lateral displacement may result from the pressure of a cyst or a fibroid growing between the layers of the broad ligament, or from cicatrization of uni-

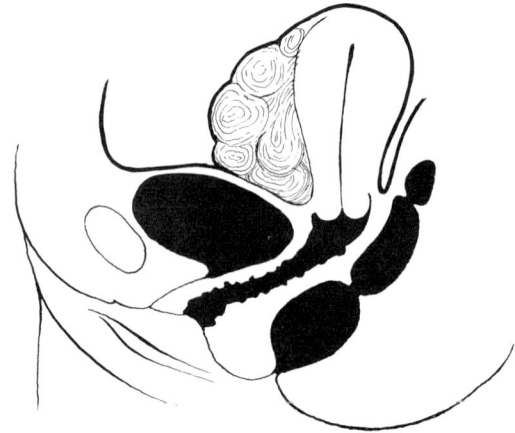

Fig. 37.1 Displacement of the uterus by an anterior wall fibroid.

lateral cellulitic exudates. Upward displacement occurs physiologically in the fourth month of pregnancy when the uterus becomes too large to be any longer contained in the pelvis; and pathologically, as a result of swellings below it, e.g. a haematocolpos or a cervical fibroid. In all such circumstances, it is the primary cause of the displacement, not the displacement *per se* which calls for treatment—at any rate in the first instance.

The anterior surface of the uterus (Fig. 37.2) rests on the upper surface of the bladder and as the latter organ fills up, the body of the

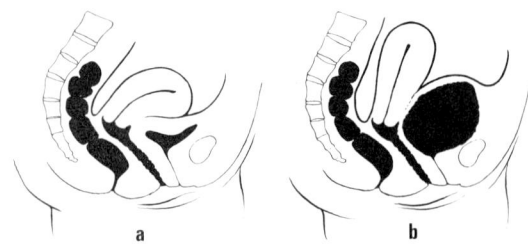

Fig. 37.2 Uterus in normal position.
(a) Bladder empty.
(b) Bladder full.

uterus is raised with it. Some coils of small intestine rest on the posterior or upper surface of the uterus. These conditions and intra-abdominal pressure prevent any sudden or extensive change of position of the uterus when the patient stands up or lies down. The urethra and the canal of the rectum, except in its last inch, run parallel to the vagina. These three canals—the urethra, the vagina and the rectum—are all supported by the fibres of the levatores ani muscle and by the processes of the pelvic fascia which encircle the walls of all three. The supports of the uterus are mainly two in number:

1. the fascial supports;
2. muscular supports.

The uterine ligaments and paracervical tissue are the main components of the fascial supports of the uterus. The ligaments are the broad and round ligaments which are already described in the anatomy chapter. The round ligament helps to keep the uterus in ante-version and the broad ligament keeps the uterus in its central position in the pelvis. The paracervical tissue is the portion of the parametrium surrounding the cervix, through which pass blood vessels including the uterine arteries, veins, nerves and lymphatics. This tissue forms a supporting framework for these vessels and nerves and constitutes the principal direct support of the uterus. The ureter also passes forward through it $\frac{1}{2}$–$\frac{3}{4}$ inch lateral to the cervix.

The paracervical tissue is composed of connective and fatty tissue with some smooth muscle fibres. Above, it is continuous with the parametrium in the base of the broad ligament; below, its fibres pass into the recto-vesical fascia. Posteriorly, two special bundles pass back to be attached to the anterior surface of the lower portion of the sacrum and form the utero-sacral ligaments. Anteriorly, a thin layer passes forward beneath the base of the bladder to be inserted into the posterior surface of the pubis—the pubo-cervical fascia. The strongest development of this tissue is found laterally—the transverse cervical ligaments—which form a chief support of the uterus in the pelvis. The spread of infection or malignant disease from the cervix to the paracervical tissue causes fixation of the uterus. At the operation of hysterectomy, abdominal or vaginal, the uterus cannot be pulled up or down freely unless paracervical tissue has been divided.

MUSCULAR SUPPORTS

1. Muscles of the pelvic diaphragm

These muscles—the levatores ani and coccygei —and the superimposed recto-vesical fascia have been described. This muscular shelf runs from each side of the pelvis in front of the rectum, vagina and urethra at some distance below the cervix. It has no attachments to the uterus and therefore does not act as a direct support of the uterus, but it maintains the rectum and vagina in position.

2. Perineal muscles

The perineal muscles keep the vaginal orifice and the anus closed—they do not act as direct supports to the pelvic viscera. They contract during sexual intercourse and defaecation, and are overstretched and frequently torn during parturition.

PROLAPSE OF THE UTERUS AND VAGINAL WALLS

Descent of the vaginal walls is so intimately associated with uterine descent that the two must be considered together. Prolapse of the uterus does not occur without some prolapse of the vaginal walls, while the uterus remains in its normal position. Many patients are referred to hospital with a diagnosis of prolapse of the uterus, when the vaginal walls alone have come down.

If the prolapse of the uterus is so marked that the body of the uterus projects outside the vagina, the term 'procidentia' is often applied.

Aetiology
The primary cause is injury to the para-cervical tissue. If the fetal head is pulled through a partially dilated cervix by the use of forceps or the Ventouse extractor, this tissue may be stretched or torn even if the cervix itself remains undamaged. The number of cases of prolapse of the uterus resulting from this type of aetiology is declining due to improvements in obstetric care. In many cases, however, prolapse occurs in women who have had spontaneous deliveries and in some this is thought to be due to bearing down efforts before the cervix is fully dilated. Furthermore, the passage of a large baby may also overstretch the vaginal tissues and result later

in prolapse. Timely episiotomy may help to prevent this. Early rising after childbirth has been cited as a cause. This is probably not the case provided that early rising does not mean the patient returns to work or household duties more quickly. Any condition which increases intra-abdominal pressure is likely to cause prolapse. These may be chronic bronchitis, or long-standing constipation.

In many cases no predisposing factors can be found and in these the general body tone may be poor and laxity of muscles is one aspect of this.

The symptoms of prolapse most usually occur after the menopause even though the structural damage primarily responsible may have occurred at childbirth many years previously. This is due to the general atrophy of supporting tissue which occurs at the time of the menopause and the supports of the uterus become inefficient and unable to support the organs.

Prolapse is also most common in the poor socio-economic groups due to a combination of excessive manual work and frequent childbearing. This causal factor is also diminishing now.

Very occasionally uterine prolapse occurs in nulliparous women. A severe accident may cause the paracervical tissue to be wrenched or torn, but more often the prolapse is due to laxity of the uterine support and tissues following the menopause. This type of prolapse often occurs suddenly after some violent movement such as moving a heavy piece of furniture.

A neoplasm in the lower abdomen may also push the uterus down. These factors may be primary causes of the prolapse but increase in severity of the condition is aggravated by increased intra-abdominal pressure. When the uterus becomes tilted backwards, as it does in the first stage of prolapse, the small intestines come to lie on its anterior surface and it is thus placed at a greater mechanical disadvantage in resisting pressure from above.

LOCAL SIGNS OF PROLAPSE

In the puerperium, the uterus, which is heavier than normal, sags in the pelvis and this stretches the paracervical supports. The fundus tends to lie backwards in the long axis of the pelvis, and this may be the first stage in the development of prolapse. Once the long axis of the uterus lies in the axis of the vagina, descent may continue until the cervix reaches

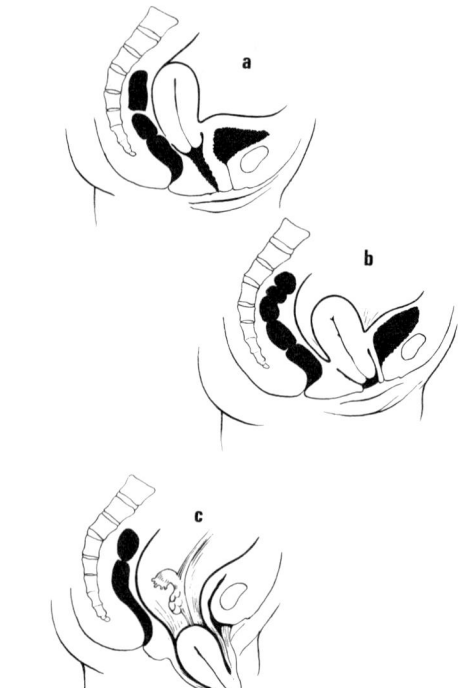

Fig. 37.3   (a) First degree prolapse.
(b) Second degree prolapse.
(c) Procidentia.

the vaginal orifice—the second degree of prolapse. When the cervix protrudes through the orifice then there exists the third degree of prolapse. If further descent occurs the uterus ultimately lies completely below the level of the vulva inside a sac of the vaginal wall. This is called the fourth degree of prolapse, but is more commonly referred to as procidentia. Anteriorly, the bladder is dragged down because of its attachment to the vaginal wall and cervix. If a sound is introduced to the urethra the tip of the bladder can be demonstrated almost at the end of the cervix in procidentia.

As the uterus prolapses, it also pulls down the posterior fornix and the vaginal wall, without necessarily dragging the rectum with it, since the posterior wall is only loosely attached to the rectum, except at its lower part. The pocket of peritoneum which forms the pouch of Douglas also descends. In procidentia, there is therefore a hernia of the uterus through the pelvic diaphragm, dragging with it the bladder in front and the posterior vaginal wall behind. Fallopian tubes, ovaries and coils of intestine may be included in the large prolapsed sac.

When the patient lies down, replacement of the procidentia into the vagina can be done, but congestion and oedema, which result from mechanical stasis or infection, may make replacement difficult. If the condition is neglected for a long time, replacement may be impossible.

The external os is at first oedematous owing to the congestion produced by the change in course of the uterine vessels; this oedema gives place later to hypertrophy. The cervix may be the seat of old lacerations and mucus from endocervical glands may flow from the external os. If the condition is persistent the vaginal skin becomes much thickened, dry and leathery. Rubbing of the patient's clothing and walking causes ulceration, especially on the lower part of the anterior vaginal wall and cervix. These ulcers associated with procidentia will heal spontaneously when the prolapse is reduced and maintained in the vagina. This can usually be achieved by keeping the patient in bed and packing the prolapse with a pack soaked in medicated solution such as Flavine and paraffin emulsion. In some cases, these ulcers may be malignant, but this is relatively uncommon. The stage in the process of uterine prolapse can best be seen by asking the patient with a procidentia to strain. When this is done the vaginal wall just behind and above the urethral orifice first appears at the vulva. It is followed by the rest of the anterior wall from below upwards and then the cervix appears. When the cervix is completely extruded the whole of the anterior wall is exposed. As the cervix passes through the vulva it pulls the upper part of the posterior vaginal wall with it and eversion of this wall is completed from above downwards.

Prolapse of the vaginal walls

We have seen that when the uterus prolapses, the vaginal walls accommodate this descent. Injury or overstretching of the fibres of the levatores muscle and of the pelvic fascia which encircle the vagina, may result in prolapse of the vaginal walls even though the uterus still remains at its normal level in the pelvis.

CYSTOCELE

Prolapse of the anterior vaginal wall, cystocele, is always associated with descent of the bladder

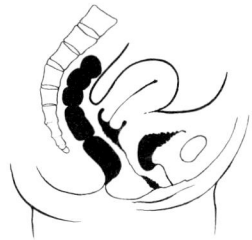

Fig. 37.4 Cystocele. Anterior vaginal wall including bladder bulging into vagina.

since the bladder wall and vagina are closely attached.

The support of the floor of the bladder is much less secure than that of the uterus. Fibres pass forwards from the paracervical tissue below the base of the bladder and are inserted into the posterior surface of the symphysis pubis. This fascial plane is known as the pubo-cervical fascia and fibres from the levatores ani muscles with the recto-vesical fascia complete the support. It is a relatively thin structure and these tissues are easily overstretched or torn during parturition. When the bladder is full during the second stage of labour, forceps extraction or even spontaneous delivery may weaken the supports of the bladder and cause cystocele.

In spontaneous delivery the protrusion of part of the vaginal wall in front of the head may be a basic cause of cystocele. In many cases the development of cystocele is encouraged by damage to the perineum. In a nulliparous woman the vagina is at an angle of 60° to the horizontal, and its anterior wall is supported by the posterior vaginal wall at the perineal body. If the perineum is torn the anterior vaginal wall loses much of its normal support and therefore tends to extend more easily. Cystocele may occur, however, with an apparently intact perineum and bearing down for an unduly long time with the head on the perineum, may be a cause of damage to the vaginal walls. This can be prevented by correct timing of episiotomy.

The extent of the cystocele can be gauged by asking the patient to strain as she lies on her back with knees apart and the labia separated. The anterior wall descends as already described.

RECTOCELE

If the perineum is torn and the supports of the posterior vaginal wall have previously been

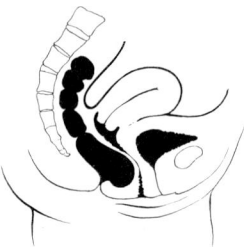

Fig. 37.5 Rectocele. Posterior vaginal wall bulging into vagina and including rectum.

stretched during childbirth, there is a tendency for the posterior vaginal wall to bulge downwards when the patient strains at stool or increases the intra-abdominal pressure in another way. The swelling (rectocele) contains bowel and if it is large may hinder emptying of the rectum. Prolapse of the uterus, however, can occur without any descent of the rectal wall. In some cases the upper part of the posterior vaginal wall and the upper part of the rectum may come down when the lower part of both remains in normal position. Usually where the cervix projects from the vaginal orifice, the pouch of Douglas descends with it and may be opened into when the cervix is amputated during operations to cure prolapse.

The conditions which aggravate rectocele are similar to those which have been described for cystocele—hard manual work, bronchitis and straining at stool.

ENTEROCELE

The pouch of Douglas and its contents may relate to the posterior fornix especially where

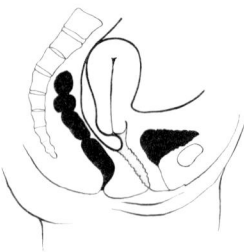

Fig. 37.6 Enterocele. Hernia of Pouch of Douglas into posterior fornix of vagina.

the pouch of Douglas is unusually long. This is usually seen in association with a prolapse of the uterus and vaginal walls, but on occasion is present alone. Sometimes it is seen after an operation for prolapse since the condition,

although present at the time, is not recognized and only becomes obvious after the prolapse of the uterus and vaginal walls has been cured. Modern operative techniques where the hernial sac is obliterated or removed and where the utero-sacral folds are approximated, will usually prevent such an occurrence.

Hypertrophic elongation of the supra-vaginal portion of cervix

In prolapse there is usually (Fig. 37.7) considerable enlargement of the cervix. This is

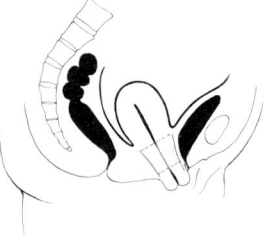

Fig. 37.7 Hypertrophic elongation of the supra-vaginal cervix.

associated, in the first place, with oedema and later with chronic inflammatory changes in the tissues. These changes affect, most particularly the vaginal portion of the cervix. As the prolapse becomes more severe, an overgrowth and/or elongation of the supra-vaginal portion of cervix may occur. This may become so marked that the external os protrudes at the vulva without descent of the uterine body occurring. This condition is sometimes wrongly diagnosed as uterine prolapse.

In this condition, the vaginal portion of the cervix is pushed down and carries with it the vaginal walls so that both the anterior and posterior fornices become shallower than normal. This condition is sometimes called vault prolapse. When the patient strains, the tip of the cervix appears at the vulva before the vaginal walls have become everted.

Clinical features and diagnosis
In the various types of prolapse the patient usually has the feeling of a lack of support in the pelvis. She complains of a 'bearing down' sensation and often a dragging pain in the back referred to the upper sacral region. She may say that she has 'something coming down', but this may also be due to other conditions. She may have difficulty in walking if the procidentia is very marked. In many cases the

discomfort does not become troublesome until she is over-tired, mainly through remaining too long in the standing position. Procidentia rarely causes pain, more discomfort, and sometimes remarkably little, so that women with very large procidentia may have little pain or discomfort. A woman may often tolerate procidentia for many years and it is frequently some other symptom such as slight bleeding which makes her consult her doctor. This bleeding is frequently due to simple ulceration but the patient is afraid that cancer may have developed.

Disturbances of micturition associated with prolapse

These may be troublesome in prolapse. The descent of the cervix causes a pocket of bladder to lie at a lower level than the urethra, thus preventing emptying of the bladder. Residual urine may result in cystitis in a patient with procidentia. Occasionally she may be unable to pass urine until she presses up the prolapsed mass with her fingers. Frequency of micturition and nocturia may also occur.

Stress incontinence

Stress incontinence (Fig. 37.8) of urine is frequently associated with varying degrees of

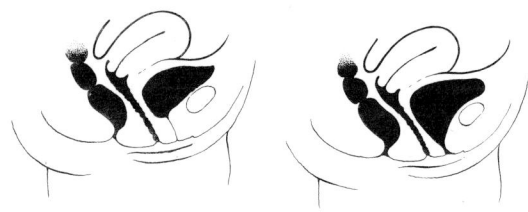

Fig. 37.8   Stress incontinence. Note absence of normal urethrovesical angle.

prolapse, although it may occur without any demonstrable laxity of the vaginal walls. The patient passes a small quantity of urine whenever her stress leads to increased intra-abdominal pressure. Coughing and sneezing, sudden movements, or even walking, may cause leakage of urine. This condition should always be asked about in all patients complaining of prolapse. It is said to be due to damage to the base of the bladder during childbirth. This results in the urethro-vesical angle function being poorly supported and more or less permanently in the position where

micturition occurs. A slight increase, therefore, in intra-abdominal pressure causes the flow of urine through the urethra.

URGENCY OF MICTURITION

The patient has a frequent and urgent desire to void urine and she may lose control if delay occurs. Sometimes the symptoms are due to chronic urinary infection and may disappear if this is treated, but recurrence may be troublesome.

In many cases, however, no cause can be found and the condition is described as functional, usually of unknown aetiology. In this condition cystoscopy is usually essential to check that there is no other abnormality of the bladder. Some cases of urgency in post-menopausal women may be due to lack of oestrogen since the bladder takes part to some extent in the post-menopausal atrophy of the genital tract. Sometimes a small dose of oestrogen for a period of one month may be helpful in treating the so-called functional conditions of the bladder in post-menopausal women.

Conditions which (Fig. 37.9) simulate pro-

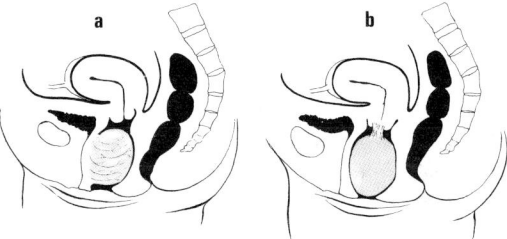

Fig. 37.9   Conditions which may simulate prolapse.
  (a) Vaginal cyst.
  (b) Cervical polyp.

lapse are a fibroid polyp, hypertrophy of the cervix and cystic or solid tumours of the vaginal walls. Prolapse of the rectum can sometimes be confused with uterine prolapse.

Hypertrophy of the cervix

Hypertrophy of the supra-vaginal portion of the cervix and its relation to uterine prolapse has already been described. Hypertrophy of the vaginal portion of the cervix may also occur and the cervix is then found to be broad and irregular. The vaginal fornices are of normal depth and the fundus is at its normal level. There is no appreciable descent of the cervix when the patient strains. In the case of hypertrophy of the vaginal portion of the cervix of congenital origin, the cervix is smooth in outline and conical in shape.

Treatment of prolapse

The surgical pathology of the various types of prolapse make it obvious that no form of treatment other than surgical can cure the condition. The cases which require special consideration here are those in which other circumstances, e.g. pregnancy, extreme debility or old age, render the operation inadvisable. In such cases palliative measures have to be employed.

Pessaries of various kinds can be used to treat the prolapse, but since the pessary is a foreign body in the vagina it may act as an irritant and cause inflammation. It does not strengthen the tissue of the vagina, but stretches them and thus probably prevents muscular contraction of the vagina. Regular visits are required to have the ring removed and cleaned and vaginal douching may sometimes be recommended. Frequently, some get tired of this requirement and even though they refuse operation at first, may change their minds later. Pessary treatment, therefore, should be reserved for only those who are unwilling or unsuitable for operation, or as a temporary measure in younger women who have not yet completed their families.

With the increasing interest in geriatrics and the attempt to keep old people mobile and independent for as long as possible, operation is much more common now in elderly women. Improvements in anaesthesia and surgical techniques have rendered such operations much safer, but the risks of vascular accident, etc., make the operation less safe than in younger women. Home circumstances, the patient's attitude and the severity of the symptoms are factors to be taken into consideration when deciding whether operation is the obvious measure to be used.

When a woman with a prolapse desires further children, special consideration has to be given as to the best form of treatment. If pregnancy follows a repair operation, especially if amputation of the cervix has been performed, there is an increased risk of abortion, early rupture of the membranes and premature onset of labour. Labour may also be prolonged if the cervical stump is fibrotic and will not dilate normally. There is also a risk of rupture if the scarred cervix tears and this rupture may extend into the lower uterine segment and cause serious bleeding. Caesarean section may therefore be indicated as the mode of delivery in a patient who has undergone a previous repair operation. This is particularly so when the operation has been done for stress incontinence since, if this type of patient has a subsequent vaginal delivery, the likelihood of recurrence of stress incontinence is very high.

During the early months of pregnancy, the prolapse may become worse, temporarily due to softening of the tissues. Pessary treatment may be helpful at this stage and the pessary can be removed by about the 16th–18th week when the uterus has become an abdominal organ and will not fall into the pelvis. Two types of pessary are available—the rigid polyethylene pessary and the soft polyvinyl pessary. The former is thin and made of rigid plastic; the latter is thick and malleable, being made of a vinyl plastic material. A flexible pessary is easy to insert as it can be compressed and is less likely to cause discomfort from pressure on the vagina. However, in some cases it is not rigid enough and readily falls out. These circular pessaries act by stretching the vaginal walls and are usually effective in relieving symptoms. If, however, the perineum is deficient, they are frequently expelled as soon as the patient bears down, particularly if she is constipated.

The rigid pessary is probably most suitable as a temporary measure in young women since the tissues are much more resilient and the vaginal orifice, even if not patulous, will stretch sufficiently to allow the pessary to be inserted. In old women, this may not be possible and the malleable pessary has to be used as it slips easily through the vaginal orifice.

Unless vaginal discharge is a problem, douching is hardly required. If a douche is recommended, plain water or a mild antiseptic solution such as 2 per cent lactic acid could be used. A strong antiseptic or an alkali should not be recommended as this may lead to vaginitis and the patient may develop a rash. A neglected pessary may ulcerate deeply into the vaginal wall and become overgrown by vaginal skin. If this occurs, it must be dissected out, a segment removed and the pessary extracted.

The surgical treatment of prolapse is a successful and safe procedure and gives a high rate of cure (about 85 per cent). The operation aims at reconstructing the vagina by removing redundant mucosa, amputating the hypertrophied cervix and reconstructing the various ligaments and fascial planes which surround the uterus. In many cases, vaginal hysterectomy is combined with a plastic repair procedure for the cure of prolapse. Particular attention must be paid to the paracervical tissue, the chief supports of the uterus and vaginal vault. Where possible, the reconstructed vagina should be of normal length and width. These operations are fully described in Chapter 45. Pelvic floor exercises may help to strengthen the supports. Following operation the patient should be advised against any heavy lifting or strenuous exercise in order to avoid recurrence of the prolapse.

Backward displacement of the uterus

These fall into three main groups: retroversion, retroflexion and combined retroversion and retroflexion.

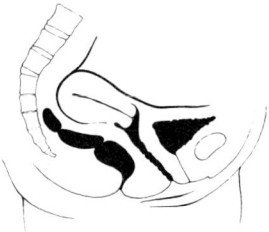

Fig. 37.10   Retroverted uterus.

Retroversion may be congenital or acquired. Retroflexion is almost invariably acquired.

Pre-pubertal retroversion—the normal position of the uterus in the child is more or less vertical. At the approach of puberty it begins to assume adult characteristics, including not only the increase in size and the change in the relative proportions of the cervix and body, but also the anteverted and slightly anteflexed attitude. It may, however, assume the ante-retroverted position and this is thought to occur in about 20 per cent of women.

Acquired retroversion is most frequently a sequel to parturition but may also be caused by shrinkage of posterior adhesions or by the pressure or weight of a tumour. Occasionally, it is caused by some accident.

1. Puerperal retroversion is due to the heavy involuting uterus combined with the laxity of uterine supports which have been stretched during pregnancy and labour.

If this retroversion is not recognized and corrected at an early stage, delay in the involution of the uterus may occur and it remains bulky and congested. Although it may be possible at a later date to antevert the uterus manually and keep it in this position with a pessary, it will frequently become retroverted again as soon as the pessary is removed.

2. The contraction of inflammatory adhesions between the fundus and the rectum, or the back of the pelvis, may draw the uterus into the position of retroversion or retroflexion.

3. The weight of a fibroid or other tumour, particularly on the posterior aspect of the fundus uteri may draw the uterus into a retroverted position.

SYMPTOMATOLOGY

Very careful review of the symptoms is necessary before attributing the complaint to retroverted uterus, since some 20 per cent of women seem to have their uterus in this position without complaint. If somebody of a neurotic temperament is told that her uterus is 'lying back', then it may be extremely difficult to help her. It should also be remembered that the retroverted uterus can function perfectly normally and only if it seems to be the likely cause of the symptoms should the condition be mentioned.

Most cases of retroversion have no symptoms at all. When possible symptoms are present, an effort should be made to find out if these are caused by the retroversion and whether correction will relieve the symptoms. Dyspareunia and backache are symptoms which are frequently associated with retroversion, but the former may be more particularly due to prolapsed ovaries, which accompany the condition. Backache may also be due to many other causes. Dysmenorrhoea is not usually due to retroversion, although it may be associated with it in conditions such as pelvic inflammatory disease and endometriosis. While some women who complain of infertility have retroverted uteri and become pregnant if the retroversion is corrected, it is doubtful whether retroversion is commonly responsible for this or for menstrual upset or abortion.

Diagnosis

At bimanual examination the cervix is directed downwards or forwards depending whether the condition is a retroversion or a retroflexion. The body of the uterus is felt in the posterior fornix and the differential diagnosis depends on the fact that it is continuous with the cervix and moved when the cervix is pressed up. Its size is not easy to assess, but if the cervix is moved backwards or forwards, some idea of the weight of the uterus and its size can be obtained. It is also important to determine whether the uterus is fixed in its abnormal position or not. This is done by trying to push up the fundus with the fingers in the posterior fornix. It may also be useful to have a finger in the rectum at this stage. If there is any tenderness it possibly suggests a degree of infection and it is better to re-examine the patient later under anaesthesia. If, under anaesthesia, the uterus springs back to its previous position after the pressure of the finger is removed, adhesions probably exist.

Differential diagnosis
The diagnosis has to be made from tumours and inflammatory masses in the pouch of Douglas or collections of blood clot. If there is any doubt about the diagnosis, the patient should be examined under an anaesthetic and a sound passed when the direction of the cavity of the uterus can be determined.

Treatment
It is essential to decide first of all whether the retroverted uterus is in fact causing symptoms. It is frequently wise not to mention the condition to the patient unless it is thought to be definitely causing symptoms. If a patient complains of infertility or dyspareunia or when the backward displacement is accompanied by prolapse of the ovaries, the position should be corrected and a pessary test applied. Only if the pessary test is positive should an operation be considered.

Replacement of the mobile, retroverted uterus—this can be done (1) digitally; (2) with the aid of a Volsellum; (3) with the aid of a sound. An anaesthetic may be necessary.

1. Digital correction is performed by placing two fingers in the posterior fornix of the vagina and pressing up the fundus of the uterus. As soon as the organ reaches the correct position, the external hand should be pressed behind it and the vaginal fingers slipped into the anterior fornix and used to bring the cervix backwards and upwards.

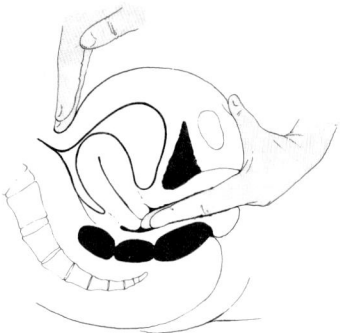

Fig. 37.11   Digital correction of retroverted uterus.

2. The procedure may be aided by gripping the anterior lip of the cervix with the Volsellum and drawing the uterus downwards. The point of the Volsellum should then be directed back into the hollow of the sacrum and made to pass upwards following the curve of the sacrum, while the external hand presses the abdominal wall over the fundus as before.

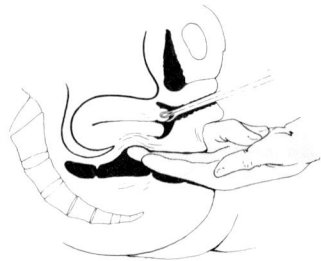

Fig. 37.12   Correction of retroversion with volsellum forceps.

3. The use of the sound is the least desirable method, as it may perforate the uterus. It should always be preceded by careful examination to make certain that no pregnancy exists. A sound is then passed

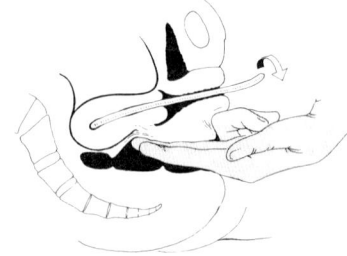

Fig. 37.13   Correction of retroversion using a uterine sound.

into the retroverted uterus with the point directed backwards (it is best to try to bring the uterus forward with a dilator of about No. 10 Hegar size. Using this, it is unlikely that perforation will occur). The handle of the dilator made to describe half of a large circle so as to minimize movement of the point. When the point is directed forward, the uterus is gently eased into the anteverted position and held there by depression of the hand on the abdominal wall.

INTRODUCTION OF THE PESSARY

The Hodge pessaries are suitable for this condition. To gauge the size of the instrument,

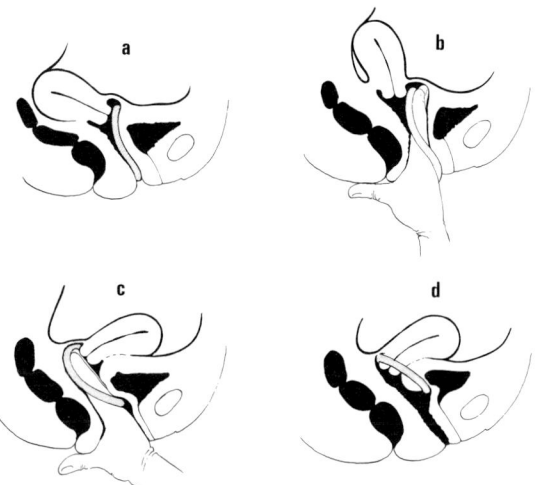

Fig. 37.14   Use of a Hodge pessary for the treatment of retroversion.

      (a) Introduction.
      (b) Insertion of the finger behind the pessary.
      (c) Finger and pessary bar in posterior fornix.
      (d) Pessary in correct position.

the length of vagina from the posterior fornix to the lower border of the symphysis pubis should be measured with the fingers. The smallest pessary which will retain the uterus in position should be used. With the instrument in position there should just be room to introduce the tip of the finger between the lower bar and the back of the symphysis pubis and when a well-fitted pessary is in position the patient should not be conscious of its presence.

Introduction of a pessary—the instrument is introduced by its transverse axis obliquely so as to pass easily through the vaginal introitus. It should then be rotated to lie trans-

versely in the vagina with its concave forwards. The finger should then be passed into the vagina behind the pessary which will now have its upper bar in the anterior fornix. The gauge slips this back into the posterior fornix where it should lie. In this position, the pessary is supported by the back of the symphysis pubis and the perineum. Its upper end gently stretches the utero-sacral ligaments and therefore pulls the cervix up towards the sacrum. The intra-abdominal pressure maintains the position of anteversion. The patient may then continue her normal work and no restriction of coitus is necessary. If she feels any discomfort or should the pessary come out, she should be asked to consult her doctor.

The operative treatment of retroversion is considered in Chapter 45.

Inversion of the uterus

This condition, when (Fig. 37.15) the uterus is turned inside out, is one of the types of displacement of the uterus. It is rare and usually

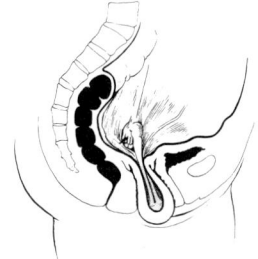

Fig. 37.15   Inversion of uterus.

occurs during the third stages of labour and at this time is called acute inversion. In a few cases, however, the complication escapes notice at that time because of the absence of symptoms and is later discovered, when it is known as chronic inversion.

Very occasionally, inversion may occur apart from pregnancy if a fibromyoma or sarcoma growing from the fundus of the uterus is driven through the cervix and drags the fundus with it.

Chronic puerperal inversion

This is a rare condition where the uterus involutes in its inverted position, but remains in the vagina as a soft swelling, which bleeds readily to touch, and shows dark areas of superficial ulceration. Its surface is usually dark in colour but in old standing cases the columnar epithelium of the uterine wall may become converted into a stratified squamous epithelium and become lighter in colour.

Sometimes one or both tubes and ovaries are dragged into the inverted sac. If infection of the endometrium spreads to the peritoneal surface of the uterus, the inner walls of the sac, tubes and ovaries may become sealed together, thereby preventing reduction. Very occasionally, a loop of intestine may enter the sac immediately after the occurrence of the inversion and become obstructed.

The patient complains of irregular bleeding and a mucoserous or mucoprurulent vaginal discharge and has a feeling of something coming down. The haemorrhage and infection lead to general ill health.

Diagnosis
A large globular body is found in the vagina.

Above the swelling, the ring of the cervix may be felt. An important sign is identification of the abdominal wall of the cup-shaped depression which represents the ring through which the fundus has descended. An anaesthetic may be required before this can be determined.

A fibroid polypus projecting through the cervix may stimulate inversion, In this case, however, the fundus of the uterus can be felt abdominally and the stock of the polyp can be found passing through the cervical canal. If there is any doubt about the diagnosis, a sound should be used. In the case of inversion of the uterus it will be arrested just inside the cervix. In such cases the diagnosis of the presence of tumour is not difficult, but on the other hand the associated inversion may be missed. The cup-shaped depression above, may be difficult to identify because comparatively little of the fundus may have passed through the cervix. As a rule, the surface of the tumour and vaginal canal are very septic and the uterine wall at the seat of the growth is usually thin. A portion of the tumour tissue should always be sent for histological examination to exclude sarcoma.

Treatment
In this variety, the treatment of chronic inversion involves replacement by a surgical operation, as described in Chapter 45.

38. Tumours

Discussed in this chapter are tumours of the female organs of reproduction. The word tumour is taken to include all forms of enlargement as well as the true neoplasms. Tumours are discussed mainly in an anatomical (organ) basis, but there are special sub-chapters on e.g. early diagnosis and special forms of investigation and therapy.

TUMOURS OF THE UTERUS

The uterine body may be enlarged by many simple conditions which are not neoplastic but which may cause difficulty or doubt in diagnosis. Pregnancy is a common cause of uterine enlargement and may be confused with carcinoma or fibromyoma particularly when there is an abnormality with bleeding such as abortion or hydatidiform mole.

The hypertrophied uterus of chronic inflammatory disease, 'sub-involution' or endometriosis or even that associated with endometrial hyperplasia can often resemble the uterus with a neoplasm. The uterus distended with blood, pus or fluid associated with a cervical or uterine neoplasm or cervical stenosis alone may cause confusion as can a distended horn of a double uterus.

True neoplasms are however relatively common.

Endometrial polyps

Polyps of endometrial glands and stroma may gradually acquire a stalk and ultimately present at the vulva. Polypoid endometrium is commonly associated with any form of endometrial hyperplasia, and single or multiple polyps of endometrial tissue can occur even in post-menopausal women. The clinical picture is intermenstrual or post-menopausal spotting or bleeding. Polyps may be seen at the cervix and may be removed with polyp forceps by curette from the uterus or by 'twisting off'. Polyps with endometrial glands and stroma in normal arrangement are essentially 'simple' in nature. Profuse or recurrent polyps should raise a suspicion of carcinoma and careful histology is essential. This also applies to polyps consisting of stroma only as sarcomatous change may be present.

Fibroid Polyps

Polypoid tumours containing muscle are fibromyomata.

FIBROIDS (FIBROMYOMATA)

This common and benign tumour of the uterus, derived from muscle tissue, has been variously designated myoma, leiomyoma and fibromyoma. Although *fibroleiomyoma* is more strictly accurate, the term which has now acquired almost universal usage is the *uterine fibroid*.

The fibroid is the most common tumour affecting the female genital tract. Because many of these tumours are symptomless and thus may remain undiagnosed it is not possible to give a precise figure of incidence. Most estimates suggest, however, that at least 20 per cent of all women who have reached the age of 35 years have fibroids in the uterus. There seem to be racial differences in incidence. For example, fibroids are found more frequently in negresses amongst whom they often occur at a much younger age. The tumour is essentially restricted to women of the childbearing age in so far as growth and development are concerned, and there is no evidence of primary growth either before puberty or after the menopause. It follows that when symptoms arise from fibroids they occur mostly towards the end of the childbearing period and are most common between 35 and 45 years. Exceptionally, symptoms arise or persist into the post-menopausal years but this is always due to some complication.

The association between fibroids and infertility has aroused much interest and conjecture with respect to the possibility of common aetiological factors. In some 60 per cent of cases of fibroids the history is that of nulli-parity or one-child sterility. The ovarian hormones, particularly the oestrogens, have been held responsible for providing the stimulus for fibroid development. Fibroids may originate from embryonic rests of muscle tissue deposited in the uterine wall during fetal life. Some evidence for these views has been derived from the experimental produc-tion of fibroids in guinea-pigs following the administration of oestrogens and the tempo-rary reduction in size of fibroids in the human following treatment by male hormones. It has to be admitted, however, that although this is such a common tumour we know very little about its aetiology.

Pathology

This benign solid tumour of the uterus is spherical in shape and firm in consistence. Its size will obviously depend upon extent and rate of growth and will vary through very wide limits. Whereas one tumour may never pro-gress from the seedling stage, another may reach such dimensions that it comes to fill the abdominal cavity; the majority are of a size somewhere between these extremes. The tumour is encapsulated; the capsule consists of flattened and condensed fibrous and muscle tissue and contains the blood-vessels supply-ing the tumour. The vessels are thus most numerous at the periphery and, with growth, the centre of the tumour becomes progres-sively less vascular and is very liable to degenerative changes.

The presence of this clearly defined capsule makes possible the enucleation of the tumour. The cut surface of the tumour presents a solid pale appearance, the muscle and fibrous elements being interlaced in a concentric fashion, giving a regular whorled pattern. On section the tumour substance bulges out from the capsule, rendering the cut surface convex. On microscopic examination the bundles of plain muscle cells are identified intermingling with fibrous connective tissue and the blood-vessels are most numerous at the periphery of the tumour. The capsule is recognized by its loose structure, its greater vascularity and the higher proportion of fibrous tissue.

Fibroids are usually multiple; as many as two hundred tumours may be found in a single uterus. Fibroids in the body of the uterus are much more frequent than in the cervix. Not

more than eight per cent of all fibroids arise from the cervix and in this situation usually occur singly.

Every fibroid arises from within the muscular wall of the uterus and may grow mainly in one of several directions (Fig. 38.1). First, although

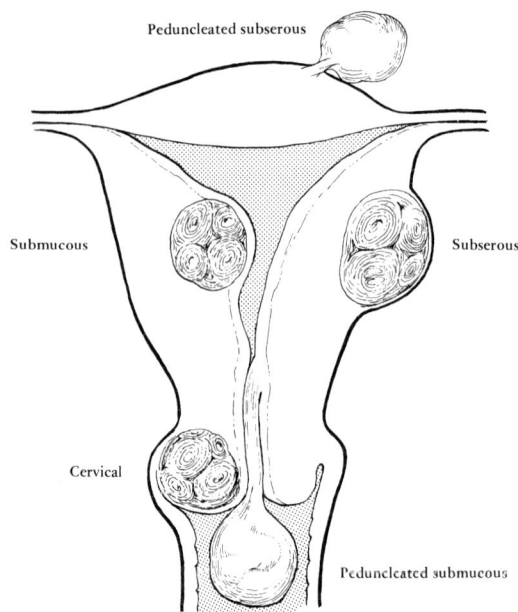

Fig. 38.1   Common sites of fibromyomata.

attaining a fair size, the tumour may remain wholly within the wall of the uterus and will continue to be completely surrounded by normal uterine wall. This *interstitial* or intramural fibroid is the most common type. It may arise at any point in the wall of the uterus but rarely in the cervix. Multiple tumours give rise to an irregular enlargement of the uterus, whereas the much less common single tumour, arising in the mid-line of either the anterior or posterior wall, results in a symmetrical enlargement of the uterus. Other tumours grow mainly out-wards in the direction of the peritoneal cavity. When the fibroid comes to lie immediately under the peritoneum, covering the uterus, it is known as a *subserous* tumour. In this case there appears to be less limitation to growth than in the interstitial type and thus the subperitoneal tumour may reach a very large size. Again, this type of tumour causes an irregular enlargement of the uterus. In some cases the subperitoneal fibroid becomes ex-truded from the uterine wall and, whilst re-taining its peritoneal covering, develops a pedicle. The blood supply is maintained through the pedicle but this becomes progressively deficient as the tumour grows and the pedicle becomes thinner. This type of tumour is described as a *pedunculated subserous fibroid*. Very rarely a pedunculated tumour may become detached from the uterus and become adherent to surrounding structures from which it obtains a blood supply and continues to survive as a *parasitic fibroid*. Other tumours grow towards the cavity of the uterus and, in time, come to lie immediately beneath the endometrium, in which case they are known as *submucous fibroids*. Such tumours cause marked distortion of the uterine cavity and lead to changes in the overlying endometrium. Contractions of the uterine wall may lead to extrusion of the submucous tumour into the cavity of the uterus and, in time, it develops a pedicle. This constitutes a *fibroid polypus*. Aided by muscular contractions of the uterine wall, the pedicle gradually becomes attenuated, and the tumour may eventually dilate the cervix and appear through the external os or, in extreme cases, even at the introitus. If a fibroid arises from the lateral wall of the uterus it may grow outwards between the layers of the broad ligament. This tumour is usually referred to as an *intraligamentary fibroid*. Finally, fibroids may arise from the cervix; if arising from the vaginal portion they tend to become polypoidal or, if arising from the supravaginal portion, they are likely to grow outwards to lie beneath the peritoneum as *retroperitoneal cervical tumours*. An important practical point to keep in mind particularly if the tumour is arising from the lateral or posterior wall of the cervix, is that it is likely to cause displacement and distortion of the ureters and uterine vessels which often lie in the *upper* surface of the tumour.

In the classical case of multiple uterine fibroids it is usual to find many of these types occurring together, but a single fibroid of any one type may develop and give rise to symptoms peculiar to its type. The various types of tumour arising in the body of the uterus are illustrated diagrammatically in Fig. 38.1.

Complications. Complications of uterine fibroids are both common and varied and include several forms of degenerative change, infection, torsion and certain associated pathological conditions.

Hyaline degeneration, typically seen in the centre of the tumour, is the most common and usually indicates that the tumour growth has outstripped its blood supply. The normal structure and regular pattern is lost. The muscle and connective tissue cells become replaced by homogeneous tissue which on microscopic examination appears as an eosiniphilic substance obliterating cellular structure in both cytoplasm and nucleii. Simple hyaline degeneration is symptom-free.

Cystic degeneration is most frequently a sequel to hyaline change. It is due to liquefaction of the hyaline tissue and occurs in one of two forms: either multiple small loculi scattered throughout the tumour or one single large space occupying the centre of the tumour. The cystic areas contain clear straw-coloured fluid in the uncomplicated case. If haemorrhage occurs the fluid becomes blood-stained or with infection it becomes purulent. A single large cystic space may so alter the physical characteristics of the fibroid that differential diagnosis from a cystic ovarian tumour may be impossible even with ultrasound.

Red degeneration, sometimes referred to as *necrobiosis,* is considered to be due to obstruction of the venous return from the tumour, the result of either thrombosis, pressure or injury. It is most commonly seen during pregnancy but is not confined to the pregnant state. Following thrombosis, haemorrhage occurs into the tumour. There is also an extravasation of haemoglobin so that these two factors share responsibility for the red discoloration which is widespread throughout the tumour. As will be seen, this form of degeneration is associated with certain characteristic clinical features.

Fatty degeneration is rare but may occur in areas of localized necrosis. The characteristic appearance of the tumour is lost since the normal constituents are replaced by yellowish-grey tissue which, under the microscope, shows the presence of fat droplets. This change is not associated with any special clinical features and the diagnosis is likely to be made only on histological examination.

Calcareous degeneration is liable to occur if the blood supply is deficient as may occur in the case of a large tumour or in the postmenopausal patient. Calcium salts are deposited in devascularized tissue and the calcified areas are recognized by their irregular greyish-white gritty appearance. If the calcareous change is extensive, the tumour may become stony-hard in consistency, hence the use of the term *womb stones* by authors in the past.

Malignant degeneration takes the form of sarcomatous change—p. 726.

Infection is largely confined to the fibroid polypus and particularly when extruded through the cervix or arising from the cervix. The predisposing factors are exposure and necrotic change due to interference with the blood supply. Very rarely a tumour of the body of the uterus may become infected, in which case infection reaches the tumour either by direct or by lymphatic spread from the bowel, by lymphatic spread from the endometrium or by way of the blood stream.

Torsion of a fibroid is rare and is confined to the pedunculated subperitoneal variety. Torsion may occur slowly or suddenly and may also be intermittent. If the obstruction to blood supply is complete, strangulation, necrosis and sloughing of the tumour will result. Even more rarely the whole uterus, containing fibroids, may undergo torsion.

Impaction of a fibroid within the pelvis may occur in the case of the retroperitoneal cervical tumour or in the case of the fundal tumour which has caused complete retroversion of the uterus. In either event, the tumour, by growth or by becoming congested may fill the pelvis completely and cause pressure symptoms of varying severity. It is a common cause of retention of urine in perimenopausal women.

Intraperitoneal haemorrhage associated with fibroids is very rare and is due to rupture of a vein coursing over the surface of the tumour. Precipitating factors include trauma, torsion and hypertension, and the clinical picture will vary according to the rapidity and severity of the bleeding.

Post-menopausal atrophy occurs in uterine fibroids, as in the pelvic organs generally, as a result of reduction in blood supply. Reduction in the size of the tumour may not be marked but at least there is no further increase in size after the menopause unless some degenerative change occurs.

Associated pathological conditions
Endometriosis and chronic inflammatory conditions frequently coexist with fibroids. The coexistence of fibroids and endometriosis is interesting from the point of view of aetiology, for it has been suggested that prolonged oestrogenic action may provide the stimulus for development of both conditions. Both are commonly associated with infertility. *Chronic tubal infection is also frequently found in association with fibroids.*

SYMPTOMS
It must be emphasized that, in many instances, fibroids develop and grow during the active childbearing period, and regress after the menopause without causing symptoms and will never be diagnosed unless they are found incidentally during pelvic examination, during laparotomy or at autopsy. This is particularly true of the interstitial type of growth. Symptoms directly attributable to fibroids depend mainly upon their number, size, and site and upon the presence and nature of degenerative changes in the tumour.

Bleeding
The presence of and nature of abnormal bleeding depends entirely on the size of the tumour and its relation to the endometrial cavity. Tumours which do not enlarge or distort the cavity *do not* cause abnormal bleeding.

The typical change is prolongation of the periods which are usually also heavier and this is caused by tumours enlarging the cavity and therefore the area of endometrium. There may also in those cases be some hormonal induced endometrial hyperplasia.

If the tumours become submucous and certainly if polypoidal, menstrual irregularity or intermenstrual bleeding occurs.

Degenerative change of any type may also be associated with irregularity of bleeding.

Post-menopausal bleeding from fibroids is due either to degenerative or sarcomatous change or to a polyp.

Pain is *not* common with uncomplicated uterine fibroids but may occur intermittently in cases of submucous tumours or fibroid polypi. The pain may be caused by powerful and painful uterine contractions endeavouring to expel the tumour from the wall or cavity of the uterus.

Pain at the site of the tumour is characteristic of red or sarcomatous degeneration, torsion or infection and generalized abdominal pain will accompany the rare occurrence of intra-abdominal bleeding.

In the case of a tumour occupying the pelvic cavity, pain may result from pressure on the pelvic nerves and may be located in the back or referred to the thighs or legs.

In the post-menopausal patient the occurrence of pain in a previously painless tumour is strongly indicative of malignant change.

Because of the frequency of coexisting diseases such as salpingitis or endometriosis it may well be that the pain is due to these conditions rather than to the fibroid itself.

Pressure

Reference has already been made to effects of pressure upon the pelvic nerves. In similar circumstances pressure may affect the other pelvic organs, especially the bladder and rectum. Gradual pressure upon the bladder causes frequency and dysuria but the sudden impaction of a retroperitoneal tumour is likely to cause acute retention of urine. Pressure upon the bowel leads to constipation or, in extreme cases, obstruction.

Vaginal discharge

When infection of a fibroid polypus occurs it is always accompanied by vaginal discharge. As the infected tissues are necrotic and sloughing the discharge is purulent and frequently blood-stained. Again, however, it should be kept in mind that such a discharge may be due to some coexisting condition such as chronic cervicitis or carcinoma and not to the fibroids themselves.

Abdominal swelling

Sometimes, the only complaint is of gradual enlargement of the abdomen. This symptom will obviously result from a fibroid of considerable size most frequently of the subserous variety. Fibroids seldom cause enough pressure on the bowel to produce abdominal distension or constipation but may occasionally cause oedema of one leg because of obstruction to the venous return. Rapid increase in the size of the abdomen signifies rapid growth of the tumour which is a feature of malignant change.

Sterility

Fibroids are most frequently encountered in the single woman or in the married woman who is either nulliparous or whose childbearing efforts have been restricted involuntarily to one child. Whilst it may be that fibroids and infertility have a common aetiology, it is clear that in some cases at least the presence of the fibroids causes the sterility. Thus a large interstitial or subserous tumour may obstruct the Fallopian tube or a submucous tumour or fibroid polypus may block the intramural or interstitial portion of the tube. The related hyperplasia and congestion of the endometrium may also contribute towards infertility. Unsatisfactory embedding of a fertilized ovum may occur in the endometrium over the fibroid and early abortion may result.

Infertility in patients with fibroids may of course, be due to coexisting disease, particularly salpingitis. It is, therefore, wise to ensure that the tubes are patent before embarking upon conservative surgical treatment of the fibroids as a 'cure' for infertility. 'Fibroids' and pregnancy are discussed on p. 722.

General health

Prolonged bleeding may cause progressive anaemia and debility. An interesting but rare association with fibroids however, is polycythaemia. Abdominal pain or vulvar pruritus from an irritating discharge may interfere with sleep. Continued failure to conceive may lead to psychological distress and malignant degeneration will eventually reveal itself by progressive cachexia.

From what has been said it is clear that, in the majority of cases, uterine fibroids will give rise to certain characteristic symptoms. However, the exceptions to this rule are summarized in the following observations: (1) fibroids do not necessarily cause symptoms; (2) symptoms, in the presence of fibroids, may be due to some associated disease; (3) unless some complication arises, fibroids do not cause symptoms after the menopause.

SIGNS AND DIAGNOSIS
The precise clinical findings depend upon many factors, including number, location and size of the fibroids and the presence of complications.

A history of excessive uterine bleeding may be confirmed by the diagnosis of anaemia. Abdominal inspection and palpation may reveal the presence of a solid tumour, of varying size and shape, arising from the pelvis. The variation in size is such that in one instance the tumour may not be palpable abdominally while in another it entirely fills the abdomen. In the typical case of large multiple fibroids the tumour mass will be mainly in the mid-line but will show gross irregularity of outline. Less commonly a single large tumour in either the anterior or the posterior wall or in the fundus of the uterus will be central and the regular contour is in keeping with a symmetrical enlargement of the uterus. The tumour is firm and dense in consistence and is not tender in the uncomplicated case. There may be considerable lateral mobility but vertical mobility is restricted. The tumour mass is dull on percussion and sometimes a souffle may be heard on auscultation: this is synchronous with the patient's pulse and is due to blood rushing through the large superficial vessels. Degeneration will alter the physical characteristics: cystic change may be sufficiently marked to give the entire tumour a cystic feel and it may even be possible to elicit a fluid thrill. Infection, torsion, red degeneration or maglinant change will be associated with localized tenderness. Vaginal examination may reveal the presence of a vaginal discharge or a firm cervic grossly displaced by a supravaginal retroperitoneal cervical tumour. A rounded, firm, fibroid polyp may be encountered at the introitus or discovered protruding through the cervix in the upper part of the vagina. On bimanual examination the uterus is found to be hard in consistence and enlarged. It may be symmetrical or, more probably, have an irregular 'knobbly' outline. It may sometimes be possible to palpate the ovaries distinct from the tumour mass.

Differential diagnosis

All other causes of irregular bleeding in a woman approaching the menopause will have to be considered, in particular, malignant disease of the genital tract. Not infrequently a degree of ovarian dysfunction coexists and this probably explains the delay in the menopause which is said to occur frequently in patients with uterine fibroids. Abdominal pain may be due to chronic inflammatory conditions of the tubes and ovaries, endometriosis or ovarian tumours, and vaginal discharge to cervicitis or vaginitis.

Uterine fibroids must be differentiated from ovarian tumours, a gravid uterus, a tuboovarian inflammatory swelling, an encysted tuberculous peritonitis, retroperitoneal or mesenteric tumours, bowel tumours, and a full bladder. In many cases the diagnosis can be made fairly easily by careful abdominal and bimanual examination but the main difficulty usually involves differentiation between an ovarian tumour and fibroids. An ovarian tumour is often mobile to a degree seen only occasionally in the pedunculated sub-peritoneal fibroid. It feels elastic and a fluid thrill can be readily elicited if it is cystic. It is only in the fibroid which has undergone cystic degeneration that this clinical sign can be demonstrated and in such cases a final diagnosis may have to await laparotomy. Other causes of uterine enlargement, including carcinoma of the body, metropathia haemorrhagica and pregnancy may have to be considered. Difficulty sometimes arises in the case of a fibroid polyp, for with necrosis and infection the appearance may well simulate a proliferative carcinoma of the cervix. The identification of a pedicle coming through the dilated cervix will clear up the diagnosis but in all such cases, irrespective of the clinical diagnosis, histological examination should be done.

Treatment

The choice of treatment depends upon the severity of symptoms, the age and general condition of the patient, the presence of complications and the type or types of tumour present.

Non-operative treatment. If the fibroid is small and causing no symptoms or minimal symptoms or if the patient is unfit for surgery then a conservative approach may tide the patient over to the menopause when symptoms should disappear. The menopause is often delayed however. Anaemia must be corrected.

Surgical treatment. In most cases operation is the treatment of choice usually by the abdominal route except where the fibroid is in the cervical canal or vagina. Pre-operative treatment, especially of anaemia, is most important. This may, in a few cases, necessitate curettage to stop uterine haemorrhage and thus allow time to give iron therapy or a blood transfusion, usually of packed cells. Such pre-operative treatment is particularly important if it is anticipated that the operation may be difficult due to the size and fixation of the tumours. Curettage will also exclude associated carcinoma of body of uterus.

The precise method of dealing with a fibroid polyp will vary with its size. It is usually possible to seize the more common smaller fibroids with ring forceps and to rupture the pedicle by twisting. Bleeding from the base of the pedicle may be controlled by diathermy coagulation. Once the obvious fibroid has been removed a careful pelvic examination and curettage of the uterus should be carried out to exclude further tumours, which may have to be removed by the abdominal route at a later date. Much less commonly the fibroid polypus is so big that it cannot be removed intact. It may be removed piecemeal by the operation of morcellation and again this may have to be followed by hysterectomy.

The choice of operation in all other types of fibroid lies between myomectomy and hysterectomy. Where it is desirable to retain the uterus, particularly when pregnancy is desired, myomectomy or enucleation of the tumours is ideal (see Chapter 45).

In the older patient and where pregnancy is not desired, hysterectomy is the best method of treatment (total or subtotal depending on the fitness and parity of the patient). Hysterectomy is specifically indicated in the post-menopausal patients with symptoms. Multiple uterine fibroids constitute one of the commoner indications for hysterectomy in the woman between 40 and 50 years of age.

FIBROIDS AND PREGNANCY

Although fibroids usually occur in the infertile patient it is, nevertheless, not uncommon for pregnancy to exist in a uterus containing such tumours. In this event, the fibroids will often complicate the pregnancy but this is not invariably the case. It is sufficient, here, to summarize the main effects of fibroids upon the course of pregnancy and the possible effects of pregnancy upon the fibroids.

1. Fibroids may cause abortion which may be due either to the associated endometrial changes, to weak placental attachments or to retroversion of the uterus.

2. Red degeneration may occur in the antenatal period and may cause acute symptoms. Treatment is symptomatic and operation is rarely indicated.

3. Obstruction in labour may be due to a fibroid which fails to rise out of the pelvis, and Caesarean section will almost certainly be indicated.

4. By interfering with the normal contractions of the uterus in the third stage, fibroids may cause incomplete placental separation and post-partum haemorrhage.

5. Following delivery the tumours may be involved in a puerperal uterine infection.

In view of these possibilities it is clear that a patient with fibroids should be supervised with particular care during pregnancy and delivered in hospital.

Carcinoma of the body of the uterus

Carcinoma occurs less frequently in the body of the uterus than in the cervix. Relative frequency was formerly 1:4, but in recent years there has been an increase in the number of cases of cancer of the uterine body and some decrease in those of cervix, so that the relative frequency of the two types in most western communities is now about 1:3 or 1:2.

Pathology

Carcinoma of the corpus arises from the columnar epithelium lining the glands and covering the surface of the endometrium, and the cells are arranged to form gland spaces and an adenomatous pattern may be present throughout the tumour, with here and there penetration into the myometrium. More often large epithelial masses are produced which infiltrate the stroma and fill up the gland spaces, transforming them into solid blocks of cells. Microscopic appearances of those anaplastic growths closely simulate squamous carcinoma.

Squamous cell carcinoma of the cervix may of course, extend upwards to the uterine body. Very rarely a primary squamous carcinoma of endometrium may follow simple squamous metaplasia of the columnar epithelium, but usually areas of squamous metaplasia exist with adenocarcinoma, the condition known as adenoacanthoma (Charles, 1965).

The degree of muscle wall penetration varies with the type and age of the tumour. Most are well differentiated with diploid chromosome characteristics and spread slowly. The lesion starts in a small localized area but by lateral expansion and deep penetration the myometrium would ultimately be completly replaced by soft thick adenocarcinomatus tissue. Lymphatic involvement is relatively late in view of the need to penetrate muscle first, but deep myometrial involvement is almost always associated with lymphatic gland involvement. Lewis, Stallworthy and Cowdell (1970) found that there was involvement of the pelvic lymph nodes in 13·2 per cent of cases, but Douglas *et al.* (1972) by lymphography have shown 26 per cent gland involvement in their case material and in half of those the spread was to *ovarian and para-aortic glands*. The glands first involved will depend on the exact situation of the primary growth within the uterus. Growth close to the fundus may rarely spread to the superficial inguinal glands via the round ligament but usually tend to spread direct to the aortic glands along the lymphatics accompanying the ovarian vessels, and also to involve ovary in secondary deposits. Lesions in the lower half of the body spread like lesions of the cervix to the glands of the broad ligament and the lateral pelvic wall. In neglected cases of course, there is gross myometrial involvement with direct spread to ovary, broad ligament, bowel and pelvic wall. Metastases to lung, bone, liver and brain occur by blood spread and are late.

The final situation is very like that of an extensive cervical disease but the ureters become blocked less frequently.

Aetiology

The condition is uncommon before the age of 45, but in some 25 per cent the woman is pre-menopausal. The disease becomes somewhat more common with advancing age as does breast and colon cancer and especially in the infertile. The condition is frequently associated with disturbance in carbohydrate metabolism, in overt diabetes, obesity or hypertension.

Clinical features

A clear watery discharge and haemorrhage are the main features. In post-menopausal women it must be remembered that discharge alone may be the presenting symptom, but in the pre-menopausal woman irregularity of bleeding or intramenstrual bleeding may be the primary sign. For this reason all women with irregularity of bleeding at the menopause, especially where bleeding occurs too often, or is too much, should be investigated, to exclude cancer of the uterine body, as should all women with post-menopausal bleeding.

Pain is a late feature, except when it occurs in association with blockage of the cervical canal and pyometra. Findings on pelvic examination vary tremendously with the extent of the disease; no abnormality may be found whatsoever, or there may be gross enlargement and fixation of the pelvic organs. The presence of post-menopausal bleeding or a clear watery discharge usually merits full investigation by brush cytology and curettage.

Diagnosis

Diagnosis can be made only following curettage, but suspicion should be raised by post-menopausal bleeding or by discharge, or intramenstrual irregular bleeding and a bulky uterus would of course, also cause suspicion. It is to be remembered that many of these ladies are nullipara or certainly infertile, and examination may not be easy. Irregular bleeding at the menopause is much more often due to hormonal disturbance, fibroids, cervical carcinoma or sometimes even to abortion. As a rule the bleeding in those conditions is more profuse than in carcinoma of the body of the uterus, but histological examination of curettings is essential. A very thorough curettage of endometrium preferably under anaesthesia should be done in case an early carcinoma exists. Sometimes endometrial carcinoma coexists with fibroids which may distort the uterine cavity and make it more difficult to explore with the curette.

A difficult situation exists when oestrogens have been given to relieve peri menopausal symptoms and bleeding has occurred. Probably it is wisest in the circumstances to do a diagnostic curettage and to have the material examined by a competent pathologist. When a polyp is present the uterus should always be curetted since it is quite possible for a double lesion to exist. A similar situation arises in association with senile vaginitis, and unless curettage has been performed senile vaginitis should never be inculpated as the sole source of post-menopausal bleeding.

It is often difficult to tell even after curettage, whether the lesion in the uterus is spreading down into the cervix or not (the *corpus cum collis* lesion) which requires a separate form of therapy. Fractional curettage is not easy to do successfully and quite often the impression of the operator is the main feature to guide therapy.

Histology may be helpful to distinguish between carcinoma of the endocervix and carcinoma of the body of the uterus, but there is a mutual zone where the distinction is impossible and not really necessary.

Therapy

It has been accepted for some time that some form of combined therapy probably gives the best results. In the modern situation most cases are seen and diagnosed early when there is minimal uterine enlargement and minimal myometrial invasion. Only some 1–20 per cent will have gland spread, and apart from a certain operative risk the main risk is of vaginal recurrence. Five year survival rates close to 80 per cent can be expected in the early lesions and an overall rate of 60–70 per cent, by total hysterectomy with bilateral salpingo-oopherectomy, but this may be enhanced and vaginal recurrence largely prevented by pre- or post-operative radiation. In general total hysterectomy and bilateral salpingo-oopherectomy is the internationally accepted therapy. If the carcinoma invades the myometrium by more than half or if the tumour is poorly differentiated, there is a serious risk of gland invasion and radiotherapy to the pelvic wall is advised. It should however, be part of the operative technique to inspect and biopsy the glands of the pelvic wall in all such cases. Where the lesion involves the endocervix it should be treated like a cervical carcinoma. A two-thirds standard radium should be given preliminarily to extended hysterectomy or full radiation as a total therapy as in cervical carcinoma. In this situation the gland spread is to the pelvic glands as in the cervix case, and lymphadectomy or pelvic wall radiation is certainly essential. In the late case preliminary radiation and simple hysterectomy may be all that is possible, with super voltage palliative therapy to the pelvis.

More recently it has been shown that such lesions are very frequently sensitive to hormone therapy and the use of high doses of the medroxy progesterones, or the caproates, 'Provera' or 'Depostat', may well suppress the otherwise helpless case or apparently deal with pulmonary, bone or other secondary deposits and may be of course, used for months or years. Survival is also dictated somewhat by histological grade and is much better in the more highly differentiated lesions, even where the spread is beyond the uterus.

Bonham and Bonham (1973) have shown that, if a computerized life table technique is used for survival studies, older patients had a higher cancer specific mortality but could also live longer with recurrence. In younger women surgery as a primary therapy was best. They also confirmed the better survival in the patients with well differentiated lesions. Premenopausal women with a well differentiated Stage 1 lesion have over 90 per cent five year survival.

IN SITU CARCINOMA OF THE ENDOMETRIUM

There is a lesion of adenomatous hyperplasia which is occasionally called *in situ carcinoma*.

It is difficult to prove that this is a lesion which might progress. It can be altered by progesterones and eradicated by simple hysterectomy.

SARCOMA OF THE UTERUS

Malignant lesions may arise from the endometrial stroma (1) stromatosis or (2) stromal sarcoma; from the muscle of the myometrium (3) leiomyo sarcoma or from the connective tissues of the uterus itself, (4) fibro sarcoma. Altogether these tumours form some 8–10 per cent of malignant uterine body neoplasms and 0·2 per cent of all gynaecological malignancies. There is a mixed group of tumours which arise from mesoderm of multi-potential type and these 'mixed mesodermal tumours' contain many different elements and cell forms. Carcino sarcomas of endometrium also occur.

The sarcoma botryoides of young children affect mainly cervix and vagina (*see* page 756).

UTERINE STROMATOSIS

Typical endometrial stroma cells infiltrate between the muscle bundles of the myometrium. This lesion has to be distinguished from leiomyo sarcoma and haemangio pericytoma by special stains and study of cellular detail and pattern. The condition was extensively reviewed by Park (1949). This tissue responds to progestogens which may be used in therapy.

Clinically the picture is nonspecific with irregular bleeding and the finding of an enlarged bulky uterus. Uterine fibromyoma is usually the first clinical diagnosis. At operation plugs of white tumour may be seen in the broad ligament veins. This disease is locally invasive and recurrence may appear after some years, but only 12 per cent are likely to die of their disease.

As there is some hormone dependence, oopherectomy is advised with hysterectomy and the progestogens Provera and Depostat may be used with effect (Baggish and Woodruff, 1972).

STROMAL SARCOMA

This group includes the diffuse stromal sarcomas, the mixed mesodermal tumours, and the carcino-sarcomas which are often highly malignant. The histology is often difficult to interpret.

They present as soft polypoid masses within the uterus and often cause the uterus to be grossly enlarged. Spread is direct to neighbouring tissues and via the usual lymphatics. Blood spread to chest, brain or bone is somewhat more common than with epithelial lesions.

The disease is commonest in the 50 to 60 age-group and the clinical features are discharge, and irregular peri-menopausal or post-menopausal bleeding. Extensive disease is associated with an enlarged tender uterus and pyrexia. Diagnosis is surprisingly often missed on curettage as the curette may slide off the tumour. The diagnosis should always be suspected in patients who have recurrent 'endometrial' polyps or in women with a large slightly soft uterus associated with irregular bleeding.

LEIOMYO SARCOMA

Malignant change in the muscle of an apparently simple fibromyoma occurs in 1–2 per cent of cases and appears as soft yellowish or haemorrhagic area. More often it is diagnosed only after careful histological examination of suspicious areas (Fig. 38.2). Clinically there

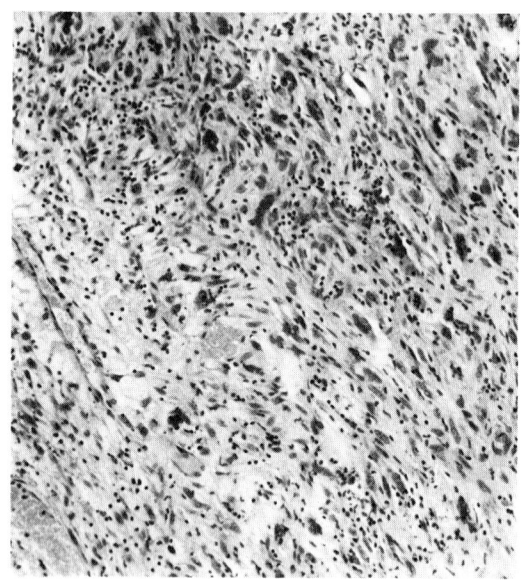

Fig. 38.2 Sarcomatous change in a fibromyoma-Leiomyosarcoma.

may be no symptoms or signs apart from those of the fibromyoma but rapid increase in size or tenderness especially in the post-menopausal women should raise suspicion.

Prognosis and therapy

In general the leiomyo-sarcomas occur in the younger perimenopausal woman and the carcino-sarcomas in the oldest. The prognosis depends on the age of the patient and on the type of growth.

In pre-menopausal women with leiomyosarcomatous change enclosed in small areas of fibromyoma the prognosis after simple removal is excellent. In older women with stromal sarcoma or mixed mesodermal tumour the prognosis is poor.

In all cases total hysterectomy with removal of all obvious tumour is the best therapy.

In view of the obviously advantageous situation of the pre-menopausal woman hormone therapy with progestogens has been suggested as an adjuvant in the post-menopausal woman. Radiation therapy seems of little advantage. Recent reports suggest that in the patient with extensive disease cyclophosphamide and actinomycin D or vincristine used in combination may produce remission (Hall, 1971).

Haemangiopericytoma arises from pericytes close to the endothelial cells of small blood vessels. They have endothelial lined capillaries surrounded by whorl-like fibrous neo-plastic pericytes. They are sluggishly malignant. They resemble fibroids in their clinical presentation and are rare.

TUMOURS OF THE CERVIX UTERI

The cervix uteri and upper vagina arise from the same Mullerian tissue as do the Fallopian tubes and uterus. The endocervix is characterized by columnar epithelium which shows minor histological changes with the menstrual cycle but rather more marked cyclical changes in the character of the mucous secretion. The *vaginal cervix* is however, like the vagina itself, covered with a skin of squamous epithelium. The behaviour of this epithelium and of the area of the squamo columnar junction creates the special characteristic of cervical neoplasia.

The association of the cervix and the vagina, and of the cell rests in both is further seen to be close by the appearance in both tissues of clear cell adenocarcinoma in adolescent girls following the administration of stilboestrol to their mothers in pregnancy.

Enlargement of the cervix may be due to hypertrophy associated with *chronic cervicitis* where there may be clinically a large thick cervix with glands pouring muco pus. Some forms of specific infection of the cervix which can cause enlargement are tuberculosis, schistosomiasis, syphilis and gonorrhoea. Herpes of the cervix causes the surface to be raised in a white ground glass appearance. *Non neoplastic tumours* include retention cysts of cervical glands (nabothian follicles) containing clear mucus. They may be single or multiple and are usually asymptomatic in themselves. *Endometriosis* may appear in the cervix.

Simple tumours

Papillomas, and *fibromas* and *fibro-adeno* and *leiomyofibromas* can occur. The most common simple tumour is the *cervical mucus polyp* consisting of a mass of distended mucus glands on a long stalk and arising from the endocervix. The mass may be long enough to protrude through the cervix, and may become necrotic and infected. It is associated with discharge and intermenstrual or post-coital or post-menopausal bleeding and is better seen with the aid of a speculum than felt.

Treatment is simple removal with cautery or diathermy to the base.

These tumours should never be accepted as the sole cause of perimenopausal or post-menopausal bleeding and uterine curettage should always be performed to exclude intra-uterine carcinoma.

Malignant lesions of the cervix

These include all forms of primary malignancy as well as malignant disease secondary to carcinoma of body of uterus, ovary or elsewhere.

Probably the commonest of all gynaecological neoplasms in any part of the world is squamous carcinoma of the cervix and its association with social and behavioural patterns is fascinating. It is also 'par excellence' the tumour with a proven long history of development and particularly suitable for early diagnosis by cytology.

CARCINOMA OF CERVIX
The majority of cases are of squamous carcinoma but in some 6–10 per cent of cases the disease is an adenocarcinoma of the mucus secreting glands (*see* page 732).

Squamous carcinoma
The lesion varies greatly in incidence throughout the world and even within people of different groups within one country. The maximum incidence is reported in Colombia where one woman in every thousand suffers each year as against 0·06 women per thousand in Israel.

In the South African Bantu it is by far the commonest type of female cancer and is some three to five times more common than cancer of the breast. In Scotland however, breast cancer is some three times more common than cancer of the cervix.

Aetiology
Those wide variations in incidence suggest environmental or behavioural differences and should perhaps offer clues to aetiology. It has been suggested that the disease is associated with the chemicals of male smegma, with the bacteria of poor hygiene, with the virus of herpes or with the protein of spermatozoa themselves.

SQUAMOUS CARCINOMA OF THE CERVIX
1. Is rare in virgins and common in the promiscuous.
2. Is related directly to early age at which regular intercourse begins.
3. Is positively correlated with poor living conditions and lack of personal hygiene.
4. Is somehow associated with a high incidence of genital herpes.
5. Is negatively related to the incidence of newborn male circumcision.
6. Has its highest incidence in women of the age of 35–55 years and decreases thereafter.
7. It is more common in the wives of men who are in occupations where promiscuity is more likely.

Prevention
In view of the direct relationship with sexual intercourse it would seem at first sight unlikely that preventative measures would be possible and especially since the increasing and earlier sexual freedom associated with the free use of the contraceptive pill and the lesser use of the barrier contraceptives, may in fact be increasing the extent of the risk. However, improved hygiene which can be taught, and active therapy to genital herpes and special attention to the dysplasias may help a great deal. As shown below—proper therapy of the *in situ* stage should virtually eradicate the clinical disease.

Pathology
Squamous carcinoma may arise anywhere in the squamous epithelium of the cervix but in

the younger woman appears to arise most commonly at the squamo columnar junction at the edge of erosions (*see* page 688). In the older woman it may arise higher in the canal in association with carcinoma *in situ* which may arise there in the older patient. Arising first as a sessile nodule or small ulcer it presents clinically as an ulcer with deep infiltration or as an exfoliative growth often with little invasion of the deeper tissues. Occasionally the cervix appears normal but is widely infiltrated by malignant tissue.

Infiltration of all surrounding tissues occurs but is mainly laterally and rarely forwards to the bladder or posteriorly to rectum in the earlier stages. Blockage of ureters occurs if there is extensive parametrial involvement. Lymphatic spread is to the glands on the pelvic wall (sacral, obturator, internal and external iliac) and thence via the iliac to the para aortic glands. Blood spread, though uncommon, occurs to lung, brain and bone.

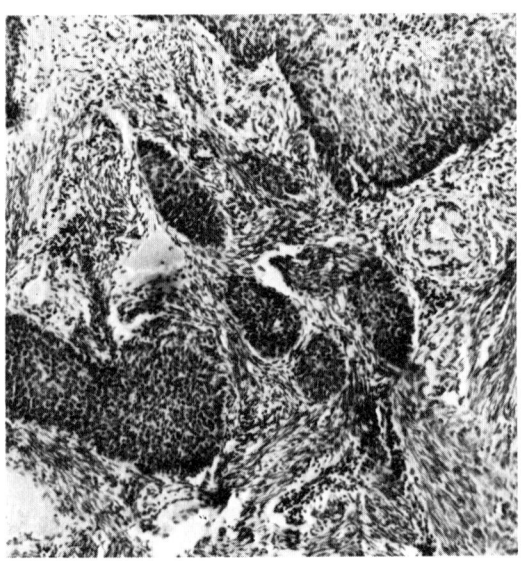

Fig. 38.3   Invasive squamous carcinoma of the cervix.

The disease is 'staged' for purposes of international comparison and therapy according to the degree of local spread diagnosed by clinical examination under anaesthesia (Fig. 38.4).

Staging of carcinoma cervix
Stage IS or O—Carcinoma *in situ*.
Stage 1a—Micro invasive or minimally invasive.

Subclinical but clearly invasive with confluences.
Stage 1b—Clinical lesion—confined to the cervix.
Stage 2a—Vagina but not lower third.
Stage 2b—Parametrial involvement but not of the pelvic wall—vagina, but not lower third.
Stage 3a—Involvement lower third vagina.
Stage 3b—Involvement of pelvic wall.
Stage 4—Bladder or rectal mucosa involved or distant metastasis.

Clinical staging is intended to be made after clinical examination. Uterine curettage, biopsy or cone biopsy may be necessary for diagnosis and cystocopy, urography, and chest skeletal survey are accepted as part of the initial clinical examination.

If a lesion is found to be associated with a blocked or non-functioning ureter, the stage allocated is Stage III even though on palpation a lesser stage might have been suggested.

Staging is required to allow the incidence of the disease and the value of various therapies to be compared between various units, districts or countries.

There is in addition a further staging made possible by more advanced methods of assessment.

Sub-groups are allowed to distinguish these with palpable pelvic wall glands or distant metastases.

Incidence of various stages
Most carcinoma *in situ* and micro-invasive lesions are diagnosed from cytology and their incidence will therefore, depend on the activity and range of cytology practised. Increasing awareness has also increased the early referral of patients so that many more early cases are seen. Ignorance and personal apathy and inadequacy of services still, however, permit many cases of Stages 3 or 4 disease to be seen. Patients often report after five or more years of post-menopausal bleeding with lesions often slowly growing and of that obvious duration.

During the years 1955–62 and 1963–67 in the Eastern Region of Scotland, the incidence by stages of carcinoma of cervix was as shown in Table 38.1. The great increase in the early lesions in the latter period coincides with an actively developed Regional cytology service.

Table 38.1   Incidence of carcinoma of cervix by stages
Eastern Region of Scotland (now Tayside Health Board) from 1955–1967

Years	Total	0	1a	1b	2a	2b	3	4
1955–62	417	15·0	2·0	19·0	18·0	18·0	16·0	11·0%
1963–67	404	30·0	10·0	16·0	12·0	13·0	13·0	5·0%

Diagnosis

In more and more cases diagnosis follows the findings of a 'positive' smear taken as a routine at some clinic in a patient who has not clinically 'complained' though she may have symptoms. Symptoms are:

Irregular vaginal bleeding which may be menstrual, intermenstrual, post-coital or post-menopausal.

Discharge which may be clear, blood stained or foul in the later stages.

Pain occurs only with nerve involvement or metastasis and then very late.

In the late and neglected case there may be massive haemorrhage, swelling of legs from venous or lymphatic blockage, uraemia from blocked ureters, incontinence from fistulae or the many signs and symptoms associated with secondary spread. Death is fortunately often associated with ureteric blockage but can be by the attrition and cachexia of advanced disease often with severe nerve pain or central pain from deep pelvic involvement.

Diagnosis should always be confirmed by biopsy since other lesions can resemble carcinoma, e.g. proliferative erosions, necrotic fibroid polyps, tuberculosis or amoebiasis (Fig. 38.4).

Treatment

Throughout most of the world the primary therapy to clinical carcinoma of the cervix is local radium (perhaps soon to be replaced by caesium).

This is then followed by radiotherapy to the parametrial tissues and to the pelvic wall so that a full cancerocidal dose is given over the whole pelvis. In many centres however, local radium is followed by extended hysterectomy with pelvic lymphadenectomy (*see* Chapter 45) in those lesions stages Ib or IIa (Schlink, 1960, Stallworthy, 1964, Currie, 1971).

In extensive lesions (IIb and III) trial is now being undertaken of a radiotherapy regime with supervoltage techniques as a primary therapy with local caesium as an item in the middle of the course. This regime is being tried on an experimental basis under conditions of hyperbaric oxygen.

Selection of therapy

In general the systems of therapy advised are:

Stage O or Stage Ia (micro invasive)—Cone or total hysterectomy with conservation of ovaries.

Stage Ia (invasive) and early Stage Ib—Caesium in 'cancerocidal' dosage followed by simple hysterectomy with lymphadenectomy. Alternatively—Primary extended hysterectomy with conservation of ovaries.

Stage Ib (clinical) and Stage IIa—Primary caesium with extended hysterectomy and pelvic lymphadenectomy with later supervoltage radiotherapy to the pelvic wall if the glands are involved.

Stage IIb and III—Radium and radiotherapy in planned regimes.

Stage IV—Each case judged individually. Extensive surgery to be considered, palliative surgery with colostomy or ureteric transplant; radiotherapy where indicated.

Post operative

Even with extended surgery there should be minimal mortality and morbidity and there is probably more immediate morbidity due to local radiation effect (*see* Chapter 45).

Follow up

The treated patient should be followed up indefinitely; four monthly for 3 years and annually thereafter. Vaginal cytology should be routine in the follow-up with vaginal/rectal examination to assess the local situation.

Occasional pyelography is advised and certainly if urinary symptoms persist since ureteric blockage with hydronephrosis does occur.

With carcinoma of the cervix it is rarely possible to give curative therapy to recurrences, but palliative therapy has a real place and ureteric transplant, internal iliac ligation, diversion colostomy and bowel resection are often necessary, as is neurosurgery for the relief of pain. A great deal can be done to help.

Therapy in special conditions

Other conditions
Where there is an associated pelvic tumour, or proven pelvic inflammation, the malignant lesion should be treated by surgery alone or the tumour, e.g. ovarian cyst, large fibroid, or the inflamed tissues removed before radiotherapy.

Poor conditions for radium placement. Where

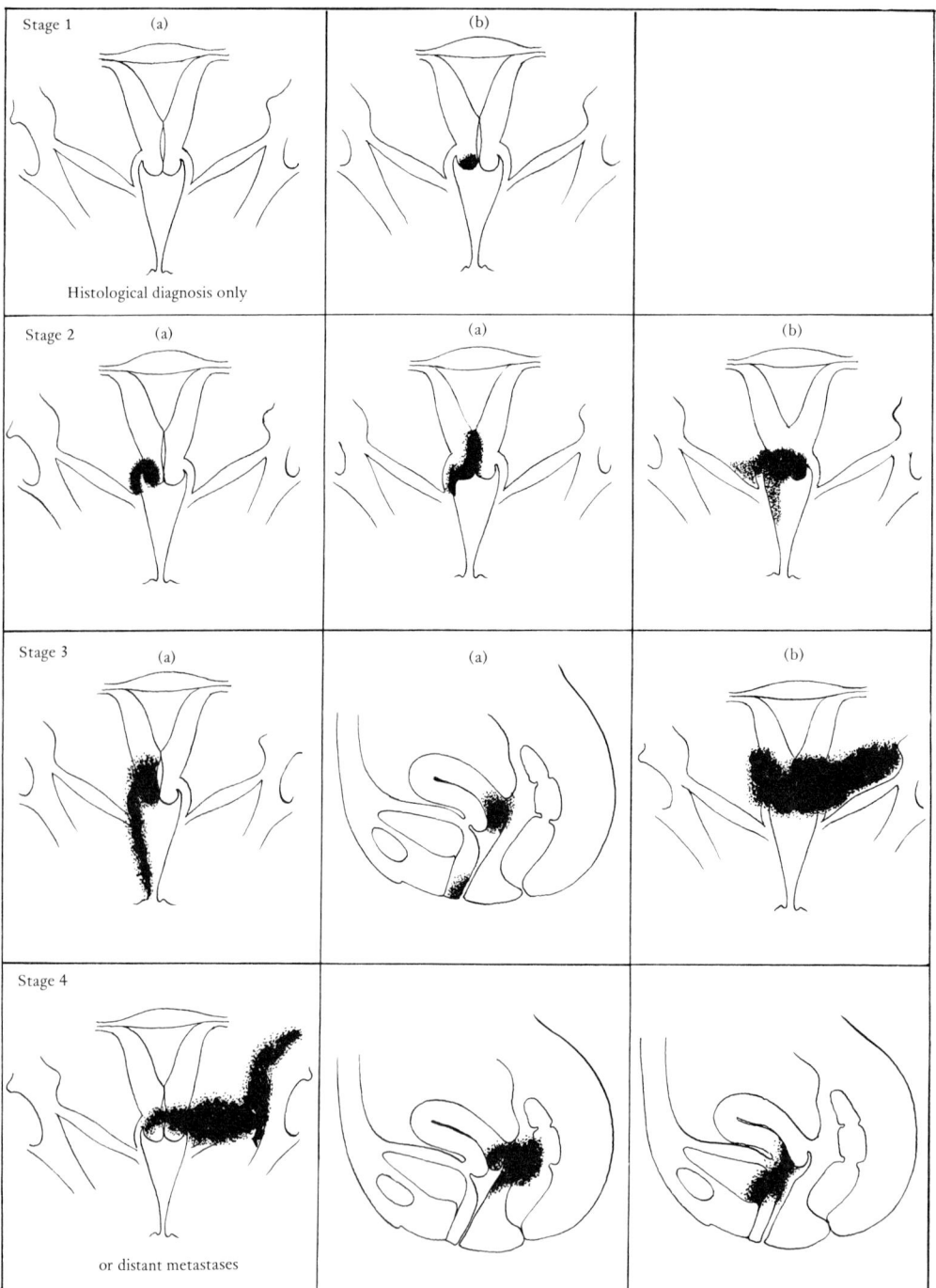

Fig. 38.4   Stages of carcinoma of the cervix. (As agreed by the Cancer Committee and General Assembly of FIGO (1971).)

radium placement is inadequate due to a narrow vagina or where the cervical lesion is bulky and unlikely to have received adequate radiation a simple or extended hysterectomy should always follow radiation.

Reaction. Where there is inflammatory reaction to radium and the radium has to be removed early surgical treatment may have to be considered as the chance of adequate radiotherapy is much less.

Pregnancy—(*see* Chapter 29).

Ureteric blockage. Evidence of ureteric blockage at preliminary assessment is a very worrying situation, and therapy is unlikely to be curative. Where there is also unilateral leg pain and oedema it is doubtful if any therapy even total pelvic clearance will succeed. Leg swelling is usually due to gland involvement on the pelvic wall.

Persisting or recurrent disease. Cure of recurrence or of tumour persisting after radiation is difficult to achieve but, of course, disease persisting in the cervix after radiation (10 per cent of Stage 1 and 20 per cent of Stage 2) is removed by the routine extended hysterectomy. Patients with positive nodes and recurrence after radiation are probably not curable but those with persistent or recurrent local disease without positive nodes may have a 25 per cent or so cure rate with exenteration but the primary mortality may be as high as 15 per cent.

Stage IV : carcinoma with bladder invasion. Despite the extent of the disease planned radiation therapy will allow 25 per cent five year cure (Miller, Rutledge, Fletcher, 1972), with exenteration reserved for the failures.

Involved nodes. Some authorities recommend that preliminary laparotomy should be routinely employed to assess the extent of disease and to remove any large node masses, and that where nodes are known or proven to be involved special therapy should be directed to those or to the areas from which nodes have been removed.

Results

Cure is usually assessed as case surviving without evidence of disease at 5 or 10 years.

The results of therapy will depend on such factors as the stage of the disease when first treated, the presence or absence of involved nodes or distal metastasis, the method of therapy, the completeness of the therapy and the patient's age and general condition.

If the results of many centres are reviewed, it would appear that:

Stage 0—lesions should be cured in 95 per cent of cases. In some 5 per cent recurrence of *in situ* or invasive lesion will appear either as a persistence or as a new growth in another site.

Stage 1a lesions—behave like Stage 0.

Stage 1b lesions; there will be a some 10–15 per cent gland involvement, but results of some 80–85 per cent five year *cure* ought to be obtained. These results are obtained in some units by radiotherapy plus surgery and occasionally by radiotherapy alone. The 10 year cure rate should be some 75 per cent.

Stage 2a lesion; the nodal involvement and the distal spread are correspondingly higher and the five year cure of 70 per cent is likely to be best achieved.

Stage 2b and 3 lesion; it is very difficult for therapy to eradicate disease and the gland involvement is up to 40 per cent. Supervoltage therapy has greatly increased expectation and it is likely that 30–40 per cent five year cure is possible.

Stage 4. Results vary from nil to 20 per cent depending on detail of disease or of therapy.

Philosophy of therapy

Many early lesions have been overtreated in the past. In general, some of the later lesions are also overtreated. All lesions may be undertreated because of inadequate experience of the practitioners in charge.

All cases should be discussed by an oncology team of gynaecological oncologist, radiotherapist, chemotherapist and pathologist at least so that the proper and adequate therapy can be given to the individual patient. *There is no place for the amateur or the occasional operator.* The gynaecologist should be able to refer the patient to such a team for assessment and for such care as is necessary, and not direct to a single discipline.

Complications of surgery

As well as all the complications that follow simple surgery, extensive surgery has the special risks of bowel, ureteric or bladder damage, massive haemorrhage from pelvic veins, sepsis and post-operative ileus or urinary tract infection. Fistulae ureteric or vesico vaginal, follow radical hysterectomy in 2–15 per cent of cases. The patient after exenteration suffers at least a 15 per cent primary mortality mostly from sepsis or biochemical disturbance due to ureteric transplant. The patient with transplanted ureters into ileal loop, colonic bladder or into colon should be cared for in the long term by a 'urinary unit'.

ADENO CARCINOMA OF THE CERVIX

Those tumours account for 6–10 per cent of carcinoma of the cervix. Except for the clear cell group they have no known special aetiology, increase in incidence with rising age, have no special relationship to parity or virginity and are on the whole less responsive to therapy. Since the lesion tends to occur high in the cervical canal it tends to be diagnosed later than squamous carcinoma.

Certain adenocarcinomas with clear cells may arise in the mesonephric rests seen in 1 per cent of normal cervices. However, recently (as in vagina) many of those *clear cell adenocarcinomas of the cervix* have been seen in adolescent girls whose mothers received diethylstilboestrol during pregnancy, usually beginning before the 18th week and continuing throughout. A recent analysis of 170 cases in the register of clear cell adenocarcinomas of vagina and cervix shows that patients currently reported are from 7–29 years of age. Most cases presented with discharge or bleeding but nearly 20 per cent were asymptomatic and in 20 per cent the cytological smear was negative. Lymphatic spread is rapid even in the smaller tumours. Lung metastases are common.

Therapy is no different from therapy of the squamous disease but if anything, radical surgery is to be preferred, Lewis, Diaz, Stallworthy and Ellis (1970).

DISEASES OF THE OVARY, BROAD LIGAMENT AND FALLOPIAN TUBES EXCLUDING INFLAMMATORY DISEASE

THE OVARIES

In this part dysfunction, pseudocysts and true neoplasms of the ovaries are discussed.

Follicular cysts

The ovary frequently contains small clear cysts bulging from the surface. These may be single or multiple, very small or as big as the ovary itself. They are not new growths but are retention cysts of follicles which have failed to produce normal ova and to rupture. They may be due to failure of the ovum to mature, or to thickening and fibrosis of the tunica albuginea, preventing rupture of normal follicles. In small cysts a layer of granulosa cells is still visible in the wall but as the cysts enlarge these cells may disappear. The fluid is clear and may in some cases still contain oestrogens.

Some degree of cyst formation is a relatively common finding at operations in women who have no apparent symptoms relative to the cysts. It is, for example, common to find such cysts in 'metropathia haemorrhagica', in association with uterine fibroids, and in the healed stage of salpingo-oophoritis.

Sometimes, however, multicystic ovaries are found in association with premenstrual dysmenorrhoea, some menstrual irregularity, dyspareunia and a dragging discomfort in the pelvis. In such cases the ovaries may be prolapsed into the pouch of Douglas in association with a retroverted uterus and are tender to palpation in the posterior fornix. In such cases much of the discomfort is due to premenstrual congestion and interference with venous return caused by the retroversion. Chronic constipation and coitus interruptus, by increasing pelvic congestion, may aggravate the symptoms. In such cases correction of the retroversion and use of a Hodge pessary to maintain the uterus in good position for four to six months may result in cure.

The association of secondary amenorrhoea, infertility, masculine type of hirsutes and, occasionally, obesity, with multicystic ovaries, has been reported by Stein and Leventhal (1935). Characteristically the ovaries are enlarged by cysts to about four times their normal size (Chapter 4). Histologically the most striking feature is a marked hyperplasia of the theca interna cells.

Corpus luteum cysts

The corpus luteum of menstruation is 1–2cm in diameter, but in early pregnancy this is increased to about 3cm. 'Corpus luteum persistens' is an uncommon condition where the corpus luteum of the menstrual cycle persists and continues to produce its hormones. Clinically there is amenorrhoea, a slightly enlarged uterus and a unilateral tender cystic swelling.

Occasionally these cysts rupture and up to half a pint of blood may escape into the abdominal cavity. The clinical syndrome before and after rupture may be indistinguishable from ectopic pregnancy. If operation is performed because of intraperitoneal bleeding the cyst alone need be resected.

Theca lutein cysts

These cysts are seen typically in association with hydatidiform mole or chorionepithelioma. They are usually multiple, rapidly growing, bilateral and, may become very large. After abortion or removal of the mole the cysts disappear (see Chapter 9).

Non-neoplastic cysts of the ovary

Endometriosis of the ovary may produce cysts as big as a melon but usually they are smaller and bilateral. This condition is discussed fully in Chapter 39.

Following chronic salpingo-oophoritis a tubo-ovarian cyst may be produced where the tube communicates with a large cyst in the substance of the ovary. This condition is fully discussed in Chapter 40.

Both endometriosis and tubo-ovarian inflammatory cysts must be carefully differentiated clinically from true ovarian neoplasms.

Neoplasms of the ovary

Since the histogenesis of many ovarian neoplasms is unknown it is not possible to offer a complete and accurate classification based on cellular origin. The classification which follows is based mainly on their clinical and pathological characteristics. Teratomata and functionally active tumours are considered

Table 38.2   Classification of ovarian neoplasms

BENIGN	
Cystic (Cystadenomata):	*Solid:*
1. Mucinous	1. Fibroma
Simple	
Papillary	
2. Serous	2. Brenner
Simple	
Papillary	
3. Cystadenofibroma	

MALIGNANT
Primary

Cystic:	*Solid:*
1. Pseudomucinous cystadenocarcinoma	1. Adenocarcinoma
2. Serous cystadenocarcinoma	2. Sarcoma
3. Mesonephric tumours	

Metastatic
Arising from genital tract:
1. Adenocarcinoma
2. Squamous epithelioma
3. Sarcoma
4. Chorionepithelioma

Arising from stomach, bowel, gall bladder, breast, kidney:
1. Adenocarcinoma
2. Krukenberg
3. Hypernephroma

Teratoma

Cystic:	*Solid:*
Teratomatous cyst (dermoid)	Malignant teratoma

'FUNCTIONALLY ACTIVE' OR 'SEX CELL' TUMOURS

Feminizing—Granulosa cell; thecoma; theca cell tumours
Virilizing—Arrhenoblastoma; hilus cell tumour.

OTHER TUMOURS

Dysgerminoma

separately, partly because of their special clinical characteristics and partly because it is not possible to classify them as simple or malignant (Janovski & Paramanandhan).

Frequency of types of neoplasms
Simple cystic tumours are most common. Malignant cysts and solid tumours are also very common. Simple solid tumours are uncommon and those in the sex cell group are rare.

At least 25 per cent of all ovarian tumours seen clinically are malignant and of these 15–20 per cent are secondary tumours.

Miller *et al.* (1962) reporting from the Eastern Region of Scotland on 214 primary malignant ovarian neoplasms classified 50 per cent as cystadenocarcinomata (the majority serous), 37 per cent as solid adenocarcinomata and 8 per cent belonged to the 'sex' cell group.

BENIGN TUMOURS

Mucinous cystadenoma (Fig. 38.5)
This is, clinically, the commonest of all ovarian neoplasms. Most of the very large ovarian

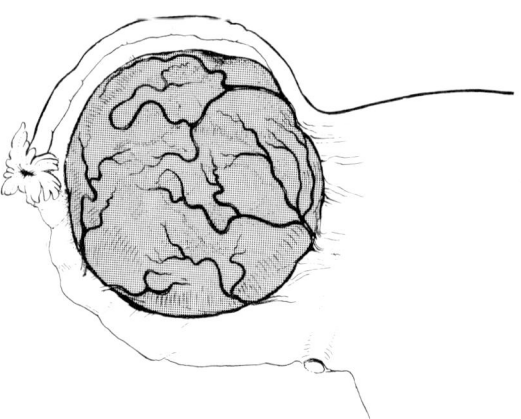

Fig. 38.5   Mucinous cystadenoma.

cysts are of this nature but in educated communities the patient usually consults her doctor and has the cyst removed while it is still relatively small. Usually unilateral, they have a lobulated appearance with a smooth, bluish-white outer surface free of adhesions. The ovarian veins on the surface are prominent. The Fallopian tube is usually stretched over the surface of larger cysts and a well-defined pedicle consisting of the infundibulopelvic ligament, the tube and the ovarian ligament usually develops, allowing the cyst to be

brought out through the abdominal wound at operation.

The cyst is almost always multilocular, the locules varying greatly in size. In some there may be only two or three large locules while in others they are very numerous. Sometimes the locules are so small and closely packed together that they produce what feels like a solid area or areas. The cysts are filled with a true mucin—a glycoprotein. This cyst is therefore a *mucinous cystadenoma*. In appearance the content varies from a clear, rather soapy fluid to very thick firm jelly, clear yellow, green or brown in colour. The epithelium lining the locules is typically tall with basal nuclei and clear cytoplasm; goblet cells are very numerous. Occasionally the epithelium is modified, due to pressure or degeneration, and in some very actively growing cysts it is cuboidal. Secondary or daughter cysts are always being formed by downgrowth of epithelium into the stroma. In many cysts careful search will disclose more solid areas. While these may be merely areas of rapid growth, some will show Brenner tumour tissue and others (5 per cent) malignant change. In a few cases there are papillae within the locules (papillary mucinous cystadenoma). Very rarely spontaneous rupture of thin-walled cystadenoma may allow dispersal of the epithelium throughout the peritoneal cavity and the transplanted cells may continue to secrete mucin, producing the condition known as *pseudomyxoma peritonei*. The abdominal cavity may be gradually filled by this jelly-like material. This is not strictly a malignant condition and there are not metastases. It is possible, by opening the abdomen at intervals, to clear away most of the jelly-like material and tumour tissue, but usually it cannot be completely removed and after many operations to remove the material the patient gradually becomes cachectic and dies. Removal of the cyst, the other ovary and any associated mucocele of the appendix does sometimes result in a complete cure.

Serous cystadenoma
These are fractionally less common than the pseudomucinous variety but are much more likely to show a papillary form. They rarely reach a large size. The *simple serous cystadenoma* is a variety of this group and is unilocular and unilateral with a thin translucent wall. It contains clear fluid and the epithelium is cuboidal. The pedicle consists of the mes-

ovarium. It is histologically impossible in some cases to differentiate this type of cyst from a large follicular cyst. In general the larger serous cystadenomata are bilateral, lobulated and multilocular, and one or more compartments show papillary outgrowths. These papillae vary greatly in form, some being flat and sessile and others profuse and feathery. In many instances, even in benign growths, the papillae perforate the capsule and may even infiltrate surrounding structures. In some cases it is impossible to distinguish between simple and malignant forms at laparotomy or even on histological examination (Fig. 38.6).

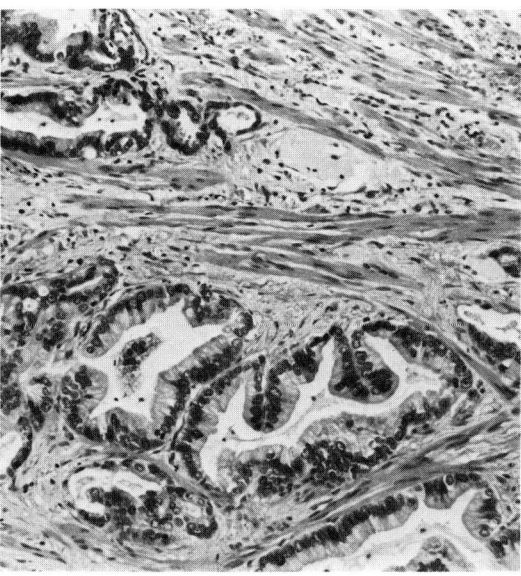

Fig. 38.6 Mucinous cystadenocarcinoma.

The epithelium may be ciliated columnar, with interspersed pear-shaped or cuboidal cells. Malignant degeneration is more than twice as common in this tumour than in the mucinous variety and many areas must be examined histologically. There is however, in both mucinous and serous cystadenomata a histologically borderline group of some 10 per cent where the exuberant histological pattern suggests borderline malignancy.

Cystadenofibroma

This is a mixed tumour with characteristics of both the serous cystadenoma and the fibroma. It is semi-solid and may be quite large. There are two distinct components. The glandular element has cyst-like spaces lined by epithelium. Tall columnar, ciliated, clear cuboidal and transitional varieties of cell may all be seen in the same tumour. The fibromatous element is of spindle-shaped cells embedded in a dense collagenous stroma. Though histologically simple, these tumours, like the papillary serous cystadenomata, may be invasive in places.

Fibroma

This solid tumour probably arises primarily from the ovarian stroma. It usually replaces the ovary completely but encapsulated and surface forms can occur. Histologically the cells are small and fusiform in some areas and in others spindle-shaped and in bundles, giving the appearance of connective tissue of varying composition. Histologically it is impossible to distinguish a cellular fibroma from a thecoma. The tumour can be very large but is usually about 4–6 inches in diameter, unilateral, dense and hard. The cut surface shows much the same whorled appearance as a fibromyoma of the uterus, but is whiter. There may be cystic degeneration in larger tumours. In the larger tumours torsion of the pedicle may occur. There is often ascites and, rarely, fluid in the pleural cavity (Meigs' syndrome). It is important to remember when examining a patient who appears to have advanced ovarian malignancy with ascites and metastases in the chest, that the symptoms may very occasionally be due to a simple fibroma the removal of which will effect a complete cure.

Brenner tumour

This is a comparatively rare tumour. It may arise from Walthard cell nests or from modified ovarian stroma. It occurs most often after the menopause and grows slowly. It causes few symptoms, does not secrete hormones, and is nearly always unilateral. The cut surface is uniformly solid and white. Histologically it is characterized by nests of epithelial cells in a fibromatous connective tissue groundwork. The cell nests may be solid, show central degeneration, or be frankly cystic. Occasionally the epithelium of these cysts may become indistinguishable from pseudomucinous epithelium and with growth large apparent pseudomucinous cystadenomata may arise with no trace of their origin apart from a small nodular area in which the typical Brenner pattern may be observed.

OVARIAN MALIGNANT DISEASE

Ovarian cancer is much less common in

Japan than in the Western countries, and very much less common in the South African Bantu than in the Afro-American. There seems to be some social class or nutritional variation as the disease is more common in the better nourished and in the upper social groups. It has been suggested that possibly the higher incidence is associated with the greater frequency of multiple ovulation which occurs in better nourished communities. In general ovarian malignancy is common in single women and in the infertile. Malignancy is not more common in intersex female, in contradistinction to a similar situation in the male. Ovarian endometriosis appears to be a predisposing factor. After hysterectomy the risk of malignant disease in retained ovaries is less than 2 per thousand, which is no higher than it would be in the normal person, and even after unilateral oopherectomy for benign disease the risk of the remaining ovary becoming malignant is very small indeed, somewhere less than 1 per cent. The disease is no more common after radium menopause.

MALIGNANCY FOLLOWING SIMPLE TUMOURS

Obviously simple tumours may show malignant change in some areas, but this is relatively uncommon in the cystadenomas, but in the benign cystic teratomas some 3 per cent become malignant mostly squamous carcinoma, but any of the cell layers may show malignant change.

MALIGNANT TUMOURS

Primary

Both primary and secondary ovarian cancer are relatively common and nearly half of the tumours are bilateral. Cystic carcinomas are somewhat more common than solid, but many of the solid tumours show large areas of degeneration and many of the cystic tumours are so filled with papillary growth that they feel almost solid. It is often difficult at operation to distinguish the histological type. Mucinous cystadenocarcinoma is less common than papillary cystadenocarcinoma.

Mucinous cystadenocarcinoma. Some 5 per cent of mucinous cystadenomata show isolated areas of malignant change. In most cystadenocarcinomata the growth is wholly malignant from the start. In outward appearance the simple and malignant tumours may look alike, but on section a malignant tumour shows spongy gelatinous areas, or areas of much firmer consistency. The gross and histological appearances depend greatly on the degree of malignancy; the least malignant most closely resemble the simple tumours and are often considered 'borderline'.

In some cases the epithelial cells, though active and with large nuclei, still resemble those in the simple type of tumour (Fig. 38.6), but in others the epithelium consists of many layers, of solid columns of malignant cells.

Papillary serous cystadenocarcinoma. It may be very difficult at operation, or even histologically, to distinguish the simple and malignant variety. It is recognized, however, that at least half of papillary tumours seen clinically are malignant. Papillary outgrowths from the cyst wall or attached to surrounding organs are not necessarily evidence of malignancy, but the more profuse and slender the papillae the more likely is the tumour to prove histologically and clinically malignant. In the typically malignant type the papillary pattern is intricate and there is obvious overgrowth of anaplastic epithelium covering and invading scanty stroma.

Primary solid carcinoma

These tumours may be small or large and are very often unilateral in the early stages, though what appears to be a normal second ovary may contain a very small metastatic deposit. The larger tumours always show cystic degeneration so that at operation their malignant character may not be appreciated. The cut surface shows soft brain-like areas with haemorrhage or necrosis. The histological picture may be that of an adenocarcinoma with a well-defined stroma or there may be large collections of malignant cells with little or no stroma. Characteristic histological patterns are seen where the carcinoma develops at the site of ovarian endometriosis.

Sarcoma. This tumour may occur primarily in the ovary, but is very uncommon. On section there is usually haemorrhage followed by necrosis. All histological types are seen, the round-celled sarcoma being especially malignant.

Mesonenephroid tumours. This group of uncommon bizarre tumours which account for less than 6 per cent of all primary ovarian malignant tumours has recently been reviewed by Hayes (1972).

The tumours are cystic with papillary and

solid areas protruding into the lumen and they are rarely bilateral.

There is a wide variation in histology (tubules, cysts and clear cells) and this allows their separation from the true adenocarcinomas.

Therapy as for malignant tumours in general shows a 50 per cent five year cure.

Metastatic

Carcinoma of the ovary, secondary to primary disease in other organs, is seen clinically almost as frequently as primary ovarian cancer. Even where the secondary tumours are very large the primary may be so small that it can be detected only at post-mortem and after careful histological search.

The pylorus, sigmoid colon, rectum, gall bladder, breast and kidney are the most likely extragenital sites of the primary tumour. Carcinoma of the body of the uterus may spread commonly to the ovary, but this is unusual in carcinoma of the cervix or vagina.

Carcinoma may spread to the ovary by direct extension, by the lymphatics, by the blood-vessels or, occasionally, by direct seeding across the peritoneal cavity.

Secondary ovarian tumours are usually bilateral and fixed and associated with free fluid, often blood-stained, in the peritoneal cavity. Cancer cells can usually be detected in fluid obtained by paracentesis. The tumours are usually solid, but rapid growth leads to central necrosis with liquefaction and the formation of pseudocystic spaces. The larger tumours are therefore semicystic. Histologically they are adenocarcinomata. A well-recognized but rare type of secondary cancer is the *Krukenberg tumour*. It arises from a mucin-secreting primary in the gastrointestinal tract. The ovarian secondaries are bilateral, solid, lobulated and yellow, with a smooth surface. They do not form adhesions. The cut surface is typically brain-like with haemorrhagic areas. Histologically the tumour cells produce mucin which distends the cell body to form typical signet-ring cells in a dense connective tissue stroma.

Teratomata

The cystic and the solid teratomata are rightly discussed together, since their histogenesis is identical, but there are certain clinical differences between the two. They arise possibly from pluri-potential cells isolated early in embryonic development.

Benign cystic teratoma or Dermoid cyst. This cyst which accounts for 10 per cent of all ovarian tumours, is found at any age, is often bilateral, multiple and multilocular, but is not very often large. Since the cyst is formed by the accumulation of sebaceous material from the glands of the neoplasm it enlarges very slowly. It is a whitish yellow colour with a thick wall and is filled with sebaceous material mixed with hair. It tends to be heavy and sink deep in the pelvis. Histologically the cyst may be lined by skin or other tissue of epithelial type on a fibrous base, but at one point the mammilla, the main tissue of the tumour is seen. Characteristically this area is composed of skin with sebaceous glands, hair follicles and sweat glands. Teeth may be found, often imbedded in rudimentary sockets. All primitive cell layers are represented and bone cartilage, pulmonary and intestinal epithelium may be seen.

Thyroid tissue is not infrequent in such cysts, but if the thyroid tissue amounts to more than 50 per cent of the total material the tumour is then called a *struma ovarii* (Fig. 38.7). Such thyroid tissue is often functional

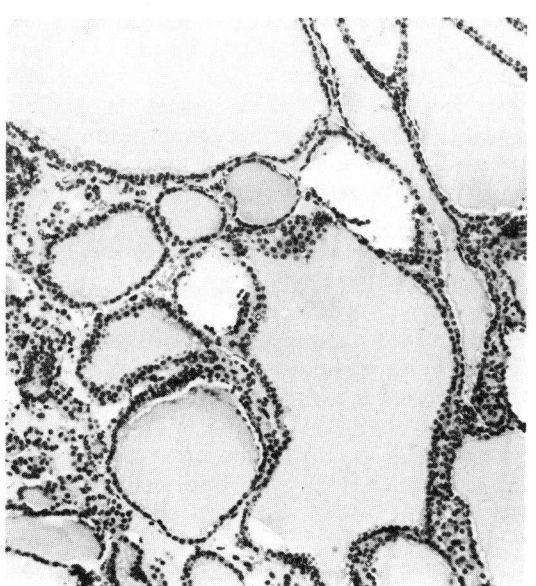

Fig. 38.7   Struma ovarii.

and some 5 per cent of patients with functioning struma will present with clinical thyrotoxicosis. The thyroid gland itself, may also be enlarged and in the unusual case the possible co-existence of an ovarian tumour must be remembered. Diagnosis can be made of course, by radioactive uptake studies of the pelvic mass.

Probably the most interesting association with cystic teratoma is the existence of *carcinoid* or *argentaffin* tumours arising in the teratoma producing the typical symptomatology of flushings due to excess bradykinin, diarrhoea due to serotonin, cyanosis, right heart failure, ankle oedema. The condition can be diagnosed by finding a raised serum 5HT. If removed before any metastises occur the results are excellent. *Autoimmune haemolytic anaemia* has been reported in association with cystic teratomas, and anti Rh Antibodies are often present which disappear once the tumour is removed.

Malignant change may occur in any of the tissues of a simple teratoid cyst.

Squamous carcinoma arising spreads by direct spread to the local pelvis. Sarcomas, when they occur, are blood spread.

When a struma becomes malignant it is no longer usually hormonally active and it spreads by local blood spread and may have very late metastasis.

Solid teratomas. These tumours are very rare and seen mainly in the adolescent. They are actively growing and may become very large. They are almost always malignant and histologically show all forms of embryonic body tissues, often with a concentration of one type. Dysgerminoma is not infrequently a main tissue material in those tumours.

The prognosis depends entirely on whether they are unilateral or free, but must be looked upon as very poor.

FUNCTIONING TUMOURS OF THE OVARY

The ovarian stroma can, during reproductive life, differentiate into the various cells of the follicle, such as the granulosa and the theca interna cells, both of which normally secrete hormones. It is not unexpected, therefore, that granulosa-cell tumours and thecomas, which have strong oestrogenic effects, should arise from it. Luteinization of these tumours may also occur with the production of progesterone. In addition, virilizing tumours, which secrete androgens, can arise.

The tumours in this group show a very varied and mixed histological pattern and endocrine activity. Some have a marked hormonal activity; others, histologically indistinguishable, appear to be inert.

Granulosa cell and thecoma

These tumours are found at any age, but more often after the menopause. They vary greatly in size and show central areas of degeneration. Occasionally atypical truly cystic granulosa-cell tumours occur. All such tumours produce oestrogens which, in children, may cause 'precocious puberty', during adult life irregular uterine haemorrhage, or amenorrhoea if the level of oestrogen production is high enough, and after the menopause enlargement of the uterus and bleeding.

In the granulosa-cell tumours the typical granulosa cells are arranged in widely varying patterns, either in clusters, cylindroids, pseudo-follicles or diffusely scattered with no attempt at organization.

The *thecoma* is usually smaller, yellow on the cut surface and histologically shows broad spindle cells. Thecoma and granulosa elements frequently coexist in the same tumour and both may become luteinized. In such cases the endometrium may show secretory activity in contrast to the oestrogenic effects more commonly seen.

Rarely granulosa or thecomas may be locally and invasively malignant from the start. Granulosa cell tumours frequently (thecomas not at all) may recur in the opposite ovary or anywhere in the abdomen 5–15 years after the first surgical removal. Recurrences having begun as single or multiple ball like tumours of friable tissue which are usually easily removed although sometimes inaccessible, persist and regular recurrence occurs every one to two years, till death.

Virilizing tumours

Arrhenoblastomas are very rare. They are of very mixed histological types and many types of sub groups are described, but they are probably of mixed mesodermal origin. They are all associated with varying virilizing effects on the woman. In the normal female the first effect is of defeminization with amenorrhoea, loss of female fat distribution and breast shrinkage. There is then virilization with loss of hair on the temples, masculine hair growth especially facial, enlargement of the clitoris and deepening of voice. The skin coarsens and acne may appear. Very rarely malignant forms appear.

Results of hormone studies will vary with the type and activity of the tumour but testosterone and androstendione may be found in peripheral blood and tumour tissue and normal female ovarian hormone production is suppressed (Hughesdon and Fraser, 1953).

OTHER TUMOURS

Dysgerminoma

This is an uncommon tumour more prevalent in young women and girls, with 80 per cent under 30. They form less than one per cent of ovarian neoplasms (Fig. 38.8).

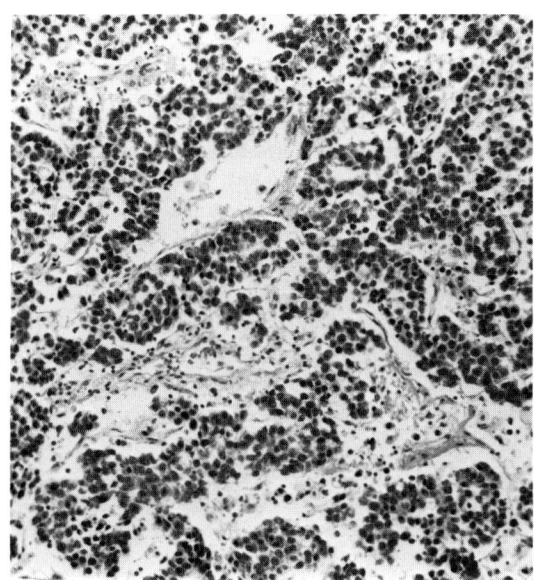

Fig. 38.8   Dysgerminoma.

Consisting classically of typical solid groups of vesicular cells separated by connective tissue strands infiltrated by lymphocytes. The tumour is histologically indistinguishable from a seminoma.

Those tumours must arise from primitive cells of the genital ridge but in several cases they have admixtures of other tumour types or are themselves only part of a teratoma.

They are most commonly unilateral but spread to the other ovary does occur. They vary in size and can become very large tumours indeed. Normally free and encapsulated they may spread widely and locally.

Where the tumour is confined to one ovary with an intact capsule there is nearly 90 per cent five year survival with simple oopherectomy. If bilateral the survival rate drops to 30 per cent. Where, however, there is an admixture of other malignant cell types, e.g. choriocarcinoma, teratocarcinoma, gonado-

blastoma, etc., or there is spread at the time of operation, the prognosis is much worse. In young women with a pure dysgerminoma, encapsulated and unilateral it may well be justified to perform simple unilateral oopherectomy. If, however, there is any suspicion of activity, mixed tumour, or spread, surgery should be followed by radiotherapy especially to the metastasis and to the pre-aortic nodes. These tumours are highly radio sensitive (Taberman et al., 1973).

Many other tumours are described including phaeochromocytoma, Burketts lymphoma, etc.

CLINICAL FEATURES OF OVARIAN TUMOURS

Ovarian tumours all tend to produce the same general clinical picture depending on whether they are benign or malignant, although certain of them produce more specific symptoms which may enable them to be diagnosed accurately before operation. Many ovarian tumours, especially simple cysts, give rise to very few symptoms and may be diagnosed only when they are large enough to cause obvious swelling of the abdomen. If they become very large such cysts produce *pressure symptoms* with general abdominal discomfort and a feeling of distension, vomiting and flatulence, or dyspnoea and palpitation from pressure on the diaphragm and displacement upwards of mediastinal contents. There may be oedema of the lower extremities and frequency of micturition. Pressure on the rectum or colon is unusual. If the patient does not seek medical advice her condition deteriorates so that she becomes very emaciated and this contrasts with the enormous size of the abdomen. A diagnosis of malignant ovarian cyst may be made erroneously in such a case. Very large cysts are almost always simple. Pain may develop because of adhesions to the parietal peritoneum or other structures and for this reason is present in nearly half of all malignant tumours. In some cases the cyst may become adherent over its whole surface and this makes removal very difficult and dangerous. Ovarian tumours of moderate size may produce abdominal pain from retention of urine, from impaction in the pelvis, or from torsion of the pedicle, with subsequent necrosis, rupture and possibly infection.

Ovarian tumours vary greatly in their *rate of growth* and even a simple mucinous cystadenoma may grow as quickly as a pregnancy. Rapid growth does, however, suggest malignancy and in many cases it will be found that some of the enlargement is the result of free fluid in the peritoneal cavity. There may be a large amount of free fluid, especially where there is a general carcinomatosis involving the omentum and peritoneal surface as well as the ovaries. The original malignant ovarian tumours in such cases may be quite small. Occasionally malignant ovarian tumours, especially if bilateral, cause *amenorrhoea*. Simple ovarian cysts, even when unilateral, may on occasion cause *menstrual irregularity* or intermenstrual bleeding.

Occasionally a large ovarian cyst is first diagnosed because the resultant increased intra-abdominal pressure has caused the uterus to prolapse.

Examination

On *inspection* of the abdomen a localized swelling may be seen rising out of the pelvis, although occasionally, with small cysts, the swelling may be wholly in the abdomen or wholly in the pelvis. Striae may be seen if the cyst has grown rapidly.

On *palpation* the typical cyst is smooth in outline and often lobulated. In mucinous cysts firm solid areas, due to collections of small daughter cysts, can often be felt. Unless the cyst is very large or adherent it can be moved from side to side. Teratomatous cysts are often extremely mobile and can be displaced anywhere in the lower abdomen. When the cyst is large a lobe may project deeply into the pelvis, but in other cases where the lower pole is rounded the cyst may not be able to enter the pelvis.

On *percussion* the cyst is dull. Usually the bowel is displaced laterally and as a result the flanks are resonant. A fluid thrill can be elicited over the cyst only if the locules are large and the contents of low viscosity.

Auscultation may help in defining the limits of the cyst, since the sound produced by a scratch on the skin changes at the cyst boundary.

On *bimanual examination* an attempt should be made to identify the ovaries and uterus since, if they can be felt clearly and are independent of the mass, then the tumour is unlikely to originate in the pelvic organs. If an ovarian cyst has a long pedicle it may be moved about without causing any displacement of the uterus, but if there is no pedicle, as in some cases of *broad ligament cyst*, the uterus and cyst will move together. It may be found on careful palpation with the vaginal fingers that such a cyst may appear to merge into the uterus, as in the case of a uterine fibroid. Some broad ligament cysts arising in the outer half of the broad ligament may be quite freely mobile.

The clinical features which point to a diagnosis of *malignancy* are bilateral tumours, ascites, semi-solid consistency, oedema of one leg, pain of sacral nerve distribution, rapid growth, immobility and the palpation of hard nodules in the pouch of Douglas or the omentum.

Solid tumours are harder than the semi-cystic tumours and, when small, usually unilateral and very mobile. Fibromata are usually very hard indeed, while malignant tumours have often softer areas due to cystic degeneration.

Differential diagnosis

An ovarian tumour may be mistaken for almost any form of intra-abdominal mass, from an enlarged spleen or an ectopic kidney on the one hand to a solid mass of faeces on the other. Most commonly, mistakes are made where adiposity of the abdominal wall makes palpation difficult. Pregnancy may be wrongly diagnosed where an ovarian cyst is associated with amenorrhoea or an ovarian cyst wrongly diagnosed where pregnancy is accompanied by vaginal bleeding. A distended bladder may simulate a soft cyst or a cyst be mistaken for a distended bladder. Small retention cysts may be felt at one examination and have ruptured spontaneously before the next. The following conditions may most closely resemble an ovarian tumour:

1. Adiposity.
2. Free fluid in the abdomen.
3. Distended bladder.
4. Pregnancy
5. Uterine fibroids.
6. Tumours of other abdominal organs.
7. Retroperitoneal cysts.

Adiposity. Careful deep palpation and percussion usually suffice to confirm the diagnosis but it can be very difficult to detect a thin-walled cyst in the abdomen of an obese woman. On pelvic examination, with or without anaesthesia, the tense lower pole of the cyst may be felt.

Free fluid. A mid-line tympanitic percussion

note and signs of shifting dullness are seen with free fluid but not with an ovarian cyst. The degree of malignancy does not determine the amount of free fluid present, for example, marked ascites may exist with an ovarian fibroma and only moderate ascites with malignant ovarian neoplasms. If the abdomen is very distended with fluid accurate diagnosis can be impossible.

Distended bladder. In the presence of any lower abdominal swelling of unknown aetiology the patient's bladder should be emptied before examination is attempted. If there is the least doubt about the state of the bladder, a catheter should be passed. This is of particular importance in the puerperium and in the aged, since in both circumstances bladder atony is common.

Pregnancy. In a normal pregnancy, between the tenth and the sixteenth week, the isthmus of the uterus is very soft and the fundus appears to be detached from the cervix and may be mistaken for an ovarian cyst. A retroverted gravid uterus may be mistaken for an ovarian cyst, especially if the history of amenorrhoea is not clear-cut. If there is, in addition, retention of urine the distended bladder will resemble a cyst, except for the fact that it is tender to palpation. Ovarian cysts may coexist with pregnancy.

Uterine fibroids. These tumours are usually hard and produce irregularities of the uterus, since they are often multiple. A single pedunculated fibroid may be difficult to diagnose, since, if the pedicle is long and the fibroid soft or cystic, it may very occasionally be indistinguishable from a mobile ovarian cyst. Bimanual examination under anaesthesia, if necessary, should clear up the diagnosis, since the ovaries may be identified by palpation or the attachment of the tumours directly on the uterus made out.

Tumours of other organs. Mesenteric, renal, omental and pancreatic cysts may be mistaken for ovarian cysts. Ectopic kidneys in the pelvis simulate solid tumours. All such conditions are much less common than ovarian lesions.

The greatest difficulty may be found in distinguishing a left-sided fixed malignant ovarine tumour from a carcinoma of the colon. Sigmoidoscopy, barium enema and examination under anaesthesia help, but the final diagnosis may be made only by laparotomy.

Echinococcal cysts. These are common in some countries and the differential diagnosis from neoplastic ovarian cysts may be difficult, if not impossible.

Complications

The most common complications are torsion of the pedicle, rupture and infection.

Torsion. Any type of non-adherent tumour may undergo torsion of its pedicle, but it most often occurs with a fibroma, dermoid, mucinous or broad ligament cyst.

Torsion may be found at operation even though no clinical signs have been present. This is due to the fact that untwisting has occurred before any vascular changes are produced or because the twisting process is not tight enough to cause any disturbance at all. Where acute symptoms develop there is severe pain over the pedicle and dull pain over the tumour, which is tense and tender. There is often a low grade pyrexia which must be taken into account in the differential diagnosis. At operation the blood supply will be found to be completely shut off and the pedicle of the cyst oedematous. The cyst itself will be dark purple in colour from extravasation of blood into the wall, caused by the fact that the venous return from the cyst is occluded before that of the artery so that the wall becomes engorged and blood is extravasated into its tissue.

Rupture. Spontaneous rupture is not uncommon. If this results in dissemination of malignant cells throughout the peritoneal cavity the prognosis is bad. With simple cysts the event is unnoticed by the patient, but occasionally pain from acute peritoneal irritation may result. If a dermoid cyst ruptures, a low-grade peritonitis follows from the discharge of sebaceous material.

Infection. This complication is now rare. It may, however, be seen in the puerperium if the cyst has been bruised during labour, or if there is associated puerperal sepsis. Cysts may become infected from coincident salpingitis, appendicitis or diverticulitis. The signs resemble those of torsion but the patient's temperature is higher and the cyst more tender. The overlying abdominal wall may become oedematous and inflamed.

Adhesions. Most large cysts form light adhesions where they are in contact with the bowel and peritoneum, but dense adhesions may follow torsion or infection.

Treatment

All ovarian neoplasms should be removed

once the diagnosis is made because of the great risk of malignancy and other serious complications. When a mobile tumour is diagnosed early in pregnancy, operation is best postponed till the 16–20th week to lessen the risk of abortion.

The type and extent of the operation performed depends on the type of tumour and the age of the patient.

With *simple tumours* in a patient under the age of 50 it is generally correct to remove the affected ovary for a simple ovarian neoplasm. After that age the uterus and the other ovary should also be removed unless the patient is frail. In young women, it is correct, even with bilateral tumours, to shell them out (ovarian cystectomy) so as to conserve normal healthy ovarian tissue.

In the *functioning* group of tumours it may be difficult to decide on the correct treatment. In young women usually the tumour alone is removed. In older women, or in women who already have children, it is wise to remove the uterus and the other ovary as well as the tumour, since there is a 10–20 per cent risk of recurrence. It must be remembered that secondaries may not appear for 10–15 years.

With obviously *malignant tumours*, both ovaries should be removed and a total hysterectomy performed, even though one ovary appears healthy. In the case of a secondary tumour or tumours the same operation should be performed, if possible, since occasionally the primary tumour may be small and removable. If the malignant ovarian tumours are fixed in the pelvis and involve peritoneum or other organs, as much malignant material as possible should be removed. Chemotherapeutic agents e.g. thiotepa may be instilled at this time and a chemotherapeutic regime continued after operation.

The most difficult cases are those where, at operation, a unilateral tumour is found in a young woman and the clinical features or the naked-eye appearance of the tumour on section suggest malignancy. Much necrosis with widespread degeneration suggests an anaplastic growth, and the uterus and other ovary should be removed. If the tumour is free, the capsule intact and the appearances of the cut surface similar to those of a simple tumour, then it is probably safe to remove the affected ovary only. Where the pathologist subsequently reports that a unilateral tumour removed alone is, in fact, malignant, further treatment must depend on the estimated degree of malignancy. If it is high, a second operation to remove the uterus and other ovary is best, if low, then there is a reasonable chance of cure and no further treatment need be given.

The use of X-ray therapy (250 kV) or supervoltage therapy should be considered, but most malignant ovarian tumours are resistant. Where, after operation, it is known that some malignant tissue has been left in the true pelvis, X-ray therapy directed at the residual tumour tissue should be tried. If malignant tissue has spread beyond the true pelvis, or if the patient is old and infirm, X-ray therapy is of little or no value and, if given to the whole abdomen, will gravely upset the patient and probably hasten her end. A supervoltage machine should be employed since there is a chance that a sufficiently high depth dose may be possible without damage to the skin.

ADVANCED OVARIAN CARCINOMA

Ascites is a grave sign but if due to mucin is somewhat less serious.

There is little doubt that in the young woman there is no statistical proof that it is necessary to remove a healthy ovary if the other is malignant. However, in some 17–20 per cent of cases the other ovary will contain metastasis and therefore should be removed in women in whom childbearing is *not* essential. The pelvic peritoneum and omentum should certainly also be removed.

Tumours with local extension to peritoneum, rectum, bladder and omentum *within the pelvis* are best treated firstly by radiotherapy (250 kV) or Cobalt to 4 500 rads. Some six weeks later laparotomy may allow complete removal of the pelvic peritoneum and all involved tissues including rectum, caecum, etc. Anterior resection permits normal bowel function and ureters and bladder are maintained. Some 10–15 per cent 'cure' may be expected.

Granulosa cell and dysgerminoma are radiosensitive, papillary and solid adenocarcinoma only moderately and mucinous tumours, not at all.

THE BROAD LIGAMENT AND FALLOPIAN TUBES

Parovarian cysts

The parovarium is the vestigial remnant of the sexual portion of the Wolffian body and lies in the broad ligament between tube and hilum of the ovary. Its main duct (the Wolffian duct) is, in the adult female, called *Gärtner's duct*. The blind outer extremity of the duct forms the small cystic structures, the hydatids of Morgagni. Occasionally one of these may become enlarged and, if on a long pedicle, may produce symptoms due to torsion.

From the main duct or from any of the subsidiary tubules cysts commonly develop. Cysts of the subsidiary tubules are usually small and may be multiple. Cysts of the main duct may become quite large. They contain clear watery fluid and are unilocular, have a thin wall, distend the broad ligament, are separate from the ovary and usually have the Fallopian tube and other structures of the broad ligament stretched along their upper surface. If they originate from the main duct close to the cervix they may have the uterine vessels and the ureter on the upper surface.

TUMOURS OF THE FALLOPIAN TUBES

Benign

CYSTS

Cystic change in one of the fimbria produces a small thin-walled cyst, resembling the hydatid of Morgagni. Torsion of this cyst may occur and produce acute, though minor, symptoms. In association with chronic inflammation small surface cysts may be seen.

SOLID TUMOURS

Fibroids and papillomata have been described, but are rare. Endometrioma is a little more common.

Malignant

Adenocarcinoma in the fundus of the uterus may spread to the Fallopian tube. Chorionepithelioma occurs occasionally, usually as a secondary deposit, but very rarely as a primary lesion following a tubal pregnancy.

PRIMARY ADENOCARCINOMA

This is a rare tumour. It is usually papillary in type and is bilateral in one-third of the cases. Necrotic tissue, serous discharge and blood distend the lumen of the tube, the fimbriated end closes early and the tube assumes the retort shape usually seen in hydrosalpinx. The affected tube may become very large. Involvement of the tube wall and adhesions are late occurrences. Spread is direct through the wall to the peritoneum, giving rise to ascites, and by the ovarian lymphatics to the para-aortic glands. Clinically there is clear discharge or bleeding from the uterus with some pain on the affected side. Treatment is unsatisfactory as most cases are inoperable when first seen. Total hysterectomy with bilateral salpingo-oophorectomy should be attempted, followed by deep X-ray therapy directed at any residual tumour tissue.

SARCOMA OF THE FALLOPIAN TUBE

Is a very rare tumour. Metastases to lung may occur but are reported to be surprisingly radio sensitive.

TERATOMA OF THE FALLOPIAN TUBE

Benign cystic teratoma is reported.

HAEMATOSALPINX

This condition, an accumulation of blood in the Fallopian tube, may be secondary to many lesions. Typically it is seen with a tubal mole. It may be part of the distended genital tract seen when menstrual blood is retained, due to an imperforate hymen or cervical stenosis. It occurs occasionally in association with fibroids or endometriosis or in some cases of chronic salpingitis.

Retroperitoneal tumours

PELVIC HAEMATOMA

Blood in the retroperitoneal tissue is seen occasionally after operation on the pelvic organs, due to capillary oozing from a large raw surface, or to the slipping of a ligature from a larger vessel. In pregnancy or after labour it may follow tears of the lower segment or cervix. Such a haematoma is usually left to absorb, unless the causal lesion itself needs operation, e.g. ruptured uterus; but if the haematoma is massive or becomes infected it may need to be drained through the vaginal vault. Very occasionally laparotomy is necessary to ligate the bleeding vessel, or if this is impossible, to tie the internal iliac artery on the affected side.

NEOPLASMS OF THE RETROPERITONEAL TISSUE

These are uncommon. Parovarian cysts are strictly retroperitoneal since they arise within the layer of the broad ligament. Ovarian cysts may grow retroperitoneally, especially in cases where salpingectomy or partial ovarian resection has been performed previously. They distend, first, the mesosalpinx, then the broad ligament; they then burrow behind the peritoneum of the infundibulo-pelvic fold and the lateral pelvic wall and finally open into the sigmoid mesocolon. Clinically and at operation they are truly retroperitoneal cysts. Removal is not usually difficult but displacement of the ureter, the ovarian vessels and the vessels supplying the sigmoid colon may complicate the operation.

Embryonic cysts in the mesentery or in the broad ligament or as simple dermoids. Traumatic cysts follow haemorrhage, inflammatory cysts are mycotic, parasitic or tuberculous, and neoplastic cysts are lymphangiomata, mesenchymoma.

Cysts may present after rupture or torsion or as a mass, normally they are smooth round and mobile. They are *not* tethered in the pelvis.

Solid neoplasms of the retroperitoneal tissue of the pelvis are fibromas, neurofibromas, chondromas, osteogenic sarcomas, chordomas, giant-cell tumours, mesenchymomas etc. Treatment depends on the type of tumour and is best done in conjunction with a general or orthopaedic surgeon.

TUMOURS OF VULVA

There are many and varied causes for vulvar swellings and ulcerations, and the differential diagnosis can be difficult.

Developmental lesions vary from inguinal hernia and accessory breast tissue to unilateral hypertrophy. Oedema may be associated with varicosity or elephantiasis or with various infections from furuncle to tuberculosis.

Simple cysts, simple solid neoplasms and malignant neoplasms may occur in the labia; urethra or associated vulvar glands.

Varices of the vulva

During pregnancy extensive varices of the vulva and of the vagina may develop, usually, but not always, in association with extensive varicosity of the saphenous veins. Despite the fact that the veins are thin-walled and may become very distended, they *seldom rupture*, even during labour. Dragging discomfort, due to varicosity of the veins of the inguinal region, may suggest a hernia. Under such circumstances the patient should be examined standing.

Rest, with the legs elevated, is the only effective palliative treatment during pregnancy. Wearing of elasticated tights may help. If the veins remain dilated after the puerperal period, excision, or obliteration by means of sclerosing fluid, is possible.

In old women permanent varicosity of veins of the mons and labia majora may cause a feeling of weight or tension. Such cases present with a provisional diagnosis of prolapse and unless they are examined standing the real cause of the symptoms may be missed.

Cysts of the vulva

Retention cysts may arise from sebaceous or pseudiferous glands. Wolffian remnants occasionally give rise to cysts and lymphangiomatous cysts sometimes occur. Implantation cysts of epithelial tissue may follow operative incisions. All such cysts are best excised. The most common type of cyst is that arising in connection with the *ducts of Bartholin's gland*. These cysts usually arise as a later result of infection (*see* Chapter 36), with blockage of a main or a subsidiary duct. The cyst may be discovered when it is quite small and can best be palpated between the finger and thumb deep in the tissues of the labium majus. Enlargement of the cyst usually takes place outwards and forwards and medially. First the labium minus and then the labium majus becomes flattened out over the enlarging cyst which may reach the size of a hen's egg, fill the posterior two-thirds of the labia and bulge across the introitus. Apart from its presence and discomfort on walking or sitting, the cyst may produce no symptoms. Exacerbation of the infection may occur and the clinical picture of an abscess develops. Abscesses should be drained by free incision and marsupialized. It may be necessary to excise the gland later. Cysts of the gland which are uninfected are best treated by marsupialization.

Hydrocele of the canal of nuck

This due to the presence of fluid between the round ligament and its associated peritoneum. It is uncommon, is congenital and presents as an elongated translucent swelling in the upper vulva. Differentiation from a hernia is difficult and somewhat academic, as, if symptoms are present, both need operative exploration of the inguinal canal.

Endometrioma of canal of nuck

This is an unusual site for endometriotic deposit.

Condylomata acuminata

Such warts associated with intranuclear papilloma virus behave like a sexually transmitted disease. They are sited at the areas most often damaged by coitus and are exacerbated by pregnancy. These warts cannot be innoculated to the general skin surface. The incubation period may be up to one year.

There may be associated seed warts from the condylomata lata of syphilis but since both are sexually transmitted both may coexist. In such patients the other sexually transmitted diseases, gonorrhoea and trichomaniasis, should be searched for. These warts rarely become malignant.

Treatment depends on size. Podophyllin resin 10 per cent in spirit can deal with most small warts. The surrounding skin should be protected in the several weekly applications. For large warts diathermy or electro cautery under general anaesthesia is used.

In the pregnant patient when warts may be extensive podophyllin should be used sparingly and then only diluted in Tinc. Benz. 60. Intravaginal warts are best treated by Tincture of Iodine followed by povidine iodine (Betadine) pessaries. Extensive vulvar warts are best treated by the expert by extreme cold applied by copper forceps cooled to $-196\,°C$ in liquid nitrogen.

Endometriotic deposits

These and cysts may appear on the vulva usually in association with endometriosis elsewhere.

Neoplasms of vulva

The simple tumours are fibroma, lipoma, fibromyoma, neurofibroma and angiomas.

HIDRADENOMA OF VULVA

This tumour appears as a nodule on the labia or perianal region probably arising from an apocrine sweat gland. Histologically it has papillary and solid components. The acini show broad irregular columnar cells with large rounded nuclei. Mitotic figures occur and some pleomorphism may suggest adenocarcinoma. The lesion is simple and simple excision is adequate therapy.

All simple tumours may be localized, excised primarily as a biopsy procedure but often as a sufficient curative therapy.

Pre-malignant and Malignant lesions of the vulva

In the vulva as elsewhere there exist a series of lesions which may progress to invasive disease. This progress as elsewhere, is not inevitable and some may even regress.

The first group are the dystrophies, kraurosis, lichen sclerosis and leukoplakia. The second group are the more specific lesions which are variously considered pre-malignant in themselves.

The chromosome pattern of condylomata acuminata, Paget's disease in situ, invasive carcinoma and malignant melanoma studied by Katayama et al. (1972) show ranges of pattern. Most cells of condylomata and Paget's disease are normally diploid but those from in situ and invasive lesions are occasionally polyploid and some triploid especially with node involvement. The melanoma had particularly bizarre patterns.

BOWEN'S DISEASE

The condition appears as a fairly well demarcated area of the vulvar skin. The skin shows some thickening, and the area may be velvety or reddened, or if there is much keratinization, be scaly and white. There is usually burning pruritus and some bleeding. Diagnostic biopsy shows typical squamous carcinoma in situ. Areas for biopsy may be outlined by painting with 1 per cent toluidin blue in 1 per cent acetic acid in water (Collins Test).

PAGET'S DISEASE

Occasionally however, a similar clinical picture is on histological examination shown to have cells with pale vacuolated cytoplasm due to the presence of mucopolysaccharides as an intracellular material. This histology is identical to that previously described by Paget in the skin of the nipple.

Paget's cells in the skin of the vulva are in a fairly large proportion of cases associated with a sweat duct carcinoma somewhat deeper in the tissues of the vulva, but in some 25 per cent of cases no such primary source of cells can be found.

In this latter case it would appear that this is a locally induced metaplasia of the epithelial cells but the significance is unknown and in those cases the cells are themselves not malignant.

Lentigo malignum or malignant melanoma in situ
This is a rare condition clinically similar to the previous two, but in this situation the cells instead of containing mucin contain melanin.

Therapy of each of the three conditions above described is simple local vulvectomy without particularly wide excision and without gland dissection. It is quite imperative that in each of the three, careful search should be made for invasive diseases, in the first as a malignant invasive squamous carcinoma, in the second as sweat gland adenocarcinoma, and the third, of course, as an invading melanoma. Fluouracil ointment is suppressive to local recurrence.

Clinical carcinoma vulva

Malignant disease of the vulva is in 90 per cent of cases squamous carcinoma, but adenocarcinoma of sweat glands may occur and also of the Bartholins gland or its ducts and of the lower urethral orifice. Rarely malignant tumours may arise in residual tissues, such as the Wolffian duct system. Melanoma or naevocarcinoma is rare.

The lesion of carcinoma may appear as a crack in a previously atrophic or dysplastic skin, as a punched out ulcer or, as an elevated nodule. The lesion is usually ulcerating, with elevated edges and a sloughing base. Where the disease is advanced there may of course, be destruction of most of the vulva, with involvement of the surrounding skin. Infiltrative spread occurs to surrounding tissues, to urethra, to rectum or to bone. Lymphatics which run postero-anteriorly to anastomose freely in the area of the mons carry cells to the superficial and deep inguinal glands of *both* sides and ultimately to the iliac system. There may be occasionally a spread direct to internal iliac glands by lymphatics following the dorsal vein of the clitoris. Lymphatic spread within the pelvis is of course, to the iliac and ultimately to the aortic gland system. In 30–50 per cent of cases the glands are involved by the time the patient is first seen. In the advanced situation the involved glands may ulcerate through the skin forming buboes in the groin.

CLINICAL FEATURES
The symptoms are those of itching, burning, pain and discharge. Such symptoms may already exist in view of dystrophy or leukoplakic changes and there may be no apparent alteration with the development of the malignant disease.

Differential diagnosis is of course from herpes, Bechet's syndrome, lymphogranuloma, granuloma inguinalae, yaws, tuberculosis and syphilis. Biopsy is therefore essential in investigation.

Except in the West Indian Negro the disease is uncommon in young women but is progressively more common with advancing age. The most distressing feature of the condition is the lateness of diagnosis in elderly single ladies who are loathe to proclaim the symptom of itching or where inadequate investigation of such a symptom has not disclosed the disease. Pruritis occurring for the first time in a post-menopausal patient certainly must be considered to have malignant origin until proven otherwise. Women known to have atrophic vulvar lesions must be regularly followed up and checked so that the earliest onset of malignancy can be diagnosed. Diagnosis is made on clinical grounds but a surface cytological scrape is certainly worth doing when first seen, and biopsy is of course, essential.

Treatment
Therapy depends on a knowledge of the normal pattern of spread of the disease and on an appreciation of the extent of gland involvement. The only reasonable curative therapy currently available is radical surgery (*see* Chapter 45), with bilateral removal of palpable superficial and deep inguinal nodes. However, in the very old or very frail the glands need not necessarily be removed, unless they are clinically palpable. Unilateral operation rarely is justified. Where the disease involves or is close to the lower urethra it is often difficult to avoid incontinence, but the attempt should be made. Very extensive surgery may be necessary in some cases.

With experienced surgeons, modern techniques of anaesthesia, the judicious use of antibiotics and application of immediate or late skin grafting, the immediate prognosis has greatly improved and it has been possible to extend the range of operation and the number of women to whom it can be offered.

However, as already said, simple vulvectomy will often remove a distressing growth and in the elderly may offer a very excellent chance of cure.

It is generally accepted that radiotherapy has no place, but consultation with the radiotherapist in the apparent inoperable situation sometimes is of real value, as new techniques are being developed.

After operation, follow-up should be meticulous and prolonged and early local recurrence or persistence can often be dealt with by piecemeal excision.

The 'cure' rates vary from 30–75 per cent depending primarily on gland involvement and to some extent on the extent of operation (Charles, 1972).

Melanoma (naevo carcinoma) of vulva

This is a highly malignant tumour which may appear anywhere on the skin of the vulva and may be associated with melanoma elsewhere. It is rare in the very young, and becomes more common with advancing years, with a peak around about the age of sixty. Usually there is a single pigmented (or multiple) mole which bleeds or is associated with pruritis or dysuria. The only possible therapy is radical surgery as described under carcinoma of vulva, pelvic lymphadenectomy may be necessary where the disease is situated near the clitoris. Fifty per cent five year survival is to be expected provided the disease is diagnosed reasonably early. The great danger is early and rapid dissemination by the blood stream and clinically positive regional nodes is an ominous finding (Morrow & Rutledge, 1972).

Sarcoma of vulva

This is obviously possible, but very rare. Most lesions appear as small nodules. They may be fibrosarcoma or rhabdomyosarcoma. Simple excision appears to cure.

TUMOURS OF THE URETHRA

Urethral caruncle

This is the commonest tumour of the vulva and may be neoplastic or inflammatory in origin. It is discussed in Chapter 36.

Prolapse of the urethral mucosa

This condition may present as a red mushroom-like fold of mucosa which protrudes through the urethral orifice on straining. It is seen mainly in old women but occasionally in young children. It may be symptom-free or be associated with frequency and dysuria. Strangulation of the prolapsed mucosa may occur and the mass becomes blue-black, is very tender and may cause retention of urine. Excision of the prolapsed mucosa is the best treatment.

Carcinoma of the urethra

Where the cancer arises at the orifice the treatment is as described under Carcinoma of the Vulva. Half the urethra can be removed without residual incontinence. Carcinoma higher in the urethra has usually spread from the bladder or from the uterine cervix. The treatment of such lesions is very difficult and involves surgical removal of the urethra and bladder, along with the uterus, cervix, vagina and the pelvic lymph glands. The ureters are transplanted into the pelvic colon as a preliminary step. Assessment of the results of these extensive procedures is not yet possible.

Diverticulum of the urethra

This a relatively uncommon condition in Britain, but comparatively common in some populations. It presents as a mid-line cystic swelling about $\frac{1}{2}$ to one inch from the urethral orifice and a sound can usually be passed into it from the urethra. The diverticulum can be excised and the urethra repaired.

TUMOURS OF THE VAGINA

Lumps or masses in the vagina arise from many reasons and may be developmental or retention cysts, or simple or malignant tumours. A rather unusual granuloma may persist in scars from various forms of vaginal repairs.

CYSTS

Cysts commonly arise in the anterior or lateral walls from embryonic remnants of Mullerian tissue or from portions of the Wolffian (Gärtner's) duct. Implantation cysts of epithelium may appear in scars following childbirth or operation. Most cysts are single, but some Gärtner's duct cysts or adenomas arising are multiple and extend along the whole length of the vagina.

Symptoms are uncommon, unless the cyst is large. There may be difficulty in intercourse or the cyst may be discovered when a contraceptive diaphragm or sanitary tampon is being inserted.

The diagnosis is usually easy but urethral diverticulum, cystocele, rectocele and enterocele should be considered. The treatment is excision.

SOLID TUMOURS

Of the vagina, these are uncommon, but fibromata and *fibroids* are seen. These may ulcerate, cause bleeding and discharge, and occasionally reach a large size. They may be technically difficult to remove without damage to the bladder, urethra or rectum.

Occasionally, vaginal deposits of *endometriosis* present as pea-sized purple nodules under the mucosa. These closely resemble the vaginal nodules secondary to *chorion-epithelioma*. These latter deposits may be the first sign of the disease.

Vaginal adenosis

This condition has become more common in recent years and is clearly associated in young women (as is vaginal adenocarcinoma) with previous maternal intake of stilboestrol in pregnancy, but it occurs in other women, usually in older age groups.

Adenosis and adenocarcinoma may co-exist. The primary complaint is commonly bleeding often with yellowish discharge and dyspareunia. The lesion usually appears as large clusters of heaped up masses of small cysts throughout the vagina (Blaikley *et al.*, 1971).

Biopsy should always be performed in case of malignant change. Local excision is sufficient as therapy.

Carcinoma of the vagina

Squamous carcinoma of the vagina, as a primary disease, is relatively uncommon. In the Eastern Region of Scotland, with some 450 000 people, 51 cases of primary invasive disease have been seen in the last 25 years (Daw, 1971). *In situ* squamous carcinoma as a single or multiple focal lesion does of course, occur in the vaginal skin and may be associated with *in situ* or invasive carcinoma of the cervix.

Clinical staging of the carcinoma of the vagina as suggested by the International Federation of Obstetrics and Gynaecology is almost identical to staging of carcinoma of cervix.

Stage 0   Carcinoma *in situ*.

Stage 1   Disease limited to the vaginal wall.

Stage 2   Disease affecting the subvaginal tissues but not yet reached the pelvic wall.

Stage 3   Disease extending to the bony pelvis.

Stage 4   Disease has extended to bladder or to the rectum or outwith the true pelvis.

Clinically the condition presents with postmenopausal or inter-menstrual bleeding or discharge and usually exists as a fungating tumour or an eroding ulcer. Most such tumours are seen in the upper vagina and have been in the past, often associated with the long time use of a vaginal supporting pessary, which may well have been forgotten. Vault lesions may of course, later follow known carcinoma of cervix and primary invasive vault carcinoma may follow *in situ* of the cervix previously treated by hysterectomy. The condition of squamous *in situ* or invasive carcinoma of the cervix and vagina is of course, multi focal and lesions which are apparent recurrences are often new growths arising in a different area of squamous epithelium.

Treatment

In situ carcinoma is beat treated by multiple local excision of the affected sites or rarely by total vaginectomy. αFluoracil ointment may suppress the disease.

Clinical lesions in the upper third of the vagina should be treated by radiation or by surgery or by a combination of both, rather as of they were lesions of the cervix. As in cervix therapy it depends on the stage of the disease.

Lesions in the lower third may, if very low down, be treated surgically as if they were carcinomas of vulva. In general lesions of the middle area of the vagina are best treated by intra-cavity radiation followed by high voltage therapy. There is however, a place for posterior exenteration, that is removal of the vagina, uterus and rectum, in cases of middle third posterior lesions which involve the rectum.

Stage 1 and very early Stage 2 lesions should have at least a 75 per cent 5 year survival; more extensive lesions have a much poorer chance and overall survival is barely 40 per cent.

ADENOCARCINOMA OF THE VAGINA

This is extremely rare. It may arise from Wolffian of Mullerian cell rests, and has recently been reported from the United States (Herbst *et al.*, 1971), but not yet from Britain; to occur in a form resembling endometrial carcinoma or as a clear cell adenocarcinoma in young women from 15–22 years of age, whose mothers had been treated by intensive therapy with diethylstilboestrol during pregnancy. There are estimated to be more than 10 000 young women at risk. Such stilboestrol therapy was almost always begun in the first trimester and given in increasing dosage until term. Such therapy was given mostly in the treatment of the pregnant diabetic or the woman with a previous history of poorly grown babies. It is likely that vaginal adenosis may also be stilboestrol related and also of course, clear cell carcinoma of cervix.

Secondary malignant disease

Of the vagina, this can, of course, follow carcinoma of the cervix, carcinoma of the body of the uterus, bladder or urethra and on occasion carcinoma of ovary has been seen to grow into the posterior fornix. Direct spread from carcinoma of the rectum is not uncommon. It will be obvious therefore, that all patients with malignant disease of the vagina should be carefully searched for a possible primary source, especially if the vaginal disease should seem unusual in any way.

Choriocarcinoma

This in the vagina is not uncommon and as a rarity *endometriosis* with conversion to adenocarcinoma has been reported.

Melanoma of vagina

This is rare but Daw (1972) has reviewed the published series.

Papillary pigmented growths usually in the lower third are associated with post-menopausal bleeding. Therapy should be similar to that for carcinoma but local and blood spread to liver or brain is rapid.

EXFOLIATIVE CYTOLOGY IN GYNAECOLOGICAL NEOPLASIA

The fact that epithelial carcinomas exfoliate abnormal cells has been long known. Papinocolaou and Traut in 1943 however, described the techniques of investigation of the fluid from the posterior fornix pool to search for cells exfoliated from the genital tract. Ayre in 1947 suggested the use of a spatula to scrape the cervix in the region of the squamo-columnar junction, and more recently it has been suggested that lesions high in the cervical canal might be best ascertained by a special brush to produce cells. It was very rapidly found that severe dysplasia of the cervix and certainly carcinoma *in situ* produced cells that could be recognized as grossly abnormal in themselves and that subclinical invasive carcinoma occurring in an apparently healthy cervix, could be discovered by cytological smear.

Throughout the world mass screening programmes to detect early cervical carcinoma have been instituted with various degrees of success and with very varied response from the women themselves and from the medical and scientific profession.

In some forms of population screening it is clear that worthwhile results are found only when population at special risk are selected for study e.g. in breast, women over 45 with late first pregnancies. In carcinoma of cervix the risk to a population reaches significance numerically only after the age of 35 and it was this fact that originally suggested to the Ministry of Health in England that screening only above that age should be instituted as a routine in the NHS. While in a total population this is a true age at which the major risk starts there are below that age some very high risk groups indeed. Recently, however, with the contraceptive pill replacing the barrier (sheath and cap), contraceptives and the increasing sexual freedom at younger age-groups the incidence of preclinical cervical cancer has doubled in the 20–24 age-group in the British Columbia programme. Stephenson (1973) reported on the colposcopic findings in women in a prison population in the age-group 15–70. Forty-five per cent showed abnormal colposcopy and 10 per cent serious histological change. He stated that preclinical precursor lesions begin in the cervix in susceptible women within two to three years of first intercourse and all young girls with a history of promiscuity already had abnormal lesions. It is clear therefore, that cervical smear cytology should be carried out routinely in all women having regular intercourse and most certainly in those where there is, in addition, promiscuity, poor social conditions or malnutrition. Carcinoma *in situ* will be found in young women in these groups.

Criticism of cervical cytology as a population screen or a valid method for reduction of clinical carcinoma is mainly along three lines. Firstly that dysplasia is rarely if at all a malignant precursor, Green (1970); secondly that many invasive lesions never have an *in situ* phase and thirdly that diagnosis of *in situ* carcinoma in the young woman leads often to therapy the results of which may be worse than the risk of later disease.

It is quite clear that dysplasia in all its forms may not proceed further and certainly most of the dysplasia associated with infection will regress with therapy. It is true that even carcinoma *in situ* may remain as such for very many years. It is also true that poor quality cytology and histopathology may over diagnose (or under diagnose and miss lesions) and that ill-conceived surgery or poor later obstetric care can have disasterous results. Bad quality care does not negative the basic value of the technique and such poor care is seen in many other situations.

Rickart (1973) in reporting the natural history of cervical neoplasia suggested that such lesions begin as single cell changes and that 'there was convincing evidence that progression from the mildest dysplasia through carcinoma *in situ* to clinically invasive cervical was continuous and accelerating. Some 40 per cent of early dysplasia did not progress but the more severe the intra-epithelial change the more likely was progression to occur'.

Worth (1973) reported on the British Columbia screening programme which started in 1949 and now includes 800 000 records. Smears were taken (mainly by general practitioners) of all women over 20 who had had intercourse. Smears taken before the use of oral contraceptives had proved that carcinoma *in situ* in young women was *not* due to the pill. Medial ages were 28 for carcinoma *in situ* (most common at 35), 41 for micro-invasion and 52 for clinically invasive cancer. The incidence of clinically invasive cancer had fallen by 1972 to one-third of that for 1955 and the mortality halved in the last ten years.

Women (age for age) in the *non screened* members of the community were seven times more likely to develop and twelve times more likely to die from invasive cancer of cervix. Similar results are reported from one other major centre Jefferson County, Kentucky which has been in operation since 1956. Cytology for cervical carcinoma in the United Kingdom owes most to the pioneer work of the University of Edinburgh Department of

Obstetrics and Gynaecology—Anderson 1953, and Anderson *et al.*, 1953.

In recent years cytological services have been established in most centres and with great success in the smaller centres of Aberdeen and Dundee where a defined population can be determined and attacked.

In Aberdeen there has been particular development of the various techniques of total population screening so that it has been possible to show results very similar to those from British Columbia (McGregor, Fraser & Man, 1971).

In Dundee, where 75·7 per cent of all married women aged 20–60 are now regularly screened, Duguid has shown that in comparing the years 1969–71 with the years 1959–61 there is now an *increase* in the frequency of Stage 1a lesions, a clear fall in Stage 1b and 2a lesions but no fall in the Stage 2b and 3 and 4. The fall in incidence of invasive lesions is almost entirely (as reported from other centres) in women in the age-groups under 50 years.

One of the problems of cytology screening and the main reason which lessens the impact is the difficulty of achieving screening in women of the lower social groups who are obviously for all reasons more highly susceptible to the disease. In Dundee for example, it has, to date, been possible to screen only a little over 60 per cent of those at risk, in social classes four and five. This is despite routine smears of all antenatal patients and a very intensive population pressure.

In Finland some 200 000 women have annual cervical cytological smears out of a total female population of 2·4 million. Some 98 per cent of the women at risk in Helsinki have been screened, and the figure is 87 per cent for the whole country. The incidence of cervical carcinoma has been clearly falling since 1967 especially in those women under 60 years of age and it is suggested that 100–120 carcinomas are annually prevented from reaching an invasive stage. There is also a clear fall in mortality. It is expected that quite soon when the screened women become older the mortality rate will fall (Timonen *et al.*, 1974).

In Auckland, where only some 20 per cent of women at risk appear to be screened, Green (1970) considers that the incidence of invasive cancer or the death rate both of which was already falling has not been accelerated by cervical screening. He also does not think that the survival rate has been improved. He has found in his own series of carcinoma *in situ*, followed over some years no little increased risk of development of invasive cancer (but longer follow-up is needed). He cannot agree that carcinoma *in situ* is a condition which commonly proceeds to invasive carcinoma.

While squamous carcinoma of the cervix is probably preventable as a clinical disease in a very large number of women by the routine use of cervical smear cytology every five years, cytology cannot be expected to eliminate the disease entirely. This is especially so where the disease progresses rapidly through its phases in less than five years. A fairly large number of women escape screening either by chance or by design and these are still seen with disease in Stage 3 to 4.

Cervical cytology for carcinoma should continue as a screening programme, but it is quite essential that the quality of the cytology, the investigative colposcopy (p. 753), the surgery and the histopathological reporting be first class and the quality constantly monitored. Failure to do this will result in over or under diagnosis and over or under treatment.

TECHNIQUES OF THE CYTOLOGIST IN GYNAECOLOGY

Cytological examination of aspirate from the posterior fornix pool (Papanicolaou), of material scraped from the cervix (Ayre, 1947), or 'brushed' from the uterine cavity is used mainly for the detection of cells which may arise from cervical or uterine epithelial neoplasia. However, those techniques frequently disclose cells from lesions elsewhere in the genital tract, vagina, tube or ovary and very occasionally from a generalized peritoneal malignancy.

Other lesions of the cervix, e.g. bilharzia or other helminth infection show special changes. The epithelial changes secondary to Vit B_{12} or folic acid deficiency are definitive and a guide sometimes to diagnosis.

Cervical or lateral vaginal wall scrape cytology is also of value in assessing the tissue response to hormones and to some extent therefore can be used to measure hormone production in menstrual anomaly or in infertility.

Vaginal smear cytology is also used to assess maturity of pregnancy and especially to discover post maturity.

Trichomonas and other infective material may be seen coincidentially in the smears.

Cellular debris, epithelial and bacterial in the background of the smear helps to evaluate the status of the epithelium.

Technique of the cervical scrape

It is customary to say that the scrape should be taken before digital examination but it may be necessary first to locate the cervix by such examination before visualization is easy. Lubrication of speculum and of rubber or plastic gloves is best done with warm water.

Most cytologists consider that (Duguid, 1974) the main cause of the dangerous false negative result is a smear that is scanty in material due to a scrape of the cervix which is much too gentle or occasionally where the smear is contaminated by blood or pus.

The cervix should be gently mopped clear of covering blood or pus and then the spatula should firmly scrape the entire squamocolumnar junction. The material is then smeared from both sides of the spatula on to a glass slide which is previously prepared with the name and identification of the patient.

The slide should then immediately be placed in fixative (95 per cent alcohol acetic acid and water soluble wax). The wax allows the slides to be removed after 10 minutes and air dried before transport to the laboratory.

Smears for hormone evaluation are best made from scrapes of the upper lateral vaginal wall.

Staining may be by a whole range of methods; the original Papinocalaou is used mostly, but special stains are used for special purposes.

Interpretation of the stained material should be undertaken only by experts. In many laboratories staff are trained to search slides for neoplastic cells only as a simple diagnostic service. In others the whole pattern of the smear is studied and interpreted.

Malignant cells show an enlarged nucleus more nearly filling the cell and there is some range of cytoplasm/nuclear ratio from cell to cell.

The nucleus is irregular and it stains dark with coarse clumps or strands of chromatin.

Dyskariotic cells are midway between simple and malignant. They have nuclear changes similar to the malignant cell but the cytoplasm has not been much altered.

Fully trained technicians can and do examine accurately some 90 per cent of slides but all cells containing selected types of abnormal cells require the opinion of an expert cytologist or a team of cytologists.

Detailed reporting of the smears will vary with the extent of the study and the purposes for which the smear is taken. The following is an example of a cervical screening service report.

Class 0 Unsatisfactory please repeat.
Class 1 Normal.
Class 2 ⎫ Abnormal—please repeat in three to six
Class 3 ⎭ months.
Class 4 Probably malignant—suggest cone.
Class 5 Clearly malignant.

Class 0 smears are those where there is obvious inadequacy of material since the scrape is badly taken, or there is little exfoliation (as in a post-menopausal woman). When the detail is obscured by blood or pus, this is the classification which should be used and further smears taken after gently cleaning the cervix.

Class 1. The smear is normal for the age and parity of the patient and presumably for the stage of the menstrual cycle at which it was done.

Classes 2 & 3. These smears show varying degrees of dyskariosis and may also demonstrate trichomonas or other infections. They are 'dirty' smears. Both indicate changes which must be further investigated by repeated smears or colposcopy if available.

In some 10 per cent of cases patients with Class 3 smears are already harbouring an *in situ* lesion. Repeat smears will become Class 4 or 5. In others treatment of infection or diathermy will return the smear to normal.

Class 4. Smears show sufficient cellular aberration to suggest severe dyskariosis or *in situ* change at least. Colposcope selected multiple punch or cone biopsy is essential.

Class 5. Smears show malignant cells and it is up to the gynaecologist to find the source.

Accuracy

If the smear reports Class 2 or 3 there is usually some clinical evidence of infection. Class 4 or 5 smears *from a first class laboratory* are very rarely false positives provided proper biopsy material is taken for review and studied by an expert histopathologist. The false negative is a more worrying situation. Some 10 per cent of cases of *clinical* carcinoma of the cervix will be 'negative' in a smear, but clinical carcinoma should never require a 'smear'. If there is suspicion or certainty of clinical disease, biopsy is essential.

A false negative report is more likely because of poor quality smears badly taken or with the cells obscured by blood or pus, or because of poor quality cytology. Very occasional scanty abnormal cells may be missed. In susceptible populations there is much to be said for two smears one taken some months after the first before the cervix is accepted as free of disease.

The incidence of positive Class 4 or 5 smears from the cervix will obviously vary with the age and social structure of the population studied.

Young women have a very low rate (carcinoma *in situ* 0·6 per cent) unless they are prostitutes or promiscuous in which case a very high incidence of abnormal smears will be found. Most of those girls will have inflammatory or early dyskariotic changes only in their cervical epithelium.

In older women of high parity from the poorer social groups a high incidence of positive smears will be found.

Overall some seven women per 1000 will show seriously abnormal smears i.e. Class 4 or 5 and of those one will prove to be an already invasive carcinoma, four will be carcinoma *in situ* and two will show some degree of dysplasia.

Significance

A Class 2 smear is the most difficult to assess but interpretation is greatly helped by colposcopy which allows areas of abnormal epithelium to be selected for biopsy. A fair number (some 10 per cent) of Class 3 smears are shown to arise from already established carcinoma *in situ* (rarely micro-invasive) and persistence of such smears despite local therapy requires action as in a Class 4 or 5 smear.

A Class 4 or 5 smear is a clear indication for further investigation, again with colposcopic examination. Except in the pregnant patient selective or multiple punch biopsy or cone biopsy is required. In all cases cervical curettage should follow so that disease high in the cervix will not be missed.

In the pregnant woman clinical assessment should be made and if the cervix is apparently normal no action should be taken until after the patient is delivered. If repeat smear is then positive cone biopsy is undertaken some three to six weeks after delivery (*see* Chapter 20).

In a significant study of some 150 000 unselected patients screened by cytological techniques Bibbo, Keebler and Wied (1971) discovered 3602 cases of dysplasia (24 per cent), 849 of carcinoma *in situ* (6 per cent) and 228 invasive cancers (1·5 per cent).

The peak prevalence for invasive disease was at age 50–60, for dysplasia 25–29. Lesions were more common in patients taking contraceptive steroids or with an IUCD fitted, possibly because they were more at risk.

Carcinoma *in situ*

The history of the recognition of carcinoma *in situ* as a lesion of importance has been outlined by Te Linde (1973). Early American and German writers had noted the existence of a histological lesion, sometimes associated with invasive carcinoma and sometimes showing an apparent superficial spread. The German writers in particular suggested that this was a superficial spread of invasive disease. Rubin (1910) suggested that this peculiar lesion might be an early form of invasive disease. It was Te Linde and Galvin who in the period of 1944–52 suggested that carcinoma *in situ* preceded invasive cancer by a period sufficiently long to allow therapy. Cytology developed about this time and because of the findings and suggestions of Te Linde and Galvin and the availability of cytology as designed by Papinocolaou and Traut (1943) a whole new possibility of screening for this lesion was made possible.

The work of Te Linde and Galvin (1944–52) and of very many others has shown clearly that there is a natural progression from early dystrophic change in the epithelium of the cervix through varying degrees of dysplasia, through the classical histological change of intra-epithelial carcinoma (*in situ*) and then through subclinical invasion and thence to clinically obvious disease.

This process may take a very long period of time perhaps as long as twenty or more years. In many women the process may regress at any of the earlier stages. In others it is never completed, while in those who have clinical disease by the age of 25 the process must be very fast indeed. It is significant that the peak age at which carcinoma *in situ* is found is 35–45 some 10 years earlier than the peak age of 45–55 for clinical disease.

It is clear therefore, that it should be possible to detect changes at some stage when definitive therapy could prevent further progress. It must however, always be remembered that natural regression does occur, that all cases in each stage do not necessarily progress into the next or later stages and these factors should be taken into account when determining the extent of therapy required. It is also important to realize that the limited extent of the disease process in early stages may allow very minimal therapy to be successful.

THE PRECANCEROUS AND EARLY INVASIVE LESIONS OF THE CERVIX

According to Coppleson & Reid (1967) the first change at the squamo-columnar junction is a metaplasia of the columnar epithelium. They consider that this change is associated with abnormal external influences (pH, oxygen tensions, etc.). Other authors suggest that this change is essentially in response to chronic inflammation. From the areas of squamous metaplasia further change may lead directly to carcinoma *in situ* but more likely to dysplasias and thence to carcinoma *in situ*.

Dysplasia is characterized by disorderly arrangement of cells which at least in the basal layers have hyperkeratotic nuclei. There is much pleomorphism and areas of the epithelium have clearly active apparently malignant characteristics. Varying descriptions are given to varying pictures. Occasionally there is much activity of the basal layers alone (basal cell hyperplasia).

The degree of dysplasia is determined by the degree of change and the extent of the change through the epithelium. A full thickness change merits the diagnosis of carcinoma *in situ*.

Carcinoma in situ

The distinction between the more severe forms of dysplasia and 'carcinoma *in situ*' is often a matter of the opinion of the histopathologist, although the distinction is said to be more easily made by colposcopy. Classically in carcinoma *in situ* there is a full thickness change and the whole or virtually the whole of the epithelium consists of cells of obvious malignant characteristics (Fig. 38.9). Occasionally the

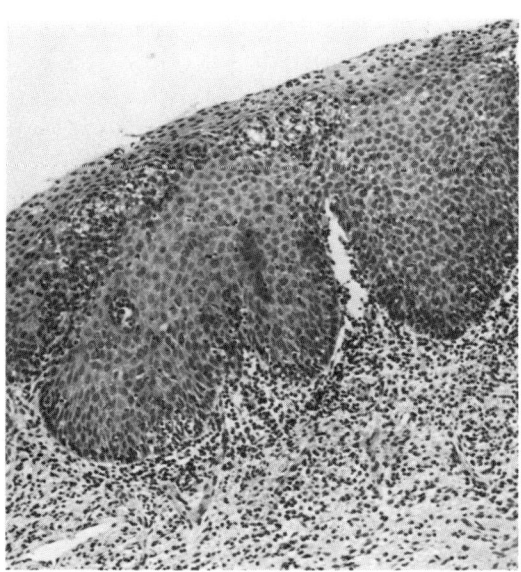

Fig. 38.9 *In situ* carcinoma.

abnormal epithelium invades and displaces the epithelium of the cervical glands. To the unwary the histology suggests invasion.

Studying of the chromosome of cells of carcinoma *in situ* Kirkland (1963) suggests that a diploid pattern indicates that progression to invasion is more likely.

Micro-invasive carcinoma (Stage 1a)

The extent of disease which can truly be called micro-invasive varies a little with the reporting laboratory, the condition where a few small tongues of malignant cells invade the stroma is sometimes reported as 'minimally invasive'. This is the first measurable stage at which the disease has spread into the tissues of the cervix. This state may remain for some time. This early stage is more often discovered since smear cytology demonstrating 'malignant cells' is followed by selective diagnostic biopsy or cone biopsy.

Subclinically invasive (Stage 1a)

This is a further stage of the disease. The scattered tongues of discrete micro-invasion become confluent and coalesce but there is still no clinical appearance of disease.

Colposcopy

The examination of the living cervix, of its epithelium and of the angio architecture in the normal and metaplastic state can be undertaken by binocular magnifying microscopy.

Colposcopy was originally developed in Europe in 1925 by Hinselmann and is a standard procedure in most European clinics.

Basically the colposcope (Fig. 38.10) provides a means of viewing with magnification the cervix, vagina and vulva, its cervical use method and each evaluates different aspects of neoplasia. Cytology evaluates changes in cells shed by or scraped from the tissue under investigation whereas through the colposcope the intact living tissue may be viewed without any pain or discomfort to the unanaesthetized

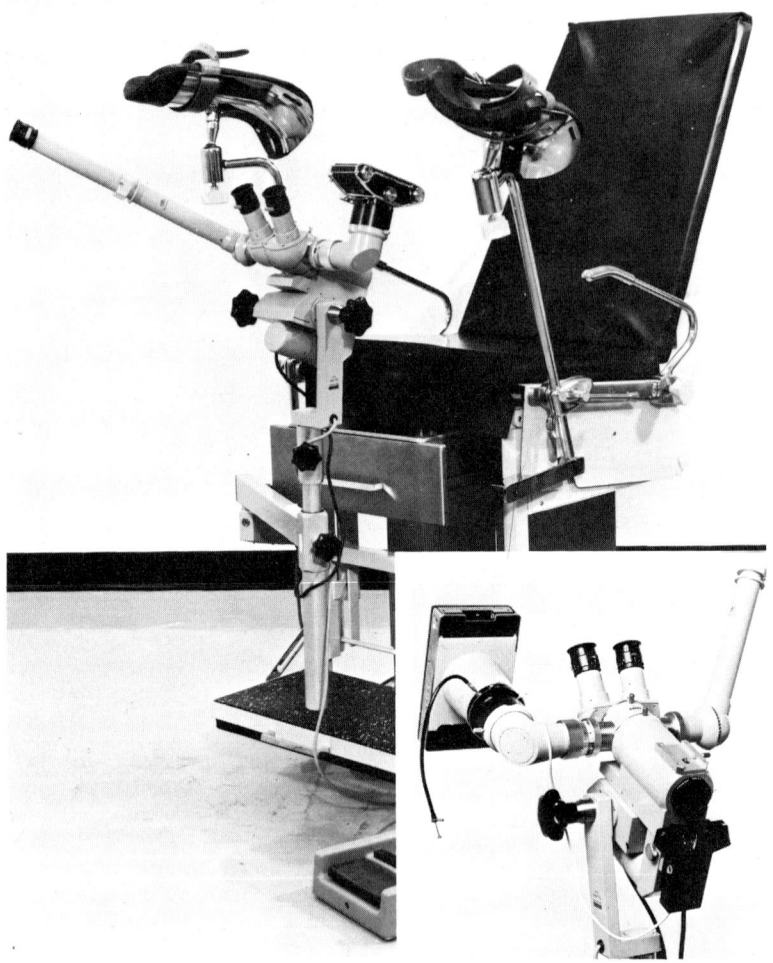

Fig. 38.10   The colposcope and Gynaemat Chair.

being the main one. During the past decade the use of colposcopy in the early diagnosis of cervical neoplasia has become increasingly widespread in the USA. The earlier evolution of cytology in Britain and the historical competition of cytology versus colposcopy in the early diagnosis of cervican neoplasia probably accounts for the slow acceptance of colposcopy in this country. Only recently has it become evident that both methods actually complement each other. Cytology is a laboratory method whereas colposcopy is a clinical patient and observation made of the epithelial vascular pattern, surface contour and colour, all of which gradually change with advance of the neoplastic process from normal through dysplasia and carcinoma *in situ* to invasive cancer.

Coppleson and Reid (1967) have shown that colposcopic appearances are abnormal in 90 per cent of women with *in situ* carcinoma or pre-clinical invasive carcinoma of the cervix. Usually all abnormal epithelial areas fail to stain with iodine. If there are abnormal smears, colposcopy should follow Schiller iodine test and abnormal areas selected by the colposcope should be taken by punch biopsy. Cervical curettage should follow so that abnormal areas within the canal are not missed. Many studies have compared cytology and colposcopy and there is general agreement that the combination of both methods increases the diagnostic accuracy over that of each method used separately—Limburgh (1958) and Navratil et al. (1958).

In the presence of abnormal cytology a tissue diagnosis should be made on which to base therapy. Random punch biopsies, even of areas which fail to stain with iodine in the absence of a visible lesion commonly result in a false negative histological diagnosis the focus or foci of abnormality being missed by the biopsy forceps. Invasive carcinoma is visible to the naked eye, *pre-malignant intra-epithelial neoplasias is visible only through the colposcope*. Since blind biopsies taken randomly are unreliable, recourse in the absence of colposcopy has had to be made to the widespread use of cold knife conization whereby a large cone of tissue is excised from the cervix for histological study. Unfortunately a cone biopsy as well as having to be performed on in-patients under anaesthesia carries with it also a notable morbidity from haemorrhage, infection, cervical stenosis and incompetence, the last two conditions possibly adversely affecting the future fertility of the patient. In pregnancy the increased chance of haemorrhage and risk of premature labour resulting from the procedure are very real. Ideally therefore, one would prefer a procedure less radical for blanket use on patients caught in the cytology screening net. Colposcopically directed biopsies have proven to be the answer in those cases where there is a colposcopically visible lesion and this lesion can be seen in its entirety. This is true in up to 95 per cent of all patients (Stafl and Mattingly, 1973). Such biopsies may be taken without anaesthesia in the out-patient clinic thereby avoiding the necessity of hospitalizing the patient for biopsy purposes alone. Conization can be reserved for those patients where it is definitely indicated. This might be when the lesion is seen through the colposcope to extend up the canal; when no lesion whatsoever is seen despite repeatedly abnormal cytology smears; or where the degree of abnormality suggested by cytology is significantly worse than the histology of the colposcopically directed biopsy. Cone biopsy as well as being diagnostic may also be therapeutic but recent reports of the use of cry-surgery (Creaseman et al., 1973) suggest an acceptable alternative, less morbid, less expensive out-patient procedure, the more-so welcome in view of the increasing numbers of abnormal cytology smears and the younger age-groups from which these smears are being obtained.

Since 1928 when Papanicolaou introduced the study of cytology, advancements in cytology laboratories and training centres have greatly influenced the clinical accuracy of this diagnostic tool. Similarly increasing experience with colposcopy will greatly fine the accuracy of diagnosis and the correctness of therapy in the very large and increasing number of women with abnormal smears.

Lymphography

Lymphography using the veins of the foot to outline the external and common iliac and aortic glands is of value in all patients with bulky tumours of whatever stage (Douglas et al., 1972). It is possible to outline fully the internal and obturator systems only by using the femoral head as a site of injection. This is very painful, requires anaesthesia and is of doubtful value in any case.

Five ml of iodized poppy seed oil (lipiodol) injected into a foot lymphatic will visualize the whole of the lymphatic chain to the supra-clavicular nodes. Excess must not be used as it becomes small fat emboli in the lung. Immediate photography show the vessels, and after at least 24 hours the nodes are visualized.

White (1971) considers that interpretation of results depends on even filling. Totally involved nodes do not fill although the peripheral sinuses may show. Micro-invasion cannot be discovered and occasionally a normal node will not fill.

Probably the technique is of value only in assessing the extent of advanced disease but much more experimental work is needed. It has been used with chlorophyl colouring of the lipiodol and therefore of the lymphatic glands to delineate the glands for dissection for the Wertheim operation moreover it can be used after surgery to decide whether any glands have not been removed and where they are.

GYNAECOLOGICAL ONCOLOGY AND THE PATIENT

The gynaecological surgeon who wishes to treat patients with malignant disease should be part of a team who can bring to the patient the investigative skills necessary for early and accurate diagnosis, not only of the existence of a lesion but of its extent and the areas to which it has spread. There must be available surgical skill for radical elimination of the disease and expert chemotherapy, radiotherapy, hormone therapy or immunotherapy, so that the treatment selected is dictated by the patient's need alone. The details of her therapy should be obtained by joint discussion of a group expert in all the requisite fields.

There seems little doubt that more extensive training and experience in gynaecological oncology is essential within the speciality and that the trained gynaecological oncologist should be an essential part of the new oncological centres.

The attitude of the oncologist should be one of total ruthlessness in cure of the disease coupled with compassion for the patient to whom should be offered only that therapy which will cure or clearly palliate to her advantage. There is no simple guide to the approach to the patient.

Very few patients wish to be told the full truth and in any case what in the given circumstance is the truth that she should be told? Need she know that she has a micro-invasive carcinoma of cervix or that she has a Stage III lesion when the word 'early' would give her much more hope and the will to live?

British doctors on the whole take part in a somewhat kind and tolerant relationship in which hope and forward plans are part of the patient's right. It is virtually impossible to select the patient who ought to be told but always with the patient and certainly with the relatives hope must not be destroyed and prognosis though guarded must always be on the optimistic side. Why should a woman who statistically has a 30 per cent chance of survival be told that her chances are poor? She should have a chance to live with life not death, for what might be very many years.

GYNAECOLOGICAL TUMOURS IN CHILDREN

In the *cervix* carcinoma is usually an adenocarcinoma or perhaps a carcinoma of apparently mesonephric origin and behaves no differently from that in the adult, or adolescent.

Sarcoma botryoides (mixed mesodermal tumour) is a rare tumour of vaginal or cervical origin and arising from one may involve the other. It is associated with a serosanguineous discharge and appears as a polypoid or grape-like mass which may or may not be pedunculated. Metastasis to the lymphatics are late; local spread is early. Recurrent polyps of the cervix are almost certainly malignant in the young. Total hysterectomy and vaginectomy are essential as a minimum therapy and radiation appears to be of limited value.

The presenting symptom of *ovarian tumours* in children is most often pain from torsion or of course, the presence of a mass, but diagnosis is difficult as the possibility is often not considered. In 81 tumours recently reported in children up to 14 years of age, some 10 were cystadenomas, 17 were simple teratoid cysts, 20 embryonal or malignant teratomas, 15 dysgerminomas, and 8 were granulosa cell tumours. Cystadenomas and the teratoid cysts should of course, be treated by simple cystectomy. Simple salpingo-oophorectomy may suffice for apparently malignant lesions limited to one ovary, but extensive surgery is necessary with bilateral lesions or lesions which have apparently spread.

Good results are reported from limited surgery even in the dysgerminoma although there is in general some dubiety about the proper therapy of this lesion (*see* Chapter 45). More recently it has been suggested that radical treatment with irradiation of the pre-aortic nodes (as in seminoma) is essential. Embryonal carcinoma and myxosarcomas may respond to radiation with associated chemotherapy.

Carcinoma of the vulva in prepubertal girls is reported from Africa. This is a hypertrophic exophytic squamous carcinoma arising on top of a chronic papilloma.

GYNAECOLOGICAL TUMOURS IN PREGNANCY

Ovarian tumours in pregnancy

In view of the fact that most pregnant woman are under 40, only two or three per cent of ovarian tumours are malignant. All types of ovarian tumour have been reported, but some but rarely, the most common tumours are the cystic teratomas and simple benign cysts. They are often associated with fairly rapid growth in pregnancy and often become very big. Diagnosis is often difficult and it is surprising how often the tumour is missed.

Gynaecological malignant disease and pregnancy

(*See* Chapter 29 for full discussion.)

Pregnant women rarely have gynaecological malignant disease probably because of the lower incidence in women under 45 years of age. More recently however, with developments of antenatal smear cytology carcinoma *in situ* has become a diagnosed antenatal complication in some two to six per thousand pregnant women and invasive disease may be seen in 0·5 per thousand.

Carcinoma of the vulva is very uncommon in the Western world in women currently pregnant, but no so infrequent in the West Indies. Women have successfully become pregnant after radical vulvectomy for vulvar carcinoma.

Carcinoma of the ovary may be expected perhaps in 1 in 10 000 women but the chance of an ovarian neoplasm in a pregnant woman being malignant is about 1 in 30.

Pregnancy and malignant disease in general

The patient who has already had malignant disease treated may well become pregnant.

Obvious examples are those with surgical excision of lesion of vulva, *in situ* of cervix, a single ovary, breast, stomach, of the central nervous system, of bone, etc., and those where chemotherapy has been used for treatment say of Hodgkin's disease or radioactive therapy for thyroid disease.

In general there is extremely little information available and much of the therapy is based on suspicion or doubt and very little on scientific evidence. In general breast carcinoma recurrence is thought to do badly if pregnancy is present. If a woman is suffering from recurrence of her malignant disease it would seem in general wise to consider termination of the pregnancy but when there is *no* recurrence a history alone of malignant disease should not preclude successful pregnancy but the extent and type of special antenatal or delivery care may have to be carefully determined.

RADIOTHERAPY

As discussed under various treatment headings radiotherapy has a wide field of application in gynaecological malignant disease. For many years the standard primary therapy for uterine cancer was radium but this is currently giving way to caesium. It is now generally agreed that the modalities of radiotherapy, surgery and chemotherapy are, in the management of the majority of cancers, complimentary the one to the other.

Pre-operative radiation

Some tumours especially ovarian may be so extensive and fixed that surgical extirpation is not possible. Pre-operative radiation carefully programmed, may so reduce the mass and extent of tumour as to render the tumour operable.

Pre-operative radiation to enhance the surgical cure rate

It is occasionally considered worthwhile to render a large fraction of the cancer cells incapable of growth. This will make dissemination at operation by seeding or by invasion of blood vessels or lymphatics less likely. The dose necessary to render 90 per cent of the cells incapable of further growth if disseminated or if already spread minimally is about 2000r or one-third of the total 'cancerocidal' dose. Irradiation of the tumour bed prior to surgery significantly lessens the number of cells which will survive if spilled or disseminated. It is difficult to decide on the ideal interval between radiation and operation or whether the radiation should be fractionated.

Post-operative radiation

Such radiation is given when the tumour has not been completely removed or where there may have been local dissemination at operation. Pre-operative radiation is theoretically better able to deal with cells which might be disseminated by suppressing their activity.

Efficacy

In general the cure rates of Stage 1 and Stage 2a lesions of the cervix are only slightly improved by X-ray therapy added to conventional radium to the local lesion.

In Stage 2b, 3 and 4 lesions supervoltage therapy would appear to have a distinct advantage over 250kV and the overall five year survival would appear to have risen.

On the whole, differentiated carcinomas respond better than undifferentiated. Mixed squamous and adenocarcinomas do badly as do clear cell adenocarcinomas.

Serial biopsy of the growing edge of a tumour under therapy is occasionally used as a test of response to radiotherapy. Cells are assessed as resulting, dividing, differentiating or degenerating and if *under therapy* the first two groups predominate, the outlook is poor. Alteration of the cell population depends not only on a direct effect of the rays on the cells but also the effect on the tumour bed and especially on its vascular supply system.

In general ovarian tumours can be expected to show response in some 20 per cent. Mucin secreting tumours and all mucin secreting secondary tumours virtually do not respond at all.

TECHNIQUES OF RADIOTHERAPY IN
GYNAECOLOGICAL MALIGNANT DISEASES

Radium was classically used for primary therapy to carcinoma of cervix or vagina although it is now being replaced by caesium. Therapy with X-ray 250kV or supervoltage over one million volts (linear accelerator) or cobalt is used in most other situations, or as an additive therapy in cervix or vagina.

The *plan* of therapy is to deliver a 'cancerocidal' dose to the tumour itself and to all areas to which the disease may have spread. In general the 'cancerocidal' dose is 5000 to 7500r. ('r' is a physically determined measure of radiation dosage received at site.)

Radium to carcinoma cervix

There are several accepted techniques but that most frequently used in the United Kingdom is the Manchester method (Tod and Meridith, 1938, 1953). In this method the therapy is fractionated into two doses 7 days apart—dosage is expressed in roetgens (r) and constant reference points are selected for dosage calculation. Point A is in the same sagittal plane as the uterus and sited 2cm from the mid-line and 2cm above the lateral fornix. Point B is 5cm from the mid-line at the same level and on the same plane.

Carcinoma cervix spreads laterally, upwards and downwards and rarely anteriorly or posteriorly.

The aim of radiation treatment is to cure the

primary local disease but it must be realized that 'cancerocidal dosage' from a standard radium application extends little more than 2cm from the mid-line and mainly laterally. So if the growth itself is greater than 2cm it will not be eradicated by radium.

The optimum dosage must be selected to give maximum dosage to the tumour without serious damage to the normal tissues. An optimum dosage to point A of 6–7500r is usually selected and the actual duration of therapy is calculated depending on the r/hour produced at point A by the radium sources (Fig. 38.11).

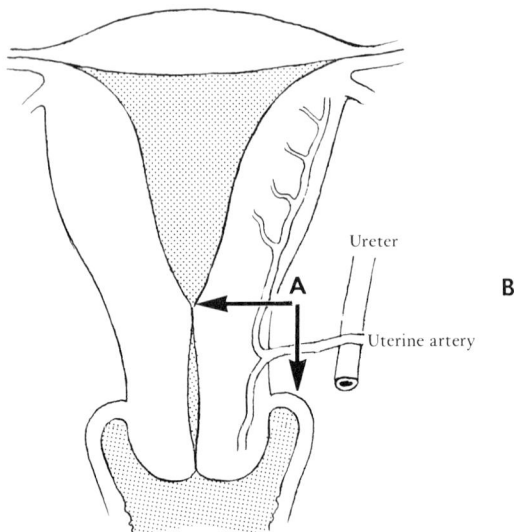

Fig. 38.11   Position of Point A. Pelvic landmarks for radiotherapy.

While the actual arrangement of the radium sources, the type and the central tube and the size of 'ovoids' varies with the case in question a standard system would be:

Intra-uterine tube—25–35mgm (15 + 10 + 10)mgm
Ovoids (Fornix)   —25mgm each

The first application gives roughly two-thirds of the total dose to be delivered. The second dose is given one week later. The time required may be something of the order of 70 and 40 hours, respectively.

Radium placed in the method shown will produce some 25–30 000r dosage at the mucosa, and 7000r at point A. Since the radiation dosage received falls off with the square of the distance from source the 'cancerocidal' effect is over a very limited area indeed (2cm or so). There is however some contribution across the pelvis even on the pelvic wall and where X-ray therapy is added allowance must be made for the contribution already made by the intracavity radium which of course falls off steadily across the pelvis. At point B the dosage is about 25 per cent of that received at point A. The rectum and bladder cannot stand high dosage and the rectum must be packed away from the radiation so that dosage received there is less than 60 per cent of that at point A.

Ideally after the radium is inserted a radiograph should be taken to determine the actual position of the radium sources so that the actual dosage to the various areas of the pelvis can be calculated. It is also possible to calculate rectal dosage by a dosimeter placed in rectum.

Calculation of the dosage given and received
Calculation is made of the dosage received by a knowledge of the physics of the system plus a knowledge of the actual planes as pre-planned by the use

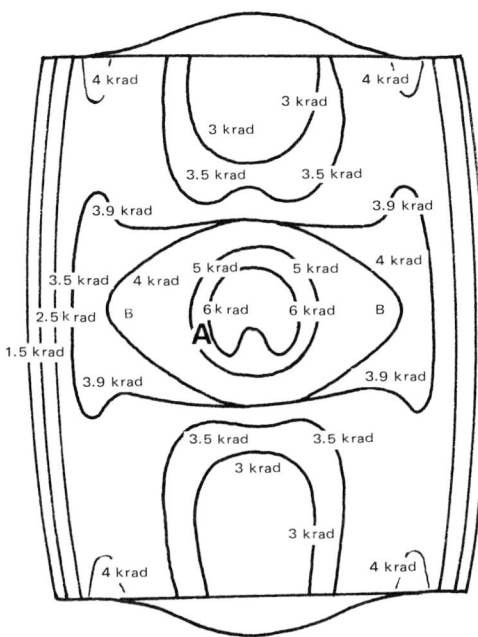

Fig. 38.12 Isodose curves. The dosimetry for a Point A dose of 6000 rads from combined intracavitary and external beam therapy, after Joslin. (This is a copy of a drawing by C. A. Joslin from 'Modern Radiotherapy—Gynaecological Cancer'. Ed. T. J. Deeley (1971), Butterworth. Fig. 8b.

of a treatment planner or simulator, or as shown by radiograph of situation of actual sources. Dosage at any point in the pelvis can be calculated by computer techniques (Fig. 38.12).

Replacement of radium by caesium
Recently there has been a tendency to replace radium by radioactive caesium (Cs^{137}) a by-product of nuclear fission. In contra-distinction to radium, caesium has no gaseous form and so is not subject to any radioactive gas leakage and it also does not emit α particles which is the main problem with any

leak. It needs less shielding and is much safer to handle and protection is less of a problem.

Its only disadvantage is that it has a half life of only about 30 years compared with radium 1700 years and this means an annual correction for dosage. Otherwise the dose distribution from both sources is almost identical.

After loading. Many modern techniques to apply radium, caesium, or cobalt use equipment which allows after loading. Applicators of various types are first placed in the uterus and vaginal vault under anaesthesia so that their correct and absolute placement can be guaranteed. The radiation source is then inserted after all the manipulation is performed. This allows minimal radiation exposure to the operator. In some, after loading is manual but in the *Cathetron, Cervitron* and *Curietron* the cobalt or caesium source is mechanically or pneumatically shot into position.

The 'cathetron' uses Cobalt 60 and the dosage times are very short (a matter of minutes), and the patient is virtually fixed in position during this time. In the cervitron or curietron (using caesium) the source can be removed temporarily into a bedside 'safe' while nursing is taking place and returned to the patient once the attendant is away from the risk.

X-ray and other therapies
Undoubtedly the most significant advance in the radiation treatment of malignant disease has been the introduction and widespread usage of High Energy (alternatively called Supervoltage or Megavoltage) therapy apparatus, that is Radiotherapy Units producing radiation of an energy over 1 000 000 electron volts (1MeV).

Prior to the advent of this type of apparatus, the radiation energy in common use was in the now called Orthovoltage range, using energies generally between 250 000 and 300 000 volts (250–300 kV), and this type of unit will always have a place in Radiotherapy, but not in the attempted cure of deep seated malignant disease, or where bone or cartilage intervene between the radiation source and tumour.

Unfortunately increase in energy means increase in cost, not only of apparatus but also of protection. It is fortunate that the cost of apparatus has not greatly increased, they have become more compact than the originals, and technology has kept both size and price fairly constant. However, building costs have increased greatly, and as high energy radiotherapy requires a concrete protective wall at least four feet thick, this will always be a major factor in cost.

In clinical practice the first widely used high energy apparatus came from the nuclear reactor by the production of radioactive cobalt (Co^{60}). This isotope emits gamma (γ) radiation, which is an electro-magnetic beam similar to X-rays with a narrow energy range between 1·1 and 1·3MeV.

Cobalt
A normal Cobalt^{60} Teletherapy unit can contain up

to 6000 Curies of cobalt compared with the original radium teletherapy unit of 100-150 Curies. Hence a great increase in the amount of radiation emitted which allows an increase in the distance between the source and subject for irradiation. X (or γ) rays, just like light, obey 'The Inverse Square Law'. In practical terms this means, double the distance, quarter the intensity or dose. So by increasing distance and source from the skin the percentage dose at depth, compared with that in the skin is increased. For example, treating a tumour at a depth of 10cm from the surface with a radiation source only 10cm from that surface would be $\dfrac{10^2}{(10+10)^2}$ or 25 per cent of skin dose reaches the tumour making no allowance for absorption. Treating the same tumour with a source of radiation 100cm from the skin surface results in $\dfrac{100^2}{(100+10)^2}$ or 82 per cent of the surface dose reaching the tumour making no allowance for absorption. So by increasing the treatment distance the percentage dose at depth is increased, and high dosage to the tumour does not increase the skin risk. Such teletherapy units will remain in many parts of the world as the principal form of high energy radiation. Co^{60} has however, several disadvantages, the main one being that it has a half life of 5·5 years which means that although the energy remains unchanged, the radiation dose rate falls (over the years), with the consequence that fewer patients can be treated per day and that the source (expensive) has eventually to be replaced about every three years.

Linear accelerator
The next stage was the introduction of electrically produced high energy radiation by units such as the *betatron* using electron or particle therapy, which was favoured on the continent of Europe and the *linear accelerator* producing *X-rays*, which was preferred in this country and *is now generally accepted as the best type of high energy radiation source available.*

High energy radiation has the following advantages.
1. First we have a unit producing a high output of short wave length radiation. High output means more patients treated due to shorter treatment times.
2. A greater distance between radiation source and tumour results in an increased percentage dose at the tumour compared with the maximum dose, which with orthvoltage (kV) falls on the skin.
3. This leads to further advantage. Radiation once it reaches a surface starts to 'scatter'. With orthovoltage this takes place in all directions—forwards, sideways and backwards. Because of this the dose falling on skin is maximum from the incident dose plus the contribution from 'scatter'. High energy on the other hand, produces 'scatter' mainly in a forward direction and so the maximum dose falls deep to the skin in subcutaneous tissue.
4. It has generally been accepted that moistness

with radiation has the adverse effect of increasing the skin reaction and this is common when the maximum dose falls on the surface as with orthovoltage, so that patients cannot wash when under treatment. But with high energy, when the maximum dose is in subcutaneous tissue, the patient being irradiated may well be allowed (with certain reservations) a daily bath.
5. Furthermore, orthovoltage therapy is of an energy just higher than that used in diagnostic radiology (which depends on the differential absorption of X-rays by different tissues for the production of pictures). In radiotherapy at orthovoltage energy this has a dual effect. Bone absorbs radiation, and as very high dosages are given, this can lead to necrosis of bone or cartilage due mainly to an endarteritis—interfering with blood supply. Also due to the high absorption by bone, there is a reduction in the dose of radiation delivered to a tumour site lying behind bone—that is to say that bone can be 'protecting' the tumour from radiation. This is not so with high energy. In this case bone absorption is less and so bone can be treated like soft tissue. In consequence, bone is at less risk of necrosis and, more important, bone does not protect underlying tumour.
6. A further major point in favour of high energy radiotherapy is that because of the increased dose at depth, fewer treatment fields are necessary. The amount of radiation that can be tolerated is related to the total *volume* of the patient encompassed by the radiation fields. So by decreasing the number of radiation fields (portals) of entry of X-rays into the patient), the dose to the tumour can actually be safely increased in some cases by 50 per cent.

The oxygen effect and radiosensitors
One paradox of radiation therapy is the fact that cells near to necrosis due to lack of blood and oxygen are those that are most resistant to the effects of radiation. This is what is called 'The Oxygen effect'. It was initially a matter of chance that a course of treatment was protracted over a period of weeks, but this is now established as a means of improving the oxygenation of the necrotic cells by reducing the number of 'healthy' malignant cells. Another method is by the use of hyperbaric oxygen chambers to increase the oxygenation of tumours. This appears to be of some value in therapy of tumours of the head and neck but has not been shown to be of value in pelvic malignancy. High energy *Neutron therapy* is now on trial as this to a certain extent reduces the 'oxygen effect', but again costs become enormous and unless, or until, there is a great breakthrough, the principal weapon of the radiotherapist against deep seated malignancy will be by high energy X or γ radiation.

There are some radio sensitizor chemicals under study. Actinomycin D in therapy of Wilm's tumour (nephroblastoma) appears to reduce the necessary radiation by 50 per cent.

COMPLICATIONS OF RADIOTHERAPY IN PELVIC MALIGNANT DISEASE

The morbidity and overall risk of surgery for malignant disease is fairly well known, but radiotherapy is often thought to be a relatively safer alternative. The treatment given to an individual patient should however, be the best that a joint gynaecological, radiotherapeutic, chemotherapeutic and pathological group have available to them and not be based only on a clinical evaluation of risk.

The risks of radiotherapy in the treatment of carcinoma of cervix have been recently outlined by Villasanta (1972), and the late risks of proctitis; vault necrosis; haemorrhagic cystitis; parametritis; fistula; bowel necrosis and obstruction are discussed. He does not mention bone absorption with fracture which can occur.

Proctitis. Diarrhoea with some tenderness may follow almost immediately after radiation while the patient is still in hospital. It is customary to treat with kaolin and opium mixtures, but lomotil (diphenoxylate hydrochlor with atropine) sometimes helps. After discharge the condition may persist. Proctitis may first appear at any time from two months to a year after treatment. The patient complains of tenderness, diarrhoea and passage of fresh blood and mucus; on rectal examination the mucosa is soft and velvety to touch. If there is ulceration this can be felt about 5–6cms from the anus on the anterior rectal wall. Treatment is with prednisolone suppository (Predsol) or with predsol retention enemata daily, along with some simple laxative to soften bowel contents. Biopsy should not be done as the typical case should be diagnosed on the history and by the findings of an experienced examiner. Treatment must be early (often within a month of discharge from hospital), active and prolonged. Most patients will recover within a few weeks or months, but occasionally treatment is necessary over a much longer period before symptoms remit. Some cases are associated with discomfort severe enough to require temporary transverse or iliac colostomy, others may develop strictures at the site and still others rectovaginal fistula.

Cystitis. Haemorrhagic cystitis follows radiotherapy in some 50 per cent of cases and is seen to be more likely after supervoltage application. Frequency, dysuria and haematuria are associated with hyperaemia of the bladder base. Sometimes there may be actual ulceration, *and biopsy renders fistula more likely.* Deposit of phosphate material and associated infection are common. The condition first appears after about 1 year and may persist to some degree for many years. Antibiotics, antispasmodics and occasional bladder lavage with prednisolone 1:1000 are worthwhile.

Vesico vaginal fistula may appear 1 year to 10 years after radiation.

Ureteric blockage. Periureteric fibrosis consequent to radiation can cause partial or complete ureteric blockage. Recovery from partial blackage can occur. The difficulty here is to differentiate radiation blockage from that due to persistent or recurrent disease, but the diagnosis can usually be made on clinical grounds. This may appear quite a few months after radiation and settle over a period of years.

Intestinal obstruction. Small bowel necrosis leading to obstruction or associated with adhesions secondary to radiation can occur and resection of necrosed areas may be necessary. Perforation may occur at sites of multiple necrosis.

Vaginal necrosis. Necrosis of the vagina may occur very soon after therapy especially if there has been associated surgery. Part or whole of the vaginal mucosa appears as a grey-green slough. While in the occasional case severe stenosis may occur, most cases respond amazingly well to oestrogen creams and prednisolone (Predsol) pessaries.

Vesico vaginal and rectovaginal fistula. Following radiation are more liable to occur if active treatment of the initial cystitis or proctitis is not early and thorough. These are necrotic fistulas through tissues which have a complete loss of blood supply. In contradistinction to surgical fistulas they rarely close themselves and ureteric transplant or colostomy are almost always necessary. Repair especially of rectovaginal fistula may be attempted after a year or so when the tissues have recovered something of this blood supply (*see* p. 829).

Parametritis. Towards the end of radiation or soon after removal an acute parametrial inflammatory response may appear. This must be treated with antibiotics and rest. There may be subsequent ureteric blockage due to scarring but the condition often settles amazingly well.

Bowel. Radiation may affect the small or large bowel which happens to be in the Pouch of Douglas or has an excessive dose for some reason. Vascular degeneration and hyaline fibrosis may produce obstruction and perforation or fistula formation many years after therapy.

Bone. Radiation absorption fracture of the femoral neck is reported. Such fractures may impact and need no therapy.

Leukaemia. There is some small risk of leukaemia induced by therapeutic radiation but this may take 25 years to develop clinically.

Immuno-suppression. There is some modern belief that radiotherapy to glands may completely destroy the ability of these glands to develop immune reaction to persisting cells and to some extent therefore lessen the ability of the body to cope with the disease.

Chemotherapy

Julianc and Woodruff (1969) in discussing the role of chemotherapy in the treatment of primary ovarian malignancy point out that the high percentage of trophoblastic tumours cured by chemotherapy had given hope that such agents could be the means by which the poor salvage rates for ovarian carcinoma might be improved. This hope has not proved well founded.

Chemotherapeutic drugs used commonly in gynaecology and of value are:

1. Alkalating agents. Thiotepa, chlorambucil and cyclophosphamide.
2. Antimetabolites. Methotrexate: 5 fluorouracil: 6 mercaptopurine.
3. Antibiotics. Actinomycin D.
4. Hormones.

Progestogens $\begin{cases} \text{medroxy progesterone} \\ \text{Progesterone caproate.} \end{cases}$

The major cytotoxic affects of those drugs appears to be on the desoxyribonucleic acid, which ultimately prevents protein synthesis. They interfere with normal mitosis and cell division in all rapidly proliferating tissues. The antimetabolites tend to act directly on the folic acid and folinic acid by competitively inhibiting folic reductives.

5-Fluorouracil is a manufactured substance produced in an attempt to interfere with nucleic synthesis.

Doses of these various drugs varies. Thiotepa for example, starts with 0·4mg per kilo of body weight intravenously per day for 2 days, and then 0·2mg weekly thereafter.

Cyclophosphamides starting off again with intravenous dosage of 15mgm/kilo may be followed by a maintenance dosage of 50–150mg per day, starting after obvious bone marrow recovery.

Mercaptopurine has a somewhat similar effect but of course, a very different dosage range, the maintenance dose being 0·1mg per kilo per day.

All these substances have serious side effects of nausea, vomiting, anorexia, leukopaenia, thrombocytopenia and possible local skin reaction. Alopaecia is more marked with cyclophosphamides. In all instances haemoglobin, red and white cell counts, platelet production may be seriously depressed and counts must be done regularly.

The response of ovarian tumours to chemotherapy depends very much on their type of epithelial growth, and to some extent on the degrees of malignancy of the various types. Serous ascites should perhaps respond best to the intra-abdominal or intravenous injections of thiotepa, but pleural effusion is little affected.

Chemotherapy has been used largely as a palliation in the inoperable or hopeless case. There is no doubt that a reasonable number of patients apparently respond by a diminution in ascites, in size of tumour and an increase in weight and wellbeing. Remission will often last for years and the chemotherapy must be permanently maintained. A 'second look' in the patient with the shrinking tumour is often justified as operability may be restored.

SENSITIVITY

There is a suggestion that it might be possible to expose tissue cultures of ovarian tumours to various cytotoxic agents to check the sensitivity of the cells before therapy is begun. Currently extensive clinical studies of forms of chemotherapy for ovarian tumours are under way.

The use of the hormones in carcinoma of the body of the uterus has already been discussed. They can be effective but hormones have not been shown to be of any value in other gynaecological neoplasms.

Bleomycin is of no proven value in squamous carcinoma.

EFFECT OF CYTOTOXIC DRUGS ON THE OOZYTE

The oozyte is protected from the mal effects of cytotoxic therapy e.g. for trophoblast disease (Chapter 9), by its resting state in prophase of meiosis. Developing and therefore metabolically active oozytes may be damaged and it is therefore recommended that at least one year be allowed to elapse between any serious chemotherapy and a subsequent pregnancy. Some 60 per cent of women who have had successful therapy for trophoblastic disease have subsequently conceived.

Before the 14th week almost all 'cancerocidal' chemotherapeutic drugs have a drastic effect on the fetus. In general terms after the 14th week chemotherapeutic drugs have very little deleterious affect on the child.

REFERENCES

Anderson, A. F. (1953) Latent cancer of the cervix. *J. Obstet. Gynaec. Brit. Emp.*, **60**, 353.

Anderson, A. F., Grant, M. P. S., McBryde, R. M., Cockburn, M. K. (1953) The place of cervical smears in the diagnosis of early cervical cancer. *J. Obstet. Gynaec. Brit. Emp.*, **60**, 345.

Ayre, J. E. (1947), Selective cytology smear for diagnosis of cancer. *Amer. J. Obstet. Gynec.*, **53**, 609.

Baggish, M. S. & Woodruff, J. D. (1972) Uterine Stromatosis. *Obstet. & Gynaec.*, **40**, 487.

Bibbo, M., Keebler, C. M. & Wied, C. L. (1971) Prevalence and incidence rates of cervical atypica. *J. Reproduct. Med.* **6**, 184.

Blaikley, J. B., Dewhurst, C. J., Ferreira, A. P. & Lewis, T. L. T. (1971) Vaginal adenosis. Clinical and Pathological. Features with special reference to malignant change. *J. Obstet. Gynaec. Brit. Cwlth.*, **78**, 1115.

Bonham, D. G. & Bonham, R. J. G. (1975) Cancer of the endometrium and improved method of assessment. *Aust. & N.Z. J. Obstet. Gynec.*, **13**, 172.

Charles, A. H. (1972) Carcinoma of Vulva. *Brit. med. J.*, **i**, 397.

Charles, D. (1965) Endometrial Adeno acanthoma. *Cancer*, **18**, 737.

Coppleson, M. & Reid, B. L. (1967) *Preclinical carcinoma of the cervix uteri.* London: Pergamon.

Creasman, W. T., Week, J. C., Curray, S. L., Johnston, W. W. & Parker, R. T. (1973) Efficacy of cryosurgical treatment of severe cervical intraepithelial neoplasia. *Obstet. & Gynaec.*, **41**, 501.

Currie, D. W. (1971) Operative treatment of carcinoma of the cervix. *J. Obstet. Gynaec. Brit. Cwlth.*, **78**, 385.

Daw, E. (1971) Primary carcinoma of the vagina. *J. Obstet. Gynaec. Brit. Cwlth.*, **78**, 853.

Daw E. (1972) Primary melanoma of the vagina. *Amer. J. Obstet. Gynec.*, **112**, 307.

Dealey, T. J. (1971) *Modern radiotherapy in gynaecological cancer.* London: Butterworth.

Douglas, B., MacDonald, J. S. & Baker, J. W. (1972) Lymphography in carcinoma of the uterus. *Clin. Radiol.*, **23**, 286.

Donald, J. & Walker, J. (1970) Carcinoma of cervix in the Eastern Region of Scotland. *J. Obstet. Gynaec. Brit. Cwlth.*, **77**, 435.

Duguid, H. (1974) *Personal communication.*

Galvin, G., Jones, H. W., Te Linde, R. W. (1952) Clinical relationship of carcinoma in situ and invasive carcinoma of cervix. *JAMA*, **149**, 744.

Green, G. H. (1970) Cervical carcinoma in situ. *Aust. & N.Z. J. Obstet. Gynaec.*, **10**, 41.

Hall, J. E. (1971) Leiomyosarcoma of the uterus. *Obstet. & Gynaec.* **38**, 629.

Hayes, D. (1972) Mesonephroid tumours of the ovary. *J. Obstet. Gynaec. Brit. Cwlth.*, **79**, 728.

Herbst, A. L., Ulfelder, H. & Poskanzer, D. C. (1971) Adenocarcinoma of the vagina. *New Engl. med J.*, **284**, 871.

Hughesdon, P. E. & Fraser, I. T. (1953) Arrhenoblastoma of ovary. *Acta Obstet. Gynec. Scand.*, **32**, Suppl. 4.

Julianc, G. & Woodruff, J. D. (1974) The role of chemotherapy in treatment of primary ovarian malignancy. *Obstet. & Gynaec.*, **24**, 1307.

Katayama, M. D., Woodruff, D. J., Jones, H. W. & Preston, E. (1972) Chromosomes of condylomata acumenata, Paget's disease, in situ invasive cell carcinoma and malignant melanoma of the human vulva. *Obstet. & Gynaec.*, **39**, 346.

Kirkland, J. (1963) Carcinoma in Situ. Diagnosis and Prognosis. *J. Obstet. Gynaec. Brit. Cwlth.*, **70**, 232.

Kirkland, J. (1969) The study of chromosomes in cervical neoplasia. Survey 24, *Obst. & Gynec.*, **784**.

Lang, W. R. & Rakoff, A. E. (1956) Colposcopy and cytology. Comparative values in the diagnosis of cervical atypism and malignancy. *Obstet. & Gynaec.*, **8**, 312.

Lewis, D. V., Diaz, P. R., Stallworthy, J. A. & Ellis, F. E. (1970) Primary Adenocarcinoma of the Cervix. *J. Obstet. Gynaec. Brit. Cwlth.*, **77**, 277.

Lewis, B. V., Stallworthy, J. A. & Cowdell, R. (1970) Adenocarcinoma of the body of the uterus. *J. Obstet. Gynaec. Brit. Cwlth.*, **77**, 343.

Limburg, H. (1958) Comparison between cytology and colposcopy in the diagnosis of early cervical carcinoma. *Amer. J. Obstet. Gynec.*, **75**, 1928.

McGregor, J. E., Fraser, M. E. & Mann, N. F. (1971) Improved prognosis of cervical cancer due to comprehensive screening. *Lancet*, **i**, 74.

Million, R. R., Rutledge, F. & Fletcher, G. H. (1972) Stage IV Carcinoma of the cervix with bladder invasion. *Amer. J. Obstet. Gynec.*, **113**, 2.

Miller, M. M., Robertson, G. T., Swanson, W. C. & Walker, J. (1962) a. Malignant Disease body of uterus. *J. Obstet. Gynaec. Brit Cwlth.*, **69**, 553. b. Malignant Disease of the Vagina. *Scot. med. J.*, **7**, 399.

Morrow, C. P. & Rutledge (1972) Melanoma of Vulva. *Obstet. & Gynaec.*, **39**, 745.

Navratil, E., Bajardi, F. & Nash, W. (1958) Simultaneous colposcopy and cytology used in screening for carcinoma of the cervix. *Amer. J. Obstet. & Gynec.*, **75**, 1292.

Ovarian Tumours in Infants and Children. (1971) *Brit. med. J.*, **ii**, 2762.

Papinocalaou, G. N. & Traut, H. F. (1943) Demonstration of malignant cells in vaginal smears and its relation to diagnosis of cancer of uterus. *N.Y.St.J. Med.*, **43**, 767.

Papinocalaou, G. N. & Traut, H. F. (1943) Diagnosis of uterine cancer by vaginal smear. *The Commonwealth Fund, N.Y.*

Park, W. W. (1949) The nature of stromatous endometriosis. *J. Obstet. Gynaec. Brit. Emp.*, **56**, 759.

Rickart, R. (1973) Cytology. *Brit. med. J.* July 1973, p. 36.

Robertson, M. A., Harington, J. S. & Bradshaw, E. (1971) a. The cancer pattern in Africans at Baragwanath Hospital, Johannesburg. *Brit. J. Cancer.*, **25**, 377. b. The cancer pattern in Africans of the Transvaal low veld. *Brit. J. Cancer*, p. 385.

Rubin, I. C. (1910) The pathological diagnosis of incipient carcinoma of cervix. *Amer. J. Obstet. Gynec.*, **62**, 668.

Sall, S., Rini, S. & Pineda, A. (1974) Surgical management of invasive carcinoma of the cervix in pregnancy. *Amer. J. Obstet. Gynec.*, **118**, 1.

Schlink, H. H. (1960) Cancer of the female pelvis. *J. Obstet. Gynaec. Brit. Emp.*, **67**, 402.

Stafl, A. & Mattingly, R. F. (1973) Colposcopic diagnosis of cervical neoplasia. *Obstet. & Gynaec.*, **41**, 168.

Stallworthy, J. (1964) Radical Surgery following radiation therapy for cervical carcinoma. *Amer. Roy. College Surg. Eng.*, **34**, 161.

Stanley, M. A. & Kirkland, J. A. (1969) Chromosome analysis in a progressive lesion of the cervix. *Acta Cytologica.*, **13**, 76.

Stein, I. F. & Leventhal, A. L. (1935) Amenorrhea associated with bilateral cystic ovaries. *Amer. J. Obstet. Gynec.*, **29**, 181.

Stephenson, M. C. (1973) Cancer screening. *Brit. Clin. J.*, **1**, 15.

Taberman, A., Huyzinga, W. T. & Kiupers, T. (1973) Dysgerminoma. *Obstet. & Gynaec.*, **41**, 137.

Te Linde, R. W. (1973) Demonstration of the relationship of carcinoma in situ to invasive carcinoma cervix. *Amer. J. Obstet. Gynec.*, **117**, 1022.

Te Linde, R. W. & Galvin, G. (1944) Minimal histological changes in biopsies to justify diagnosis of cervical cancer. *Amer. J. Obstet. Gynec.*, **48**, 774.

Timonen, S., Nieminen, U. & Kaureanieme, T. (1974) Cervical screening. *Lancet.*, **i**, 401.

Tod, M. C. & Meredith, W. J. (1938) A dosage system for use in the treatment of cancer of the cervix. *Brit. J. Radiol.*, **71**, 809.

Tod, M. C. & Meredith, W. J. (1953) Treatment of carcinoma of the cervix uteri—a revised 'Manchester Method'. *Brit. J. Radiol.*, **26**, 252.

Ulfelder, H. (1973) Stilboestrol adenosis and adenocarcinoma. *Amer. J. Obstet. Gynec.*, **117**, 6.

Villasanta, U. (1972) Complications of radiotherapy for carcinoma of the uterine cervix. *Amer. J. Obstet. Gynec.*, **114**, 717.

White, D. F. (1971) in *Modern Radiotherapy in Gynaecological Cancer*. Ed. Deeley, T. F. p. 284. London: Butterworth.

Worth, A. (1973) Screening Programmes. *Brit. med. J.*, **ii**, 36.

FURTHER READING

Adenosis and Clear-cell Adenocarcinoma of the Vagina (1975) An Invitation Symposium. *J. Reproduct. Med.*, **15**, 2.

Barber, H. R. K. & Graber, E. A. (1973) Gynaecological tumours in childhood and adolescence. *Obst. & Gynaec.*, **28**, 357.

Bibbo, M., Al-Maqueeb, M., Baccarni, I., Gill, W., Newton, M., Sleeper, Kay, Sonek, M. & Wied, G. L. (1975) Follow-up study of male and female offspring of DES-treated mothers. *J. Reproduct. Med.*, **15**, 29.

Boyes, D. A., Worth, A. J. & Fidler, H. K. (1970) The results of treatment of 4389 cases of preclinical cervical squamous carcinoma. *J. Obstet. Gynaec. Brit. Cwlth.*, **77**, 769.

Creasman, W. T. & Rutledge, F. (1972) Carcinoma in situ of the cervix. *Obstet. & Gynaec.*, **39**, 373.

Cancer uterine and ovary (1966) *Eleventh Commonwealth Clinic Conference*, University of Texas. Chicago: Year Book Pub.

Coppleson, M. & Reid, B. L. (1967) *Preclinical carcinoma of the cervix uteri*. London: Pergamon.

Dealey, T. J. (1971) *Modern Radiotherapy in Gynaecological Cancer*. London: Butterworth.

Easson, E. (1973) *Cancer of the uterine cervix*. London: Saunders.

Janovski, N. A. & Paramanandhan, T. L. (1973) *Ovarian Tumors*. London: Saunders.

Kolstad, P. (1966) Carcinoma of the cervix, Stage 0. Diagnosis and treatment. *Amer. J. Obstet. Gynec.*, **96**, 1098.

Kolstad, P. & Stafl, A. (1973) *Atlas of Colposcopy*. Oslo: Universitats farlaget.

Malignant Tumours in Children (1975) A symposium. *Proc. Roy. Soc. Med.*, **68**, 653.

Vaeth, J. M. (1969) *The interrelationship of chaemotherapeutic agents and radiation therapy in the treatment of cancer*. Basel: Karger.

Vaeth, J. M. (1970) *The interrelationship of surgery and radiation therapy in the treatment of cancer*. Basel: Karger.

39. Endometriosis

In this interesting condition there is growth of endometrial tissue in sites other than the mucus lining of the uterine cavity. The condition can arise in many sites of the body. When it occurs outside of the uterus it is sometimes called endometriosis externa and in the uterine wall endometriosis interna, but more usually it is termed adenomyosis, when it is in the myometrium.

Pathology
Because of the glandular component of endometrium, the areas of endometrium are, to some extent, cystic and contain altered blood. In some instances, particularly in the ovary, the cysts become quite large and are usually called chocolate cysts. The epithelial lining may be compressed and flattened because of the pressure of the blood inside and in such cases may not be recognizable on histological examination. In others the glandular pattern may be of proliferative or secretory pattern and in some lesions there is the appearance of cystic glandular hyperplasia. The glandular spaces are surrounded by endometrial stroma. Histological confirmation of the diagnosis is difficult if the endometrial glands have become flattened and this is quite often the case in chocolate cysts. In adenomyosis a direct connection between the mucosal layer or uterine endometrium and the tumour can be seen on serial section. The glands are surrounded by stromal cells and by myometrial cells.

There may be only a few small areas or the uterus may be markedly enlarged and containing many areas of adenomyosis. It is noteworthy that unlike a fibromyoma an adenomyoma has no capsule but they both have a striated and whorled appearance.

There is a rare type of tumour which is thought by some to be a form of *stromal endometriosis*, but by others to be a low grade sarcoma. The macroscopic appearances of this tumour are fleshy and softer than a fibromyoma or adenomyosis. Histologically the cells resemble endometrial stromal cells but cannot readily be distinguished from sarcoma arising from metaplasia of myometrial cells. The tumour is locally malignant and pulmonary metastases have been reported. The tumours can arise after the menopause.

Incidence of endometriosis
The incidence is difficult to determine because, on the one hand, it may be quite easily missed even at laparotomy if it is a small lesion or, on the other hand, it may not be diagnosed unless laparotomy or laparoscopy are performed. The condition is much more common in nulliparous women than those who have had pregnancies and it tends to be found in the age group between 30 and 40 years but can occur at any time between the menarche and the menopause. It is said to occur more commonly in upper social class women but this may be due to family limitation and later child bearing.

Theories on aetiology
There are two main theories on the causation of endometriosis. These are Samson's implantation theory and Meyer's serosal metaplasia theory. This rather academic argument has been going on for many years and is not yet resolved but the implantation theory is probably in the ascendancy at the moment. According to the implantation theory there is a reflux of endometrial tissue along the Fallopian tubes into the peritoneal cavity at the time of menstruation and this endometrium becomes implanted and grows on the peritoneal surfaces. It is well known that menstrual bleeding can occur into the peritoneal cavity but the proponents of the serosal theory argued that the endometrium was dead and

necrotic and would not become implanted. They believe that there is a metaplasia of the peritoneal mesothelium. As the epithelium of the Mullerian system is derived from the primitive mesothelium of the coelom its conversion to endometrial type tissue will cause chocolate cysts and other types of pelvic endometriosis. The serosal theory can explain endometriosis in all sites where peritoneal

(b) extra uterine pelvic and (c) extra pelvic, *see* Fig. 39.1.

UTERINE ENDOMETRIOSIS

This is commonly called adenomyosis and the clinical features are very similar to those caused by fibromyomata but it is much less common than fibroids. It occurs in the same age group, that is, women of about 40 and gives rise to

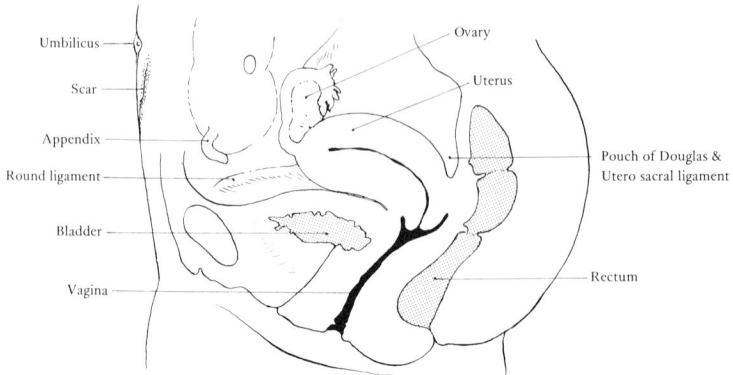

Fig. 39.1   Sites of endometriosis

mesothelium is present or even in laparotomy scars into which it may have been displaced. It does not however explain adenomyosis. The implantation theory was given a considerable boost by the experimental work of Te Linde and Scott (1950) on rhesus monkeys. In this they have shown that menstrual endometrium produced endometriosis when it flows into the peritoneal cavity or into the abdominal muscles.

The hormonal influence on the development and maintenance of endometriosis is also of interest. Oestrogens are necessary for the continuance of the condition but progesterone is not necessary. However, the endometriosis can show secretory activity under the influence of progesterone. In spite of the very large amount of oestrogen produced during pregnancy, however, there is a marked tendency for the condition to regress and to be apparently cured by pregnancy. The explanation of this is not clear but it would appear that the marked decidual reaction in the endometriotic areas during pregnancy may in some way cause the regression when there is a marked fall in hormones after delivery.

Sites of endometriosis

These are usually divided into (a) uterine,

menorrhagia and usually dysmenorrhoea. Dyspareunia can also sometimes occur. On pelvic examination the uterus will be found to be enlarged, the swelling may be diffuse and symmetrical or there may be one or more discreet tumours on the uterus. It is sometimes possible to differentiate an adenomyoma from a fibromyoma because the former tends to be associated with pain, the uterus is rarely larger than 12 weeks pregnancy and the uterus is more often uniformly enlarged. The diagnosis is often, however, only made after a hysterectomy or when a myomectomy is being attempted and it is found that the tumour is not encapsulated.

Treatment

As most of the women with adenomyosis are in the older reproductive age group, hysterectomy is performed. The ovaries are not removed unless there is evidence of endometriosis elsewhere. In younger women it may be possible to exercise the area of endometriosis if she is particularly anxious to have a pregnancy or alternatively hormonal therapy is tried.

PELVIC ENDOMETRIOSIS

This may be limited to a few pinhead sized

areas in the Pouch of Douglas or it can involve most of the structures of the pelvis.

The minor degress of pelvic endometriosis are usually only discovered at incidental laparotomy and do not necessarily produce any symptoms. These small areas of endometriosis usually occur under the peritoneum in the region of the utero-sacral folds. The peritoneum around these small black spots may appear puckered. In more advanced cases fibrosis is more marked and adhesions may form between the various organs in the pelvis. The lesion may spread to involve the recto-vaginal septum and infiltrate the wall of the rectum. This can give rise to an anular type of stenosis of the rectum which closely simulates carcinoma. The lesion can also extend from the recto-vaginal septum into the vault of the vagina producing bluish cystic swellings in the posterior fornix. These cysts can sometimes rupture giving rise to ulcerated bleeding areas and this can be confused with a carcinoma of the cervix.

Although adhesions to bladder are fairly common, it is very unusual for endometriosis to penetrate the bladder wall and give rise to haematuria. Although rectal involvement is not infrequent, it is unusual for the small bowel to be involved. Occasionally the appendix or ileum may be affected by endometriosis.

Endometriosis of the ovary may present with small black areas of endometriosis or more usually as the typical chocolate cysts of the ovaries. These chocolate cysts are formed by the coalescence of nodules of endometriosis in the ovary forming cysts which contain thick dark fluid blood. The ovary is enlarged and the surface is thickened. It is usually adherent to the back of the uterus and to the back of the broad ligament. The adhesions are typically dense and relatively avascular. Both ovaries may be involved in dense adhesions to the other structures in the pelvis. The cysts are usually between one and five centimetres in diameter but rarely they may fill the pelvis or extend into the abdomen.

Endometriosis of the Fallopian tubes may occur as part of the general pelvic involvement and in these cases the small black areas may occur on the surface of the tubes which may also be adherent to the other structures. A form of adenomyosis of the tube or endosalpingiosis has been described. These usually occur when the tubes have been removed and there is a mass of epithelium formed in the stump at the uterine cornu. The epithelium is tubal in type in these cases.

Pathology of pelvic endometriosis

Although the characteristic small black or purple dots found in the peritoneum are highly suggestive of endometriosis, it is not always possible to confirm this on histological examination but usually endometrial epithelium which may or may not have undergone cyclical change will be identified. This, however, is unfortunately not true of the chocolate cyst of the ovaries. In these cases the diagnosis may be extremely difficult because the typical configuration of the endometrial epithelium is lost due to the pressure of the blood in the cysts. These chocolate cysts can be confused with haemorrhagic corpora lutea particularly as there are often cells in the tissues under the epithelium which closely resemble luteum cells. These are pigment laden macrophages and are large polyhedrals containing haemosiderin which gives them the brown or yellow colour. The surface epithelial lining is usually formed from flattened endothelial cells but the cells may become columnar in the pockets in the walls. The presence of typical endometrial epithelium lining the cysts is rare but is of course diagnostic.

Symptoms of pelvic endometriosis

As already mentioned there may be no symptoms with small lesions but this can also be true of lesions where there is fairly extensive disease with adhesions. Some of these cases are only detected when they are being investigated for infertility which is one of the common features of endometriosis. The cause of infertility in these cases is obscure because the tubes are not usually blocked. Pain is the most important symptom. This may be a fairly constant dull ache in either or both iliac fossae or in the lower abdomen or back or may present as typical dysmenorrhoea restricted to the immediate premenstrual and menstrual phases. Acute pain is rare but such attacks are probably due to the rupture of small cysts in the pelvis. The dysmenorrhoea is secondary in type and tends to be progressive. Dyspareunia is a common complaint also in these cases and is probably due to the nodules in the Pouch of Douglas or in the ovaries. It is sometimes surprising, however, that some women with extensive pelvic endometriosis may have had no complaint of pain at all. Menstrual irregularities are common and the periods are often heavy. It is not clear, however, whether menstrual disturbance is due to the endometriosis itself or whether it is an underlying hormonal dysfunction which is the cause. Sometimes fibromyomata are present and these contribute to the menstrual irregularities. Bowel symptoms are common when the recto-vaginal septum is involved. Pain on defaecation, tenesmus, constipation or diarrhoea may be present. If the rectal mucosa is involved and ulcerated cyclical bleeding may occur. Bladder symptoms are uncommon but frequency, dysuria and even haematuria may occur.

Signs of pelvic endometriosis
These depend on the extent and location of the lesion but it is important to remember that very small nodules can produce marked symptoms while lesions producing swellings, adhesions and fixity of the pelvic organs may produce very little if any symptoms. A very careful palpation of the likely areas of the pelvis, particularly along the utero-sacral ligaments should be carried out and any tenderness in them elicited. The size, position and mobility of the uterus must be determined because in many cases the uterus will be fixed in a retroverted position. The ovaries may be enlarged and fixed because of chocolate cysts. A combined rectal and vaginal examination is very useful in suspected cases of endometriosis as this allows a more detailed examination of the recto-vaginal space where endometriosis very commonly occurs, and palpation of multiple small nodules in the Pouch of Douglas and in the utero-sacral ligaments is more easily performed.

Differential diagnosis
The symtomatology and findings on examination particularly if there are tender nodules in the recto-vaginal space, will usually make a presumptive diagnosis possible but there are some conditions from which it is difficult to differentiate endometriosis without laparotomy or laparoscopy.

The following conditions can give rise to difficulty:
1. *Chronic salpingo-oophritis*. The findings on pelvic examination are so similar in pelvic endometriosis and salpingo-oophritis that errors in diagnosis are often made. If the history is not sufficiently helpful in both there is usually tenderness, swelling and fixity of the uterus and appendages. Again in both there is usually pelvic pain, dysmenorrhoea, dyspareunia, menstrual irregularity and infertility. A history of acute infection at some time in the past will of course be very helpful in making the diagnosis.

2. *Pelvic cellulitis*. The differential diagnosis is particularly difficult in these cases if there is cellulitis of the utero-sacral ligaments as well as of the paracervical ligaments. This will give rise to tenderness and thickening which is found in endometriosis. The symptomatology in pelvic cellulitis is of pain, worse at menstruation. Another feature common to both is that on moving the cervix pain is elicited. The diagnosis may only be possible on laparoscopy or laparotomy.

3. *Ovarian carcinoma with metastases* in the recto-vaginal septum can be confused on vaginal examination with endometriosis but usually the history helps to differentiate.

4. *Rectal carcinoma*. This can easily be confused with endometriosis involving the rectum and it is extremely important that the two conditions should not be confused. Although it is obviously undesirable that rectal endometriosis should be dealt with by radical surgery and radiotherapy it is worse that a rectal carcinoma be dealt with by hormone therapy.

Treatment of pelvic endometriosis
Hormone therapy. Endometriosis regresses during pregnancy and on the assumption that this was due to the effect of progesterone a conservative approach to the treatment of endometriosis by inducing a pseudo pregnancy with synthetic progestational agents has been introduced. The early hopes of producing a permanent cure in all cases have been unfounded but complete relief from symptoms can be obtained in some cases while they are on therapy or even for many months after they complete the treatment. It is particularly desirable to try this therapy in younger women especially if they wish to have a pregnancy. It is, of course, desirable to confirm the diagnosis possibly by laparoscopy before embarking on the treatment. Although in some cases hormone therapy can be used as an aid to diagnosis this can be particularly useful in cases where the differential diagnosis is between endometriosis and chronic pelvic inflammatory

disease. In such cases it is possible that an extensive surgical procedure might be avoided by giving a high dose of a gestogen for a month, this will probably produce relief of symptoms and a reduction in the size of the pelvic mass in cases of endometriosis.

The hormone therapy may be given as a continuous treatment for nine months or a year or may be given cyclically. The gestogen is given in increasing doses from 10mg daily up to 40mg daily over a two month period. Norethynodral or norethisterone are commonly used. This is now commonly given in combination with an oestrogen in a contraceptive pill. As symptoms and signs can clear up even when the hormone therapy is given cyclically and menstruation is occurring, it is difficult to understand how this controls or eradicates the endometriosis. This also occurs even though a progesterone alone is given cyclically and ovulation is not suppressed.

It is well worth trying hormone therapy in cases of pelvic endometriosis particularly in young women but it has to be remembered that not all of them will be relieved and those that are will probably not be relieved permanently and also some of the women will abandon the hormone therapy because of side effects. Surgical treatment is therefore often required in cases of endometriosis.

Surgical treatment of pelvic endometriosis. Surgical treatment will depend not only on the site of the endometriosis but also on the age of the patient. In the older woman who is approaching the menopause and has no desire for a pregnancy the disease can be controlled by removing the ovaries. It is not necessary to remove other tissues in the pelvis unless the oophrectomy is made easier by doing, for example, a hysterectomy. In most cases it is usual to do a total hysterectomy but if there is dense adhesion between the cervix and the recto-vaginal septum a subtotal hysterectomy should be performed rather than risk damaging the rectum. Conservative surgical treatment in the younger patient who is anxious to retain her reproductive function is indicated and the precise type of operation will depend on the findings. The pelvic organs are mobilized by dividing the adhesions and any affected ovarian tissue is excised. Nodules of endometriosis in the pelvic peritoneum are coagulated with diathermy. A ventro-suspension

of the uterus is performed to prevent recurrence of adhesions on the pelvic floor. This surgical treatment is followed by progestagen therapy.

EXTRA PELVIC ENDOMETRIOSIS
Endometriosis can occur in many unusual situations outside of the pelvis. They can sometimes be explained by implantation of endometrial tissue as in abdominal or perineal wounds but in some the explanation must be due to coelomic metaplasia as for example at the end of the round ligament in the inguinal canal, in the umbilicus or in the perineum. Another explanation might be that there is lymphatic spread of endometrium to these sites.

1. *Endometriosis of the umbilicus*
This causes a small nodule in the umbilicus which enlarges, becomes tender and dark blue in colour at the time of menstruation. Some may bleed externally at the time of menstruation. A simple excision is curative and the diagnosis is confirmed on histological examination of the specimen.

2. *Endometriosis of the round ligament*
This presents as a small firm nodule similar to a lymphatic gland in the inguinal canal. The swelling enlarges and becomes tender and some may even become discoloured at the time of menstruation. Areas of endometriosis can also occur in hernial sacs in the inguinal and femoral canals.

3. *Endometriosis in scars*
This is most likely to occur after operations involving the uterus when endometrium can become implanted in the abdominal or perineal wound. This can occur after Caesarean section or hysterotomy or episiotomy. Endometriosis in abdominal scars can, however, recur following operations in which the uterus has not been opened as for example the removal of ovarian cysts or even appendicectomy. A tender nodule appears in the scar sometime after the operation and at the time of menstruation the endometriotic area is removed surgically.

Endometriosis and pregnancy
It is well known that pregnancy has the effect of curing endometriosis but the mechanism of this is obscure. It would appear that a marked

decidual reaction which occurs in pregnancy in some way causes such a marked regression after the pregnancy is completed that the condition is cured. On the other hand it is also known that women with endometriosis are less likely to become pregnant. It is not clear, however, whether the infertility predisposes to the endometriosis or whether it is the endometriosis which prevents conception.

REFERENCES

Te Linde, R. & Scott, R. B. (1950) *Amer. J. Obstet. Gynec.*, **60**, 1147.

40. Other Gynaecological Conditions

CONGENITAL ABNORMALITIES

These developmental abnormalities can affect the whole genital tract or any part of it. Abnormalities of the genital and renal systems often occur together. Some of the abnormalities are very minor and do not cause any clinical problems, but the degree of abnormality is not necessarily related to the amount of clinical trouble caused, for example, complete duplication of the genital tract may not cause any functional disturbance whereas a simple imperforate hymen can cause very considerable symptomatology.

IMPERFORATE HYMEN

The hymen is formed from the urogenital sinus by invagination of the posterior wall. It covers over the lowest part of the vagina and is normally open at birth. Failure to canalize gives rise to the condition of imperforate hymen. This does not initially give rise to any symptoms and it is not usually until some time after puberty that the condition is discovered. There is a history of recurrent abdominal pain usually at monthly intervals, but as menstruation is quite often irregular at the commencement of the reproductive cycle, the rhythmic nature of the pain may be missed. The pain initially is due to dysmenorrhoea and it is only after a few menstrual cycles that distension of the uterus begins to cause the pain. If the condition is still not diagnosed then the vagina becomes filled with blood (*haematocolpos*) and at this time inspection of the vagina will show the imperforate hymen as a bluish membrane and the diagnosis becomes obvious. If this condition is still not diagnosed then the uterus becomes distended and the girl may be brought with an abdominal swelling due to *haematometra* or even with distension of the Fallopian tubes with blood (*haematosalpinx*). The presenting symptom is sometimes acute retention of urine.

It is obviously important that this condition is borne in mind when a young girl is brought with an abdominal swelling or with abdominal pain, as the condition is very easily treated if it is recognized. However, if the diagnosis is not made and laparotomy is performed a greatly distended uterus and tubes may not be recognized as such and cases are on record where they have been removed. The treatment of an imperforate hymen is by a simple cruciate incision of the membrane. The dark altered blood is simply allowed to drain away without any other interference which might lead to infection and subsequent infertility. Normal menstruation usually occurs thereafter.

IMPERFORATE VAGINA

The upper part of the vagina may be absent because of failure of canalization of the lower part of the Mullerian ducts and the lower part may be absent because of failure of canalization of the urogenital sinus. Complete absence of the vagina is due to the failure of canalization of both parts; a transverse septum can occur at the junction of the two areas. A medial vaginal septum may be present in uterus didelphys, uterus bicornis and uterus septus. The symptomology in such cases is the same as in imperforate hymen if the patient is menstruating. A medial septum, of course, does not interfere with menstruation. The treatment of imperforate vagina depends on the amount of canal present. The operations for creating artificial vaginas are referred to in Chapter 45.

Uterine abnormalities

These may be due to absence or failure of development or to deficient fusion of the two Mullerian ducts (Fig. 40.1). The uterus may be completely absent if the Mullerian ducts have failed to develop. If the ducts have failed to canalize then there will be absence of the upper four-fifths of the vagina and there will be one or two fibrous cords instead of the uterus.

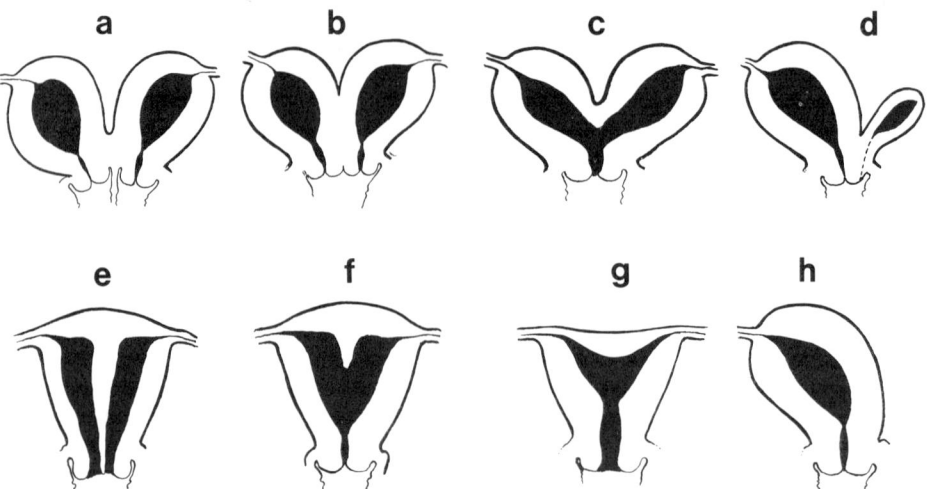

Fig. 40.1   Diagram to illustrate the main forms of developmental abnormalities of the uterus.

a. Uterus didelphys.
b. Uterus duplex bicornis bicollis vagina simplex.
c. Uterus bicornis unicollis vagina simplex.
d. Uterus bicornis unicollis with rudimentary horn.

e. Uterus septus.
f. Uterus subseptus.
g. Uterus arcuatus or cordiformis.
h. Uterus unicornis.

UTERUS DIDELPHYS

There is complete separation of the two horns of the uterus and duplication of the cervix and vagina. This may cause no symptoms at all and only be discovered during a pregnancy or even at delivery. During labour the empty horn of a uterus didelphys can cause obstruction. Uterine dysfunction is common in such cases and Caesarean section is often required. Cases of superfetation have been reported with a baby in each uterus.

UTERUS BICORNIS, BICORPUS, BICOLLIS

In this there is also complete duplication of the body and cervix of the uterus but not of the vagina although there is sometimes a septum present in the vagina. There may be some dyspareunia from the septum between the two vaginas. The condition is very similar to uterus didelphys.

UTERUS BICORNIS, BICORPUS, UNICOLLIS

There are two uterine bodies but only one cervix. Sometimes one corpus is less developed than the other forming a rudimentary horn. The condition may be diagnosed because the patient complains of dysmenorrhoea, dyspareunia or menorrhagia, but it may not be diagnosed until the patient becomes pregnant. They tend to be relatively infertile, and abortion or premature labour is likely to occur. Rupture of a pregnant rudimentary horn

produces signs and symptoms of ectopic pregnancy. Uterine dysfunction and obstruction of labour may occur. If Caesarean section is performed the type of abnormality should be carefully assessed and any other abnormalities, particularly of the urinary tract should be noted. In cases of repeated abortion a plastic operation can be performed. This was described by Strassman (see Chapter 45).

CORDIFORM UTERUS

The uterus is heart shaped and this is due to a partial duplication of the two horns. This condition is also usually diagnosed with pregnancy. There may be recurrent abortion or persistent breech presentation, or transverse lie. Excision of the fundus of the uterus may be done in cases of recurrent abortion.

SEPTATE UTERUS

In this there is a septum extending from the fundus of the uterus to the internal os. This gives rise to symptoms and signs similar to that in a uterus bicornis bicorpus unicollis. In the sub-septate uterus the septum extends from the fundus and only part of the septum is inside the cavity. It causes the same problems as the cordiform uterus, and is treated by excision of the septum. Another complication which arises in both subseptate uterus and the cordiform uterus is retained placenta on the septum.

UNICORNUATE UTERUS

This arises when one Mullerian duct fails to develop or to be canalized, so that there is absence of one half of the uterus. The ovary and kidney on the same side may also be absent. Pregnancy can occur in the unicornate uterus but abortion and premature labour may occur.

Abnormalities of Fallopian tubes and broad ligaments

If the Fallopian tubes are absent then the rest of the genital tract is also absent because canalization of the Mullerian tract occurs from above downwards. The Fallopian tube on one side may be absent and in such a case there will be a unicornuate uterus.

Abnormalities of ovaries and broad ligaments

Unilateral absence occurs with a unicornuate uterus and the absence of the Fallopian tube and kidney on that side. Both ovaries are rarely completely absent and it is more likely that there will be a streak of rudimentary ovarian tissue. This is found in Turner's syndrome (ovarian dysgenesis) in which there is infantilism, amenorrhoea, cubitus valgus and webbing of the neck (*see* Chapter 7). There are only 45 chromosomes and as there is no Y chromosome, they appear female.

Supernumerary ovaries are sometimes present and may or may not be functioning. They are usually found retroperitoneally.

GÄRTNER'S DUCT CYSTS

This is formed from the Wolffian duct which is in the broad ligament below the Fallopian tubes. The duct sometimes extends down alongside the uterus to the level of the cervix or to the antero-lateral wall of the vagina. The end of the duct forms a cystic swelling which is in the antero-lateral part of the vagina. This can be mistaken for a cystocele, but is usually symptomless and is found on vaginal examination. It may sometimes cause dyspareunia. As the duct goes upwards into the broad ligament the cyst may be difficult to remove. If it is symptomless it is best left alone. The epoophoron are a few tubules connecting the Gärtner's duct to the hilum of the ovary. The paroophoron consists of a few tubules in the broad ligament close to the uterus. They are the remains of the mesonephros and are not connected with the Gärtner's duct.

INTERSEX

Sex is difficult to define and can be on the basis of gonadal, chromosomal or hormonal factors. The extreme appearances are such that males are usually easily differentiated from females because of the hair distribution, body contours and external genitalia. There are many cases, however, where boys have been brought up as girls or vice versa and they may develop the mental attitudes of the opposite sex. Psychological factors also play an important role in sex and transvestism is the term given to someone who believes himself or herself to be of the opposite sex in spite of the gonadal, chromosomal, endocrine and external genital development clearly indicating which sex they belong to. This is a different condition from the child brought up as the wrong sex and is referred to on page 585. Although there is no absolute division into completely male or completely female, the term intersex is used when there is obvious failure to differentiate into the male type or the female type. Problems of sex determination may arise at birth or as a secondary feature later in life. It is extremely important that full investigations are carried out if there is any doubt about the sex of the baby at birth, and should include chromosomal examination. Chromosomal sex is referred to in Chapter 7. Cases of intersex can be divided into true hermaphrodites or pseudo-hermaphrodites.

True hermaphroditism

In this condition there are both ovaries and testes. This can occur either as an ovary on one side and a testis on the other or as a combined ovary and testis on each side. There is a phallus present and the uterus and tubes are also usually present. Facial configurations may be male and the breasts female. This is not usually diagnosed until the child has grown and the treatment is aimed at maintaining and perfecting the sex which seems most natural and normal to the patient.

Pseudo-hermaphroditism

In this condition the gonads are of one sex but the secondary sex characteristics are those of the other sex. In male pseudo-hermaphrodites the gonads are testes and in the female pseudo-hermaphrodites the gonads are ovaries.

MALE PSEUDO-HERMAPHRODITISM
(TESTICULAR FEMINIZATION)

The chromosomal sex of these cases is male XY. They are usually reared as females and indeed they appear externally to be completely female until puberty. At this time the breasts grow normally but the nipples are under-developed and there is hypertrophy of the clitoris and development of hair on the face. There may be a mixture of male and female external genitalia and pelvic organs. Usually there is a small penis with hypospadias and a small vagina with a cleft scrotum. The testes may be in the scrotum but are commonly in the pelvis. There may be quite well developed tubes and uterus present in the pelvis. The distribution of hair tends to be male.

If there is doubt about the sex of a baby at birth efforts should be made to determine the true sex and the child should be reared according to this. If there is doubt it is probably better to raise the child as a male until puberty when the secondary sex characteristics appear. The investigations at this time will include nuclear sexing, smearing of the vagina to determine hormonal effects and hormone determinations including 17 ketosteroids. If the condition is detected in early childhood chorionic gonadotrophin can be given in the hope of causing descent of the testes. Once it has been decided which sex the patient should adhere to various plastic operations may be carried out. If it is decided that this should be as a female then a vagina can be fashioned and an enlarged clitoris can be excised. Similarly in the male a pseudo-vagina can be removed and undescended testes either brought down and fixed in the scrotum or removed if it is thought that there is a danger of malignancy developing in them.

FEMALE PSEUDO-HERMAPHRODITISM

The sex chromosome pattern of these cases is female XX. During early fetal life abnormal male hormones cause some degree of sex reversal and in addition of development of the ovaries. The uterus and tubes are also under-developed. The clitoris is enlarged, the vagina is usually absent and the urethra opens at the base of the clitoris. The diagnosis and treatment are along the same lines as for the male pseudo-hermaphrodite.

ADRENO-GENITAL SYNDROME

This is a congenital condition in which there is a deficiency in production of hydrocortisone with a resultant excessive production of ACTH, which in turn causes hyperplasia of the zona-reticularis of the adrenal cortex. Excessive amounts of androgens are therefore produced and this causes virilism. This may or may not be associated with electrolyte disturbances and hypertension. In female babies there is pseudo-hermaphroditism with hypertrophy of the clitoris and the urethra and vagina formed from the uro-genital sinus open behind like a hypospadias. Later there is hirsutism, acne and primary amenorrhoea. The children grow rapidly but as the epiphyses close early they stop growing and become short adults. Male babies do not show any evidence of abnormal sex development at birth but virilism occurs early causing rapid growth of the long bones and premature appearance of hair on the face, axillae and pubis. There is also enlargement of the penis, but the testes remain small and immature. The epiphyses again close early so that adults are short. Urinary 17 ketosteroids and pregnanediol are found to be in excess. In some cases there is also excessive secretion of desoxycorticosterone by the adrenal cortex resulting in hypertension. This may be also associated with the disturbance of sodium and potassium metabolism. In both female pseudo-hermaphrodites and cases of adrenal virilism administration of cortisone will diminish the hyperplasia of the reticular zones and thus cause a reduction in the amount of ACTH being produced. The treatment should be started as early after birth as possible and in the female it is possible by treatment to restore the patient completely to normal and pregnancy may be possible. The dose of cortisone should be sufficient to reduce the 17 ketosteroids to normal. Usually 50mg intramuscularly are given daily to start with and reduced to 25mg daily after a month. The cortisone therapy will also correct the hypertension and electrolyte disturbance. Plastic surgery may be required to correct the external genital abnormalities.

Intersexuality due to abnormal numbers of sex chromosomes as in Turner's syndrome (gonadal dysgenesis), Klinefelter's syndrome and the human superfemale are discussed in Chapter 7.

TRAUMA OF THE GENITAL TRACT

Injuries to the genital tract may be acute due

to blows or lacerations or burns, or can be chronic as for example the result of foreign bodies. Many of the injuries of the genital tract occur in pregnancy and particularly in labour or abortion.

Vulval injuries

Probably the commonest injury in this area is the tearing of the hymen and this may occur at the first coitus. Usually there is only slight bleeding but sometimes a larger vessel is torn and the bleeding can be profuse and necessitate ligation of the bleeding points. Vulval lacerations and haematomata usually occur from direct trauma as for example falling astride a hard object such as a chair back or due to the trauma of childbirth. Haematomata are painful and can attain a large size. They are very painful and the patient can be markedly shocked. Usually it is necessary to incise and evacuate the blood clot and to ligate bleeding points. It is preferable to avoid packing if possible as this is more likely to cause infection and scarring. Sometimes if a vaginal tear or episiotomy is sewn up without effective haemostasis a large haematomata can form. The repair should be undone and the bleeding points ligated before re-repairing the laceration or episiotomy.

Ritual circumcision as practised by some North African tribes can cause gross scarring and distortion of the vulva.

Vaginal injuries

These are quite often associated with vulval injuries and as well as those described above the vagina may be injured by instruments used for procuring abortion. Coitus can also cause tearing of the vaginal walls and in cases of rape of young girls there may be extensive lacerations involving not only the vagina but the bladder and rectum. The repair of such lacerations may be difficult because of the problems of access.

Burns of the vagina can be caused by douching with strong antiseptic solutions or by the insertion of plastics. Potassium permanganate crystals were at one time used in the belief that they cause abortion, but they only cause vaginal bleeding and can lead to extensive cicatrization of the vagina.

Lacerations of the vagina can be caused by instruments used to procure abortion such as crochet hooks, slivers of wood or knitting needles. Injuries from these sources can often be overlooked because of bleeding coming through the cervix from a threatened abortion.

Foreign bodies in the vagina can be irritant and cause ulceration of the vaginal walls. There is often an offensive discharge which may be blood stained. If the object has been in the vagina for a long time it may become completely covered over by the vaginal tissues. This can happen with vulcanite or rubber pessaries but is less likely to happen with plastic pessaries. A great variety of objects may be found in the vagina. These can range from swabs left in at the time of delivery, forgotten tampons, bougies or catheters introduced as abortifacients and a wide variety of objects put into the vagina by small girls or by women practising masturbation or sexual perversions. Removal of the foreign body is usually sufficient treatment, but in some cases antiseptic douches or pessaries may be required.

Cervical lacerations

These most commonly occur at delivery but can also occur during operative dilatation of the cervix particularly in pregnancy. Small lacerations of the cervix do not require treatment but if there is bleeding then it is necessary to ligate and if there is extensive laceration the cervix has to be repaired. Extensive laceration and cicatrization of the cervix can occur when abortion or labour occurs in women who have had a suture inserted for incompetence of the cervix. This is only likely to occur if the suture is not removed promptly when abortion or labour commences.

Uterine injuries

Rupture of the pregnant uterus is described in Chapter 32. It is very unusual for the non-pregnant uterus to rupture spontaneously and the commonest cause is a carcinoma of the endometrium. Perforation of the uterus is most commonly caused by a uterine sound, cervical dilator or uterine curette. It is more liable to happen if there is an endometrial carcinoma particularly in an atrophic uterus or if it is a pregnant uterus. If this should happen no further attempts are made at dilating the cervix or curettage and the patient is kept under observation. A laparotomy is performed, however, if there is evidence of bleeding or if there is prolapse of bowel contents. If the operation was for evacuation of an abortion then the operation must be completed by hysterotomy. Cases of endometrial carcinoma are usually treated by hysterectomy if the uterus is perforated. Lacerations of the uterus or the cervix can cause haematoma of the broad ligament. As there is little resistance from the peritoneum the blood can spread extensively and immediate treatment to stop bleeding is necessary.

Other vaginal injuries

Recto-vaginal and vesico-vaginal fistulae usually result from obstetrical tears. A recto-vaginal fistula usually arises from faulty repair of complete perineal tears. The perineum itself heals but there is an opening left higher up between the vagina and the rectum. Recto-vaginal fistulae can also rarely follow a colpo-perineorrhaphy. The patient usually complains of uncontrolled passage of flatus and sometimes there may be a discharge of faeces from the vagina. Sometimes carcinoma, diverticulitis or tuberculosis can cause fistulae between the intestine and the uterus. The treatment of recto-vaginal fistulae is either by direct repair or by opening up the perineum again and repairing as for a complete perineal tear.

Urinary fistulae

These can occur from the ureter, bladder or urethra and can communicate with the uterus, cervix or vagina. The commonest are between the ureter or the bladder and the vagina. Fistulae can also occur between the bladder or ureter and the cervix, intestine or abdomen. Urinary fistulae are mostly due to obstetrical causes in the developing countries such as tropical Africa, but in western countries the majority are caused either by gynaecological operations or by radiotherapy or by carcinoma usually of the cervix but sometimes of the vagina. Most of the obstetrical fistulae are vesico-vaginal whereas the uretero-vaginal fistulae are usually due to operative trauma. Occasionally, vaginal trauma may involve the bladder, particularly if there has been impalement or a fracture of the pelvis. The bladder, of course, may also be damaged at the time of hysterectomy or vaginal repair. Obstetrical injuries may be caused by direct trauma with instruments, for example during forceps delivery but it is more often caused by pressure as in prolonged labour which results in slough-ing so that incontinence of urine does not appear for several days after delivery. Bladder fistulae can also occur at symphysiotomy. Urinary fistulae cause true incontinence and there is usually little difficulty in differentiating them from other causes of urinary incontinence such as that due to stress incontinence or neurological diseases. There is a continuous flow of urine from the vagina and it is not related to any effort on the part of the patient. Fistulae are usually easily diagnosed if they are large but if there is only a pin-hole fistula it may be difficult to locate. The 'three swab test' is very useful in such cases. In this test three large swabs are placed in the vagina one above the other and methylene blue solution is run into the bladder through a urethral catheter. This will not only locate the fistula but will differentiate between a vesico and a uretero fistula. The fistula is ureteric if none of the swabs is stained but the top swab is wet with urine. The fistula is vesical if the middle or upper swabs are stained and urethral if only the lowest swab is stained. Cystoscopy and intravenous pyelography should be performed before embarking on repairs to fistulae. Injuries of the ureter or bladder should be repaired immediately if they are not noticed at the time of operation or delivery. If they are not noticed during operation or delivery then conservative treatment should be carried out when the urinary leak is detected. A vesico-vaginal fistula, provided it is not too large will often close if continuous drainage is carried out for three weeks. Most vesico-vaginal fistulae can be closed by the vaginal approach but this should be delayed for two months after the fistula has developed. While awaiting operation the patient should be kept as dry as possible by inserting a large Foley catheter either into the bladder in the case of a vesico-vaginal fistula or into the vagina in the case of a uretero-vaginal fistula. The tissues must be mobilized as much as possible so that they can be sutured without tension. The after care is probably as important as the operation and it is essential that the bladder should be continuously drained for two or three weeks.

Uretero-vaginal fistulae can be repaired or the upper cut end can be transplanted into the bladder. More elaborate operations may be required in some cases depending on the extent of loss of tissue. The treatment of urinary fistulae is described in Chapter 45.

41. Tropical Gynaecology

Strong taboos and traditional beliefs to do with health, disease and childbirth are part of every culture. Those in the tropics will be unfamiliar to doctors trained in Europe, but nevertheless they must be studied and understood because they form an important background to clinical practice. In gynaecology, for instance, a hysterectomy for menstrual dysfunction may be unacceptable if the woman would lose her status in a polygamous marriage if she ceased to menstruate. By contrast, this radical treatment is often welcomed by a woman in Britain who has completed her planned family.

Underdeveloped countries are always under-doctored and, worse still, such medical facilities as are available may be under-used when the local population hesitates to accept their value. This is particularly relevant to gynaecology, as confidence in modern scientific medicine is least common amongst middle-aged and elderly women, always the least emancipated and most superstitious group anywhere.

Delay in seeking medical aid leads to patients coming late to hospital with tumours such as fibroids and ovarian cysts which may therefore be very large. Obstructed labour, too, is common in the tropics because of delay in seeking treatment; the resulting injuries of the bladder and rectum are considered in this chapter.

The risks of gynaecological surgery are increased in the tropics by the poor general health of many women. Careful pre-operative 'work-up' is therefore essential, especially the correction of anaemia. Shortage of skilled anaesthetists, modern anaesthetic equipment and medical gases may also increase the risks of operation. Furthermore, in the dark-skinned races cyanosis is difficult to detect, and in the humid tropics excessive sweating contributes to post-operative dehydration.

Tropical gynaecology provides constant reminders that inheritance as well as environ-ment influences the incidence of disease. For instance, the Negro peoples characteristically have a high proportion who form keloids, and this greatly influences the reaction of their tissues to trauma and infection and may spoil the result of the most careful reparative surgery.

Some gynaecological conditions are confined to the tropics because they are caused by infections which occur only there, such as genital schistosomiasis and elephantiasis of the vulva secondary to filariasis. Other infective conditions which, although they have a world-wide distribution, are particularly common in the tropics, are lymphogranuloma venereum and granuloma inguinale. Other world-wide infections such as syphilis and gonorrhoea not only have a high incidence in the tropics but delay in treatment commonly produces very florid lesions. Gonococcal infection, for instance, is responsible for widespread pelvic inflammatory disease with pelvic abscesses and much irreversible infertility.

Within the tropics, variations in incidence are striking. Thus, utero-vaginal prolapse is a major problem in south India, but it is surprisingly uncommon in tropical Africa. Chorionepithelioma, a very rare tumour in Britain, is much more common in South-east Asia, with the incidence in tropical Africa lying between these two extremes.

Endometriosis is very rare in Africans and in most other tropical peoples, which may be related to their almost universal early start to childbearing. Endometrial carcinoma, even allowing for differences in parity and age-structure of the population, is much less common in Africans than Caucasians.

Carcinoma of cervix is very common throughout the tropics, particularly in Africa where it occurs more frequently than malignant tumours of the breast or bowel, which are much rarer than in Britain. Unfortunately, delay in coming for treatment has a particularly serious effect in carcinoma of cervix: very few cases at present reach tropical hospitals when still in a curable stage. Epithelioma of the vulva, a rather rare disease of old women in Britain, is seen at a much younger age in the West Indies, which may be related to the high incidence of granuloma inguinale.

In general, then, most gynaecological conditions have a world-wide distribution, but their incidence in the tropics may be very different from that in Europe. Tropical gynaecology is the gynaecology of poverty and ignorance, with important exotic conditions added.

PELVIC INFLAMMATORY DISEASE

Subacute and chronic infection of the tubes, ovaries and neighbouring pelvic peritoneum are exceedingly common in the tropics and pose very difficult problems. Most cases are probably of gonococcal origin but a proportion follow puerperal or post-abortal infections.

Presentation in the acute phase of salpingitis is relatively rare. Usually, the patient presents with subacute or chronic pelvic infection with abdominal pain, irregular bleeding, malaise and recurrent fever. Those who present at a later stage may complain of dyspareunia, dysmenorrhoea, menorrhagia and infertility, a chronic picture punctuated by occasional exacerbations. Not infrequently a patient with this history develops a pelvic abscess which causes an acute and desperate illness. Collapse may follow as a result of bacteraemic shock if the abscess ruptures into the peritoneal cavity.

Management
When salpingitis is diagnosed in the acute phase, the treatment is conservative. Most cases will resolve completely with ampicillin or tetracycline in high dosage, although residual abscesses should be watched for and drained when they occur.

The management of subacute or chronic pelvic inflammatory disease is much more difficult. Antibiotic treatment is not likely to secure complete resolution and surgery has to be considered. To be completely effective this has to be radical, but as most of the patients are young, pelvic clearance is a very serious step which should be deferred as long as possible. In the meantime drainage of recurrent abscesses will be necessary, usually per abdomen although occasionally a collec-

tion in the pouch of Douglas can be drained very simply through the posterior fornix.

Eventually the infection may die down, leaving the patient irremediably sterile. Even the recurrent cases settle down after the menopause, so in older women an attempt should be made to temporize until this occurs.

However, chronic ill-health often forces the surgeon's hand before this. In these cases removal of the uterus with the chronically inflamed adnexa is necessary, but if possible some functioning ovarian tissue should be conserved. The most difficult pelvic surgery which the gynaecologist in the tropics ever has to attempt is the removal of densely adherent masses of fibroids and chronic pyosalpinges, so this should not be lightly undertaken by the beginner.

EXTRA-UTERINE PREGNANCY

In most tropical communities extra-uterine pregnancies are much more common than in Europe: in tropical Africa and the Caribbean ruptured ectopic pregnancy is the commonest surgical emergency in women. This high frequency is no doubt because gonococcal, puerperal and post-abortal pelvic infections, which predispose to tubal implantation of the ovum, are so common.

Although the pathology of ectopic pregnancy is the same in the tropics as elsewhere, the clinical presentation is often very different. The diagnosis may therefore be missed (with disastrous results) unless the possibility is always borne in mind whenever a woman in the childbearing years presents with abdominal or pelvic symptoms.

The acutely exsanguinated type with a massive haemoperitoneum forms a smaller proportion of cases than in Europe. The chronic type, in which pelvic haematomas may mimic fibroids, ovarian cysts or pelvic abscesses, is relatively more common. Cases in which the extra-uterine fetus continues to develop either in the peritoneal cavity or between the leaves of the broad ligament are also seen more frequently. These different features all result from delay in presenting for treatment, either because of stoicism or mistrust of modern medicine or difficulty in reaching medical aid. As a result of this delay some of the acute cases die at home, and the survivors may present a chronic picture by the time they reach hospital.

Diagnosis

Culdocentesis, aspirating the pouch of Douglas through the posterior fornix with a needle and syringe, is a most useful diagnostic procedure in these cases. Although a negative aspiration does not exclude ectopic pregnancy, the appearance of *old* blood confirms the diagnosis and indicates immediate laparotomy. It is a useful way of distinguishing a pelvic haematoma from an abscess, as the pus which is obtained from the latter indicates drainage per vaginam by posterior colpotomy.

In doubtful cases laparoscopy is useful if the necessary equipment and expertise are available. If not, diagnostic laparotomy may be indicated. Above all, no patient who might conceivably have an extra-uterine pregnancy should be allowed to leave hospital with the diagnosis still in doubt. If she bleeds again after she has gone home, she may not get back to the hospital in time.

Autotransfusion

However collapsed and exsanguinated by a ruptured ectopic pregnancy, most patients can be salvaged in Britain because stored blood is readily available, but blood banks are rare in the tropics. Autotransfusion, in which freshly-shed blood is collected from the peritoneal cavity and returned to the circulation intravenously, is therefore a very useful technique in the tropics.

At its simplest, the method consists of baling the haemoperitoneum into a transfusion bottle through a funnel containing sterile gauze to filter off the clots. The blood should not be transfused if there is any evidence of haemolysis or infection: some degree of contamination is inevitable, so storage is dangerous and the blood should be given immediately or not at all.

ACQUIRED GYNATRESIA

Stenosis of the lower genital tract follows traditional gynaecological procedures in many parts of the tropics.

Female circumcision

The custom of female circumcision is mainly confined to Africa. Although it is officially discouraged and is now on the wane, it is still widely practised.

The severity of the vulval stenosis which may follow circumcision depends on how much of the vulva is removed and the degree of scarring and contracture which follows. At one end of the scale, among the Yoruba of Western Nigeria, the procedure is confined to a limited trimming of the labia minora and tip of the clitoris, so vulval stenosis is rare.

The more radical circumcision of the Nile Valley has more serious after-effects because it includes infibulation. This is a deliberate attempt to make the raw surfaces of the vulval wound adhere across the mid-line, which results in obliteration of the anterior part of the vulval cleft and sometimes almost completely closes it. Dyspareunia, interference with the urinary stream and dystocia may result. During delivery the anterior bridge of scar tissue has to be divided (by 'anterior episiotomy') to permit delivery, and the patient and her husband usually demand that this is repaired afterwards: the same procedure is then necessary at each subsequent delivery.

Scarring following chemical vaginitis

The insertion of medicaments into the vagina is a common feature of folk medicine the world over (including Britain, where the custom of douching for 'hygiene' is still firmly established). Irritants introduced into the vagina damage the epithelium by producing chemical vaginitis which may result in necrosis of the full thickness of the vaginal wall. The ulceration is likely to be annular as the vaginal wall is in contact with the irritant all the way round, so healing will be followed by circumferential contracture of the scar and thus vaginal stenosis.

In parts of Arabia, particularly amongst the Bedouin, lumps of rock salt are still inserted into the vagina during the puerperium. The purpose is to shrink down the vagina to its nulliparous state and thus increase the sexual gratification of the husband. If the resulting stenosis is marked, severe dyspareunia or even apareunia may follow. Occasionally the lumen of the vagina is totally occluded, as a result of which the menses accumulate above the block.

Vaginal stenosis following chemical vaginitis is also found in Western Nigeria, where caustic herbal pessaries are inserted to treat a variety of gynaecological symptoms. The herbal content is probably harmless but the base, a crude soap made by mixing palm oil with potash, is highly alkaline and causes severe chemical vaginitis.

Scarring following difficult labour

In obstructed labour the presenting part may be arrested in the vagina for so long that pressure necrosis of the vaginal wall occurs. Some days after delivery the affected part of the wall sloughs, in many cases including the underlying wall of the bladder or rectum. After the sloughs have separated, the unlined vaginal cavity heals by granulation. The fibrosis which follows produces scarring: when the scar contracts, stenosis follows if a wide annular area is involved.

Repair of concurrent vesico-vaginal or recto-vaginal fistulae in these cases is likely to exaggerate the stenosis, a result which may be difficult to avoid.

Management

In the acute phase of a chemical vaginitis, thorough cleansing (if necessary under anaesthesia) to remove all remaining traces of the caustic is the first step. The depth of sloughing may be limited by controlling infection with frequent vaginal douches of weak antiseptic and parenteral antibiotics. Replacement of the sloughed vaginal skin by fibrosis is inevitable, although cortisone packs may limit this.

Contracture of the scar tissue occurs very rapidly, so the best method of preventing this in severe cases is to insert a skin graft on a large mould as soon as the vaginal cavity is lined by clean granulations.

Later, after stenosis of the vagina by scarring is established, plastic reconstruction is made difficult by the density of the scar tissue. In some cases a Williams' vulvoplasty may lengthen the vagina enough to permit satisfactory coitus. However, when the lower half of the vagina is involved in the stenosis or menstrual fluid is retained above the block, this will not be effective.

In these circumstances a modification of MacIndoe's procedure should be performed, in two stages (Lawson 1968). The vaginal cavity is first reopened widely, excising all scar tissue, and is then packed temporarily with gauze bandage soaked in Whitehead's varnish. When this is removed three or four days later,

all oozing has ceased and a clean, granulating, raw surface is revealed which is ready for grafting. A mould of appropriate size is covered with a Thiersch graft taken from the thigh, and after insertion is kept in place by a high perineorrhaphy.

VESICO-VAGINAL FISTULAE

Urinary incontinence following damage to the bladder in obstructed labour is unfortunately still common in many parts of the tropics. Prolonged and unrelieved pressure between the fetal head and symphysis pubis causes ischaemic necrosis of the intervening soft tissues. Usually between the third and tenth days of the puerperium, the slough separates and a vesico-vaginal fistula results. Less commonly, the bladder may be torn when the neighbouring lower uterine segment ruptures as a result of obstruction, or it may be damaged during operative procedures such as craniotomy or symphysiotomy performed to relieve obstruction.

Whatever the cause, the resulting urinary incontinence is a disaster for the woman who, usually deserted by her husband, lives in stinking misery. The condition is often thought to be incurable, so sufferers will travel enormous distances to seek help from doctors who acquire a reputation for successfully treating incontinence.

Early treatment

When bladder fistulae first form they should always be treated conservatively. Natural healing will reduce their size and some will close completely. This may be encouraged by continuous drainage of the bladder through a urethral catheter. It is worth continuing with drainage for up to six weeks after delivery so long as most of the urine drains through the catheter (but not if it does not).

Definitive repair should not be attempted until at least three months have elapsed since the causative labour. During this time all sloughs will separate, effusions into the tissues will reabsorb and infection will subside. In the tedious waiting period the skin of the vulva and neighbouring thighs should be protected with a simple barrier cream such as zinc and castor oil, and the patient's general health should be built up by the treatment of any residual sepsis and the correction of anaemia and malnutrition. Other sequelae of obstructed labour which may be present, such as sacral bed sores or foot drop, should be dealt with and the patient's morale should be sustained by constant encouragement and the promise of eventual cure.

When the time comes for definitive repair, or if the patient first presents long after the causative labour, exact localization of the fistula by preliminary examination under anaesthesia is necessary to plan the best procedure.

Sites of vesico-vaginal fistulae

Vesico-vaginal fistulae may be classified into the following four anatomical groups: each poses different problems (Fig. 41.1).

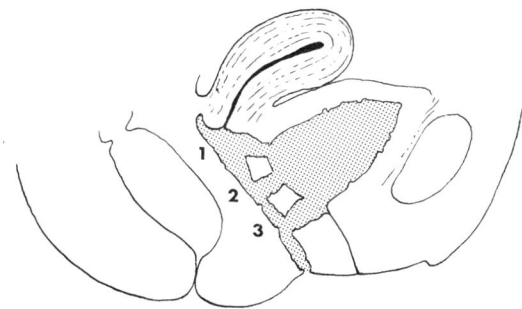

Fig. 41.1 Sites of vesico-vaginal fistulae. (1) Juxta-cervical fistula. (2) Mid-vaginal fistula. (3) Juxta-urethral fistula. Massive fistulae combine all three types.

1. *Juxta-urethral fistulae*. These involve the bladder-neck and proximal part of the urethra, and fixation to the back of the symphysis or pubic rami is common. The urinary sphincter mechanism is usually damaged, so urethral incontinence may be a serious problem after successful closure of the fistula.

2. *Mid-vaginal*. These fistulae are easiest to repair as they are usually readily accessible and fixture to bone is unusual. Neither the trigone above nor the sphincter below is involved. Unfortunately, they are the least common type.

3. *Juxta-cervical*. These fistulae open either into the anterior fornix or into the cervical canal. As they are close to the trigone, the ureteric orifices may be in the edge and some are inaccessible per vaginam if the cervix is fixed high in the pelvis.

4. *Massive fistulae*. Called circumferential

by Chassar Moir, these fistulae are a combination of the above three types. The tissue loss extends from the bladder-neck to the trigone, the ureteric orifices are usually in the edges of the fistula and inverted bladder-wall may prolapse through the defect.

PRINCIPLES OF MANAGEMENT

The repair of some of these fistulae can be very difficult, and success depends on good nursing as well as on correct surgical technique. Most important of all is personal experience: as every fistula is different, the necessary versatility and skill only develop with practice. It is therefore desirable that patients with urinary fistulae should be transferred to the care of gynaecologists with special expertise who work in well-staffed and well-equipped centres. However, referral for specialist treatment may involve a long and expensive journey, so the easier fistulae may have to be tackled in peripheral hospitals, only the more difficult cases being referred. The guiding principle should be that the first attempt at repair must be successful, as each further attempt provokes more scarring and makes success less likely.

Surgical technique

For a detailed description of the technique of fistula repair the reader is referred to Moir (1967) and Lawson (1967). The following principles are important:

1. *Approach and exposure*. Most obstetric fistulae are best repaired per vaginam, the abdominal approach being preferable only for high fistulae which cannot be drawn down under anaesthesia to allow access from below. For juxta-urethral and mid-vaginal fistulae, the knee-elbow position gives the best exposure: it is particularly valuable for massive fistulae, as prolapse of the bladder-wall through the fistula is thereby reduced. High fistulae which can be reached per vaginam are best repaired in exaggerated lithotomy position with strong traction on the cervix.

2. *Dissection and mobilization*. In general the flap-splitting method of repair is preferred, in which the vagina is separated from the underlying bladder and the edges of the bladder defect are widely mobilized. Occasionally, however, smaller fistulae can be closed by saucerization without dissecting the layers.

3. *Accurate closure*. The defect in the bladder is closed with interrupted catgut

sutures which invert the edges into the bladder. Tension must be avoided and the closure should be with at least two layers of sutures. It is not always possible to close the overlying vaginal wall defect.

4. *Secure catheter drainage.* After completing the repair, an indwelling urethral catheter should be inserted into the bladder. Provided the repair does not involve the bladder-neck, a self-retaining Foley's catheter is satisfactory, but after the repair of a juxta-urethral fistula a simple whistle-tip catheter should be stitched to the vulva, thus avoiding traction on the suture line.

POST-OPERATIVE CARE
Continuous bladder drainage is essential for at least 10 and preferably 14 days after the repair to keep the suture line at rest. The catheter should drain into a closed-circuit system to prevent infection, and drainage bags containing a non-return valve are best. Appropriate chemotherapy is also necessary.

The success of the repair should be proved by examining the patient under anaesthesia about four weeks after the operation, instilling a dilute solution of methylene blue into the bladder to detect any leak.

The patient should be advised to avoid coitus for at least three months, and all subsequent deliveries should, of course, be by elective Caesarean section to prevent breakdown of the repair.

Alternative procedures
Unfortunately not all repairs will be successful, but a practised operator should achieve success at the first attempt in at least 80 per cent. If a further operation to close a residual fistula is necessary, this should be deferred for at least two months after the previous repair.

A few very severe cases may be judged to be irreparable, in which case a urinary diversion procedure will be necessary to secure continence. However, this is a serious decision and diversion should not be performed until the most practised operator in the locality has failed to close the fistula.

Transplantation of the ureters into the rectum has been the main stand-by for these cases in the tropics because of the almost universal dislike of an abdominal stoma. However, recurrent ascending urinary infection and eventually death from renal failure inevitably follows this procedure. Transplantation of the ureters into an isolated loop of ileum undoubtedly gives better long-term results, or transplantation of the ureters into the rectum after it has been isolated from the faecal stream by a terminal colostomy. These procedures are therefore preferable if an abdominal stoma can be accepted.

RECTO-VAGINAL FISTULAE

The commonest cause of recto-vaginal fistula in the tropics is obstructed labour. Pressure necrosis of the soft tissues between the presenting part and the posterior pelvic wall is followed by sloughing, in the same way as anteriorly the more common bladder injuries are produced. A recto-vaginal fistula may also result from the breakdown of the upper end of the repair of a third-degree tear. Ulceration of the recto-vaginal septum due to lymphogranuloma venereum may also produce recto-vaginal fistulae (often associated with rectal stricture) and this is a relatively common cause in some tropical areas.

Not all recto-vaginal fistulae produce total faecal incontinence. This depends on whether the defect is above or below the pubo-rectalis sling, so defects in the recto-vaginal septum are classified into two types, depending on whether they involve the upper half of the vagina or not (Fig. 41.2).

Lesions confined to the lower half of the vagina (either short third-degree defects or low recto-vaginal fistulae) are responsible for incontinence of only flatus and fluid faeces. Contraction of the pubo-coccygeus muscle kinks the rectum forwards and prevents the escape of solid faeces.

Lesions involving the upper half of the vagina, either recto-vaginal fistulae high in the posterior fornix or third-degree defects involving the whole of the posterior vaginal wall up to the cervix, are far more serious. They result in the continuous passage of faeces per vaginam because the defect is above the pubo-rectalis sling. Access is often difficult because the upper end of the defect is high up the vagina and tethering by scar tissue to the sacrum is common.

GENERAL MANAGEMENT
Before a recto-vaginal fistula is repaired at least two months should be allowed to elapse

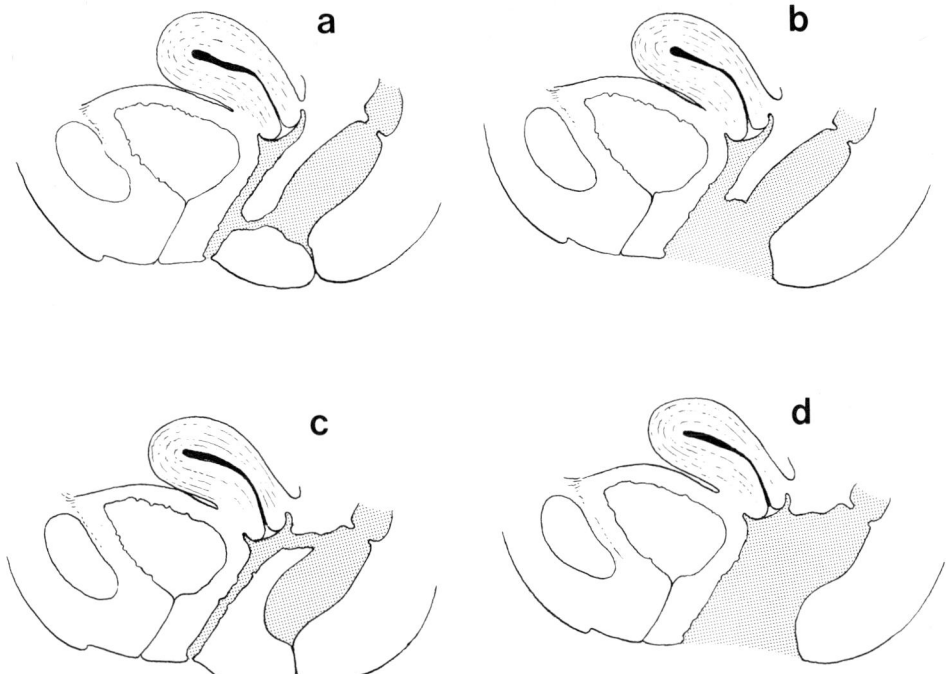

Fig. 41.2 Sites of recto-vaginal defects. (a) Low recto-vaginal fistula. (b) Short third-degree defect. (c) High recto-vaginal fistula. (d) Loss of whole recto-vaginal septum.

since the causative labour or previous attempt at closure.

Pre-operatively, clearance of the large intestine by cathartics and repeated rectal wash-outs is important, and it is customary to attempt to reduce bacterial activity in the bowel with neomycin or pthalyl-sulpha-thiazole.

Management of low recto-vaginal fistulae

Low recto-vaginal fistulae and short third-degree defects are not usually difficult to repair in layers as they are easily accessible. A preliminary colostomy is not necessary.

Post-operatively, the healing tissues should be kept at rest for as long as possible by confining the bowels, and the first stools should be softened with liquid paraffin. The temptation to examine the rectum digitally to see if the repair has healed should be resisted for at least three weeks after the operation.

Management of high recto-vaginal fistulae

High recto-vaginal fistulae may be repaired per vaginam or per abdomen, and the decision should be made at preliminary examination under anaesthesia. Most can be reached from below, but if the upper edge of the defect is too high to be accessible per vaginam, repair by the abdominal route is indicated.

A preliminary transverse colostomy is required when the rectal defect is larger than 1cm in diameter, and always before repair by the abdominal route.

Before a vaginal repair is embarked upon, a deep Schuchardt incision which splits the vaginal tube up to the lateral fornix may be needed for access, particularly if the vagina has been narrowed by scarring.

The mobilization of the upper border of the high fistula is greatly facilitated by deliberately opening the pouch of Douglas behind the cervix. The rectal fistula is closed transversely in the usual two layers, and intact vaginal wall is then drawn up over the repair. To close the peritoneal cavity, the anterior wall of the rectum above the repair is attached to the back of the cervix, which leaves an area of rectal wall covered with peritoneum in the posterior fornix.

Inaccessible high fistulae which have to be approached per abdomen are usually tethered to the sacrum. In some cases the depths of the pouch of Douglas can be reached after releasing adhesions between the cervix and the sacral promontory. Access to the fistula can then be gained by incising the peritoneum of the cul-de-sac and dissecting between the rectum and vagina.

However, when the fibrosis and scarring is very dense and the cervix and vaginal vault are completely fixed in solid scar tissue, this technique is impracticable. A method which involves preliminary subtotal hysterectomy (Lawson, 1972) is advised in these circumstances.

Combined fistulae

Obstetric injuries involving both the rectum and the bladder follow exceptionally severe pressure necrosis. The difficult high recto-vaginal fistulae are nearly always associated with vesico-vaginal fistulae and severe scarring.

It is tempting to try to repair the defects in the bladder and rectum at the same time. This should be resisted, however, as too much tissue has to be borrowed and the suture lines, being under tension, are therefore likely to break down.

It is usually best to close the bladder defect first and, after this has been proved to have been successful, to close the rectum later.

Conclusion

Vesico-vaginal and recto-vaginal fistulae of obstetric origin are, of course, readily preventable by good obstetrics. However, until effective maternity services are available to all tropical communities, women with contracted pelvis will continue to go into obstructed labour when far from help, and fistulae will remain the chief gynaecological challenge of the tropics.

SCHISTOSOMIASIS

The trematode parasites of the genus Schistosoma depend on certain varieties of fresh-water snails as intermediate hosts, so the disease occurs in the tropics where these snails are found. In the human host *S. haematobium* and *S. mansoni* worms migrate into the pelvic veins: the gravid females travel against the blood stream towards an excretory viscus to deposit their ova in the wall of the bladder (*haematobium*) or the bowel (*mansoni*). Some of the ova are ultimately extruded into the lumen of the viscus to escape with the host's excreta into fresh water, where the ova hatch into miracidia which lodge in snails of the appropriate species. After further develop-

ment in the intermediate host, cercariae escape into the water and enter human hosts through the skin, or less commonly through the mouth, to continue the cycle.

The lesions of schistosomiasis result from tissue reaction to the ova. In *S. haematobium* infections particularly, the female genital tract is invaded when ova spill over from the neighbouring bladder wall which is the preferred site. The ova first cause hyperaemia and an inflammatory reaction and later become surrounded by areas of granulation tissue. When close to the skin these produce raised, flat or papillomatous masses which frequently ulcerate. Before puberty, schistosomal lesions are commonest on or near the vulva and take the form of dry, flat, indurated papillomata. In young adults, vaginal and cervical lesions develop. Papillomata in the vagina usually ulcerate, and on the cervix they closely resemble carcinoma. The corpus uteri is less commonly involved: the tubes, ovaries and bases of the broad ligaments may be the site of dense fibrosis provoked by massive deposition of ova.

The main symptom of vulval schistosomiasis in young girls is pruritus. The vaginal and cervical lesions cause discharge, dyspareunia and post-coital bleeding. Genital schistosomiasis is almost always associated with urinary tract involvement, and a history of this can be obtained even if no evidence of active schistosomiasis of the bladder can be found in the urine. The diagnosis of lower genital tract lesions is easily made by biopsy, which will distinguish them from malignant or tuberculous lesions.

The ulcers and papillomata usually clear up rapidly with appropriate medical treatment, and surgery is seldom required. Trivalent antimony compounds given by injection have been the main standby in the past: nowadays Ambilhar (Ciba) is preferred.

LYMPHOGRANULOMA VENEREUM

Lymphogranuloma venereum (sometimes confusingly called lymphogranuloma inguinale) is caused by an organism of the Chlamydia genus, half way between a large virus and a small bacterium, very similar to the causative organisms of psittacosis and trachoma. The disease is transmitted by sexual contact and is common in the West Indies, Central and West

Africa, South India, Indonesia and Central and South America.

The primary lesion is a small, painless, shallow ulcer. It usually heals quickly and spontaneously and is therefore only observed occasionally in this phase on the female genitalia. In the male, a similar primary lesion on the penis is frequently followed by suppurative inguinal adenitis. These 'buboes' are much less commonly seen in females, but when involvement of the inguinal lymphatics has been widespread, subsequent fibrosis may cause obstruction to the lymph drainage of the vulva.

In some cases the primary lesion slowly progresses to extensive deep ulceration of the vulval structures, which is surprisingly painless. This may destroy the urethra, leading to severe stress incontinence, or the perineal body so that the end result looks like an old third-degree tear. Ultimately the process burns out and the ulcers heal, leaving bridges and tunnels of uninvolved vaginal skin and notching and fenestration of the labia, which are characteristic.

Sometimes the infection spreads through the recto-vaginal septum to involve the rectal wall. Chronic proctitis may follow, and severe stricture of the rectum due to peri-rectal fibrosis is a common sequel which is often associated with recto-vaginal fistulae. Although the rectal stricture hardly ever causes intestinal obstruction, severe constipation is common: the constant straining at stool may result in a procidentia.

The diagnosis of an established case of lymphogranuloma venereum is usually not difficult because more than one of the clinical features described above is nearly always present. Confirmation of the diagnosis may be obtained by the Frei test, in which an antigen prepared from infected material is injected intradermally. Unfortunately, however, false negatives are not uncommon and a positive result does not prove a recent or active infection because sensitization persists for many years.

Treatment of lymphogranuloma venereum in the acute phase is with sulphonamides or, preferably, with tetracycline. The disabling long-term effects of the destructive lesions pose very difficult surgical problems. For a detailed description the reader is referred to Annamunthodo (1962) and Stewart (1962).

DONOVANOSIS

Donovanosis (granuloma inguinale) is caused by *Donovania granulomatis*, a small, encapsulated, gram-negative cocco-bacillus. The disease is transmitted by sexual contact but is probably not very infectious as the conjugal partner of a sufferer often escapes. It is found in widely-scattered areas of the tropics, notably the Caribbean, South India and New Guinea.

Donovanosis is primarily a disease of the skin and mucous membranes. The earliest lesions are discrete, raised papules on or near the external genitalia or in the vagina. These break down into irregular destructive ulcers with rolled edges: their base is beefy-red granulation tissue covered with offensive exudate. The ulcers are tender and painful (unlike lymphogranuloma venereum) and may extend along the crural folds to the groin and over the perineum to the perianal skin.

In the healing phase, massive swelling of the distorted genitalia is fairly common and the ulcers are replaced by leathery depigmented scars.

Diagnosis
Examination of a tissue smear from an active ulcer reveals typical Donovan bodies within large mononuclear cells. These are found below the surface, so the superficial layer of the ulcer is removed with a knife before squeezing the exudate onto a slide. This may be stained either with Giemsa or Leishman stain, or by the standard Papanicolaou technique.

Treatment
The active ulcerative phase is very rapidly controlled by streptomycin, which should be given daily for 20 days, or by tetracycline.

In the inactive, healed phase, trimming of the swollen vulval tissues may be necessary if they are causing inconvenience or discomfort.

Prognosis
There is little doubt that the lesions of donovanosis predispose to carcinoma. An ulcer which heals incompletely or recurs should therefore be viewed with caution. Follow-up of treated cases is essential, with biopsy of suspicious areas.

AMOEBIASIS

Infection of the vulva and vagina with *Entamoeba histolytica* is not common but has been reported from India, Central America and New Guinea.

There is nearly always a previous history of intestinal amoebiasis, and in some cases clinical evidence of this may be found at the same time as lower genital tract lesions.

The presenting symptom is a very offensive blood-stained vaginal discharge. Scattered, friable, oozing ulcers are found on the vulva and in the vagina and, occasionally, in the groin folds.

The diagnosis is confirmed by finding active amoebae in a warm stage preparation of the discharge or of scrapings from the ulcers.

The response to treatment with systemic amoebicides such as metronidazole is rapid. This is usually combined with vaginal douches of one of the hydroxyquinoline drugs.

CHRONIC LYMPHOEDEMA AND ELEPHANTIASIS OF THE VULVA

Since the lymph vessels of the vulva drain through the superficial inguinal nodes, obstruction to the flow of lymph by fibrosis of these nodes results in subcutaneous oedema of the vulva. Puffy swelling of the labia results, and vesicles may appear on the skin which leak lymph and keep it constantly moist. Later, when the deeper layer of the dermis becomes converted into a myxomatous mass in a fibrous matrix, elephantiasis may develop. The thickened leathery epidermis is tightly stretched over the mass and warty excrescences appear.

In the tropics three main causes of obstruction to the lymph drainage of the vulva are found: filariasis, tuberculous inguinal adenitis and lymphogranuloma venereum.

Filariasis

The adult forms of the parasitic nematodes *Wuchereria bancrofti* and *Brugia malayi* inhabit the lymphatic tissues. *W. bancrofti* is commonest in the Pacific islands of Samoa, Fiji and Tahiti, and *B. malayi* only occurs in Asia, from the west coast of India to as far north as Japan. The parasites are transmitted by mosquitoes infected by ingesting human blood containing micro-filariae. After a short cycle in the vector, larval forms are injected into the host where they reach maturity in the larger lymphatic channels: they may survive for many years in the lymph nodes. After mating, large numbers of micro-filariae reach the peripheral blood and the life-cycle is repeated when they are taken up by the intermediate host.

By the time the fibrosis caused by dead adult worms has caused inguinal lymphatic obstruction and thus vulval elephantiasis, the infection is usually no longer active and micro-filariae have disappeared from the peripheral blood.

Tuberculous adenitis

With the rapid decline of tuberculous infections in Europe due to effective chemotherapy, protection with BCG and improved social conditions, tuberculous adenitis has virtually disappeared. However, in the tropics a similar improvement has not yet occurred and widespread tuberculous infection of the lymph nodes is therefore still common.

Particularly in Africa, sclerosis of the inguinal lymphatics after chronic tuberculous adenitis not infrequently leads to lymphoedema and elephantiasis of the vulva.

Characteristically, the scars of multiple sinuses are found overlying lymph nodes in the neck and axillae as well as the groins, and lymphoedema of the leg, arm or breast may be found associated with lymphoedema of the vulva.

Lymphogranuloma venereum

As has already been mentioned, lymphogranuloma venereum causes suppurative inguinal adenitis in the male more commonly than in the female. Lymphoedema and elephantiasis of the vulva due to this infection is therefore not often seen and is seldom severe. When it does occur, other lesions of lymphogranuloma are present, such as fenestration of the labia, rectal stricture and recto-vaginal fistulae.

Treatment of elephantiasis

Although the original infection has usually burnt out by the time elephantiasis of the vulva develops, it is customary to give a course of appropriate chemotherapy to complete the eradication of the causative tuberculous, filarial or lymphogranulomatous infection. Unfortunately the obstruction to the lymphatic drainage of the vulva is permanent. The results of surgical treatment of elephantiasis of the vulva are therefore disappointing, as recurrence is common.

However, when the vulval masses are large enough to cause inconvenience and discomfort they have to be removed. The incision should be well clear of the tumour so that it goes through healthy skin whose lymphatic drainage is still intact. The patient should be warned that further surgery may be required in years to come.

REFERENCES

Annamunthodo, H. (1962) Intestinal Lymphogranuloma. In *Lymphogranuloma Venereum*, Ch. 5. Edited by M. M. Sigel. University of Miami Press.

Lawson, J. B. & Stewart, D. B. (1967) *Obstetrics and Gynaecology in the Tropics and Developing Countries*. London: Edward Arnold.

Lawson, J. B. (1968) Birth canal injuries. *Proc. roy. Soc. Med.*, **61**, 369.

Lawson, J. B. (1972) Rectovaginal fistulae following difficult labour. *Proc. roy. Soc. Med.*, **65**, 283.

Moir, J. C. (1967) *The vesico-vaginal fistula*. London: Baillière, Tindall and Cassell.

Stewart, D. B. (1962) Lesions of the vulva, vagina and urethra associated with lymphogranuloma venereum. In *Lymphogranuloma Venereum*, Ch. 6.

42. Surgical Conditions in Gynaecology

The two circumstances in which the gynaecologist is faced most commonly with surgical conditions are in cases of acute abdomen and abdomino-pelvic tumours. It is sometimes possible from a carefully taken history and planned investigation to arrive at a correct diagnosis, but in some cases this can be achieved only after laparotomy has been performed. Where the gynaecologist is presented with a surgical finding at laparotomy he should seek the help of a specialist surgeon if one is available or be prepared to deal with the situation himself. He may, however, find that after careful inspection of the situation, it is best to close the abdomen and deal with the condition after more thorough investigation and preparation of the patient has been carried out. Obviously if the condition is acute or intestinal obstruction is present the situation must be dealt with before the abdomen is closed.

The 'acute abdomen' may be due to inflammation, haemorrhage or distension of a viscus, usually due to obstruction or to torsion, or it may be due to perforation of some part of the alimentary tract.

Appendicitis

Appendicitis in pregnancy is discussed in Chapter 12.

This can cause considerable difficulty in diagnosis and may be mistakenly diagnosed as salpingo-oophoritis, ectopic pregnancy or torsion of an ovarian tumour. In acute appendicitis the pain commences around the umbilicus and across the abdomen, and then shifts to the right iliac fossa. Pain is unilateral and is not associated with pyrexia or vomiting at first. There is usually anorexia and maybe vomiting later, but no disturbance of menstruation and there is absence of vaginal discharge. If, however, a considerable time has elapsed since the onset of the illness then the characteristic picture becomes obscured.

Instead of localized muscle rigidity with hyperaesthesia and tenderness in the right iliac fossa there will now be generalized lower abdominal pain and tenderness. There will be pyrexia and tachycardia and evidence of generalized pelvic peritonitis. In the early stages of acute appendicitis pelvic examination will not reveal tenderness in the lateral fornices, but moving the cervix from side to side may cause pain on the right side. If the appendix occupies a pelvic position there will be tenderness in the posterior fornix and this should be confirmed by rectal examination. If the appendix is retrocaecal or pelvic in position there may be no localized tenderness. Pressure over the left side of the colon causing pain on the right side (Rovsing's Sign) can be helpful in these cases.

In late cases where an appendix abscess is forming there may be tenderness in both fornices, but the tenderness will usually be so severe that an accurate assessment of any swelling cannot be made. In the early phase of acute appendicitis the diagnosis is more likely to be confused with an ectopic pregnancy, and in the later stages with salpingo-oophoritis, but in the doubtful case laparoscopy may be helpful. In both acute appendicitis and ectopic pregnancy laparotomy is indicated, and in the female in the reproductive age-group the incision should always be *mid-line or para-median*, and not grid-iron. Salpingo-oophoritis is best treated conservatively with antibiotic and analgesic therapy, and laparotomy is best avoided. Acute salpingo-oophoritis is almost always bilateral and is associated with pyrexia from an early stage of the disease, a high leucocyte count and a high erythrocyte sedimentation rate.

If a presumptive diagnosis of salpingo-oophoritis has been made, but conservative therapy has failed to cure the condition then a laparotomy must be carried out. If an appendix abscess is found, it is emptied by suction and a corrugated drain is inserted. The appendix should only be removed if it is possible to do so without gross disturbance of the abscess site and spreading of pus. Interval appendicectomy is carried out in about three months' time.

Acute diverticulitis

This may also be confused with acute gynaecological conditions. There is acute pain and tenderness with rebound tenderness usually in the left iliac fossa. There may be a history of constipation or diarrhoea. On vaginal examination there may be tenderness and fullness in the Pouch of Douglas or in the left iliac fossa. The condition is best treated with antibiotics and the patient is maintained on a fluid diet until all inflammation has settled. Occasionally perforation can occur in diverticulitis and this carries a high mortality. Laparotomy is performed and drainage and a transverse colostomy carried out. Better results are now obtained by emergency colectomy, but this should only be performed by surgeons experienced in the procedure and faecal peritonitis must be avoided. Occasionally in older women a left sided tender mass is due to subacute diverticulitis with associated tubo ovarian abscess formation. Removal of the tubo ovarian abscess with conservation or radical treatment of the diverticulitis is necessary—a similar tubo ovarian lesion often accompanies sigmoid carcinoma.

Rupture of aneurysms

Splenic, renal or aortic aneurysms may rupture and produce haemoperitoneum which may cause confusion with a ruptured ectopic pregnancy. Rupture of a splenic aneurysm is rare but the incidence is increased in the third trimester of pregnancy, and the symptoms and signs are largely upper abdominal in the first instance. Blood loss must be replaced as quickly as possible prior to and during operation, and the bleeding artery is controlled by the best means possible.

Perforation of carcinoma of the colon

Full investigation will not usually be possible in cases of perforation of carcinoma of the colon so that the diagnosis will not be made until laparotomy has been performed. There will be evidence of localized or even more commonly generalized peritonitis and treatment will be aimed at draining the site of the perforation and diverting the faeces by performing a defunctioning colostomy. A transverse colostomy is usually performed in the transverse colon, if the primary lesion is in the rectum or sigmoid.

Intestinal obstruction is discussed in Chapter 14.

Ureteric calculus

Due to the anatomical relations between the nerve supply to ovary and ureter ureteric colic due to calculi produces symptoms very similar to that of torsion of an ovarian cyst. The pain is usually vice-like in character and lasts in its acute form for a matter of minutes wearing off to a dull ache and then there is recurrence of the acute pain. There is tenderness along the line of the ureter and no swelling suggestive of a cyst is palpable. An X-ray of the ureter will usually reveal a calculus and examination of the urine may reveal red blood cells.

The treatment is aimed initially at the relief of the acute symptoms and morphine and pethidine are given preferably by the intravenous route. An anti-spasmodic such as Buscopan may be helpful. If the stone is considered to be small enough to pass spontaneously then copious fluids are given and full movement is encouraged. With larger stones the treatment will depend to some extent on the site. If the stone is in the lower part of the ureter then expectant treatment should be continued for some time in the hope that the stone may be passed, but if the stone is in the lumbar part of the ureter, ureterolithotomy should be carried out without too much delay.

Perforated peptic ulcer

This condition which usually occurs in the duodenum is very much commoner in males than in females. The onset of pain is sudden and the whole abdomen is found to be tender. When a comparatively small perforation occurs the escaping fluid sometimes travels alongside the ascending colon to the right iliac fossa. The symptoms then simulate closely those of acute perforated appendicitis. Usually the site of onset of the pain distinguishes the condition from an acute gynaecological lesion, although the diagnosis may be made difficult if the fluid from the perforation has tracked down into the pelvis and tenderness is found on vaginal examination.

ABDOMINO-PELVIC TUMOURS

Carcinoma of the colon

This usually occurs after the fifth and sixth decades but it is not exceptional for it to occur earlier. Growths of the caecum occur at an earlier age than those in the rest of the colon. Constipation and diarrhoea sometimes alternating are the usual presenting complaints, but in some cases the first symptom is lower abdominal pain with a fixed mass in the iliac fossa and in others the first complaint is of a lower abdominal swelling. The diagnosis is usually made by barium enema and sigmoidoscopy. If found at laparotomy surgical opinion if sought usually advises later specific designed therapy after adequate bowel preparation unless active obstruction is present when defunctioning colostomy is required—although more recently primary resection is being advised.

Tumours of small bowel

Leiomyoma and leiomyosarcoma of small bowel do exist and may present as lobulated tumours mistaken for ovarian tumours.

Mesenteric cysts

These are usually simple cysts and present as fluctuating swellings in the abdomen near the umbilicus. There is usually a zone of resonance round the cysts. The swelling moves freely in a plane at right angles to the attachment of the mesentery. The complications which may arise are intestinal obstruction, rupture, haemorrhage into the cyst, torsion of a pedunculated cyst and pressure on the pelvic organs. Enucleation of the cyst is usually possible, and fortunately resection which must include the involved segment of intestine is seldom necessary. Mesenteric cysts are often mistaken for pedunculated ovarian cysts.

Retroperitoneal tumours

Lipoma is a benign tumour which can reach an immense size and can be mistaken for ovarian tumours. Mesenchymoma and sarcoma present similar signs, but the growth is more rapid.

Ectopic kidney

The kidney is arrested in some part of its normal ascent from the pelvis. This is usually at the brim and a palpable swelling is felt which appears to be arising from the pelvis and is often mistaken for an ovarian cyst. Care should be taken that a kidney is not removed in mistake for a solid ovarian tumour. Sometimes such ectopic kidneys are solitary.

Ascites

Distension of the abdomen by fluid can be mistaken for ovarian cysts (Fig. 42.1), but there is an area of resonance centrally and

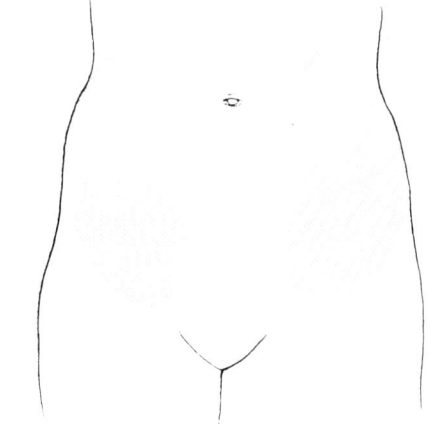

Fig. 42.1 Area of resonance centrally and dullness in the flanks with ascites.

dullness in the flanks with ascites. Confusion can arise when it is thought that there is a small tumour of the ovary associated with ascites and an unnecessary laparotomy may be performed in such cases where the ascites is due to a non-surgical condition such as in cardiac or renal failure or in cirrhosis of the liver or some other forms of portal obstruction.

Other rarer conditions giving rise to ascites are enlargements of the spleen, tuberculous peritonitis and polyserositis. In the last as well as peritoneal effusion there are effusions into the pericardium and the pleural cavities, and there may be confusion with Meig's Syndrome due to ovarian fibroma or with an ovarian carcinoma. Ascites can occur when there is carcinoma of the colon, or other intraperitoneal organs including the ovaries. The peritoneum both parietal and viceral may be studded with secondary tumour and the peritoneal cavity becomes filled with ascitis fluid. Examination of fluid removed by paracentesis will reveal malignant cells in these cases.

DISEASES OF THE BLADDER

Cystitis

Acute cystitis does not usually cause difficulty in differential diagnosis from gynaecological conditions because the symptoms are usually clear cut. The painful, difficult and frequent micturition and the presence of numerous red and white cells and many desquamated epithelial cells in the urine make the diagnosis relatively easy. Cystoscopy should be part of the investigation.

Chronic cystitis is important in differential diagnosis because the condition might be confused with the symptoms due to a cystocele. It is essential to remember that a cystocele is not associated with dysuria unless cystitis co-exists.

Hunner's ulcer

This is a non-specific ulcer of the bladder which is usually found in post menopausal women. The cause of this ulcer is unknown. The ulcers are usually multiple and are found over the vault but not on the trigone. The ulcers are star-shaped and there may be some induration around them. At first there is frequency with a little discomfort, but later there is pain in the supra-pubic region which is relieved by emptying the bladder. The diagnosis is made on cystoscopy. There is no specific treatment for this condition, but good results are obtained by repeated dilatation of the bladder and treatment of any secondary infection. In intractable cases cystoplasty is indicated.

Bladder calculus

Bladder stones may arise secondary to bladder pathology such as urethral obstruction, diverticulum of the bladder and chronic cystitis or they may have come down from the kidneys. They cause frequency of micturition, pain and haematuria. The diagnosis may be made by radiography or cystoscopy or the use of a sound. If the stones are small they can be removed through an operating cystoscope but may require to be crushed before removal if larger. If the stone is the size of a hen's egg then crushing should not be attempted and a supra-pubic operation should be performed.

Tumours of the bladder

These are usually papillomas, adenocarcinomas or squamous carcinomas. They usually give rise to painless haematuria which may be confused with vaginal bleeding, particularly in the post-menopausal women. Cytoscopy should be part of the investigation of post-menopausal bleeding, especially where no obvious lesion is found in the vagina or uterus. Frequency of micturition and dysuria can also occur. Radiological and cystoscopic examinations should be carried out and Papanicolaou staining of a urine specimen may be helpful. A biopsy of the tumour can be taken at cystoscopy. Depending on the type and extent of the tumour the treatment may be simple excision or cystectomy or radiotherapy.

Secondary ovarian tumours

When bilateral ovarian tumours are found at laparotomy some search should be made of large bowel (at least) and upper abdomen for possible primary growth. This is especially important when the tumours of ovary are free and removable as an undisclosed primary elsewhere would then certainly merit treatment.

Tumours of the rectum

Haemorrhoids, anal and ano-rectal tumours are frequently disclosed at gynaecological examination. Rectal bleeding is sometimes mistaken for vaginal bleeding, rectal mucus is found with pelvic inflammatory disease and high rectal tumours may mimic ovarian tumours.

FURTHER READING

Simmons, S. C. & Luck, R. J. (1971) *Surg. Cond. Obstet. Gynaec.* Oxford: Blackwell.

43. Termination of Pregnancy

When Sir Dugald Baird wrote about *The Fifth Freedom* (1965), he was referring to the freedom of women to control their fertility and to be able to decide whether they wished to continue with an unwanted pregnancy or not. Attitudes towards abortion in Britain had been deeply entrenched and it was only under exceptional medical circumstances that an abortion was done. The law in Scotland is based on common law practice whereas in English law it is defined by statute so that it was possible for Baird who was a pioneer in the field of liberal abortion to take advantage of this fact and terminate pregnancies on what would by most people be considered to be mainly social grounds. He felt strongly that women who had had five or six children should be allowed to have a termination of pregnancy and sterilization and he carried out this policy in Aberdeen.

The Law on abortion

Before the Abortion Act of 1967, a doctor who had carried out an abortion on a woman in Scotland could not be charged with any crime unless a definite complaint was made. Even then the matter would be investigated by doctors chosen by the procurator fiscal and if they were satisfied that the operation had been carried out in good faith and in a proper manner the case would then be closed. Dugald Baird was never challenged by the legal authorities in Scotland for his liberal interpretation of what constituted a hazard to the health of the women, and indeed it was not possible for him to challenge the law on abortion as was done by Alec Bourne in England. The famous Bourne case in 1938 in which a well known London gynaecologist carried out an abortion in a hospital and was then charged with the crime of procuring an abortion, was done as a test case to try to have the law in England altered.

The law on abortion in England and Wales was based on the Offences Against the Person Act of 1861, which made abortion an offence carrying a maximum sentence of penal servitude for life. This antiquated law had provoked several test cases particularly the Bourne case and gradually a more relaxed interpretation was put on the law by the Courts, but in general the law still remained hostile to the idea of abortion in England and Wales. Although it was possible in Scotland to adopt a much more liberal attitude very few obstetricians were willing to terminate unwanted pregnancies. It was against this background that agitation for Abortion Law Reform was started. Several attempts had been made in the past to introduce a change in the law but public interest was not really roused until 1966 when Mr David Steele introduced the Medical Termination of Pregnancy Bill in the House of Commons. The Abortion Act was passed in 1967 and became operative in 1968. It applies to England, Wales and Scotland but not to Northern Ireland. There was considerable resistance to the Bill from many quarters, particularly religious and medical. No other subject has caused such intense and often acrimonious discussion in medical circles. Fears were expressed that abortion would replace contraception, that the hospital service would be overwhelmed both in terms of bed usage and of availability of consultants to carry out the investigation and termination of the cases, that abortion was merely encouraging and condoning the permissive society, that abortion rackets would develop and that there would be a high morbidity and mortality from the terminations. There were some grounds for some of these fears as it turned out and in 1971 a Royal Commission of Enquiry was set up (The Lane Committee) to inquire into the working of the Act.

The working of the Act appears to be very different in Scotland compared to England and Wales. The very high percentage of private terminations performed in approved places other than in NHS hospitals in England and Wales compared to Scotland (Table 43.1) is only partly due to the influx of foreign cases, and either reflects unwillingness on the part of hospital doctors to do the operation or of some doctors taking advantage of the situation. There are undoubtedly difficulties in some regions because of shortage of hospital beds and because gynaecologists have conscientious

Table 43.1 Percentage National Health Service Abortions in Britain

	1968†	1969	1970	1971	1972	1973*
England and Wales	62 (35 000)	62 (55 000)	55 (87 000)	42 (127 000)	36 (157 000)	33 (169 000)
Scotland	97 (1500)	98 (3500)	99 (5000)	99 (6500)	98 (7500)	98 (7500)

Total abortions in brackets
† Based on eight months April–December 1968
* Based on six months January–June 1973

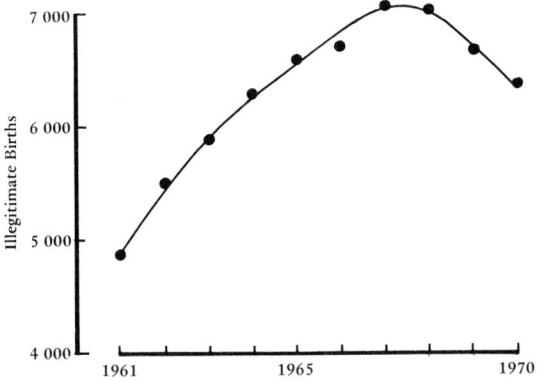

Fig. 43.1 Showing the illegitimate births in England and Wales from 1961–70. The peak number (69 928) occurred in 1967 with a slight fall in 1968 to 69 806.

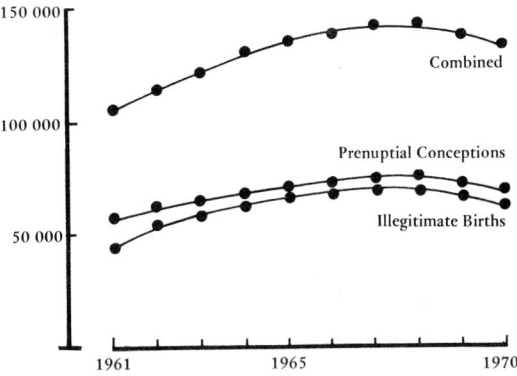

Fig. 43.3 Prenuptial conceptions and illegitimate births, England and Wales, 1961–70. The peak in the combined figure occurred in 1968 (144 337).

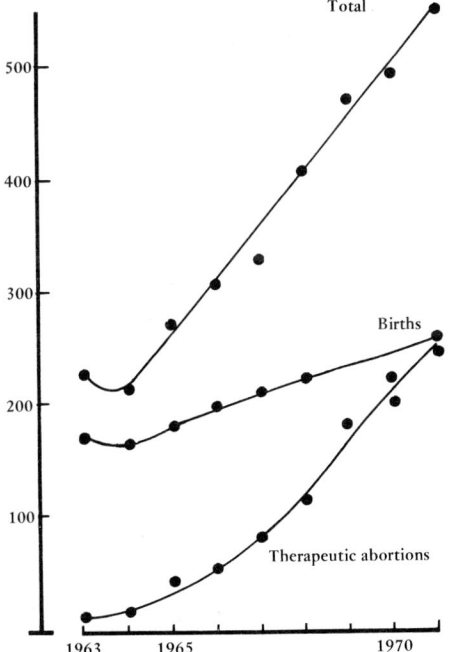

Fig. 43.2 Aberdeen City illegitimate pregnancies 1963–71. The total of illegitimate pregnancies rose steeply but the births rose only slightly because of the increase in therapeutic abortions.

objections to terminating pregnancy. Not least of the problems is that of the vast number of unwanted illegitimate pregnancies. There was a steady increase in the numbers of illegitimate births in England and Wales until 1968 but thereafter with the introduction of the Abortion Act there was a fall (Fig. 43.1). The total number of illegitimate pregnancies in Aberdeen has risen steadily until 1972 (Fig. 43.2) (Fig. 43.3), but it can be seen that the number of illegitimate births has been kept down because of the increasing number of terminations. It seems clear that if large numbers of terminations were not being done there would be vast numbers of illegitimate babies being born. It is often said that the Abortion Act has encouraged women to have unwanted pregnancies because they could have them terminated, but as can be seen from the figures the illegitimate pregnancy rate began to rise long before the Abortion Act came into force.

Although Britain was ahead of such countries as America, Australia and Germany in introducing a more liberal Abortion Act the liberal attitude to abortion was developed in the communist bloc countries some years before.

In Japan too there has been a liberal attitude to abortion for many years. Many state laws in America had recently been made very liberal and in some abortion had become virtually on request by the patients. In 1973 by an order of the Supreme Court abortion on request became legal in all states.

The laws relating to abortion in different parts of the world are summarized in Table 43.2.

Basically the new Abortion Act of 1967 has made little difference to the law in Scotland apart from making all terminations of pregnancy notifiable to the Chief Medical Officer of the Home and Health Department and the registration of nursing homes. The law has, however, been quite radically changed in England as it has been changed from case law to statute. Abortion is now legal in England, Wales and in Scotland as described in the following abstract from the Abortion Act, 1967.

Table 43.2   Legislation on Abortion

Africa	Illegal	Legal	Asia and Oceania ctd.	Illegal	Legal
Gambia		M	Malaysia	*	
Ghana		M	New Zealand		L
Guinea		L	Pakistan		L
Ivory Coast		L	Singapore		L&H, Eug,
Kenya		M			Eth, MS, S.
Malawi		M	Thailand	*	
Mauritius	*				
Nigeria		L&H	*Europe*		
Sierra Leone		L&H			
Somali		L	Austria		L
South Africa		L(L&H2)	Belgium	*6	
Sudan		L	Bulgaria		L&H, Eug,
Swaziland		M			Eth, MS, S.
Tanzania		L	Czechoslovakia		L&H, Eug,
Uganda		L&H			Eth, MS, S.
Zambia		M	Denmark		L&H, Eug,
					Eth, MS, S.
Americas			Finland		L&H, Eug,
					Eth, MS, S.
Argentina		L&H, Eth	`France		L
Canada		L&H	Germany, Democratic		L&H, Eug,
Honduras		L&H	Republic		Eth, MS, S,
Jamaica		L&H			R.
Mexico		L, Eth	Germany, Federal		L
Trinidad & Tobago		L&H	Republic		
USA		L&H, Eug,	Greece		L&H, Eth
		Eth, MS4	Hungary		L&H, Eug,
					MS, S, R.
Asia and Oceania			Irish Republic	*	
			Italy		L, Eth
Australia		L&H, Eug,	Luxembourg	*	
		MS5	Malta	*	
Burma	*		Netherlands		L
Ceylon		L&H	Norway		L&H, Eug,
China, People's		L&H, Eug,			Eth, MS
Republic		Eth, MS,	Poland		L&H, Eth, MS,
		S, R.			S.
Cyprus		L	Portugal	*	
Fiji		L	Rumania		L&H, Eug,
Hong Kong	*				Eth, MS, S.
India		L&H, Eug,	Spain	*	
		Eth, MS,	Sweden		L&H, Eug,
		S3			Eth, MS
Indonesia	*		Switzerland		L&H, MS4
Japan		L&H, Eug,	United Kingdom		L&H, Eug, MS
		Eth, MS.	USSR		L&H, Eug, Eth,
					MS, S, R.

1. (1) Subject to the provisions of this section, a person shall not be guilty of an offence under the law relating to abortion when a pregnancy is terminated by a registered medical practitioner if two registered medical practitioners are of the opinion, formed in good faith—

(a) that the continuance of the pregnancy would involve risk to the life of the pregnant woman, or of injury to the physical or mental health of the pregnant woman or any existing children of her family, greater than if the pregnancy were terminated; or

(b) that there is a substantial risk that if the child were born it would suffer from such physical or mental abnormalities as to be seriously handicapped.

(2) In determining whether the continuance of a pregnancy would involve such risk of injury to health as is mentioned in paragraph (a) of subsection (1) of this section, account may be taken of the pregnant woman's actual or reasonably foreseeable environment.

(3) Except as provided by subsection (4) of this section, and treatment for termination of pregnancy must be carried out in a hospital vested in the Minister of Health or the Secretary of State under the National Health Service Acts, or in a place for the time being approved for the purposes of this section by the said Minister or the Secretary of State.

(4) Subsection (3) of this section, and so much of subsection (1) as relates to the opinion of two registered medical practitioners, shall not apply to the termination of a pregnancy by a registered medical practitioner in a case where he is of the opinion, formed in good faith, that the termination is immediately necessary to save the life or to prevent grave permanent injury to the physical or mental health of the pregnant woman.

2. (1) The Minister of Health in respect of England and Wales, and the Secretary of State in respect of Scotland, shall by statutory instrument make regulations to provide—

(a) for requiring any such opinion as is referred to in section 1 of this Act to be certified by the practitioners or practitioner concerned in such form and at such time as may be prescribed by the regulations, and for requiring the preservation and disposal of certificates made for the purposes of the regulation;

(b) for requiring any registered medical practitioner who terminates a pregnancy to give notice of the termination and such other information relating to the termination as may be so prescribed;

(c) for prohibiting the disclosure, except to such persons or for such purposes as may be so prescribed, of notices given or information furnished pursuant to the regulations.

(2) The information furnished in pursuance of

Definitions of the terms used in classification are those used by WHO (1971)

Medical indications	L	To save the life of mother.
	L&H	To preserve the health of mother (in some countries this covers mental health as well as physical).
	M	Unspecified medical grounds.
Eugenic indications	Eug	To prevent the transmission of hereditary diseases and to avoid the birth of children liable to be affected by physical or mental disorders as a result of intra-uterine damage.
Ethical indications	Eth	Where the pregnancy results from a criminal act such as rape, incest, or sexual intercourse with a minor or a person suffering from a mental disease or deficiency.
Medico-social indications	MS	Several previous deliveries in close succession, the period of time since the last delivery, domestic difficulties resulting from the presence of infants in the household, a difficult financial situation, or the ill-health of other persons living in the same household.
Social indications	S	Number of children, death or disability of husband, illegitimacy.
Abortion on request	R	A statute which enables a woman to have her pregnancy terminated on request, without having to show evidence of any indications.

1	In practice.
2	Reduced penalty in certain cases.
3	Includes contraceptive failure.
4	Some states or cantons are more liberal.
5	South Australia only.
6	Not strictly enforced.

From International Planned Parenthood News, March, 1972.

regulations made by virtue of paragraph (b) of subsection (1) of this section shall be notified solely to the Chief Medical Officers of the Ministry of Health and the Scottish Home and Health Department respectively.

The Act states that no person shall be under any legal obligation to participate in any treatment authorized by the Act to which he has a conscientious objection unless the treatment is necessary to save the life, or prevent grave permanent injury to the physical or mental health of a pregnant woman. The conscience clause does not, however, absolve a practitioner from his general obligations to his patient, and the practitioner should refer the patient to another doctor if (a) he considers that it might be lawful to recommend or perform an abortion if he did not have a conscientious objection, or (b) he feels that he cannot form an opinion in good faith because of his conscientious objection. The conscience clause does not apply only to members of a particular religion or faith. In Scotland a statement on oath in a Court by any person is considered sufficient proof of conscientious objection. In England and Wales a person must prove his conscientious objection in any legal proceedings.

In ordinary cases certificate A is used and in emergency cases certificate B. Certificate A must be completed and signed by the two practitioners giving the opinion, one of whom will usually, though not necessarily, be the gynaecologist who carries out the termination. Certificate A must always be completed before the commencement of the operation. Certificate B must also be completed before the commencement of the operation, unless this is not practicable and in such an event it must be completed within 24 hours of the termination of the pregnancy. The certificates must be preserved by the operator for three years after the termination of the pregnancy and then may be destroyed. Notification of every termination of pregnancy must be submitted by the operator within seven days of the termination to the Chief Medical Officer of Health of the Ministry of Health and Social Security, in England and Wales or to the Chief Medical Officer of the Scottish Home and Health Department.

The Chief Medical Officer may at his discretion permit disclosure of information on the notification forms in the following circumstances:

1. To an officer of the Ministry authorized by the Chief Medical Officer or to the Registrar General or to a member of his staff authorized by him for the purposes of carrying out their duties.
2. For the purposes of carrying out his duties in relation to the offences against the Abortion Laws to the Director of Public Prosecutions or a member of his staff authorized by him.
3. For the purposes of investigating whether an offence has been committed against the Abortions Laws to a police officer not below the rank of superintendent or a person authorized by him.
4. For the purpose of criminal proceedings which have begun.
5. For bona fide scientific research.
6. To the practitioner who terminated the pregnancy or to any practitioner with the written consent of the patient.

A gynaecologist is not under any obligation to perform an abortion on a patient for whom a certificate has been signed by two other practitioners if, in his opinion, an abortion is not indicated.

It is obviously a matter for individual judgment whether continuation of the pregnancy or termination constitutes the greater risk to the mother's physical or mental health. The methods of abortion which can be employed and the possible risks are referred to in detail in Chapter 27, but it is sufficient to say here that a suction termination using a Karman plastic curette and local anaesthesia for a pregnancy of less than eight weeks will carry less physical risk than a full-time pregnancy and delivery. On the other hand a hysterotomy on a mid trimester pregnancy possibly carries more physical risks.

Many factors must be taken into consideration before making a decision about termination of pregnancy including the previous obstetric history, physical health, mental well-being, and socio-economic circumstances. In the case of the unmarried woman the possibility of a successful marriage to the putative father should be explored. The possibility of her keeping the baby herself should be discussed but this is very difficult unless she receives a lot of help as our society does not as yet accept or give much support to the unmarried mother so that many who start out anxious to keep their baby have to reluctantly give it up for adoption or fostering after a few months because they cannot cope. Adoption is another alternative which can be offered to the girl with an illegitimate pregnancy but most reject this as being too emotionally traumatic and prefer to have an abortion.

The risks that the baby will be seriously handicapped can usually be fairly accurately judged from the previous history or by examination of liquor amnii obtained by amniocentesis or, as in the cases of rubella, by testing the maternal serum (see Chapter 16).

The written consent of the patient who is to undergo termination of her pregnancy should always be obtained. If the patient is married and living with her husband the proposed abortion should always be fully discussed with him if time and circumstances permit. This is particularly important if the physical or mental health of any existing children of the family is the reason for the proposed termination. If the pregnancy is to be terminated because its continuance would involve a risk to the mother's life or her physical or mental health it is not essential in law for the husband's consent to be obtained. If the patient is unmarried consent is not required from the putative father. It is not considered necessary in law to obtain the consent of the parents to terminate the pregnancy of an unmarried girl

the parents could sue for assault upon their daughter in such cases, but it seems highly improbable that such a claim would be upheld. If on the other hand the girl herself was opposed to termination it would not be permissible to carry it out even if the parents demanded it.

Striking features in the statistics relating to abortion since the Abortion Act, 1967, came into effect in April, 1968 are first that there are very many more abortions carried out in private accommodation in England and Wales than in Scotland, and secondly that the number of pregnancies aborted has been going up both in Scotland and in England and Wales (Table 43.3). Also there is a marked

Table 43.3

Year	Country	In NHS Hospitals	In private accommodation i.e. approved places under the Act
1968	Scotland	1 448	44
	England and Wales	14 500	9 030
1969	Scotland	3 475	69
	England and Wales	33 728	20 943
1970	Scotland	4 962	74
	England and Wales	46 355	37 282
1971	Scotland	6 248	84
	England and Wales	53 706	73 071

who is of 16 years of age or more. If the girl were living with the parents it would be considered prudent practice to try to obtain such consent, but the girl's authority must be obtained before seeking such consent from the parents. If the girl had left home with her parents' agreement and was living independently of them it would not be necessary to obtain their consent. The parents of girls under 16 years of age should always be consulted even if she does not give consent. If possible written consent should be obtained from the parents, but if they refuse to do so, and the patient herself consents a termination would be lawful if in the gynaecologist's opinion it was clinically necessary. It has been suggested that

regional variation in abortion rates (Table 43.4).

Mortality and morbidity from abortion
The Report on Confidential Enquiries into Maternal Deaths in England and Wales, 1964–66, showed that there were 579 deaths directly due to pregnancy and 176 deaths due to associated causes. The main causes of maternal death were abortion (133 cases), pulmonary embolism (91 cases), haemorrhage (68 cases), toxaemia (67 cases), cardiac disease (50 cases), complications of anaesthesia (50 cases), uterine rupture (30 cases), amniotic fluid embolism (30 cases) and ectopic pregnancy (42 cases). When, however, the causes

Table 43.4   Regional Variations in
Abortion Rates per 100 live
births in Britain

	1972
Newcastle	11·0
London and Home Counties	10·6
Wales	9·5
South West	9·5
Scotland	9·4
East Anglia	8·1
Manchester	7·2
Oxford	6·6
Wessex	6·1
Liverpool	5·4
Sheffield	5·3
Leeds	4·5
Birmingham	3·2
Britain	7·9

of death from abortion are reclassified according to whether they were due to haemorrhage, sepsis or embolism, the causes of death are then changed to haemorrhage (152 cases), sepsis (123 cases), embolism (95 cases) and toxaemia (67 cases). This illustrates the point that most abortions are due to haemorrhage or sepsis. Some of the deaths of abortion cases occurred when it was carried out for therapeutic reasons. In such cases many were seriously ill when the therapeutic abortion was performed.

It is very difficult to get accurate figures on deaths from abortions. This is due to many deaths not being clearly defined as abortion deaths, or a reluctance to classify a death as being due to abortion unless this was obviously the case. Nine cases which were classified as deaths from natural causes turned out to be criminal abortions in an analysis of 5038 unnatural deaths at the London Hospital between 1963 and 1967 by Johnson (1969). He concluded that in many cases of death in young women the attending doctors did not consider the possibility of pregnancy and abortion. Simms (1971) pointed out that in 1969 the Office of Population Censuses and Surveys gave 10 deaths as resulting from legal abortion from a total of 55 000 legal abortions,

eight from spontaneous abortions and 17 from other causes. What seems to be significant, she says, is that the legal abortion death rate at 19 per 1 000 000 is about the same as the maternal mortality rate for that year, and at the very least it can be said that there is no evidence to suggest that legal abortion is more dangerous than childbirth. It has been pointed out that if sterilization is done concurrently with hysterotomy the death rate is more than nine times the rate for abortion by dilatation and curettage, and it is higher than for hysterotomy alone. It must be remembered, however, that the women who are having a hysterotomy and sterilization are older, more parous and physically less fit than the women having hysterotomy alone, and that the sterilization probably adds nothing to the risk of the operation of hysterotomy. It is obviously preferable, however, to empty the uterus by curettage or suction, rather than hysterotomy, and many operators prefer to do vaginal terminations followed by either a laparoscopic or small abdominal incision sterilization rather than do a hysterotomy and sterilization.

The Annual Report of the Chief Medical Officer (1970) indicates that the greatest danger of death occurs in the age-group 35–44 years and also women terminated by hysterotomy (8·4 per 10 000) and by hysterectomy (12·6 per 10 000). The figure for uterine aspiration techniques was 2·2 per 10 000.

The figures for mortality from abortion are usually lower than the overall maternal mortality, but the figures are slightly higher when legal abortion is first introduced into a country. This may be because the gynaecologists are relatively inexperienced in the procedures but another factor is that many of the cases will be late when first presenting for abortion.

Soskice (1973) calculated that even though the deaths from legal abortion had risen between 1961 and 1970 the overall deaths from abortion had fallen because of the decline in deaths from illegal abortions (Table 43.5).

In many of the eastern European countries in which abortion was legalized a policy of

Table 43.5   Adjusted Abortion Deaths (England and Wales)

	1961–63 (average)	1964–66 (average)	1967	1968	1969	1970
Illegal	34	41	31	32	19	14
Legal	4	4	1	5	10	10
Total	38	45	32	37	29	24

contraception and family planning had not been developed. In such countries, for example, Hungary, Poland and Czechoslovakia, there is now much concern about the introduction of preventive measures such as sex education in schools and education for planned parenthood with the possible issue of free contraceptives. In this way they hope that the number of pregnancy terminations will decrease. They would prefer to see abortion replaced by efficient contraception.

These opinions are in part due to the known morbidity which is associated with abortion and in some eastern European countries the abortion laws are being tightened up. In the last few years Bulgaria and Rumania have changed their abortion laws. In Bulgaria one of the main effects is to prohibit induced abortion in the case of women with no living children, except for serious medical indications. The restrictions in the Rumanian legislation have been much more marked. When the law was liberalized the number of induced abortions rose markedly and in 1959 there were 220 000 or 60 per 100 live births and the figure rose to 1 115 000 in 1965 or four abortions for every live birth. Now abortion is only permitted on health grounds or if the woman is over 45 years of age, or has more than three children.

Japan is another example where the abortion law was very liberal and has now been restricted.

Although the number of deaths is few there is the immediate risk of haemorrhage and sepsis. Both can now fortunately be treated with blood transfusion and antibiotics respectively, but some long term morbidity seems likely.

There are no long term reports as yet of follow-up studies in this country. Because of the different standards it is doubtful if the results of follow-ups in eastern European countries can be applied to this country. Some studies there have shown an increased incidence of chronic inflammatory conditions, sterility, ectopic pregnancy and cervical incompetence. They do not quote any figures for the long term results of confinements and there are no figures available for the results from illegal abortions. In this context it is worth noting that the numbers of so-called spontaneous abortions which probably included illegally procured abortions admitted to hospital have fallen in Britain. Account has to be taken of

the fact that if the pregnancies were not being terminated legally in this country there would be morbidity from illegally procured abortions. The number of discharges from hospital after septic abortion fell markedly in England and Wales from 2950 in 1965 to 2100 in 1970 (Fig. 43.4).

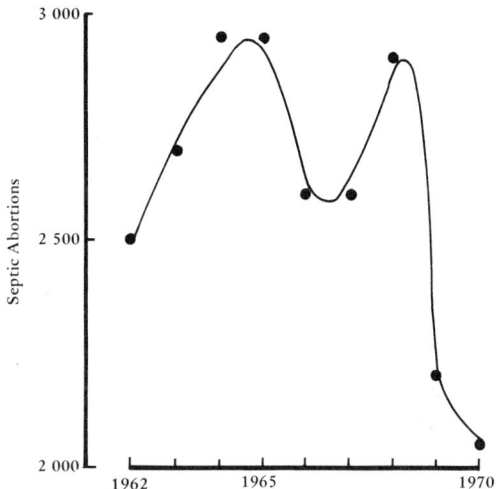

Fig. 43.4   Septic abortions from the Hospital Inpatient Enquiry, England and Wales, 1962–70.

Long term studies have not yet been carried out in this country to show whether there is a reduction in procured abortions, and to compare the incidence of late morbidity after full time pregnancies with the incidence of morbidity after therapeutic abortions.

In the Aberdeen study (Horobin, 1973) which was retrospective from 1963–67 and prospective from 1967–70 the women were referred by general practitioners for consideration of abortion and were seen by a sociologist and psychologist before being seen by the gynaecologist. It showed that the wave of illegitimacy which travelled from the south reached Scotland in the early 1960s and it affected the better educated, upper socioeconomic group girls earliest. Requests for abortion were, therefore, multiplying before the abortion act became an issue. The rate of abortion of illegitimate pregnancies did not change until after the act was passed in 1967, when there was an increase in the numbers referred and a proportionate increase in the abortions performed. There has been a greater proportion of illegitimate pregnancies and abortions and fewer live births among the total pregnancies. There were 3640 total pregnancies in 1963 to 3370 in 1971. As well as the abortions the fall in total pregnancies was due to sterilizations and the introduction of oral contraception to Aberdeen family planning clinics in 1964. Oral contraception has been provided free in Aberdeen since 1966 by the Local Authority.

The gynaecologists in the City of Aberdeen could be divided into conservatives and liberals. The refusal rates for the City cases for eight years, 1963–70 combined, divided the eight consultants into three categories. Three conservatives with refusal rates between 37 and 40 per cent, four liberals with the rate of 16–20 per cent and one ultra-liberal who refused only 4 per cent. The general practitioners referring the women also had varying attitudes. A random selection of 34 practices in Aberdeen run by 79 doctors was made in 1971, and in most of the practices between 30 and 40 per cent of their female patients were aged 16–44. Referral rates in this group ranged from 1·3 per cent to 5·5 per cent.

About three-quarters of referrals for the years 1963–69 fell into the category of social or one of the three combined categories in

primarily medical declined although the absolute numbers remained fairly stable.

In order to try to assess the morbidity following termination a comparison was made between the women who had a termination at a point in time when they would have been 34 weeks pregnant and women who were refused termination at six to eight weeks after delivery. Assessment of the physical wellbeing after termination was limited by doing a single assessment at one point in time only. Had it not been carried out with a number of control subjects who were also pregnant, but whose pregnancy was not terminated the conclusion that pregnancy termination caused ill health in a large proportion of cases would have been inescapable. There have been several reports (Stallworthy et al., 1971 and Sood, 1971) which have quoted high risks of morbidity following abortion, but others, notably the very large study of Titze and Lewitt (1972) showed much lower rates particularly when cases with pre-existing pathology or sterilization were excluded. They classified the degree of morbidity in the various types of abortions (Table 43.7). None of these reports, however,

Table 43.7   Complications per 100 Abortions

	Total	Major
Suction	4·2	0·4
D & C	6·0	0·5
Amniocentesis	23·4	1·7
Hysterotomy	33·3	6·2

From Titze, C. & Lewitt, S. (1972) Studies in Family Planning, 3, 97.

which there was a strong social component (Table 43.6). The proportion in these categories increased from 57 per cent in the earlier to 79 per cent in the last year of the series. At the same time the proportion classified as

Table 43.6   Referrals by Indications (1963–69)

	Number Referred	Percentage
Medical	118	7·1
Social	421	25·2
Eugenic	58	3·4
Psychiatric	272	16·3
Medical/Social	143	8·6
Psychiatric/Social	636	38·1
Not Stated	23	1·3
	1671	100

Percentage with social component 71·9

had any control series comparing the abortion cases with full time deliveries. In the Aberdeen study the changes in symptomology appeared to be due to the fact that the subject had recently been pregnant rather than that she had had a pregnancy terminated. The two exceptions to this generalization appeared to have been that in approximately 6 per cent of pregnancy terminations significant urinary symptoms were present and that menstruation frequently deteriorated following hysterotomy and sterilization in the elderly multiparous women.

A psychological part of the study showed the unmarried women to have a different personality structure to the married women. Both groups seeking termination showed abnormal psychological characteristics compared to the control groups. Neurotic personality patterns were more prevalent among the ever-married whereas more psychopathic features with 'accident prone' tendencies were prominent in the single women cohort. Although the majority presented in a state of depression major mental illness both in the past and at the time of referral was uncommon in the cohorts. Women who were aborted were significantly more depressed at the time of referral and especially in the case of the ever-married had more vulnerable personality characteristics than women who continued the pregnancy.

A follow-up of cases referred for consideration of abortion was carried out about 15 months later. The balance of evidence indicated that it tended to be the more vulnerable and maladjusted women who were selected for abortion and the more stable who continued the pregnancy. At the time of the follow-up severe depressive reactions were few, but moderate degrees of depression were not uncommon. Depression among those who continued with their pregnancies was more often associated with regrets at going to term. At follow-up the aborted women were no more depressed than women who had continued the pregnancy despite the fact that the former group were significantly more depressed at referral and displayed more vulnerable personality traits. Both aborted and non-aborted groups had improved psychologically since the time of referral, but the aborted group showed the greatest change. Regrets about continuing with the pregnancy were more common than regrets about abortion in both single and ever-married groups, but especially so in the former. Adoption for single women appeared to be generally unsatisfactory as far as the woman was concerned. There was more psychological distress occasioned by going to term with an unwanted pregnancy than by having an abortion, and the worst affected were the single women.

Termination of pregnancy must be looked upon as an undesirable procedure but is in many instances preferable to the alternative of allowing the pregnancy to continue. Unwanted pregnancies should be avoided and abortion should not be used as a form of family planning or contraception. The emphasis must be on education of adolescents in contraception, but probably even more important is to motivate women to avoid unwanted pregnancies.

REFERENCES

Annual Report of the Chief Medical Officer (1970).

Baird, D. (1965) The Fifth Freedom. *Brit. med. J.*, **ii**, 1141.

Horobin, G., Ed. (1973) *Experience with Abortion—A case Study of North-East Scotland.* Cambridge: Cambridge University Press.

Johnson, H. R. M. (1969) The incidence of unnatural death which might have been presumed to be natural in coroners autopsies. *Medicine, Science and Law*, **9**, 102–106.

Simms, M. (1971) The abortion act after three years. *The Political Quarterly*, **42**, 278.

Sood, S. V. (1971) Some operative and post-operative hazards of legal termination of pregnancy. *Brit. med. J.*, **iv**, 270.

Soskice, D. W. (1973) Effects of the Abortion Act. *Brit. J. Hosp. Med.*, **7**, 299.

Stallworthy, J. A., Moolgaoker, A. S. & Walsh, J. J. (1971) Legal Abortion—A critical assessment of its risks. *Lancet*, **ii**, 1245.

Titze, C. & Lewitt, S. (1972) *Studies in Family Planning*, **3**, 397.

FURTHER READING

Abortion Laws. A Survey of Current World Legislation. Geneva: World Health Organisation, 1971.

Experience with Abortion. A case study of North-East Scotland. G. Horobin, J. Aitken-Swan, C. Farmer, C. McCance, P. Olley, I. MacGillivray & K. J. Dennis. Cambridge: Cambridge University Press, 1973.

44. Family Planning and Population Control

INTRODUCTION

In 1877 Charles Bradlaugh, M.P., and Annie Besant were prosecuted for publishing a pamphlet on birth control, but they won their case. In 1921 Dr Marie Stopes founded the first birth control clinic in Britain and by 1924 there were 16 clinics. In 1930 the Minister of Health advised Local Authorities that they could give advice to 'women to whom further pregnancy would be detrimental to health' and in the same year, the Family Planning Association (FPA) was formed. Family planning is now done in three ways, by Family Planning Clinics in hospital, and in the community, and by General Medical Practitioners. It is now Government policy to have free family planning under the National Health Service.

There is very little evidence that in Britain today women are less capable of bearing children than they were 50 years ago. The fall in the average family size is almost certainly by design. With the present low death rates amongst children a return to the large family would mean a rapid rise in the total population, a serious problem in a small island like Great Britain, which is overcrowded at present. One of the factors responsible for the low infant mortality and the improvement in health and physique of children, is the fall in the size of the average family. In mothers of all ages, the infant mortality rises as the size of the family increases. It is highest in the lowest socio-economic group where many children are born to young mothers, i.e. where the interval between births is very short and the standard of living tends to be low in any case.

Many factors influence the size of the family, but whether the number is large or small, each individual child should be desired by its parents and not grudgingly accepted because its conception was not prevented. It is sometimes held that the parental instinct is not sufficiently strong to maintain the population. If in any country too few children are born, it would be better to try to bring about conditions which will make parents glad to have a reasonable number of children than to promote involuntary parenthood by withholding contraceptive knowledge.

There is danger in too much as well as in too little planning. On the one hand the mother may be over anxious and fussy with her children and should an unplanned pregnancy occur, may find it difficult to accept the fact and insist on termination. On the other hand the couple who do not plan may find the family growing beyond their means so that standards fall and the health of both parents and children suffer.

The doctors' role in the area of contraception is in helping the couple with advice and counselling. He will be able to put the case for and against the use of contraceptives at the start of marriage, before the first pregnancy and, while pointing out the value of proper spacing of children, will also point out the value of youth for efficient and successful childbearing, and the disadvantages of having children with too big a difference between their ages. Perhaps the doctors' most significant role is in helping the couple to a sound choice of method. Contraceptive advice to the unmarried is still a controversial subject but it is much better that young girls, who are likely to expose themselves to the possibility of pregnancy, should have advice on how to protect themselves than that they should become pregnant and request termination. The health education of young people both male and female should include adequate advice on the responsibilities associated with sexual intercourse and also in methods of preventing unwanted pregnancy from occurring. Contraceptive advice should be sought before marriage so that the couple have been advised in the most suitable method and possibly the woman has already started on the pill and adjusted to it by the time marriage occurs.

After the first child is born, advice on contraception should be routine. Most women wish to know when sexual intercourse can be resumed and how soon a pregnancy could occur. Post-partum sterilization is now a common method of family planning when the couple feel that their family is complete. It is best discussed early in the antenatal period so that the decision about this important step is not hurried or unwisely made.

The family doctor should be prepared to discuss these problems with the patient and give the best advice he can, not only on the detailed technique of contraception but on the wider aspects of sex in marriage. Some young couples still hesitate to consult their family doctor on the subject of sex and marriage and it is important that he should be sympathetic and understanding of the problem and be willing to help.

METHODS OF CONTROL OF CONCEPTION

Contraception is not a recent innovation and various methods have in fact been used for thousands of years. The chief method of preventing births in primitive societies was abortion but other measures were also used. Soranus, the Greek gynaecologist, used wool plugs soaked in various astringents and acids inserted into the vagina—the forerunners of the modern chemical contraceptives. The Chinese, in early times, used salt intravaginally as this was considered to be highly spermicidal. The condom was first described by Fallopius, the great Italian anatomist. In mediaeval times the chastity belt was popular and douches of lemon juice, vinegar and other substances were used. Throughout the ages, therefore, various types of contraception have been practised but it is the widespread use of more effective contraceptive methods that has taken place in recent times.

Until the discovery of the contraceptive 'pill' no fully satisfactory method of contraception was available. To be satisfactory, a contraceptive must be easy to use, reliable, cheap, harmless and acceptable aesthetically. Up till now there have been serious objections to all the methods in use, but since the alternative was repeated unwanted pregnancies, most husbands and wives tried to make the best use they could of the methods available. It has been shown by experience that where a couple have a strong desire to prevent pregnancy and use a standard technique carefully, they are usually able to avoid pregnancy. Other couples find the techniques too much trouble and the desire to avoid additional future burdens conflicts with the unimpeded pleasure of the moment. Some become resigned to having large families which often means drudgery and financial hardship and become so dejected and numbed emotionally that they give up trying and may eventually make little or no effort to prevent pregnancy. This usually happens in the semi-skilled and unskilled social classes.

In spite of great advances in contraceptive methodology the basic problems of successful contraception and the successful practice of

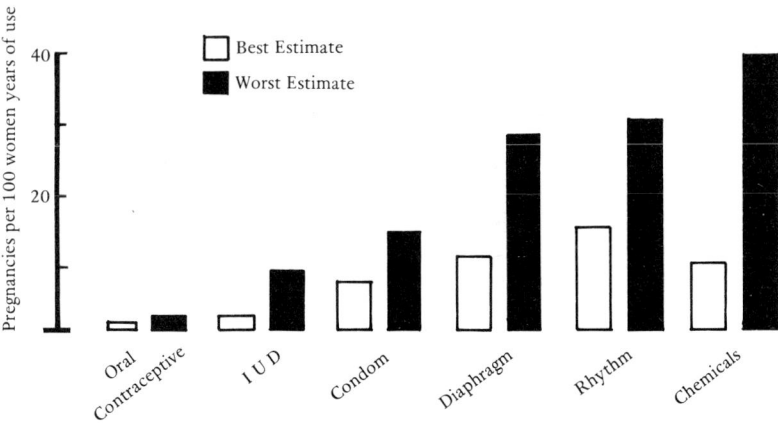

Fig. 44.1   Failure rates of contraception methods (Peel & Potts, 1969).

contraception remain. The contraceptive needs of a couple during their reproductive years vary from time to time.

The effectiveness of a contraceptive method is its capacity to prevent unwanted pregnancy.

The calculation of this is based on the Pearl Index and is expressed thus:

Failure rate per hundred woman years

$$(HWY) = \frac{\text{Total accidental pregnancies} \times 1200}{\text{Total months of exposure}}$$

When this formula is applied the total accidental pregnancies shown in Figure 44.1 should include all known conceptions whatever the outcome. It is perhaps easiest to think of the index in terms of the number of unplanned children which would occur either in 100 women using a particular technique for 1 year or more hypothetically the number of children one woman would have in 100 years using a particular method.

Oral contraceptives

In the 1950s oral steroid contraceptives were first introduced. In 1954 Djerassi synthesized the first oral progestogens which, with added oestrogen were used in the now famous oral contraceptive trials in Puerto Rico in 1956, published by Garcia, Rock and Pincus in 1958.

It is estimated that in the UK 2 million women and some 20 million women throughout the world are using oral contraceptives. About 65 per cent of women attending Family Planning Association clinics choose oral contraceptives as the method of choice at the first visit. The synthetic progestogens which are used as oral contraceptives are of two types. The most commonly used type is a Nortestosterone derivative (Fig. 44.2). Nor-testosterone derivatives are not chemically closely related to progesterone and do not mimic its biological actions exactly. Although, as the name indicates, they are related to testosterone they are not androgenic in normal use. They should, however, be avoided in pregnancy as cases of virilization of a female fetus have been reported where the mother took this compound in early pregnancy. The other type of oral contraceptive is derived from 17 α hydroxyprogesterone and is chemically much closer to the hormone of the corpus luteum

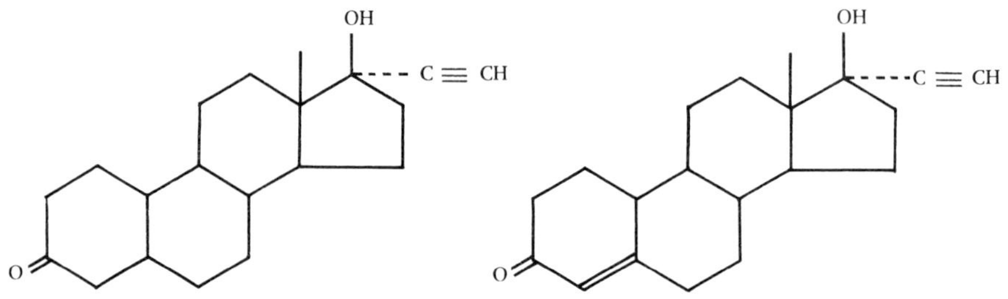

Norethynodrel   Norethisterone

Fig. 44.2 Structural formula of 19 nortesterone derivatives.

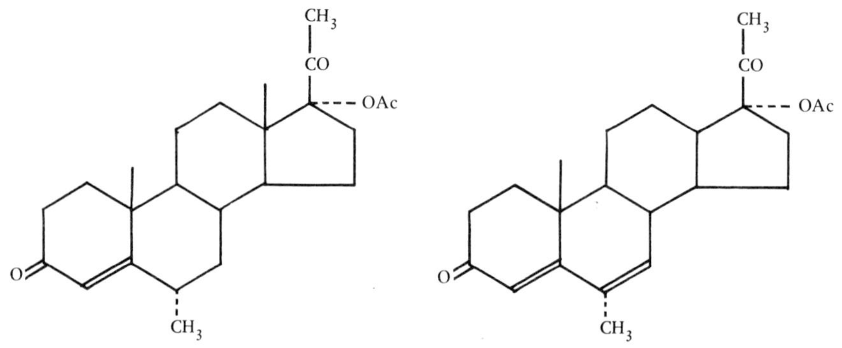

Medroxy progesterone acetate   Megestrol Acetate

Fig. 44.3 Structural formula of 17 hydroxyprogesterone derivatives.

(Fig. 44.3). Both types are broken down to simpler compounds in the body and excreted in urine but neither gives rise to the same metabolites as progesterone. Part of the breakdown products of nor-testosterone derivatives are in fact potent oestrogens, so that, although dispensed as progestogens, these compounds are also oestrogenic. The 17 α hydroxyprogesterone derivatives do not yield oestrogens when metabolized. Two main oestrogens are used in the pill. These are ethinyl oestradiol, and its 3 methyl-ether, mestranol. Of the two, ethinyl oestradiol is the more potent and the more frequently used.

MODE OF ACTION OF STEROIDAL CONTRACEPTIVES
Naturally occurring oestrogen and progesterone have an effect on the output of Follicle Stimulating Hormone (FSH) and Luteinizing Hormone (LH) by a feedback mechanism—see Chapter on ovulation. In women on the combined pill, the high circulating levels of synthetic oestrogen and progestogen are thought to inhibit ovulation by a similar feedback mechanism. This effect is probably mediated through the hypothalamus. It is also possible that progestogen alone may have a direct action on the reproductive tract itself. There are four possible sites where progestogen may act. At the endometrial level progestogens may produce changes which interfere with implantation of the ovum. Thickening of the cervical mucus may inhibit sperm penetration. There is also some evidence that progestogen may have a direct action on the ovary and a number of gestagens have been shown to depress the function of the corpus luteum. A fourth possible site of action may be on the Fallopian tubes changing the dynamics of sperm and ovum transport but evidence for this so far is scanty.

TYPES OF PILL
1. Combined oestrogen-progestogen pill: This is the most commonly used type at present. The dose of oestrogen is standard and does not exceed 0·05mg. The most usual gestagen in the combined pill is nor-ethisterone or its acetate but 17 α hydroxyprogesterone has also been used.

2. Progestogen-only pills: Much of the unwanted effects of oral contraceptives are attributed to the oestrogen component and pills have been introduced with only the progestogen component. These pills are usually composed of 19 nor-steroids and nor-ethi-

sterone or its acetate are again the most commonly used chemicals.

3. The Post Coital Pill: High doses of oestrogen of the order of 25mg daily for 5 days have been used as the 'morning after' pill particularly as an emergency measure in victims of rape or failure of some other method or unprotected intercourse at times of risk. These doses of oestrogen prevent implantation of the ovum and increase tubal motility. Oral tolerance of high doses of oestrogen is usually poor.

4. Injectable progesterone: The compounds used are long acting progestogen compounds given at intervals of 3, 6 or 12 months and particularly in the post-partum period. The major drawbacks of this method are the episodes of prolonged amenorrhoea and a very unpredictable bleeding pattern. Injectable compounds for use as contraceptives have been found valuable for national family planning programmes and where clinic service is difficult for one reason or another.

Prescribing the pill
Before prescribing the pill the doctor must take a detailed history, examine the woman and decide whether or not she is suitable for this method of contraception. Family history, obstetrical and gynaecological history and details of previous illnesses must be checked and consideration given to age and intelligence of the woman. Fears that the woman may have must be allayed. The weight and blood pressure should be recorded and routine examination of the breasts and pelvic organs including a cervical smear should be performed. Some specific tests such as glucose tolerance or liver function tests may be indicated. With this information the doctor can decide whether or not a woman is suitable for oral contraception.

It is possible to get a general indication as to which type of pill may be most suitable in the individual case. Some women tolerate any preparation and some tolerate none so no method of selection is foolproof. The effect of a particular pill on a particular woman will depend on her inherent hormone balance and methods of assessing this are indefinite.

It is best to select a pill with the lowest dose of each hormone in it and if this preparation proves unsuitable, others with different progestogens can be tried. Most pills are dispensed in packs containing 21 pills. The woman is instructed to start taking the pill on the fifth day of her menstrual period whether or not the menstrual flow has ceased. She then takes one pill each day at approximately the same time for 21 days followed by 7 pill free days. On the eighth day she starts on her next packet of pills and so the sequence is repeated. It does not matter at what time of the day pills are taken provided they are taken regularly as near to 24 hour intervals as possible. When starting oral contraceptives additional precautions are advised for the first 14 days. It is no longer necessary to wait until menstruation is re-established post-partum before starting oral contraception. Ovulation may occur as early as the thirty-third day after delivery and it is wise to start on the pill earlier where intercourse is taking place. Oral contraception should therefore be started 28 days after delivery to ensure completely effective contraceptive cover. Patients taking oral contraceptives should be seen 3 months after starting therapy. Weight and blood pressure should be recorded. At this visit a check should be made on cycle control, side effects assessed and the patient reassured. If no problems presents six-monthly visits are adequate thereafter.

SIDE EFFECTS OF ORAL CONTRACEPTION
Since oral contraceptives act systemically and therefore produce a wide variety of changes in the body, women taking the pill may find that their health is actually improved or they may develop clinical symptoms which they find unacceptable. Some of the side effects may even be detrimental to her health. Sometimes side effects may also be due to emotional factors such as guilt over taking the pill, desire for another baby, etc., and may therefore be very difficult to treat. Minor side effects are very common during the first two months of oral contraceptive therapy but after that time about 80 per cent of women settle down happily on their oral contraceptive pill. The incidence of side effects in different studies is so variable that in many cases it is meaningless to quote them.

Many women actually feel better while taking the pill and they experience a feeling of wellbeing knowing that they will not become pregnant. The menstrual cycle becomes regular even in those who previously had irregular periods. In more than 50 per cent menstrual blood loss is reduced resulting in raised haemoglobin and serum iron levels. Dysmenorrhoea, mid-cycle pain and premenstrual tension disappear.

Minor side effects
Nausea. Nausea is a common complaint and is thought to be due to the woman's sensitivity to oestrogen. It may recur at the beginning of each cycle. It is less troublesome if the woman takes her pill at bedtime. It is most common in the first few cycles and if nausea develops for the first time in later months it is unlikely to be due to the pill and some other cause should be sought. Vomiting is not common. If a woman vomits for any reason within one hour of taking the pill, she should take another one.

Weight gain. Weight gain can be a troublesome side effect especially in the first six months. It may be the result of eating too much due to an increase in appetite or due to fluid retention. A feeling of abdominal distension can cause great discomfort. Any weight gain of more than 14 lb should be watched with care.

Headache. Women may complain of headache for the first time after they start taking the pill but generally headaches do not start until after several months of therapy. Women who suffer from migraine can be given the oral contraceptive pill but the resultant headache pattern should be watched carefully. If migraine attacks become frequent and severe, and certainly if they are associated with motor or sensory disturbances, the pill should be stopped.

Breakthrough bleeding. Slight vaginal spotting may occur during the first few cycles on taking the pill. These symptoms can be ignored for 2 or 3 cycles but if they persist, a pill containing a larger dose of progestogen should be prescribed.

Amenorrhoea occurs in about 9 per cent of cycles in women who are taking oral contraceptives. This is a source of great concern to them unless they have been warned of this possibility. If amenorrhoea occurs in more than two consecutive cycles, pregnancy must be excluded. If it persists for more than three consecutive cycles the pill should be stopped and not restarted until regular menstruation is established.

Premenstrual tension. This is relieved in the majority of women but a few will develop it for the first time or find that the pre-existing symptoms are exaggerated. The breasts may also become tender, fuller or even enlarged in size in the first cycle but these changes generally disappear in later months. The enlargement and fullness may be reduced by reducing the progestogen content of the pill while pain and tenderness will respond to an increased dose of progestogen. There is no evidence that women taking the pill are more or less liable to develop breast cancer.

Libido. This is a very subjective symptom and it is difficult to assess the effect of oral contraceptives. Some women report no change in their sex drive and response. Some find it enhanced while others report diminution or complete loss of libido.

Depression. This is a frequent complaint by women taking the pill but in most cases it is a mood swing rather than a true depressive state although the latter condition can occur. It may be sufficient to necessitate stopping all oral contraception.

Major side effects and contra-indications

Cardiovascular system. The relationship between the pill and a rise of blood pressure is well known. Few women develop hypertension on the pill but nevertheless the blood pressure should be recorded before the woman starts taking the pill and repeated at intervals during treatment. Hypertension itself is not a contra-indication to oral contraceptives but when it rises progressively during pill taking, the pill should be discontinued. There is no evidence that coronary artery disease is more common in women taking oral contraceptives except when other predisposing factors are present. Varicose veins may become more prominent and painful. Their presence is not a contra-indication to the use of the pill but oral contraceptives should be stopped one month before injection or ligation and not restarted for a month after treatment is complete.

Thrombo-embolic disease. The combined oral contraceptives produce disturbances of certain coagulation mechanisms particularly an increase in factors VII and X and an increased platelet adhesiveness. Progestogen-only preparations do not appear to cause similar platelet and clotting changes. There is now much evidence supporting the view that combined oral contraceptives can be a cause of thrombo-embolic disease. Doll and Vessey (1970) have shown that the incidence of deep venous thrombosis, pulmonary embolus and cerebral thrombosis among hospital admissions is 8–9 times greater in those women using oral contraceptives than in women who do not take the pill. The mortality from these conditions was greater, particularly among women over the age of 34. In 1969 the Committee on the Safety of Drugs correlated the incidence of thrombo-embolism with the dose of oestrogen in the pill and recommended that the dose of oestrogen should not exceed 50μg. As a result of these findings oral contraceptives should not be prescribed for patients with a history of deep venous thrombosis whether or not they have had a pulmonary embolus. Although the incidence of superficial thrombo-phlebitis is higher in women taking the pill, oral contraceptives are not definitely contra-indicated in all women who have had superficial thrombo-phlebitis and each case should be judged on its merits. It is most important, however, to put this whole question into proper perspective. In women between the ages of 20 and 24 the annual risk of death from thrombo-embolism due to oral contraceptive use is about one-third of that from a road accident, one-ninth of that from a latent disease and one-fifteenth of the risk of death from all causes associated with pregnancy. In fact a woman under the age of 35 in Scotland today has the same chance of dying from the pill as she has of being murdered. It must be remembered that this risk is not an iatrogenic risk thrust on a previously healthy population but is a hazard accepted by women who would otherwise run the risk of pregnancy and death from pregnancy. For the women, therefore, who find oral contraceptives the *only* satisfactory method of contraception and in whom there are no other contra-indications to its use, the thrombo-embolic hazard should prove acceptable.

Effect on glucose tolerance. Abnormal glucose tolerance tests have been reported in 18–46 per cent of women taking the pill and this abnormality is greatest in women with a family history of diabetes. It is therefore necessary to be careful in supervising women with such a history and also those who are grossly overweight and have had babies over 9lb or glycosuria in pregnancy. Oral contraceptives are not contra-indicated in the diabetic patient but it is necessary to recognize that insulin requirements may need adjusting at the start of treatment. It is very often important for such patients to have efficient contraception and the pill may be the best method in a well controlled diabetic. Serum lipid changes occur in women on oral contraceptives. These may be important in the possible development of atherosclerosis in women on long-term therapy.

Effect on hepatic function. The liver plays a vital part in the metabolism of both oestrogens and progestogens and these drugs produce a variety of changes in liver function. Abnormal serum transaminase levels have been reported. Infective hepatitis is not a contra-indication to the pill but it should not be prescribed for at least six months after an attack unless there are no symptoms and liver function tests are normal. If a woman on oral contraceptives develops jaundice, the pill should be stopped. A history of idiopathic jaundice of pregnancy, cirrhosis of the liver and hereditary disorders of hepatic function contra-indicate the use of oral contraceptives.

Effect on the thyroid gland. The levels of protein bound iodine, thyroid binding globulin and T3 uptake all rise during oral contraception. It is therefore important to know whether a patient is on oral contraceptives when evaluating tests of thyroid function. The patient with a past history of thyrotoxicosis or a thyrotoxic patient well controlled may take the pill safely.

Effect on the genital tract. Many changes occur in the genital tract. The ovaries and uterus decrease in size, the endometrium becomes hypoplastic and pseudopregnancy changes occur in stromal tissue. Fibroids may enlarge rapidly and red degeneration has been reported. The presence of fibroids is not a contra-indication to the pill but merely an indication that a careful watch be kept on their size. Cervical erosion is more common on the pill but is less evident since high dose oestrogen pills were stopped. Monilia infection may be resistant to treatment in women taking oral contraceptives. There is no evidence that the pill is carcinogenic and oral contraceptives may be prescribed for patients who have had a cone biopsy of the cervix for carcinoma *in situ* provided they are followed up by serial cervical smears.

Effect on fertility. There is some evidence that after taking the pill, fertility may not return to normal immediately. Amenorrhoea after stopping oral contraceptives is associated with failure of ovulation and may be associated with galactorrhoea. Most were found to respond to treatment with Clomiphene or Gonadotrophins. There is no evidence that fertility is increased after discontinuing the pill or that multiple pregnancies are more common.

Effect on the menopause. The onset of the menopause is neither delayed nor accelerated by the pill. Withdrawal bleeding should cease when the woman reaches the menopause even if she is taking the pill. If, however, it continues when there is other evidence that she has reached the menopause, the pill should be stopped to see if her periods have in fact ceased. If they have not, oral contraceptives should be prescribed for another two years if she has not yet reached 50 and one year if she has.

Effect on lactation. The pill inhibits lactation in a proportion of women and can alter the quantity and quality of breast milk though the hormones themselves will not harm the baby.

Masculinization effect. There is no evidence of masculinization or any increase in congenital abnormalities in babies born to women who have taken the pill.

The pill is the most acceptable and most effective of all methods of contraception in use at present. There has been much adverse publicity particularly in connection with thrombo-emobolic disease. This should be put in proper perspective when considering contraceptive advice to a patient and in many cases taking the pill is better than risking the possibility of a pregnancy.

The intra-uterine device

The intra-uterine device or IUCD is made of plastic and is inserted into the uterine cavity to prevent conception. These devices have become popular in recent years but are not new. In the 19th century, in the USA and in Europe, intra-uterine devices were first used in the treatment of gynaecological disorders and later as a means of contraception. During the 1920s Graffenberg, a German gynaecologist, used a ring made of gold or silver wire which was inserted into the uterus. This ring was never popular and fell into disrepute when a few cases were associated with chronic infection and subsequently carcinoma. In 1959 two physicians working independently, revised the idea of intra-uterine contraception —in America, Oppenheimer described a device made of silkworm gut and Ota in Japan, a metal one. The next year Margulies produced an intra-uterine device made of polyethylene.

Since then a great number of devices of different shapes and sizes have been produced made of polyethylene. In the United Kingdom the most popular devices are the Saf-T-coil, the Lippes Loop, and the Gravigard (Fig. 44.4). The Lippes Loop has been very widely

has shown that the pregnancy rate is inversely proportional to the amount of copper (Zipper and Tatum, 1971). However, the long term effect of copper on the endometrium has not yet been assessed. The effectiveness of any intra-uterine device is thought to relate to the

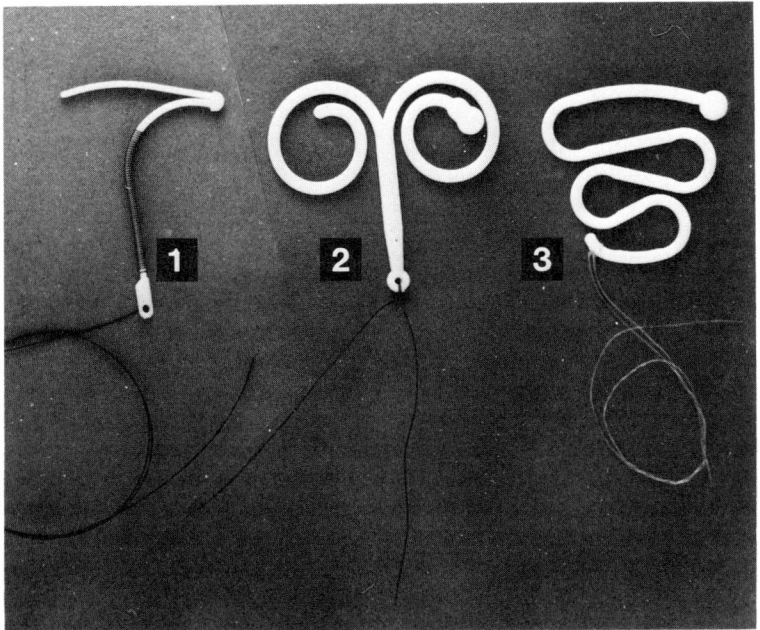

Fig. 44.4   Types of intra-uterine devices in common use: (1) Copper-7; (2) Saf-T-coil; (3) Lippes Loop.

used and more than 7 million have been inserted throughout the world. It is available in four sizes A–D. The Saf-T-coil is also made of polyethylene but comes in only one size. Both devices are flexible and can be straightened within an introducer. The introducer is then inserted through the cervical canal and once it is in position the device is extruded into the uterine cavity where it regains its original shape. In order that the device may return to its original shape in the uterus it should not be kept straightened out in the introducer until immediately prior to insertion. (The Dalkon Shield* is made of plastic ethyl vinyl acetate and also contains trace elements of copper. Its lateral fins and flexibility make it 'fundal seeking' counteracting the natural tendency to expulsion. It cannot be straightened out within an introducer and is therefore more bulky to pass through the cervical canal.) The Gravigard or 'Copper 7', as it is sometimes called, is shaped like a 7 with copper wire wound round the shank. Experimental work

* N.B. The Dalkon Shield is now being withdrawn (1975).

amount of physical contact it has with the endometrium and to the presence of copper. Each device has a nylon tail attached to it which provides a means of knowing whether the device is still *in situ*.

Mode of action. Intra-uterine devices are thought to work by preventing nidation but how this occurs is not entirely clear. The contraceptive effect of an intra-uterine device on the human is immediate and the rate of conception within one week of introduction of the device is no higher than the rate for the first three months. The contraceptive effect is rapidly reversible. The removal of an IUCD within one week of ovulation has been followed by conception even when coitus has only taken place while the device was still *in situ*. This rapidity of action and rapid reversibility suggests a biochemical rather than a cellular effect. The endometrium adjacent to an IUCD shows tissue oedema, stromal fibrosis and increased vascularity. Subsequently chronic infiltration with plasma cells and lymphocytes may occur and the endometrial maturation may be delayed. In some cases there appear to be no significant changes. There is no evidence that the IUCD prevents ovulation and biopsies suggest that normal ovulatory cycles occur (Eckstein, 1970).

Insertion. The best time for insertion is two months post-partum when the cervix is still patulous. The longer the interval since childbirth the more difficult the insertion may be but intra-uterine devices may be inserted at any time.

Insertion is best accomplished during or very soon after menstruation. Most devices now come presterilized by gamma radiation. If this is not the case, they may be sterilized by placing them for a minimum of 24 hours in a 1 in 750 aqueous solution of Benzalkonium Chloride.

The patient should lie supine with the buttocks raised on a firm pillow near the end of the couch. Lithotomy stirrups may be used but are not essential. The size and position of the uterus should be determined by bimanual examination. It is important to know whether it is ante or retroverted or deviated laterally. Under aseptic precautions with the speculum in place, a sound is passed to find the depth and direction of the uterine cavity. It may be necessary to insert one or two dilators but this is not usually required. A long handled Volsellum forceps should be applied to the cervix and gentle traction on this straightens out kinks in the cervical canal. Loading of the introducer should be postponed until one is sure of entry as plastic devices when stretched soon lose their power to recover their original shape. The actual technique of introduction varies with the device used. In the case of the Lippes Loop, the shaft of the introducer has to be rotated 90° after introduction so that the loop can be placed in the wide frontal plain. In the case of the Gravigard for example no such rotation is required.

It is possible to insert IUCDs without any discomfort to the patient but dilatation and handling of the cervix may cause pain and shock. Mild abdominal cramp is relatively common during insertion. Shock rarely happens without warning and often the patient will have complained of feeling faint and there will have been something difficult or unusual about the insertion such as repeated attempts to find the cervical canal. In rare cases it may be necessary to give general anaesthesia for insertion of an IUCD.

SIDE EFFECTS

1. *Pain.* Pain is usually manifested as mild discomfort similar to dysmenorrhoea which can be relieved by mild analgesics and reassurance. This type of pain is most commonly present just at the time of insertion. Dysmenorrhoea may be associated with a device which is too large for the uterine cavity. This is most common in a nulliparous woman. A previous history of painful periods is frequently found in these cases. It may be reduced by inserting a softer or smaller device. Another kind of pain sometimes found is backache and low abdominal discomfort. These patients should always be examined to exclude gynaecological disease, in particular pelvic inflammation. This has been reported in women with intra-uterine devices and in some series has been as high as 2 per cent.

2. *Bleeding.* Most patients after insertion of an IUCD report longer and heavier menstrual loss in the first few months. Menstruation tends to occur more frequently and may be irregular. In the majority of patients this will settle down at the end of the third month to tolerable limits. Severe persistent bleeding, persisting beyond the three months' period, may require the removal of the device. If the patient is anxious to persist with this method it is worthwhile replacing the device with a smaller and more pliable one. If this is not effective in patients where the intra-uterine device is the only effective method of contraception, a progestogen such as norethisterone may be tried. It is important to remember that a patient with severe persistent bleeding may become anaemic and require oral iron for correction of the anaemia. The possibility of gynaecological disease causing heavy irregular and particularly intermenstrual bleeding has always to be borne in mind.

3. *Expulsion.* This is known to be a troublesome risk with all forms of device. Depending upon the type of device used, between 4 and 30 per cent are expelled in the first year after insertion. Expulsion is particularly common at the time of menstruation and the highest incidence is at the first post-insertion period. The purpose of the cervical tail is to allow the patient or doctor to check that the device is in place and each patient should be instructed how to feel this device so that she can check its position following each period.

4. *Perforation.* Perforation is uncommon. With the majority of devices it only occurs in

about 1 in 4000 insertions. Perforation is most likely to occur post-partum in the soft uterus and for this reason insertion may have to be delayed until 8 weeks after delivery. However, in certain patients it is necessary to insert the device at once otherwise pregnancies will occur. Perforation is frequently silent and not suspected at the time but subsequent examinations reveals the absence of the threads although the device can be detected radiologically in the peritoneum. If it should be expelled it is worthwhile trying to insert a device of another type which may be more suitable to the configuration of the uterine cavity.

5. *Infection.* This is a late effect of the intrauterine contraceptive device. Infection usually occurs where there has been pre-existing infection in the cervical canal. Some workers insist that an intracervical swab should be taken for culture before insertion. If gonorrhoea is present the disease should be treated before the coil is inserted. The presence of trichomoniasis, candidiasis, mild cervicitis or an erosion should not prevent insertion if this is urgent pending treatment of the condition. If patients develop pelvic inflammation with an intra-uterine device *in situ* then it should be removed. The incidence of infection is probably in the region of 2 per cent.

6. *Pregnancy.* Although pregnancy can hardly be described as a side effect, it may occur either because the device has been extruded unknown to the patient or because it fails to prevent nidation. There is a wide range of pregnancy rates for the different types of IUCDs. It would appear that the larger devices, those with the greatest surface areas and those containing metallic copper, are most effective in preventing pregnancy. If pregnancy does occur with a device *in situ*, there is a slightly increased tendency to miscarriage. The incidence of ectopic pregnancy, however, does not seem really to be increased and there is no increase in the rate of congenital defects if the pregnancy continues.

Careful selection of patients, devices, operator and time of insertion can greatly minimize the side effects. At the time of insertion a calm, well run clinic where insertion of IUCDs is a daily routine procedure helps greatly in reassuring the patient and reducing side effects. The presence of a good nurse exuding confidence and who can distract the patient appropriately is of the greatest value.

The patients most likely to have difficulties at the time of insertion are the over-anxious women who dislike vaginal examination, nulliparous women whose cervical canal is tighter and uterine cavity narrower than the parous, menopausal women who have not been pregnant for many years or any woman who has a stenosis of the cervical canal perhaps as a result of a D & C or cauterization of the cervix. Precipitation of an epileptic fit in a susceptible person has also been known during insertion and it is essential to ask this in the history taking.

Contra-indications. Menorrhagia and recent acute pelvic infection provide contra-indications to the IUCD. Cervical erosion need not be a contra-indication as the patient's need of contraception may take priority but cauterization of a grossly infected cervix should first be performed. Trichomonas and monilial infections may be treated with the loop *in situ*. There is no evidence that the IUCD is carcinogenic or that they impair future fertility unless infection occurs in which case tubal blockage may result.

The IUCD is of great value where oral contraception cannot be used or is unacceptable to the patient and is particularly helpful in protecting mothers in the poorly motivated, lower socio-economic group who have hitherto benefited little from previous methods even including the 'pill'. In developing countries is is widely used as a means of population control.

These two methods are probably the most widely used and most effective at the time of writing. However, it is necessary to have a wide variety of contraceptive methods available so that all tastes may be satisfied. The other and more traditional methods will now be described.

The safe period

The safe period depends on estimating the time of ovulation and avoiding intercourse during the days of the month when conception is most likely. Difficulties arise over finding out the exact time of ovulation since not only is one woman different from another but the same woman may have a different length of cycle from one month to another. In spite of these difficulties, many women wish to use this method, especially as this is the only form of contraception advocated by the Roman

Catholic Church. It is therefore important to make it as reliable as possible.

In the average 28 day cycle, ovulation occurs about the 14th day. 24 hours are allowed on one side of this for ovum survival, and 48 hours on the other side for sperm survival. In practice, a further 48 hours are added on either side for extra safety. Therefore, in the 28 day cycle the unsafe period would be from day 10 to day 17. Evidence suggests that coitus before the 10th day of the cycle sometimes results in pregnancy either because coitus acts as a stimulus to ovulation or because a short cycle might result in ovulation occurring early in the cycle, soon after the cessation of menstruation i.e. what is normally a safe time. On the other hand, in a long cycle ovulation will be delayed and pregnancy might occur in what would normally be the safe time several days before the onset of menstruation. In women with cycles of irregular length, the total period of risk is from the first unsafe day of her shortest cycle to the last unsafe day of her longest cycle. For example, in a woman with a short cycle of 26 days and a long cycle of 31, intercourse should be avoided from day 8 to day 20.

It is also possible to use the basal body temperature as an indication of the time of ovulation. If intercourse does not take place until 72 hours after the rise, conception is very unlikely. The temperature should be taken first thing in the morning under the tongue with the mouth closed for four minutes. The woman should not have been out of bed, eaten or drunk anything or smoked. A specially calibrated and easily read thermometer is available for use with this method. The safe period works best in highly motivated couples where coitus is restricted to the post ovulatory phase after the temperature has been raised for three days. The failure rate here is claimed to be 6·6 per 100 woman years. The advantages of the safe period are that it requires little equipment or medication except a thermometer and it has no side effects except frustration.

As to the disadvantages, it requires a great deal of consistent and persistent motivation. The temperature method, particularly, is not practical with people of limited education and poor standards of living. It demands abstinence for a considerable part of each month which one partner may tolerate but the other may not. It is unsuitable for women with very irregular cycles. It is important to remember that the 'safe period' is not really safe but its use may give a longer gap between pregnancies than would otherwise occur and this will be beneficial both to the woman herself and to her children.

Barrier and spermicidal methods of contraception

1. *Coitus interruptus.* This is probably the oldest and most commonly used method and consists of withdrawal by the husband before ejaculation occurs so that no seminal fluid is deposited in the vagina. This method is not efficient as some seminal fluid may escape before ejaculation. It requires considerable care and control on the part of the man and it also causes anxiety lest control will not be maintained and may interfere with the attainment of complete orgasm especially for the wife. Since it does not, however, require the use of any appliance and costs nothing, it is popular among the casual, uneducated and relatively unintelligent section of society.

2. *Spermicidal methods.* These are substances which kill spermatozoa and are placed in the vagina before intercourse. Pessaries, concentrated tablets of spermicide, are placed high in the vagina immediately before intercourse. Some dissolve spontaneously but others called 'foaming tablets' have to be dipped into water before insertion. They then produce a spermicidal foam within one or two minutes. Other spermicidal agents used are in the form of creams or jellies which are inserted high into the vagina with the help of an applicator. None of these agents are very reliable. A sperm can reach the cervico-mucous plug and pass through into the cervical canal almost immediately after ejaculation where they are beyond the reach of spermicides. Allergy may also be a problem in either partner. The disadvantages of chemical barriers are that they are unreliable, unaesthetic and may lead to the development of allergy. However, they are better than nothing, are easily obtained and relatively cheap. If used with a mechanical barrier they provide an effective method of contraception but alone they are unsatisfactory.

Recently a new type of spermicidal contraceptive has been introduced from Hungary. This is known as the C-film and consists of a square of water-soluble plastic material which is impregnated with a potent spermicide. The device can be used by either the man or the woman. In the case of the man the C-film is placed over the tip of the erect penis just prior to intercourse. The substance adheres to the glans and is therefore carried to the top of the vagina during intercourse. The woman places the C-film on the cervix prior to intercourse. This method has the advantage of ease of application, and would be suitable for the act of casual intercourse and investigations have shown this method to have a potent spermicidal action in the vagina (*IPPF Medical Handbook*, 2nd ed. 1967).

3. *The condom.* This is a rubber sheath worn by the husband. They are made of rubber and may be plain or lubricated and may or may not have a teat at the end. The modern condom with its rigorous testing is a very reliable device. Most of the failures in the past were due to poor quality of rubber or irregular use because of cost. They are not always aesthetically acceptable and many couples, especially men, dislike using them mainly because the act of intercourse is interrupted both before and after coitus. Coital difficulties may therefore arise both in husband and wife. The failure rate with the condom is between 5 and 15 per 100 woman years.

4. *Vaginal diaphragm.* Before oral contraception, the Dutch Cap or vaginal diaphragm, in existence for over 80 years, was the main method used in clinics. The modern diaphragm is a saucer shaped appliance of latex rubber with a flat spring or coiled spring rim. The diameter in millimetres is used as a means of identifying size which may be from 45–105mm. Correct positioning of the diaphragm is essential. The proximal part is inserted into the posterior fornix so that the cervix is properly covered. The distal part then lies behind the symphysis pubis which in most women is recognizable as an easily felt shelf or recess $\frac{1}{2}$–1 inch along the anterior vaginal wall. In this way the diaphragm forms a false roof to the vagina. It is absolutely essential that the correct size is used. If the diaphragm is too small it does not cover the cervix properly and if it does not lie snugly in the retropubic shelf the rim can sometimes be felt by the man. If it is too large and projects from the vaginal orifice it is felt by the woman who rapidly becomes aware of the discomfort. Within practicable limits the best fit is the largest consistent with comfort. Recent work by Masters and Johnson (1970) have changed some of our preconceived ideas about the

importance of exact fit since it is now known that the vagina can dilate enormously during intercourse thus making the question of millimetres in the fitting of a cap rather nonsensical. A professional check on the correct size is therefore necessary at regular intervals of about one year. This is particularly important if there has been a pregnancy.

Sterilization

Sterilization is a means of family limitation not of family spacing. It is an attractive method of birth control offering, as it does, a permanent and in most cases an irreversible alternative to other methods.

FEMALE STERILIZATION

Sterilization can be done for many reasons, the indications falling into three main groups which in many cases are closely related—the medical, the social and the socio-medical.

Under the medical indications conditions such as cardiac disease, hypertension, renal disease, diabetes, malignancy and psychiatric disease are common. The question here is whether another pregnancy will be more likely to make the disease worse or indeed lead to a fatal outcome. When considering advice on this, in addition to the management of the condition in pregnancy it is also necessary to consider whether the woman will be able to look after the baby in the following months and years. For example, some women with heart disease may well be able to cope with the pregnancy but looking after the baby with disturbed nights may cause her cardiac state to deteriorate.

Most sterilizations are now done for social or socio-medical reasons. The basic social reason is that the woman does not wish any more children and has completed her family. Socio-medical indications are multiparity and debility, the patient not wishing to go on taking contraceptive measures for years and the failure or unsuitability of other methods of contraception. It is essential not to be too rigid about age and parity and to consider the possibility of sterilization when requested even if the woman has only one child. The techniques of the operation will be described in the chapter on operations.

Timing of sterilization. This may be done at a number of different times, in the puerperium, at Caesarean section, at termination of pregnancy or in the non-pregnant state when it is called interval sterilization.

Sterilization during the puerperium is very suitable for many women, particularly parous women. The subject should be discussed during the antenatal visits so that it can be well aired by the time the confinement takes place. It is usually done about two days after delivery when the patient has recovered from her confinement and the state of the baby is known. It suits most women, particularly those with a family, to have the operation while they are already in hospital and have arrangements made for their children to be looked after. This type of patient finds it very difficult to come back into hospital for interval sterilization and is usually delighted to have the operation and then go home completely protected at the end of her stay in the maternity unit. For these reasons post-partum sterilization is a very acceptable method for many women but it should be realized that the failure rate is greatest when the operation is done at this time.

When a woman has had two or more Caesarean sections, or does not wish any more children and is having a Caesarean section, the matter should always be raised and discussed. The problem here is if something happens to the baby after its delivery and this must always be discussed with the patient. Many women who are having a termination of pregnancy do so because they do not wish any more children. It is therefore unwise just to terminate the pregnancy without considering sterilization at the same time. It should never be made a condition of termination but the question should always be discussed when the reason for termination is that the patient does not wish any more children.

Interval sterilization, i.e. in the non-pregnant state, is usually done where the woman has decided that she does not want any more children or is dissatisfied with her method of contraception. She has usually completed her family and has fear of a further pregnancy.

Counselling for sterilization. A couple contemplating sterilization want information on a wide range of practical questions and adequate counselling should be provided. Hostile or unsympathetic handling by those discussing the problem can have an important effect on the outcome. One must therefore be careful to consider each couple on the basis of their personal and social circumstances. They will want to know what in fact is done, what kind of anaesthetic will be required, whether the procedure will be painful, how long the woman will have to be in hospital and they will wish to know details of the outcome and reliability of the operation. Their main worry is usually about femininity and in all strata of society there is no doubt that many women equate sterilization with castration. The effect of the operation on libido, sexual performance, menstruation and on general health must be discussed. A few husbands feel that their wives may become promiscuous and this suggestion must be aired. All the circumstances of the case have to be carefully weighed up and of course the written consent of both husband and wife should be obtained. The operation is not 100 per cent successful and although reversible by tubal anastomosis or reimplantation if the tubes have been tied at the uterine end, no guarantee can ever be given to an individual woman that she will achieve pregnancy. It therefore has to be assumed that the operation will result in permanent sterility.

Results of sterilization. Evidence shows that the vast majority of women, in fact over 90 per cent, are satisfied with the operation. They report unchanged or improved health, better sex life and increased coital frequency at an age when it is normally decreasing in the general population. Good marital and socioeconomic adjustments are attributable to freedom from fear of pregnancy. Not all women, however, are satisfied with sterilization. About one-third report menstrual upset, usually heavy periods. This may be due to psychogenic maladjustment to sterility. A few women report frigidity after sterilization but may be very satisfied because of its other advantages. On average, less than 10 per cent express regret or guilt. There are three main reasons for unsatisfactory results. First, unsatisfied maternal feelings. Some of the most difficult cases of dissatisfaction and regret involve women who have been sterilized on account of medical conditions but who would have liked more children had they been well. Many of these women do in fact accommodate reasonably well if treated with sympathetic understanding and adequate social support. Secondly, changed circumstances such as the death of a husband or child should always be brought up in discussion before sterilization is done for it is always a possibility however unlikely it seems at the time. Thirdly, women with abnormal or unstable personalities, e.g. schizophrenia, often regret being sterilized. Problems arise where women with pre-existing psychological disturbances expect sterilization to solve their underlying problems. Each couple must be considered on the basis of their personal and social circumstances. Sexual, psychological, social and economic factors all need to be considered. The aim of counselling is to help the couple to decide what is likely to be best in their circumstances, to ensure that they are fully informed in what is involved and to allay any unnecessary fears.

MALE STERILIZATION

Vasectomy. The interest in vasectomy is increasing and a significant number of operations are now performed in both developed and developing countries. It is imperative that the doctor should explain the nature and consequences of the operation to the patient. The general counselling is similar to that described in female sterilization but there are certain questions that the man will wish answered. As in the case of the woman, the man frequently equates sterilization with castration and wonders what his potency will be like following the operation. In some men there seems to be a slight reduction in potency but in general terms it is unaltered. Questions like—'what happens to the sperm that continue to be formed?'—will also be asked. Vasectomy is a simple, safe and effective procedure but has the mild disadvantage of not

being immediately effective. In contrast to tubal ligation it involves no measurable risk to life and when a normal, stable, happy couple request sterilization, vasectomy is probably preferable to tubal ligation. If there is any condition in the wife which might lead to her death, then vasectomy is probably not the best method for use in this particular couple but is especially suitable where the husband is the unwell partner in the marriage.

It is essential for the doctor who provides a contraceptive service to be familiar with all the methods of contraception so that he can give the advice most appropriate to the needs of the individual man and woman who consult him.

POPULATION CONTROL

For hundreds of thousands of years, man has multiplied slowly and now he is multiplying fast. This is the basic problem. It is not that we have become more fertile in recent years, but just that more of us are remaining alive. In former days, deaths were nearly as numerous as births, but today for every one person that dies two are born to take his place. One of the main reasons for this change is that an immense effort has been put into the prevention or postponement of death, but very little into the prevention of birth.

Many countries have huge natural resources, but their development is jeopardized by the excess speed with which they are multiplying. Economic progress becomes difficult or

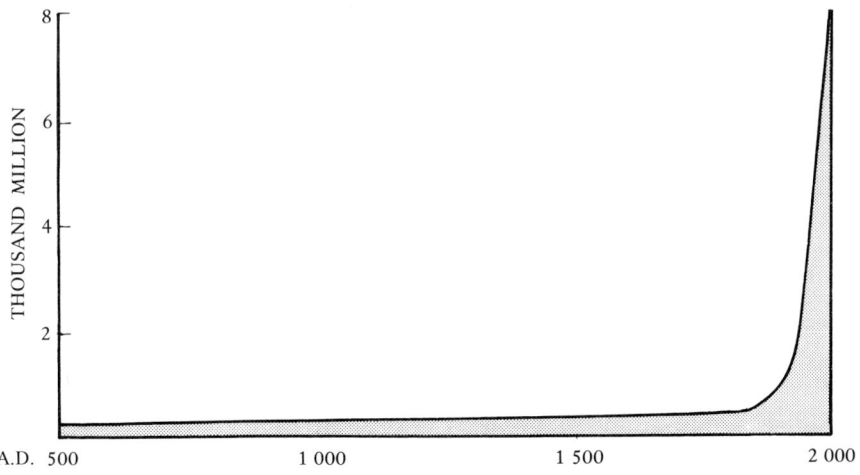

Fig. 44.5   Population growth from AD 500–AD 2000.

impossible when a population doubles in 20 to 30 years and when perhaps 45 per cent are dependent children. In some countries, e.g. South America, the social consequences include a dangerous immigration from countryside to city and the great capitals are now enlarged by shanty towns where inhabitants too often live in squalor and chronic underemployment. It is impossible for authorities to build houses fast enough to cope with this problem.

Whether we like it or not, we must consider the matter wherever we live, if we are to survive. Figure 44.5 shows the world population change from AD 500 to AD 1960 and the projected increase to AD 2000. The great increase in recent times and the projected increase is mainly accounted for by death checks, such as control of endemic disease, control of infection, etc.

Great changes in death rates have occurred over the last twenty years (Table 44.1). Many

Table 44.1   Change in Death Rate

	1940	1960
Mexico	23·2	11·4
Venezuela	16·6	8·0
Singapore	20·9	6·3
Japan	16·8	7·6

areas show a fall of 50 per cent in this period and in some areas such as Singapore, the fall is even more than this. This marked change is due mainly to advances in medical and related sciences. In comparison—Table 44.2—the

Table 44.2   Birth Rates

Guinea, Mali, Niger	55–60
Africa, Asia, Latin America	35 +
North America & Europe	25 −
United Kingdom	18·8

birth rates in many countries, particularly Africa, are very high.

An active and successful family planning policy in these areas is essential if living standards are to be maintained, let alone increased. Successful policies in individual cities in developed countries has been shown to have great benefits to the community. In the city of Aberdeen in Scotland where there has been an active policy over many years and in which sterilization and therapeutic abortion were included, the medical services could be redeployed and were able to concentrate their resources on those needing most care.

There is little doubt that every country requires a population policy and the aim should be to achieve population stability which means a family of two children. More than this means an increase in the population.

One of the tasks of family planning in the population context is to achieve this aim as far as possible. Any programme of family planning must fulfil four criteria:

1. There must be available to the population, an acceptable method of contraception for the particular group of people at risk. If the method is not acceptable it will not be used and therefore will be useless.

2. The methods used should be relatively cheap when prescribed in a large scale. This in general means that methods requiring a lot of medical or other supervision are not so suitable since staffing is expensive in money terms and training may be difficult. Some developing countries are relatively poor and the cost of a method must include bringing the knowledge required to the people.

3. The methods prescribed must be effective. If methods used are not effective, (a) they will fall into disuse since the patients will have no confidence in them, and (b) they will make no impact on the problem.

4. The methods must be safe. If patients are made ill or changes occur as the result of using a particular method, they will become apprehensive and stop.

Methods suited to large scale care

Most of the methods which are available have been used in fertility control programmes in developing countries. Some are obviously more appropriate than others and no method is outstandingly superior for every situation. Nations, like individuals, can be confused and inconsistent in their birth control practices. In Japan, the legalization of abortion in 1949 resulted in a drastic reduction in the birth rate, but it was accompanied by a very uneven programme of family planning. The government of India has favoured voluntary male sterilization with a cash payment to volunteers and have found this an acceptable method for that country. In Korea and Taiwan the family planning programme has been based on the mass fitting of IUCDs. Elsewhere the pill and the condom have been successfully used, although it has been argued that the assumed need for continuing medical supervision of women using the former and the high cost of the latter make these methods less suitable for developing countries.

The great need for the future is to extend the range of cheap, acceptable and moderately effective forms of birth control, to make these more widely available and to improve the quality of family planning services.

The problem is, however, not limited to Asia and Latin America; it is a world problem and it is essential, if it is to be tackled on a global scale, to raise the level of contraceptive practice in the Western nations. During the past 150 years, it is possible that European and American medical research and clinical practice has been more successful in increasing individual well being and happiness than has any other communal activity in human history. The single outstanding exception of the potential achievements is that it has failed to provide and has often opposed rational methods of lowering the birth rate and of contributing to the universal desire of women to restrict their fertility—what Sir Dugald Baird called the Fifth Freedom—the freedom from the tyranny of excessive fertility.

REFERENCES

Djerassi, C., Miramontes, L., Rosenkranz, G. & Sondheimer, F. (1954) Syntheses of 19-Nor-17α ethynyl testosterone and 19-Nor-17α methyl testosterone. *J. Amer. Chem. Soc.*, **76**, 4092–4094.

Doll, R. & Vessey, M. P. (1970) *Brit. med. Bull.*, **1**, 33–38.

Eckstein, P. (1970) *Brit. med. Bull.*, **1**, 52–59.

Garcia, C-R., Pincus, G. & Rock, J. (1958) *Amer. J. Obstet. Gynec.*, **75**, 82

I.P.P.F. Medical Handbook, second edition (1967), p. 74.

Masters, W. H. & Johnson, V. E. (1970) Human Sexual Inadequacy. London: J. & A. Churchill.

Zipper, J. and Tatum, H. J. (1971) *Amer. J. Obstet. Gynec.*, 1 March, p. 772.

FURTHER READING

Loraine, J. A. (1970) *Sex and the Population Crises*. London: W. Heinemann Medical Books Ltd.

Peel, J. & Potts M. (1969) *Textbook of Contraceptive Practice*. Cambridge University Press.

Population and its Problems (1974) ed. Parry, H. B. Oxford: Clarendon Press.

Potts, M. & Wood, C. (1972) *New Concepts in Contraception*. Lancaster: Medical & Technical Publishing Co. Ltd.

Tatum, H. J. (1972) *Amer. J. Obstet. Gynec.*, 1 April.

45. Pre-operative, Operative and Post-operative Care

In gynaecology, as in most disciplines, surgery is to a large extent elective and often decided upon to relieve discomfort, or nuisance, or selected to improve the quality of life. It is therefore obvious that the most meticulous care should be taken to ensure maximum safety of the procedure contemplated and the best available condition of the patient before surgery. The responsibility is entirely that of the operator and must be accepted by him. In the last few years there has been a great improvement in the safety of surgery and this is in large measure due to improvement in techniques of, and facilities for, pre-operation evaluation, in the science of anaesthesia, in the development of biochemical profiles to assess progress, in systems of central sterile supply, in the range of antibiotics, and in the availability of blood and intravenous fluids of all kinds. The surgeon has become more skilful, more gentle and more adventurous but only because other advances have made this possible. A very large number of experts and a large range of services and equipment are necessary to ensure surgical safety.

PRE-OPERATIVE

The most minor procedure even without the necessity of anaesthesia poses a risk to the patient and cautery, curettage, or biopsy should never be undertaken lightly in the outpatient clinic without some explanation and without thought for the patient's condition and possible responses.

Patients for day case surgery with anaesthesia should be carefully selected not only for the minor gynaecological condition but also for their fitness for short anaesthesia, their likely ability to recover fast, the ease with which they can get home in the evening and the home facilities to which they return. Extensive use of day surgery requires first class anaesthesia, a high nursing standard for supervision of the recovery area, availability of in-patient beds as a back up, and close liaison with general practitioners to ensure follow up.

At the other extreme radical surgery for malignant disease requires the total resources of a large teaching hospital to ensure maximum safety and minimum morbidity.

In gynaecology, many patients are young and fit and routine surgery poses no real danger. Others may suffer from hypertension, diabetes, gross obesity, or have a history of coronary infarction or cerebral vascular accident.

The operative mortality from pelvic floor repair is higher than for simple hysterectomy because of the older age and poorer physical quality of many patients with prolapse.

The surgeon is responsible for a full explanation to the patient of the reason for and the extent of the operation. The patient must understand what is to be done. Most hospitals now have a 'permission form' for signature by the patient and confirming that such explanation has been given and that it is understood.

Where possible full discussion and explanation minimize the fear of the unknown and create the confidence necessary to allow the patient to make an intelligent choice and to face surgery at least with understanding and hope in success.

Pre-operative assessment

A routine history is taken and conditions likely to make surgery hazardous specially searched for, e.g. epilepsy; cardiovascular or respiratory disease; anaemia; obesity; metabolic disorder (diabetes or thyroid); malnutrition; sepsis. A history of 'allergies or sensitivity' or previous adverse response to medication is sought.

The contraceptive pill should be, if possible withdrawn some 4–6 weeks before *major gynaecological surgery* and *other suitable measures of contraception advised.*

The patient should be advised and encouraged to stop cigarette smoking.

Before an elective procedure an attempt should be made to correct any risk situation, e.g. anaemia, minor sepsis, bronchitis, obesity, urinary infection or vaginal sepsis.

Examination and investigation

The extent of the examination will depend to some extent on the likely extent of surgery but as an absolute minimum the patient's height, weight and blood pressure should be noted, the haemoglobin level ascertained, the urine checked for albumin and sugar, and the heart, lungs, and nasopharynx and mouth, examined.

Before extensive radical procedures full blood studies including plasma volume, red cell mass, blood urea and electrolyte levels, electrocardiogram; intravenous pyelogram and skeletal survey may be amongst the other assessments essential to determining fitness or suitability.

Pre-operative preparation

General. Patients should not be in hospital too long before surgery and a maximum of 24–48 hours before major procedures is advised. However, the patient may require a longer hospital stay for the necessary investigation or to have her condition improved before surgery, but as far as possible this should be done as an outpatient.

Respiratory function. All patients for major surgery should be visited by the physiotherapist and instructed in controlled respiration.

Anti thrombosis. Heparin 5000 units subcutaneously 5–6 hours before surgery and twice daily for 7 days or Macrodex 500ml IV during the operation and on the second and fourth post operation days will lessen greatly the incidence of deep vein thrombosis.

Bowel preparation. Sulpha guandine 250mgm q.i.d. for 4 days, or neomycin for 48 hours should be given to all patients likely to sustain bowel damage or if the bowel is to be opened. A diet of 'vivonex' before operation should allow minimum bowel content at surgery.

Blood volume. Many women requiring surgery have a deficiency in circulating red cells or plasma. If these levels are more than 20 per cent below ideal, transfusion of blood or certainly maintenance of plasma volume during operation will be necessary. Blood loss will be of course, monitored during surgery.

Premedication

Anaesthesia and pre-anaesthetic medication should be selected by the anaesthetist who will, of course, visit and examine the patient the day or evening before, so that he can determine fitness and suitability for the anaesthetic, select the correct plan of anaesthesia and discuss his procedures with the patient.

Following premedication reduction in anxiety allows a fall in the cortico steroid production in the patient's blood. The level rises rapidly in response to surgery but the rise is very much less when epidural block is associated with sleep anaesthesia and minimal in the post operative period when the epidural is prolonged and topped up. Gordon, Scott and Robb (1973).

Immediate pre-operation

For virtually all gynaecology procedures the bladder must be empty.

Asepsis and antisepsis

True asepsis and ideal condition of temperature and air flow for surgeon and patient and others in the theatre are difficult to attain but various forms of special device, e.g. laminar flow are being used experimentally. In some instances total asepsis is designed for the isolated procedure such as the delivery of a baby with agammaglobulinaemia.

Modern theatre design still falls short of the ideal for total asepsis and some antisepsis is essential.

Skin. The skin of surgeon, of patient and of other ward and theatre staff is a potent source of infection, especially with Staph. aureus. In lower abdominal groin and perineal operations there is the further contamination with E. coli on the patient's skin.

Although rubber gloves are normally worn, the surgeon's hands are still a potential danger since minute holes or damage to gloves can occur.

Surgeons hands respond poorly to scrubbing and the longer the scrub the larger the number of bacterial colonies that can be grown from the skin.

Washing with soap and water and the use of brushes to clean nails should be used only for the removal of overt dirt. The hands should then be thoroughly rinsed since the modern scrubs are incompatible with soap. Two minute hand washing with chlorhexidine 1 per cent in 4 per cent detergent (Hibiscrub) or with povidone iodine (Betadine) are probably best. Both have some residual effect and will kill Staph. aureus or E. coli.

Antibiotic gentamycin cream will clear the nostrils of staphylococcal carriers.

Hand bowls in theatre should have 1:10 000 chlorhexidine or 3 per cent hexochlorophane in saline.

The need for preparation of the *patient's skin for surgery* depends on the operation to be undertaken. For minor vaginal procedures including pregnancy termination it is unnecessary to shave the patient but the vulva should be washed with soap and water some time before and then in theatre labia and vulva and vagina cleansed with a chlorhexidine solution. Any obvious vaginal discharge should be clearly removed.

In pelvic floor procedures and in vulvectomy shaving is advised but should be limited to the area to be operated upon. Great care should be taken to avoid injury to the skin.

Skin preparation should begin with soap and water washing to remove dirt, epithelial scales and exudate. In lower abdominal procedures only the hair of the mons and lower abdomen, as late as possible, need to be shaved. In theatre several applications of 0·5 per cent chlorhexidine or 1 per cent iodine in 70 per cent alcohol or Betadine swabs should be applied. In particular risk situations this could be preceded by a hibiscrub wash.

There is some virtue in washing the wound with 1:5000 chlorhexidine before closing but adequate wound haemostasis, gentleness with tissue and use of non-irritant suture material are more important. Wounds contaminated by infected material are difficult to keep clean, Lowbury (1973).

Incisions

The incisions commonly used in gynaecology are:

1. *Mid-line subumbilical.* This incision which is strictly mid-line ideally transverses the mid-line fascia without opening either rectus sheath. This is difficult and usually one or other sheath is opened, but the rectus muscle does not need to be separated from its sheath.

2. *Right or left paramedian.* The incision 1–2cm from the mid-line and opens the rectus sheath. The rectus muscle is separated and the posterior sheath and peritoneum incised in the line of the original skin incision. The idea is that the rectus muscle will fall back and so separate the incision and anterior and posterior sheath. This incision is usually subumbilical but may be extended past the umbilicus when access is required (as in extended hysterectomy) to the glands of the lower aorta.

3. *Low transverse or pfannenstiel.* This incision is usually made in the hair line just above the symphysis. The sheath of rectus and the transversus abdominis fascia and muscle and the internal oblique are incised on the line of the skin incision. The rectus muscles are, however, separated to allow access to the peritoneum. Greater access to the pelvis may be obtained by cutting the rectus muscles in the line of the incision and later uniting the cut ends. If this is planned the sheath should not have been previously separated as it is used to support the united muscle and to hold the sutures.

4. *Special incisions* are used for extra peritoneal approaches, for colostomy, for supra pubic operations, and for appendicectomy in later pregnancy, etc.

THE OPERATIONS OF GYNAECOLOGY

Descriptions here are simple outlines of the operations expected in routine gynaecological practice. Details of techniques should be studied in specialist manuals.

Examination under anaesthesia (EUA)

The urinary bladder is emptied and careful inspection is made of the external genitalia, the vagina and cervix. Combined examination by vaginal (or vaginal/rectal) fingers and an abdominal hand allows consideration of the shape, size and mobility of uterus and/or any other mass. Much information can be obtained. Such examination is an essential preliminary to all gynaecological surgery. It is, combined with cystoscopy, an essential preliminary in all cases of suspected or proven malignant disease, and with laparoscopy in many cases of infertility or doubtful pelvic pain.

Cystoscopy

This investigative procedure is required in many cases of post menopausal bleeding (especially if no vaginal or uterine lesion is

Equipment consists primarily of an inspecting telescope with operating instruments combined or inserted through separate trocars, the lighting system is fibre optic (Fig. 45.1). Anaesthesia should be general with intubation,

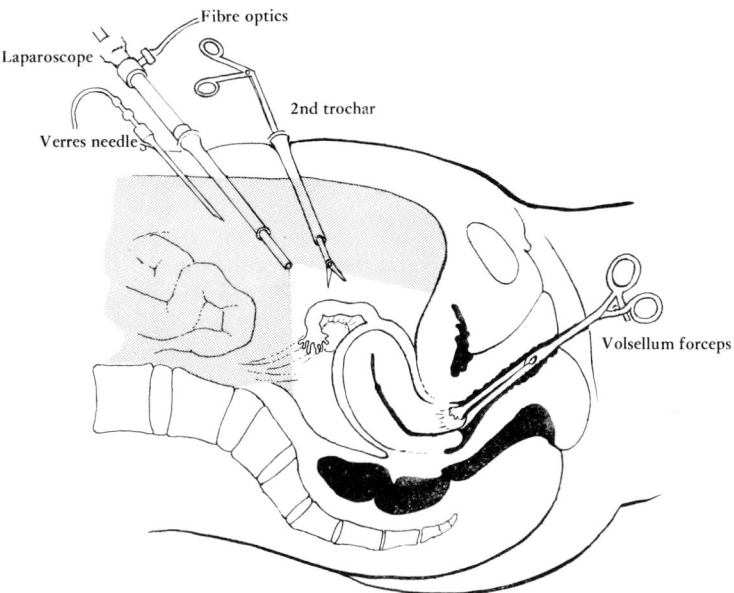

Fig. 45.1   The technique of laparoscopy.

found), in all cases with bladder or ureteric damage, and routinely in gynaecological malignant disease for preliminary assessment and often in follow up. Modern fibre optic equipment is, of course, advised, and operating telescope with facilities for catheterization of ureters, and biopsy of tumours are essential. It is often easier to examine the inside of the bladder while it is being filled. Catheterization of ureters is best done whenever a clear view can be obtained and this is often when the bladder is only half full.

Laparoscopy

This procedure has very recently become deservedly much more popular and this is due largely to the work and stimulation of Steptoe (1967 and 1973). There is a concern, however, over the dangers of using diathermy particularly for sterilization through the laparoscope (see page 839). Instruments vary and the extent of operation possible varies from operator to operator and many new techniques have limited and short applicability.

a cuffed tube, good muscle relaxation and controlled respiration.

The patient is best placed in the semilithotomy position (Lloyd Davies leg supports). The bladder is emptied, a volsellum placed on the cervix to control and manipulate it, or a cannula locked in the uterus. The uterus is sounded and after dilatation curettage may be performed. The operator inserts a guarded Vorhees needle *without* the gas lead attached, into the abdomen probably best in the mid-line just below the umbilicus and directed towards the pelvis. Once clearly in the cavity and not in bowel (odour) the gas lead is attached and some 3-4 litres of gas (CO_2) are run in slowly (10-15 minutes) at controlled pressure from a suitable source with the patient tilted head down. Once the lower abdomen is suitably distended the main trocar with sheath is inserted. This trocar is again probably best inserted in the mid-line although left or right lateral insertion are sometimes used. A crescentic incision 1cm is made just below the umbilicus and the subcutaneous tissue and sheath are incised.

The point of the trocar is inserted directed towards the pelvis and firmly (with some rotation) pushed through into the abdomen. The telescope is inserted, lights are connected and the pelvis inspected. An area to one or other side in the region of the rectal muscle is trans-illuminated so that an area clear of vessels can be selected and if necessary a second trocar inserted at least 7cm from the main trocar to carry probes; cautery, forceps, needle or other operating instrument. There are dangers associated mainly with damage to vessels, or to bowel especially if previous scars with adhesions are present. Contra-indications include difficulty in obtaining an adequate pneumoperitoneum, acute abdominal conditions and medical contra-indication to pneumoperitoneum.

Dilatation of the cervix

This operation is performed frequently, usually as a preliminary to curettage. Although it is a minor operation all precautions should be taken to prevent sepsis since in some cases the cervix is torn and spread of infection to the parametrium can occur.

After the patient is anaesthetized, a careful bimanual examination should be made, to determine the exact condition of the pelvic organs, and particularly to exclude the possibility of early pregnancy, or of latent inflammatory conditions in the adnexa. The latter, if overlooked, may be stimulated into an acute phase by any pelvic operation, however trivial.

The patient having been placed in the lithotomy position, a speculum is introduced into the vagina to retract the posterior vaginal wall. The anterior lip of the cervix is grasped with a volsellum and a sound passed into the uterus to mark the length of the cavity and the direction of the canal. Graduated dilators are then gently introduced one after the other. For many purposes only minimal dilatation is necessary. It is rarely necessary or advisable to dilate beyond 10–12 Hegar. In cases of inevitable or incomplete abortion a wider dilator may be passed or it may be possible to insert the forefinger into the uterus to separate placental tissue and thus empty it. This is only possible because the cervix in such cases is soft and partly dilated before the operation is undertaken. Suction curettage may make wide dilatation unnecessary. The cervix,

especially in nulliparous women, is more easily dilated immediately before a menstrual period.

Although usually a simple procedure, dilatation may be difficult owing to rigidity of the cervix or if the point of the dilator is caught by the ridges of the cervical mucosa. To avoid damage to the cervical canal dilators must be introduced gently and slowly and each one should be allowed to remain in the canal for some seconds. To estimate the amount of pressure being exerted by the dilators against the cervical canal, it is advisable that the volsellum be held by the operator himself. Force should never be used as it may easily cause splitting of the cervix. Tears may extend through the internal os to the body of the uterus; they may be repaired from the vagina but it may be necessary to perform a laparotomy to deal with bleeding into the broad ligament. Another danger is perforation of the uterine wall, and this risk is high in post-menopausal women, in pregnancy or where the uterine body is sharply flexed upon the cervix. Smaller and narrow pointed dilators are particularly liable to pass straight through the wall of the uterus immediately above the level of the internal os instead of following the cavity of the uterus. Great care is especially necessary in the pregnant uterus (*see* page 823).

Curettage of the uterus

The indications for curettage are (1) diagnostic and (2) therapeutic.

1. Diagnostic

Diagnostic curettage is required to obtain tissue for histological examination mostly in patients with menstrual irregularity, or abnormal bleeding. Curettage for diagnostic purposes is also carried out in cases of sterility, amenorrhoea and oligomenorrhoea. The tissue removed should *always be sent for histological and occasionally for bacteriological examination.*

2. Therapeutic

In cases of incomplete abortion and in some cases where the endometrium is hyperplastic or polypoid, thorough curettage will stop the bleeding.

In biopsy curettage, a single whole length strip of the anterior and posterior walls is often sufficient. In suspected malignant disease and in therapeutic curettage, in the non-pregnant, the whole of the cavity should be curetted by steady, gentle strokes from above downwards. If the curette is employed too vigorously muscle tissue will be removed.

Perforation of the uterus is particularly liable to occur in (a) an infected uterus; (b) malignant disease of the body of the uterus; (c) hydatidiform mole; (d) pregnancy; (e) the small uterus of an elderly woman. In most cases perforation (except of the pregnant uterus) is not followed by serious sequelae and careful observation of the patient for a few days is all that is necessary. The risk of intra-peritoneal haemorrhage is much greater after perforation of the pregnant uterus and laparotomy is always necessary to assess the damage, which must be repaired.

Aspiration curettage

Curettage may be performed by aspiration through a fine 3–5mm firm plastic suction curette. Suction may be obtained by a 20mm syringe or by a vacuum pump. Curettings are sucked into the syringe or into a reservoir for histology. The system is said to be of value in avoiding anaesthesia in diagnostic curettage of multipara as an outpatient procedure. It has also been used to terminate very early pregnancy. The term 'Menstrual Regulation' is applied to this type of vacuum curettage, p. 840. ('Menstrual Extraction' is the term applied by the US Supreme Court), when used to terminate possible or doubtful early pregnancy.

OPERATIONS ON THE CERVIX

The cervix

During labour the cervix is exposed to trauma which predisposes to chronic inflammatory changes and to cervical discharge and pelvic pain. Thorough treatment of cervical lesions may not only cure the immediate symptoms but may lessen the risk of later malignant change.

In many cases treatment by cauterization with the electric cautery or with diathermy is sufficient; but when deep lacerations, or hypertrophy of the cervix, are present repair, conization, cryosurgery, amputation or hysterectomy may be necessary.

DIATHERMY TO THE CERVIX

The cervix is held with volsella and the canal well dilated. The diathermy point is then employed to make linear strokes over each lip

of the cervix and to open all the Nabothian follicles that can be seen or felt (Fig. 45.2). In two or three days the cervix is covered by a thick, whitish slough which separates in ten to fourteen days' time. Healing proceeds slowly and it may be seven to eight weeks before the area is covered by healthy epithelium.

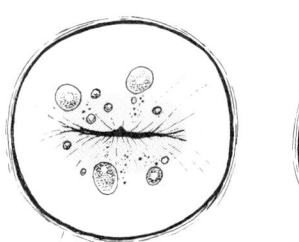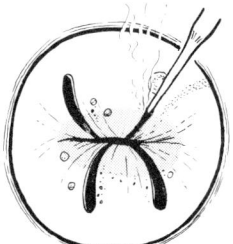

Fig. 45.2   The technique of diathermy.

After deep diathermy the patient should be kept at rest for a day or so, and she should be warned that a discharge, bloodstained at times, will be present for a time. Bleeding is seldom very profuse. Intercourse should be prohibited for 7–10 days.

Adequate diathermy of the cervix requires anaesthesia, especially since it should be preceded by dilatation. Superficial diathermy causes little pain and can be carried out without anaesthetizing the patient but is probably of little therapeutic value.

CRYOSURGERY

Recently chronic cervicitis has come to be treated by the intense cold of a cryosurgery probe (refrigerated by carbon dioxide or nitrous oxide) which by freezing destroys the tissues which form a slough some days later.

It can be used without anaesthesia and as an out-patient. Some 50 per cent of patients have some 'cramps' at the time of operation. There is a watery discharge for 7–10 days. It is eight weeks before the healing is complete and the lesion must not be packed or touched (e.g. tampax or intercourse) during the healing process or bleeding may occur.

CONIZATION

This operation may be performed as a therapeutic procedure in chronic cervicitis (instead of diathermy) to remove the 'infected' areas without limiting childbearing but, as a 'cure' of the chronically infected cervix, is less useful than hysterectomy because of the parametritis which is often associated.

The main use, however, is as a 'cone biopsy'

in cases where a cervical cytological smear has been reported as 'positive for malignant cells' (*see* Chapter 38). With the patient in a lithotomy position and after a routine pelvic examination the vagina and cervix are painted with lugols iodine. The cervix and vagina are then searched for areas which fail to take up the iodine and are therefore still pink or white. This is the 'Schiller test' and selects epithelium with metabolic abnormality sufficient to justify biopsy. After biopsy of any unstained areas of the vaginal wall the anterior lip of the cervix is grasped by a single-toothed volsellum and postero-lateral sutures are inserted at 4 and 8 o'clock to close off the cervical branch of the uterine cavity and to act as stay sutures. A cone of cervical tissue to include all non-iodine staining areas of the vaginal cervix sometimes 'shallow' (Chapter 38) and sometimes up to, almost, the internal os is then removed; preferably by a knife. The raw area may be cauterized, over-stitched or closed by suture (*see* Fig. 45.3). The cone must then be

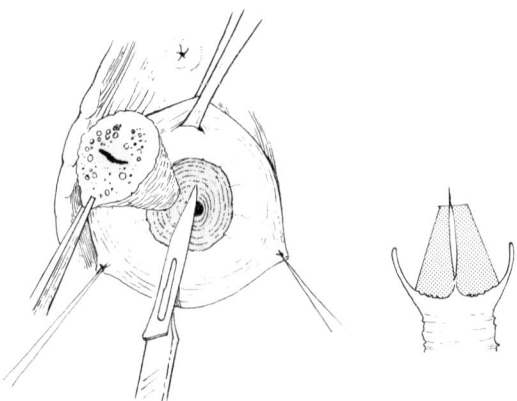

Fig. 45.3   Technique of cold knife cone biopsy.

thoroughly examined histologically. Examination of very many sections in various planes, may be required before the type of lesion, its extent and in malignant conditions the degree of 'invasion' can be assessed. Complications of the operation are haemorrhage which may be quite severe but usually occurs within 24 hours. Subsequent pregnancy and delivery are usually relatively normal after this operation especially where a 'shallow' cone has been possible (Chapter 38). Occasionally incompetence or stenosis of the internal os may occur leading on the one hand to premature onset of labour or to cervical dystocia on the

other, for which Shirodkar suture or Caesarean section may be required. Antenatal care and delivery should always be arranged under specialist supervision.

TRACHELORRHAPHY
This operation is now seldom performed possibly because severe tearing of the cervix is much less common. The usual indication is suspected cervical incompetence and the Emmett operation is usually selected.

Emmett's operation
The cervix is held with volsella and thoroughly cleansed to remove all mucus, and an antiseptic is then applied. The laceration is incised so as to get beyond the scar tissue at the angle of the tear. On either side of the cervical canal areas of mucous membrane are dissected off the everted lips of the cervix, leaving a narrow strip of mucosa in the middle line. Chromicized

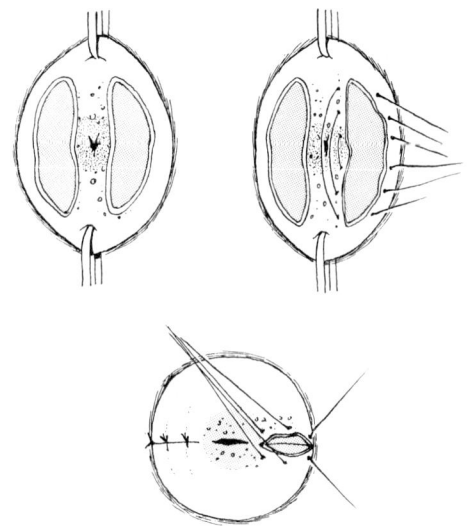

Fig. 45.4   Technique of trachelloraphy.

catgut stitches are then inserted from the lateral aspect of the cervix in such a way that no dead space is left between the united lips (Fig. 45.4).

AMPUTATION OF THE CERVIX
This operation itself is very rarely advised and has been largely superseded by conization. It is still, however, part of the operation for pelvic floor repair which is more fully discussed on page 825.

VAGINAL REPAIR OPERATIONS

Genital prolapse

The principles underlying the surgical treatment of genital prolapse have been discussed in Chapter 37. It has been explained that while descent of the uterus, bladder and rectum may occur together in the same individual, each of these organs may 'prolapse' separately. Marked descent of the uterus is associated nearly always with elongation of the supravaginal portion of the cervix, and the close relationship of the bladder to the cervix means that some descent of the bladder will usually accompany uterine prolapse. A large cystocele may be present with practically no prolapse of the uterus; or rectocele may be present without herniation of other pelvic organs. In parous women the levator ani muscles may be separated to a considerable degree and the perineal body deeply lacerated, with the result that the vaginal introitus gapes widely. There is often an associated urethrocele with stress incontinence. An enterocele may accompany a rectocele or occur alone.

All these features must be borne in mind when operation for genital prolapse is undertaken. The surgical procedure is adapted to the needs of each case though the most usual steps are: (a) the elongated cervix is amputated; (b) the parametrial tissues supporting the uterus are shortened to raise the uterus to its normal position; (c) the fascia supporting the bladder and bladder-neck is tightened across the mid-line; (d) the pelvic floor muscles

and fascia are brought together and the perineal body is reconstructed; (e) the excess skin of the relaxed vaginal walls is removed to leave a vaginal canal of normal dimensions.

The extent of the various procedures is influenced to some extent by the age of the patient. In young women high amputation of the cervix should be avoided since it predisposes to abortion and premature labour in a subsequent pregnancy. In addition, there could be risk of rigidity of the cervix in labour and of rupture into the lower segment should the cervix tear rather than dilate, Caesarean section is often necessary. It is most important not to narrow the vagina unduly in patients where coitus is still occurring and often in young women posterior repair is omitted. The whole position should be discussed with the patient beforehand. Improved obstetrics and more frequent resource to episiotomy and forceps delivery have greatly lessened the need for extensive plastic vaginal surgery.

Pelvic floor repair

Carcinoma of the cervix should have been excluded previously by examination of a cervical smear. At the beginning of the operation a thorough pelvic examination should be made to allow full assessment of the situation and to exclude other gross pathology.

The detail of operation depends to a large extent on the pathology to be corrected and on the technique preferred by the operator (Fig. 45.5).

In general, however, all techniques used

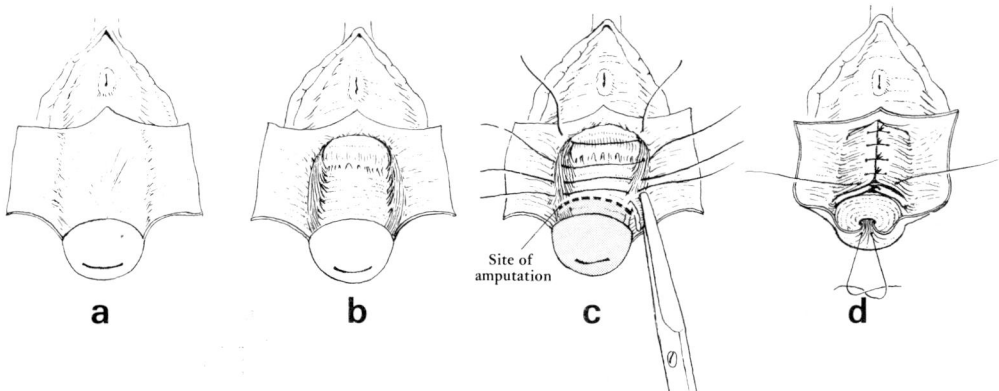

Site of amputation

a　　**b**　　**c**　　**d**

Fig. 45.5　The techniques of repair of the anterior vaginal wall with some degree of cervical prolapse. (a) Vaginal mucosa separated—fibro-muscular tissue exposed. (b) Bladder reflected from cervix. (c) Parametrial bundles cut. (d) Parametria transposed—bladder platform closed—posterior Sturmdorf stitch inserted.

begin by stripping the vaginal skin from the bladder and then stripping the bladder from the cervix to expose the supravaginal cervix and the insertions of the parametral bundles.

Support for the uterus in a higher position is achieved by clamping and cutting the transverse parametral bundles at their insertion into the cervix and, after amputation of a varying length of cervix, re-attaching the bundles in front of the cervix itself. Support for the bladder and bladder neck are achieved by bringing fibromuscular tissue from the side underneath the bladder and bladder neck or where necessary plicating the fibromuscular supporting fascia of the bladder itself. Following this or sometimes as part of those techniques the anterior wall is trimmed and closed.

Occasionally as a routine, and certainly if enterocele is suspected, the Pouch of Douglas should be opened at the time of amputation of the cervix, the enterocele sac dissected free, ligated, the excess excised and the gap closed by approximation of the cervical and vaginal end of the uterosacral ligaments.

Where vaginal hysterectomy has been performed the technique of repair just described is applied where relevant, but the parametrium bundles and the ends of the round broad ligaments and utero sacral ligaments are fixed together in the mid-line together to form a new pelvic diaphragm.

The posterior wall may not need repair and in young women repair of minor rectocele may be omitted. In posterior colpoperineorrhophy the general principles are to strip skin from underlying rectum, to support the prolapsed rectum by plication of the pre-rectal fascia and by bringing in fibro fascial support from the side to form a new pelvic fascia. The perineal body is reconstituted by stitches approximating the levator group of muscles and later the superficial muscles and fascia. The perineal skin is sutured vertically with a subcuticular fine catgut stitch, or with interrupted stitches.

The bladder is catheterized and a gauze pack may be placed in the vaginal canal to be removed in twelve hours.

The operation described comprises anterior colporrhaphy, amputation of the cervix, posterior colporrhaphy and perineorrhaphy. Many variations of the operation are practised, but the underlying principles are the same in all.

Le fort operation

This operation is used occasionally in old frail ladies who have vaginal wall prolapse with or without uterine prolapse. It may be used instead of other forms of repair or as an adjunct to vaginal hysterectomy.

The anterior and posterior walls of the vagina (and cervix) are denuded over an area two-thirds of their length and about 1cm wide. The walls are then sutured together in such a way that the raw areas are opposed and adhere, thus forming a thick central supporting septum.

Vaginal hysterectomy

The operation is most easily performed where some prolapse of the uterus allows the cervix to be pulled down to or through the vaginal orifice. The anterior wall of the vagina is opened up from the cervix and the bladder stripped free. If there is stress incontinence, support sutures to the bladder neck are best inserted at this time. The parametral bands are exposed and the uterovesical pouch identified but not opened at this time. The posterior vaginal wall is opened and the posterior pouch located and opened. The uterosacral ligaments are located within the Pouch of Douglas and clamped and cut close to the cervix. Sutures are left long. The uterus is then gradually removed by clamping, cutting and tying firstly the parametral bundles and then the uterine vessel and later the tube, round and ovarian ligaments close to the uterus. The anterior pouch is usually identified and opened after the uterine vessels have been cut to allow the tubes to be located. Care should be taken at this time that the ureters are clear. The fundus may be delivered through the anterior pouch and the upper part of the broad ligament clamped. Ovaries at this time can be inspected or removed. The operator is then left with an opening into the peritoneal cavity with four pedicles, the tube and round ligament/uterine artery/parametrium/uterosacral in pairs from front to back. The peritoneum is closed by a purse string suture and the pedicles are then joined together extraperitoneally in the mid-line. The uterosacral ligaments may be united over a fair length to close any herniation of the Pouch of Douglas. Routine anterior repair is then performed. The bladder may be plicated and finally the bladder platform stitched to the

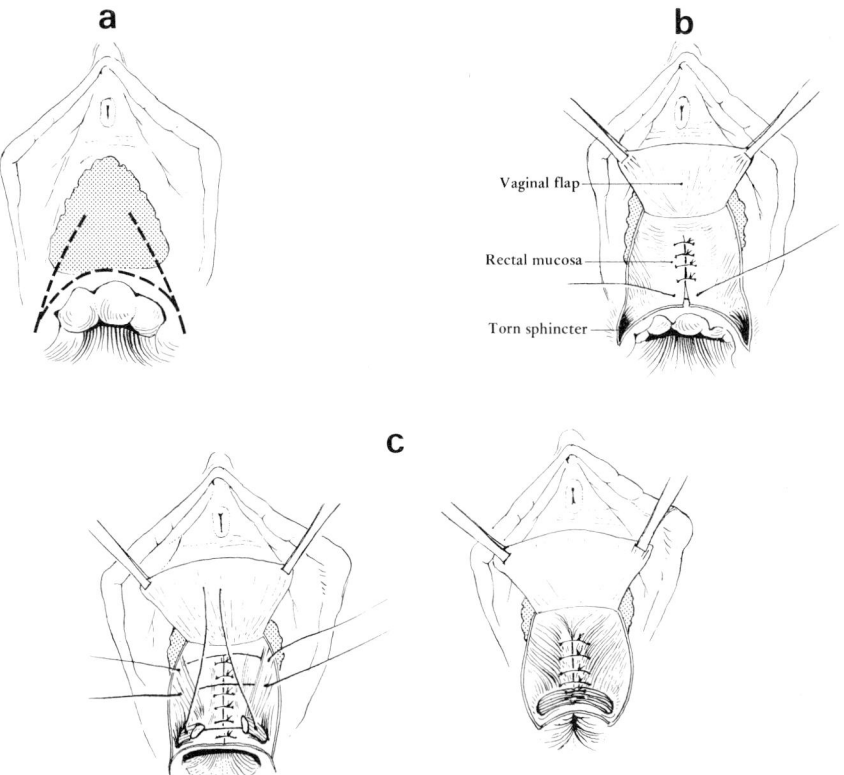

Fig. 45.6   Repair of a 'complete' tear. (a) Separation of vagina from rectum. (b) Exposure torn ends of sphincter and closure of rectal mucosa. (c) Approximation of ends of sphincter and closure of perineal muscles.

mid-line of the pedicles. An area of the vaginal skin is then selected as the top of the new vault and this is sutured to the pedicles and the anterior vaginal wall closed. Routine colpoperineorrhaphy completes the operation. A small pack is normally inserted and a foley catheter drains the bladder for some days.

COMPLETE LACERATION OF THE PERINEUM

When damage has occurred at parturition the tear may involve the sphincter ani alone, or it may extend to the anal canal and rectum. If the primary repair becomes infected and breaks down, it is advisable not to attempt a second repair until three months or so have elapsed, to allow time for the congestion, oedema and infection to subside.

Pre-operatively the bowel should be sterilized by sulfasuxidine, streptomycin or neomycin. The first step in the operation is to separate the vaginal wall from the rectum, and then to carry the skin incision backwards on each side of the anus to expose the torn ends of the sphincter muscle (Fig. 45.6).

The bowel wall is repaired from the apex of the tear downwards by inserting a fine submucosal catgut continuous Lembert suture. The edges of the torn rectal mucosa are thus turned into the lumen of the bowel. The torn retracted sphincter muscle is brought up and repaired over the closed anal canal with chromic catgut. The rest of the operation to reconstitute the pelvic floor is carried out as described for colpoperineorrhaphy.

Liquid paraffin may be given from the third day to soften the motions, but emptying of the bowel should be discouraged for a week after the operation.

For the next delivery a wide episiotomy and guided forceps are imperative or Caesarean section may be necessary.

STRESS INCONTINENCE OF URINE

Stress incontinence due to incompetence of the sphincter mechanism must be distinguished from urgency and frequency of micturition, for the causes and treatment are different. All three symptoms may occur together, but stress incontinence frequently occurs alone. In nearly every case the outrolling of the urethra and sagging of the neck of the bladder, following coughing or increase in intra-abdominal pressure is the result of weakening of the supporting tissues during

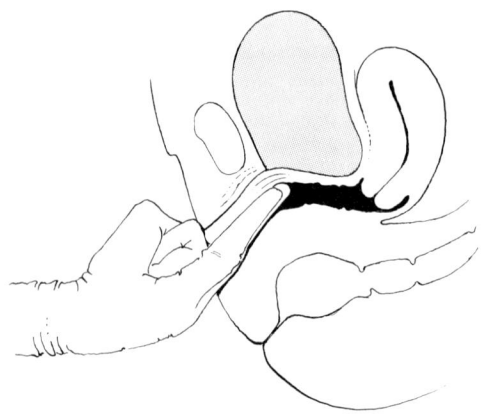

Fig. 45.7   Pressure lateral to bladder neck to demonstrate support.

pregnancy and labour. Incontinence can occur when there is a marked increase in intra-abdominal pressure in nulliparous women but it is rare for treatment to be requested or be necessary. If pressure is exerted on either side of the neck of the bladder by two fingers introduced into the vagina to stop descent of the bladder neck on coughing and thus stops the leak of urine, the case is probably a suitable one for operation (Fig. 45.7).

Work by Jeffcoate and others has shown that in many cases of 'stress incontinence' the main abnormality is a sagging of the area of the bladder neck and a loss of the posterior vaginal angle on straining. The posterior vaginal angle is normally lost during micturition and a similar loss of angle in straining allows urine to leak under 'stress'. Many cases however, require very full investigation with micturating and stress cystograms measurement of intra bladder pressures, cine radiography of detrusor action and other radiological expert investigation before full information is obtained.

In true stress incontinence where bladder neck sagging or loss of angle is determined, operation to restore the angle will be either

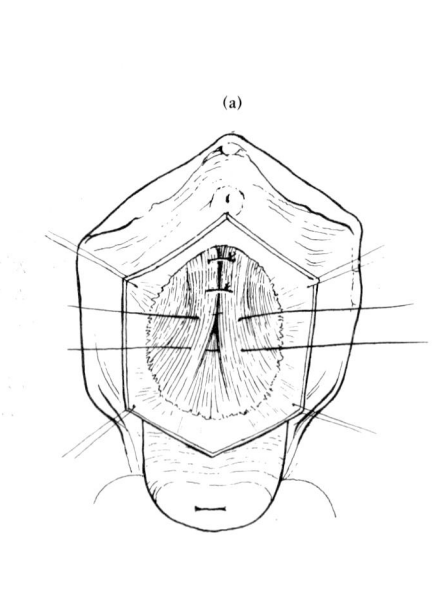

(a)

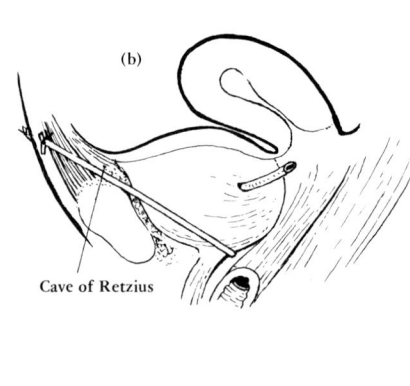

(b)

Cave of Retzius

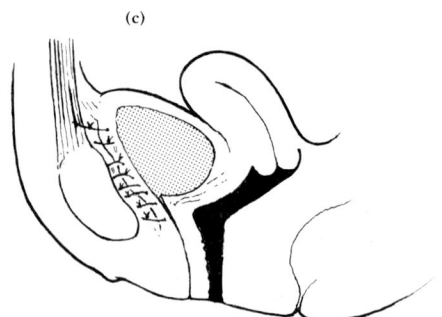

(c)

Fig. 45.8   (a) Kelly buttress. (b) Position of sling. (c) Marshall-Marchetti urethropexy.

partially or wholly curative. The simplest method is to perform an anterior wall repair and to buttress the bladder neck with supporting tissues from the side (Kelly stitches) (Fig. 45.8a). The bladder may then also be advanced on the cervix. Alternatively the bladder neck may be supported by transversalis fascia (Aldridge) or nylon slings placed under the bladder-neck and led through the cave of Retzius and through the rectus muscle (Fig. 45.8b). More recently, nylon net has been used in the sling from the rectus muscle to the under aspect of bladder-neck. Another method is to suture the peri urethral tissues and bladder to the back of the symphysis pubis and lower rectus sheath (Marshall Marchetti 'urethropexy') (Fig. 45.8c). There are however, other techniques of value in individual cases.

FISTULAE

These may result from:

1. Extension to the bladder of carcinoma of the cervix.
2. Injury during hysterectomy.
3. Injury during labour or delivery.
4. Radiation injury.

In malignant cases, closure of the fistula is impossible; but if the patient's condition is good transplantation of the ureters into the bowel may be undertaken as a palliative procedure or as part of the operation of anterior pelvic exenteration which involves removal of the uterus, tubes and ovaries, parametrium and bladder.

Bladder or ureteric fistulae following hysterectomy may heal if the condition is recognized quickly and the bladder drained continuously by catheter for one or two weeks.

Fistulae acquired during labour, as a result of direct trauma from instruments, should be closed at once and usually heal very well. If a fistula is discovered in the puerperium resulting from pressure necrosis, continuous drainage should be tried, but if this fails operation should be postponed for several weeks until any pelvic sepsis has subsided. Fistulae resulting from radiation are very difficult to treat and at least one year must be left to allow the radiation effect on the tissues to settle before attempts are made to close the fistula. The great majority of fistulae can be repaired by the vaginal route (see Chapter 41). The first step is to determine by cystoscopic examination the relative positions of the ureters and the fistula. The essential feature of the operation lies in the separation of the bladder from the anterior vaginal wall sufficiently to allow the fistula to be closed in layers *without tension*. Chromicized catgut is usually employed throughout, but in difficult cases the *vaginal* wall may be closed with silver wire or other non-absorbable suture material, which is removed some three weeks later. Special reviews should be consulted (see Chapter 41), and Lawson and Stewart (1967).

Ureterovaginal fistula

This usually results from injury at operation, e.g. removal of a broad ligament tumour or extended hysterectomy. If long enough the cut ureter can be satisfactorily implanted into the bladder; failing this, implantation into the colon is usually indicated. Joining the two ends of the ureter over a ureteric catheter, which is passed upwards from the bladder, may be successful. Occasionally, nephrectomy may be advisable provided the function of the other kidney is satisfactory.

Rectovaginal fistula

The fistula is usually low in the vagina and is most commonly the result of imperfect healing after repair of a complete tear of the perineum. It is, as a rule, best corrected by incising what remains of the perineal body, thus forming a complete tear which is repaired in the manner already described (p. 827).

Radiation fistulae follow the application of vaginal radium for carcinoma of the cervix. They are usually preventible if the proctitis which precedes them is properly treated (see Chapter 38). The fistula itself can rarely be closed and colostomy or surgical closure of the vagina may be necessary. However, occasionally the fistula may close itself after some months if relieving colostomy has been performed.

RETROVERSION OF UTERUS

Retroversion found in a woman without gynaecological symptoms scarcely requires treatment. Particularly when enlarged, the retroverted uterus may be associated with such symptoms as menorrhagia, pre-menstrual backache and a history of recurrent abortion and it may be thought necessary to secure it in the anteverted position by operation. Operation may be indicated in cases of infertility or dyspareunia, especially if an ovary has been carried down to the pelvic floor by the retroverted uterus. The surgical anteversion of the uterus may be part of an operation performed to treat endometriosis, chronic pelvic sepsis, to remove fibroids or after tubo uterine implantation.

Retroversion of the uterus frequently accompanies genital prolapse; but although the vaginal operation for prolapse will usually correct the position of the uterus, *abdominal operation for retroversion will not cure prolapse* of the uterus or vaginal walls.

Backache is seldom, if ever, caused by an uncomplicated retroversion. The pessary test, after manual correction of the displacement, will be of value in assessing the significance of the retroversion.

After manual correction of a retroversion a correctly fitting Hodge or ring pessary will often maintain the uterus in the anteverted position and the uterus may even stay forwards after the pessary has been removed. This is most likely to happen when the pessary is used in cases of puerperal retroversion.

The pessary can be used to find out whether the retroverted position of the uterus is causing symptoms or not, by observing what happens to the symptoms: (1) when the uterus is held in the anterior position by means of a pessary; (2) when the pessary is removed and the uterus falls backwards again. The result of this pessary test may help to determine whether operation should be undertaken or not. A number of operations have been devised to keep the uterus anteverted but the simplest method is to plicate both round ligaments with silk or linen sutures, so shortening them. This technique is particularly useful at the end of plastic operations on uterus or tubes. A Hodge pessary should be fitted to the vagina for 2–3 months to help support the uterus in its new position.

THE UTERUS

Myomectomy

The operation consists of the enucleation of fibroids from the uterine wall and reconstruction of the uterus. In the reproductive period

of life myomectomy is, as a rule, to be preferred to hysterectomy when the tubes and ovaries are healthy. Successful pregnancy may follow the procedure, and there is very little risk that the scar will rupture during labour. During pregnancy, however, myomectomy should be performed only under the most exceptional circumstances, for example, for severe and persistent pain due to degeneration of the fibroid, for the operation is apt to bring on premature labour, and haemorrhage may be so profuse and difficult to control that hysterectomy may be necessary.

Vaginal myomectomy
This is usually a simple procedure consisting of the removal of a pedunculated fibroid (fibroid polypus) lying in the cervical canal or hanging down into the vagina (Fig. 45.9). The pedicle is grasped and twisted until the tumour is separated or is cut as near as possible to its base.

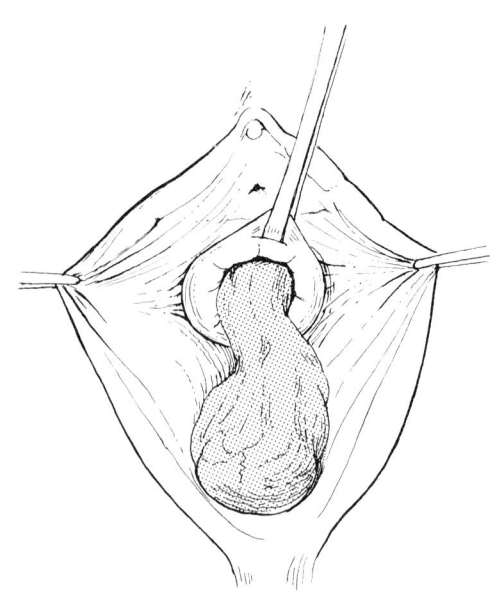

Fig. 45.9   Fibroid polyp.

If the fibroid polypus is infected, any operation necessary to remove other fibroids should be postponed for some time to allow the infection to subside.

Abdominal myomectomy
This operation may be easy or difficult according to the number, size and situation of the fibroids in the uterus (Fig. 45.10). As many of the fibroids as possible should be

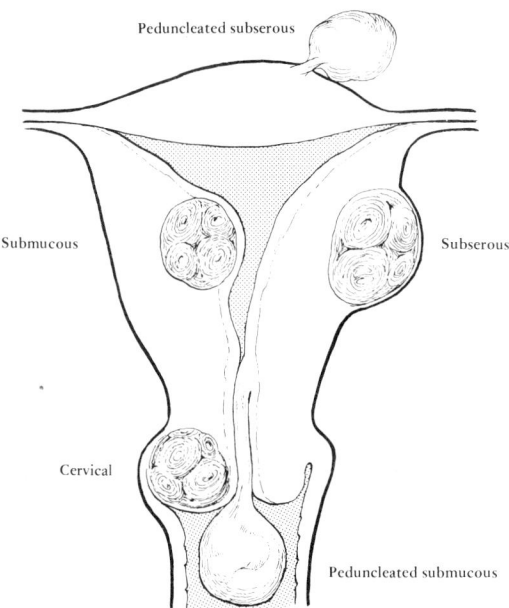

Fig. 45.10   Type and situation of fibromyomata.

removed through one main incision in the uterine wall, to diminish the risk of post-operative adhesions of bowel to the uterus. The cavity of the uterus should be opened so that a finger can be inserted to explore for the presence of small fibroids which might otherwise be missed.

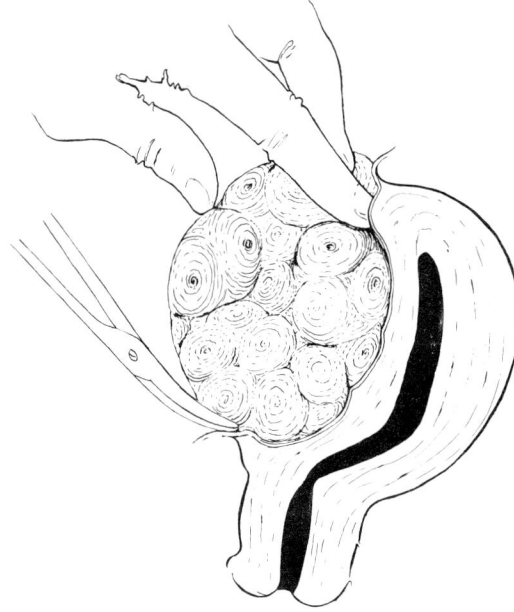

Fig. 45.11   Technique of myomectomy.

The incision in the uterine wall should be sufficiently deep to cut through the capsule of the tumour and thus disclose the plane of cleavage between it and the uterine muscle; the tumour is then enucleated with the finger and scissors (Fig. 45.11). It is essential to effect complete haemostasis in the bed of each fibroid since, if blood collects, it may become infected and a weak scar result. Interrupted sutures of catgut should be employed to obliterate the cavity rather than a continuous suture which may cause ischaemia of the muscle and necrosis. To lessen bleeding during the operation, a specially designed myomectomy clamp may be placed round the isthmus of the uterus to occlude the uterine vessels, and intestinal clamps on the infundibulopelvic ligaments to occlude the ovarian vessels. Alternatively a rubber tourniquet can be placed low down on the uterus so as to occlude the uterine vessels and the ovarian vessels in the infundibulopelvic ligaments. Occlusion of the vessels for the time required for myomectomy does not appear to increase liability to thrombosis and embolism, but the tourniquet may be loosened if necessary to flush the vessels if the period of occlusion is more than 30 minutes.

Hysterectomy

Indications

Hysterectomy may be performed for benign and malignant tumours of the uterus and also when malignant tumours of the ovaries are being removed. In some cases of pelvic endometriosis or inflammatory disease, the uterus may have to be removed. Hysterectomy is often the best treatment for excessive menstrual haemorrhage at or near the menopause. Many other indications are discussed in association with the text.

Varieties of hysterectomy

1. Total hysterectomy.
2. Subtotal hysterectomy.
3. Extended or 'Wertheim' hysterectomy.
4. Pelvic exenteration.
5. Vaginal hysterectomy.

1. *Total hysterectomy.* In the operation of hysterectomy the cervix is best removed, even in benign conditions, unless there is good reason to the contrary. This is particularly so in women who have borne children because of the risk of cancer of the cervix and because the cervix may be infected and remain a source of

discharge. A 'smear' should always have been previously examined to exclude the risk of a hidden carcinoma. The total operation is the more difficult procedure and the risk of injury to the bladder or ureters or of haematoma is greater.

The essential steps of the operation are shown in Figure 45.12. The upper parts of the broad ligaments and the round ligaments are clamped and cut, the ovaries being removed or not as indicated. The peritoneum across the lower part of the front of the uterus is incised and the bladder pushed down from the cervix and the top of the vagina. The uterine arteries are clamped close to the side of the uterus at the level of the isthmus, care being taken to avoid the ureters which lie just beneath them. The utero-sacral ligaments are next divided and the peritoneum dissected and pushed down from the back of the cervix. The vascular cellular tissue lateral to the vault of the vagina is clamped close to the cervix and cut, the vagina is then opened, and the incision is extended right round the cervix till the uterus can be lifted out. All the vessels are tied, the vaginal angles and vault closed, the para-metrial bundle attached as a support to the angle of the vaginal vault, and the pelvic peritoneum stitched together to cover the raw areas. In some cases an opening is left in the vaginal vault to allow drainage from the retro-peritoneal space, or preferably vacuum suction drainage is established where exceptional oozing is to be expected or where large raw areas are left.

2. *Subtotal hysterectomy*. Subtotal hysterectomy may be preferred when total hysterectomy would be technically very difficult or would

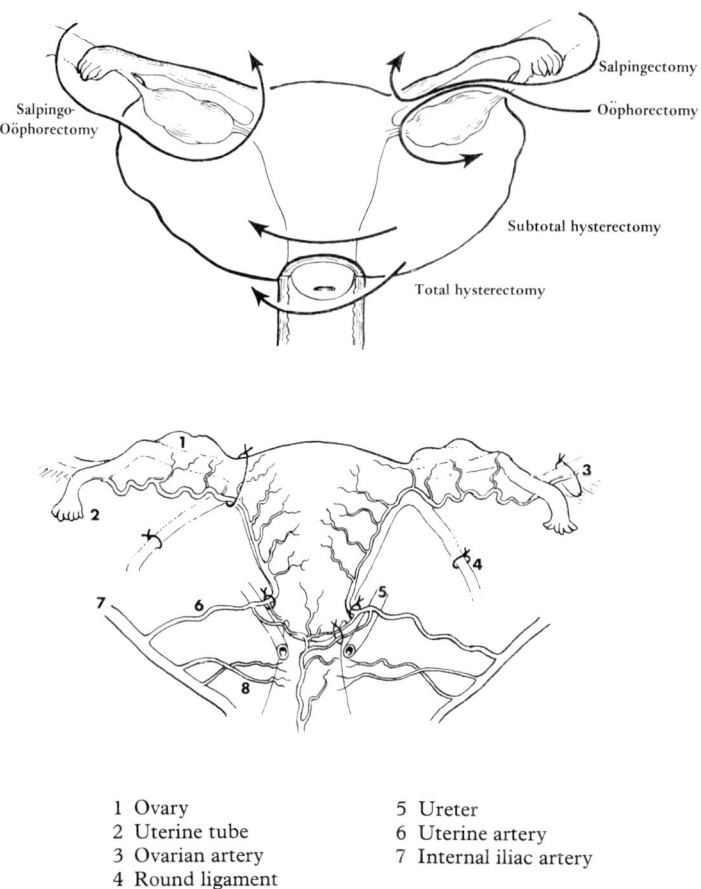

1 Ovary
2 Uterine tube
3 Ovarian artery
4 Round ligament

5 Ureter
6 Uterine artery
7 Internal iliac artery

Fig. 45.12   Extent of various operations associated with hysterectomy.

carry undue risk to bladder or bowel, or in the virginal woman where the risk of cervical carcinoma is negligible. In this operation the cervix is amputated just below the isthmus of the uterus and the edges of the cervix stump are oversewn. The bladder is not separated from the vaginal wall as in the total operation, nor is the dissection so deep in the pelvis (Fig. 45.13).

3. *Extended hysterectomy.* The operation of total hysterectomy is 'extended' in various either or both of the other organs (Fig. 45.15). Operation is limited to cases *without* gland involvement and where there is only early invasion of the other organ, or occasionally where there are bladder and rectal fistulae or where radiotherapy has failed. In the 'total' operation which carries a primary mortality of 5–15 per cent the ureters are transplanted to an ileal or colonic bladder, or into the descending colon; and the bladder, uterus, vagina, parametrium, rectum and anal canal are removed.

a   **b**

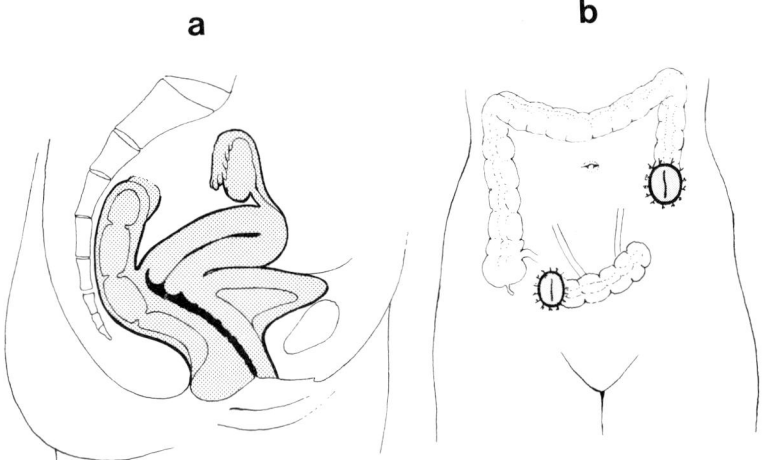

Fig. 45.13   The extent of exenteration. (a) The organs involved. (b) Colostomy and colonic bladder.

ways and in various degrees to meet different situations. In cases of carcinoma *in situ* of the cervix (especially where conization has not cleared the growth): in micro-invasive carcinoma of the cervix, or in carcinoma of the body of the uterus, it is customary to extend the operation to include a small area of parametrium, a length of uterosacral ligaments and about one inch of vagina. This operation may necessitate dissection and exposure of lower end of the ureters. In clinical cases of carcinoma of the cervix a very much wider dissection and removal of parametrium is performed and nearly half of the vagina is removed. Dissection and wide displacement of the ureters is necessary and the bladder has also to be deeply freed. Lymphadenectomy is also performed. This is the standard 'Wertheim' hysterectomy (Fig. 45.14).

4. *Exenteration.* The operation of pelvic exenteration is performed occasionally when there is extensive *local* malignant disease of uterus, bladder, vagina, or rectum involving

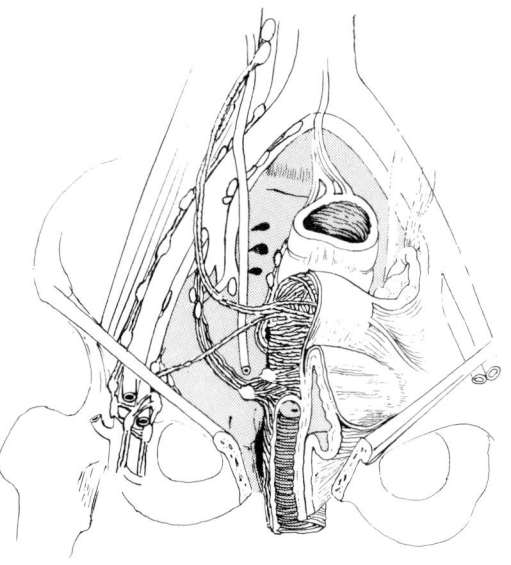

Fig. 45.14   Anatomy of the main pelvic structures.

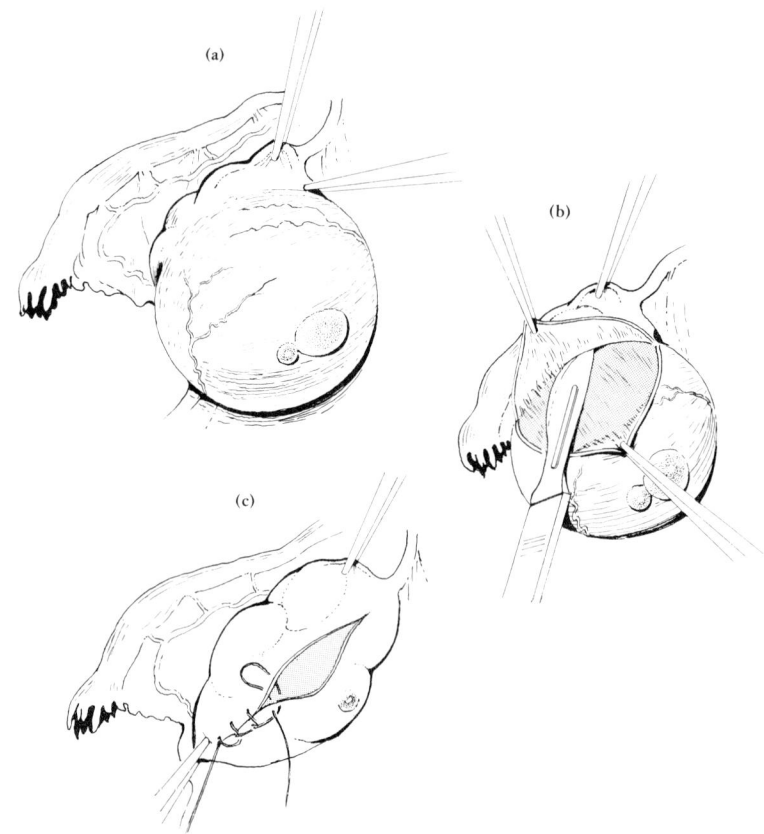

Fig. 45.15   Ovarian cystectomy.

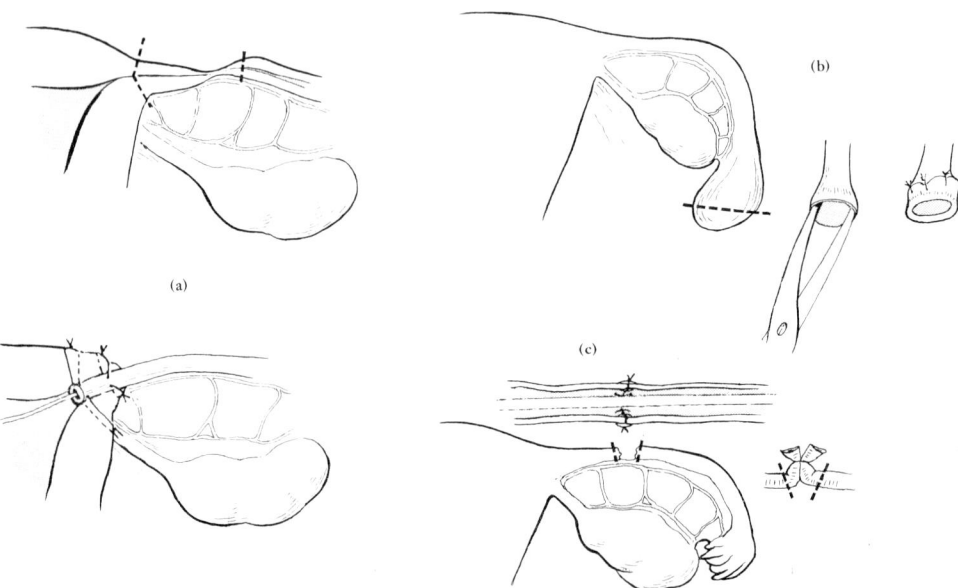

Fig. 45.16   Operations to restore tubal patency. (a) Implantation after cornual block. (b) Cuff salpingostomy for fimbrial block. (c) Anastomosis.

The anterior operation leaves the rectum and anal canal but has nearly as high a primary mortality since ureters are again transplanted. The posterior operation which is used when the vagina and rectum are involved has a much lower primary mortality, and is comparable with that of the abdomino-perineal resection of rectum for cancer of the rectum alone.

There is a very limited place for these operations; primary mortality is due to renal infection, peritonitis or occasionally to ileus and or haemorrhage or leaks from uretero-bowel anastomosis.

5. *Vaginal hysterectomy.* Removal of the uterus by the vaginal route may be performed as an alternative to abdominal hysterectomy in many cases. It is, however, specially indicated where hysterectomy and pelvic floor repair are both required. Vaginal hysterectomy is sometimes necessary as part of the technique to permit an adequate repair of the pelvic floor.

6. *Pelvic lymphadenectomy.* In most cases of malignant disease of uterus, vulva, or vagina, biopsy of pelvic lymph glands may be performed as a diagnostic procedure and where radical surgery is intended an attempt at total pelvic lymphadenectomy is made. The main gland groups involved are: parametrial, obturator, internal and external iliac, common iliac, lower aortic and sacral. In carcinoma of the body of the uterus the first glands involved may be those lying on the lower end of the inferior vena cava just lateral to the bifurcation of the aorta. In ovarian carcinoma the para aortic glands at the site of insertion of the renal vein are the first involved but no attempt is made to remove them (Fig. 45.16). It has recently become customary to inspect routinely para aortic glands before attempting radical curative surgery for carcinoma cervix or body.

THE OVARY

Ovarian cystectomy

This operation is performed for simple cysts of the ovary. Normal ovarian tissue should always be retained if possible provided the blood supply is intact. This situation applies in inflammatory conditions, endometriosis, ectopic pregnancy, etc., but especially with simple ovarian cysts which displace and do not

replace ovarian tissue. (The solid tumours, Brenner, fibroma etc., replace ovarian tissue.) Even with very large cysts the capsule is composed of compressed thickened ovarian tissue and the cyst itself can be shelled out and the ovary reconstituted by infolding the capsule etc. (Fig. 45.17). Simple serous cysts

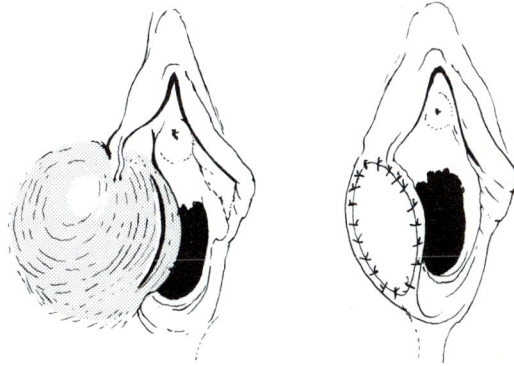

Fig. 45.17 Marsupialization of a 'bartholins' cyst or abscess.

are easily enucleated but there may be difficulty with large cysts such as pseudomucinous cystadenomatos or cysts associated with adhesions such as endometrial cysts.

Ovariotomy

This term is applied only to the operation of removal of the ovary for neoplasm. It was first performed successfully by Ephraim MacDowell of Kentucky in 1809 and led to the development of abdominal surgery.

If malignant disease is suspected the abdominal incision should be long enough to allow the tumour to be removed intact; in those circumstances tapping of a cyst is rarely advisable. The tumour should be lifted out so that its pedicle may be clamped and cut. The pedicle consists of the infundibulopelvic ligament, the upper part of the broad ligament, the Fallopian tube and the ovarian ligament. These structures are transfixed and tied with catgut; the round ligament is then sutured to the back of the uterus to cover the raw stump of the pedicle.

If torsion of the pedicle has occurred, the structures are swollen and engorged with blood. The pedicle should be untwisted before clamps are applied, otherwise haemorrhage may occur when clamps are replaced by ligature. A retroperitoneal haematoma may collect quickly if this precaution is neglected. If there are large vessels in the infundibulo-pelvic ligament double clamps should be applied and the external clamp first removed when the ligature is applied. A careful inspection should be carried out to see if there is any evidence that the tumour is malignant especially of the peritoneum, omentum, liver and other ovary.

Every ovarian tumour should be inspected after removal and if it is obviously malignant the uterus and other ovary should be removed. If the patient is young or the nature of the tumour in doubt, the abdomen should be closed and the histological report awaited. If malignancy is proved, the wisest course may be to reopen the abdomen and remove the uterus and remaining ovary. Frozen section is of little value for identifying malignancy in ovarian tumours. There is a special problem with 'sex cell' tumours (*see* Chapter 38).

THE FALLOPIAN TUBES

Operations to restore the patency of known occluded tubes may be carried out if no other reason for infertility exists in the wife and if the fertility of the husband is proved. The best results follow the separation of adhesions surrounding the outer end of tubes which are otherwise healthy; from plastic operations where the block is at the uterine end of an otherwise healthy tube (30 per cent pregnancy), or from re-anastomosis of healthy tubes where minimal resection has been performed as a sterilization procedure (40–50 per cent pregnant). Tubal infection often results in pathological changes in the muscle wall as well as in the mucous membrane and may cause blocking at either the inner or outer end of the tube, but the associated pathological change makes operation less successful. Correction of tubal occlusion by operation does not guarantee normal tubal function, but pregnancy may follow operation if the tubes are not grossly abnormal. Ectopic pregnancy is a real risk. The operation may be carried out if the patient is keenly desirous of pregnancy, though the proportion of successes is small.

Tubal implantation, tubal reconstruction and salpingostomy

Following sterilization or infection the Fallopian tubes may be blocked at the uterine

cornu, or in any part of the tube out to the fimbrial end. In inflammatory conditions the tubal patency may be totally disrupted as in tuberculosis and no reparative surgery is possible. Where the block is in the cornu or close to it and there is a length of healthy tube the tubes may be implanted within the fundus through small openings bored or cut where the tubal orifice normally exists. When the tubes have been blocked or separated elsewhere anastomoses of the cut ends may be possible (Fig. 45.18). Blockage at the fimbrial ends

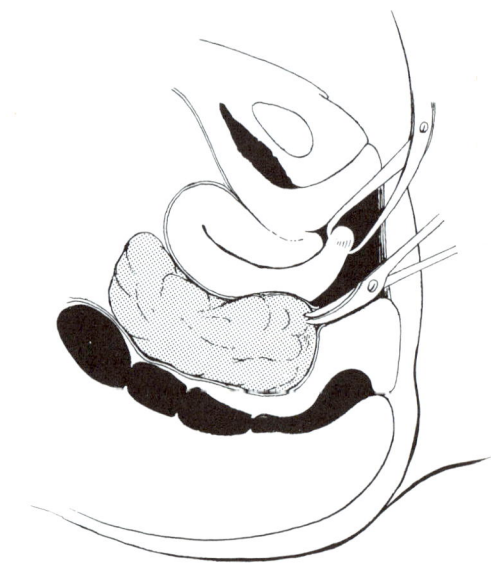

Fig. 45.18   Posterior culdotomy.

may be opened and the mucosa turned back as a cuff or specially designed plastic hoods used to maintain patency in healing. Hydrotubation with 25mg of hydrocortisone in 10mm saline daily through plastic tubes left *in situ* helps after the first 5 days and some 40 per cent may get pregnant.

In all cases plastic rods are used within the tubes to maintain patency and to support the repair for some 6 weeks. These operations are moderately successful, and the success rate may reach 30–40 per cent when the tubes are healthy and a sufficient length is left to allow ovum maturation during transport. Salpingo-stomy of blocked fimbria is less often successful since such closure is usually due to inflammatory disease which interferes with tubal peristalsis and cilial action.

Salpingectomy—removal of tubes

Salpingectomy for tubal pregnancy
When the tube containing an ectopic gestation is removed care should be taken to avoid injuring the blood supply to the ovary, which can usually be conserved. Removal of the ovum with conservation of the tube may occasionally be carried out, but if its patency has not been destroyed the risk of a second pregnancy in the tube is considerable. With a few exceptions, therefore, the tube should be removed.

If intraperitoneal haemorrhage from *tubal rupture* has been severe, blood transfusion should be commenced immediately before the operation and continued during it. There may be so much blood in the abdomen that the source of the bleeding cannot be identified. The uterus should therefore be located by touch and raised so that the tubes can be seen. If the affected tube is grossly swollen it is quickly recognized; but when rupture occurs early, as in isthmic pregnancy, the tube is little enlarged and the site of the rupture is more difficult to see and no mass is palpable on pelvic examination. The tube and ovary should be removed if bleeding has been severe and there would be difficulty in separating and conserving the ovary.

In *tubal abortion*, where the ovum may be protruding through the dilated abdominal ostium, the operation may not take place for days or weeks after the onset of the initial symptoms. In such cases the swollen tube will be found embedded in a mass of dark clotted blood filling the pelvis (haematocele), often with small bowel lightly adherent.

The tube is removed after clamping the mesosalpinx and the inner end of the tube, the clamps being replaced by ligatures which are understitched to prevent slipping. All manipulations should be performed very gently as the tissues may be very friable. The stump of the tube may be covered over by stitching the round ligament over the cornu of the uterus. The blood clot is then removed from the pelvis and abdomen, but in acute cases where the blood is mostly fluid it is unnecessary to remove the blood as it is rapidly absorbed. In any case, since the patient may be collapsed, speed is essential. Before the abdomen is closed the other tube and ovary should be examined and a careful description of their condition recorded in the case notes; in some cases light adhesions may have formed round blood clot and these should be separated.

Salpingectomy and salpingo-oophorectomy for inflammatory lesions
These operations are rarely indicated in *acute* infections of the tube and ovary, but may be necessary to relieve symptoms due to chronic inflammatory lesions. Inflamed tubes and ovaries quickly become adherent to surrounding structures. When there is pus in the tube it may track into the ovary and a tubo-ovarian abscess may be formed. In such cases adhesions to the pelvic wall and bowel may be so dense that surgical removal may be very difficult.

THE VULVA

Benign lesions calling for operation include simple abscess, urethral caruncle, Bartholin's duct cyst or abscess, and various simple tumours where surgery is local. Total vulvectomy may be needed for skin disease and radical or extended vulvectomy for cancer.

Urethral caruncle. A simple adenomatous polyp is removed and the base cauterized lightly. A malignant caruncle is investigated by biopsy and then suitably treated. The commonest type of caruncle is the granulomatous caruncle at the posterior aspect of the urethral orifice which is often associated with chronic infection of the Skene's para urethral ducts. The caruncle itself may be cauterized or excised. The Skene's ducts should be opened with the incision or cauterized with a fine point.

Bartholin's cyst or abscess. This is a cyst or abscess of the gland duct with the gland itself in the wall. In both cases marsupialization is performed. The cyst is opened just on the vagina/vulvar skin junction with a long vertical incision. The walls of the cyst are then stitched to the opened skin edges. If an abscess is present hot baths may be needed for a few days. When the gland is chronically infected it may need to be excised.

Perineotomy. Enlargement of the vulvar orifice may be necessary to allow intercourse or to permit access for proper examination or for surgery high in the vagina. Access can usually be obtained by wide episiotomy, usually mediolateral, and the incision is later closed to restore the perineum to its original state or carefully repaired to permit later access.

To permit intercourse when the perineal body is tight from congenital reasons or after too enthusiastic repair it is necessary to retain the vaginal skin without scar and to incise deeply into the superficial perineal muscles to obtain an adequate opening.

The skin at the vaginal orifice is incised transversely, the vaginal skin made loose and free for about one inch—the perineal muscles and perineum incised in the mid-line vertically and the intact mucosa then drawn down and the whole wound stitched transversely.

Posterior culdotomy. Most abscesses in the pelvis whether para-tubal or tubo-ovarian tend to settle in the Pouch of Douglas and can be drained through the posterior fornix where the peritoneum is separated by aveolar tissue only from the vaginal skin. The cervix is held well up and forward by a volsellum on the posterior lip. The abscess is located in the mid-line with a large syringe held needle (if proof be required) and then opened with blunt pointed scissors which nibble (strictly in the mid-line) through vagina and abscess wall. The incision should be opened widely and a tube drain inserted to maintain patency (Fig. 45.19).

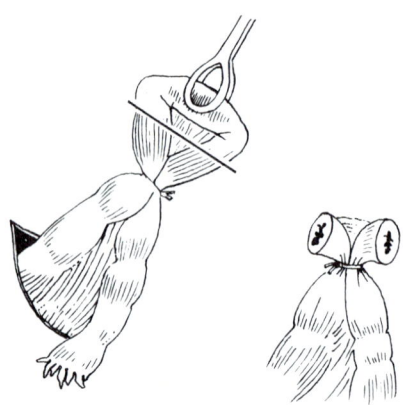

Tubal sterilization

Fig. 45.19   Tubal sterilization—Pomeroy.

Simple vulvectomy. This operation is occasionally required for atrophic or other non malignant changes of the vulvar skin. Incision extends round the labia majora and the inner incision is just external to hymen and urethra. The skin is removed alone and the extent of excision depends on the extent of the lesion.

Radical vulvectomy. It is primarily to Way (1954) that we owe the development of extensive and radical surgery for carcinoma of the vulva. Modern techniques are somewhat less extensive than those originally advocated Charles (1972).

The operation removes the whole of the labia majora and minora and the mons and all superficial tissues down to bone and fascia. If the lesion is posterior the perineal body also may need to be removed. The superficial and deep inguinal glands are removed and the gland of Cloquet is used as a marker of the extent of spread. If it is involved then the external iliac nodes may require removal extra peritoneally through an extension of the inguinal incision. Modern anaesthesia, subdermal post-operative suction drainage and skin flap or grafting techniques allow the operation to be well tolerated by the older women in whom it is frequently required.

PAIN RELIEF

Much pelvic pain arises from disease which is amenable to therapy but occasionally surgical cure is not possible, and pain relief alone is required. There are two operations currently of value:

Pre-sacral neurectomy may be used in severe untreatable dysmenorrhoea in some cases of endometriosis, and rarely in malignant disease.

It is performed by removing the presacral or hypogastric nerve elements which lie in the triangle formed by the common iliac arteries and the promontory of the sacrum. After opening the posterior peritoneum the whole wedge of tissue down to bone is removed. The middle sacral artery should be preserved. There may be temporary interference with bladder function.

Antero lateral cordotomy. All patients with intractable pain due to malignant disease should be discussed with a neurosurgeon who can frequently offer much help especially for unilateral pain in the legs or occasionally for central pain.

The sensations of pain and temperature run separately in the antero-lateral tracts of the spinal cord. Division of the antero-lateral tracts may be undertaken by open or closed techniques and are usually unilateral or rarely bilateral. Open operation requires general anaesthesia and removal of one lamina and transection is made on the contralateral side to the pain. Pelvic pain is often not relieved except by bilateral cordectomy with permanent retention of urine and/or constipation in 10 per cent of cases.

Percutaneous cordotomy is achieved by a sharp pointed electrode passed through a lumber puncture needle introduced into the subarachnoid space between C1 and C2.

Cervical cordotomy carries some risk of interference with respiratory pathways.

Intrathecal injection of hypertonic saline (20ml 7·5 per cent) into the subarachnoid space under general anaesthesia is followed by hyperventilation and tachycardia for some 20 minutes.

STERILIZATION

It is relatively easy to render a woman infertile by operations on the Fallopian tubes or a man by vasectomy but it is difficult to restore fertility, therefore sterilization should be done only after careful consideration of the long as well as the short term consequences. The demand however, for permanent infertility is rising and many thousands of patients request operation. As a post-partum procedure performed on the first day after delivery or at the end of a Caesarean section operation it is a very worthwhile procedure and should be more frequently performed provided it has been calmly discussed with the patient during the pregnancy. It should not be done post-partum in a woman with a history of venous thrombosis or with extensive varicose veins.

Many abdominal operations for sterilization have been advocated.

1. *Pomeroy method*
This has proved successful in at least 98 per cent of cases. It is a simple procedure and is, therefore, particularly suitable when sterilization is carried out soon after childbirth. Patients with a history of extensive varicosites of leg veins or phlebitis should not be done in the puerperium.

The tube is lifted up near its uterine end and a loop of the thin area of tube ligated with plain catgut *without* preliminary crushing with forceps. The loop of the tube is then cut off. This is later followed by retraction and fibrosis of the ends so that they become incorporated into the free margin of the broad ligament. Catgut should be used for the ligature and not silk or linen, for the latter may cut through the tube wall and allow the tube to become patent again. The only risk is that the tube may slip out of the ligature and, some surgeons use a stitch through the mesosalpinx.

2. *Other method*
In other techniques the tube is sectioned between ligatures and the cut ends left free or alternatively buried beneath the round ligament. This is particularly useful for the outer free tubal end as it prevents ultimate torsion. In the Madlener technique the tube is crushed and ligated in two places without section.

Obviously salpingectomy, hysterectomy, vaginal hysterectomy and even Caesarean hysterectomy can be used to achieve sterilization and are used where indicated. There is some virtue in the older parous patient in offering hysterectomy which eliminates the risk of later cervical or body carcinoma. There is also a high incidence of menorrhagia requiring later hysterectomy in such patients.

3. *Laparoscopy*
Sterilization by laparoscopy is probably best done by diathermy of the tubes about 1cm from the cornu *without* section (Fig. 45.1).

Methods using clips have in general not been a success (Wortman, 1974), but recently instrumental ligation has been successfully achieved (Clarke, 1972).

It is extremely important that the operation be done under clear vision with the tube lifted clear of bowel and other vulnerable tissues at the time of burning or section. The diathermy current should not be applied except for the brief moment of actual burning and preferably the leads should be disconnected except when actually required. It is also recommended that it is quite unnecessary to burn in more than one place and that should be at the site where the tube is thinnest.

The hazards are, burn damage to bowel, damage to blood vessels of mesosalpinx and abdominal wall, air insufflation of bowel or tearing especially if old scars are present and of course damage to major vessels from the trochar.

Laparoscopy can be undertaken with the simplest equipment in the tropical or primitive setting, but in general the patient should rest for 6 hours or overnight after such procedure.

Failure results from inadvertent coagulation of the round or ovarian ligaments, inadequate coagulation of the tubes or the patient may already be pregnant at the time of operation. *Operation should be done early in the cycle or routine curettage should precede it.*

Laparotomy should be used for post delivery sterilization but laparoscopic techniques are suitable for post abortion or interval cases.

Temporary sterilization by plugging the tubes with little plastic plugs vie the laparoscope has been suggested but this is very experimental.

Vasectomy or male sterilization

This has clearly emerged as one of the simplest, most popular and available forms of voluntary family planning and it is of special use in the countries of the Asian sub continent (Wartman & Piotro, 1973) (Richart & Drager, 1969). The operation does not significantly affect male hormonal balance, desire, capacity for erection or ejaculation of semen. The operation which involves the cutting, tying, coagulation or clipping of the vas deferens through a small incision in the scrotum. If done under local anaesthesia the patient ought to be able to go home after a brief rest for 15–30 mins. It is important when considering this operation to understand that preliminary counselling is required so that the male can understand the procedure and definitive consequences of the operation. He should also understand there are certain minor risks. It should also be made very clear that vasectomy does not provide sterilization until sperm already stored in the reproductive system are ejaculated and this may take some days, weeks or months. The sperm within the male tract have a very long life and can remain capable of fertilization. Three negative sperm tests are essential before the patient may consider that he is sterile. Depending on techniques the operation may be reversible but it should not be used in any case where he wishes further children. The operation may not be of value in communities where the ability of the male to make women pregnant is looked upon as an essential part of his masculinity.

In most vasectomy techniques both vasa are cut, the ends are then sealed by ligating, coagulation or clipping and a segment may or may not be removed.

Ninety-five per cent of patients are sterile within ten weeks of operation. Ninety-eight per cent of patients are sperm free after twenty-four ejaculations.

The complications of operation are haematoma and sepsis, occur in a moderately small percentage of cases (Calderone, MS, 1970).

OPERATIONS FOR TERMINATION OF PREGNANCY

Uterine aspiration

The bladder is emptied and bimanual pelvic examination performed to assess the size of the uterus, its position and its mobility and to exclude other anomaly. Uterine size less than 12 weeks' size are suitable.

The vaginal vault and cervix may be cleaned with chlorhexidine or provodine iodine solution.

General anaesthesia may be used or paracervical block (3–12ml of 1–2 per cent Xylocaine injected into the base of the broad ligament and lateral walls of the lower uterine segment, sites at 3, 5, 7 and 9 o'clock). Intravenous pethidine valium is very useful if out-patient operation is required in early cases. Ergometrine 0·25mgm *must* be injected intravenously before commencing operation.

Vagina and cervix are cleaned, cervix is grasped with volsella and the uterus sounded. The cervix may need to be dilated before the necessary plastic suction curette can be inserted. Fine curettes 3–5mm can be used for the very earliest pregnancies up to a firm curette of 10cm for later pregnancies. The curette is moved back and forth and rotated through 180 degrees. The entire aspiration takes 2–10 minutes, at pressures up to 20 inch of mercury (50cm). The uterus is then curetted to guarantee that it is empty.

Menstrual regulation to terminate pregnancy

This procedure which advocates suction by a fine suction curette 4 or 5mm in diameter from the week before to 14 days after the missed period (3–6 weeks from LMP) has a wide following in the lay press. It is sometimes advocated as a method for personal use by the patient as an alternative to contraception (van der Glut, 1973).

There is little doubt that such techniques used as a routine aspiration technique of an early pregnancy are valid and acceptable, but should be used only as pregnancy termination methods with all the preliminary pre-operative checks of haemoglobin, Rhesus, general disease check, cervical smear, and (in the United Kingdom) with the permission and abortion recommendation forms signed.

Hysterotomy

Abdominal hysterotomy with a classical

anterior wall incision (or a low transverse where possible) in the uterus may be used. It is usually confined to pregnancies later than 12 weeks and where sterilization is coincidentally performed. It may be required preparatory to radiation or surgery in cervical carcinoma or in some other situation where vaginal delivery is undesirable. It carries a greater maternal risk than other forms of termination and there is some risk of scar rupture in subsequent pregnancy.

Dilatation and curettage
This may be used similarly to suction in very early pregnancy and sponge holder or ovum forceps will succeed in termination up to 8 weeks. It is, however, likely to produce more bleeding than aspiration.

Risks are blood loss, uterine perforation in some 1–2 per cent of patients requiring laparotomy.

Prostaglandin
The use of prostaglandin techniques are described in Chapter 43.

CORRECTION OF CONGENITAL ANOMALY

Hermaphroditism, transsexualism and other anomalies of development or behaviour occasionally call for reconstructive surgery to convert the external genitalia to confirm with the elected sex. Occasionally atrophic testes may require removal to allow proper feminization or to avoid the risk of malignant change.

Imperforate anal canals and other *cloacal* anomalies require careful assessment and surgical correction but usually this is best done by someone who has a special interest or experience in such reparative surgery in the very young.

Imperforate hymen. In this situation there is a stout membrane closing the vagina just above the introitus. In the young child fluid may collect to form a hydrocolpos but usually the condition presents with retained menses (Chapter 34). A cruciate incision right down through the hymen ring is best. The blood should be allowed to drain and no douching used.

Vaginal septae. A longitudinal anteroposterior complete or partial septum may co-exist with a double uterus and double cervix and it is rarely necessary or advisable to deal with this surgically.

A transverse septum producing blind pockets or a diaphragm high in the vagina may be best ignored or dilated with graduated dilators. Surgical excision tends to leave a tight ring. If such a septum is found at the time of delivery it is usually best to perform a Caesarean section rather than disrupt with forceps delivery.

Doubling of uterus. All degrees of doubling exist from total failure of fusion of the Mullerian ducts to total fusion except for a mid-line uterine fibrous fundal dip. Occasionally one horn is atrophic, or blind and forms a menstrual blood cyst and must be removed.

Totally double and single horn uteri rarely cause serious difficulty in reproduction although the first pregnancy may abort. Partial doubling, however, often seriously interferes with pregnancy with at the best retained placenta and at the worst regular early abortion. Uteroplasty to remove the septum or unite two horns may be worthwhile, where some two to three abortions are associated with a proven lesion. It is often not easy to be certain before operation whether there are two separate horns or a thick septum. The operation is most successful where there is a single vagina and single cervix (Fig. 45.20c).

Subsequent delivery should be by Caesarean section and hospital rest for the last 6–8 weeks is advised.

Absence of vagina. May occur as simple congenital anomaly because of failure of formation or of canalization of the vaginal buds (Chapter 6) and is of course seen in 'testicular feminization'. Occasionally the uterus, tubes and ovaries are normal and the condition presents as a haematometra with no vagina on inspection. A vagina can be formed by burrowing in the perineal body between rectum and urethra and the space opens fairly easily up to cervix or peritoneum. The space may be maintained by a mould covered with a split skin graft or by a mould alone.

Williams (1964) has recently developed a simple operation using the labia minora and the perineal skin to construct a pocket vagina which is an alternative and can be used especially where the vagina has been shortened after surgery.

Urethral diverticulum. Removal of a urethral

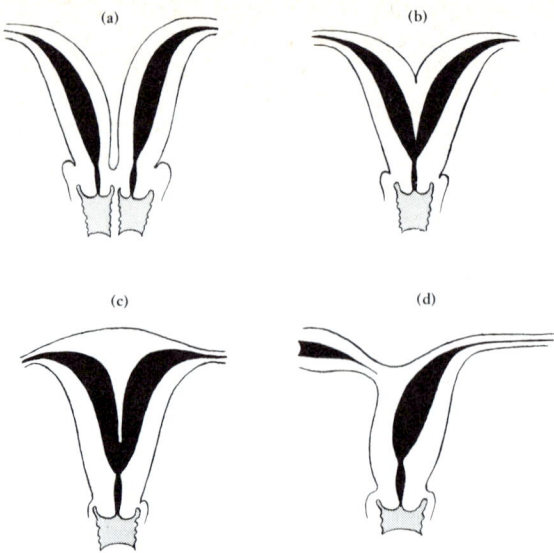

Fig. 45.20 Uterine anomalies. (a) Double uterus and vagina—didelphus. (b) Double uterus with single cervix—bicornus unicollis. (c) Subseptate. (d) Uterus with rudimentary horn.

diverticulum is best achieved by incision over and into the diverticulum itself, to expose the narrow neck as it arises from urethra. The excess diverticulum wall is then removed and the neck closed by transverse sutures supported by fibro muscular peri urethral tissue.

OTHER OPERATIONS

Repair of incisional hernia

Incisional hernia may occur in mid-line wounds or where there is a serious degree of devarication of the rectus muscles. The low transverse incision is rarely associated with herniation except occasionally at its outer ends.

In repair the edges of the hernia should be approached from the lateral aspects, the sheath having first been exposed. Great care should be taken in opening the hernial peritoneal sac which often contains adherent bowel or omentum.

Once the sac is exposed and opened and adherent bowel or omentum made free the excess sac is excised and the peritoneum closed. The muscles are then brought together to close the wound making certain that the apposing edges are raw and will adhere.

The anterior sheath is then closed in an overlapping technique to form a firm support.

Occasionally through and through muscles and peritoneum sutures will be advisable.

Rarely it is necessary to use foreign material, e.g. tantalum gauze or mesh to support the wound.

Bowel damage

During pelvic surgery the bowel wall may be damaged or torn. Superficial damage or minimal rents may be dealt with by oversewing or closure in two layers with interrupted fine catgut or linen. Extensive damage may require resection with or without relieving colostomy, but this should be very rare.

Resection of small bowel may be necessary on occasion when the bowel is involved in inflammatory adhesion or in malignant disease. Where the risk is expected pre-operative bowel preparation is mandatory and surgical help should be arranged.

Damage to large pelvic veins may occur during major pelvic surgery especially where gland dissection is being undertaken. Adequate equipment to allow temporary occlusion of veins is often life saving and will allow repair to be calmly undertaken or time to call for help from a vascular surgeon. Such venous bleeding can always be temporarily arrested by pack pressure.

OTHER PROCEDURES

Depending on his attitudes or experience the gynaecologist will look upon colostomy (permanent or temporary), ureteric transplant to bladder, colonic or ileal conduit, repair of a wound hernia, and ligature of ileac veins as part of his routine or will refer cases to a surgical or urological colleague. Certainly these operations are all required in gynaecology and should be part of the routine training of the gynaecologist. They are so rarely required, however, that it is often best to call for help from a colleague more experienced in the particular field.

POST OPERATIVE CARE

All operations are hazardous and especially so when the patient is already debilitated from anaemia, chronic disease, or infection, or has cardiac or pulmonary disease. No operation should therefore be undertaken lightly and adequate recovery supervision is necessary even when no anaesthetic is used.

The immediate post operative recovery of the patient is greatly facilitated by the provision of an *intensive care recovery unit* staffed by experienced personnel and constantly supervised by the anaesthetist.

This is a unit separate from the coronary care unit or the unit offering respiratory support or for that matter the unit responsible for resuscitation from major trauma although it resembles all three.

Facilities for cardiovascular and respiratory resuscitation must be fully available although probably rarely used. However, dehydration, bacteraemic shock and severe post-operative acidosis can create immense and urgent problems even though they are rare (*see* Chapter 31).

Mainly in such a unit respiratory and cardiovascular responses are checked, intravenous fluids are given and preliminary antibiotic therapy stated. Once the patients are clinically recovered from anaesthesia and respiratory and cardiovascular functions are normal they can be returned to the ward.

Post-operative care after pelvic floor repair
The patient is encouraged to move the legs from the first day and also to turn gently from side to side. She should be encouraged to get out of bed as soon as she feels able to do so, at the latest by the second or third day.

Deep breathing exercises should be given. The bladder may be catheterized six-hourly if the patient cannot void, or alternatively a catheter may be kept in the bladder for the first two or three days. The bowels should move on the fourth or fifth day but violent purgation should be avoided. The perineal area must be kept dry till the part has healed. Vaginal douches should be given only if discharge is present. This sometimes occurs when the vaginal catgut stitches separate about two weeks after operation. The patient may leave hospital after 10-12 days and fourteen further days convalescence is advisable. Full heavy duties should not be resumed till about 2-3 months after the operation. She should be given clear instructions regarding rehabilitation.

CONVALESCENCE
Day case patients should be early to bed that night and many will return to full duty the next day. Other patients should probably convalesce if possible, for a period similar in length to that spent in hospital. Many patients after hysterectomy for menorrhagia or pelvic inflammatory disease are slower to recover and radical extensive surgery, however, requires 3-4 months gradual convalescence before full convalescence is achieved.

SEDATION
Any pain should be relieved post operatively by aspirin, panadol or if necessary by morphia or pethidine. Patients with epidural or spinal anaesthesia usually have little pain in the first few hours especially if top up is used. Many surgeons use routine four or six hourly morphine or pethidine for 36 hours. Respiratory depression should be watched. Even patients after minor surgical conditions benefit from sedation on the first evening.

DIET
In many cases intravenous fluid is continued for the first post-operative 24 hours, and then fluids to light diet are gradually introduced.

BED REST
Most patients after major surgery are up by the first 48 hours and walking by the fourth to fifth day and home on the eighth or ninth day. Older women and patients after extensive pelvic floor repair, or extensive radical surgery should be mobilized a little slower and a little more gently but 12-14 days in hospital is usually adequate even after such surgery.

FOLLOW UP

After minor surgery especially termination or if curettage has been performed there may be short term menstrual upset. After major abdominal or pelvic surgery vault or wound haematomas may discharge especially if sepsis has supervened. These conditions should have been noted before the patient left the ward.

Healing of vaginal wounds is slow and it may be some three to four weeks before discharge ceases. Extensive surgery takes, of course, longer.

After extended surgery for malignant disease thick oedematous bands exist in the parametrium for many months and even after some years may still exist.

After laparoscopy, especially with diathermy sterilization, some infection may arise and pelvic pain and tenderness may exist and require rest and antibiotic therapy.

Many minor conditions do not require follow up except, of course, to discuss further therapy, say for menorrhagia, but all major and all laparoscopy cases must be seen by the surgeon six to eight weeks after discharge. Cases of malignant disease in all its stages will, of course, be followed indefinitely by the oncological group.

Techniques of wound repair and wound healing

It is essential to avoid haemorrhage into the healing wound as clot will liquefy and a cystic haematoma will form. If it is likely to be unavoidable the wound should be drained by suction. Retained foreign material will inhibit healing and if non-absorbing sutures become infected a sinus may result.

Suture material and techniques of suturing vary and change with much rapidity. In general, catgut is used for peritoneum and fat and non-absorbing material for sheath and skin. In pelvic floor repairs catgut is usually used throughout.

There is no difference in the tensile strength of wounds sutured by interrupted or continuous sutures provided that the continuous sutures do not strangle the blood supply to the edges.

Wound healing depends on the local tissue response to injury, Douglas (1963).

The basic principles are fibroplasia in the depths and epithelial migration on the surface, but this actual healing process follows a preliminary period of traumatic inflammation for the first 2–3 days.

Protein leaks from the venules and the capillaries between the endothelial cells and this plasma protein forms the basis of the inflammatory exudate. This is followed by a phase of invasion by leucocytes and then by macrophages from the circulation which clean up the wound. Fibroblast development follows over the next 14 days and normally a quickly healed scar results.

Wound healing is disturbed by protein deficiency, ascorbic acid deficiency and, of course, is less likely to be efficient in the patient with malignant disease.

WOUND CARE

It is customary to apply no dressing to the wound or at the most a light dressing to protect from bed clothes. The wound should require no special care. Sutures can be removed any time from the fifth to seventh day or as late as the twelfth day when the wound has been resutured.

Haemorrhage from the wound may respond to pressure or require suture. Wound haematoma may discharge after 4–5 days or if infected, earlier.

Wound infection

The factors responsible for wound infection are diverse. It would appear that the infection rate in clean wounds, e.g. elective hysterectomy should be less than 2 per cent. Where the wound is associated with open pus or spillage from bowel the infection rate may rise to nearly 40 per cent.

The rate rises with—increased pre-operative hospital stay, open or stab wound drainage, coagulation to surface bleeders, longer operation times, excessive shaving, poor haemostases.

Wound dehiscence

Abdominal wounds are said to lose their integrity in 2 per cent of cases and this is, of course, much more likely if associated with—haematoma, sepsis, or abdominal distension. Careful repair of the peritoneum and sheath should usually make dehiscence more unlikely.

Wound disruption may involve skin only or be complete. Abdominal wounds may suddenly burst open with bowel loops or omentum appearing where the sutures are removed. This event is almost always preceded by a period of 'serous' staining and some signs of obstruction.

Haematomas and abscesses should be drained and disruption repaired immediately by single layer thro' and thro' closure with non-absorbable sutures. Great care is required to avoid damage to bowel but such cases usually do extremely well.

SEPSIS

Some degree of wound sepsis is unfortunately moderately common especially where a septic lesion has been dealt with or bowel is damaged.

Pelvic sepsis itself is rare after surgery. If it occurs or is suspected the possibility of bowel damage may have to be considered.

Sepsis in a vault haematoma may appear as a malodorous discharge from the fault at the seventh to eighth day after hysterectomy or vaginal hysterectomy. It may have declared itself sooner. If drainage is not free the infected area should be gently opened with a finger.

Osteitis pubis may follow operation in the retropubic space especially those like Marshall Marchetti procedures which require sutures through the periostium.

General body response

The constitutional response is discussed by Walker & Johnston (1971), and Shoemaker & Walker (1970).

After major abdominal surgery up to 400mg of protein can be lost per day for the first four to five days from breakdown of tissues and blood clot. A high calorie intake, e.g. carbohydrate will minimize this loss.

Potassium loss is maximum in the first 24 hours, magnesium later, while sodium is retained especially with trauma in older patients. The normal energy needs after trauma are met in most cases by the reserve created by the bed rest, but the patient's carbohydrate and later fat stores will be used if not replaced.

Cortisol levels in the blood rise mostly during operation but the rise can be greatly controlled by the use of nerve block anaesthesia, e.g. epidural. Similar responses can be helped by simultaneous correction of circulating blood volume.

Water loss. The loss of circulating water may be quite great from respiration or from the skin in conditions of heat, or if there is diarrhoea, or if post-operationly the gut is distended by ileus. There is, of course, a close relation between water, sodium and other ions

which should be monitored by constant check of electrolyte levels.

Other ions; chloride, calcium and phosphorous and magnesium are important to the gynaecologist only in those patients who have suffered utero-colic anastomoses (in the main centres those patients will be supervised by the renal units).

The pH level (normally 7.4 ± 0.04), expresses the hydrogen ion concentration and with the pO_2 and pCO_2 and standard bicarbonate enable assessment of the degree of acidosis (respiratory or metabolic), in the ill patient to be assessed and corrected.

Urea and 'electrolyte' levels allow some measure of the general homeostasis and should be available in all patients post-operative from major surgery.

In all ill patients correction of abnormal levels may need discussion with the clinical biochemist.

Haemoglobin, haematocrit, CVP and blood volume may require to be determined pre- and post-operation and certainly the shocked patient or the patient who has lost blood should have a central venous pressure (CVP) line as a routine monitor for fluid replacement (*see* Chapter 31).

The CVP is not, however, an absolute measure of loss but only of the immediate response to the loss. A normal CVP may still be present after a blood loss of two or more litres.

BOWEL

Two major lesions may follow routine gynaecological surgery or, of course, follow surgery involving bowel itself, (1) Intestinal obstruction due to kinking or band adhesion may involve small or large bowel. It usually becomes evident by the fourth or fifth day and is characterized by distension, nausea, vomiting, usually excess tinkling bowel sounds with painful spasms and clear fluid levels in X-ray (standing). (2) Obstruction due to adynamic ileus often associated with sepsis manifests itself a little sooner about the second to fourth day and is characterized by a rapid pulse and also by distension, vomiting, fluid levels, but no bowel sounds are heard. In classical cases the abdomen is very silent indeed.

Treatment of both is by intravenous therapy

controlled by regular checks of electrolytes by the use of nasogastric tube to relieve stomach distension and by sedation. There is no place for bowel stimulation in such situations. Antibiotic therapy is usually indicated and both conditions usually settle. If distension fails to settle and the general condition of the patient fails to improve after three to four days then laparotomy with relief of the adhesion or band is essential. Very rarely caecostomy or colostomy will be required.

The bowel may be damaged during operations for sterilization by laparoscope and cautery or at laparotomy tears or rents may not be noted. Clinical peritonitis appears after three to five days. Unless the condition settles very rapidly with rest and antibiotic therapy laparotomy is indicated.

Foreign bodies

Material may be left in the abdomen after surgery, and contraceptive devices or laminaria tents may be extruded through uterine rupture. As soon as the diagnosis is made laparotomy should be undertaken. Contraceptive devices may be removed through a laparoscope.

Pulmonary complication

Collapse of basal lobes, or acute respiratory insufficiency due to bronchial mucus plugs can occur and are the province of the anaesthetist. They may be prevented by planned respiratory instruction pre-operatively by a physiotherapist or greatly relieved by physiotherapy post operatively. Bronchoscopy may be necessary.

Thrombo-embolism

Superficial thrombo-phlebitis of the external saphenous system is less common in gynaecology than in obstetrics. The reddened oedematous areas are painful but responds to local heat and oral butazolodine may be used.

Thrombosis in the deep veins of the legs or in the internal iliac vein system is said to follow pelvic surgery relatively frequently and can be detected in 25–30 per cent of cases by studies of fibrinogen uptake. At least two-thirds of cases have no clinical signs and early friable emboli from the legs causing pulmonary emboli may leave no signs in the legs (Browse, Clemenson & Croft, 1974).

Thrombosis in the deep vein is difficult to prevent totally. Active mobility before operation and very early ambulation are obviously helpful but recently active preventative therapy is advocated. Heparin 5000 units subcutaneously 6 hours before and daily after surgery for 5 days is said to be most useful. Dextran 40 per cent 500ml during operation and 500ml daily for 2–3 days is also advocated (*Brit. Med. J.*, 1973).

Deep vein thrombosis may be routinely searched for by Doppler ultrasound scan. Normally there is no reverse flow in those veins. Flow velocity increases during inspiration and decreases with Valsalva manoeuvres. Partial obstruction is seen by poor or absent respiratory change.

All thrombi clinically or on detection extending past the knee must be treated, as should all patients with the clinical signs of deep vein thrombosis, i.e. calf tenderness, oedema, and a positive Homans sign.

Therapy ranges from surgical thrombectomy to fibrinolysis by Heparin or Dindevan.

Heparin should certainly be begun immediately as an intravenous drip followed quickly by Dindevan. Thrombectomy should be considered in extreme situations or if there is failure of early response to medication.

If pulmonary embolism occurs or is suspected active drug therapy is certainly indicated. Discussion or action by a vascular surgeon may be called for.

Minor degrees of pulmonary embolism have usually a good prognosis unless they are continuous and repetitive and lead to blockage of multiple fine pulmonary arterioles and to pulmonary hypertension. However, minor emboli may be followed by a massive embolus which by blocking off one-third to one-half of the pulmonary tree creates an acute life threatening situation. Minor degrees of embolism are characterized by chest pain, breathlessness, perhaps a pleural rub, minor ECG changes and are very difficult to be certain of or to interpret. Therapy with intravenous heparin 5000 to 10 000 units should be begun if there is a strong suspicion of embolus. It is then difficult to decide whether or not further action is required except that a search for an unsuspected deep vein source is advisable.

Collapse from massive pulmonary embolus is usually obvious with cyanosis, extreme breathlessness, hypotension and coldness of extremities (the myocardial infarct patient is usually *not* cyanosed), and a raised jugular pressure. If the condition is life threatening, the first treatment is active external cardiac massage, oxygen by mask, and immediate 15 000 intravenous units of heparin to block the action of serotonin released from platelets. Acidosis should be corrected.

If pulmonary arteriography or lung scan are possible the full extent of the embolus and the infarction can be judged. Heparin may be given up to 100 000 units in 24 hours to avoid further extension of clotting followed by oral anticoagulants, plus Streptokinase 200 000 units IV stat. in 100ml 5 per cent dextrose followed by a drip of 100 000 units hourly acts as a thrombolytic. Hydrocortisone 100mg 6 hourly avoids reaction to the strepto-kinase. Thrombin clotting time (prolonged × 2) is used as a check on the degree of lysis.

If bleeding occurs in either medication it should be controlled by fresh blood, plasma or fibrinogen infusion.

Lesser degrees of embolus will settle on much less definite therapy and streptokinase is not indicated in these patients.

Embolectomy under cardio pulmonary by-pass despite its great risks (especially if vaso dilation is allowed in induction) is indicated in those cases who are resistant to streptokinase, where streptokinase fails or if death is likely within a few hours and before any other therapy can help (Miller, 1972).

Ureteric or bladder injury

Damage to ureter may be by cutting, by inclusion in a stitch or by bruising. The bladder may be damaged by surgery.

Care should be taken to search for and identify the ureter were it is at special risk so that damage can be seen when the abdomen is still opened, otherwise retroperitoneal urine collection may occur with nausea and some shock or there may be a leak from the vault immediately. Leaking from the vault on the fifth or later day follows bruising or slough or stitch damage.

Cystoscopy and ureteric catheterization is essential to locate the site and level of damage.

High ureteric damage should be immediately repaired if possible by anastomosis over an indwelling ureteric catheter. Low damage (close to bladder) or a small bladder fistula should be given a chance to close for one to three weeks, unless detected immediately.

Haemorrhage

Immediate haemorrhage or continuing haemorrhage is always declared by a rising pulse rate or a failure of the pulse rate to fall rapidly post operatively. Such haemorrhage is seen from pedicles or from large bladder veins below the peritoneum after hysterectomy, and occasionally after pelvic floor repair. Once diagnosed exposure of the bleeding area is essential, i.e. repeat laparotomy or exploration of abdominal or vaginal wounds. Occasionally such signs follow termination of pregnancy and are due to uterine perforation or laceration and again immediate operation is indicated.

Post lumbar puncture headache

This distressing complication is due to extra vasation of spinal fluid into the peridural space. It lasts five days and then disappears. Supine bed rest with adequate analgesics is required.

REFERENCES

Brit. med. J. (Editorial) (1973) Prevention Pulmonary Embolism. April, p. 1.

Browse, N. L., Clemenson, G. & Croft, D. N. (1974) Fibrinogen-detectable Thrombosis in the legs and Pulmonary Embolism. *Brit. med. J.*, **i**, 603.

Calderone, M. S. (Ed.) (1970) *Manual of Family Planning and contraception practice.* Baltimore: Wilkins.

Charles, A. H. (1972) Carcinoma of Vulva. *Brit. med. J.*, **i**, 397

Clarke, H. C. (1972) Laparoscopy—new instruments for suturing and ligation. *Fert. Steril.*, **23**, 274.

Douglas, D. M. (1963) *Wound healing and management.* Edinburgh: Livingstone.

Falk, H. C. (1964) *Urologic Injuries in Gynaecology.* Oxford: Blackwell.

Gordon, M. H., Scott, D. B. & Robb, I. W. P. (1973) Modification of plasma corticosteroids concentration during and after surgery by epidural blockade. *Brit. med. J.*, **i**, 581.

Lawson, J. B. & Stewart, D. B. (1967) *Obstet. & Gynaec. in the Trop.* London: Arnold.

Lowbury, E. S. L. (1973) Skin preparation for operation. *Brit. J. Hosp. Med.*, **10**, 627.

Miller, G. A. H. (1972) Pulmonary Embolus. *Brit. J. Hosp. Med.*, **8**, 259.

Richart, M. M. & Drager, D. J. (Ed.) (1969) Human sterilization. (*Proc. of a Conference*). Springfield: Thomas.

Shepard, M. K. (1974) Female Contraceptive Sterilization. *Obstet. & Gynaec. Surv.*, Vol. **29**, No. 11, 739–787.

Shoemaker, W. C. & Walker, W. F. (1970) *Fluid and electrolyte therapy in acute illness.* Chicago: Year Book.

Steptoe, P. (1967) *Laparoscopy in Gynaecology.* Edinburgh: Livingstone.

Steptoe, P. (1973) Gynaecological Laparoscopy. *J. Reprod. Med.*, **10**, 211.

Van der Glut, T. (1973) Menstrual Regulations what is it. *Pop. Rep. Ser.*, F2 p. F9. George Washington University Medical Center.

Way, S. (1954) Carcinoma Vulva. *Brit. med. J.*, **ii**, 780.

Williams, E. A. (1964) Congenital absence of the vagina—a simple operation for its relief. *J. Obstet. Gynaec. Brit. Cwlth.*, **71**, 511.

Wortman, J. (1974) Laparoscope sterilization with clips. *Pop. Rep. Ser.*, C No. 4 p. C45. George Washington University Medical Center.

Wortman, J. & Piotro, P. T. (1973) Vasectomy old and new techniques. *Pop. Rep. Ser.*, D1 p. D1. George Washington University Medical Center.

46. Sexuality, Sexual Difficulties and Sex Education

Sexuality is the awareness of gender. This awareness is largely based on the response, real or imagined, of the individual to his or her recognition by the opposite sex. This response to recognition process is the basis from which one of the most powerful drives emanates, namely heterosexual attraction, mutual to a greater or lesser degree, which is so efficient that it guarantees the reproduction of the species. The spread of factual knowledge of sexuality has been impaired by the embarrassment of the seekers and the restrictions placed on the better informed and potential teachers by powerful influences in society. Thus it is found at this time that there is no general agreement regarding education in sexuality, and in sexual behaviour and responsibility. Consequently while world population exhibits mushroom growth debate continues. Who should be taught, what, by whom and when? Whenever this subject is introduced the question of morality is raised. Morality strictly means the conduct of man which has come to mean more 'the discrimination between right and wrong'. Thus the moral aspects of a situation are arbitrary depending on the arbiter and at best a medical practitioner can act only as educationalist and not as judge. It is, however, the duty of the educationalist to state the facts clearly and without bias. This is an immense responsibility to be shouldered by family doctors or specialists and paramedical workers engaged in this field and should not be undertaken lightly. Voluntary amateur organizations should have their scope restricted to that of operatives in the business of referral of those in need to professionals.

CHROMOSOMAL AND HORMONAL BASIS OF SEXUAL BEHAVIOUR

Except in the rare situation of XY androgen-insensitivity (testicular feminization), the presence of the Y chromosome determines maleness. Whereas the XX or the XO embryo develops ovaries which are inactive in fetal life, the XY fetus develops testes which secrete testosterone. From animal studies it has been clearly shown that early exposure of the fetal brain to male gonadal hormones affects sexual activity in adult life. For example, genotypic female rhesus monkeys have been observed to exhibit male behaviour in later life when their mother has received testosterone injections in early pregnancy. However, genotypic males require to be castrated before exogenous oestrogen and progesterone can produce feminine sexual behaviour.

Thus in genotypic males with the testicular feminization syndrome where cell insensitivity to androgen occurs, behaviour has been found to be feminine. In contrast in genotypic females with the rare congenital adrenogenital syndrome frank homosexual attitudes are manifest in some and in others sexual arousal from stimuli more characteristic of the male pattern has been found.

From adolescence the male is dependent on androgen secretion for his sexual drive and behaviour but women may be castrated without loss of libido or sexual response and these are not increased by oestrogen replacement therapy. Indeed excessive oestrogens in some instances appear to decrease libido.

DEVELOPMENT OF HETEROSEXUALITY

Before adolescence there is little difference in endocrine secretion between boys and girls although in emotional and behavioural terms characteristic masculine or feminine preferences may be seen, e.g. mechanical and military toys preferred by boys, and dolls and clothes by girls; although much may be determined by the opportunity and exposure provided, and customs of the society in which they find themselves. However, children of this age are not without sexual interest although the pleasure experienced in physical contact play between two 8-year-old children of unlike and like sex is similar. However, it is thought that conditioning may occur in childhood which will produce homosexual rather than heterosexual inclinations and conduct later. The influence of the parent or guardian during this emotionally vulnerable period in development may contribute to the development of homosexuality, e.g. if the concept of marriage as an eventual goal is discouraged, if the parent figure of the like sex is so cruel or so ineffectual as to prevent the child identifying and expressing the similarity of gender, if the parent figure of the unlike sex is so unpleasant to the child as to produce a revulsion of that sex in the child, or if the parent produces conflict in the child's own gender identification, by instilling and encouraging contragender attitudes and behaviour. Nevertheless later childhood before adolescence is usually an asexual or a sexually neutral phase and there is a body of opinion which considers it to be the optimal time for comprehensive health education including sex education (p. 861).

ADOLESCENCE AND PUBESCENCE

By definition adolescence is simply the process of growing up and pubescence the period of sexual development. Adolescence is an ill-defined and variable period when the child reaches adult sexual maturation with its accompanying psychological transition recognizable by the expression of awareness and interest in the opposite sex. Although at the time of the onset of menstruation or menarche, the reproductive system in the girl has not attained full maturation, she is capable of sexual responsiveness. The changes in her body associated with puberty characterized by protuberant enlargement of the breasts and nipples, rounding of the hips and thighs accentuating the waist, produce the womanly contours. It is a natural reaction that she should take an introspective interest in these changes and anxiously evaluate the reaction to them from male society. At puberty fat is deposited in the labia majora and the vaginal orifice becomes hidden. Subcutaneous fat is also increased over the mons veneris and pubic hair growing there is one of the earliest signs of

puberty. This serves to promote her sexual awareness and curiosity, but, in some girls may be accompanied by symptoms of difficulty with adaptation and readjustment to a new found awareness of sex which may be expressed as negativism or social withdrawal. Expressions of empathy and effective counselling by an understanding parent, health visitor or family doctor may foreshorten this period of uncertainty.

In boys, adolescence is similarly determined in time by the secretion of the anterior pituitary gonadotrophins. In the male these are follicle stimulating hormone (FSH) and interstitial stimulating hormone (ITSH), the former stimulates the seminiferous tubules in the testicles to produce spermatazoa, and the latter stimulates the augmented release of the androgens, testosterone, and androsterone from the interstitial cells. These androgens produce the typically male secondary sex characteristics namely hair growth on the pubic area, chest, face, and axillae, skeletal muscular development, and deepening of the voice. Erection of the penis follows sexual arousal, spontaneous nocturnal emissions of seminal fluid occur, and at masturbation ejaculation follows the experience of orgasm. According to Kinsey data, approximately 75 per cent of boys have experienced orgasm through masturbation before puberty. Other authors suggest that 95 per cent of boys will masturbate at some time and failure to do so indicates abnormality (Jeffcoate, 1969). Feelings of guilt may be engendered by this practice of masturbation. There is no evidence that masturbation causes any ill effects. Nocturnal emissions can be regarded as a normal body function, the spontaneous expulsion of excess secretion.

Sexual Behaviour in Adolescence

It is difficult to review this in a world-wide context because adolescents are conditioned in their sexual behaviour and role in society by a variety of influences—economic, moral, religious, legal, and cultural. In the western world there has been recently a move towards accepting sexual intercourse as a means of heterosexual communication, rather than as an expression of love between two people. This is a far cry indeed from the belief that sexual intercourse should take place within marriage only, which is an ethic accredited to Victorian

Britain. Much of this change has occurred in the last two or three decades. Adolescents strongly stimulated by their new found sexuality are often bewildered. The boy finds that some sociological opinion condones if not encourages him to seek sexual gratification before marriage. Near his zenith of sexual drive he experiences an urgent need for this. On the other hand the adolescent girl also strongly sexually motivated finds society ambivalent. She is still encouraged to have heterosexual social relationships, to take pride in her appearance, to learn the techniques of home-making and courtship but she is expected to reach marriage *virgo intacta*, not only by her elders, but frequently also by her bridegroom. Even if the husband-to-be encourages her to have pre-marital sexual intercourse with him, pre-marital relationships with others is unacceptable and may prove a recurring topic of annoyance to him and regret for her for the rest of their married lives. The sexual behaviour of the girl is conditioned by her desire to allure and retain the interest of the chosen male. It seems however that more frequently now she deems that this must include sexual intercourse. However as a significant but unknown percentage of males are attracted principally by 'the chase rather than the kill', she finds herself rejected soon afterwards, particularly if pregnancy follows. It is now becoming recognized that women have sexual intercourse for a variety of reasons often quite unrelated to affection, such as boredom, loneliness, pique, rebellion, competitiveness, frustration, despair, comfort, hero worship, and often of course hunger and monetary gain—by prostitution. However there is no good evidence that true promiscuity is more common now than formerly (Bulloch and Drummond, 1975), but accurate data are impossible to collect and the wider availability of more effective contraception makes objective estimations highly speculative. However there is no doubt that pre-marital intercourse with a single partner is on the increase, especially in the very young.

The media suggest that some sort of sexual revolution is taking place and even the most reticent male or female must consider that perhaps he or she is missing something. Behavioural patterns in adolescents are not set and can be moulded easily by influences which make a direct intimate appeal as the mass media do now, and as religious organiza-

tions used to do effectively. It is too early yet to evaluate the effect of the contraceptive pill, antibiotics, psychotherapy, and the comparative safety of therapeutic termination of pregnancy on the code of sexual behaviour that has been gradually evolved.

Sexual response in the female

The attributes of the male to attract and sexually stimulate the female are difficult to define but self-confidence of manner and assured behaviour may be more important than stature, elegance, intelligence, or socio-economic status. While for generations females have expected males to exhibit aggressive traits and be masterful in their sexual role, the cult of 'women's liberation' seeks to neutralize this differential, or indeed bring about a reversal of roles. Female sexual response is not governed by a gonadal endocrine response but by conscious reception and evaluation of perceptual stimuli. Appreciation of this stimulus and communication of this sexual response to the male is commonly transmitted consciously by the look in the eye, movement of limbs and body and word of mouth. This is voluntary and can be inhibited or restrained by conscious effort. Encouragement to the male may be rejected or interpreted as a signal for further social intercourse which through time and opportunity will lead through fondling, petting and love play to sexual intercourse unless conscious interruption of the progress is made by either partner. Many areas of the female body are erogenous and although there is an individual quantitative variation, generally speaking contact with lips, tongue, back of neck and ears, shoulders, lumbo-sacral spine, breasts, thighs, mons veneris, clitoridal shaft, glans, and vagina may evoke sexual excitement. Thus kissing, caressing and love play should be the usual preludes to sexual intercourse.

It is only comparatively recently that the female anatomical and physiological adaptations for coitus have been studied in a clinical sense (Masters and Johnson, 1966). From this work it was concluded that it was justifiable to divide the female response into 4 stages:

1. *Excitement* during which the vaginal epethelium becomes moist, the upper two-thirds of the anterior and posterior vaginal walls lengthen and distend, the nipples become erect and there is flushing of the skin on the ventral aspect of the trunk.

2. *Plateau*. This phase is characterized by venous engorgement of what these workers describe as the 'sexual platform'. This comprises the lower one-third of vagina and the clitoris and surrounding structures. The clitoris although enlarged actually retracts away from penile contact. The Bartholin's glands actively produce some lubricating secretion in this phase.

3. *Orgasm*. This short phase is the most pleasant physical sensation the woman can experience and is associated with strong contractions of the pubococcygeus, myometrium, and voluntary muscles of the pelvic girdle.

4. *Resolution*. This is the phase of an exponential diminution of venous engorgement, muscle and nervous tension which may last 10–15 minutes. During this time the breasts become notably soft, the nipples retract, and the woman experiences an 'after-glow' of calm, release of nervous and physical tension with a pleasant lethargy of sleepiness. Immediate further fondling of the erogenous areas produce a different sensation from the excitatory one of the first three phases but persistence beyond the phase of resolution can produce a repeat response of the excitement phase.

It is possible for a woman to achieve an orgasm by extragenital caressing of her erogenous areas notably the breasts and nipples, but some women never achieve orgasm even with regular coitus or may require clitoridal stimulation after coitus in order to experience it. By and large it is the man who educates the woman in the art of achieving orgasm, and it is his responsibility to co-ordinate his response to hers because while the normal male has little difficulty in reaching orgasm, the woman may require a longer period of stimulus to achieve gratification.

Sexual response in the male

The woman can evoke a sexual response in the male in a variety of ways. She has her natural physical endowments which can be used adorned or unadorned. She learns of the power of allure of dress and make-up. She may study and follow assiduously the trends in fashion and the properties of the contemporaries sex sirens. Visual, olefactory, and auditory stimuli can cause sexual stimulation in the male and particularly with the lingual stimuli of kissing or the tactile stimuli of fondling the female, through the S2 and S3 parasympathetic plexus, venous congestion of the penis is caused with resulting erection. Fantasy of these stimuli can have a similar effect and fantasy is frequently used to enhance the quality of perception of the actual sexual stimuli.

Tactile stimulation of the male genitalia by the female can lead to a compulsive desire for intercourse which is frequently underestimated by the uninitiated female who may find herself subjected to unexpected aggression by the male. Failure of orgasm for the male at this stage frequently leads to intense pelvic discomfort due to unrelieved venous congestion and acute tenderness in the testicular region. However the natural progress of the sexual excitation preliminaries is penetration by the penis of the vagina and progressive activity therein until orgasm when seminal fluid is discharged through the urethral meatus over the cervix and upper vagina. Detumescence of the penis follows rapidly and seminal fluid may pass along the vagina to the introitus and it is at this time when condom contraception can become ineffective. As with the female a period of resolution ensues which is accompanied by a pleasurable lethargy or sleepiness and during which caresses produce a different response from their sexual excitation effect experienced so recently before.

FREQUENCY OF SEXUAL INTERCOURSE

The frequency of sexual intercourse varies widely according to age, opportunity, and pre-occupation although basically there is also a wide individual variation. There is no evidence to suggest that women with the greatest overt sex appeal to the male have a more frequent desire for sexual intercourse nor are more accomplished in the act. Equally there is no objective feature of the male by which the female can accurately prognosticate his sexual appetite or quality as a sexual partner. A partnership of healthy young people may have coitus more than once per day, a mature marriage of middle-aged partners 2–3 times per week while after later middle life coitus is often less frequent. However, the frequency of coitus in marriage is much less a reflection of intensity of sexuality, mental or physical health, or well-being, but much more an indicator of pre-occupation with more pressing demands such as earning a living, mothering young family or looking after aged relatives within the home. Thus a woman who is near despair with her apparent lack of libido which she ascribes to her age or ill-health and who reluctantly tolerates coitus approximately once per month, may surprise herself by having pleasurable coitus several times during a single weekend spent remote from her usual daily environment and routine. It is this escape rather than the exhibition of any particular gift in the act of coitus by the lover, which usually provides the extra sparkle of 'affairs'.

Coitus in relation to the menstrual cycle

Coitus during menstruation is usually avoided although some women may have strong sexual desire at that time not entirely attributable to it being a 'safe period'. Jewish law forbids coitus during menstruation, indeed to a total of 12 days from the onset of the period. From the medical point of view only the possibility of introducing an endometrial infection or possibly, as some believe, the risk of promoting squamous metaplasia of the cervix have theoretical grounds for consideration as contra-indications. These medical and aesthetic objections can be overcome by the temporary use of a vaginal diaphragm or cervical cap before vaginal toilet and during coitus. It is generally held that libido in the female has no particular cyclic pattern in women during reproductive life. It is doubtful if this holds for women with premenstrual tension who may have become very irritable with their sexual partner at this time and libido may not only be totally absent but sexual contact may be repulsive to them. However orgasm at this time does relieve premenstrual tension temporarily, and may represent a physiological method whereby this distressing condition may be relieved. A tablet of methaqualone 250mg and diphenhydramine 35mg may relieve the premenstrual tension sufficiently to allow pleasurable sexual intercourse.

Nuptial coitus

Traditionally and legally a marriage is not consummated until sexual intercourse has been effected. When neither partner has experience of the technique of coitus the first attempt may be best delayed until after the first night when the tensions of the wedding day are over. Clumsy first attempts when the female is insufficiently relaxed in mind and body may be a traumatic event. Vaginismus may engender a feeling of sexual inadequacy and incompetence by producing embarrassment and fear. The risk of such a background for future sexual activity should be avoided. The male may react with embarrassment also and impotence or premature ejaculation may occur. The danger of the bridegroom not pressing for consummation on the first night in the absence of the bride's agreement is that she may feel that she has offended, or that he is less fond of her than she had believed. These difficulties can be avoided if there is sensible preparatory discussion and agreement has been reached in advance. Particular difficulties may be encountered by a tight hymen or by a severe haemorrhage from hymenal rupture for which gynaecological aid should be sought and both matters treated as emergencies. When coitus results in tearing the hymen bruising may occur with subsequent tenderness, and the bridegroom must be advised to delay further coitus until the swelling and tenderness have subsided.

'Honeymoon cystitis' is due to a urethritis thought to be caused by the penis traumatizing the urethral meatus and vestibule. It may be associated with some degree of vaginismus, and sometimes with the later appearance of asymptomatic bacteruria. The clinical symptoms are those of frequency, urgency and dysuria. A clean catch midstream specimen of urine should be cultured and the appropriate chemotherapy given where it is bacteriologically indicated. Women should be advised to empty the bladder after intercourse as this reduces the tendency to 'cystitis'. Alkalinizing the urine by means of the oral administration of a mixture of potassium citrate and sodium bicarbonate may provide some degree of symptomatic relief but spontaneous cure is usually effected during abstinence from coitus for a few days as normally occurs during the first menstrual period.

Coitus in relation to pregnancy

During pregnancy the average woman has some loss of sexual desire but this is often tempered by her recognition that her mate has not lost his. Husbands may react to the effects of pregnancy on their wives in different ways.

Some may find the changes due to pregnancy make her more voluptuous and desirable while others find the pregnancy changes unattractive and may seek sexual partners elsewhere. Certain complications of pregnancy do contra-indicate coitus such as placenta praevia, and other ante-partum haemorrhage, a history or presence of cervical incompetence leading to mid-trimester abortion or extreme prematurity, premature rupture of the membranes, pre-eclampsia, monilial vulvo-vaginitis, and threatened, or history of recurrent, abortion. Generally speaking it is customary to advise against coitus until the end of the third month and again in the last eight weeks of pregnancy, but the scientific basis for this is obscure. Coital advice should be individualized as part of good comprehensive antenatal care.

In the early puerperium a return of intense sexual desire can be expected in some women and counselling is an essential part of post-natal care. The potential risks are uterine infection or perineal or vaginal epithelial injury where trauma has occurred at childbirth. It is very unlikely that these risks remain relevant after the 10th post-natal day but again individualization is important and it can be assumed that in many cases coitus occurs before that without detrimental sequelae and probably with important emotional benefits for both partners. Some authorities reckon that coitus aids involution of the uterus and improves muscle tone, and it is a popular belief that regular sexual intercourse helps to restore and maintain the female figure, and women professionally concerned in such matters support this view. Lactation is no contra-indication to coitus. Milk may be expressed from the nipples in the puerperium during orgasm even when lactation has been suppressed but this is of no clinical significance.

LIBIDO AND FRIGIDITY AND SEXUAL INADEQUACY

Libido is a word used to express the sex urge. It is probably a function of the mind, unrelated to gonadal hormone levels and is largely conditioned by environmental circumstances. Only the strongest libido can surmount adverse factors such as harassment, fatigue and preoccupation. The problems arising from lack of libido are so similar to those of frigidity that both will be discussed together.

Frigidity is a term used to express a subconscious inability on the part of the female to respond sexually to competent stimulation.

One of the advantages of the relaxation of the taboos surrounding discussion of sexuality has been the increase in the number of women distressed by sexual problems coming forward for help and being prepared to give a sufficiently valid account that valuable help can be given. It is important for the physician to project a genuine interest and to discuss this without personal embarrassment. It has also become obvious that both partners in the marriage should be involved in evaluation of, and progress in the resolution of, the psychosexual problem. The woman may present with a complaint which she finds less embarrassing such as pelvic pain. The sexual problem may by symptomatic of a social distress such as marital strife due to economic pressures and indeed sexual intercourse may be avoided deliberately as a form of retaliatory punishment. Only a detailed and accurate sexual history can form the basis for the correct diagnosis and effective treatment. Such a history should elicit early sexual education and experience, attitudes of the family and influential friends regarding sex, the expressions of affection within the family, and an account of what marriage means to the individual particularly in the sexual sense, and how the partner in the marriage is considered. Finally details of past and present sexual behaviour and any sex orientated traumatic experience should be noted.

It is currently advocated that both partners should be seen at the initial interview but this is usually impractical. The term frigidity should never be used in the presence of the patient because it may add a sense of shame or fear of her sexual capacity or capabilities. Masters and Johnson describe three positive situations related to the development of female psychosexual inadequacy

1. attitude towards sex and its significance within the marriage;
2. degree of personal regard for the marital partner;
3. fear of pregnancy.

It is likely that competent history taking will make an assessment of the relative influences these factors play in the synthesis of frigidity. If the primary basis of the problem is that the marriage is foundering and sexual disharmony is only secondary, then it is apposite to recommend referral for marriage guidance counselling. The fear of pregnancy has the best prognosis and this problem should be dealt with by full discussion of the methods of family planning including male and female sterilization with a particularly detailed explanation of the effect of such procedures on sexual desire and coitus.

If the reason for psychosexual inadequacy is her attitude towards sex then it is recommended by Masters and Johnson that the approach should be as follows: Possible anatomical and physiological abnormalities which could cause discomfort during coitus should be investigated and treated. A knowledge of the respective anatomies of the genitalia may have to be acquired by direct palpation and visualization by both partners to achieve a satisfactory physiological response. It should be emphasized that sexual expression is a natural element in the partnership of marriage but that female orgasm is not necessarily essential in every sexual encounter. The qualities of the male technique should be improved with respect to sensitivity and gentleness in order to achieve greater effectiveness.

However in many cases the kernel of the problem is found by the gynaecologist on pelvic examination when the lesion responsible either through fear of pain e.g. Lipschutz ulcer, or through fear of embarrassment at not being 'normal' e.g. Gartner's duct cyst, may be found.

Basically the role of the physician is to help the couple to learn how to have sexual intercourse and to enjoy rather than to fear it, so that coitus can become a means of natural expression of affection in their partnership. It may be necessary to teach the partner of the frigid woman suitable techniques for stimulation in the clitoridal region. It is not widely appreciated for example that the mons veneris and the shaft of the clitoris are the most sensitive erogenous areas to gentle friction. It is important for the female to let her partner know which are her most erogenous zones, preferred sequence of stimulation, the optimal moment for penetration, the choice of coital position and an indication of the imminent orgasm. Moreover the context of the proposed sexual experience is important and different times, places, situations and surfaces should

be tried—planned by the male so that it appears spontaneous opportunism to the female. Yet success may not be forthcoming if the woman is harassed, pre-occupied or fatigued. The male can help by promoting an aura of security and affection around the partnership.

A further basic cause of sexual disharmony is a disparity between the degree of sexual interest shown by the two partners. This may lead to a conscious withdrawal of sexual interest by the less strongly sexually motivated partner. The originally higher sexual tension partner may interpret the disparate motivation as an expression of rejection by the other. Thus feelings of sexual inadequacy may follow in either partner and resolution of this problem can only result from understanding by each partner of the other's individual personal sexual requirements. This can usually produce a relatively satisfactory compromise situation in which the lower response individual may show preparedness to increase sexual activity even though there is no increase in sexual drive.

Apareunia

This term describes failure of penetration of the vagina by the penis leading to an inability to practise coitus. This inability may be due to a fault in the male, or in the female or in both. The consistent failure to achieve or maintain an erection arising from impotence or premature ejaculation may be the reason. Alternatively the fault may lie with the woman through anxiety, fear or embarrassment causing vaginismus, which is constriction of the lower vagina by involuntary muscle spasm. Sometimes it is due to a mechanical barrier for example imperforate hymen, congenital absence of the vagina, vaginal septum or band, scarred introitus which may follow scalding or burns, usually found in the young, and chronic epithelial dystrophy of the vulva or atrophic vaginitis which are usually found in post-menopausal women.

Annulment of marriage

Apareunia constitutes grounds for the annulment of marriage. The medical practitioner may be called upon to provide evidence in court that his findings on physical examination of the woman are or are not consistent with the claim of apareunia. A practitioner called upon to make such an examination in order to provide an expert opinion should have proof of the woman's identity and her informed consent for pelvic examination freely given before a third party. All findings should be recorded at the time. Her general appearance should be noted carefully so that certain identification of her can be made in court. In Scotland the law is Common Law and the medical aspects of this concerns only non-consummation, and the factors of impotence in the male and inviolability in the female. The defect present must be irremediable, present at the time of marriage, and not made known to the spouse before marriage. Moreover pregnancy may be no bar to an action where *fecundation ab extra* has taken place e.g. in the absence of a vaginal introitus capable of allowing coitus.

In England and Wales there is Statutory Law also which provides other grounds of a medical nature in addition to these applicable in Scotland. These are briefly wilful refusal, insanity, a communicable form of venereal disease at the time of marriage, pregnancy to another man unknown to the spouse at the time of marriage and with sexual relations terminated by the husband forthwith on his knowledge. Proceedings instituted on these grounds must be taken within one year of the marriage.

Dyspareunia

Dyspareunia refers to difficult and/or painful coitus in the female. This symptom may, in fact, represent apareunia—the spectrum of difficulty varying from mere discomfort with coitus to complete failure. True dyspareunia *per se* is conveniently divided into superficial and deep in relation to aetiology, and by the same token, primary and secondary are also useful subdivisions with the latter designating the presence of an acquired cause dating from a specific event.

SUPERFICIAL DYSPAREUNIA

Primary
The first attempt at intercourse may well be accompanied by dyspareunia due to a combination of circumstances e.g. an inexperienced or impatient partner, the environment ill-suited, poor orientation towards the anatomy of the vulva and vagina, and the presence of a tight hymen, even when the female is totally uninhibited by fear or apprehension. This can

lead to traumatic inflammation of the introitus and honeymoon cystitis and may engender apprehension of future attempts due to local tenderness and general embarrassment. Pyogenic infection of the vagina can cause superficial dyspareunia. Attempted penetration before adequate sexual stimulation of the woman may result in the insufficient relaxation and lubrication of the introitus and vagina. A lubricant such as KY jelly can help with the latter, it contributes nothing to the former and thus is a poor substitute for considerate loveplay, and the need for the use of a lubricant generally reflects a failure in psychosexual counselling. Occasionally the introitus is found to be unnaturally small and the operation of Fenton's perineoplasty is necessary which is, in essence, incision of the introitus vertically and resuture of the incision transversely (Chapter 45).

SECONDARY SUPERFICIAL DYSPAREUNIA
The common causes are atrophic vaginitis, vaginismus usually due to fear of further pregnancy, fungal, trichomonal and bacterial vaginitis, Bartholin's gland duct abscess, post-traumatic adhesions and scars following vaginal and perineal repair procedures, Behçet's syndrome, Lipshutz ulcer, chronic epithelial dystrophy of the vulva, urethral caruncle and fissure *in ano*.

DEEP DYSPAREUNIA
This is only experienced on deep penetration and can be demonstrated by careful internal pelvic examination. Sometimes women state this does not accompany intercourse or does so only slightly but manifests itself some hours later as low backache or dragging lower abdominal pain. Many gynaecologists attribute this to lack of proper orgasm but this is difficult, if not impossible, to prove.

Primary deep dyspareunia
This is uncommon in young women because the underlying pathological conditions causing deep dyspareunia are found usually in older women. However adhesions of the right salpinx and ovary may follow appendicitis, pelvic tuberculosis may occur in the young, threadworms may settle in the salpinges, and chronic inflammatory changes in the Fallopian tubes attributed to talc are not unknown in the younger age-group.

Secondary deep dyspareunia
On pelvic examination there may be found one

of several loci of varying degrees of tenderness from exquisite to slight on digital pressure and this simulates the dyspareunia. By far the most common is seen in parous women and is in the area of the utero-sacral ligament and parametrium (transverse cervical ligaments) which would justify the diagnosis of para-metritis. The left side is more commonly affected than the right and there is frequently a laceration in the cervix which is not remark-ably tender on the ipsilateral side. In addition to deep dyspareunia, unilateral or bilateral iliac fossa pain demonstrated by synchronous convergent movement of the palms towards the symphysis pubis and sacral backache demonstrated by lateral movement of the dorsum of the hand across the sacrum make up the characteristic picture. The cause of this condition is ill-understood and bacteriology is notably unhelpful. Sodium fusidate 500mg taken orally with meals three times a day for seven days improved many in a double blind crossover trial (Sutherland, 1975). Hysterec-tomy is curative in the remainder.

On other occasions the cervix is found to be acutely congested and exquisitely tender and appropriate chemotherapy dependent on bacteriology with subsequent diathermy or cryosurgery of the cervix is curative. The presence of a tubal ectopic pregnancy or acute salpingitis is sometimes betrayed by the complaint of recent severe deep dyspareunia, while women with chronic salpingo-oophoritis and endometriosis commonly present with a longer history of dyspareunia and vaginal examination and diagnostic laparoscopy or laparotomy are helpful in the differential diagnosis of these two conditions. Bulky tumours e.g. fibroids and ovarian neoplasms which occupy the Pouch of Douglas and the vaginal lateral fornices may distort the pelvic anatomy sufficiently to obstruct pain-free coitus. Not only excessive size but also torsion, ischaemia, haemorrhage and degenerative changes may render a tumour tender to pressure and thus pain is produced at coitus. It is frequently stated that retroversion of an other-wise healthy uterus causes deep dyspareunia because the ovaries are prolapsed into the Pouch of Douglas. Formerly, large numbers of operations were done to elevate the gonads. In the absence of all the conditions so far described here only rarely is this an entity demanding of surgical interference. A trial of change in coital position e.g. male inferior

may be diagnostic and therapeutic. On the other hand a fixed retroversion giving rise to dyspareunia signifies additional pathology and further investigation and treatment is manda-tory. Occasionally with chronic constipation, megacolon, or with faecal impaction of the rectum the posterior vaginal wall is displaced anteriorly firmly against the anterior vaginal wall and coitus is not possible without evacuation of the bowel. Rarely bowel lesions such as Crohn's disease or carcinoma may cause difficulty or pain with intercourse.

There is no reason why coitus following abdominal or vaginal hysterectomy should be difficult or painful. Radium treatment however does lead to diminution of the elasticity and lubrication of the vulva and vagina. Generally speaking the use of a vaginal obturator to increase the size of the vagina is rarely of value except following plastic operations to create an artificial vagina. On the other hand the reassurance gained by a patient at the sight of the dimensions of a skilfully and painlessly passed vaginal dilator makes such an exercise worthwhile in many psychosexual problems, and in a few who have had recent local obstructive difficulties rectified or after other forms of gynaecological surgery in which the patient suspects the capacity of the vagina has been diminished.

Continence

Continence is not harmful physically although it is possible that it may produce irritability in the high sexual tension male accustomed to regular coitus. However healthy male adults who do not practise sexual intercourse may have nocturnal emissions (p. 850) which occur about every three or four weeks. Nocturnal orgasms occur mainly in women who have experienced sexual intercourse e.g. widows, and are thought to be usually associated with vivid erotic dreams.

Masturbation

This can be defined as self stimulation of the genitalia leading to orgasm. This practice in boys has been discussed (p. 850). In men it is much less common although its practise in individuals will vary enormously according to circumstances, for example in an all-male situation. By and large contemporary writers regard it as an uncommon practice in adults in a mixed society.

Girls admit to masturbation in a lower incidence, around 30 per cent, than do boys but it is estimated that over 50 per cent produce orgasm by this practice. Female children practise genital stimulation about a year earlier i.e. age 6–7 than do boys, and the highest incidence appears to be in the lowest socio-economic class groups (Elias and Gebhard, 1974). Self-stimulation in the female is usually achieved by gentle digital friction of the clitoridal shaft associated with fantasy. On occasions phallic objects are introduced into the vagina and this practise can cause vaginal laceration, chemical irritative vaginitis, and introduce vaginal infection. There is no good evidence that abnormalities of menstruation are caused in the absence of pelvic inflammatory disease. Many of the previously suggested effects can also be discounted, such as, excessive loss of energy, loss of intelligence, loss of fertility, premature old age, and adverse effects on future children; and physical appearance is not altered. The main consequence may be a feeling of guilt or depravity both of which proper education should dispel. There is no good evidence at the present time that masturbation causes congestive dysmenorrhoea or varices of the veins in the broad ligament.

Nymphomania

Nymphomania is the morbid incessant and uncontrollable sex desire in women. It can reach obsessional proportions and lead to soliciting. The nymphomaniac is not necessarily accomplished in sexual gratification, indeed many are incapable of orgasm and in those women it is thought to be causally related. Some deliberately avoid coitus because it enhances the sex urge without fulfilling the need even temporarily. It is not dependent on ovarian hormone secretion for this psychosexual manifestation is seen in post-menopausal women. Many background motivations have been attributed to its aetiology e.g. frustration with the domestic scene, as a demonstration of rebellion against the dominant sexual role of men, or for reassurance of sexual capacity or attraction which is sometimes seen transiently at the time of menopause. No satisfactory treatment of nymphomania is known. It is certainly not gynaecological surgery, and hormone therapy even with progestogens, has been disappointing. Encouragement to

undertake new all-absorbing interests and advice helpful in resolving domestic problems are worthwhile. Sexual counselling of both partners in marriage should be undertaken so that the problem is taken clinically and seriously and an informed understanding results between them. The use of mild sedatives may be evaluated and found helpful in some instances but clearly this line of therapy does not provide a satisfactory long-term solution.

Homosexuality in the female

Homosexuality means sexual attraction to the same sex.

Lesbianism (also sapphism and tribadism)— a Lesbian is a woman who is sexually attracted to another woman. It has been suggested that the prevalence is approximately 1 in 45 of the adult female population (Kenyon, 1970). It is estimated that 25 per cent of all women have had homosexual contact at some time although the practice can become widespread in institutions such as prisons. This leads to 'situational' or 'facultative' homosexuality as opposed to 'obligatory' homosexuality. There is a spectrum of homosexual identity from a subject expressing homosexual behaviour to the practising lesbian. Indeed it is believed that all individuals have the potential for homosexual as well as heterosexual urges.

Lesbianism is practised by kissing, naked body contact particularly genital contact, and mutual masturbation. The use of an artificial phallus is less common and orgasm is usually achieved by clitoridal stimulation. Physical lesbian practice is harmless but feelings of guilt, depravity and jealousy may cause mental disturbances. It is usually found among the unmarried, but when associated with a conventional marriage it can be a cause for frigidity. In view of the susceptibility of young unmarried girls to be encouraged into lesbian practices and acquire homosexual habits caution should be exercised in the encouragement of apparently innocent adolescent relationships especially with older women.

Trans-sexuality and transvestism

Trans-sexuality refers to an overpowering desire to change sex. Evidence suggests that this occurs in response to activity in the temporal lobe. Dressing in the clothes of the other sex, transvestism, is part of this urge.

Trans-sexuality may be associated with a psychosis but the majority have no gross psychiatric deficit. The sex chromosomes have been shown to exhibit no abnormality and the genitalia are anatomically and functionally normal. The trans-sexualist strongly identifies with the opposite sex, most commonly male with female, although homosexual practices are not invariable, and indeed trans-sexualists usually have low sexual tensions. Their belief is that they have been given the wrong anatomy in development, and come pleading for removal of their sex organs all of which offend them. The outlook for the sufferers of trans-sexualism at the present time is poor. To acquiesce to the surgical demands may be extremely ill-advised because a demand for restoration to former anatomical configuration may follow (Jeffcoate, 1969) and it is argued that the basic defect is in the psyche and psychiatry is the proper approach, however 'a marked improvement in social and psychological readjustment' was noted in at least two-thirds of 29 males who underwent sex-reassignment surgery (Randell, 1969).

Not all transvestites are trans-sexualists, some cross dressing may be practised for the singular occasions of masturbation and this seems to be a harmless and somewhat unusual perversion.

Male coital problems

IMPOTENCE

Impotence is the term used to describe failure to perform coitus. This is not an uncommon condition particularly after the age of 60. Three major types are described:

1. failed erection with or without sexual urge;

2. fleeting or incomplete erection achieved only, and usually without ejaculation;

3. Non-emissive erection in which the ejaculation cannot be effected with the penis within the vagina and orgasm does not occur. This last type is not be be confused with retrograde ejaculation into the bladder in which orgasm does occur which is in no way a form of impotence.

Impotence in the male like frigidity in the female usually has a psychosexual basis. The more often impotence occurs because self-confidence is undermined, the more likely impotence will follow on the next occasion. Important aetiological factors are business anxieties, fatigue, pre-occupation, and in some men a strict upbringing during which the idea that sex is evil or dirty is engendered from an early age. Maternal domination of an only son with the inculcation that women should be avoided is also thought to be causative. The relationship with the wife may be important either because he cherishes her so much that he does not wish to hurt her or cause her the discomforts of pregnancy and labour, or share her attention with children, or because the relationship is superficial or has broken down with a lack, or loss, of mutual respect. Frigidity can beget impotence and impotence can beget frigidity. Mechanical contraceptive techniques particularly fiddling about with condoms can produce impotence. Mockery of sexual technique to an apprehensive male could cause lasting uncertainty with impotence. Excessive alcohol intake is one of the most widely recognized factors. Anti-depressive or hypotensive drugs may have a similar effect. Some central nervous system and endocrine diseases particularly where the pituitary is involved may be a cause but, somewhat surprisingly, castration does not lead invariably to impotence, nor is impotence caused by testicular radiation, orchitis, cryptorchidism or hypoplasia of the testes. Any physical or psychiatric disease leading to debility can cause impotence and this should be excluded when the diagnosis is made. In a healthy subject a sexual history, and if appropriate, counselling along the lines described for frigidity should be undertaken. In order to raise the husband's morale and self esteem where infertility is the problem, artificial insemination (AIH p. 660) of the wife may be tried and sometimes the use of a penile splint to facilitate penetration and, it is hoped, ejaculation thereafter. For the situation of the non-emissive erection associated with infertility, AIH is indicated.

PREMATURE EJACULATION

This is a common condition on occasions in perfectly normal males who are relatively inexperienced or have had infrequent coitus and who are excessively sexually stimulated by accident or design by their sexual partner. As a persistent phenomenon it is usually associated with impotence and the wife fails to have orgasm for ejaculation occurs before or immediately following penetration. The line of treatment should be the same as for impotence except in the situation where over-stimulation has occurred and the avoidance of excessive love play will effect a cure. The use of a condom is sometimes advised to reduce the stimulation of the penis in the vagina. The monoamine oxidase inhibitors have been successfully used in this condition but their therapeutic value has to be weighed against the limitations imposed by their side effects.

SEX EDUCATION

This subject as a formal circumscribed entity in the education curriculum of children is in its infancy. It has had much adverse publicity, is highly controversial and at the present time is badly programmed or not included at all in many school curricula.

The educationalist

Principal among the many claimants for this role are parents, school class teachers, biology teachers, social workers, family doctors, gynae-cologists, and nurse/health visitors.

Certain criteria of suitability and aptitude can be used to draw a profile of the individual best placed to supervise the educational process of children in the nature and respon-sibilities of their sexuality. It should be a person with the following qualities: strongly motivated; appreciative of the responsibility for its consequences for the individual child; possessing a depth of knowledge of reproduc-tion, anatomy, physiology, and endocrinology so that penetrating questions from children can be answered correctly and authoratively; experienced in dealing with children as indivi-duals, if possible as a parent; professionally aware of, and experienced in the handling of medical and psychological problems of child-hood; trained in teaching methods; widely experienced in handling social problems in the home; and one who is completely free from embarrassment in discussing sexual matters. The married health visitor or female doctor who has had children of her own and who has received special training in health education is specially suited for this role including sex education as part of the course in health education. It is difficult to believe that people without medical training and experience could acquire the degree of insight, the knowledge or the understanding of human biology required for competent sex education. 'No adult, be it teacher or parent, should attempt the task with insufficient knowledge or self-confidence' (Jones, 1970).

The need for sex education

The need for sex education is argued on the basic assumption that some of the ills of contemporary society would be favourably modified or cured by sex education. The medico-social aspects of life on which sex education is hoped to have a favourable impact are the steeply rising prevalence of venereal diseases and therapeutic abortion rate, the high illegitimate pregnancy rate, the high premarital conception rate, the increased interest in obscenity and pornography, the rising divorce rate and the increasing demand for psychiatric help. Some authorities also look for a diminution in certain types of crime as a consequence of competent sex education. At the present time it is possible neither to quantify nor qualify the actual future advan-tages but most authorities now seem to accept that overall favourable medico-social effects will result.

The recipients

It goes without saying that anyone giving sex education should have had sex education, thus strictly speaking all parents should have had it, and until they have, runs the argument, its propagation should be supplemented by designated professionals.

Over the long term school provides a suitable opportunity for sex education and the children find the subject of interest and are used to learning in this environment. At what age should it begin? Two popular answers to this question are that it depends on when the child asks a suitably provocative question or that 'it depends on the child'. Both views represent pleas for individualization and as such demand respect, but the first does not necessarily mean that the child is intellectually or emotion-ally sufficiently mature to take in more than what is requested, namely an answer to a single question, although such an opportunity should not be missed if the child manifestly is so; and with the second, it is to be remembered that the process of growing up is conditioned by a reaction to environmental physical, intellectual and emotional experiences. Moreover a sensitive and competent teacher will anticipate out of depth situations in individuals provided that the size of the class is not excessive.

The author fully supports the view of Professor K. J. Dennis, who was responsible for the first edition of *Living and Growing*, the sex education series produced by Grampian Television, that sex instruction should be started in primary school children age 5–9 'before the embarrassments at the onset of puberty begin'. There should be no division in time between the teaching of the mode of human reproduction and its context of interpersonal relationships, nor between conception and contraception. Special consideration should be given to physically and mentally handicapped children.

Context

The most suitable context for an introduction of matter of fact sex education for primary school children is inclusion in a course of health education. This course stimulates interest and educates the children in such matters as dental and general hygiene, communicable disease and vaccination, nutrition, care of the feet, posture, vision, hearing, taste, and accidents within and outside the home, and smoking and drug-taking. This provides an opportunity for promoting discussion in human functional anatomy and elementary physiology, and the excretory and reproductive systems fall naturally and unremarkably into such a course. There is a view that the topic of sex education should be treated in the curriculum where it may be apposite, e.g. illegitimacy rates during mathematics, interpersonal relationships during English literature, etc. My view is that sex education would go by default during school days because, for example, the mathematics teacher is primarily interested in teaching mathematical aspects of statistics not the psychosexual motivations which produce illegitimacy. It is also a view that sex education should be introduced with biology but this is rarely programmed in the curriculum sufficiently early and references to human reproduction would be better regarded as complementary to a specifically designed course rather than an alternative to it.

Optional?

This question is only of practical relevance where sex education is scheduled at specific times in the curriculum. Where this is so it should be possible for the child to be given alternative work and forgo the instruction if both parents demand it. However, such a parental demand may betray the very child for whom proper sex education could be of particular value.

Content

Clear and simple instruction in the physiology and functional anatomy of the influential endocrine glands, genitalia, breasts, and pregnancy forms the basic curriculum but it can be anticipated that questions will arise in discussion on such matters as puberty, menarche, menstruation, premenstrual tension, conception, baby care, fertility and sterility, contraception, handicap, twins, screening for sub-clinical disease, menopause, male and female sterilization, illegitimacy, termination of pregnancy and venereal disease. Topics which may worry the adolescent such as masturbation, homosexuality and nymphomania should be dealt with in response to questions at a later stage. Greater discretion and knowledge is required to answer these questions than to present the basic facts.

Presentation

This subject should be presented to small classes on as informal a basis as possible and preferably without other teaching staff members present so that the child will feel no restraint in asking questions. Continuity with the class teacher can be maintained in the staffroom afterwards. It is important to try to achieve continuity of the tutor throughout the whole course. The subject lends itself particularly well to the use of audio-visual aids but slides, film, or videotape should never be shown to a class unsupervised by the tutor.

At present sex education in Britain is in a state of disarray due to a lack of clear direction as to whose responsibility it should be. In Scotland a Report commissioned by the Secretary of State for Scotland (Curriculum Paper 14 Health Education in Schools, 1974) deserves wide and deep consideration and if implemented should meet the needs. It recommends that 'the primary headteacher must ensure that within the programme for health education in his school the basic facts of reproduction are adequately explained' . . . 'In the secondary schools young people should be given the opportunity to have all the information they want regarding the psycho-social aspects of sex' . . . 'Many pupils in SIV and upwards are of an age to be married and preparation for a happy marriage is as important for them as preparation for academic success'.

REFERENCES

Bulloch, J. & Drummond, A. L. (1975) *The Church in Victorian Scotland, 1843–74*. Edinburgh: St. Andrews Press.
Curriculum Paper 14. Health Education in Schools (1974). Scottish Education Department. HMSO.
Elias, J. & Gebhard, P. (1974) In *Sex Education Rationale and Reaction*, p. 145. Ed. Rogers, R. S. Cambridge University Press.
Jeffcoate, T. N. A. (1969) *Principles of Gynaecology*, 3rd ed., p. 729. London: Butterworths.
Jones, W. T. (1970) Sex Education Today. *Brit. J. Hosp. Med.*, **3**, 53–55.
Kenyon, F. E. (1970) Homosexuality in the Female. *Brit. J. Hosp. Med.*, **3**, 183–206.
Masters, W. H. & Johnson, V. E. (1966). In *Human Sexual Response*. Boston: Little, Brown & Co.
Randell, J. (1969). In *Trans-Sexualism and Sex Reassignment*. Eds. Green, R. & Money, J. Baltimore: John Hopkins Press.
Sutherland, H. W. (1975). Unpublished.

FURTHER READING

Health Education in Schools. Curriculum Paper 14. Scottish Education Department. HMSO.
Health Principles and Practice. C. L. Anderson. 6th ed. The C. V. Mosby Company, St. Louis, 1970.
Human Sexual Inadequacy. W. H. Masters and V. E. Johnson. Little, Brown & Co., Boston, 1970.
Human Sexual Response. W. H. Masters and V. E. Johnson. Little, Brown & Co., Boston, 1966.
Sex Education: Rationale and Reaction. Ed. Rogers, R. S. Cambridge University Press, 1974.
The New Sex Therapy. H. S. Kaplan. Balliere Tindall, London, 1974.
The Sexual Behaviour of Young People. M. Schofield. Longmans, London, 1965.

TEACHING FILM

Sexuality and Communication. Ortho Pharmaceuticals Ltd.

Index